A DICTIONARY OF THE
HISTORY OF
MEDICINE

A DICTIONARY OF THE
HISTORY OF
MEDICINE

Anton Sebastian

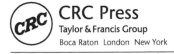

CRC Press
Taylor & Francis Group
Boca Raton London New York

CRC Press is an imprint of the
Taylor & Francis Group, an **informa** business

CRC Press
Taylor & Francis Group
6000 Broken Sound Parkway NW, Suite 300
Boca Raton, FL 33487-2742

First issued in paperback 2019

© 2011 by Taylor & Francis Group, LLC
CRC Press is an imprint of Taylor & Francis Group, an Informa business

No claim to original U.S. Government works

ISBN-13: 978-1-85070-021-0 (hbk)
ISBN-13: 978-0-367-39967-2 (pbk)

A CIP record for this book is available from the British Library.

Library of Congress Cataloging-in-Publication Data available on application

Visit the Taylor & Francis Web site at
http://www.taylorandfrancis.com

and the CRC Press Web site at
http://www.crcpress.com

Preface

The idea of this book came to me nearly ten years ago when I started cataloging my antiquarian and rare medical and science books for my personal library of 3000 volumes. The vast amount of material available for reference on the history of medicine only confused the issue. Often I had to spend a lot of time looking through several books before I obtained any specific information on a subject. As I went on I became more and more convinced about the need for a single book that could give specific information on any topic in history of medicine, as the Oxford Dictionary is to the English language. I wanted this book to serve medical researchers, presenters and clinicians who could not afford to spend their valuable hours in the library looking for specific historic information on their topics. I also intended the book to be of interest to laymen, paramedics, medical students and anyone else concerned in anyway with health care.

The task of producing such a book I knew was formidable as I realized that the story of medicine is in essence a recapitulation of man's attempts at survival since his first appearance on Earth. This brought a prehistoric element into my book. In order to survive, early man had to hunt and gather, and for this he had to be fit and healthy, which led to the concept of health and disease. The study of paleopathology has shown that disease affected the hunter and hunted alike, leaving tell-tale marks in the skeletons of dinosaurs and prehistoric man. The beginnings of medicine probably started with hunting and gathering. During the pursuit of his prey, early man had the opportunity to study its locomotion, and he learned of the fatality of wounds and signs of death when he killed for food. He unintentionally began his dissections when he cut up his game for food. A cave painting of a mammoth drawn by Cro-Magnon man and estimated to be over 39,000 years old reveals that he knew the position of the heart in the animal.

The study of normal and morbid human anatomy probably began with the practice of embalming by the Egyptians, who excelled in medicine for nearly 3000 years until overtaken by the Greeks around 600 BC. The Greek temples of Aesculapius built around this time were probably the first inpatient institutions for treatment of disease. Hippocrates around 400 BC dispelled the myths of medicine and started treating it as a science. Around this same period, contemporary Ayurvedic medicine in India and Chinese medicine in the East were developed independently. The Romans accepted medicine as a respectable profession around 100 BC. The Arabs, around 750 AD, translated and modified Greek medicine and adapted it to suit their religion and climate and their influence lasted until the end of the Middle Ages. During the 15th century in Europe Paracelsus developed the art of alchemy into chemotherapeutics. The French surgeon Ambroise Paré revolutionized surgery in the next century. William Harvey announced his discovery of blood circulation in the early 17th century. Several other important discoveries and rapid progress were made in the next few centuries. Most modern scientific principles and concepts were established in the 19th and 20th centuries. The atomist theory of the universe proposed by Democritus over 2000 years ago was revived on a scientific basis by Ernest Rutherford. Gregor Mendel's work was revived by William Bateson, establishing genetics as a separate science. The birth of modern physics gave explanation to electricity, heat, light, sound and magnetism which were previously observed as natural magic. Geology unfolded the origin and development of Earth and its life forms. The relatively new sciences such as anthropology contributed to evolution theory and paleopathology established the antiquity of diseases. Archeology unearthed the evidence of ancient cultures and knowledge. These are only a few examples of the progress that occurred.

Modern inventions and improved travel brought cures as well as diseases. The miracle cure for malaria, cinchona bark, was brought from Peru to Spain from where it reached the rest of Europe in the early 17th century. Sea travel spread the bubonic plague and the discovery of the New World may have brought syphilis to Europe. Epidemics became pandemics causing a domino effect on lives. Industries brought occupational disease, pollution and overcrowding. Airplanes removed the remaining barriers to disease, and cars introduced health problems resulting from road accidents, pollution, road rage and lack of exercise. With man's achievement of ample production of food and comfortable living, diseases such as atherosclerosis, hypertension and diabetes became common in affluent society. On the other hand, with division of wealth came the diseases of deficiency and famine.

Apart from the fact that medical history makes interesting reading why should we study it, especially in this era of high technology and specialization? In not doing so we are in danger of losing the wisdom that has been handed down to us since the time of Aristotle. We may also lose the sense of medical ethics proposed by Hippocrates. We may fail to realize how contemporary gurus failed great men like Mendel, Semmelweiss and Henry Hickman in the past. Most of all, we may lose the sense of gratitude to our predecessors, lose ourselves in our own achievements and fail to learn from the past. The pride and glory of medicine enjoyed by doctors today belongs in essence to those men of the past such as Hippocrates, Galen, Celsus, Harvey, Vesalius, Malpighi, Bernard, Pasteur, Lister, and others whose discoveries have stood the test of time. They laid the framework upon which others have worked to make medicine a marvel of today. In the present world of specialization where we know more and more about less, we are in danger of intellectually isolating ourselves from the knowledge of other walks of life. Today, politics controls medical policies and threatens medical ethics. Market forces undermine our efforts to curb tobacco smoking and pollution. Disintegration of social and family units compound the problems of drug and alcohol addiction. Pollution by industries and cars increases the incidence of chest diseases. Mass media such as television and radio mold people's concepts of health and disease. Ready access to computers and faxes may undermine patient confidentiality. Genetic engineering has also produced several ethical dilemmas. Specialized surgery, such as cardiac transplant, saves relatively few lives but take a large share of the pooled funds. I believe that an historical understanding of the genesis of these factors will help us understand the complexity of our profession.

Throughout the preparation of this book over the past ten years I had to keep reminding myself that it is a dictionary of the history of medicine, and not a dictionary of medicine. In doing so I have minimised the use and explanation of technical language and definitions which otherwise could be found in hundreds of available medical dictionaries. The portraits used in this book emphasize those leaders of medicine as human beings and not just names. The other illustrations, mostly taken from my library, are for the readers to relate to the subject more effectively.

I have used over 5000 volumes and hundreds of journals as sources of primary and secondary references. Although I have endeavored to cover every aspect through over 10,000 key entries covering more than a dozen specialties, my book can never do full justice to the subject of the history of medicine because it is vast and almost endless. An element of judgment has been used in the selection. Hopefully, future editions will benefit from and incorporate reader's comments.

In summary, I must thank my colleagues at the Berkshire and Battle Hospitals who took part in the audit of my work during the early stages seven years ago. I am indebted to David G.T. Bloomer, the Managing Director of Parthenon Publishing who painstakingly guided his skilled team over the past year to bring my book to publication. A big thank you to the Parthenon editor for her meticulous scrutiny of my work and skillful editing. I am also grateful to the graphics team for assembly and reproduction of the illustrations

Last but not least I dedicate this book to my wife Vasanthi and my two children, Chuchi and Kevin, whose time with me over the past decade I stole to complete this monumental task.

Anton Sebastian
April 1999

Anton Sebastian MBBS MRCP is a consultant physician in general medicine with a life-long interest in the history of medicine and related sciences. He has developed one of the finest private collections of antiquarian books in these fields, currently totalling over 3000 volumes, including many original editions dating from the early sixteenth century onwards. Following the completion of his postgraduate training at the Charing Cross Hospital, London and Kingston Hospital, Surrey, he has held a number of appointments both in Great Britain and overseas. He is currently a consultant physician at the Victoria Infirmary, Glasgow.

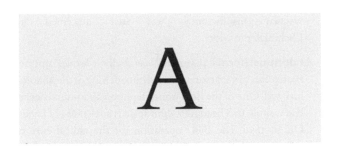

Aaron of Alexandria Jewish physician and presbyter in the 7th century, who is supposed to have written 30 books on medicine in Syrian, many now lost. Most of his remaining works compiled, from Greek, were called the *Pandects* of Aaron and were translated into Arabic by the Syrian Jew, Maserjawaihi, in AD 683. Some of Aaron's work was cited by the Arabian physician, Rhazes (850–932) who mentioned Aaron as one of the first to describe smallpox and measles, which were brought into Egypt following the conquest by the Arabians in AD 640. The first three chapters of the first tract in Haly Abbas (930–994) famous book *Al-Kitabul-Maliki* also contains some discussions on the writings of Aaron along with those of Hippocrates (460–377 BC), Galen (AD 129–200), Oribasius (325–403) and Paul of Aegina (625–690).

Abactus [Latin: *abigere*, to drive out] Term used by Roman physicians for miscarriage.

Abadie sign Spasm of levator palpebrae muscle of the eye as a sign in exophthalmic goiter, described at Paris, France in 1877 by Charles A. Abadie (1842–1932), ophthalmologist.

Abaptiston or Ababtista [Greek: *a*, negative + *babtiston*, to sink under] Ancient surgical instrument in the form of a circular saw described by Galen (129–200), Fabricius ab Aquapendente (1537–1619) and Johann Schultes (1595–1645). It was used to trephine the cranium. An earlier form of the instrument was cone-shaped so as to prevent the instrument sinking into the dura mater, hence its name.

Abbasides Second line of rulers and descendants of Abul Abbas, the first Saracen Caliph of the Eastern Caliphate of Baghdad, from AD 750–1250. Abul Abbas on his accession transferred the Caliphate to Baghdad which became a great city of science and literature. At one time it had 860 licensed physicians with numerous hospitals. The dynasty of Abbasides included Harun-Al-Rashid, Al-Mansur and Al-Mamun (AD 813-833) who encouraged the collection and translation of Greek and Roman medical classics into Arabic. Their efforts, especially those of Almamon or Al-Mamun, the son of Caliph Harun-Al-Rashid, resulted in the preservation of the earlier works of Hippocrates (460–

377 BC), Galen (AD 129–200), Paul of Aegina (625–690), Ptolemy and Euclid through turbulent times in history. According to the Fihrist (Index of Sciences), compiled in AD 987, ten of Hippocrates' works were translated by Hunayan ibn Ishaq or Johannitus (809–873) and his pupil Isa ibn Yahya and the 16 books of Galen were translated by Hunayan and his pupil, Hubaysh ibn el-Hassan, who was also his nephew.

Abbe, Ernest (1840–1905) A German physicist from Eisenach who became professor at the university of Jena in 1870 before he was made director of the Astronomical and meteorological Institute in 1878. He was partner at the optical company of Carl Zeiss (1816–1888) who first brought the improved microscope to the market. Abbe modernised the microscope by adding the apochromatic objective, and the oil immersion method (first suggested by John Ware Stephenson) in 1878. He also introduced the sub-stage condenser in 1886. At the death of his partner Carl Zeiss in 1888, Abbe became the owner of the optical works. He improved the technique of phase contrast microscopy in 1892.

Abbe technique *See Abbe, Robert.*

Abbe, Robert (1851–1928) Surgeon from New York, USA who introduced the use of catgut for suturing the intestines in 1889. He also devised the method of dilating the esophageal stricture in a retrograde fashion by opening the stomach to receive a 'string saw' from the buccal end and cutting the remaining tissue that contributed to the stricture. The Abbe technique was named after him.

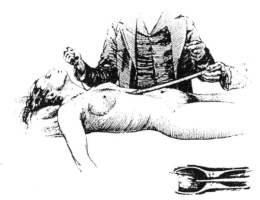

Abbe technique for division of esophageal stricture. Hochberg, LA, 1960, *Thoracic Surgery before the 20th Century*. Courtesy of Vantage Press, New York

Abbott Laboratories *See Abbott, Wallace Calvin.*

Abbott, Alexander Crever (1860–1935) Bacteriologist from Philadelphia, USA who designed a process for detecting spores in bacteria with the help of methylene blue and fuchsin.

Abbott, Edville Gerhardt (1871–1938) Orthopedic surgeon from Portland, Maine, USA who designed a treatment for scoliosis using bandages and a frame, followed by a series of plaster jackets.

Abbott, Maude Elizabeth Seymour (1869–1940) Canadian pioneer in the field of pediatric cardiology. She published the results of a study into congenital heart disease that showed that it was associated with an 18% risk of other malformations. Soon after the death of Sir William Osler (1849–1919) in 1919, Abbott published a memorial volume to his work. She is also famous for her promotion of medical education for women in Canada.

Abbott, Wallace Calvin (1857–1921) Founder of the Abbott Laboratories. Born into poverty in Vermont, USA, Abbott was able to fulfill his ambition of going to medical school only at the age of 22. After obtaining his medical degree from Michigan University in 1885 he borrowed a small sum of money from a friend and started The People's Drug Store in Ravenswood. He sold his own preparations, such as toothache powders, laxatives and cold remedies and in the early 1900s introduced a sugar-coating technique for tablets. His company later expanded to become the Abbott Alkaloidal Company and by 1930 it had grown into the pharmaceutical giant, Abbott Laboratories.

Abderhalden, Emil (1877–1950) Pupil of Emil Fischer (1852–1919) and professor of physiology at the University of Halle, Germany. He completed a bibliography of alcoholism in 1897 and was the first to describe familial cystinosis in 1903. He edited the series *Handbuch der biologischen Arbeitsmethoden*, 1920–1939.

Abderhalden–Fanconi Syndrome or Familial cystinosis was first described by Emil Abderhalden (1877–1950) in 1903. The occurrence of glycosuria and phosphaturia in the condition was described by Guido Fanconi (1892–1979) in 1936. *See cystinosis, Fanconi syndrome.*

Abdominal [Latin: *abdomen*, belly].

Abdominal aneurysm [Latin: *abdomen*, belly; Greek: *aneurysma*, a dilatation; French: *eurys*, wide] A sac formed by the dilatation of the wall of the abdominal aorta. The first successful resection of an abdominal aneurysm and repair with a homologous graft was performed by Charles Dubost (b 1914) of Paris, France in 1948. *See aortic aneurysm.*

Abdominal angina [Latin: *abdomen*, belly + *angere*, to strangle] A form of spasmodic abdominal pain due to mesenteric vascular insufficiency was first described by J. Schnitzler in 1901.

Abdominal hernia [Latin: *abdomen*, belly + *hernia*, rupture] Protrusion of a structure through an opening in the abdominal wall. One of the first monographs on abdominal hernia was written by Thomas Pridgin Teale (1801–1868) of Leeds, UK in 1846. The Ball operation for the radical cure of abdominal hernia was described in 1887 by Charles Bent Ball (1851–1916), surgeon and proctologist from Dublin, Ireland.

Abdominal hysterectomy *See hysterectomy.*

Abdominal injuries [Latin: *abdomen*, belly; French: *in*, negative + *jus (jur-)*, right] Henri de Mondeville (1260–1320), a surgeon to King Philip-le-Bel of France, was one of the first to write on abdominal injuries *c.*1306. In his treatise he advised that if the large intestines were wounded they should be sutured 'as ferriers sew a skin'. The explorer and doctor, David Livingstone (1813–1873), in his experience during his African travels, described the successful surgical treatment of extruded abdominal viscera due to injury by placing a gourd shell or calabash and sewing it to the abdominal wall. Many of the patients treated in this manner were observed to do well and return to their normal life. The repair of abdominal injuries has also been described by the ancient Hindus, who excelled in surgery. The works of the Hindu Brahmin Susruta, written *c.* AD 500, amongst its hundreds of surgical procedures, describes the surgical treatment of protrusion of intestines. Abdominal injuries became a focus of interest owing to their common occurrence during the wars in the preceding three centuries. Sir Cuthbert Wallace's *Abdominal Wounds* (1918) is considered to be a classic on the subject and his *Surgery of the Abdominal Wounds* (1922) is a treasure store of historical information. Another important book, *Abdominal Injuries of Warfare*, was published by G. Gorden-Taylor in 1939.

Abdominal pregnancy *See ectopic pregnancy.*

Abdominal surgery [Latin: *chirurgia;* Greek: *cheir*, hand + *ergon*, work] The era of modern abdominal surgery started in the 19th century. The first splenectomy was performed by Carl Friedrich Quittenbaum (1793–1852) of Germany in 1826, but his patient died of shock within six hours. The first splenectomy in England was performed by Sir Thomas Spencer Wells (1818–1897) in 1865 and his patient lived for 6 days. The first successful long-term result of the procedure was achieved by Jules Émile Pean (1830–1898) of Paris, France in 1867. One of the first successful abdominal operations for intussusception was performed by Sir Jonathan

Hutchinson (1828–1913) while he was at London Hospital in 1874. The first resection of the stomach for carcinoma was performed by Pean in 1879, but his operation was not successful. The first successful gastric resection was performed by Theodor Billroth (1829–1894) in 1881. Phineas Sanborn Conner of Cincinnati, USA did a complete resection of the stomach in 1884 but his operation was also unsuccessful. Carl Bernhard Schlatter (1864–1934), a Swiss surgeon, performed the first successful total gastrectomy for carcinoma of the stomach in 1897. A procedure of partial gastrectomy for carcinoma of the pyloric end of the stomach was devised by William James Mayo (1861–1939) in 1900. Pólya operation, which is a modification of Billroth operation II, was performed in 1911 by a Hungarian surgeon, Jenö Eugene Alexander Pólya (1876–1944). His operation involved gastrectomy combined with side-to-side anastomosis of the gastric remnant and the duodenum. Pólya is supposed to have been killed by Nazis, although his body was never recovered.

Abdominocentesis [Latin: *abdomino-* ; Greek: *kentesis*, puncture] *See paracentesis abdominis.*

Abdominoperineal resection [Latin from Greek: *perineon, perinaion*] Combined abdominoperineal resection for carcinoma of the rectum was introduced by William Ernest Miles (1869–1947) in 1908. (syn. Miles resection). *See Miles operation.*

Abducent nerve [Latin: *ab*, away from + *ducere*, to lead] (Syn. nervus abducens) The sixth cranial nerve, deriving its name from its relationship to the abductoris oculi or lateral rectus muscle. It was first described by Bartolommeo Eustachio (1524–1574), Italian anatomist.

Abdul-Latif or Abu Mohammed Abdul Latiff ibn Jusuf (AD 1161–1231) Arabian scientist and traveler in Egypt during the time of Saladin (1137–1193), the Sultan of Egypt and Syria. He taught medicine at Damascus, Aleppo and Egypt and has been credited with 166 treatises, some of which are on medical topics. He also studied human osteology and found that many of Galen's (129–200) writings on the subject were inaccurate. During his stay in Egypt he wrote a comprehensive account of the country's flora and fauna.

Abegg, Richard (1869–1910) Chemist from Danzig, Germany. One of the first to realize the chemical significance of electrons. In 1897 he proposed that the outer electron shell governed the chemical properties of the atom. He also did important work on osmotic pressures and freezing point of dilute solutions. Abegg died in a ballooning accident at Koszalin, Poland.

Abel Method The first chemical extraction of the active principle of the suprarenal gland, performed by John Jacob Abel (1857–1938) of Johns Hopkins Medical School in 1898. He gave the name epinephrine to this extract which is known as adrenaline in Britain.

Abel, Frederick Gottfried (1714–1794) Physician and poet from Halberstadt, Germany who took his medical degree at Königsberg. He published a German translation of Juvenal in 1788.

Abel, John Jacob (1857–1938) Biochemist born in Cleveland, Ohio, USA who graduated from the University of Michigan. After obtaining his PhD from the same university in 1883 he went to Europe where he spent 7 years studying under the foremost scientists in Austria and Germany. He returned to America in 1891 and became professor of therapeutics at Michigan. Aged 36 years he was appointed as the first professor of pharmacology at Johns Hopkins University. His notable contributions to medicine include: construction of the first membrane for artificial kidneys; first extraction of epinephrine (adrenaline), posterior pituitary hormones, hirudin and specific amino acids from the blood; and the first determination of the molecular weight of cholesterol. He was also the first to obtain a crystalline form of insulin, in 1926.

Abella A woman surgeon of the Middle Ages from the School of Salerno, Italy during the reign of Charles of Anjou around AD 1059. She wrote several medical treatises including *Treatise de Atra Bili* and *De Natura Seminis Hominis.*

Abengnefil or Aben-Guefit (997–1075) Arabian physician. He wrote a medical treatise which was translated under the title *De Virtuitibus Medicinarum et Ciborum* and printed at Venice, Italy in 1581.

Aberavon Skull In 1910 Arnalt Jones presented the frontal part of a skull belonging to the Neolithic Period, or later Stone Age, found at Aberavon, south Wales, to the Museum of the Royal College of Surgeons in London, UK. This and a similar skull found in the same region earlier in 1840, provided additional evidence for the presence of Neolithic man in England. *See skull.*

Abercrombie, John (1780–1844) Born in Aberdeen, Scotland, he graduated in medicine from Edinburgh University. He had a successful practice in Edinburgh and became surgeon to the Royal Public Dispensary in 1805. He published *Observations on the Diseases of the Spinal Marrow* (1818), *Pathological and Practical Researches on Diseases of the Brain and Spinal Cord* (1828), the first book on neuropathology and several other important medical works.

Abercromby, David (1621–1695) London physician who in 1684 first suggested a parasitic cause for syphilis. Works include *Opuscula Medica hacteneus edita* (1689).

Abercromby, Patrick Thomas (1656–1726) Physician from Angus, Scotland who qualified from St Andrew's University in 1685. He became physician to James II and wrote *Treatise on Wit* (1686).

Aberdeen Medical Society Founded as a debating society by two physicians, Sir James McGrigor (1771–1858) of Inverness, Scotland, his companion James Robertson and ten medical students from Marischal College in 1789. McGrigor became Director General of Army Medical Service in 1815.

Aberdeen Medico–Chirurgical Society *See Aberdeen Medical Society.*

Aberdeen Royal Infirmary Founded in 1739 with James Gordon, Professor of Medicine at Marischal College, as its first physician in 1741. It contained six beds at the start in 1742 and had expanded to 19 beds by 1749.

Aberdeen University Third of the Scottish universities to be founded (1494). Although St Andrews and Glasgow were founded earlier (in 1411 and 1451, respectively), Aberdeen was the first to organize regular medical teaching in Britain. It awarded its first medical degree in 1630. Marischal College was founded in 1593 by Earl Marischal and the two merged in 1860.

Abernethian Society Inaugurated at St Bartholomew's Hospital, London, UK in 1795. It's principal figure was John Abernethy (1764–1831) and the Society functioned as a Medical and Philosophical Society with regular presentation of papers followed by discussions. It was revived in 1832 and renamed the Abernethian Society.

Abernethy Fascia The fascia covering the external iliac artery is named after the surgeon, John Abernethy (1764–1831) of St Bartholomew's Hospital, who first described it in 1828.

Abernethy Tumor A fatty growth of the body, described in 1817 by John Abernethy (1764–1831), who was a surgeon at St Bartholomew's Hospital.

Abernethy, John (1764–1831) From Little Moor Fields, near Finsbury Square, London, UK he was a pupil of John Hunter (1728–1793), who later became a surgeon at St Bartholomew's Hospital. He founded the Medical School at his Hospital with David Pitcairn (1749–1809). He ligated the external iliac artery for aneurysm, in 1796, advocated drainage of lumbar abscess by incision and ligated the common carotid artery to arrest brain hemorrhage in 1798. His *Surgical Observations on the Constitutional origin and Treatment of Local Diseases and on aneurysms* was published in 1809.

Aberrant Conduction [Latin: *ab*, from + *errans*, wander] *See Wolf–Parkinson–White syndrome, Lown–Ganong–Levine syndrome, ablation catheter.*

Abetalipoproteinemia (Syn. Bassen–Kornzweig syndrome) Abetalipoprotein deficiency causing acanthocytosis, retinitis pigmentosa and multiple neurological deficits. First described by a Canadian-born American physician at Mt Sinai Hospital New York, Frank A. Bassen (b 1903) and an American ophthalmologist at the same hospital, A.L. Kornzweig (b 1900) in 1950.

Abiogenesis [Greek: *a*, without + *bios*, life + *genesis*, origin] The doctrine of the origin of living things from inorganic matter. First proposed by Anaximander around 570 BC. *See germ theory of disease.*

Abiotrophy [Greek: *a*, without + *bios*, life + *trophe*, nourishment) During the late 19th and early 20th century almost any disease tended to be explained by an infective process. Sir William R Gowers (1845–1915) introduced the term abiotrophy in 1902 to denote and focus attention on diseases not due to infection. This group included hereditary and idiopathic disorders. Hereditary abiotrophy or Leber optic atrophy is one example.

Ablation [Latin: *ab*, from + *latum*, carried] Removal. The ablation of various parts of the brain served as an experimental tool that greatly contributed to the identification of specific functions of the brain in the field of neurology at the turn of the 19th century. Homonymous hemianopia was first demonstrated by experimental unilateral ablation of the occipital cortex in monkeys by Edward Alfred Sharpey-Schafer (1850–1935) in 1888. *See pituitary ablation.*

Ablation Catheter G. Giraud, P. Puech and H. Latour used an electrode catheter in humans in 1960. Benjamin Scherlag of Columbia University developed a catheter for recording electrical activity of the bundle of His in 1969 and an experimental method for injecting formaldehyde to block the bundle of His and produce complete heart block. This work formed the basis for electrophysiological studies of the heart and development of electrode catheter ablation by R. Gonzalez and co-workers in 1981. A transvenous catheter to deliver high energy direct electrical current for ablation of the aberrant pathway in Wolff–Parkinson–White syndrome was devised by F. Morady and M.M.

Scheinmann in 1984. A laser balloon catheter was developed by J. Richard Spears in 1987. *See Wolf–Parkinson–White syndrome.*

Ablepharon [Greek: *a*, without + *blepheros*, lid] or cryptophthalmus. A congenital abnormality in which there are no eyebrows or palpebral fissure and the skin is continuous from the forehead to the cheek. Described in a child who died at 9 months by W. Zehender in 1872. Further cases were recorded with dissections and numerous drawings by H. Otto in 1893 and by Van Duyse Bruxelles in 1899.

ABO Blood Groups Blood transfusions were hazardous and risky prior to the discovery of blood groups in 1900. The important observation that the serum from animals caused lysis of red blood cells when cross reacted with red blood cells of another species was made by Leonhard Landois (1837–1902) in 1875. The unpredictable outcome of blood transfusions, ranging from success to violent reactions and sometimes death, led to the virtual abandonment of the procedure around 1890. In 1900, Samuel G. Shattuck (1852–1924) noted that the serum from some patients caused clumping of red cells from other patients. The significance of this finding was not realized until Karl Landsteiner (1868–1943) of Vienna made the discovery of the three groups of blood through agglutination reactions in the same year. He migrated to America in 1922 and became the first American to win the Nobel Prize in 1930 for his discovery. A fourth group was discovered by Alfred von Decastello (b 1872) and Adriono Struli (1873–1964) in 1902. In 1909 Jan Jansky (1873–1921) of Prague classified blood into A, B, AB and O groups. Although a similar classification was proposed by American pathologist William Lorezo Moss (1876–1957) around the same time, Decastello's work was the first to be published. They were shown to be inherited according to Mendelian laws by Emil von Dungern (1876–1961) and Ludwik Herszfeld (1884–1954) in 1910. The exact method of inheritance was worked out by Felix Bernstein (b 1878) of Germany in 1924. Landsteiner in 1927, while working at the Rockefeller Institute with Philip Levine (1900–1987), also discovered minor blood groups M and N, which played a part in establishment of paternity and the study of racial characteristics. Landsteiner, while working with a Brooklyn physician Alexander Solomon Wiener (1907–1976), discovered the rhesus or Rh factor in 1940. The S group, based on isoaglutinins subdividing the M and N groups, was discovered by Robert John Walsh and Carmel M. Montgomery in 1947.

Abortin A substance analogous to tuberculin, it was introduced by veterinary surgeon, J. McFadyean of Edinburgh and S. Stockman during their attempt in 1909 to devise a test for the diagnosis of brucellosis.

Abortion [Latin: *aboriri*, to miscarry) Abortion has been practiced since ancient times, whenever a child was not wanted. During the time of Hippocrates (460–377 BC) mostly midwives performed abortions. Greek physicians considered it necessary only to preserve the health of the mother or save her life. The ethics of that time are reflected in the Hippocratic oath, which states, 'to no woman I will give a substance to produce abortion'. Soranus of Ephesus who lived around AD 200 has stated that 'the fruit of conception is not to be destroyed at will because of adultery or care of beauty, but is to be destroyed to avert danger appending to birth'. The church upheld this view and abortion was condemned with eternal damnation. Juvenal (AD 100) the Roman poet referred to the common practice of abortion amongst higher class women in Rome. Among the ancient Incas abortion was a crime punishable by death. The various methods of performing abortion for therapeutic reason such as a small pelvic outlet have been described by Avicenna (980–1037) and Rhazes (850–932). Methods described include bleeding especially from the ankle, leaping from heights, application of pessaries medicated with helabore or similar substances and forcible dilatation of the cervical os with a roll of paper, polished wood or a quill. Avicenna also described fumigation of the uterus and this was practiced abundantly in the 16th century. A fumigation apparatus for this purpose has been drawn and described in Ambroise Paré's (1510–1590) works. Law on abortion in England was set out in sections 58 and 59 of the Offences Against the Person Act of 1861. The position of therapeutic abortion was more clearly defined in the Infant Life Preservation Act of 1929 which recognized the right of the child to live as soon as it has reached the 28th week of gestation, but it had an important provision which stated that abortion 'in good faith and for the purpose only of preserving the life of the mother' was lawful. The later Abortion Act of 1967 liberalized the criteria for therapeutic abortion.

Abortus Fever [Latin: *aboriri*, to miscarry] Sir David Bruce (1855–1931), a physician of Scottish origin in Australia, isolated minute forms of Gram-negative organisms from patients with Malta fever in 1887 and he named the species *Micrococcus melitensis*. Bernhard Laurits Frederik Bang (1848–1932) obtained a similar organism from the uterine discharge of aborting cows in 1897. He named it *Bacillus abortus* and the illness came to be popularly known as abortus fever. Similar organisms were obtained later from pigs, cows and goats. Karl Friedrich Meyer and E.B. Shaw of America introduced the generic term *Brucella* to this species in 1920 in honor of its discoverer, David Bruce.

Abraham, Karl (1877–1925) Born in Bremen. Assistant to Eugene Bleuler (1857–1939) at the Burgholzli Asylum in Zurich. He founded the Berlin Psychoanalytic Society in 1908.

Abraham, Sir Edward Penley (b 1913) English chemist born at Southampton. He graduated from Queen's College, Oxford and was professor of chemical pathology there in 1964. While working with Sir Ernest Boris Chain (1906–1979), a biochemist from Germany, Abraham demonstrated the production of penicillinase by Gram-negative bacilli, in 1940. He also reported the therapeutic action of penicillin on humans in 1941 and isolated the first cephalosporin antibiotic from *Cephalosporium* in 1954.

Abrams, Albert (1863–1924) Medical graduate from Heidelberg in 1882 who practiced in San Francisco. He invented, in 1910, spondylotherapy in which he applied pressure or percussion to various points in the spine as treatment for a variety of illnesses. He experimented on other forms of fringe medicine and introduced a bizarre machine called a 'dynamiser' to diagnose diseases. This was later proved to have no scientific basis. He founded the American Association of Medico-Physical Research which pursued an unscientific approach to fringe medicine.

Abreaction [Latin: *ab*, from + *reaction*] Josef Breuer (1842–1925), who helped Sigmund Freud (1856–1939) in his early career, provided the incentive and basis for Freud's psychoanalytic theories. Breuer, using hypnosis, brought out the experiences of one of his patients which explained her symptoms. His method was initially called the 'talking cure' and the expression of emotions related to the patient's past experience was termed 'abreaction'. In 1882 Freud recognized the significance of this phenomenon of discharged repressed emotions under hypnosis, but at the same time also realized its limitation as a permanent cure, as it was only a transient state under hypnosis. In 1895 Freud devised the method of bringing out these repressed emotions by a process of free association where the patients, through their unmeditated words, unconsciously provided a link to their past experiences. Freud interpreted these in relation to repressed emotions and named his method psychoanalysis in 1896.

Abrikosov Tumor Also called granular cell myoblastoma, is a painless tumor occurring in the tongue, axilla and mandible in the above order of frequency. It was described by Aleksei Ivanovitch Abrikosov or Abrikossoff (1875–1955) of Moscow in 1926.

Abruptio Placenta [Latin: *ab*, from + *ruptus*, broken] Premature separation of normally implanted placenta with a fatal outcome. First described by American Joseph Bolivar Dee Lee (1869–1942) in 1901. The same condition accompanied by albuminuria, azotemia and shock was described by Alexandre Couvelaire (1873–1948) of Paris in 1911.

Abscess [Latin: *abs*, from or away + *cedere*, to depart] Aulus Cornelius Celsus (25 BC–AD 50) recommended incision of the abscess before it hardened. Superficial scarification and cataplasms were advocated as treatment by Galen (129–200). Aetius of Amida (AD 502–575) recommended application of barley meal or boiled bread in a decoction of figs before suppuration took place and incising the abscess where the skin was thinnest when suppuration was complete. Arnold of Villanova (1234–1311) realized the importance of surgical treatment and stated 'to postpone opening an abscess is dangerous'.

Absence Term introduced by Louis Florentine Calmeil (1798–1895) to describe a minor form of epilepsy in 1824.

Absinthe [Greek: *absinthion*, wormwood] An active extract from the plant *Artemisia absinthium* or wormwood. It has been used since ancient times for a variety of conditions, as a tonic, as an antihelmintic or narcotic and for gastric complaints. It was a social drink amongst the elite in Paris in 1860 and absinthe parlors became a vogue. It is said to have inspired famous poets and artists in France and became so popular that 25 distilleries in France produced it on a mass scale in the late 19th century. It was banned in 1915 by the French government owing to its injurious effects on health and disruption of social life.

Absorbent Dressings [Latin: *absorbere*, to suck up] *See Gamgee tissue.*

Absorption of Heat [Latin; *ab*, from + *sorbeo*, suck in] Robert Hooke (1635–1703) discovered that glass absorbed radiant heat. M de La Roche demonstrated the loss of heat by radiation and conduction through a glass medium, in 1812 which was fundamental to study of laws related to heat.

Absorption Spectra Isaac Newton (1642–1727) described the spectrum in his book *Opticks*. Melville, a Scotsman, in 1752 observed that metals gave a discontinuous spectra. Dark bands in the spectrum of sunlight were observed by William Hyde Wollaston (1766–1822) in 1802. Joseph von Fraunhofer (1787–1826) in 1814 studied this phenomenon and mapped about 400 dark lines. John Herschel (1792–1871) in 1823 suggested that these lines could be used to identify various metals. Robert Bunsen (1811–1899) and Gustav Robert Kirchhoff (1824–1887) concluded in 1829 that the dark lines were due to the absorption of certain wavelengths by the atmosphere. Analysis of the three primary colors of light was done by David Brewster (1781–1868) in 1831 and later applied to develop spectrometry for analysis of elements. *See dispersion, spectroscopy.*

Absorption *See digestion.*

Abstemius [Latin: *abs*, from + *tementum*, drink] An ancient Latin term for a person who abstains from meats and drinks according to his physician's instructions.

Abu, Bakr Muhamed ibn Zachariya *See Rhazes* (850–932).

Abu, Musa Jabir ibn Hayyan *See Geber.*

Abu, Zaid Hunayn ibn Ishak al-Ibadi or Johannitus (AD 809–873) Arab physician born at Alhira in Iraq. He studied medicine under Mesue Senior. He translated 10 Hippocratic treatises with his pupil Isa Ibn Yahya. The 16 books of Galen (129–200) were also translated by him with his nephew Hubaysh, another of his pupils. Most of the Galenic system of medicine was introduced into Arabia by Hunayan with his *Isagoge* which was translated into Latin by Marcus of Toledo in the 12th century. Abu Yaqub Ishaq (AD 910), a son of Johannitus, was also a physician who translated several Greek works into Arabic. *See eye, vision.*

Abul, Walid Muhammad ibn Ahmed ibn Ruschid *See Averrhoes.*

Abulcasim *See Albucasis.*

Abulfaragius, Gregory (1226–1286) Armenian physician, born in Malatia near the source of the Euphrates. He wrote a universal history in Arabic which was published in Latin in 1663.

Acacia Genus of leguminous trees producing many medically important substances. Intravenous administration of acacia solution was used as routine treatment for nephritic syndrome in the early 1900s.

Academia dei Lincei of Rome Named after the lynx, an animal with keen vision. It was formed by Duke Federigo Cesi in 1603 to serve as a forum to stimulate scientific discussions. The great astronomer and physicist, Galileo was one of its founder members. *See Academia Secretorum Naturae.*

Académie des Sciences *See Académie des Sciences.*

Academia Secretorum Naturae Founded by Italian physicist, Giambattista della Porta (1535–1615) in 1560. It was suppressed by the inquisition and replaced by the Academia de Lincei in 1603.

Académie des Sciences Gatherings of a group of eminent mathematicians and philosophers including Rene Descartes (1596–1650), Blaise Pascal (1623–1662), Pierre de Fermat (1608–1665), Edme Mariotte (1620–1684) and Pierre Gassendi (1592–1655) at Paris in the mid-17th century formed the basis of the Academy. It was initiated as a regular institution by French statesman, John Baptist Colbert (1619–1683) under the sponsorship of Louis XIV in 1666. The French writer, Bernard le Bovier de Fontenelle (1657–1757) developed it and was its secretary for 40 years. The Paris Observatory was established as a part of the Académie des Sciences in 1667 and its building was completed in 1672. Jean Piccard Huygens (1620–1682) and Giovanni Cassini (1625–1712) were members of the observatory. It underwent reorganization in 1699 and was abolished in 1793. It was replaced by Institut National des Sciences et des Arts in 1795.

Académie Royal de Chirurgie Paris Founded by Royal Charter of King Louis XV in 1731. It was suppressed during the Revolution but revived as the Societe National de Chirurgie in the early 19th century.

Académie Royal de Médicin Paris Founded by Royal Charter in 1820 by incorporating the old Académie Royal de Chirurgie. The new Académie was divided into medicine, surgery and pharmacy.

Academy of Psychoanalysis Formed in 1955 by a group of psychoanalysts in America who wanted to break away from the conformist views of the American Psychoanalytic Association. Its meetings expressed ideas from the smaller psychoanalytic institutes.

Academy Derived from 'academia' a grove in Athens where Plato taught his pupils. The academies of Plato and Aristotle continued for several centuries until they were closed by emperor Justinian in AD 529. The modern term, academy denotes a place of learning. The Academy of the secrets of nature in Italy was the first of the scientific societies to be established, around 1450. Though it initially consisted of physical scientists, it was later suspected to advocate magic and illicit arts and was banned by Pope Paul III. The Accademia del Cimento, one of the first important scientific academies, was founded in Florence, Tuscany, in 1657. It had many distinguished members such as Torricelli, Borelli,

Nicolaus Steno and Redi. The academy at the time of closure left a volume on *Natural Experiments*. The Berlin Academy was formed in 1700 through three decades of effort by the mathematician Gottfried Wilhelm Leibniz (1646–1716). The Academy of Sciences at St Petersburg in Russia was founded by Peter the Great in 1724. The Schemnitz Mining Academy, the first technical college in the world, was founded at Schemnitz, in Hungary in 1733. The Royal Danish Academy of Sciences was founded by Christian IV at Copenhagen in 1742. The National Academy of Sciences in America was founded as a private organization dedicated to science and chartered by Congress in 1863. *See Academia dei Lincei, Cimento.*

Acanthabolus [Greek: *akantha*, thorn + *bolus*, lump or cast out] Ancient instrument to remove thorns from the body.

Acanthocytosis [Greek: *akantha*, thorn + *cytos*, cell] Crenation or thorn-like projections of erythrocytes. Described as a feature of abetalipoproteinemia by Canadian-born American physician, F.A. Bassen (b 1903) and New York ophthalmologist, Kornzweig (b 1900) in 1950.

Acanthoma Adenoides Cystecum *See Brooke disease.*

Acanthosis Nigricans Diffuse hyperplasia of the skin with black pigmentation. Described by Sigmund Pollitzer (1859–1937) of Hamburg and Viktor Janowsky (1847–1925) in 1890. A modern description was given by R. Degas of Paris in 1964.

Acarus scabiei Mite sometimes called Sarcoptes Hominis causes scabies and antedates the appearance of humans by millions of years. Aristotle (384–322 BC), Zan-yun-fang (AD 700), Avenzoar (AD 1070), Hildegard of Bingen (AD 1050) and At-Tabari (AD 970) are all credited with having seen and described the mite. English physician, Thomas Moffet (1553–1604) recorded the relief of symptoms by extracting the mite from the skin with a needle in his work which was published in 1634. Pierre Borel (1620–1689) saw this mite under the microscope in 1653 and a microscopic description was given by Italian physician, Giovanni Cosimo Bonomo (1663–1696) in 1687. A drawing was done by August Hauptmann in 1657. Giovanni Bonomo and Giacento Cestoni (1637–1718), a pharmacist, established it as the cause of scabies in 1687. This discovery was a landmark as it was the first time a microscopic organism had been established as the cause of a specific disease. Johan Ernst Wichmann (1740–1802) wrote a monograph on scabies which established the parasitic nature in 1786. The Acarus mite was rediscovered in 1834 by a student, Simon

François Renucci, of Paris. He showed it without a magnifying glass and specified its site in the skin.

Accadians or Akkadians Inhabitants of Babylon who belonged to the earliest civilization in Eastern Asia. They believed that all diseases were caused by evil spirits and depended on priests and sorcerers for their cure.

Accessory Chromosomes Also know as X chromosomes. Noted by Hermann Henking (1858–1942) in 1891. They were suggested to be the determinants of gender by Ervin Clarence McClung (1870–1946), an American cytologist, in 1902. This was proved by Edmund Beecher Wilson (1856–1939) of Illinois in 1935. The presence of an extra X chromosome that determined the female sex was pointed out independently by American biologist, Nettia Maria Stevens (1861–1912) at Bryn Mawr College, Pennsylvania. These chromosomes were subsequently renamed sex chromosomes. One of the two X chromosomes in females was suggested to become inactive, as sex chromatin, in the normal female by English biologist, Mary Frances Lyon (b 1925) in 1961.

Accessory Food Factors Additional dietary factors required to maintain health. Found by Sir Frederick Gowland Hopkins (1861–1947) in 1906, who named them accessory food factors. The first of these, which prevented beriberi, was discovered by Casimir Funk (1884–1967) in 1911 who named it 'vitamine'. *See vitamins.*

Accident and Emergency Services The development of an accident center in every major city was urged by English orthopedic surgeon, Sir Robert Jones (1858–1933) soon after World War I. The first accident service in England was started at Birmingham by an Australian, William Gissane (1898–1981) in 1941. Known as Birmingham Accident Hospital the service was expanded later to include other emergencies. Widespread dissatisfaction with the poor quality of accident services and their poor level of staffing later led to two reviews: *Casualty Services and their Setting*, by Nuffield Provincial Hospitals Trust in 1960 and *Accident Services of Great Britain and Ireland*, by the British Medical Association in 1961. Anton Freiherr von Eiselberg (1860–1939) of Austria was a pioneer in establishing accident departments in Europe. He founded several accident and emergency departments within the university surgical clinics in Vienna in 1909. Ironically he died in a railway accident.

Accident Services Started in England with the establishment of Birmingham Accident Hospital in 1941 and the service was expanded later to include other emergencies. *See Accident and Emergency Services.*

Accident-Prone Personality The tendency of some individuals to have repeated accidents on a statistical basis. Observed by Major Greenwood (1880–1949) and C.V.Yule in 1920. E. Farmer and E.G. Chambers used the term 'accident proneness' in 1926. It was described in more detail by American psychoanalyst and pioneer in psychosomatic medicine, H. Flanders Dunbar (1902–1959) of Yale School of Medicine in 1954. A modern account was given by A.M. Freedman and co-workers in 1975.

Accommodation of Eye [Latin: *ad*, to + *commodus*, fitting] The pupillary changes in the eye in response to light. Observed by Fabricius ab Aquapendente (1537–1619) in 1600 and the original hypothesis for its mechanism was put forward by René Descartes (1596–1650) in 1655. Alteration of the curvature of the crystalline lens during accommodation was demonstrated by Jesuit astronomer, Christoph Scheiner (1575–1650) in 1619. Hermann Helmholtz (1821–1894), using his ophthalmometer, explained the mechanism brought about by contraction of ciliary muscles, affecting an increase in curvature of the anterior surface of the lens. English physician, Thomas Young (1773–1829) in 1801 demonstrated that changes of accommodation were always associated with the lens.

Accoucheur Male midwife during the Renaissance period when they were rare. King Louis XIV, after watching a male midwife attending his mistress, gave them official recognition. In 1670, Julian Clement, a French male midwife attended Madame de Montespan at the birth of the Duc de Main and in 1682 he delivered the Dauphin. Clement also attended three times on the wife of Prince Philip V of Spain and was honored with the title 'Accoucheur' which later became the official name for a male midwife. A physician, John Duppy of New York, was the first recorded male midwife in America in 1745.

Accum, Frederick (1769–1838) German chemist from Buckeburg who emigrated to London in 1793, where he became the chemical operator of the Royal Institution of Great Britain. He pioneered gas lighting and published *Treatise on Adulteration of Food and Culinary Poisons* (1820) and a *System of Theoretical and Practical Chemistry*.

Acephalocystis endogina [Greek: *a*, without + *kephale*, head] Headless bag-like hydatid cysts of the cestoid worm, named by René Theophile Hyacinthe Laënnec (1781–1826) in 1804. A detailed account of histology and treatment of acephalocysts was given by Richard Bright (1789–1858) in his treatise on abdominal tumors in 1824.

Acetabulum [Latin: vinegar cruet, from *acetum*, vinegar] Described as 'a cavity in the huckle bone which is appointed to receive the head of the thigh bone within it' in the first dictionary on medicine published in the Britain by Stephen Blancard (1625–1703) in 1684. Also a plant with a round leaf, *Umbilicus rupestris* or navelwort. It was used in treatment of inflammation and St Anthony's fire since the time of the ancient Greeks up to the 17th century.

Acetanilide or Antifebrin Prepared by French chemist, Frederic Gerhardt (1816–1856) in 1852 and introduced as an antipyretic by Arnold Cahn and Paul Hepp in 1886.

Acetazolamide The fact that sulfanilamide could produce alkaline diuresis was observed by R. Pitts and R. Alexander in 1945. This led to the discovery of a new diuretic, a compound of bicarbonate and sulfonamide in 1952.

Acetone Noted in urine by Wilhelm Petters in 1857 and Adolf Kussmaul (1822–1902) observed the same substances in the blood in 1874. A test for acetone in urine was designed by Viktor Frommer of Berlin in 1905 and another, using nitroprusside, known as Rothera test, was devised by Arthur Cecil Hamil Rothera (1880–1915) in 1908. *See acidosis.*

Acetum Pyrolignosum Crudum *See wood vinegar.*

Acetyl Salicylic Acid or Aspirin The term A-S-Pirin was coined in 1839 by Bayer chemists in 1899 to denote A – for acetyl group, S – for salicylic group and SPIR – for *Spiraea* plant which was the source of salicylic acid. Herman Kolbe (1818–1884) of Göttingen obtained salicylic acid from carbolic acid in 1853. Another chemist around the same time synthesized acetyl salicylic acid, but the therapeutic significance of this finding was not realized and it was discounted as a worthless relative. Later, Felix Hoffmann, a chemist at the Bayer Company, looked for a less irritant compound to treat pain in 1899 synthesized acetyl salicylic acid and presented it to Heinrich Dresser, head of the drug research department. Soon after this discovery, aspirin was hailed as a new antipyretic and a wonder drug for relieving pain. Bayer reaped the rewards of its discovery by holding the patent to manufacture and sell aspirin for the next 17 years.

Acetylcholine The hypotensive effect of this choline derivative was described by Reid Hunt (1879–1948) in 1906. Otto Loewi (1873–1961), a German pharmacologist at Strasburg, demonstrated in 1921 that a substance liberated from the stimulated vagus nerve ending, when perfused into a second heart, was capable of slowing down the rate of heart beat. This substance was the first neurotransmitter to be isolated and was identified as acetylcholine by British physiologist Sir Henry Hallet Dale (1875–1968) in 1929. Its role in transmission of neuron to neuron impulses of the sympathetic ganglia was demonstrated by Wilhelm Siegmund Feldberg (b 1900) and Sir John Henry Gaddum (1900–1965) in 1965. The mechanism of release by nerve impulses was discovered by Sir Bernard Katz (b 1911), a biophysicist who escaped from Nazi Germany and worked at University College, London, in 1969.

Achalasia [Greek: *a*, without + *chalasis*, relaxation] Failure of smooth muscle sphincters to relax at the gastroesophageal junction. The term was used by Sir Arthur Hurst (1879–1944) in 1915. A classic description of the symptoms and its treatment was given by Thomas Willis (1621–1675) in 1674 in his *Pharmaceutica Rationalis*. He designed and constructed a dilator from a whale bone and used it intermittently to dilate the cardiac sphincter on a young male. Other early descriptions were given by: Friedrich Hoffmann (1660–1742) in 1733, T. Purton in 1821 and A.J. Hannay in 1833. A large series of 17 patients was presented by F.A. Zenker (1825–1898) and colleagues in 1878. A surgical method of treatment was described by German surgeon, Ludwig Ernst Heller (b 1877) of Leipzig in 1913. The histological changes of the plexus were described by Geoffrey William Rake (b 1904) in 1926.

Achard, Charles Emile (1860–1944) Physician at Paris who coined the term arachnodactyly for the spider-like appearance of the fingers seen in Marfan syndrome in 1902. He also coined the term paratyphoid fever. *See Achard–Thiers syndrome.*

Achard–Thiers Syndrome A collection of several cases of virilism in females with diabetes, mostly taken from pre-existing literature by two French physicians, Charles Emile Achard (1860–1944) and Joseph Thiers (b 1885) of Paris formed the basis for recognition of this polyglandular syndrome.

Acheulean Culture Weapons and other utilities from the Paleolithic Age or drift age were found at St Acheul near Amiens in 1853. The Paleolithic culture which existed at St Acheul is commonly referred to as Acheulian culture.

Achilles Tendon The tendon that connects the calf muscle to the heel. Named after the ancient Greek warrior Achilles who, according to Greek mythology, was dipped in the river Styx by his mother, the nereid Thetis, to make him invincible. Apollo revealed this to Paris who mortally wounded Achilles in his heel during the Trojan war. The term was used in anatomy in 1693 by Phillipe Verheyen (1648–1710), a professor of anatomy at Louvain. He later had to have his leg amputated.

Achillini, Alexander (1463–1512) Celebrated anatomist from Bologna in Italy who described the part played by the small bones of the ear in hearing. He wrote seven important anatomical and medical treatises. His most famous, *Annotationes Anatomica*, was published in 1520. He gave the names 'hammer' and 'anvil' to two of the auditory bones.

Achlorhydria *See achylia.*

Achmet Arabian philosopher in the 4th century. He wrote on the interpretation of dreams. Although his original work was lost, a translation in the 9th century is extant and was published in Greek and Latin in Paris by Nicolas Rigault in 1603.

Acholuric Jaundice Hereditary spherocytosis accompanied by hemolytic anemia due to increased osmotic fragility of the red cells. Described by Oskar Minkowski (1858–1931) in 1900. *See congenital spherocytosis.*

Achondroplasia [Greek: *a*, without + *chondros*, cartilage + *plasis*, molding] Hereditary disturbance of epiphyseal cartilage and bone formation. Ancient paintings of Greek clinics show the existence of achondroplastics around 400 BC and a statue of an achondroplastic, Seneb of the fifth Egyptian dynasty, is exhibited in the Cairo Museum. It was described with illustrations by Samuel Thomas von Sommering (1755–1830), a Polish-born professor of medicine at the University of Mainz, Germany in 1791. Another description was given by the neurologist, Moritz Hienrich Romberg (1795–1873) in his graduation thesis. A study of the changes in the cartilage in achondroplasia was done in Berlin by German physician, Eduard Kaufmann (1860–1931) in 1892.

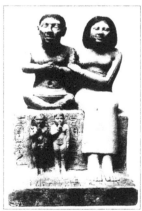

Model of achondroplastic court official Seneb, normal wife, one achondroplastic and one normal child (Fifth Dynasty). Courtesy of the Cairo Museum

Achorion schonlenii [Greek: *achorn*, watery discharge] The fungus causing favus was named *schonlenii* by Robert Remak (1815–1865) in honor of Johann Lucas Schonlein (1783–1864) who described it in 1839. Herman Lebert (1813–1878) of France described the same species under a different name earlier in the same year. David Gruby (1810–1898) established it as a cause of disease in 1841. *See favus.*

Achroma [Greek: *a*, negative + *chroma*, color] *See albino.*

Achromatic Lens [Greek: *a*, without + *chroma*, color] Lens for overcoming chromatic aberration. Produced by Chester More Hall of More Hall, Essex, who used it to construct a telescope around 1730. However, he failed to publish or patent his invention and a patent was obtained by John Dolland (1706–1761), an instrument maker in London in 1755. The achromatic objective was also mentioned by Harmanus van Deijl (1738–1809), of Danish origin, in 1807. It was adapted for the microscope by Italian physicist, Giovanni Battista Amici (1786–1863) of Modena, in 1812.

Achylia Absence of acid secretion in the stomach. Considered by F. Martius in his treatise *Achylia Gastrica*, published in 1897, to be due to an inborn error of metabolism. He postulated that gastritis was secondary to achylia rather than achylia being the cause of gastritis. Frederick Arthur Hurst [1879–1944], a physician at Guy's Hospital, supported this theory in 1923 and subsequent finding of achylia in some families with Addison anemia (pernicious anemia) also favored the familial theory. Hurst and J.R. Bell also found that it was a constant in patients with Addison anemia, presenting as subacute combined degeneration of the cord. Helge Knud Faber (1862–1956) in 1920 postulated that it was secondary to pathological changes of gastritis, which was later proved to be incorrect.

Acid-Fast Bacteria Certain bacteria are resistant to decoloration when stained with fuchsin. This was noted by Paul Ehrlich (1854–1915) in 1882. German bacteriologist Franz Ziehl (1857–1926) confirmed this and developed the method of acid-fast staining in 1883. The bacillus of leprosy (Hansen bacillus), later noted to have acid-fast properties, was discovered by Gerhard Henrik Armauer Hansen (1841–1912) in 1874. A second group of acid-fast bacilli, the tubercle bacilli, was discovered by Robert Koch (1843–1910) in 1882. The peculiar property of acid-fastness was studied by Edwin Klebs (1896), Robert Koch (1897) and Tamura (1913). Tamura isolated an alcohol from these bacteria which gave them the property of acid-fastness and named the substance 'mykol'. *See tubercle bacillus.*

Acid Phosphatase W. Kutscher and H. Wolberg demonstrated in 1935 that acid phosphatase was present at a higher concentration in the prostate gland than in any other tissue of the body. Benjamin Stockwell Barringer (b 1878) and Helen Quinsy Woodard (b 1900) in 1938 showed that metastatic lesions of cancer of the prostate led to the elevation of serum levels of acid phosphatase. In 1941, Charles Brenton Huggins (b 1901) noted that serum levels of acid phosphatase in metastatic carcinoma of the prostate could be further elevated by administering androgens and could be diminished by giving estrogenic substances. It was designated as a diagnostic marker and indicator of therapeutic response in carcinoma of the prostate.

Acid Serum Test *See Ham test.*

Acidosis Formation of acid in diabetic coma. Bernard Naunyn (1839–1925) of Berlin noted it in 1906 and named it. A minimal pH of 6.95 below which coma occurs was proposed by American biochemist and pioneer in blood gas analysis, Donald Dexter van Slyke (1883–1971). *See Kussmaul, acetone.*

Acinesia [Greek: *a*, negative + *kinesis*, movement] Term used by Galen (129–200) to denote an interval of rest which takes place between contraction and expansion of the pulse.

Ackee Poisoning Jamaican vomiting sickness. The cause was discovered by Henry Harold Scott in 1916 to be ingestion of unripe fruits from the tree, *Blighia sapida*.

Ackermann Angle The degree of inclination of the base of the skull. Use of this angle in the diagnosis of kyphosis and hydrocephalus was proposed by German physician, Conrad Theodor Ackermann (1825–1926).

Ackermann, John Christian Gottlieb (1756–1801) Professor of medicine at Altdorf, born in Upper Saxony and wrote *Institutiones Historiae Medicinae* in eight volumes in 1792. He was also an authority on Hippocratic treatises.

Acme [Greek: *acme*, from a point] The highest pitch of a disease.

Acne [Greek: *kneo*, I scrape or gnaw] Ancient Greek physicians, including Aristotle, recognized and described acne. Roman physicians used the word *varus* for the same condition, which was also mentioned by Pliny. The word is also thought to be a corrupted version of a Greek term for bloom or puberty. The term *akut* was used by ancient Egyptians for pustules and carbuncles which also raises the possibility of an Egyptian origin for the term.

Aconite *Aconitium napellus*, commonly called wolfsbane, blue rocket or monkshood. Named after the Black Sea port of Aconis. The plant has been in use for medicinal purposes from ancient times in China and India and the Gauls used the alkaloid extract (aconitine) as an arrow poison and the Romans learnt its use from them. Nicander, around 100 BC, proposed quicklime and honey as an antidote for aconitine. Apothecaries in England used it as a medicine in the 12th century and it was included in the pharmacopoeia for its poisonous nature as well as for its medicinal values in 1615. Roots and leaves were used up to the 19th century for various medical purposes, including the common cold, apoplexy and as an antipyretic. The first murder trial in England because of aconitine poisoning took place in 1881. *See Lamson, George Henry.*

Aconitine *See aconite.*

Acosta Disease *See altitude sickness.*

Acoustic Neuroma [Greek: *akouein*, to hear] The feasibility of radiologically demonstrating the local intracranial effect (widening of internal auditory meatus) of acoustic neuroma was pointed out by F. Henschen of Germany in 1912. E. B. Towne of America defined a projection that could clearly show the tumor and internal auditory meatus on X-ray in 1926.

Acquired Immune Deficiency Syndrome *See AIDS.*

Acrel Ganglion Pseudoganglion on the posterior interosseous nerve at the back of the wrist. Described by Swedish surgeon, Olaus Acrel (1720–1801) in 1779.

Acrel, Olaus (1720–1801) Surgeon at Stockholm who pioneered ophthalmic surgery in his country. He became the Director General of all the hospitals in Sweden and wrote several important treatises including *A Treatise on Fresh Wounds* (1745), *On the Operations of Cataract* (1756) and *On the Reform of Surgical Operations* (1767).

Acriflavin [Latin: *acer*, pungent] A dye. Synthesized by Benda in 1912 and introduced as an antiseptic by Carl Hamilton Browning (1881–1972), a pupil of Paul Ehrlich (1854–1915) in 1913. It was given intravenously as treatment for encephalitis lethargica by American surgeon Hugh Hampton Young (1870–1945), J. H. Hill and William Wallace Scott in 1925. British pathologist, Ewart William Gye (1884–1952) studied the neutralizing action of acriflavin on the agent of Rous sarcoma to determine its carcinogenic nature in 1931. His findings were more in favor of a living organism rather than an inanimate substance producing the sarcoma.

Acrobystia (Syn. circumcision) *See circumcision.*

Acrodynia [Greek: *acro*, extremity + *dynia*, pain] Mercury poisoning, Pink disease. Manifests as painful dermatitis affecting the extremities. Described by Erasmus Wilson (1809–1884), founder of the chair of dermatology at the Royal College of Surgeons in 1847. An account (Feer disease) was given by Swiss pediatrician, E. Feer (1864–1955) in 1923. A major cause of Pink disease in England was use of mercury-containing tooth powders and their withdrawal in 1954 led to an abrupt fall in the incidence of the disease. It was later noted to also occur in pyridoxine (B_6) deficiency or pellagra.

Acromegalic Gigantism Folk tales about giants may be of pituitary origin. An extreme case due to an overactive anterior pituitary was noted in a schoolboy giant, Robert Wadlow of Illinois. He was 5 years old when he reached a height of 5 feet 4 inches. He died at 22 years in 1940, having reached 8 feet 10 inches. Gigantism in acromegaly was observed and studied by Harvey Cushing (1869–1939) of Johns Hopkins Hospital in 1910. His patient was 35 years at the time of presentation. Despite surgery to relieve the pressure on the chiasma, his symptoms deteriorated and he died at the age of 40 years. This and three other autopsied cases are described by Cushing and Leo Max Davidoff (1898–1975) in a monograph published at the Rockefeller Institute of Medical Research in April 1927. Transphenoidal microsurgery for pituitary tumor was introduced by Jules Hardy in 1968. *See pituitary, acromegaly.*

Acromegaly [Greek: *acro*, extremity or tip + *megalon*, large or great] A clinical description was given by Nicholas Saucerotte (1741–1814), a French army surgeon, at the Academy of Surgery in Paris in 1772. Another was given by Sir Samuel Wilkes (1824–1911) in 1869. Pituitary disorder associated with gigantism was pointed out by Charcot's pupil, Pierre Marie (1853–1940), who described the clinical features of two female patients and named it in 1886. He published a series of 17 cases in 1888 but did not ascribe any specific cause to the disorder. Hyperactivity and enlargement of the pituitary as a cause were identified by Oskar Minkowski (1858–1931) in 1887. The first attempt to treat it by operative decompression was made by Richard Caton (1842–1926) and Frank Thomas Paul (1851–1941) in Liverpool in 1893, but was unsuccessful. An increase in the number of eosinophils in the anterior pituitary was demonstrated by Carl Benda (1857–1933) in 1900. Herman Schloffer (1868–1937) performed the first successful operation for pituitary tumor on a man with acromegaly in 1906. Harvey Cushing (1869–1939) described the anterior pituitary as 'the keystone of the endocrine arch' and did extensive studies on acromegaly and gigantism. Viennese endocrinologist and gynecologist, Bernhard Aschner (1883–1960) demonstrated that the anterior pituitary produced a substance that influenced growth, in 1910. American endocrinologist, Herbert McLean Evans (1882–1971) and Joseph Abraham Long (b 1879) discovered the growth hormone in 1921 and demonstrated gigantic overgrowth of rats treated with the hormone. Cushing finally established that eosinophils are the source of the growth hormone in 1927. *See growth hormone, pituitary.*

Acromian [Greek: *akros*, highest point + *omos*, shoulder] Term used by ancient Greek anatomists to denote the area between the neck and the highest point in the arm. Galen (129–200) introduced it in its current sense for a bony projection of the scapula into surgery in AD 180.

Acron (444 BC) Physician from Sicily who introduced fumigation as a method to control pestilence during the plague in Athens. His work was published at Basel in 1527.

Acropathos [Greek: *akros*, highest point + *pathos*, suffering] Extreme involvement of the surface of the body by cancer or disease.

Act for Parish Poor Infants High infant mortality rates prevailed in England in the years 1741 and 1742 and the number of deaths greatly exceeded the number of births. The appalling number of deaths of infants due to neglect and infection continued until a strong lobby prevailed to legislate an Act of Parliament in 1767. *See infant mortality rates.*

Acta Medicorum Berolinensium The first medical journal (in Latin) to be published in Germany in 1717.

ACTH or **Adrenocorticotropin** [Latin: *ad*, to + *renes*, kidney + *cortex*, bark] Hypophysectomy or the removal of the anterior pituitary was shown to prevent further development of adrenal glands by Philip Edward Smith (1884–1970), professor of anatomy at the College of Physicians and Surgeons at Columbia University in 1930. His finding started the search for an adrenocorticotropic hormone. Pioneering work was done by Choh Hao Li (b 1913) and co-workers at the University of California who obtained a homogeneous protein from extract of sheep pituitary in 1942 and also identified the 39 amino acids in sequential order in it in 1956. George Sayers (b 1914) of Yale University obtained the same protein with similar hormonal action from pig pituitary in the following year. The sequence of amino acids in ACTH was worked out by Paul H. Bell and others in 1955. Synthesis of ACTH was performed by Klaus H. Hoffmann from the University of Pittsburgh and R. Schwyzer of CIBA in 1960.

Actinobacillus Non-motile, non-branching, Gram-negative bacillus, isolated from lesions in cattle by Joseph Leon Marcel Lignieres (1868–1933) and G. Spitz in 1902. The name was proposed by Alexandre Joseph Emile Brumpt (1877–1951) in 1910.

Actinometer [Greek: *actina*, ray + *meter*, to measure] Instrument for measuring heat from the Sun. Invented by Sir John Herschel (1792–1871) in 1825 and improved by Robert Bunsen (1811–1899) and Henry Ruscoe in 1856.

Actinomyces asteroides Isolated from a brain abscess in a glass grinder by Hans Eppinger (1856–1916) of Prague in 1890.

Actinomyces bovis A detailed mycological account of actinomycosis, a common disease in cows, was given by Otto Bollinger (1843–1909) in 1877. He found that the disease presented as granulomatous lesions containing yellowish granules in the tongue of affected animals. The fungus was isolated in 1891 by Max Wolff (1844–1923) and James Israel (1848–1926). The latter also described the human form of actinomycosis.

Actinomyces caprae Isolated from the lung of a goat suffering from tuberculosis by Silberschmidt in 1897.

Actinomyces graminis Isolated by Eugen Bostroem (1850–1928) from a case of human actinomycosis in 1891.

Actinomyces madurae Madura disease or mycetoma of the foot caused by this fungus was observed by Engelbert Kaempfer (1651–1716) in 1712 and described by Henry Vandyke Carter (1831–1897) in 1874. A parasitic cause for Madura disease was suggested by George Balingall (1780–1855) in 1855. Jean Hyacinthe Vincent (1862–1950) identified the causative agent as *Streptothrix madurae* in 1894. It was present in India in ancient times and was described as padavalmika meaning foot-ant-hill in the *Athara Veda* of the Brahmins written around 1000 BC.

Actinomyces muris-ratti Isolated in 1914 by Hugo Schottmuller (1867–1936) from human patients bitten by rats.

Actinomyin [Greek: *aktis*, ray + *mykes*, fungus] The study of actinomycete fungi from the soil was pioneered by Selman Abraham Waksman (1888–1973) who emigrated from Russia to the USA in 1910. His team observed that tubercle bacilli died when exposed to a slow stream of sewage water. The bacilli were also unable to survive in unsterilized or manured soil. The significance of these findings were not grasped until 1940 when extracts of actinomycete fungi were isolated at Rutgers University in America. The toxicity of actinomycin limited its use as an antibiotic and this led to the search for similar but less toxic substances.

Streptomycin, which was less toxic, was isolated from *Actinomyces griseus* in 1943 and was renamed *Streptomyces*.

Actinomycin C Used in the treatment of acute rejection reactions following organ transplants. Isolated from *Streptomyces chrysomallus* by R. Brockman in 1960.

Actinomycin D Has marked anticancer properties in post-operative treatment of Wilms Tumor. Discovered by Selman Abraham Waksman (1888–1973) in 1940.

Actinomycosis One of the first human cases of actinomycosis was described by William Osler (1849–1919) in 1886. *See Actinomyces bovis.*

Actinotherapy [Greek: *aktis*, ray + *therapeia*, medical care] The short wavelength rays, showing least penetration of tissues, were identified as ultraviolet in the 19th century. Johan Wolfgang Dobereiner (1780–1849) used light therapy on a scientific basis in 1816. Sir Arthur Henry Downes (1851–1938) and Thomas Porter Blunt showed that these rays killed bacteria in 1877. Danish physician, Niels Ryberg Finson (1861–1904) also demonstrated the bactericidal effects of sunlight and developed a method of treating lupus vulgaris with ultraviolet light in 1890.

Action Potential The basis for the electrical wave that passes through a muscle or a nerve when it is stimulated. Demonstrated at the Paris Academy by Carlo Matteucci (1811–1868) in 1842. He observed that the leg of a frog twitched when it was placed on another frog leg which was electrically stimulated. In the same year Emil du Bois Reymond (1818–1896) detected electrical changes in injured muscle during contraction and this transient measurable electrical change was named action potential. The resting potential and the action potential in healthy nerves were recorded by a physiologist, Sir Alan Lloyd Hodgkin (b 1914) of Banbury, England and Andrew Fielding Huxley (b 1917) of London in 1939. Their dependency on sodium concentration was demonstrated by Sir Bernard Katz (b 1911) in 1949.

Active Chronic Hepatitis Also called lupoid hepatitis and accompanied by markers of autoimmune disease. Described by I. R. Mackay, S. Weiden and J. Hasker in 1965. The presence of antibodies against smooth muscle in two-thirds of patients with active chronic hepatitis was demonstrated by Glynn in the same year. Occurrence of anti-mitochondrial antibodies in 28% of patients with active chronic hepatitis was shown by D. Doniach in 1966. Steroids as treatment were suggested by. Mackay and I.J. Wood in 1961 and azathioprine and 6–mercaptopurine as

immunosuppressives were introduced by Mackay while working with Weiden and B. Unger in 1964.

Active Immunization *See Anthrax, inoculation.*

Actomyosin Albert Szent-Györgyi (1893–1986), Hungarian scientist and Nobel laureate, demonstrated the joint action of the proteins actin and myosin in bringing about muscle contraction in 1942. He said 'to see actomyosin contract for the first time was one of the most exciting experiences of my scientific career'.

Actuarius, John Zacharias (AD 1300) Jewish physician to the Court of Constantinople who recommended mild purgatives such as manna and senna and distilled water as a part of general treatment. A Latin version of his therapeutics was published in 1544 in Venice. His other works include *On Animal Spirits* (1557) published in Greek at Paris, *On Urines* and *A Treatise on Composition of Medicines.*

Acuity *See vision.*

Acupressure [Latin: *acus*, needle + *pressura*, pressure] A procedure in which a pin or needle is passed across the blood vessel in order to anchor it and apply pressure so as to promote hemostasis. Devised by Sir James Young Simpson (1811–1870) in 1864. This method was controversial and James Syme (1799–1870) became an opponent, while Thomas Spencer Wells (1818–1897) practiced it and supported Simpson's views. When Lord Lister introduced sterile catgut suture, acupressure was mostly abandoned.

Acupuncture [Latin: *acus*, needle + *punctura*, prick] The earliest record of acupuncture is found in the *Nei Ching*, written by the Emperor Huang Ti of China around 2700 BC. The theory is based on the balance of energy between *yin* and *yang* within an overall energy system called 'Chi'. The vital energy from *yang* and *yin* circulates along meridians in the body to nerves, blood and lymphatics. In the disease process this flow is said to be unbalanced. The method utilizes over 365 points in the body along 12 meridians to restore the harmony of these fundamental forces. Needles made of gold and silver were used in the past for this purpose. It was introduced into England about 300 years ago and a treatise in England was written by James Morss Churchill (d 1863) in 1821. An American book (1825) was a translation of a French work by J. Morand. The translator was Bache Franklin, grandson of Benjamin Franklin (1706–1790).

Acute Anterior Poliomyelitis (Syn. acute atrophic paralysis, infantile paralysis, Hein–Medin disease) The first disease of the nervous system to be attributed to a viral etiology.

A picture of a young boy suffering from infantile paralysis found in an ancient Egyptian stele, about 3500 years old, helped to establish its antiquity. Poliomyelitis presenting as paralysis following a brief illness in children was described by Michael Underwood (1737–1820), an English physician in 1793 and his was probably the first scientific study on poliomyelitis. A localized outbreak of flaccid paralysis was reported by another English physician, John Badham (1807–1840) in 1835 and it was described as 'essential paralysis of the children' by two French pediatricians, Frederick Rilliet (1814–1861) and Antoine C.E. Barthez (1811–1891) around 1839. Jacob von Heine (1799–1879) of Stuttgart wrote a monograph on paralytic conditions of the lower extremities which followed an acute febrile illness in 1840 and the term infantile paralysis was coined by Heine G. Colmer, who reported a similar outbreak amongst children in 1843. It was described in more detail in 1870 by Jean Martin Charcot (1825–1893), who believed that the primary lesion in poliomyelitis was in the anterior horn cells of the spinal cord. A clear clinical description including its infectious nature was given by Oskar Medin (1847–1927), who studied a large number of cases during an outbreak in Sweden in 1887. Scientific evidence for the communicability was provided by Swedish neurologist, Otto Ivar Wickman (1872–1914), during his investigation of a large epidemic involving 1200 cases in Sweden in 1905. The virus was obtained in a pure culture by Peter Kosciusko Olitsky during his work with Albert Bruce Sabin (1906–1993) in 1936. *See polio virus.*

Acute Ascending Paralysis or Landry disease *See acute infective polyneuritis.*

Acute Glomerular Nephritis   *See glomerular nephritis, nephritis.*

Acute Infective Polyneuritis (Syn. Guillain–Barré syndrome) Two cases of ascending neuropathy were described by Adolf Kussmaul (1822–1902) in 1859. A French physician from Limoges, Baptiste Octave Landry (1826–1825), also described it as 'ascending paralysis' later in the same year. Two French neurologists, Georges Guillain (1876–1971) and J.A. Barré (1880–1971) described it in 1916.

Acute Intermittent Porphyria One of the earliest observations of the symptomatology has been constructed from voluminous manuscripts related to the treatment of King George III. Although the king's illness was thought to be primarily a psychiatric illness by his physicians and others for a long time, a careful retrospective analysis during the five major episodes from the period 1765 to 1810 proved it to have been acute porphyria. The different forms were classified by Jan Gosta Waldenstrom (b 1906) in 1933.

Acute Interstitial Nephritis *See glomerular nephritis, nephritis.*

Acute Yellow Atrophy of the Liver Term coined by Viennese pathologist Karl Rokitansky (1804–1878) in 1843. He described it in postmortem findings of acute atrophy of the liver which resulted in acute failure. It is also eponymously known as Rokitansky disease. However, an earlier description was given by Richard Bright (1789–1858) in 1836.

Acyclovir [Greek: *a*, without + *kyclos*, circle] An acylic nucleoside. Synthesized by a team of American biochemists, George Herbert Hitchings, Gertrude Belle Eliot and colleagues around 1976. The discovery of its action against alpha herpes virus by H.J. Schaffer, U. Beauchamp and S. Miranda in 1978 is a landmark in the battle against the virus. When its patent in Germany expired in 1994, the drug became an over the counter topical treatment for cold sores. Within 10 weeks of its availability, over 1.3 million tubes were sold in England alone.

Adair, Robert (1711–1790) Surgeon to Chelsea Hospital, mostly known through the song *Robin Adair* written about him by Lady Caroline Keppel.

Adam's Apple The prominence caused by the projection of the larynx. It derives its name from the belief that it was caused by the forbidden fruit stuck in Adam's throat.

Adamantius of Alexandria (AD 500) Greek physician and a convert from the Jewish religion who dedicated his work on physiognomy to Emperor Constantine.

Adamkiewicz, Albert (1850–1921) Professor of pathology at the University of Cracaw who described the arterial supply of the spinal cord (Adamkiewicz arteries) in 1882.

Adams, Francis (1796–1861) Surgeon from Banchory, Scotland who made valuable English translations of Greek and Roman classics, including the works of Hippocrates (460–377 BC) and Paul of Aegina (625–690).

Adams, James (1818–1899) Glasgow physician who wrote *Burns Chloris, a Reminiscence* on Robert Burn's works.

Adams, Robert (1791–1875) Dublin physician who gave a classical description of heart block associated with syncopy, in 1827. The condition was later named Stokes–Adams syndrome. *See Stokes–Adams syndrome.*

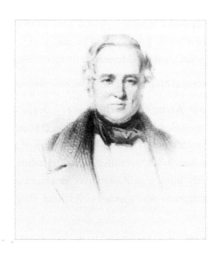

Robert Adams (1791–1875). Courtesy of the National Library of Medicine

Adams, Sir John (1920–1984) British nuclear physicist from Eltham and a founder member of the Centre Européane pour la Recherche Nucléare (CERN) at Geneva. He developed the first major post-war accelerator (180 MeV cyclotron) in 1949.

Adams, Sir William (1783–1827) London ophthalmologist who designed the original iridotasis operation for glaucoma. He also described an operation for ectropion.

Adamson Fringe Seen as a fringe in the hyphal involvement of dermatophytosis of hair without involving the bulb of the hair. Described by London dermatologist Horatio George Adamson (1865–1955). David Gruby (1810–1898) described the condition in 1895.

Adams–Stokes Syndrome *See Stokes–Adams syndrome, Adams, Robert.*

Adaptation [Greek: *ad*, to + *aptare*, to fit] *See alloplastic adaptation.*

Addenbrooke Hospital Physician, John Addenbrooke who died in 1719, left part of his estate to establish a hospital at Cambridge and Addenbrooke's Hospital was formed with these proceeds 4 years before the establishment of the Radcliffe Infirmary at Oxford, in 1766.

Addiction *Addicti* is an ancient Roman term for those who were handed over to their creditors as slaves in order to pay their debts. Aristotle forbade wine for nursing women with his statement 'it is the same whether the nurse or the child drink it'. Alcohol addiction and dependence has been recognized since that time. Addiction to alcohol became a state-recognized problem in England in the 17th century and it continued to be a major problem well into the 19th century. A treatise on alcohol addiction in English was written by John Coakley Lettsom (1744–1815) in 1779 and a book on alcoholism was published by Thomas Trotter (1761–1832) in 1804. G.B. Grinrod, the author of *Bacchus,* recognized and described alcoholism as a disease in 1838. The effects of alcohol such as dementia, neuropathy, delirium tremens and acute intoxication were also recognized during this time. One of the earliest descriptive post-mortem findings in acute alcohol intoxication was given by James Kirk of Scotland in 1830. He stated that the brain and ventricles of the deceased contained a fluid that smelt and burnt like alcohol. Later, in 1839, Percy from Nottingham observed the affinity of alcohol for the nervous tissue in animals which explained the predominant nervous effect of alcohol. Lord Ashley Cooper (1801–1885) in his evidence before the Select Committee on Lunatics, said that 50% of cases admitted to British asylums were due to chronic alcoholism. At his request, Thomas John Barnardo (1845–1905) prepared statistics on the causes of destitution in England and was moved by the fact that more than 85% of destitute children reached their plight owing to the drinking habits of their parents and grandparents. Several other reports of asylum wardens in England and America during this time gave similar findings. The earliest breathalyzer to detect the amount of alcohol in the breath was devised by Lallamand, Perrin and Duroy of Paris in 1860. Alcohol still remains a major cause of social, physical and mental ill health and Alcoholics Anonymous, which is a fellowship promoting abstinence amongst alcoholics, was founded in Ohio in 1935. Addiction to other substances and drugs became a problem mostly in the 19th century. The addictive properties of cocaine were first realized by Josef Breuer (1842–1925), a colleague of Sigmund Freud (1856–1939) in Vienna in 1884. *See alcohol, drunkenness.*

Addis Count A time-consuming method of counting various elements formed in urine, such as epithelial cells, erythrocytes and white cells. Introduced by T. Addis (1881–1945) of Edinburgh in 1925, but, owing to impracticality, it was abandoned after a few years. He was professor of medicine at Stanford University in 1921.

Addiscombe College Near Croydon, England, it was established for scientific training of the members of the East India Company in 1809. It closed in 1861.

Addison Disease Described by Thomas Addison (1793–1860), physician to Guy's Hospital in 1849, in an address to the South London Medical Society in his paper, *On Anemia: Disease of the suprarenal capsules.* Six years later, with the help of his junior colleague, Samuel Wilks (1824–1911), he produced another clinical monograph on the subject *On the Constitutional and Local Effects of the Supra-renal Capsules.* William Hunter (1861–1937) used the term 'Addison disease' to denote the condition. Addisonian crisis in situations of stress owing to surgery or infection were recognized from the early 1930s. L.G. Rowntree (1883–1959) of Rochester, Minnesota and Albert Markley Snell (1896–1960) in their monograph on the disease in 1932 pointed out the prohibitive risk involved in performing surgery in patients with adrenal insufficiency and no major surgery was performed successfully in patients with Addison disease until the synthesis of deoxycortisone in 1938. *See adrenal insufficiency.*

Addison Transpyloric Plane Surface marking of the abdomen which accurately points to the disc between the first and second lumbar vertebrae. Described by Christopher Addison (1869–1951), professor of anatomy at Sheffield in 1899.

Addison, Christopher (1869–1951) Viscount Addison of Stallingborough was professor of anatomy at Sheffield. He was appointed as Dean of the Medical School at Charing Cross Hospital in 1901 and was anatomy lecturer at St Bartholomew's Hospital in 1907. He was elected Member of Parliament for Shoreditch in 1910 and was the first Minister of Health, an office which he held from 1918 to 1921.

Addison, Thomas (1793–1860) Physician from Newcastle who graduated from Edinburgh University with his inaugural thesis *De Siphilide* in 1815. He started his career at Guy's Hospital in 1820 and was a physician to the hospital in 1837. He described a disease of the suprarenal capsules (Addison disease) in 1849. *See adrenal insufficiency.*

Addison, William (1802–1881) Medical practitioner from Malvern, England who later became physician to the Duchess of Kent. He wrote on blood and inflammation in seven sections in the *Transactions of the Provincial Medical and Surgical Association* in 1843. He gave a description of leukocytosis and diapedesis of blood cells. His theory on the role of white blood cells in inflammation was confirmed by Julius Friedrich Cohnheim (1839–1884) in 1867.

Addisonian Anemia Thomas Addison (1793–1860) described a form of anemia in 1849, which he mistakenly attributed to a disease of the suprarenal capsule. He later differentiated this condition from suprarenal disease when he defined the clinical syndrome of adrenal insufficiency in 1855.

Adductor Muscles [Latin: *ad*, to + *ducere*, to lead] The three adductors of the thigh were considered to be one muscle by ancient anatomists. Because of its action in pressing the thighs together, the adductor muscle was named *cystos virginitatis.*

Adech The inner spiritual man who is the lord and thought of imagination and influences the outer material man. Theory postulated by Paracelsus (1493–1541) in the 16th century.

Adelmann Operation Disarticulation of the finger with the attached head of the metacarpal bone. Described by German surgeon, George Blasius Franz Adelmann (1811–1888).

Aden Fever *See Dengue Fever.*

Adenia [Greek: *aden*, gland] The term used for generalized hypertrophy of superficial and deep lymphatic glands by Armand Trousseau (1801–1867). The disease was, however, described in 1832 in England by Thomas Hodgkin (1798–1866) and the name Hodgkin disease was given to it by Samuel Wilks (1824–1911) of Guy's Hospital in 1856. *See Hodgkin disease.*

Adenine [Greek: *aden*, gland] A base found in DNA. Isolated from an extract of pancreas by Albrecht Kossel (1853–1927) professor of physiology at Hamburg in 1885.

Adenoid [Greek: *aden*, gland + *oidos*, shape] Observed in humans by Albert von Kölliker (1817–1905) in 1852. Wilhelm Meyer performed the first adenoidectomy in 1868 in the belief that removal of adenoids would improve impaired hearing. Gottenstein devised a curette for adenoidectomy in 1885. The obstructive effect of enlarged adenoids, particularly during sleep, was observed by Ambroise Arnold Guillaume Guye (1839–1904) of Amsterdam in 1884.

Adenoma Sebaceum (Syn. Pringle disease, Bourneville disease) Skin condition associated with epiloia or tuberous sclerosis. Described by French neurologist, Désiré Magloire Bourneville (1840–1909) in 1880. Another account was given later by English dermatologist, John James Pringle (1855–1922). A detailed description of the skin tumors and their association with mental retardation and epilepsy in epiloia was given by John Thompson in 1913.

Adenomyomata [Greek: *aden*, gland + *myos*, muscle] Term used by Friedrich Daniel von Recklinghausen (1833–1910) to denote tumors consisting of gland-like cavities in a mass of smooth muscle. He found these in the uterine cavity

Adenosine Monophosphate *See AMP.*

Adenosine Triphosphate (ATP) Important derivative of adenosine-5–phosphate that plays a key role in cell energy. Isolated from muscle independently by Lohman of Heidelberg, Germany and American biochemist Fritz Albert Lipmann (1899–1986) in 1929. Cyrus Hartwell Fiske (1890–1978) and Yella Pragada Subbarow (1896–1948) also isolated it around the same time. It was shown to be the key factor in supplying energy for muscle contraction during *in vitro* studies by Hungarian scientist Albert Szent-Györgyi (1893–1986) who described it as a cogwheel in the mechanism of muscle contraction in 1938. It was synthesized by Baron Alexander Robertus Todd (b 1907) in 1947. The structure was confirmed by J. Baddiley in 1949. The mechanism of the chemiosmotic gradient involving a proton gradient across the inner mitochondrial membrane in the synthesis of ATP from ADP was proposed by English biochemist and Nobel Prize winner, Peter Dennis Mitchell (1920–1992) of Mitcham, England in the 1960s.

Adenovirus Discovered by Wallace Prescott Rowe and colleagues in 1953. They subjected fragments of adenoids and tonsils removed during surgery to tissue cultivation. The cytopathogenic properties of the cells were then observed and the fluid medium was found to contain an antigen capable of fixing complement in the presence of human serum. A strain of adenovirus was recovered from patients with respiratory illnesses by M.R. Hillemann and Werner in 1954. Many further antigenic types were found by Wallace Prescott Rowe and others in 1958.

Ader, William Physician from Toulouse who lived in the early 17th century. He published a book in 1621, *De Aegrotis et Morbis Evangelesis,* in which he attempted to prove that the diseases cured by Jesus were incurable by medicine.

Adermin [Greek: *a*, without + *derma*, skin] Old term for vitamin B_6 or nicotinic acid in 1938 because of its action in preventing dermatitis. *See nicotinic acid.*

Adherent Pericardium Constrictive pericarditis. Described by English physician Norman Chevers in 1842. Sir William Broadbent, although he observed the physical signs in 1878, published his findings only 20 years later in 1898. Some of the physical signs in the adherent pericardium described by him include diastolic fixation of the apex, diastolic shock on palpation, systolic retraction and indrawing of the posterior lateral aspect of the ribs during systole – now known as Broadbent sign. The occurrence of cirrhosis of the liver with ascites secondary to constrictive pericarditis was described by Friedel Pick (1867–1926) of Germany in 1896. Pericardiectomy as treatment was performed by Paul Hallopeau (1876–1924) of Paris in 1921. Franz Volhard (1872–1950) and Viktor Schmieden (1874–1945) of Germany performed complete excision of the pericardium for treatment in 1923.

Adie Syndrome Holmes–Adie syndrome. Myotonic pupils and absent tendon reflexes. Described by London ophthalmologist, James Ware (1756–1815) in 1813. Myotonic pupils were also described in 1902 by Strassburger and the complete syndrome was recognized by Charles Markus in 1905. Robert Foster Moore (b 1878) later reported 15 cases of tonic pupils which he referred to as 'non-lutic Argyll Robertson pupils'. Dublin-born London neurologist, Gordon Holmes (1876–1965), described 19 cases, all females, under the title 'partial irridoplegia associated with other diseases of the nervous system' in 1931. He also introduced the term, tonic pupils. William John Adie (1886–1935), an Australian-born English physician, after whom the syndrome is named, described it independently first under the title 'pseudo-Argyll Robertson pupils with absent tendon reflexes' in 1931 and later as 'tonic pupils with absent tendon reflexes'. Adie graduated in medicine from Edinburgh in 1911 and worked at several hospitals in London.

Adipocere [Latin: *adeps*, fat + *cera*, wax] French chemist and physician, Antoine François Fourcroy (1755–1809) gave an account of the lumpy tissues which he found in a body on opening a grave at the Cemetery of Innocents in Paris in 1787. He named this tissue 'adipocere' and presented his findings to the Académie des Sciences in Paris in 1789. The fatty nature of the adipocere was shown by Michel Eugene Chevreul (1786–1889) in 1812.

Adipose Tissue [French: *avoir*, to have + *de*, of + *pois*, weight; or Latin: *adeps*, fat] *See adipocere.*

Adiposis Dolorosa Dercum syndrome. Subcutaneous connective tissue disorder resulting from deposition of fat giving rise to painful symptoms in post-menopausal women. Described by American neurologist, Francis Xavier Dercum (1856–1931) of Philadelphia in 1889.

Adipsia [Greek: *a*, negative + *dipsia*, thirst] Term found in Cullen's *Nosology* to denote the want or absence of thirst.

Adler Theory of Psychology In 1920, Alfred Adler (1870–1937) of Vienna proposed a theory that differed from other psychoanalytic and psychological approaches. In 1929 he held that neurosis is a defect or failure in adjustment to the social environment. He said that normal social development is composed of a perfect balance between ego feeling and community feeling brought about by adjustment in three spheres: society, vocation and love. Neurosis arises as a defensive reaction against an obstacle in an endeavor to defend the ego. He also proposed the concept of the inferiority complex and mechanisms involved in overcoming it, in 1907.

Adler, Alfred (1870–1937) Founder of the School of Individual Psychology. He was born in Vienna and graduated in medicine there in 1895. He was president of the Vienna Psychoanalytical Society founded by him, Sigmund Freud (1856–1939) and others, but later broke away from it and formed the Society of Free Analytic Research. He moved to the USA in 1932 and was appointed professor of medical psychology at the Long Island College of Medicine in 1935. *See Adler theory of psychology.*

Adonis Greek god of fertility and the lover of Aphrodite. According to mythology, he was turned into a flower by Venus after he was killed by a wild boar.

Adoption Act of 1926 Passed, following the Tomlin Committee report in 1925, to regulate conditions for adoption of children. The first register for adoption of children was established following these acts. It was superseded by the Adoption Act of 1950 and the amended Act of 1958.

Adoption [Greek: *adoptio*] Practice amongst Romans and Greeks where a man made another person his son giving him the privileges and rights of that relationship. During the 19th century in England the number of abandoned children increased to alarming proportions mainly due to poverty. Adoption became common during this time and the motive varied according to circumstances. Many of the classics of literature such as *Oliver Twist*, *Mansfield Park*, and *Wuthering Heights* reflect the adoption culture during this era. Often children were adopted into poorer families to provide for them by working in the factories and farms. With the implementation of the Abortion Act the number of abandoned children and adoptions drastically reduced. *See Adoption Act.*

ADP, Adenosine diphosphate High-energy compound in cellular respiration synthesized by Baron Alexander Robertus Todd (b 1907) in 1947. *See ATP.*

Adrenal Glands [Latin: *ad*, to + *renes*, kidneys] Described by Bartolommeo Eustachio (1520–1574) whose work was published later by Giovanni Maria Lancisi (1654–1720) of Rome in 1714. A clear distinction between adrenal cortex and medulla was given by an anatomist, Emil Huschke (1797–1858) of Jena. *See adrenal insufficiency, adrenaline, adrenal tumor.*

Adrenal Insufficiency [Latin: *ad*, to + *renes*, kidneys] Thomas Addison (1793–1860) described a clinical syndrome of general fatigue, hyperpigmentation and hypotension associated with disease of the adrenal glands in 1855. The vital function of the adrenal glands required to maintain life was demonstrated by his contemporary, Charles E. Brown-Sequard (1818–1894) in 1856. Occurrence of an active substance in the adrenal medulla was shown in the same year by Edme Felix Alfred Vulpian (1826–1887) of Paris. Effective treatment of Addison disease with fresh adrenal extracts from the hog was introduced by William Osler (1849–1919) in 1896. More specific use of adrenocortical extracts in treatment was introduced independently by two Americans, Julius Moses Rogoff (1883–1966) and Frank Alexander Hartman of Buffalo in 1927, and by Leonard George Rowntree (1883–1959) in 1930. Use of bovine adrenal extract as an established form of treatment followed the work of Rowntree and Hartman. A more purified form of hog adrenal extract was introduced by M. H. Kuizenga in 1943. The importance of the sodium content of the diet of patients with Addison disease was demonstrated by Robert Frederick Loeb (b 1895) and George Argale Harrop (b 1890) of America through experiments in 1933. The deleterious effect of high potassium intake in patients with adrenal insufficiency was demonstrated by Russel Morse Wilder (in 1937) and R. Truszkowski in 1936. An active crystalline compound with effects similar to those of the extracts but more potent was isolated by Swiss chemist Tadeus Reichstein (b 1897) in 1938 who named it 'corticosterone'. Reichstein shared the Nobel Prize in Physiology or Medicine with Edward Calvin Kendall (1886–1972) and Phillip Showalter Hench (1896–1965) for his work on adrenal hormones, in 1950. *See water excretion test.*

Adrenal Rest Tumors [Latin: *ad*, to + *renes*, kidneys] Tumors of the kidney, were thought to arise from cells of the adrenal glands or 'adrenal rests' in the kidney by German surgeon, Paul Albert Grawitz (1850–1932) in 1883. Subsequent work in the following decade showed that these tumors in fact represented adenocarcinoma of the kidney.

Adrenal Tumor Radiological visualization of adrenal tumors by introducing air around the perinephric area was introduced by G. F. Cawhill in 1935. The practical application of this method became limited owing to the risk of air embolism. *See retroperitoneal pneumatography.*

Adrenaline [Latin: *ad*, to + *renes*, kidneys] George Oliver (1841–1915) and Edward Sharpey-Schafer (1850–1935) in 1895 demonstrated that extracts of the suprarenal gland, when injected intravenously, produced contraction of arteries and acceleration of the heart rate, thereby increasing blood pressure. The active substance in the extract was named adrenaline in Britain. Jacob Abel (1857–1938) of

Johns Hopkins Medical School isolated this substance in 1899 and called it epinephrine [Greek: *epi*, upon + *nephros*, kidney] in America. An oral form of crude adrenaline extract was used in treatment of hay fever by an otorhinologist, Jacob da Silva Solis-Cohen (1838–1927) of Jefferson Medical College in 1898. The first pure chemical form was obtained from adrenal extract by Jokichi Takamine (1854–1922) of Japan while he was working at New Jersey in 1901. It was synthesized from organic compounds by Friedrich Stolz (1860–1936), a German chemist, in 1903. This was a landmark in endocrinology and the first time a hormone had been synthetically produced. Subcutaneous administration in asthma was employed by Bullowa and Kaplan in 1903. *See Henry Dale, Ulf von Euler, norepinephrine.*

Adrenergic Blockade *See alpha-adrenergic drugs, beta blockers.*

Adrenocortical Hormones [Latin: *ad*, to + *renes*, kidneys + *cortex*, bark] *See steroids.*

Adrenocorticotropic Hormone *See ACTH.*

Adrenogenital Syndrome An early case was described by English physician, Henry Sampson (1629–1700) from Cambridge. William Bulloch (1868–1941) and James Harry Sequira (1865–1945) described the relationship between suprarenal glands and sex organs in 1905. British endocrinologist, Arthur Carleton Crooke and N.H. Callow described four cases due to adrenocortical dysfunction associated with adrenal tumors, in 1939.

Adrian Committee Appointed in 1956 by the Secretary of the State for Scotland and Minister of Health to review the practice and safety of diagnostic radiology and radiotherapy. The Committee published its report, *The Radiological Hazards to the Patients* in 1960.

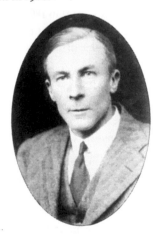

Lord Edgar Douglas Adrian (1889–1977). Courtesy of the National Library of Medicine

Adrian, Lord Edgar Douglas (1889–1977) Pioneer in neurophysiology. Born in London and received his medical education at St Bartholomew's Hospital. He did valuable work on the activity of the nervous system which later paved the way for the development of the electroencephalogram in clinical practice. He shared the Nobel Prize for Physiology or Medicine with Sir Charles Scott Sherrington (1857– 1952) in 1932. *See nerve conduction.*

Adson Sign *See cervical rib syndrome.*

Adsorption Phenomenon occurring on the surface of bacterial cells described by Willard Gibbs in 1878.

Adulteration of Food [Latin: *adulterare*, to defile] Prohibited by law in England in 1272. Frederick Accum (1769–1838), a German-born chemist in England, focused public attention on the subject with his *Death in the Pot* published in 1820. This was followed by Hassel's book *Food and its Adulteration* in 1855. Food analysis was started by the Analytical Sanitary Commission and *The Lancet*, under the editorship of Thomas Wakeley, began publishing its results on food analysis in 1851. Analysis of bread during this time showed that most contained alum to make it heavier during weighing. Similarly, milk contained flour and chalk. The law for preventing adulteration during modern times was passed in England in 1860. The battle against adulteration in America was taken up by a physician and food chemist, Harvey Washington Wiley (1844–1930) of Indiana, and his efforts led to the enactment of the Pure Food and Drug Act of 1906.

Adynmia [Greek: *a*, negative or without + *dynemia*, potency or movement] Term proposed by William Cullen (1710–1790) for one of the conditions in the four orders or groups of neuroses mentioned in his *Nosology*: A disorder of involuntary nerve actions.

Aeby, Christopher Theodor (1835–1885) Professor of anatomy at Bern who described the muscle rectus labi proprius in 1878.

Aedes aegypti Species of mosquito described by Carl Linnaeus (1707–1778) in 1762. It was later proved, by Carlos Finlay (1833–1915) in Cuba in 1881, to be the carrier of arbovirus, which causes yellow fever. *See mosquitoes.*

Aediles A group of public health officials in Rome around AD 70. They looked after the cleanliness of public roads, suitability of food items for consumption, burial methods and other matters of public health. They maintained a high standard of preventive medicine that was not repeated until modern times.

Aedosophia Ancient Greek medical term for the symptom of the passing of flatus, through vagina, uterus or urinary bladder, in cases of rectovesical fistula.

Aegidius, Atheninesis Greek physician in the 8th century who later became a Benedictine monk. He wrote *De Pulsibus et De Venensis* and several other medical works.

Aegineta, Paulus (625–690) *See Paul of Aegina.*

Aegophony [Greek: *aego*, goat + *phony*, voice] Physical sign in which a peculiar resonance of voice is heard during auscultation of the chest. Named and described by the inventor of the stethoscope, René Théophile Laënnec (1781–1826).

Aelianus A physician quoted by Galen (129–200) with respect. He used treacle against plague with apparent success.

Aepinus, Franz Ulrich Theodosius (1724–1802) German physician and physicist from Rostock who graduated from Jena. He worked on electricity and natural philosophy and was Director of the Berlin Observatory in 1755, before he became professor of physics at St Petersburg in 1757. He wrote *Tentamen Theoriae Electricitatis et Magnetisimi* and *Action of Heat* and *Experiments on Tourmalin*.

Aerootitis Media Otitic barotrauma. The first instance of aerootitis media occurred during a balloon journey by French physicist, Jacques Alexander in December 1783. A scientific description was given by S. Scott in his *The Ear in relation to Certain Disabilities in Flying* in 1920.

Aerosol Production of a fine suspension of droplets of liquid or solids in a gas was suggested by Erik Rotheim of Norway in 1926. A device to achieve this was invented by American Julius S. Khan in 1939. The commercial use of aerosol insecticide was introduced by L.D. Goodhue and W.N. Sullivan of America in 1941.

Aerosporin Antibiotic also known as polymyxin. Discovered by Geoffrey Ainsworth (b 1905) and co-workers in England in 1947.

Aesclepiads Guild of physicians who were followers of the Greek god of medicine, Aesculapius. Galen (129–200) referred to them as 'a clan of Aesclepiadae who taught their sons anatomy, who in turn transmitted their learning to the next generation'.

Aesculapiades or Asclepiades (110– 40 BC) Physician from Bithynia who studied medicine in Greece and Alexandria before he came to Rome. He was also an orator and he originated the phrase, 'to cure safely, swiftly and pleasantly'. He was one of the most successful physicians in Rome and is supposed to have founded a new sect to include the

descendants of Aesculapius and also established a medical school in Rome. He differentiated hallucinations from delusions and acute from chronic diseases. He also proposed a theory that the body was composed of atoms that were in constant dynamic action.

Aesculapius [Greek: *askalabos*, snake] Greek god of medicine who, according to legend, was the son of Apollo, the sun god of healing and Coronis, a mortal woman. He was probably a man who lived around 1200 BC. Homer also refers to him as a man and not a god in his *Iliad*. Amongst the hundreds of temples built to him, the chief was built around 600 BC at Epidaurus. His priests glorified and personified Aesculapius and practiced medicine. The practice at the onset was mainly mysticism and magic, but later gave way to physical medicine, with mineral baths, massage, blood letting and the use of therapeutics such as iron, milk and honey. The grounds of the temple contained large nonpoisonous yellow snakes which were allowed to lick diseased parts of the body to effect healing. Owing to this practice, Aesculapius was depicted with a serpent around his staff. His daughter, Panacea, was the deity for treatment of diseases, and his other daughter, Hygeia, was the deity for health and prevention of disease. His two sons, Podalirius and Machaon, were also physicians and the latter is mentioned in the *Iliad* as a blameless physician.

Aesthenia *See asthenia.*

Aesthesiometer Instrument to detect the degree of tactile sensation of the skin. Devised by E. H. Sieveking in the 19th century.

Aethrioscope [Greek: *atheros*, clear + *scopein*, to view] Instrument to measure radiation in the sky. Invented by Sir John Leslie (1766–1822), professor of physics at Edinburgh in 1819.

Aetius of Amida (AD 502–575) Royal physician to the Court of Byzantium. He left a compilation of his works on the medical practice of his celebrated predecessors such as Rufus of Ephesus, Leonides and Soranus. Many of his treatments were accompanied by religious chanting related to the Old and the New Testaments.

Afferent Stretch Fibers [Latin: *afferre*, to bring] *See Ruffini corpuscles.*

Afflatius, Johannes (1040–1100) Saracen pupil of Constantinus during the Salernital period. He wrote *De febribus et urinis.*

Affusion Application of hot or cold water for the treatment of disease. Hippocrates (460 377 BC) in his *Aphorisms* stated 'in a fever that is not of a bilious nature, a copius affusion of hot water upon the head removes the fever'. A pioneer of affusion therapy in Scotland was James Currie (1756–1805), a physician in Dumfries. He published a medical treatise on the subject, *Medical Reports on the Effects of Water, Cold and Warm as a Remedy in Febrile Diseases* in 1797.

Aflatoxins During 1960 hundreds of thousands of deaths involving turkeys, ducklings, sheep and pigs occurred in the farming industry. The cause of these deaths was suspected to be an unidentified toxin in nuts, but subsequent research proved that this toxin came from a fungus, *Aspergillus flavus* and it was named AFLA-toxin and the disease was aflatoxicosis. An assay was devised by K. Sargent and J. O'Kelley in 1961. Liver damage and cancer caused by eating peanuts contaminated with the fungus was noted by Michael May and B. Sporn and co-workers in 1966.

African Lymphoma *See Burkitt lymphoma.*

African Medicine Callie and Mungo Park, in their descriptions of their travels in Africa, mentioned the use of writing as medicine. Some medicine men made their living by writing prayers and incantations on a board and selling the water which was used to wash them. Similar practice amongst the Africans was described by Sir John Lubbock. The Bantu tribe selected their witch doctors through dreams. Those who became witch doctors had to reveal their dreams, make self sacrifices and observe taboos before they were ordained. However, they also made some scientific observations on the passage of food through the body and treated over indulgence in food with herbal laxatives. Zulu medicine men offered three explanations for disease. Either it was caused by the ghosts or *amadhlozi* in which case a sacrifice must be offered to them, or it was the work of a sorcerer. The third possibility was that it is an ordinary illness. Congo witch doctors wore carved wooden masks in their dances to drive away diseases from villages. They treated mental illness by getting patients to dance to a rapid drum rhythm in a state of trance accompanied by hysterical convulsions. Fetish figures were commonly used by the Congo medicine men. Protection against smallpox by the application of material taken from smallpox blisters to the skin, was practiced by some tribes in Africa before the colonial period. The surgeon and missionary explorer of Africa, David Livingstone (1813–1873), described several areas of medical practice during his travels in Africa. *See abdominal injuries, arrow wound, trypanosomiasis.*

Agammaglobulinemia Sex-linked familial condition, reported in an 8-year-old boy with recurrent infection by American pediatrician, Ogden Carr Bruton (b 1908) in 1952.

Agar [Malaysian: *agar-agar*, seaweed] A polymer of galactose units, derived from seaweed. It was introduced as an alternative to gelatin, as a solid culture medium for bacteria, by the wife of the Berlin bacteriologist Walter Hesse (1846–1911) in 1883.

Agassiz, Alexander (1835–1910) American engineer and son of Jean Agassiz (1807–1873) who improved the apparatus for oceanic studies. He made a complete study of deepwater animals and plants of the Caribbean and Pacific on the *Albatross* in 1880.

Agassiz, Jean Louis Rodolphi (1807–1873) Born in Motieren-Vuly, Switzerland. A glaciologist who emigrated to America in 1846 and settled in Massachusetts. He wrote *The Fishes of Brazil* while he was a student in 1829. His *Lectures on Comparative Embryology* intended for the laymen was published in a Boston newspaper in 1854. He described over 1000 species of fossil fish from 1833 to 1844 and discovered 'the Great Ice Age'. He was an opponent of Darwinian evolution and an advocator of the recapitulation theory. He founded a museum of comparative zoology at Harvard to which he gave his collections in 1859. *See glacial period.*

Agathinus of Sparta (*c.* AD 100) Contemporary of Plutrach, who practiced medicine in Rome in the 1st century. He wrote on cold baths as a cure and Galen (129–200) quoted him in his treatises.

Age In ancient Rome and Greece, 25 years was fixed as the full age required to attain majority, although a higher age was prescribed for certain positions. The royal family at certain times waived the age requirement for their heirs so that they could assume royal status and responsibility at an earlier age if needed.

Age Concern The National Old People Welfare Council (NOPWC) was set up to address the problems of elderly at the initiative of the National Council for Social Services in 1955. NOPWC became independent from the social services and was renamed Age Concern in 1974.

Ager or Aegerius, Nicholas Physician and botanist during the 17th century who was professor of medicine at Strasbourg. A friend of Caspar Bauhin (1560–1624), he published *De Anima Vegetative* (1629) and *Disputatio De Zoophytis* (1625).

Agglutination [Latin: *ad*, to + *glutinare*, glue] Described by Max Gruber (1853–1927) of Vienna and his pupil Edward Herbert Durham (1866–1945) following their observations in 1894 that clumping of bacteria occurred as a result of mixing a bacterial suspension in serum with its homologous antiserum. This was applied by French micro-biologist, Isidore Widal (1862–1929) to develop a diagnostic test for typhoid or enteric fever.

Agglutinogens [Latin: *ad*, to + *glutinare*, glue] Complex antigenic factors that stimulate antibodies in the body. Their presence was discovered by Edmund Weil (1880–1922) and Arthur Felix (1887–1956) in 1916, following their observation that the 'O' and 'H' factors of *Proteus* bacteria had specific antigenic properties.

Aggression Studied by Austrian zoologist, Konrad Zacharias Lorenz (1903–1989). He developed the study of animal behavior called 'ethology' and in his book *On Aggression* (1963), he argued that behavior in man is inherited and could be channeled to other productive activities.

Aging Alchemists searched for the elixir of life to attain eternal youth. Their search was rewarded with many serendipitous discoveries but the elixir of life remained elusive. A book related to therapeutics in old age, *The Cure of Old Age* was written by Roger Bacon in AD 1200. Another on preserving good health in old age was written by a Venetian, Luigi Cornaro (1467–1566) in 1550. He was 83 years old when he wrote this book and it contained many sensible suggestions for living healthily in old age. He wrote rules for maintaining health and prolonging life when he was 86 years and a third book on the joys of old age when he reached 95 years and he died in his 99th year. In 1724, Sir John Floyer (1649–1734) wrote a monograph on geriatrics *Medicina Gerocomica*. The first organized course on geriatrics at the Sâlpetrière was inaugurated by Jean Marie Charcot (1825–1893) in 1867. *See geriatrics, gerontology, old age.*

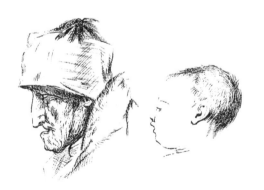

Infancy and old age. Sir Charles Bell, *The Anatomy and Philosophy of Expression*. George Bell & Son, London

Agnew Splint Splint for fracture of the patella devised by Philadelphia surgeon, David Hayes Agnew (1818–1892).

Agni An ancient fire god of the Hindus, who used fire for performing rituals in weddings and burning the dead. He was also called upon to cure fever.

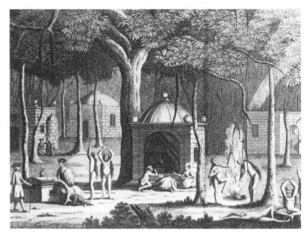

Hindus worshipping fire. Thomas Maurice, *Indian Antiquites* (1744). W. Richardson, London

Agnodice A midwife and female physician who studied under Herophilus in Alexandria around 300 BC. In her days, women were forbidden by law to practice any form of healing and she had to disguise herself as a man. For this she was brought to trial before Arcophagus. Most of her Athenian patients appeared on her behalf, and this resulted in her acquittal. The law was repealed.

Agoraphobia [Greek: *agora*, market place + *phobia*, fear] A description was given by the neurologist Carl Friedrich Otto Westphal (1833–1890) of Berlin in 1871.

Agranulocytosis [Greek: *a*, without; Latin: *granulum*, small grain; Greek: *kytos*, cell] Complete disappearance of polymorphonuclear leukocytes from the blood. Described by Werner Shultz in 1907 and in his description of a case of necrotic ulcerative lesions of the throat in 1922.

Agraphia [Greek: *a*, without + *graphein*, to write] Inability to express thoughts in writing because of a central lesion in the brain was described by French physician, Jean Albert Pitres (1848–1928) in 1884.

Agregator de Medicinis Simplicibus One of the earliest known medical *incunabulas*. Published by Adolf Rush at Strasbourg in 1470.

Agricola, Georgius (1494–1555) Georg Bauer, a German physician, was born at Glauchau in Saxony. He studied at the Universities of Bologna, Leipzig and Venice and wrote several treatises on medicine, geology, weights, measures and metals. He was official physician to Joachimsthal in Bohemia, a mining district, where he did most of his work on metallurgy. His *De Re Metallica* was published in 12 books at Basel in 1556, *De Peste* was published in 1554 and a book on physical geology, *De Ortu et Causis Subterraneorum* was published in 1546.

Agriculture For millions of years man lived by hunting and gathering. Man's ability to control the ecological conditions to produce food determined his survival. The ancient Greeks probably learnt their farming methods from Egyptians and Hesiod, a Greek poet who lived during the 8th century BC gave a description of the three principal parts of the plow. A primitive form was also known to the Chinese around 3500 BC. The threshing machine was invented by a Scottish millwright, Andrew Meikle in 1787. Corn was cut with the sickle and the scythe for many centuries until the invention of a reaping machine by a clergyman, Patrick Bell in 1826. An improved version was made by McCormick in 1833. An experimental farm was founded by English agriculturist, Sir John Bennet Lawes (1814–1900) at Rothamsted in 1843. Pioneering work in England on nitrogen fertilizers was done by Sir Joseph Henry Gilbert (1817–1901) from Hull. A scientific facility was built at the Rothamsted Experimental Farm in 1885 and was manned by 40 agricultural scientists headed by Sir John Edward Russell (1872–1965) in 1912. He wrote *Soil Conditions and Plant Growth* in 1912. The Haber process for making cheap fertilizer by extracting nitrogen from the air to make ammonia was invented by Polish professor, Fritz Haber (1868–1934) in Germany in 1908.

Agriothymia [Greek: *agros*, wild + *thymos*, mind] Insane ferocity.

Agrippa A Greek name for one who is born feet first.

Agrippa, Cornelius (1486–1535) From a noble family in Cologne, Germany. He was interested in occult science, but later studied medicine. He was in eternal conflict with himself and everybody around him, which drove him to wander across Europe. He was physician to the Queen Regent in Lyons for a brief period. His controversial treatise *The Vanity of Sciences* brought intense opposition, resulting in his persecution and a prison sentence. He died as a pauper at the Grenoble Hospital in France.

Agrypnia A nervous disorder accompanied by disturbance of sleep.

Ague Intermittent fever or malaria. *See malaria.*

Ague Drops Medicine containing arsenic in water used for cure of ague.

Ague-Cake Chronically enlarged spleen, owing to malaria.

Ahlquist, Raymond Perry (1914–1983) *See beta blockers.*

Ahmes Papyrus The oldest existing mathematical manuscript copied from an earlier manuscript (1825 BC) by Ahmes of Egypt in 1650 BC. It was bought by Egyptologist Henry Rhind at Cairo in 1858 and was brought to London. *See mathematics.*

Ahura Mazda or Ormuzd Mythical god of goodness amongst the Persians around 2000 BC. He delegated the art of healing to an angel called Thrita who later became the god of medicine and healing.

AIDS Acquired Immune Deficiency Syndrome. In 1981 the Center for Disease Control (CDC) at Atlanta, Georgia started receiving reports of an unusual number of chest infections due to *Pneumocystis carinii* in young men who were not known to have any risk factors for acquiring an opportunistic infection. At the same time a rise in the incidence of Kaposi sarcoma was noted and the only common factor between these infections was found to be homosexuality. The illness were mainly found in homosexuals and was renamed AIDS when other groups such, as hemophiliacs and Haitian immigrants, were also noted to be at increased risk. Research focused on the HTLV-1 virus as a possible cause. A new retrovirus, HIV, was isolated in Paris by a French molecular biologist, Luc Montagnier (b 1932) and colleagues at the Pasteur Institute in 1983 and an American team led by Robert Gallo also claimed credit for the discovery in *Nature* in 1983. Later findings have suggested that Gallo's sample originally came from Montagnier's laboratory. Montagnier was made head of the department of AIDS and retroviruses in 1990.

Aikin, John (1747–1822) Physician from Great Yarmouth who wrote several poems, biographies and translations from Tacitus.

Ainhum [African: *ainhum*, to saw] Disease that affects the toes and forms a constriction leading to natural amputation. Described amongst people of Sudan by Clarke in 1860 in *Dry Gangrene of the Little Toe Among the Natives of the Gold Coast*. It derives its name from an African word for 'to saw'. The same disease, where a concentric ring appeared in one of the digits leading to dry gangrene, was described amongst the Hindus of India by A. Collas of Paris in 1867.

Ainsworth, Geoffrey *See aerosporin.*

Air Anaximenes, Greek philosopher and disciple of Thales proposed that air is the essence of all things including life around 570 BC and he called it 'pneuma' to mean 'breath'. Empedocles of Agrigento demonstrated that air had mass in

450 BC. A study of the physical properties, including compressibility, elasticity and mass was done by Robert Boyle (1627–1691) and Robert Hooke (1635–1703) in 1660. John Mayow (1643–1679), an English physician in 1674, showed that when a substance was burnt in a closed vessel the volume of air diminished and combustion stopped. His study also included one of the early experiments on respiratory physiology. Nitrogen was obtained from air by Daniel Rutherford (1749–1819), a pupil of Joseph Black (1728–1799) in 1772. Carl Wilhelm Scheele (1742–1786) demonstrated the presence of oxygen in air in 1773. Cavendish published his treatise on the composition of air in 1784. Gay-Lussac (1778–1850), a French chemist, took several samples of air from a balloon at different altitudes and formulated the law of combination of gases. Lavoisier published his *Elementary Treatise on Chemistry* describing the properties of hydrogen, nitrogen and oxygen in 1789.

Air Balloon Proposed by Albert of Saxony, an Augustinian monk in the 14th century. The principle was demonstrated to the King of Portugal by a Jesuit priest, Laurenco de Guzmon in 1709. Two brothers, Joseph Michael Montgolfier (1740–1810) and Jacques Etienne Montgolfier (1745–1799) flew a 35 m diameter balloon in 1783. Later in the same year a flight carrying a live cargo, a sheep, a cock and a duck, was performed before Louis XVI. The first balloon crossing of the English Channel was achieved by an American physician from Boston, John Jeffries (1744–1819), who emigrated to England. Aviation medicine started with medical problems related to air balloon travel. Jacques Alexander Charles, a French physicist, was the first casualty. He suffered aerootitismedia during a balloon journey in December 1783 and never flew again. Scientific observations and physiological data were recorded by Glashier and Coxwell flying to a height of 29,000 feet in 1862. Emission of toxic gases was a problem and many unexplained deaths occurred amongst air battalions in Prussia and other countries around 1884. A detailed description of high altitude anoxia experienced by James Glashier who performed several balloon flights at a height of over 26,000 feet at the Wolverhampton base in England, started research into high altitude anoxia.

Air Filter Filter made of powdered charcoal for purifying air was devised by Stenhouse in 1854. They were used in 1920s to provide allergen-free air to patients with asthma.

Air Hunger *See Kussmaul breathing.*

Air Pollution Hippocrates (460–377 BC) in his treatise on air mentioned that those cities in the west were so influenced by those from the east that winds had no access

to blow away noxious vapors, making their inhabitants unhealthy and subject to bad distempers. An early treatise on the pollution of air in London, *Fumifugium: or the Inconvenience of the Aer and Smoake of London Dissipated*, was written by John Evelyn (1620–1706) in 1661. English physician, George Bodington (1799–1882) of Sutton Coldfield, pointed out the value of fresh air in pulmonary complaints. In 1927, Willem Storm van Leeuwen (1882–1933) of Holland did extensive studies on the effect of allergens in air on asthma. He devised allergen-free chambers that drew air from 35 m above the ground and were airtight. These were housed in buildings called van Leewen houses. The air pollution from burning coal was noted by Charles Proteus Steinmetz in 1910. *See air sampling, ozone, smog.*

Air Pump Devised by Otto Guericke (1602–1686), Mayor of Magdeburg in Prussia in 1656 and published by a Jesuit priest, Kasper Schott (1608–1666) in his *Mechanica Hydraulico-Pneumatica* in 1657. This was studied by Robert Boyle (1627–1691) and Robert Hooke (1635–1703) who modified and improved it in 1659. Boyle conducted experiments on gases and air and demonstrated that air was essential for life by creating a vacuum and studying the effect of it on small animals and on combustion. His *New Experiments Physico-Mechanical touching the spring of the Air* was published in 1660.

Air Sampling A biological study was done in 1748 by J.G. Gleditsch, a botanist in Berlin. He obtained samples of air and showed that they could still propagate growth of molds despite being introduced into a sterile closed container. Christian Gottfried Ehrenberg (1795–1876) of Berlin did further extensive studies around 1840 to prove that air contained contagious organisms. The presence of organisms in air was also shown by Angus Smith of England in 1846. In 1861, Louis Pasteur (1822–1895) demonstrated microbes in air taken from different areas. The presence of spores in air was demonstrated by John Tyndall (1820–1893) in 1881. Pierre Miquel of Paris developed the quantitative technique for estimating spore contents in the air in 1883 and similar work was carried out independently around the same time by Walter Hesse of Berlin.

Air Sickness Due to vertical acceleration and excessive rotatory movements during aircraft flights was described independently by F. Dammart and E. Everling of Germany in 1930. An English treatise, *Air Sickness and Sea Sickness* was published by M. Flack in 1931.

Air Travel Regulations were drawn up in 1944 to curb the spread of disease through air travel by the International Convention for Aerial Navigation. The methods proposed included immunization against the five diseases: yellow fever, smallpox, plague, cholera and typhus. An English treatises *Epidemiology in Relation to Air Travel* was written by A. Massey in 1933. A treatise dealing with medical fitness to travel and the transport of invalids was written by F. Rohrer in 1915.

Air Ventriculography Introduction of air into the ventricles of the brain for visualizing them radiologically. Practiced by Walter Edward Dandy (1886–1946) of Missouri who was professor of neurosurgery at Johns Hopkins in 1918. Erik Lysholm (1891–1947) improved the technique by introducing new apparatus and taking 12 different projections in 1938. His method required minimal introduction of air, thereby reducing the risk. A technique of encephalography using less air was described by Edward Graeme Robertson (b 1903) in 1941.

Airy, Sir George Biddle (1801–1892) Northumberland Astronomer Royal who modernized the observatory at Greenwich. He applied photography to astronomical research and founded the magnetic department of Greenwich Observatory in 1834. He did research on optics and corrected astigmatism using lens in 1824. He performed a series of pendulum experiments to determine the mean density of the Earth at Harton Colliery, South Shields near Newcastle and published over 500 papers.

Aitken, John (1839–1919) Scottish physicist from Falkirk who did extensive studies on climatology, dealing with atmospheric dust, dew and cyclones. His collected works were published posthumously by Knott in 1923.

Aitkin Pill A remedy containing reduced iron, quinine, strychnine and arsenic. Prepared by Scottish physician, Sir William Aitkin (1825–1892).

Aitkin, John (d 1790) Edinburgh surgeon who wrote *A System of Anatomical Tables with Explanation* in 1786 and designed the operation, which now bears his name, of double pelviotomy for a narrow pelvis.

Aka Mushi [Japanese: *mushi*, red insect] (Syn. *Shima mushi*, Japanese river fever, flood fever) Seasonal fever along the rivers of certain regions in Japan was described independently by T. A. Palm (1878) and E. Balz (1879). A trombeculoid tick, known as *aka mushi* in Japan was identified as the transmitter.

Akakia, Martin (d 1551) Native of Champagne and professor of physick at Paris who changed his name to the Greek, Akakia. He translated Galen (129–200) *De Ratione Curandi.* His son Martin became physician to King Henry III and wrote *De Morbis Mulieribus* and other treatises.

Akenside, Mark (1721–1770) Physician and poet who rose to be physician to the Queen. He was a son of a butcher at Newcastle-upon-Tyne and studied divinity at Edinburgh at the age of 18, changed to medicine which he studied for 18 months. He practiced as a surgeon in 1743. His poetical talents were revealed in his *The Pleasures of Imagination.* With the rewards from his poetry he proceeded to Leiden to complete his medical degree with a dissertation on the human fetus in 1744. On his return he rapidly advanced to become a member of the Royal College of Physicians and fellow of the Royal Society in 1753. He was appointed physician to the Queen in 1761. His other poetry includes *Love, an Elegy* and *An Ode on the Winter-Solstice* published in 1740.

Akut *See acne.*

Alastrim [Portuguese: to spread or strew about] Variola minor, a mild form of smallpox.

Albarrán, Joaquin Dominguez (1860–1912) Born in Cuba and emigrated to France, where he became professor of medicine. He made significant contributions to renal medicine. He also devised the Albarrán lever found in early cystoscopes. *See Albarrán gland, Albarrán operation, Albarrán test.*

Albarrán Gland The portion of the median lobe of the prostate immediately underlying the uvula vesicae. First described by Joaquin Dominguez Albarrán (1860–1912) in 1891.

Albarrán Operation Nephropexy. Designed by French surgeon of Cuban origin, Joaquin Dominguez Albarrán (1860–1912).

Albarrán Test Oral water-load test for assessing kidney function. Devised by Joaquin Dominguez Albarrán (1860–1912).

Albee, Houdlett Fred (1876–1945) Born in Maine, he employed living bone grafts for internal splints and transplanted tibia into spine diseased with Pott Disease. He also introduced anterior spinal fusion in the treatment of Pott disease in 1906.

Albers-Schönberg, Heinrich Ernst (1865–1921) German radiologist who graduated from Leipzig University in 1891. He described an inherited disorder of bone, osteopetrosis accompanied by leukoerythroblastic anemia and hepatosplenomegaly in 1903. The disease, also known as marble bone disease, was later named Albers-Schönberg disease.

Albert Disease Form of bursitis of the achilles tendon

accompanied by pain. Described by Austrian surgeon Eduard Albert (1841–1900) in 1893.

Alberti, Solomon (1540–1600) Born in Nuremberg and studied anatomy under Fabricius. He became the professor of medicine at Wittemberg and wrote *Historia pleramque Humani Corporis partium Membratim Scripta* and *Tres Orationes*.

Albertini, Ippolito Francisco (1666–1746) Italian physician at Bologna who described bed rest and abstinence from food as treatment for aortic aneurysm.

Albertus Magnus (1192–1280) Dominican priest, philosopher and scientist who studied astrology and alchemy. His compilation of botanical plants in 1250, *De Vegetabilibus*, remained popular for many centuries. He was a follower of Aristotle and wrote voluminous commentaries on his works. He described arsenic in detail.

Albini, Guiseppe (1827–1911) Professor of physiology at Naples who described the minute nodules at the margins of the tricuspid and mitral valves of the heart (Albini nodules) in 1856.

Albinism *See albino.*

Albinolo, Felix Italian who established himself in London around 1880 selling his own brand of ointments and supplying leeches. Thomas Holloway (1800–1883), the founder of Holloway Sanatorium, got the idea of making ointments from him, and made his fortune. *See Holloway, Thomas; Holloway pills.*

Albino [Latin: *albus*, white] Aristotle (384–322 BC) mentioned this as *leuce*, a disease in which all the hairs of the body turn white. It was previously called 'snow white leprosy' by ancient Jews. It was defined as a change of skin to a white color by a viscid and glutinous phlegm, by Paul of Aegina (625–690). He pointed out that *alphos* is similar to *leuce*, but the former produced a deep color change in the skin. Aulus Cornelius Celsus (25 BC–AD 50) described a variety of vitiligo which resembled leuce. Islamic physicians treated the condition as 'morphoea alba', a name which Guy de Chauliac (1300–1370) also used. Paul of Aegina stated that Negroes affected with the condition were called 'albinos'.

Albinus, Bernard Siegfried (1697–1771) Anatomist whose anatomical museum in Leiden was visited and admired by many eminent men, including William Hunter (1718–1783) who visited in 1746. He published a three-volume work on anatomy in 1744, 1749 and 1753. Several muscles in his treatises were named after him.

Albinus, Christian Bernard (d 1778) Also known as Weiss or White. Professor of medicine at Utrecht in 1702. He published a history of spiders and insects with engravings and also wrote several treatises in medicine. He was a brother of Bernard Siegfried Albinus (1697–1771).

Albiruni (AD 973–1048) Physician, astronomer and physicist who used the principle of Archimedes to determine the specific weight of 18 metals and precious stones. He wrote *Chronology of Ancient Nations.*

Albrecht, Karl Martin Paul (1851–1894) Hamburg anatomist who described the basal ossicle between sphenoid and occipital bones (Albrecht bone) in 1878.

Albright Syndrome Patchy areas of skin pigmentation, bone change, endocrine dysfunction and precocious puberty in females. Described by Fuller Albright (1900–1969), Alan Marcy Butler (b 1894), A.O. Hampton and P. Smith in 1937. It was described independently in the same year by D. McCune and H. Bruch, as osteodystrophia fibrosa.

Albright, Fuller (1900–1969) Father of endocrinology in America. He graduated from Harvard Medical School in 1924 and did most of his work at the Massachusetts General Hospital. His main interests were bone diseases and the parathyroid glands. He described vitamin D-resistant rickets, osteomalacia of steatorrhea, idiopathic hypoparathyroidism, bone changes in kidney disease and several other important endocrinological entities. He observed the symptomatology of Parkinson disease on himself for over 10 years and became incapacitated by it.

Albucasis or Abul Qasim uz-Zahrawi (936–1013) Author and surgeon, born at El-Zahara near Cordova and appointed physician to Abdar Rahman III (912–961). He wrote an encyclopedia of medicine and surgery, *Altasrif*. The surgical portion was published separately and became the first independent illustrated work on the subject. It contained illustrations of a remarkable array of surgical instruments and described operations for fractures, dislocations, bladder stones, gangrene and other conditions. It replaced Paul of Aegina's (625–690) *Epitome* as a standard work and remained as the most used textbook of surgery for nearly 500 years. The Latin translation of *Altasrif* was printed in Venice in 1497. He wrote *Liber Servitorus* which described medical preparations obtained from plants, animals and minerals – an early example of chemotherapeutics. He described the obstetric position now known as Walcher position.

Albumazer Arab physician in the ninth century who studied astronomy. His wrote *Introductio ad Astronomium* published in 1489 and other treatises.

27

Albumin [Latin: *albumin*, white of egg] Egg white was first commented upon by Aristotle. Pliny called it *ovi albus liquor* and Palladius named it *albumentum*. A preparation of crystalline egg albumin was made by Franz Hofmeister (1850– 1922) in 1899. The term 'albumin' for proteins that are soluble in water and salt solutions is based on the proposal of the British Physiological Society (1907) and the American Physiological Society (1908). The molecular weight of egg albumin was calculated at 34000 d by P.L. Sorenson (1868– 1939) in 1917.

Albuminuria Albumin present in the urine. White clouds in the urine were noted by Hippocrates (460–377 BC). Albumin in the urine was shown by boiling and the addition of acetic acid by Fredericus Dekkers (1648–1720) of Leiden in 1694. Dominic Cotugno (1736–1822) of Vienna rediscovered it in the urine by a similar method in 1764 and the term albuminuria was introduced by Martin Solon of Paris in 1838. English physician John Blackall (1771–1860) demonstrated it in cases of dropsy in 1813. The relationship between albuminuria and renal disease was established by Richard Bright (1789–1858) in 1827. Its occurrence in fevers was described by Martin Solon in 1838 and named febrile albuminuria by Carl Gerhardt (1833–1902) of Germany in 1868. The presence of albumin in the urine of mothers with puerperal convulsions or eclampsia was observed by John Charles Lever (1811–1858), a lecturer in midwifery at Guy's Hospital in London in 1843. The presence of massive albuminuria in subarachnoid hemorrhage was noted by French pathologist and microbiologist, Georges Fernand Isidore Widal (1862–1929) in 1903. *See benign albuminuria.*

Alcadinus A native of Salerno and a celebrated physician of the 12th century. He was physician to the French Court and his works in Latin include *De Balneis Puteolanis* and *De Trumphis Henrici Imperioris* which he wrote after he cured Emperor Henry of a rare malady.

Alcandrius A Latin document on astrology of Arabic origin dating back to AD 950 bearing the name of Alcandrius has provided evidence for Arabic influence in Europe during that period. It also has occasional use of Hebrew script in it which suggests that it must have passed through Jewish hands.

Alchemy [Greek: *chemia*; Arabic: *kimiya*, art of counterfeiting gold or silver + *al*, the] Its origin is difficult to trace but it is supposed to have been practiced by the Chinese in 133 BC. Documented literature dates to the fourth century written in Alexandria by Zosmismus of Papolis. The fundamental of alchemy is to obtain the 'essence' which would change base

metals into gold, cure all diseases and give eternal youth. The guardian or possessor of this mythical essence or 'philosopher's stone' was a mythical personality, Hermes Trismegeastos. The pursuit of this goal contributed to the development of methods of experimentation in chemistry and metallurgy. Some of the works on alchemy are found in the writings of, Geberius in the Middle Ages; Albertus Magnus (1206–1280), a Dominican monk; Roger Bacon (1214–1294), and a Benedictine monk, Basilus Valentinus (AD 1500). Paracelsus (1493–1541) proposed that the true aim of alchemy should be to cure diseases and the preparation and study of drugs should be the main object of the chemist.

Alcmaeon Philosopher and a pupil of Pythagoras who founded the Sicilian School around 500 BC. He dissected animals and studied their brains. He proposed the balance of body fluid in health and disease which probably formed the basis for the Hippocratic theory of the four humors. He is credited with the discovery of the optic nerve and the Eustachian tube.

Alcock, Benjamin (b 1801) Irish professor of anatomy, born at Kilkenny and graduated from University of Dublin in 1827. He was the first professor of anatomy at Queen's College, Cork in 1849. He described the fascial canal lying on the obturator internus in the lateral wall of the ischiorectal fossa which is named after him. He was forced to resign over a dispute on the Anatomy Act in 1853. After an unsuccessful petition to the Queen, he left for America.

Alcock, Nathan (1707–1779) English physician, born at Runcorn, Cheshire. He studied under Herman Boerhaave (1668–1738) in Leiden and took his doctor's degree in 1737. His *On the Effects of Climate* was unfinished at the time of his death.

Alcock, Sir Rutherford (1809–1897) Ealing surgeon who trained at Westminster Hospital. He became the British Consul in China and helped to establish the port at Shanghai. In 1858 he moved to Japan as the Consul General but resigned in 1871 and returned London. His *Notes on the Medical History and Statistics of the British Legion of Spain* was published in 1838.

Alcock, Thomas (1784–1883). The father of Sir Rutherford Alcock (1809–1897), a surgeon who became British Consul in China. He was a surgeon at St James' Workhouse in London. He contributed several scientific essays to medical journals.

Alcocke, Nicholas (d 1550) Surgeon to King Edward VI.

Alcohol [Arabic: *alkohl*] Term adopted by alchemists for fermented grapes. It is the oldest drug known to man and the Chinese were probably the first to make wine. Scottish diplomat Sir John Malcolm (1769–1833) in his *History of Persia* credited the Persians with the discovery of alcohol. In Greek mythology, the god Dionysos is credited with the discovery of wine making. The earliest charge of drunkenness was documented around 1300 BC. Pliny described over 100 varieties of wine made in ancient Rome. Alcohol, mainly in the form of wine, was used as a medicine, aphrodisiac, social stimulant and chemical. Arabian alchemist Geberius, who lived around the 8th century at Seville, called it aqua vitae. An attempt at producing absolute alcohol was made by Arnold of Villanova (1234–1311) in 1300, who introduced brandy into the pharmacopoeia. German Benedictine monk, Basil Valentine obtained absolute alcohol in the year 1400. Alcoholism was recognized as a problem in England in the 18th century during the gin-drinking era (1740–1742). Legislation to curb the use of foreign alcohol fueled by a nation of excessive gin drinkers was passed by Parliament in 1736 but was ineffective and was followed by a prohibitive tax on alcohol. Lavoisier discovered that alcohol contained carbon, hydrogen and oxygen and the proportion of these elements was estimated by Nicolas T. de Saussure (1767–1845) in 1814. Production of beer was known to ancient Chinese and Egyptians and became popular in Germany around 1600. A microchemical method of measuring small quantities of alcohol in blood using a photoelectric colorimeter was devised by J.G. Gibson in 1938. *See alcoholism.*

Alcohol Dehydrogenase Enzyme crystallized from yeast by E. Negelein and J. Wulff in 1937.

Alcohol Injection Treatment for neuralgia introduced by French physician Jean Albert Pitres (1848–1928) in 1887. Injection into the deep foramina of the exit of the main fifth nerve in the skull as treatment for trigeminal neuralgia was performed by Jean Pitres and Henry Verger (1873–1930) of Paris in 1902 and French ophthalmologist, Joseph Louis Jean Abadie (b 1873) advocated the same treatment. Ferdinand Levy and A. Baudouin devised another approach for injection from outside the cheek to the foramen ovale and foramen rotundum in 1906 and this was established over the previous intra-oral route. An alcohol injection into the Gasserian ganglion through the sigmoid notch was performed by Wilfred Harris (1869–1960), a neurologist at St Mary's Hospital in 1910.

Alcoholic Polyneuritis The earliest account of this condition was given by John Coakley Lettsom (1744–1815) in

Some remarks on the Effects of Lignum Quassiae Amarae published in 1786. James Jackson (1777–1867) of Boston Medi-cal School described the clinical features in *On a Peculiar Disease Resulting from the Use of Ardent Spirit* in 1822. An account of alcoholic paraplegia was given by Samuel Wilks (1824–1911) in 1868. Julius Dreschfield (1845–1907) of Manchester divided the clinical presentation of alcoholic neuritis into paralytic and ataxic groups in 1898 and it was also known as pseudotabes of alcoholics. Patrick Manson (1844–1922) in 1898 pointed out the association with thiamine deficiency and G.C. Shattuck in 1928 and other workers confirmed the part played by nutritional deficiency.

Alcoholic Psychosis Associated with delirium tremens and described by Thomas Sutton (1767–1835) in 1813. The neurological manifestation of chronic alcoholism, characterized by polyneuritis and marked memory loss with confabulation, was described by Russian physician, Sergei Korsakoff (1853–1900) in 1887.

Alcoholics Anonymous A worldwide fellowship to promote abstinence and rehabilitation amongst alcoholics. Originated in Ohio in 1935.

Alcoholism Described by Pliny (AD 23–79) as 'pallor, pendulous cheeks, bloodshot eyes, tremulous hands which spill the full cup and an ever-present penalty, sleep disturbed by furies, restlessness at night and lastly monstrous passions and even crimes which in their eyes have become supreme delight. The next day the wine infects their breath and their memory is dead'. *See addiction, drunkenness, temperance.*

Alcola A secret remedy offered by the Physicians Cooperative Association of Chicago as treatment for drunkenness in the late 19th century. Three kinds of tablets were prescribed to be taken in a complicated ritual manner. These were later found to contain lactose, calcium and traces of strychnine.

Alcuin (AD 735–804) English monk from York who had considerable influence on Emperor Charlemagne which helped to bring about educational reforms and establishment of schools in many parts of France. He helped to transmit knowledge and learning of the earlier ages into the Middle Ages.

Aldehyde Named by German chemist, Johann Christian Poggendorf (1796–1877), professor of chemistry at Berlin. He produced a collection of biographies of over 8000 physicists from all countries in two volumes, which has since been extended to 18 volumes. He discovered a multiplying galvanometer (1821) and a magnetometer (1827).

Alderman Nerve The auricular branch of the vagus nerve. Named because of the practice of applying cold water to the external auditory meatus by aldermen to induce vomiting after excesses.

Alderotti, Taddeo (1223–1303) Professor of medicine in Bologna who wrote *Della Conservazione Della Satue* and *Consilia*, or a collection of clinical cases.

Aldinol A drug used as an anti-obesity agent in America in the 1930s. *See dinitrophenol.*

Aldolase Enzyme crystallized from rabbit and rat muscle by J.F. Taylor and co-workers in 1948.

Aldomet a-methyl dopa, the first effective inhibitor of the synthesis of norepinephrine. Discovered by Theodore R. Sourkes of McGill University in 1954. It was introduced into clinical practice for treatment of hypertension by Oates and Sjoerdsma in 1960 and remains the longest surviving antihypertensive drug.

Aldosterone Sodium-retaining factor in venous blood from the adrenal glands. Identified through chromatography by S.A. Simpson, J.F. Tait and P.G.G. Bush in 1952. It was isolated from beef renal extract by Hillary Grundy in the same year. The clinical syndrome due to excessive secretion of aldosterone was described by William Jerome Conn (b 1907) of Michigan in 1955 and it was named Conn syndrome.

Aldosterone Antagonist The 17–spironolactone, a compound with the reverse effects of aldosterone, was produced by C.M. Kagawa and J.A. Cella in 1957. Its sodium diuretic effect was explained by G.W. Liddle in the same year. The beneficial effect in treating ascites of cirrhosis was demonstrated by D.N.S. Kerr, A.E. Read, R.M. Haslam and Shiela Sherlock in 1958.

Aldrich Syndrome *See Wiskott–Aldrich syndrome.*

Aldrovandus, Ulysses (1527–1605) Professor of medicine and philosophy at Bologna. He wrote *Ornithology* (1599) in three volumes, *Quadrupeds which Divide the Hoof, Insects* (1602) and other works on biology and natural science.

Ale Egyptians were supposed to be the first to have made liquor from corn by fermentation. It was known as a beverage as early as in 404 BC. Ale-houses are mentioned in the laws of the King of Essex in AD 688 and were regulated in 1551. In 1603 during the reign of James I, the price and the measure of ale were specified and duty was introduced in 1643.

Aleppo Boil Due to endemic leishmaniasis in Aleppo. Described by Jean Louis Alibert (1766–1837) in 1829 and by Alexander Russel in 1856.

Alexander of Tralles or Trallianus (525–605) Philosopher and physician, considered one of the best Greek physicians after Hippocrates (460–377 BC). He described parasitic worms for the first time in his work on medicine which was published in Paris in 1543.

Alexander the Great (356–323 BC) The symptoms of Alexander during his last illness are described in Greek royal journals. Much speculation has taken place regarding its nature and his symptoms fit the description of Ardent fever for which there are many possible causes. The two commonly proposed causes of his death are yellow fever and malaria.

Alexander, Benjamin (1735–1768) Irish physician who graduated from Leiden in 1761 and was elected physician to the London Hospital in 1765. He is remembered for his English translation of Morgagni's *De Sedibus et Causis Morborum.*

Alexander, G. Franz (1891–1954) A student of the Berlin Psychiatric Institute and co-author of the *History of Psychiatry* published posthumously in 1966.

Alexander, Nicholas (d 1728) Benedictine monk and medical writer in the early 18th century. His *Physic and Surgery for the Poor* (1738) was published after his death.

Alexanderini de Neustain, Julius, (1505–1590) Physician from Trent who was physician to Maximilian II. He wrote *De Medicina et Medico, Paedotrophia, Methodus Mendi* and *Salubrium sive de sanitate tuenda.*

Alexandrian College or Museum Linked the culture and education from Egypt to Macedonia, was founded by Alexander the Great in 331 BC. It became a great university where scholars from all over the world such as Euclid the mathematician, Archimedes the physicist, Herophilos the anatomist, Erasistratos the physiologist and scores of others came to study and participate. It consisted of four departments: literature, mathematics, astronomy and medicine and its library was the largest and the most famous in the world, counting over 400,000 volumes. It was supported by descendants of Ptolemy, who was general to Alexander the Great. Though the Ptolemic dynasty ended in 30 BC the university lasted until AD 600 until Rome replaced Alexandria as the learning center. Its library was partly destroyed by Bishop Theophilus in AD 390 and was fully burnt by the Mohammedans in AD 640.

Alexin Eduard Buchner (1860–1907) noted a thermolabile substance in the serum which promoted the killing of bacteria. He named it alexin. Paul Ehrlich (1854–1915) and Jules Vincent Bordet (1870–1961) did further work on bacteriolysis in 1901 and alexin was renamed 'complement' by Ehrlich and Julius Morgenroth in the same year. The complement fixation reaction in immune hemolysis was described by Martin Manfred Mayer (1916–1984) and Lawrence Levine (b 1924) in 1954.

Alexipharmaca [Greek: *alexein*, to ward off + *pharmakon*, poison] A poem on poisons and antidotes was written by the Greek poet Nicander in 200 BC. Euricus Cordus translated it into Latin in 1532.

Alfonso X, King of Castille (1223–1284). He studied astronomy and the *Alfonso Tables* in astronomy were completed under his auspices in 1253. Four volumes of Alphonsine tables were reprinted by the Spanish Government in 1863

Algae An early study was done by German botanist, Nathaniel Pringsheim (1823–1894) in 1823.

Algazirah (d 1004) Abu Jafar Ahmed ibn-Abraham Abu Chalid was physician at Kairouan in Tunisia and a prolific writer. His *Viaticum peregrinantis*, a compendium of medical symptoms and treatment, was translated into Latin by Constantinus Africanus (d 1087).

Algebra Mohammed ibn Musa al-Khowarisimi, an Arab who lived around AD 825, introduced letters in place of numbers and figures in calculation in his treatise *al-jabr wa l muqabalah* ('joining the parts to make a whole'). Diophantus, an Alexandrian mathematician during the time of Nero, wrote 13 books on arithmetic which led to the establishment of the present system of algebra. Brahmagupta, a Hindu mathematician from Ujjain around 7th century, assigned rules for negative numbers in algebra. The use of letters in algebra to designate known quantities was popularized in Europe by French mathematician, Francis Vieta (1540–1603). A treatise in English was written by English physician Robert Recorde in 1542. The concept of group, which is the cornerstone of modern algebra, was proposed by French mathematician, Evariste Galois (1811–1832) around 1829.

Alghizi, Thomas (1669–1713) A lithotomist from Florence who wrote *Lithotomia Overodel caver la Pietra*.

Algid Extreme coldness of the body associated with a morbid state such as cholera or remittent fever.

Algophily [Greek: *algos*, pain + *philos*, love] A collective term for masochism and sadism. *See sadism, masochism.*

Algorism Derived from 'al-Khowarisimi', an Arab who invented algebra. It is related to the exposition of Hindu–Arabic numerals which were popular in the 14th century. Besides containing discussion of numerals, they included application of arithmetic to problems and business. An anonymous algorism written in the 14th century gives the puzzle of a wolf, a goat and a cabbage that must be ferried across a stream by a boatman.

Alhazen or ibn Al-Haitham (AD 965 –1038) Arab mathematician of Basra who studied the properties of light and used convex lenses. His *Kitab Al-Manazir* (Book of Optics) included refraction, reflection and study of lenses, formed the basis for the invention of spectacles, telescopes and microscopes. A Latin translation of his mathematical works was done by Robert Grosseteste (1175–1253), Bishop of Lincoln, around 1210. His treatise on astrology was printed in Latin at Basel in 1572.

Alibert, Jean Louis Marc le Baron of Villafranche de l'Aveyron (1766–1837) Considered the founder of modern French dermatology. He described mycosis fungoides as *piors fungoide* in 1806 and *cancroide* (keloid) in 1810. *See Aleppo boil.*

Alimentary Canal [Latin: *alimentary*, nourishment] A series of organs, the names of which are derived from Latin, Greek and other languages. Pharynx denotes throat or gullet in Greek, lumen is a term for 'windows' in Latin, esophagus means 'food carrier' in Greek and anus means 'a ring' in Latin. The word 'gut' is an Anglo-Saxon term.

Alison, William Pulteney (1790–1859) Graduated in medicine from Edinburgh in 1811 and appointed physician to the New Town Dispensary in 1815. His special interest was study of fevers and he made several contributions with his articles in the *Edinburgh Medical Journal* from 1817 to 1819. He was professor of jurisprudence in 1820 and promoted health for the poor. His pamphlet *Observations on the Management of the Poor in Scotland and its Effects on the Health of the Great Towns* was published in 1840. Two of his other important publications were *Outlines of Physiology* (1831) and *Outlines of Pathology and Practice of Medicine* (1844). He was later appointed professor of medicine at University of Edinburgh.

Alizarin Red dye used as biological stain was isolated by French entomologist, Jean Henri Fabre (1823–1915) of Aveyron.

Alkali Act To control the emission of toxic gases into the atmosphere by factories or 'alkali works' in England was enacted in 1863. It was amended in 1874.

Alkali [Arabic: *alqaliy*, potash] Defined in early dictionaries of medicine as a salt without an acid. The modern definition considers such substances to have properties which turn litmus paper blue and neutralize acids.

Alkali Disease In horses, due to selenium poisoning from industrial waste was described by Madison, an army surgeon from South Dakota, in 1856. It was named due to the mistaken notion that it was caused by alkali in waste from factories.

Alkaloid Clinic A publication originally devoted to pharmaceuticals, started by Calvin Abbott (1857–1921), the founder of Abbott Laboratories. It later became the *American Journal of Clinical Medicine.*

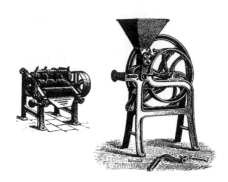

Apparatus for extracting alkaloids from plants. R A Cripps, *Galenic Pharmacy* (1893). Churchill, London

Alkaloid [Arabic: *alqaliy,* potash] Nitrogen-based substances found in plants. The transition from herbal medicine to scientific pharmacology started with the discovery of several alkaloid extracts in the 19th century. The alkaloid quinine was extracted from cinchona bark by Pierre Joseph Pelletier (1788–1842) and J.B. Caventou (1795–1877) of Paris in 1820, and ephedrine, one of the earliest of the alkaloids known to the Chinese, was extracted by Nagajosi Nagai (1844–1929) in 1887. The Nobel Prize in Chemistry for the study of plant alkaloids was won by Sir Robert Robinson (1886–1975) of England in 1947.

Alkalometry Alkaloidal therapy or dosimetry denotes a method of prescribing practiced by doctors during the late 19th century. They determined the dose of the active ingredient on an individual basis and prepared medications in the form of pellets, granules or liquid, suited to individual patients.

Alkaptonuria Metabolic disease that causes urine to turn black on exposure to air. Described by Alexander John Gaspard Marcet (1770–1822) in 1822. The presence of homogentisic acid in urine in the condition was noted by Carl Wilhelm Boedeker (1815–1895) of Germany in 1859. Archibald Garrod (1857–1936), a physician to St Bartholomew's Hospital and the Hospital for Sick Children at Great Ormond Street, London, observed its frequency in

the progeny of first cousin marriages in 1904. He introduced the concept of inborn errors of metabolism with his theory that this defect was inherited according to Mendel's laws.

Alkindi (813–873) Abu Yusuf Yaqub ibn Ishaq Al-Kindi of Basra, also known as Alkindus, was a physician to the court of Al-Mamun at Baghdad. He is considered as the first Arab philosopher and is credited with over 200 works out of which 22 are on medicine. Several were translated into Latin by Gerard of Cremona. He wrote on optics, dealing with the reflection of light and translated Ptolemy's *Almagest.*

Alkindus *See Alkindi.*

All-or-None Phenomenon Found in muscle contraction and proposed in 1871 as a mechanism by American physiologist at Boston, Henry Pickering Bowditch (1840–1911). In his work on the animal heart, he proved that if a stimulus was adequate to provoke a response in a motor unit the response became independent of the size of the stimulus. He demonstrated the refractory period following response during which no stimulus was effective. It was further described and demonstrated by Keith Lucas (1879–916) from Cambridge and Lord Edgar Douglas Adrian (1889–1977). A summary of their work is found in *The Conduction of Nerve Impulse* published in 1917.

Allan Anti-Fat A secret cure for obesity sold by the American 'Botanic Medicine Company' based in London at the turn of the 19th century. On analysis it contained mainly glycerin and potassium iodide.

Allantois [Greek: *allas,* sausage + *oeides,* shape] Term used by Galen (129–200) to denote the embryonic structure presently known as the allantois. Its structure and formation in the embryo was described by Wilhelm His, Senior (1831–1904) in 1887.

Allbutt, Sir Thomas Clifford (1836–1925) Clinician from Dewsbury and a medical historian. He invented the short-stemmed clinical thermometer in 1866, wrote an early description of joint symptoms in locomotor ataxia in 1858 and gave the Goulstonian Lecture on diseases of the heart in 1896. He was professor of physics at the University of Cambridge in 1902. His publications on medical history include *Science and Medieval Thought* (1901), *The Historic Relations of Medicine and Surgery* (1905) and *Greek Medicine in Rome and other Historical Essays* (1921). He edited *The System of Medicine* in eight volumes from 1896 to 1899 and was President of the British Medical Association from 1916 to 1921.

Allelomorph or allele [Greek: *allelon*, of one another + *morphe*, form] One of two or more dissimilar genes was studied by Gregor Mendel (1822–1884) in 1865 and his work led to the postulation of the Mendel's first law of inheritance. *See genetics*

Allen and Hanbury Early Quaker pharmaceutical establishments founded by Sylvanus Bevan, grandson of William Bevan, a merchant from Swansea. He established an apothecary shop and a laboratory at Lombard Street, London in 1725 and acquired a good reputation. The business was taken over by his brother, Timothy, and was passed on to his son, Joseph Bevan, in 1775. He took William Allen from another eminent Quaker family into the business, and two of his nephews Cornelius and Daniel Hanbury and the firm was named Allen, Hanburys and Barry in 1824. It became Allen and Hanbury and produced quality medical products including medical and surgical instruments.

Allen Cement Made of silica, to join porcelain teeth to a plate. Formulated by New York dentist, John Allen (1810–1892).

Allen Starvation Treatment for diabetes proposed in 1913 by Frederick Madison Allen (b 1876), a leading Boston diabetologist. He used starvation as a method to lower blood sugar. He was born in Iowa and studied medicine in California before he joined Harvard as a research fellow on the study of sugar metabolism.

Allen Test A test for peripheral vascular disease of the hand, by compressing and relieving the ulnar and radial vessels and observing color changes. Described by E.V. Allen (1900–1961), a medical graduate from Nebraska. He became professor of medicine at the Mayo Clinic and wrote a treatise on peripheral arterial disease.

Allen, Edgar (1892–1943) Biochemist from St Louis who did extensive work on ovulation and hormones and isolated the active principle of the ovarian hormone (estrin) in 1928. *See ovulation, hormones.*

Allen, Harrison (1841–1897) Anatomist from Philadelphia who became the President of the Association of American Anatomists in 1891. He described Allen fossa on the neck of the femur in 1882.

Allen, John (1771–1843) Born in Edinburgh, he took his medical degree in 1791. He was a lecturer in physiology in Edinburgh but chose to let politics and his interest in philosophy and metaphysics overshadow his medical career. He accompanied Lord Holland abroad as his family physician.

Allergic Alveolitis (Extrinsic alveolitis) Farmer's lung. The symptoms were noted by Bernardino Ramazzini (1633–1714) in 1700 and Manchester physician, Charles Blackley (1820–1900) wrote a treatise on it in 1873. It was known as *heymaedi* in Iceland in the late 18th century. J.H. Salisbury of Ohio developed a skin test for diagnosing it in 1861. Five cases were presented by J.M. Campbell in 'Acute symptoms following work with hay' in the *British Medical Journal* in 1932. It was registered as an occupational disease in 1965 under the National Insurance Industrial Injuries Act of 1945. The causative organism, which belongs to a group of aerobic thermophilic actinomycetes, was named *Micropolyspora faeni* in 1968. *See bagassosis, paprika-splitters lung.*

Allergic Granulomatosis Involving the lung. Described by New York pathologist J. Churg (b 1910) and L. Strauss in the *American Journal of Pathology* in 1951. It was later named Churg–Strauss syndrome.

Allergic Rhinitis Hay fever (Syn: Bostock catarrh, catarrhus aestivus, vasomotor rhinitis) Described by John Bostock (1773–1846) of Guy's Hospital, London in 1817. *See allergy, John Bostock, hay fever.*

Allergy [Greek: *allos*, other + *ergon*, activity] The term means 'altered activity' and was coined by a pediatrician, Clemens Peter Pirquet von Cesenatico (1874–1929) of Austria in 1904. The common allergic condition now called hay fever was described by John Bostock (1773–1846) of Guy's Hospital, London in 1817. He called it 'catarrhus aestivus' and was himself affected. Pollen was identified as a cause of hay fever by John Elliotson (1791–1868) of University College, London in 1831. *See hay fever, asthma, pollen.*

Allingham, William (1829–1908) A surgeon during the Crimean war at the Scutari Hospitals. On his return he became a specialist on fistula and diseases of the rectum at St Mark's Hospital, London.

Allopathy [Greek: *allos*, another + *pathos*, suffering] Doctrine of counteractive treatment which has been practiced since ancient times. Treatments such as cooling for fever and laxatives for constipation were originally based on this concept. Hippocrates (460–377 BC) in his treatise on *Airs* declared 'contraries are the cure of contraries'. The term was defined and described by Christian Friedrich Samuel Hahnemann (1755–1843), the founder of homeopathy, in 1810.

Alloplastic Adaptation [Greek: *allos*, another + *plassein*, mold + *ad*, to + *aptare*, to fit] Term used by Sandor Ferenczi

(1873–1933), a friend of Sigmund Freud (1856–1939), to denote the conscious adaptive efforts of man, such as making fire to keep warm and building shelters to protect himself. He named the natural adaptation of animals like growing fur and feather to warm themselves, autoplastic adaptation.

Allopurinol Used in the treatment of gout, and developed by George H. Hitchings of New York in 1943.

Allotransplant [Greek: *allos*, another + *trans*, across] Transplantation of tissue between members of the same species. Italian surgeon, Guiseppe Baronio (1759–1811) demonstrated the fundamental principle that a graft from the same animal was successful, whereas a graft from another animal was rejected, in an experiment on skin grafting in 1804. Alexis Carrel (1884–1947) made a major advance by performing a successful allotransplant in dogs in 1906. *See renal transplant, heart transplant.*

Allotrophy [Greek: *allos*, another + *trophos*, habit] Substances which have different sets of properties but are of the same origin.

Almagest Written by Ptolemy of Alexandria in AD 130 is considered to be the greatest work on astronomy. It was named *Al magiste* by the Arabs to mean the greatest. Its contents include illustrations of ancient astronomical instruments and elaborate astronomical tables. It was translated into Latin in the 12th century and printed in Basel in 1538.

Almaliki *See Abbas, Haly.*

Almamum Al-Meiamun Son of Harun-al-Rashid for whom the tale of *Arabian Nights* was written. He founded the Academy of Bagdad during his reign (815–833). He was an astronomer who measured the Earth by measurements of the meridian. He encouraged the collection and translation of Greek and Roman medical classics into Arabic. *See Abbasides.*

Almanac [Arabic: *al*, the; Hebrew: *munach*, to count] Ptolemy produced almanacs in Alexandria around AD 100. The first almanac of Europe, *Kalendarium Novum,* was produced in Budapest, Hungary in 1475 and thereafter almanacs became common.

Al-Mansur Hospital One of the earliest hospitals, established in Cairo in 1276. It was a marvel of medicine at that period, containing wards for special diseases, clinics, lecture rooms, a library and many other parallels of a modern hospital.

Almeloveen, Thomas Jassend Dutch physician and botanist in the 17th century. His *Hortus Malabaricus* and *Flora Malabarica* were published in 1678.

Almenar, Juan Spanish physician during the 15th century who wrote on venereal diseases. His *De Morbico Gallico* was published in Venice in 1502. He recommended mercury for the treatment of syphilis but his religious faith made him believe that the mechanism of transmission of syphilis in the clergy was different, in that it was through air.

Almoner Name given to an official in ancient Rome who distributed the King's alms.

Almshouses Built to provide shelter, food and medical care for the poor, aged, disabled and insane. Conditions in many such institutions were appalling with all patients, including those with contagious diseases and the insane, being housed together, with little or no segregation of sexes. The first Almshouse in America was opened in Boston in 1665. The Red Lion Almshouse at Westminster, Whittington's Almshouse at Highgate Hill and the London Almshouse at Brixton were founded in 1577, 1826 and 1833, respectively.

Al-Nafis of Damascus Medical writer and surgeon in the 13th century. He was one of the first to dispute Galen's (129–200) works and gave a description of the 'lesser circulation' or pulmonary circulation. He wrote a comprehensive work on medicine (80 volumes).

Alopecia [Greek: *alopex*, fox] Disease in which the hair falls out. Described by Pliny in the 1st century as 'patchy shedding of hair from a fox whose urine is said to make places barren and bald for an year'.

α-1-Antitrypsin Deficiency Deficiency of a plasma protein produced in the liver that inhibits trypsin, a proteolytic enzyme, thus contributing to the development of emphysema. The electrophoretic pattern of the serum proteins was described by C. B. Laurel and S. Erikson in 1963. Its association in liver diseases in children was pointed out by M. Odievre and colleagues in 1976.

α-Adrenergic Drugs The anti-hypertensive agents, phentolamine and piperoxan were used in the late 1940s. However, they were soon abandoned as main-line drugs but continued to be used as test drugs for differentiating essential hypertension and pheochromocytoma until the 1960s.

α-Chain Disease A case was noted in the serum of a young Arab patient who had marked plasma cell infiltration of the gut wall, by M. Seligman and co-workers in 1968. Patients were also noted to have steatorrhea, weight loss and finger clubbing. It was first called Mediterranean lymphoma, as it was thought to be restricted to Arabs and Jews, but it was later detected in other races.

α-Fetoprotein The possibility that adult malignant cells may revert to production of primitive embryonic constituents has been raised intermittently since 1930. The synthesis of α-1–fetoprotein in chemically induced hepatomas of mice was demonstrated by G.I. Abelev in 1971. Later in the same year he demonstrated its appearance in the sera of patients with hepatoma, testicular teratomas and viral hepatitis. Its increase in amniotic fluid during the last tri-mester of pregnancy in cases of anencephaly was reported by D.J.H. Brock and R.G. Sutcliff in 1972.

α-Hemolytic Streptococcus Since the name 'streptococcus' was introduced by Anton Julius Friedrich Rosenbach (1842–1923), a German surgeon in 1884, a long drawn out debate and controversy continued regarding the classification of streptococci. In 1920 Brown published a monograph in the medical researches of the Rockefeller Institute which classified the group into A, B, A' and G, based on the type and degree of hemolysis produced in a blood agar plate. Those producing greenish discoloration or partial hemolysis were assigned to the alpha group. *See streptococci, Lancefield group.*

α-Methyl Dopa Effective inhibitor of the synthesis of norepinephrine. Discovered by Theodore R. Sourkes of McGill University in 1954. It was introduced into clinical practice for treatment of hypertension by Oates and Sjoerdsma in 1960 and remains the longest used antihypertensive on the market.

α-Rays Term used in 1899 by Ernest Rutherford (1871–1937) of Cambridge, to refer to radiation rays from radium which could pass through aluminum foil of more than one-fiftieth of a millimeter in thickness.

α Rhythm *See Berger rhythm.*

α Tocopherol Vitamin E. Isolated from wheat germ oil by Herbert McLean Evans of California in 1935. Its formula was determined by Fernholtz of New Jersey and its synthesis was completed by Paul Karrer (1889–1971) of Switzerland in 1938.

Alphonso or Alfonsine Tables *See Alfonso X.*

Alpine Scurvy Pellagra in Italy was described as 'alpine scurvy' by Odoardi in 1776.

Alpini, Prospero (1553–1617) Physician and botanist from Venice. In 1580 he was physician to the Venetian consul in

Egypt and wrote *De Medecina Aegyptorum* (1591), *Historia Naturalis Egypti, De Medicina Methodica* and other works. He discovered sex and generation of plants and the genus of plants *Alpinia* is named after him.

Alport Syndrome Hereditary hemorrhagic nephropathy associated with loss of hearing and vision. Described by South African physician and graduate of Edinburgh University, A.C. Alport (1880–1959), in 1927. He included a family of 19 individuals, through three generations, which was originally studied by L. Guthrie in 1902. He was professor of medicine at Cairo from 1937 to 1944.

Al-Rhazi *See Rhazes.*

Alsaharavius Another name for Albucasis, an Arabian physician who lived around AD 980. He wrote an important textbook on surgery, *Altasrif.*

Alston, Charles (1683–1760) Scottish physician who practiced in Edinburgh. He opposed the system of classification of Linnaeus and wrote *Tyrocinium Botanicum Edinburgense* (1753) and *Lectures on Materia Medica* (1770).

Altamira Cave Paintings Painted by Cro-Magnon man and discovered by Maria Sautuola in Spain in 1879. The paintings of bison were the first Paleolithic art works to be discovered. *See cave drawings.*

Alternating Current The theory of alternating current was proposed by a Polish electrical engineer, Charles Proteus (b 1865). A successful commercial generator was built by Belgian electric engineer, Zenobe Theophile Gramme (1826–1901) in 1867. A study on the effects on the heart was performed in a dog by W.B. Kouwenhouven, D.R. Hooker and O.R. Langworthy in 1932. The advantage of direct current over alternating current, and a direct current capacitor discharge capable of depolarizing the myocardium transthoracically was developed by B. Lowen and R. Amarasingham in 1962. *See cardioversion.*

Alternative Medicine The present scientific system of medicine has evolved from sorcery, magic, religious rituals and herbal medicine, practiced since ancient times. Hippocrates (460–377 BC), considered to be the father of medicine, established medicine on a scientific basis. The medicine of the ancient Brahmins is still practiced as Ayurvedic medicine in parts of India and Sri Lanka. Some effective ancient medicines were investigated scientifically and embraced into modern medicine. The Chinese herbal drug *Ma Hung* used as treatment 5000 years ago, was found to contain ephedrine. Hundreds of other ancient remedies such as foxglove, St John's wort, rye fungus and *Ammi* *visnaga* have had their active ingredients identified and been incorporated into the modern pharmacopoeia. Those methods which are not scientifically explained, although they may be effective, still remain as alternative medicine, fringe medicine or complementary medicine. Bone setters have evolved into chiropractors or osteopaths and their field remains complementary or on the fringes of medicine. *See acupuncture, aromatherapy, bone setters, herbal medicine, spondylotherapy, hypnosis, chiropractic medicine.*

Altitude Sickness [Latin: *altus*, high] The symptoms of mountain or altitude sickness were described by a Jesuit priest, Jose de Acosta (1539–1600) who himself experienced the symptoms while he crossed the Peruvian Andes in 1590. It was known to the people of Peru as *puna* or *sorache*, and later named Acosta disease. Nicholas Theodore de Saussure (1767–1845) described the symptoms of anoxemia in 1786 during his ascent of Mont Blanc, the highest peak in western Europe. An account was also given by a Peruvian physician from Lima, C. Monge (1884–1970). Anoxemia as the cause of the symptoms was shown in 1878 by Paul Ebert, a physiologist and successor to Claude Bernard at Paris.

Altmann, Richard (1852–1900) Professor at Leipzig who detected peculiar granules within the cell with his special staining methods in 1894. These were later named mitochondria.

Altounyan, Roger Edward Collingwood (1922–1987) British physician of Armenian origin born in Syria. In 1967 he obtained sodium cromoglycate from the *Ammi visnaga* plant, which has been used for centuries as a treatment for asthma. He developed the spinhaler, based on the aerodynamic principles of the aircraft, for the delivery of drug to the lungs via inhalation. He himself had asthma.

Alum Used during ancient times to prepare leather and mentioned in the Ebers papyrus written around 2000 BC. Sir Thomas Chaloner of Longhull Manor, Yorkshire started its manufacture in 1600. An economic way of producing it on a large scale, using sulfuric acid, was invented by Scottish chemist Peter Spence in 1845.

Aluminum The word *alumen* was used by the Romans to denote substances with astringent properties. Its presence in clay was demonstrated by German chemist, Sigismond Marggrafe (1709–1782) in 1754 and Oerstedt (1777–1851) obtained the chloride of aluminum in 1826. The pure metal was extracted by F. Wohler in 1827 and the mode of obtaining aluminum metal was later simplified by Robert Bunsen (1811–1899). Production in commercial quantities was achieved in 1855 by Henri Etienne Saint-Claire Deville

(1818–1881), a French chemist of West Indian origin. The effect on health of using aluminum vessels for cooking was investigated by Plagge and Lebbin in 1893. This and further work, published in *The Lancet* in 1913, concluded that aluminum was safe for cooking.

Alvarez, Walter Clements (b 1884) Worked at the Mayo Clinic, Rochester, Minnesota. A pioneer in the use of X-ray cinematography in 1934 for investigation of stomach lesions.

Alveolus [Latin: *alveus*, hollow] Word used by Andreas Vesalius (1514–1564) to denote the socket for the tooth, in 1550. It was used to describe the lung by Rossignol in 1846. Marcello Malpighi (1628–1694) used *cellulae pulmoni* for the alveoli in 1670.

Alzaharavius *See Albucasis.*

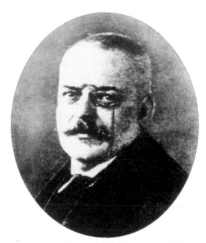

Alois Alzheimer (1864–1915). Courtesy of the National Library of Medicine

Alzheimer Disease A form of presenile dementia described (1907) by German psychiatrist, Alois Alzheimer (1864–1915), who was born in Markbreit and educated at Würzburg. During his research on neuropathology at the Emil Kraepelin Psychiatric Clinic in Munich, he studied the brains of demented and senile patients and correlated his histological findings with the signs and symptoms in dementia. He was professor of psychiatry at Breslau in 1912 and died of rheumatic endocarditis 3 years later.

Amaas Term used for smallpox in South Africa. Derived from the Dutch words 'masel' or 'mazelen'.

Amalgam [Greek: *malakos*, soft] Term introduced for alloys of various metals by Thomas Aquinas (1225–1274) in 1240.

Amaltheus, Jerome (1507–1574) Italian physician and poet born in Venice. He was a professor at Padua and became a scholar in Latin.

Amanita muscaria Scarlet fly cap fungus. Hallucinogenic fungus, known to the northeastern Siberian tribes since the 17th century who used it to produce intoxication, hallucinations and uncontrolled excited dancing. As the active principle was excreted in urine, the participants collected their urine and drank it to prolong intoxication. The first fungal toxin, muscaria, was isolated by O. Schmiedeberg of Germany in 1869.

Amanita phylloides Death cap fungus. Said to be the cause of death in 90% of cases of mushroom poisoning. In 1909 William Webber Ford estimated that at least 15 deaths occurred in America from this species. It was investigated by Letellier, who isolated 'amanatin' which was thought to be the poisonous substance, in 1826. A powerful hemolysin was extracted by Eduard Rudolf Kobert (1854–1918) who named it 'phallin' in 1891. John Jacob Abel (1857–1938) and William Webber Ford (1871–1941) demonstrated two different poisons in the lungs in 1908.

Amanita verna Destroying angel fungus. A poisonous mushroom described by Buillard of France in 1791.

Amatus Portuguese physician in the 16th century whose real name was John Rod de Castelbranco. He wrote a commentary on Avicenna (980–1037) and Dioscorides.

Amaurosis [Greek: *amaurosis*, obscuring] (Syn. gutta serena) Hippocrates (460–377 BC) mentioned it. It usually refers to blindness without apparent disease of the eye, brought on by lesions in the brain or the optic nerve. A condition of the eye, involving a diminution or total loss of sight, was described by Galen (129–200) and Aetius of Amida (502–575). If it occurred suddenly, they referred the cause to obstruction and paralysis of the optic nerve; if it was gradual, they believed the cause was either thickening of the coats of the optic nerve or change of the spirits or humors of the eye. In the acute stages they recommended bleeding from the back part of the head and purging. Later Arab physicians, including Haly Abbas (930–994), followed the same methods.

Amaurotic Family Idiocy Tay–Sachs disease and its ocular manifestations. Described by British ophthalmologist and surgeon, Warren Tay (1843–1927) at the London Hospital in 1880. Steinthal gave an accurate description in 1884 and the cerebral manifestations occurring almost exclusively amongst Jewish children were described in detail in 1887 by New York physician, Bernard Parney Sachs (1858–1944), of Bavarian origin.

Amazia Absence of the mammary gland. A rare congenital condition. John William Ballantyne (1861–1923) presented a case of 28-year-old woman to the Edinburgh Obstetrical Society in 1890. Other associated malformations were presented by W. Wylie in 1888 and L. Remfry in 1896.

Ambard Coefficient Formula to determine the concentrating power of the kidney, using blood and urea ratios. Proposed in 1910 by a physiologist, Leo Ambard (b 1876) of Strasbourg. However, owing to its practical inaccuracies and technical difficulties, the method was abandoned.

Amber [Arabic: *Anbar*, Greek: *elektron*] Fossil gum. The first substance noted to produce electricity by Thales in 600 BC. The Greeks called white amber electrum and it was held in esteem as a medicinal cure. Theophrastus (370–287 BC) wrote about its medicinal values.

Ambidextrous [Latin: *ambo*, on both sides or both ways + *dexter*, right hand] Hippocrates (460–377 BC) in his *Aphorisms* states that 'a woman does not become ambidextrous'. This notion arose from the assumption that women were of a feeble constitution.

Ambivalence [Latin: *ambo*, on both sides or both ways + *valens*, having strength or worth] Psychiatric term to denote contradicting emotions such as love and hate experienced by psychotic patients. Coined by Eugene Bleuler (1857–1939), professor of psychiatry at Burgholzli Hospital.

Amblyopia [Greek: *amblyos*, dull + *opius*, eye] Hippocrates (460–377 BC) used the term to mean dullness of eyesight in old age and Paul of Aegina (625–690) used it to describe incomplete amaurosis. *See amaurosis.*

Amblyopia Toxica (Syn. nicotinic amblyopia, tobacco amblyopia) A condition of dimness of vision due to tobacco smoking described by William Mackenzie (1791–1868) in England in 1835. A more accurate description was given by Jonathan Hutchinson (1828–1913) in 1864 and it was discussed exhaustively by Carl Friedrich Richard Forster (1825–1902) of Germany in 1868.

Amblyoscope Stereoscopic instrument designed to train the eye to overcome squint. Developed by London ophthalmologist, Claude Worth (1896–1960) around 1906.

Amboreceptor or amboceptor [Latin: *ambo*, both + *capere*, to take] A term given by Paul Ehrlich (1854–1915) in 1904 to the heat-resistant immune bodies which facilitated the fixing of complement to the immune complex.

Ambrosini, Bartholomew (d 1657) Professor of physics and director of the botanical garden at Bologna. He wrote *De Pulsebus* (1645), *Theorica Medicina in Tabulas Digesta* (1632) and several other treatises. He was succeeded by his brother, another great botanist.

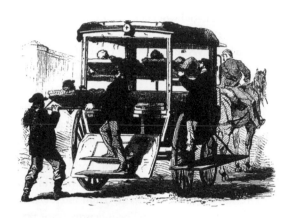

Early French ambulance. L Legoueste, *Traité de Chirurgie d'Armée* (1872). Bailliére et Fils, Paris

Ambulance [Latin: *ambulare*, to walk] The concept of walking or ambulant hospital was proposed by the French, but Queen Isabella of Castille developed the idea of field hospitals and ambulances in 1487. Her hospital, the Queen's Hospital, had over 400 wagons called *ambulancia*, which led to the current term. Later, Dominique Jean Larrey (1766–1842), the great army surgeon of France, employed carts drawn by horses, which were called 'flying ambulances' to transport the wounded and the sick, in 1781. The modern ambulance service was initiated by the Order of St John of Jerusalem in England in 1831. They established the St John's Ambulance Association in 1877. It served to spread instruction in first aid and organized the transport of helpless patients. It was recognized by a Queen's charter and the St John's Ambulance Brigade was formed in 1888. Surgeon Major Hutton was appointed to organize the ambulance work on railways in Britain in 1890. A motorized ambulance, an electromobile, was presented by the Brigade to St Vincent's Hospital in New York in 1900. The use of motorized ambulances gradually became established around 1913.

Ambulativa Ancient Greek term for herpes.

Ameba [Greek: *amoibe*, change] First drawn accurately by the portrait painter Rosel von Rosenhof in 1773 and described in detail by O.F. Muller in 1773. The living nature of substance or sarcode (protoplasm) was recognized by French zoologist Felix Dujardin (1801–1860) of Tours in 1835. A scientific monograph, *Ameba Living in Man* was published by Clifford Dobell (1886–1949) in 1919. *See amebic dysentery, ameboid movement.*

Amebic Dysentery The ameba was isolated from the stool of a patient with intestinal disease by Friedrich Losch (1840–1903) in 1875, who called it *Ameba coli*. Robert Koch

(1843–1910) found the same organism in the stools of patients with dysentery in Egypt and proved it to be the causative organism. Fritz Schaudinn (1871–1906), who discovered *Treponema pallidum* inoculated himself with *Entamoeba histolytica* and was said to have died of its effects. William Thomas Councilman (1854–1933) of Harvard University introduced the term in 1890. Modern work was done by Clifford Dobell (1886–1949), an eminent protozoologist. He wrote *Ameba Living in Man* (1919) and *Intestinal Protozoa of Man* (1921). The organism was successfully grown in culture by Boeck and Drbohlav in 1925. The pathogenicity of *Entamoeba histolytica* was demonstrated by London pathologist, Sir Leonard Rogers (1868–1962) who prescribed emetine as treatment.

Amebic Hepatitis Mild cases of hepatitis in patients with amebic dysentery were reported by A.M.M. Payne in 1945. The occurrence of parenchymal liver damage in patients was shown by D. Shute in 1947.

Ameboid Movement [Greek: *amoibe*, change + *oidos*, shape] Characteristic movement in lower organisms such as the ameba was noted by Rosenhoff (Rosel) in 1755. A description of the granular movement of protoplasm in the pseudopodia of rhizopods was given by Felix Dujardin (1801–1860) of Paris in 1841. The observation of ameboid movements in the protoplasm of higher animals was made by Wharton Jones during his studies on the movements of the white blood cells of fish in 1846.

Ameboma Mass produced by inflammation in amebiasis. Ameboma presenting as carcinoma and vice versa was noted by C.N. Morgan in 1946.

Amenorrhea A symptom exploited by quacks in the 19th century. Hundreds of secret remedies appeared in the market during this period were really camouflaged abortifacients. Their names include: Dumas' Paris pills, Nurse Powell's corrective pills, Nurse Mann's remedy, Dr John Hooper's female pills, Dr Davis's female mixture, Jefferson Dodd's corrective, Martin's apiol and Monaid tablets. The use of estrogenic hormones for the treatment was documented by Carl Kaufmann in 1933.

Amentia [Greek: *a*, without; Latin: *mens*, mind] Old term for mental diseases in childhood.

American Academy of Orthopedic Surgeons Founded in 1933. *See American Orthopedic Association.*

American Association for Cancer Research Founded in 1907. Prior to this time funds and facilities for cancer research were poor in America although the Buffalo

Cancer Laboratory managed to obtain some state funds in 1898 to continue their research. Later, in 1914, a group of physicians met in New York City and formed the American Society for the Control of Cancer.

American Association for the Advancement of Science Founded in 1847, with William Redfield (b 1789) of Connecticut as its first president.

American Association of Medico-Physical Research *See Abrams, Albert.*

American Board of Obstetrics and Gynecology Around 1920 the quality of obstetric standards in America caused considerable concern owing to the alarming statistics on maternal deaths. This led to political intervention and the Sheppard-Towner Act was passed to provide postnatal and antenatal care. A strong lobby, initiated by a professor of obstetrics at the Johns Hopkins Hospital, John Whitridge Williams (1866–1931), led to the establishment of the American Board of Obstetrics and Gynecology. It was the third board of specialty to be established in America in 1930.

American College of Physicians Founded in 1915 in New York after the efforts of Heinrich Stern, who was inspired by his visit to the Royal College of Physicians in London in 1913.

American College of Surgeons Initiated in 1913 by Chicago surgeon, Franklin Martin, following a series of successful clinical congresses attended by American surgeons in 1911 (Philadelphia) and 1912 (New York).

American Gastroenterological Association One of the first specialized associations in America was founded in 1897.

American Hospital Association Started as the Association of Hospital Superintendents in 1899. It was given its present name in 1906. It developed into an influential institution representing hospitals on national matters and maintaining standards.

American Journal of Clinical Medicine *See alkaloid clinic.*

American Journal of Obstetrics The first specialized journal to be published in America, in 1868. Its name was later changed to the *American Journal of Obstetrics and Gynecology* in 1920.

American Journal of Pharmacy *See American Pharmaceutical Association.*

American Journal of Physiology Founded in 1898 by a group of physiologists from the American Physiological Society.

American Journal of Science Founded in 1818 by an American chemist, Benjamin Silliman (1779–1864) of Connecticut. He was the father of Benjamin Silliman (1816–1885), professor of chemistry at Yale who showed that petroleum was a mixture of hydrocarbons.

American Medical Association Although this was founded in 1847, it remained ineffective for its first 50 years, failing to exert any influence at the state or national level. In 1899 it created the Committee on National Legislation to represent it before Congress. In 1901 a reformed constitution was brought about by a committee which consisted of Joseph N. McCormack of Kentucky, P. Maxwell Foshay of Cleveland and George H. Simmons of Chicago. For the next decade it expanded rapidly in terms of membership, leading to its increased influence on health care and medical education at a national level. This was spearheaded by William James Mayo (1905), William C. Gorgas (1908) and William H. Welch (1909), who served as presidents.

American Medical Books Although printing was invented in Europe in the 15th century it did not reach America until the late 16th century. *Opera Medicinalia* by Francisco Bravo was printed in Mexico in 1570 and only three copies have survived. *Summa y recopilcion de Cirugia* by Lopez de Hinozoso and *Tracto breve de Medician* by Fray Augustin Farfan were printed in Mexico in 1578 and 1592, respectively. An American treatise on smallpox was written by Thomas Thacher (1620–1678) in 1677 and a book dealing with smallpox vaccination was written by Benjamin Colman (1673–1747) of Boston in 1721. A book on tumors was published by American surgeon, John Collins Warren (1778–1856) in 1837. A textbook of pediatrics, *A Treatise on Physical and Medical Treatment of Children,* was written by William Potts Dewees (1768–1848) of Philadelphia in 1825. A treatise on pathological anatomy was written by William Edmonds Horner (1793–1853) in 1829 and a book on toxicology was written by Theodore George Wormley (1826–1897) in 1867.

American Medical Journals The first was *Medical Repository,* edited quarterly in New York by Elihu Smith, Samuel Mitchill and Edward Miller. It remained as the only medical journal in America for 5 years and ceased in 1824. The *New England Journal of Medicine and Surgery* was started in 1812 and merged with the *Boston Medical Intelligencer* as the *Boston Medical and Surgical Journal* in 1828. It later became the *New England Journal of Medicine.* The *Philadelphia Journal of Medical and Physical Sciences* was published in 1820 and the *American Medical Journal of Sciences* commenced in 1838. A journal in psychology, *American Journal of Psychology,* was published by Granville Stanley Hall in 1887.

American Medical Schools and Hospitals The oldest hospital in America appears to be the Bellevue Hospital in New York City. It is supposed to have descended from a hospital built by the West India Company in 1650. The Blockly Hospital, currently known as the Philadelphia General Hospital, began as an almshouse in 1720. It is probably the oldest hospital in America to have functioned continuously since its formation. The Pennsylvania Hospital received its charter in 1751. The first medical school in America was formed at the College of Pennsylvania in 1765. The first regular medical degree of Bachelor of Medicine in America was given to ten men who graduated from the College of Philadelphia in 1768. Two more were awarded medical degrees at King's College, New York in 1769. The Harvard Medical School, the third medical school to be established in America in 1783, was planned by an army surgeon who also served as its first professor of anatomy. The Yale Medical School was established in 1810.

American Neurological Association Founded at the suggestion of William Alexander Hammond (1828–1900), with Roberts Bartholow (1831–1904) of Cincinnati, Meredith Clymer, J.S. Jewell, Edward Constant Seguin (1843–1898) of Columbia University, James Jack Putnam (1846–1918) and T.M.R. Cross as founder members in June 1875. Silas Weir Mitchell (1829–1914) was its first president.

American Ophthalmological and Otological Society Founded in 1864. The otologists later withdrew and formed their own American Otological Society in 1868.

American Orthopedic Association Founded in 1887 with Virgil P. Gibney (1847–1927) as its first president. He graduated from Bellevue Hospital Medical College, and was the first professor of orthopedics at the Columbia University College of Physicians and Surgeons from 1894.

American Otological Society *See American Ophthalmological and Otological Society*.

American Pharmaceutical Association William Proctor (b 1817), from an eminent Quaker family who emigrated from Yorkshire and settled in New Jersey, was a major figure in its foundation. He is considered the father of American pharmacy, and edited the *American Journal of Pharmacy* in 1837.

American Physiological Society Initially a society for hygiene and health founded in 1837. The present Society was founded in 1887 with Newell Martin (1848–1896) as a founder member. *American Journal of Physiology* was first published in 1898.

American Psychiatric Association Founded in 1844 in Philadelphia as the Association of Medical Superintendents of American Institution for the Insane by 13 superintendents of mental hospitals. The initial object was to streamline the administration and day-to-day care at mental hospitals. It later became the American Medico-Psychological Association and its name was again changed in 1944.

American Public Health Association Founded through the efforts of Lemuel Shattuck of Boston. He presented an exhaustive account of the poor sanitary conditions in America in *Report of the Sanitary Conditions of Massachusetts* in 1850, which initiated sanitary reforms.

American Scientific Journals The *American Journal of Science and Arts* was founded by a chemist, Benjamin Silliman (1779–1864) of Connecticut in 1818. *Scientific American* the first American scientific magazine for the general reader was founded by Alfred Beach in 1845.

American Society for Pharmacology and Experimental Therapeutics Founded by John Jacob Abel (1857–1938) in 1908.

Amiadarone Antiarrhythmic drug obtained in 1961 as a result of research on the medicinal effects of khellin, from the plant *Ammi visnaga*.

Amici, Giovanni Battista (1786–1863) Italian physicist from Modena. He constructed the reflecting microscope and improved the achromatic objective of the microscope in 1812. He invented the water immersion objective in 1840 and produced the first high-power objectives using meniscus lenses in 1844. He was professor of astronomy at the University of Pisa in 1835.

Amidopyrene Introduced as an antipyretic and analgesic in 1889. Owing to its serious side-effect of agranulocytosis, its use was prohibited in England in 1936.

Amiloride or MK 870 Introduced as a diuretic by A.F. Lant and co-workers in 1969.

Amines [Greek: *ammoniakon*, resinous gum] *See catecholamine, amphetamine, protamine, antihistamine, histamine*.

Amino Acids Glycine was recognized as a hydrosylate of gelatin (protein) by Henry Braconnot in 1820. Albrecht Kossel (1853–1927), professor of physiology at Hamburg, Germany, postulated in 1898 that proteins are made up of polypeptides, which in turn are composed of amino acids. Asparagine was discovered by Louis Nicolas Vanqueline (1763–1829) in 1806; William Hyde Wollaston (1766–1822) discovered cystine in 1810; leucine was discovered by J.L.

Proust (1754–1826) in 1819; and Bopp discovered tyrosine in 1849. German chemist Emil Fischer (1852–1919) in 1902 linked 18 amino acids. Their importance in human digestion and metabolism was not recognized until 1906 when Otto Folin (1867–1934) of Harvard University and Willey G. Dennis of Massachusetts General Hospital demonstrated that they appeared in blood after a protein meal. Specific amino acids were isolated from blood by John J. Abel (1857–1938) in 1913. He also isolated epinephrine and antidiuretic hormone. The 'nitrous acid' method of estimation by measuring the volume of nitrogen liberated was invented by Donald Dexter Van Slyke (1883–1971) in 1912. A few years later Thomas Burr Osborne (1859–1929), Lafayette Benedict Mendel and others distinguished between essential and non-essential amino acids. The study was advanced by the introduction of electrophoresis in 1930 by Swedish chemist, Arne Wilhelm Kaurin Tiselius (1902–1971). His principle was used for the development of chromatography by A.H. Gordon, R.L.M. Synge and John Porter Archer Martin. They used water on cellulose (filter paper) as a medium for electrophoretic analysis in 1944. This technique was used by Charles Dent to identify 60 different amino acids in 1948. The solid phase method of synthesizing peptides and peptones was devised by Robert Bruce Merrifield (b 1921), a professor at Rockefeller University, New York, in 1959. The sequence of nucleic acids in each of the 20 amino acids of the human body was determined by Har Govind Khorana (b 1922) from Raipur, Pakistan while he was at the Institute of Enzyme Research at Wisconsin.

Aminoaciduria The presence of amino acids in urine and cystine crystals in bone marrow of patients with cystinosis was demonstrated by Dutch pathologist, G.O.E. Lignac (1891–1954) in 1924. A form of renal tubular dysfunction (Fanconi syndrome) leading to aminoaciduria and cystic fibrosis of the pancreas was described by Guido Fanconi (1892–1979), a Swiss professor of pediatrics at the University of Zurich in 1946. Routine diagnostic examination of urine for different forms of aminoaciduria was made possible by the application of chromatography by C.E. Dent in 1946. *See chromatography.*

Aminocaproic Acid Synthetic fibrinolytic inhibitor discovered by Okamoto and colleagues in 1957.

Aminoglycosides *See actinomycin, streptomycin, gentamycin.*

Aminopterin Antifolic acid agent. Introduced as treatment for leukemia by Sidney Faber, an American cancer scientist, in 1948. It was introduced as treatment for psoriasis by R. Gubner of America in 1951. A closely related compound,

methotrexate, was found to be more effective in treatment of leukemia. *See methotrexate.*

Aminorex Introduced as an appetite suppressant in Switzerland as Menoril in 1965. It was found to be the cause of an epidemic of pulmonary hypertension from 1965 to 1968 and was withdrawn in 1968.

Amitosis [Greek: *mitos*, thread + *a*, negative prefix] Direct method of cell division such as that found in ameba, investigated by Walther Flemming (1843–1905) of Leipzig in 1882 but later found to be a misinterpretation.

Amman, John Conrad (d 1730) Swiss physician who devoted his time to teaching the deaf to speak in France and Holland. He published *Surdus Loquens* in 1692.

Amman, Paul (1634–1691) German physician and botanist who became professor of natural history, philosophy and botany at Leipzig. He wrote *Archaeus Syncopticus, Irenecum Numae Pompilii cum Hippocrate, Character Naturalis Piantarum* and many other works.

Ammi visnaga A plant from the eastern Mediterranean used for centuries to treat asthma. Its active ingredient, khellin, was found to increase coronary blood flow and was tried as treatment for angina in 1936. Sodium cromoglycate, currently used in the prophylactic treatment of asthma, was obtained from its seeds in 1967.

Ammon Fissure Pear-shaped aperture in the sclera at an early fetal stage. Described by Friedrich August von Ammon (1799–1861), professor of pathology at Dresden.

Ammon, Friedrich August von (1799–1861) Professor of pathology at Dresden. He described the cilia on the inner surface of the ciliary body of the eye (Ammon filaments) in 1858.

Ammon Horn The pes hippocampi. In transverse section it resembles a ram's horn. The ram-headed Egyptian god is Ammon.

Ammonia Supposed to have been obtained by burning camel dung in the temple of Ammon in Libya. The composition, a mixture of nitrogen and hydrogen, was suggested by a chemist, Joseph Priestley (1733–1804) from Leeds in 1774 and it was shown by C.L. Berthelot (1827–1907) in 1875.

Ammonius of Alexandria or Lithotomos (283–247 BC) A surgeon who performed lithotrity for stones in the urinary bladder. He used a hook to hold the stone in the bladder and a blunt instrument to break the stone.

Ammotherapy [Greek: *ammos*, sand + *therapeia*, healing] Treatment of disease by sand bath.

Amnesia [Greek: *a*, negative + *mnasthai*, remember] Loss of memory. Mnemosyne, the mother of the Muses, was the Greek goddess of memory.

Amniocentesis *Contributions to the Theory of Liquor Amnii and its Origin* was written by L. Prowchownick of Germany in 1877. He obtained amniotic fluid samples using an egg membrane piercer. Application of this procedure to humans was suggested by F. Schatz in 1882. The procedure was performed by M. Henkel of Germany in a case of polyhydramnios in 1919. The next documented use was for the amniography by three radiologists T.D. Menees, J.D. Miller and L.E. Holly in Michigan in 1933. Owing to fetal deaths, the interest in amniography tailed off until it was revived in 1952 by Douglas C. Bevin of England who used it to diagnose or predict hemolytic disease of the newborn. Studying chromosomes of cells in amniotic fluid was introduced by Steele and Breg in 1966. Prenatal diagnosis of Down syndrome by amniocentesis was made in 1968 and has become an important tool in antenatal diagnosis.

Amniography [Greek: *amnion*, bowl + *graphein*, to write] Method introduced in 1930 by T.D. Menees, J.D. Miller and L.E. Holly for localizing the placenta. It was further developed by Munroe Kerr and Makay in 1933 but, owing to reports of several fetal deaths following the procedure, it was gradually abandoned.

Amnion [Greek: *amnion*, bowl] Introduced into anatomy by Galen (129–200) to refer to the fetal membrane.

Amnioscopy [Greek: *amnion*, bowl + *skopein*, to look] A method of assessing the color and volume of the liquor amnii before the onset of labor when the membranes are still intact. Introduced around 1964. In 1966, E. Saling published a series of 894 patients who had undergone amnioscopy and his work showed the risk of perinatal mortality from the procedure to be 9 per 1000 births.

Amniotic Fluid Embolism Reported by J.R. Meyer of Brazil in 1926 in a 21-year-old woman with a dead fetus who suddenly died during labor. A detailed account of *Maternal Pulmonary Embolism by Amniotic Fluid As a Cause of Obstetric Shock and Unexpected Deaths in Obstetrics* was given by two Americans, Paul Steiner (1902–1978) of Chicago and a medical student C.C. Lushbaugh (b 1916) in 1941.

Amniotic Fluid *See amniocentesis.*

Amok [Malay: *amok*, impulse to murder] A disorder of mind amongst Malays and Indians, where the affected person, after a period of withdrawal or depression, made violent attempts to kill people. According to official colonial reports of 1893 most cases occurred in the provinces of Rembang and Madura.

Amontons, Guillaume (1663–1705) French mathematician and instrument maker at Paris who invented: an air thermometer (1702); conical nautical barometer (1695); hygrometer (1687); and a folded barometer (1688). He proposed the relationship of air to pressure and temperature in 1707.

AMP or Adenosine Monophosphate Discovered by Earl Wilbur Sutherland (1915–1974) during his research on hormones at Washington University, St Louis around 1950. He received his medical degree from the University School of Medicine in St Louis in 1942 and became Director of the Western Reserve University in Cleveland in 1953. He was awarded the Nobel Prize for Physiology or Medicine for his work on hormones in 1971. *See ATP.*

Ampere, Andre Marie (1775–1836) Lived during the time of French Revolution and his father was guillotined. He deduced the formula for measuring electricity while professor at the Ecole Polytechnique of Paris in 1775 and the SI unit of current is named in his honor.

Amphetamine Synthesized in 1927 and amphetamine sulfate was introduced into clinical use for treatment of narcolepsy in 1935. Dexamphetamine and methylamphetamine became available a few years later. Dependence on amphetamines was recognized as a problem after World War ll. Early abusers were mainly women who were prescribed it for slimming or for depression. Following the demonstration of the psychotic and addictive properties of amphetamines by Connell in 1958, their use became restricted.

Amphimixis [Greek: *amphi*, both ways + *mixis*, mingling] Reproduction by fusion of two gametes during fertilization was described by August Friedrich Leopold Weismann (1834–1914) of Jena in 1891.

Amphioxus A lancet-shaped marine creature discovered in British waters in 1824. It has been used extensively in embryology due to features common in the lowest vertebrates and all vertebrate embryos. An early work was done by Hackel's pupil, Alexander Kowalewsky (1840–1901) in 1866.

Amphoric Breath Sounds [Greek: *amphora*, vessel] Sounds similar to those of blowing air through the mouth of a vessel. Noted on auscultation of the chest by René Laënnec (1781–1826) in 1819.

Amphotericin B Potent antifungal agent obtained from a culture of *Streptomyces nodosus* from Venezuela by W. Gold,

H.A. Stout and others in 1956.

Ampule Container for sterile solutions used for injections. Invented by Stanislaus Limousin of Paris in 1886.

Ampulla of Vater [Latin: *ampulla*, drinking vessel with a bulge in the center] The ampulla of the bile duct was described by Abraham Vater (1684–1751), professor of botany, anatomy, pathology and therapeutics at Wittenberg in 1720.

Amputation The Greek surgeon Archigenes, who lived around AD 100, amputated limbs for indications such as gangrene, malignant tumors, life-threatening injuries and severe deformities of the limb preventing its use. Red-hot iron was applied to stop bleeding and he suggested ligature to stop bleeding. Hippocrates (460–377 BC) and Galen (129–200) recommended that it be performed at a joint. Paul of Aegina (AD 625–690) recommended amputation for the same indications as suggested by Archigenes. French surgeon Ambroise Paré (1510–1590) revolutionized surgery by introducing ligation. The circular method of amputating limbs was used by English naval surgeon, John Woodall (1556–1643) in 1617 and his technique was later improved by another English naval surgeon, James Yonge (1647–1721) of Plymouth. Dominique Jean Larrey (1766–1842), the famous French army surgeon, performed three amputations at the hip joint, two in Egypt and one in France, around 1760.

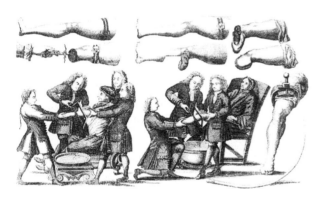

Amputation. Lorenz Heister, A *General System of Surgery* (1757). Innys, Richardson, Clark, Mansby, Whiston, Whyte, Cox & Reymers, London

Amsingiu, John Asseur or Ampsingius (1559–1642) Dutch physician who became professor of medicine at Rostock. He wrote *Dessertio Iatromathematica, De Theorica* and *De Morborum Differentiis.*

Amulet [Arabic: *hamalet*, pendant] Charms or talismans have been used as protection and cures of diseases since ancient times. The symbol of the eye of Horus was used in amulets

5000 years ago by the Egyptians. Bezoars (goats) were supposed to prevent melancholia and precious stones were used as amulets by high priests. Parts of animal bodies and metals were also used as cures. *See folklore.*

Amussat Operation Jean Zullena Amussat (1796–1856) a surgeon at Paris, performed a lumbar colotomy for obstruction of the colon in 1839. He later adapted the procedure to treat atresia of the anus. During this latter operation the mucous membrane was brought down and sutured to the margin of the new anus. *See artificial anus.*

Amygdaloid [Greek: *amygdale*, almond + *oeides*, shape] Term for swollen tonsils during the translation of Avicenna's works in AD 1000. The inferomedial parts of the cerebella hemispheres lodged within the foramen magnum were later termed amygdalae, owing to their similarity to swollen tonsils.

Amyl Nitrate Discovered by Jerome Antoine Balard (1802–1876) of Paris in 1844. Samuel Guthrie (1782–1848), a well known chemist, described its inhalational effects. Sir Benjamin Ward Richardson (1828–1896) and Arthur Gamgee (1841–1909) observed the vasodilator and hypotensive effects. It was tried as a treatment for angina pectoris by Thomas Lauder Brunton (1844–1916) of St Bartholomew's Hospital in 1867 and proved to be very effective. It remained as the only effective drug for treatment for angina until nitroglycerin was introduced by William Murrell (1853–1912) in 1879.

Amylase [Greek: *amylum*, starch] Enzyme identified by Gottlieb Sigismund Constantin Kirchhoff (1764–1833) in 1811. French chemist Anselme Payen (1795–1871) extracted a substance from germinated barley seeds that was capable of breaking down starch to sugar in 1833 and named it. Julius Wohlgemuth (1874–1948) of Germany detected it in urine of patients with pancreatitis in 1908. This was the first instance of the diagnosis of a disease through detection of an enzyme and it formed the basis for diagnostic enzymology. Estimation of serum amylase as a routine diagnostic test for pancreatitis was advocated by R. Elman in 1937.

Amyloidosis Described in 1842 in the kidney by Karl Rokintansky (1804–1878) who called it the 'bacon kidney'. The characteristic reaction of amyloid to iodine and sulfuric acid was demonstrated in 1853 by J. Meckel, who mistook amyloid for cholesterol. Rudolph Virchow (1821–1902) considered it to be cellulose and coined the term in 1854. The clinical features of amyloid kidney were described by Robert Bently Todd (1809–1860) of King's College,

London in 1857. Secondary amyloidosis of liver, spleen, intestines and kidneys arising as a result of empyema, hepatic abscess or pulmonary phthisis was described by C. Neumann of Germany in 1861. A case of primary amyloidosis was reported by Carl Wild in 1886.

Amyotonia Congenita *See Oppenheim disease.*

Amyotrophic Lateral Sclerosis Wasting palsy. Guillaume B.A. Duchenne (1806–1875) described it in 1849 and French physician, François Amilcar Aran (1817–1861) later described it as progressive muscular atrophy in 1850. Aran's view that it was a primary disease of the muscle was shared by Duchenne in 1853. French pathologist, Jean Cruveilheir (1791–1874) described it in 1853 and it came to be known as Cruveilheir disease. Lockhart Clarke (1817–1880) described the changes in the anterior horn cells of the spinal column in 1861. Wasting of the ganglion cells was described by Jean Martin Charcot (1825–1893) who differentiated it into two conditions: the Aran–Duchenne type, manifesting primarily as muscle wasting; and another type showing degeneration of the pyramidal tract of the spinal cord.

Amytal Sodium Synthesized in 1923. One of the first intravenous barbiturates used for anesthesia by Leon Grotius Zerfas (b 1897) and J.T.C. MacCallum of Indianapolis in 1929.

ANA or Antinuclear antibodies Their detection by the fluorescence technique was described by E.J. Holborn, D.M. Weir and G.D. Johnson in the *British Medical Journal* in 1957. The different nuclear patterns of staining seen in various disease conditions by fluorescence was published by J.S. Bech in *The Lancet* in 1961.

Anabolism [Greek: *ana*, up + *bolos*, throw] Constructive stage of metabolism. *See metabolism.*

Anaerobic Bacteria [Greek: *a*, without + *aer*, air + *bios*, life] Term used by Louis Pasteur (1822–1895) to refer to a group of bacteria that existed without oxygen and were harmed by its presence. He made this discovery during his experiments on the resolution of tartaric acid into racemes in 1848.

Anaerobic Metabolism Decisive experiments linking muscle contraction with anaerobic glycolysis were performed by William Fletcher and Frederick Gowland Hopkins (1861–1947) in 1907. While working on isolated frog muscles they found that contraction of the muscles caused by electrical stimulation, in the absence of oxygen, led to accumulation of lactic acid. If the anaerobic stimulation was continued the muscle eventually failed to respond and was said to be fatigued. They also noted that on exposure to oxygen the lactic acid disappeared.

Anal Fissure The causes, mechanism of production and treatment of the condition were described in detail by French surgeon, Alexis Boyer (1757–1833) in 1819.

Anal Fistula Surgical operations are described by Susruta, (AD 500), in a book belonging to the Brahmins of India. Hippocrates (460–377 BC) in his *de Fistulis*, considered it to be the result of a tubercle (abscess) or contusion accumulating in the nates near the anus, specially owing to activities such as rowing or horse riding. He advised early incision to prevent it opening in to the rectum. Aulus Cornelius Celsus (25 BC–AD 50) also described an operation for it. British surgeon John of Ardane (1307–1390), who practiced as a specialist in rectal disorders in London, operated on anal fistula. He excised the wall of the fistula while he controlled bleeding by applying pressure. He later wrote an illustrated treatise on the subject which is probably the first surgical monograph on proctology.

Analgesic Nephropathy The association between prolonged analgesic use and chronic renal failure was pointed out by O. Spuhler and H.U. Zollinger of Germany in 1953. Phenacetin was the first drug to be incriminated in this.

Analgesics Aulus Cornelius Celsus (25 BC–AD 50) wrote *De Medicina* which mentioned the use of mandrake and poppy for relief of pain in his fifth book on drugs. Myrrh, a substance obtained from *Commiphora*, was used as an analgesic by ancient Greeks and Romans. The bark of the white willow, *Salix alba*, containing salicylic acid, remains an ancient remedy for pain. Modern analgesics started to be discovered in the 19th century. The first analgesic drug, salicylic acid, was obtained in a pure form in 1853 and acetanilide followed in 1875. Phenacetin was introduced in 1886. *See aspirin.*

Anamnestic Reaction The production of antibodies in an animal remains dormant until it is challenged by the same antigen. Noted by Clemens E. von Pirquet (1874–1929) in 1911.

Anaphase [Greek: *ana*, up + *phasis*, appearance] Used to describe the third phase of cell division by mitosis [Greek: *mitos*, thread] by Walther Flemming (1843–1905) of Prague in 1882. It was popularized by German botanist, Eduard Adolf Strasburger (1844–1912) in 1884.

Anaphrodisiacs [Greek: *a*, without + *phrodesia*, venus] Medications and methods used to diminish sexual passion. Some used in the past include cold baths, ice, flagellation and warm underclothes. Bromide of potassium and ammonium, iodide of potassium, camphor, digitalis, purgatives, nauseates and bleeding were tried in the 19th century.

Anaphylaxis [Greek: *ana*, backward or up + *phylax*, protection or guard] Term used to denote an allergic reaction by Robert Charles Richet (1850–1935), professor of physiology at Paris in 1902. It has been known since ancient times and a Chinese herbal drug called *Ma Hung*, containing ephedrine, was used as treatment 5000 years ago. The fatal effects of injecting albumin into rabbits that were already sensitized to this protein by previous injections was demonstrated by François Magendie (1783–1855) in 1839. In 1894 Simon Flexner (1863–1946) reiterated this finding by demonstrating the fatal effect of the second dose of dog serum in animals which had previously received a dose of the same serum. Richet found that extracts from sea anemones and other sea organisms did not produce any ill effects when injected into the dogs for the first time. The same substance when injected for the second time produced a severe life-threatening reaction. These observations led to the concept and early understanding of sensitization, leading to understanding of the antigen–antibody reaction. The physiological mechanisms of anaphylactic death were studied by John Auer (1875–1948) and Paul Lewis (1879–1929) in 1910. Samuel James Meltzer (1851–1920) extended these findings to clinical studies by proving that similar physiological mechanisms were involved in asthma. Richet later received the Nobel Prize for his work on anaphylaxis in 1913. The phenomenon of passive anaphylaxis was demonstrated by Maurice Nicolle (1862–1932) of the Pasteur Institute in 1907.

Anarguori [Greek: *a*, without + *arguor*, silver] Physicians who practiced without fees or any other form of reward. St Cosmos and St Damien of Syria were two such physicians in the 5th century.

Anasarca [Greek: *ana*, through + *sarcx*, flesh] Massive generalized edema of the body. *See dropsy.*

Anastomosis [Greek: *ana*, up or through + *stoma*, mouth] Connection of one vessel to another. The fact that severed arteries and veins could be reunited by end-to-end anastomosis was demonstrated by John Benjamin Murphy (1857–1916) in 1897. The modern method of vascular anastomosis was introduced by Alexis Carrel (1884–1947), a pioneer in transplantation surgery in America. *See intestinal anastomosis.*

Anatomical Society of Great Britain and Ireland Founded by Charles Barrett Lockwood, a surgeon at St Bartholomew's Hospital, London in 1887.

Anatomy [Greek: *ana*, through + *temnein*, to cut] The ancient Chinese believed that the trachea opened into the heart and the spinal cord into the testicles. The Egyptians learnt most of their anatomy through embalming bodies. Most of the anatomical knowledge of the Jews during this period was obtained through inspection of meat at slaughterhouses. Herophilus of Chalcedon and Erasistratus who was a teacher at the University of Alexandria, were the first to do human dissections, around 250 BC. Human dissections were banned in the Roman Empire around 150 BC, and from this period up to the time of Andreas Vesalius (1514–1564), the knowledge of anatomy remained patchy and inaccurate. Galen (129–200) based most of his deductions from dissections of apes and other animals. Some notable anatomists of the Middle Ages in Europe include Thaddeus of Florence (1223–1303), his pupil Mondino di Luzzi (1270–1336) and Henri de Mondeville (1270–1320). Leonardo da Vinci (1452–1519) made accurate anatomical drawings of muscles, heart, nerves, bones, blood vessels and other organs. Vesalius produced his magnificent textbook of anatomy in 1543. He was the first to challenge the erroneous statements on anatomy by Galen. After Vesalius, anatomy became a regular part of the curriculum in medical studies and anatomical theaters were established at Padua (1549), Montpellier (1551) and Basel (1588). The first anatomy book in English, *A Treasure for Englishmen, Containing the Anatomie of Man's Body* was written by a surgeon from Maidstone, Thomas Vicary (1495–1561) in 1548. A law was passed in England in 1540 allowing barbers and surgeons to dissect four bodies of executed criminals each year in order to promote anatomy. Following the establishment of the study of anatomy as a regular subject in the English medical curriculum, an acute shortage of bodies for dissection emerged, which led to body snatching and murders. The supply of bodies for dissection was later regularized by the Anatomy Act of 1832. The study of anatomy related to diseases (morbid anatomy) was established by Giovanni Battista Morgagni (1682–1771) who was a professor at Padua in the early 18th century.

Anatomy Act When the study of anatomy became a regular part of the medical curriculum in England around 1700, there were no organized sources of cadavers for anatomical dissections. Body snatching from burial grounds was a common method of obtaining bodies and murders began to take place in order to supply bodies for profit. In 1829, the exposure of 16 murders committed by William Hare and William Burke in Edinburgh, in order to supply bodies, dictated the need for the control of the supply of bodies for dissection. Later, in 1832, Lord Henry Warburton

(1784–1858) brought in the Anatomy Act, which made provision for all unclaimed bodies to go to the medical schools. *See burking, William Burke, Burke and Hare murders.*

Anatomy, Private Schools Many private anatomy schools, which also taught physiology, were established during the period 1740–1840. The Great Windmill Street School started under Samuel Sharp (1700–1778), a London surgeon and pupil of Cheselden. It was taken over by William Hunter (1718–1783) in 1746 and then existed at Covent Garden. John Hunter (1728–1793) also lectured at the school and when William died in 1783, Matthew Baillie (1761–1823), his nephew, took over. A complete course of anatomy, surgery and medicine started at the school around 1800. Charles Bell (1774–1842) joined it in 1812 and with the foundation of University College in 1828 the Windmill Street School ceased to exist. John Bell (1763–1820), a brother of Charles Bell, opened the first private anatomy school at Edinburgh in 1790. The Webb Street School in London, started by Grainger of Birmingham in 1819, provided courses in anatomy, surgery, midwifery, medicine and chemistry. It had several hundred students and lasted until 1842. Joseph Carpue (1764–1846) started his school in Dean Street, Soho around 1800 and it lasted until 1830.

Anaudos [Greek: *a*, negative or without + *audos*, voice] Ancient term for loss of voice.

Anaxagoras (488–428 BC) Greek scientist who gave explanations for eclipses, meteors, rainbows, sun, moon and stars, although some of his theories were obscure and bizarre. He considered the sun to be a mass of metal reflecting the light of the moon, and stars to be heavenly bodies made white hot by heat. Despite some of his other rational explanations he was prosecuted on religious grounds and had to leave Athens.

Anaximander of Miletus (611–547 BC) He mapped the Earth giving details of its surface and speculated on the size and distances of the heavenly bodies or stars. He proposed that man evolved from aquatic animals.

Anaximenes (570 BC) Greek scientist and philosopher who proposed that the essence of all things was air which he named 'pneuma' to denote 'breath'.

Anazoturia Reduced excretion of urea and solids in the urine. Term coined by R. Willis in 1838.

Anconeus [Greek: *ancon*, elbow] Galen (129–200) used the term 'ancon' for the olecranon. Jakob Benignus Winslow (1669–1760) named the muscles attached to the olecranon 'anconeii' around 1740.

Ancrod or arvin Proteinase obtained from the venom of the Malayan pit viper, *Agkistradon rhodostoma*. The clinical features of patients following the bite were described by H.A. Reid and co-workers in 1963. A predominant systemic feature was a hemostatic defect which Reid and others attributed to defibrination caused by the venom. A purified fraction of the venom was obtained as a therapeutic agent for anticoagulation as 'ancrod' and was tried as treatment for deep vein thrombosis by W.R. Bell and colleagues in 1968.

Anchylostoma duodenale [Greek: *ankylos*, crooked or hooked + *stoma*, mouth] (Syn. anemia of Ceylon, tropical chlorosis, mal de coeur, dirt-eating disease) The symptoms of hookworm disease were known to the ancient Egyptians and described in the Ebers Papyrus. It was described as *opilatio* by Willem Piso (1611–1678) who observed it in Brazil in 1648. *Anchylostoma* was described as an intestinal parasite by Angelo Dubini (1813–1902) in 1838, who also gave the parasite its present name in 1843. It was identified as the cause of Egyptian chlorosis by Wilhelm Griesinger (1817–1868) in 1854. The fecal test for diagnosis of hookworm disease was devised by Giovanni Battista Grassi (1854–1925) of Italy in 1878, before which time it was diagnosed only at postmortem. The mode of entry of the parasite through the skin was demonstrated by Charles Albert Bently (1873–1949) in 1902. The American variety of the hookworm, *Necator americanus*, was discovered by Allan J. Smith and named by Charles Wardell Stiles (1867–1941) of the US Public Health Service in 1902. *See miner's anemia.*

Ancylostomiasis *See Ancylostoma duodenale.*

Andernach, Johann Winther von (1487–1574) Professor of medicine at Louvain who described the wormian bones or ossa suturarum (Andernach ossicles) in 1536.

Anders, James Mescheter (1854–1936) American physician and graduate (1877) of the University of Pennsylvania, Philadelphia, where he became professor of medicine. He described small fatty subcutaneous tender nodules in the extremities or on the abdomen (Anders disease).

Andersen Syndrome *See cystic fibrosis.*

Anderson, Elizabeth Garrett (1836–1917) The first woman to qualify in medicine in England. She was born in London and brought up in Aldburgh, Suffolk. She obtained her diploma from the Society of Apothecaries in 1865 against much opposition and established a dispensary for women in London in 1866. She started medical courses for women at her dispensary at Euston Road under the name New Hospital for Women, later renamed the Elizabeth Garrett

Anderson Hospital. She was elected the first woman mayor in England, at Aldeburgh in 1908.

Anderson Operation A procedure for lengthening a tendon. Devised by Roger Anderson (b 1891), an orthopedic surgeon from Seattle, Washington. He also devised an external fixation splint (Anderson splint) for fracture of long bones in 1934.

Anderson Scots Pills A secret remedy offered by Patrick Anderson, a physician at Edinburgh in the 17th century. He published the virtues of the pills in *Grana Angelica* in 1635. After his death his pills were marketed by his daughter Catherine who communicated the secret to an Edinburgh surgeon, Thomas Weir. The pills remained in popular use for well over 200 years until 1910. Analysis showed that they contained 40 ingredients but no specific therapeutic value could be determined.

Anderson Syndrome Bronchiectasis and vitamin A deficiency in children with cystic fibrosis of the pancreas, often leading to a fatal outcome. Described by New York pediatrician, Dorothy Hansine Handerson (b 1901).

Anderson, Sir Thomas McCall (1836–1908) Professor of physics at the University of Glasgow and a founder of the Hospital for Skin Diseases which started as a clinic at Elmbank Street. He published *Diseases of the Skin* (1887) and *Diagnosis and Treatment of Syphilitic Affections of the Nervous System*.

Anderson, Tempest (1846–1913) Ophthalmic surgeon from York who was educated at University College, London. He returned to York as ophthalmic surgeon to the York County Hospital.

Anderson, W. (1842–1900) English physician who graduated from St Thomas' Hospital in 1864 and served as head of the Naval Medical College in Tokyo for 7 years until his return to St Thomas as a surgeon in 1880. He described the sex-linked disorder characterized by skin lesions and renal failure, angiokeratoma corporis diffusum universale (Anderson–Fabrey disease) in 1898. The same condition had been described earlier by a German dermatologist, J. Fabrey (1860–1930).

Andral, Gabriel (1797–1876) French physician at Paris. He described the characteristic posture (Andral sign) in pleurisy, in which the patient assumes a supine position, resting on the healthy side.

Andre, Nicholas (1658–1742) *See Andry, Nicholas.*

Andree, John (1739–1785) Physician from Switzerland who graduated from Rheims in 1739. He settled in London and

was instrumental in establishing the London Hospital, in which he was a senior physician. He wrote *An Account of the Tilbury Water* (4 editions) in 1737, *A Case of Epilepsy Hysteria and Fits and St Vitus Dance, with the Process of Cure* (1746) and *Observations Upon a Treatise on the Virtues of Hemlock in the Cure of Cancers* (1761).

Andrews Operation A method of treating inguinal hernia with the application of overlapping sutures. Designed by American surgeon, Edward Wyllys Andrews (1856–1927) of Chicago in 1895.

Andrews, Thomas (1813–1885) Physician from Belfast who studied chemistry and became professor of chemistry there in 1849. He did a remarkable series of experiments with carbon dioxide from 1863 to 1869 and was the first to establish the true nature of ozone as an allotrophic form of oxygen. In his experiments with carbon dioxide he found the critical temperature of gases above which they cannot be liquefied, in 1869.

Androgenesis or Male Parthenogenesis Asexual reproduction of male gamete without fertilization. Described by American professor of zoology at Columbia University, New York, Edmund Beecher Wilson (1856–1939) from Illinois in 1928.

Androgen [Greek: *aner*, male + *gennan*, to produce] The use of testicular tissue as treatment for impotence was described in the *Ayur-Veda* of the Hindus. A scientific demonstration of the remote effects of an internal secretion from the testis was given by Arnold Adolph Berthold (1803–1861). He transplanted the testis of a rooster to another part of the body in a different bird which had been castrated. He was able to prevent the sequelae of castration and maintain the normal growth of the comb in 1849. The first active male hormone extract was obtained from the lipoid fraction of bull testis by Lemuel Clyde McGee (b 1904) of America in 1927. He injected this fraction into capons and demonstrated its effect in correcting the sequelae of castration (capon-comb test). A crude active male hormone was extracted from male urine by Casimir Funk (1884–1967) and Benjamin Harrow (1888–1970) in 1929. A quantitative physiological assay of this was designed by Frederick Conrad Koch, T.F. Gallagher and Carl Richard Moore (1892–1955). The pure crystalline form was obtained in 1931 by Adolf Friedrich Johan Butenandt (b 1903) of Germany, who named it androsterone. He established the structural formula for it in 1933 and extracted dihydroandrosterone from male urine in 1934. Testosterone from the testicular tissue was isolated by K. David, E. Emanse, F. Freud and E. Laqueur in 1933. It was prepared artificially from cholesterol by Swiss chemist, Leopold Ruzicka (1887–1976) from Croatia and Albert Wettstein of Switzerland in 1935. Butenandt and Ruzicka shared the Nobel Prize in Chemistry in 1939. The orally active preparation of testosterone, methyltestoster-one, was produced by K. Miescher and E. Tschopp in 1938.

Andromachus of Crete (AD 60) Physician to Emperor Nero. He invented a cure-all remedy or panacea, *Thericae Andromachi*, composed of 60 different medicines. His fo mula was used by Greek and Arab physicians for over 1500 years.

Androsterone *See androgen.*

Andry, Nicholas (1658–1742) French surgeon from Lyons who became professor and Dean of the Royal College at Paris. His works include *Traite de la generation des vers dans lecorps de l'homme, Remarques de medicine sur differents sujets* and *Examen de differents points d'Anatomie.* He suggested the germ theory of disease, coined the term 'orthopedics' and wrote a textbook on orthopedics in 1741. He described infraorbital neuralgia in 1756.

Anel Operation *See Anel, Dominique.*

Anel, Dominique (1679–1725) French surgeon from Toulouse who was the first to catheterize the lachrymal duct in 1712. He devised the procedure (Anel operation) of tying the aneurysm at the proximal end, before John Hunter (1728–1793), in 1710.

Anemia [Greek: *a*, without + *haima*, blood] Hippocrates (460–377 BC) noted the clinical features of anemia, the first clinical description was given only in 1620 by Varandal or Johannes Varandaeus. Various names such as icterrius am anterium, morbus virginius and cachexia virginium were given to it with no apparent cause. Anemia in young women during puberty, commonly called 'chlorosis', was described by Johann Lange (1485–1565) in 1554. Hippocrates also described a condition similar to chlorosis in his book on the diseases of virgins. This type was later recognized to be due to iron deficiency. Pernicious anemia was described by James Scarth Combe (1796–1883) in 1824 but its cause and treatment remained unresolved for nearly a century. George Hoyt Whipple (1878–1976) and Robschet-Robbins made the observation in 1925 that raw or lightly cooked liver could treat pernicious anemia. George Richard Minot (1885–1950) and William Parry Murphy (1892–1987) further established the treatment of anemia with a raw liver diet. The anti-pernicious factor or B_{12} was identified and isolated in 1948. A clear and accurate description of anemia in pregnancy was given by Hermann Nasse in 1836. *Anchylostoma duodenale* and other chronic infections such as syphilis and malignant diseases were recognized as a cause of anemia in the early 1900s, but the mechanism of production remained obscure. A classification based on red cell morphology was proposed by Maxwell Myer Wintrobe (b 1901) in 1930. *See hemolytic anemia, pernicious anemia.*

Anesthesia [Greek: *a*, negative + *aisthesig*, sensation] The term was used in a philosophical sense by Plato around 400 BC. Dioscorides used it to denote the absence of physical sensation. From ancient times up to the Renaissance anesthetic drugs used to relieve pain were obtained from herbs such as hemlock, mandragora, opium, hellebore and others. Wine was used liberally and mandrake wine was used for surgery by Dioscorides. Mandrake was also a popular anesthetic during the Middle Ages. The method of compression of the carotid artery until the patient became unconscious to perform surgery or relieve pain is mentioned in Aristotle's *Historia Animalorum.* Herbal narcotics were less used in the late Renaissance period and induction of stupor by herbal narcotics was banned in France during this period. Valerius Cordus (1515–1544) wrote the first European pharmacopoeia and obtained ether from sulfuric acid and alcohol in 1540. He called the substance *oleum dulci vitrioli,* which meant sweet vitriol. The name 'ether' was given two centuries later by Frobenus of Germany in 1730. Its anesthetic property was not recognized until 1842, when Crawford Williamson Long (1815–1878), a physician from Georgia, used it successfully to remove a tumor from the neck of a patient. Sadly, his failure to report his results in time denied him the credit. Inhalation gas therapy with nitrous oxide was demonstrated by Humphry Davy (1778–1829) in 1799, although its value was not realized for another 50 years. Henry Hill Hickman (1800–1830), an English surgeon from Shropshire, began experimenting with the inhalational effects of carbon dioxide and published his findings in *A Letter on Suspended Animation* in 1824. His discovery was ignored by his peers thus further delaying its advent. American, Horace Wells (1815–1848), a dentist in Boston, learnt in 1844 of the inhalational effect of nitrous oxide from Gardner Q. Colton, a traveling lecturer in chemistry. After achieving a successful tooth extraction under nitrous oxide, Wells arranged a demonstration at the Massachusetts General Hospital on December 12, 1844. Unfortunately for no apparent reason, his method failed and he was subjected to ridicule. He continued using nitrous oxide with success for a few years, but eventually gave up and later committed suicide. William Thomas Green Morton (1819–1868) an assistant of Wells and later a medical student, gave a successful demonstration of the effects of ether in surgery on 30 September 1846 and was hailed as its discoverer. Oliver Wendell Holmes (1809–1894) in the same year, gave the name anesthesia to what had previously been called suspended animation or etherization. James Young Simpson (1811–1870), an obstetrician from Scotland, while searching for a better agent than ether for anesthesia, began successfully using chloroform in 1847. Controversy over the use of chloroform ended when John Snow (1813–1858), a physician who specialized in anesthesia, administered it to Queen Victoria during her delivery of Prince Leopold. Ether was first used in England by Robert Liston (1794–1847) at University College Hospital in 1846. Anesthetic record charts were advocated by E.A. Codman and Harvey Cushing (1869–1939) in 1894. Introduction of endotracheal anesthesia by Samuel James Meltzer (1851–1920) and John Auer (1875–1948) in 1909 ushered in the modern era. It was recognized as a specialty in England at Oxford when Lord Nuffield created the first Chair at the Radcliffe Infirmary in 1922 and Robert Reynolds Macintosh was appointed first professor. The first diploma in anesthesia in England was awarded in 1935. *See ether, chloroform, local anesthesia, nitrous oxide, regional anesthesia, rectal anesthesia, endotracheal anesthesia, inhalational anesthesia, closed- circuit anesthesia, electrical anesthesia, epidural anesthesia, intravenous anesthesia, spinal anesthesia.*

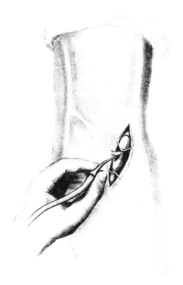

Intravenous administration of saline. P.J. Flagg, *The Art of Anaesthesia* (1916). Lippincot, Philadelphia

Aneuploidy [Greek: *a*, without + *eu*, well + *aploos*, one-fold] A state in cell division in which an incorrect number of

chromosomes is produced. Described by Tackholm in 1922.

Aneurin [Greek: *a*, without + *neuron*, nerve] Anti-beriberi factor isolated and identified as an essential food factor by Barend Coenraad Petrus Jansen (1884–1962) and Willem Frederick Donath (1889–1957) in Jakarta in 1926. They named it 'aneurin' because of its antineuritic properties. It was renamed vitamin B_I or thiamin [Greek: brimstone]. Synthesis was achieved by R.R. Williams in 1936, and Alexander Robertus Todd (b 1907), professor of chemistry at Cambridge in 1937. *See beriberi.*

Aneurysm [Greek: *ana*, through + *eurus*, broad] Galen (129–200) was the first to describe and treat aneurysm. He observed the development from an accidental puncture during venesection and advocated applying pressure over it with sponges and bandages. Applying pressure continued to be practiced for the next 17 centuries. Aneurysms of peripheral vessels were described by Antyllus in AD 250 and Aetius (AD 500) gave an account describing causes, signs and surgical treatment. He also recognized the risk of treating an aneurysm in the neck and advised the avoidance of operative interference. Paul of Aegina (625–690) advised against incision of an aneurysm in the armpit, groin or neck. Albucasis (936–1013), Rhazes (850–932) and Haly Abbas (930–994) also described the nature of the aneurysm and its surgical treatment. Their surgical method of tying it at the proximal end was practiced in the 18th century by Dominique Anel (1679–1725), John Hunter (1728–1793) and John Abernethy (1764–1831). Ante-mortem diagnosis of an aortic aneurysm was made by Andreas Vesalius (1514–1564) in 1555 and his diagnosis was confirmed 2 years later at autopsy. Abernethy, a pupil of John Hunter, ligated the external iliac artery in 1796. The use of elastic dacron in modern arterial surgery including the repair of aneurysms was introduced by D. Emerick Szilagyi (b 1910) and co-workers in 1958. *See cardiac aneurysm, intracranial aneurysms.*

Aneurysmorrhaphy [Greek: *ana*, through + *eurus*, broad + *rhaphe*, sewing] Partial excision of the aneurysmal sac of a traumatic left brachial artery aneurysm was performed by Rudolph Matas (1860–1957) of America in 1888. Use of elastic dacron in modern arterial surgery was introduced by D. Emerick Szilagyi (b 1910) and co-workers in 1958.

Anfinson, Boehmer Christian (b 1916) American biochemist, born at Monessen, Pennsylvania and educated at Harvard. He lectured at the National Institutes of Health at Bethesda, Maryland from 1950 to 1982 and did research on chromatographic identification of peptides. This led to the conclusion that 128 amino acids of ribonuclease were formed into a single peptide chain with four disulfide bonds with a single N-terminus. He was awarded the Nobel Prize for Chemistry for his work on the molecular biology of disulfide bonds in 1972.

Angelucci Syndrome Conjunctivitis, tachycardia and vasomotor lability. Described by Italian ophthalmologist and professor at Naples, A. Angelucci (1854–1933).

Angelucci, Theodore Italian poet and physician in the 15th century. He was professor at Padua and a member of the academy of Venice. He wrote *Sententia quod metaphysica, Ars Medica, De Natura et curatione malignae Febris* and other treatises.

Angina Pectoris [Latin: *angere*, to strangle + *pectoris*, of the breast] The classic symptoms of acute myocardial ischemia were described by William Heberden, the elder (1710–1801) who named it 'angina pectoris' in 1768. Thomas Lauder Brunton (1844–1916), while resident medical officer, noticed the relief of symptoms by inhalation of amyl nitrite in 1867 and this opened the door for use of coronary vasodilators in treatment. Nitroglycerin was introduced by William Murrell (1853–1912) in 1879. Sympathectomy was tried by Thoma Jonnesco (1860–1926) of Romania in 1916. The characteristic changes in the electrocardiogram during an attack were recorded by Guy William John Bousfield (1893–1974) in 1918. Paravertebral nerve injection was performed by Mandl of Austria in 1925. Samuel Levine (b 1891) and Herman Ludwig Blumgart (b 1895) tried total thyroidectomy in 1933 and functional thyroidectomy with thiouracil was tried by W. Raab in 1945. Khellin, from the plant *Ammi visnaga*, was introduced as a vasodilator for treatment by G. V. Anrep in 1949 but its use was short-lived. *See coronary atherosclerosis, coronary artery bypass graft, smoking.*

Angina Suffocativa [Greek: *angere*, to strangle] The term used to refer to diphtheria by Samuel Bard (1742–1821) of Philadelphia in 1771.

Angina, Ludwig *See Ludwig angina.*

Angina, Vincent *See Vincent angina.*

Angiocardiography [Greek: *angeion*, vessel + *kardia*, heart + *graphein*, to write] X-rays were used to assess the systolic and diastolic phases of the heart and aorta by H. Guilleminot in 1899 and this remained the only radiological method of studying the cardiovascular system until the invention of angiocardiography. Werner Forssman (1904–1979) of Germany, in 1929, was the first to insert a catheter into a living human heart and he performed the first angiography in 1931. He first catheterized himself and took X-rays to confirm his technique. The first cinefluorographic

visualization of cardiac chambers by injecting contrast into the veins was described by George Porter Robb (b1898) and Israel Steinberg (b1902) in 1938. *See cardiac catheterization, left ventriculography.*

Angiogram *See angiography.*

Angiography [Greek: *angeion*, vessel + *graphein*, to write] The visualization of blood vessels by injection of a radio-opaque substance was done by E. Haschek and O.T. Lindenthal in 1896. The method was introduced into clinical radiology by Barney Brooks (b 1884) who used sodium iodide in 1924. Pulmonary angiography was introduced by Antonio Egaz Moniz (1874–1955), L. de Carvalho and A. Lima in 1931. The technique of thoracic aortography was demonstrated by Bror Leonhard Johan Broden (b 1910) in 1948. *See angiocardiography.*

Angiology [Greek: *angeion*, vessel + *logos*, treatise] The term was used by Galen (129–200) to denote a procedure of bleeding or excision of the temporal artery in order to cure resistant headache. Paul of Aegina (625–690) used it to refer to varicose veins. It was used to denote the study of blood vessels by the German surgeon, Lorenz Heister (1683–1758), in 1720.

Angioneurotic Edema (Syn. Milton disease, giant urticaria) A description was given by Marcello Donati (1538–1602) of Italy in 1586. The next account was given by Stolpertus in 1778. A classic description was given in 1876 by London dermatologist, John Laws Milton (1820–1898) who named it 'giant urticaria'. German professor of medicine at Bern in Switzerland, Heinrich Iranius Quincke (1842–1922) described it in 1882 and the name was suggested by Strubing in 1885. The hereditary form was described by William Osler (1849–1919) in 1888 and the absence of alpha-globulin, the inhibitor of C'-1A esterase as a cause was shown by V.H. Donaldson and R.R. Evans of America in 1963.

Angioplasty [Greek: *angeion*, vessel + *plasein*, to mold] The relief of atherosclerotic intraluminal obstruction of the ilio-femoral arteries using a percutaneous catheter was achieved by C.T. Dotter and Melvin P. Judkins in 1964. Their technique was modified and improved by T.W. Stable in 1968. The use of a balloon-tipped catheter was introduced by two Americans, Andreas R. Gruentzig (d 1985) and D.A. Kumpke in 1974. Gruentzig used this method for treating renal artery stenosis in 1977 and established it as a form of treatment for coronary artery stenosis in 1979. Balloon angioplasty as a treatment for aortic valve stenosis was advocated by J.T. Walls and colleagues in 1984.

Angiotensin Converting Enzyme Inhibitor The South

American arrowhead viper, *Bothrops jararca*, was noted to produce venom that contained a potentiator of bradykinin by Sergio H. Ferreira in 1965. The effectiveness of this in inhibiting angiotensin converting enzyme was demonstrated by Y.S. Bakle in 1968. The amino acid sequence and the structure were identified later and led to the development of substance YS 980, known as captopril. This was followed by the introduction of M421 or enalapril.

Angiotensin Discovered by Irwin Henley Page (b 1901) and O.M. Helmer in 1939. It was found independently around the same time by E. Braun Menendez and co-workers in Argentina, and they named it 'hypertensin'. The two different forms, angiotensin I and angiotensin II, were identified by Leonard T. Skeggs and J.R. Kahn of America. The pure form was isolated by W.S. Peart in 1955. The structure of both angiotensin I and angiotensin II and their amino acid sequence was described by Peart in 1956. Synthesis was accomplished by F.M. Bumpus, H. Schwarz and Page in 1957.

Angle Classification Classification for various modes of malocclusion of teeth. Proposed by American orthodontist from St Louis, Edward Hartley Angle (1855–1930).

Angle of Louis Between the manubrium and the body of the sternum. Described by Pierre Charles Alexandre Louis (1787–1872), a physician and a leading authority on tuberculosis in Paris.

Anglicus, Gilbertus English physician in the 13th century. He wrote a compendium of physick in which he gave an original description of leprosy, which remained as the main source of information during the medieval period. He also suggested the contagious nature of smallpox. He died in 1230 and his work was published in 1507.

Anglicus, Ricardus English medical writer who lived around 1230. He was educated at Oxford and Paris and wrote several medical treatises.

Anglo-Saxon Medicine Few records exist on medicine at this time. An early book is the *Leech Book of Bald* written around AD 950. Others include *Peri Didaxeon* and *Lacnunga* (recipe or medications). Several versions of *Lorica* were written including that by Aethelwold, Bishop of Lichfield, around AD 820. *Lorica* comes from the Latin for a leather coat or a metal breastplate and is used for a book of prayer in which several anatomical parts of the human body are mentioned while praying for protection. Rational medicine was introduced to England through missionaries around AD 600. The school at Canterbury was established around AD 800 by Theodore, the Greek Archbishop of Canterbury.

Records show that medicine was part of its curriculum. Following the Viking invasion towards the end of the 9th century, many libraries and monasteries were destroyed and learning declined. *See Leech book.*

Angstrom, Anders Jonas (1814–1874) Swedish physicist from Lodgo who introduced the unit for the wavelength of light, ten millionth of a millimeter, the Angstrom unit. He was awarded the Rumford medal of the Royal Society in England in 1872. He also discovered hydrogen in the solar atmosphere and published a map of the solar spectrum in 1868.

Aniline An extract from coal tar used as a dye, and later recognized as a cause of methemoglobinemia. Its precursor, nitrobenzene, was found to be carcinogenic. Robert Koch (1843–1910) used aniline dyes for microscopic staining in 1877. *See bladder carcinoma.*

Anima [Latin: *anima*, breath or life] The theory that considered the soul as the vital moving force of the body was proposed by a chemist and professor of medicine at the University of Halle, George Ernst Stahl (1660–1734). He considered the characteristics of the body to be governed not by chemical and physical laws but by the laws of the soul. This was essentially the same as the concept of *psyche* proposed by Aristotle (384–322 BC). The *anima* is synonymous with *archaeus* or *pneuma*.

Animal Dissection Animal dissections were promoted during the time of Galen (129–200) as ecclesiastical and secular authorities did not approve of dissection of human corpses. Many of his observations on animals were applied to humans and went unchallenged for over 1000 years. The study and development of comparative anatomy through animal dissections has contributed significantly to our present knowledge of physiology, embryology and evolution.

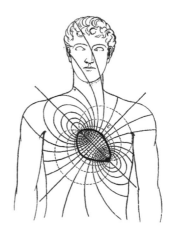

Studies on animal electricity related to the heart. Augustus Waller, *An Introduction to Human Physiology* (1893). Longmans, Green & Co., London

Animal Electricity The phenomenon was known in the ancient world through the electric properties of fish. Aristotle in his *Historia Animalium* (340 BC) studied the Mediterranean torpedo fish and stated that it 'narcotizes the creatures it wants to catch by the strength of the shock that is resident in its body'. John Walsh (1725–1795) in 1774 studied the electrical nature of the torpedo fish and established the existence of animal electricity. Luigi Galvani (1737–1798) in 1786 studied bioelectric effects using frog's legs. Electric current in organic tissues was shown by the German physiologist Emil Heinrich DuBois-Reymond (1818–1896) in 1843. He showed that a flow of electric current took place from injured to surrounding non-injured tissue. *See action potential, electrophysiology.*

Animal Experiments A large list of contributions such as William Harvey's (1578–1657) discovery of blood circulation, Humphry Davy's (1778–1829) demonstration of the inhalational effects of gases, and Matteo Realdo Colombo's (1516–1559) discovery of the pulmonary circulation were made possible through animal experiments. The use of live animals for experiments, some causing great suffering, was common in the 19th century and guidelines had to be laid down. Benjamin Ward Richardson (1828–1896) and others realized the importance of animal experiments for the advancement of science but were concerned about the way in which they were done. He devised a lethal chamber for the painless slaughter of experimental animals in 1866. *See antivivisection.*

Animal Heat Around 350 BC, Aristotle (384–322 BC) equated the heat of the body with vitality, and considered the heart as the heat center. Joseph Black (1728–1799) of Glasgow studied the phenomenon scientifically. In 1779 Adair Crawford (1748–1795) conducted experiments and proposed a theory in which the disengagement of caloric heat occurred following generation of carbon dioxide in the breath. Muscles were shown to be the principal source by Hermann Helmholtz (1821–1894) in 1848.

Animal Magnetism or Mesmerism The ancient Hindus knew that snakes and fowls could be hypnotized with sound. Study was revived by Hehl, a Jesuit in Vienna in 1774. Franz Anton Mesmer (1734–1815) called it 'animal magnetism' in the belief that hypnosis was due to an effect similar to that of a magnet and he gave a demonstration in Vienna in 1776. Although his theory was incorrect, its practice later formed the basis for hypnosis. It became an important topic in the 18th century and Louis XVI appointed a commission chaired by Benjamin Franklin (1706–1790) to inquire into it in 1784. Other members included Jean Bailly, Antoine Lavoisier (1743–1794) the chemist and Joseph Ignace Guillotine (1738–1814), who devised the method of execution. It was discredited by the Academy of Sciences, but two of Mesmer's students, the Marquis de Puysegur (1751–1825) and his brother, continued to practice it. The term 'mesmerism' was used by a German philosopher and friend of Mesmer, Karl Wolfhart. It was revived in 1830 by John Elliotson (1791–1868), professor of surgery at the University of London, who later resigned because of opposition to his practice. James Braid (1795–1860), a Manchester surgeon, substituted the word 'hypnotism' in 1843 and used it to produce surgical anesthesia. It was introduced to America by Charles Poyen in 1836. *See hypnosis.*

Animal Spirit Erasistratus, a teacher at the University of Alexandria around 300 BC, studied the brain and described the fluid in the cerebral ventricles as 'animal spirit'. He explained (erroneously) that muscular contractions were brought about by distension of the animal spirit from the brain, transmitted through the nerves. This view was held by philosophers and physicians up to the time of the Renaissance.

Anion A Greek term meaning 'that which goes up' used by Michael Faraday (1791–1867) to denote electronegative bodies.

Anisophygmia Old term to denote the inequality of pulse pressure and pulse volume.

Ankle Clonus or foot clonus Diagnostic physical sign described by Otto Westphal in 1875.

Ankylosing Spondylitis [Greek: *ankylos*, crooked + *spho-ndylos*, vertebra] (Syn. spondylitis of Marie–Strümpell and von Bekhterev, spondylitis ankylopoetica, spondylitis rhizomelique) A mention involving the vertebrae an sacroiliac regions was made by Bernard Connor (1666–1698) of Ireland in 1691. A clinical description associated with bony ankylosis of the spine and polyarthritis was given by Sir Benjamin Brodie (1783–1862) in *Pathological and Surgical Observations on the Diseases of the Joints* published in 1818. Jacques Mathieu Delpech (1777–1832) described it in 1828, and James Paget followed in 1877. It was described at necropsy as 'poker back' by Charles Hilton Fagge (1838–1883) of Guy's Hospital in 1877. Adolf von Strümpell (1853–1925) of Germany described two cases in 1884 and Russian neurologist, Vladimir Bekhterev (1857–1927) at St Petersburg described it detail in 1897. He also described the superior vestibular nucleus in 1885. Pierre Marie (1853– 1940) of France described it as 'la spondylose rhizomelique' in 1898.

It is also known as Strümpell–Bekhterev–Marie syndrome.

Ankylosis [Greek: *angchein*, to press tight] Contractures of joints arising from impacted humors or nervous tension were called 'ancylae' or 'ancylosis' by ancient Greek physicians. An osteotomy in the USA for ankylosis of the hip joint was performed by John Rhea Barton (1794–1871) of Lancaster in 1826.

Ankylostomiasis *See Anchylostoma duodenale.*

Annals of Internal Medicine First journal of the College of American Physicians, the *Annals of Medicine*, was published in 1921, but was discontinued after three issues. *Annals of Clinical Medicine* was published in 1922 but response was also poor and its name was changed to *Annals of Internal Medicine* in 1927.

Annals of Medicine, Edinburgh The earliest British medical journal, published in 1796. It became the *Edinburgh Medical and Surgical Journal* in 1805 and continued until 1855, before it combined with the *Monthly Journal of Medicine* to become the *Edinburgh Medical Journal*.

Annandale, Thomas (1838–1909) Surgeon from Newcastle-upon-Tyne who succeeded Symes as the professor of surgery at Edinburgh. He wrote *Malformations, Diseases and Injuries of the Fingers and Toes* (1864). He performed surgery for displaced semilunar cartilage of the knee in 1884.

Annulus Migrans or geographical tongue Physical sign described by Bridou Gubler of Paris in 1872.

Anodyne [Greek: *a*, negative + *dyne*, pain] Substance used to relieve pain. Aulus Cornelius Celsus (25 BC–AD 50) described several sleep-inducing drugs which could be obtained from herbs as anodynes.

Anomalous Conduction *See atrioventricular anomalous conduction.*

Anomalous Coronary Artery *See Bland–White–Garland syndrome.*

Anopheles [Greek: *anophele*, hurtful] A genus of mosquito. Their role as transmitters of malaria was mentioned in the Sanskrit works of the Brahmin, Susruta (AD 500). The suggestion that it carried the malarial parasite was made by French parasitologist, Charles Louis Alphonse Laveran (1845–1922) in 1880. A surgeon in the Indian Medical Services, Ronald Ross (1857–1932) traced the parasite to mosquitoes while working in the Niligiri mountains in India in 1897. He later demonstrated transmission to birds through bites of infected mosquitoes. The extracorporeal development of the malarial parasite in the *Anopheles*

mosquito was shown by Amico Bignami (1862–1929) and Giovanni Battista Grassi (1854–1925) in 1899. Mosquitoes were also shown to be carriers of yellow fever by Carlos Finlay (1833–1915) in Havana in 1889. *See mosquito.*

Anorexia [Greek: *a*, without + *orexis*, a longing for] Greek physician, Paul of Aegina (625–690) defined it as 'loathing of food, either from prevalence of intemperance of stomach, or a collection of humors' and advocated melca, a mixture of milk and garlic, as treatment. Aulus Cornelius Celsus (25 BC–AD 50) recommended undiluted wine to restore appetite. *See appetite, anorexia nervosa.*

Anorexia Nervosa [Greek: *a*, without + *orexis*, a longing for] Simone Porta (1496–1554) gave a description in a 10- year-old girl who refused to take food. John Reynolds described it as prodigious abstinence in 1669. In 1694 Richard Morton (1637–1698), physician to James II, gave a classic description in two patients and named it 'nervous atrophy'. He also noted the triad of anorexia, wasting and amenorrhoea. A case of anorexia in a male, *A Remarkable Case of Abstinence*, was written by London dermatologist, Robert Willian (1757–1812) in 1790. This was also noted by William Gull (1816–1890) in 1868 who called it 'apepsia hysterica'. A case of extreme cachexia associated with pituitary destruction was found by a pathologist from Hamburg, Morris Simmonds (1855–1925) in 1914 and thereafter it became confused with Simmonds disease, especially with its new term 'pituitary cachexia'. Between 1930–1940, it was gradually recognized as a separate entity due to work of several endocrinologists in Europe and the USA.

Anosognosia Term coined in 1914 by Joseph François Felix Babinski (1857–1932) to denote the denial of a striking neurological disorder by a patient.

Anoxemia *See altitude sickness, aviation medicine.*

Anoxemia Test Diagnostic test for angina in which the patients breathe oxygen-poor (10%) air to provoke angina. Test in use in the early 20th century.

Anrep, Vasili Konstaninovich (1852–1918) Physician who suggested the use of cocaine as a local anesthetic in 1880.

Antabuse or disulfiram In 1949 when tetraethylthiuram disulfide was tried as a worm treatment, those who took it became very ill if they consumed alcohol. This observation led to the development of disulfiram for treatment of chronic alcoholism.

Antacid Therapy Treatment of peptic ulcer disease with frequent milk feeds and compounds such as magnesium hydroxide Popularized by American gastroenterologist, Bertram Welton Sippy (1866–1924) in 1915.

Antefebrin *See acetanilide.*

Antenatal Care [Latin: *ante*, before + *natalis*, pertaining to birth] Eucharius Rosslin of Germany devoted a chapter to diseases in pregnancy in his *Rose Garden for Pregnant Women and Midwives*, published in 1513. This was translated into English as *Byrth of Mankind* in 1540. François Mauriceau (1637–1709), the French obstetrician, included several chapters on diseases of pregnancy in *Des Maladies des Femmes Grosses et Accouches* published in 1668. The Hôtel Dieu of Paris, founded in AD 650, was one of the first hospitals to adopt a policy of admitting women who presented themselves after they had reached the 9th month of pregnancy. The Hôpital de la Salpêtrière admitted pregnant women before the last month of pregnancy. A monograph on antenatal care in England, *Hints to Mothers for the Management of Health During the Period of Pregnancy and in the Lying Room, with Common Errors in Connection with these Subjects* was written by Thomas Bull in 1837. This was so popular that it under went 25 editions by 1877. Adolphie Pinnard (1844–1934), professor of obstetrics at Paris, wrote on malpr esentation in 1878. A shelter for abandoned pregnant wome was esta lished in Paris at the initiative of Madame Becquet in 1892. A similar establishment connected to the Royal Maternity Hospital, Dublin opened in 1899. James Haig Ferguson (1862–1934), an obstetrician at this hospital, started the first antenatal clinic in 1915. The father of antenatal care in Britain, John William Ballentyne (1861–1923), published *A Plea for a Pro-Maternity Hospital* in 1901 and established antinatal care and antenatal diagnosis. Funds for promoting bed for antenatal care were donated by Freeland Barber, a co-author of the *Manual of Gynaecology* published in 1882. The first bed was named after Hamilton, who founded the Edinburgh Maternity Hospital in 1791. In America antenatal visits were started at the Boston Lying-in Hospital in 1901 and by 1912 it was allocating three antenatal visits per patient. It was one of the first to expand to provide complete antenatal care in America.

Antergan *See antihistamines.*

Anterior Pituitary Hormone *See gonadotropic hormone.*

Anterior Pituitary-like Hormone In 1926 Selmar Aschheim (1878–1965) of the Women's Hospital, Berlin and professor of gynecology at Berlin, Bernhardt Zondek (1891–1966) found a substance in urine of pregnant women similar to gonadotropic hormone from the anterior pituitary. They called it 'Prolan'. American workers named it 'anterior pituitary-like hormone'. The main source was found to be the placenta.

Anterior Spinal Artery Syndrome (Syn. Beck syndrome) Occlusion of the anterior spinal artery resulting in complex neurological signs. Described by Karl Beck of Germany in 1951.

Anterior Spinal Fusion *See scoliosis.*

Anthimius Byzantine physician to Theodoric the Great in the 5th century.

Anthocyanin *See acidity.*

Anthracosis Term coined in 1837 by Thomas Stratton of North Shields, England to denote a form of lung disease. It manifests as abundant expectoration of black sputum, and was shown to be due to inhalation of soot by J. Wiesner of Germany in 1892.

Anthrax (Syn. carbuncle, wool sorter disease, bacteridie du charbon) Considered by the ancients to be a product of bad humors and dangerous. Major epidemics occurred in Rome around AD 80 causing nearly 50 000 deaths. The Greeks named it as it consumed victims like a burning fire. In 1849 French physician, Casimir Joseph Davaine (1812–1882), found rod-shaped organisms in the blood of sheep that had died of anthrax. The same organism was found in the spleen by Aloys Pollender (1800–1879), a German physician, in 1855. Robert Koch (1843–1910) of Germany demonstrated in 1876 that these organisms were capable of producing the disease in experimental animals. In 1881 Louis Pasteur (1822–1895) showed the protective effect of inoculating small doses of anthrax bacilli in animals. This successful experiment opened the way for active immunization. The thermoprecipitin reaction for diagnosis of anthrax was devised by Alberto Ascoli (1877–1957) of Germany in 1911. *See Bacillus anthracis.*

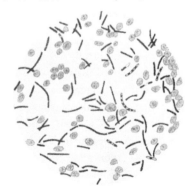

Bacillus anthracis. Illustration from G. Sims Woodhead, *Pathological Mycology* (1885), one of the first English books on systematic microbiology. Young, J. Pentland, Edinburgh

Anthropology [Greek: *anthropos*, man + *logos*, discourse] Study of the human race in relation to its origin, evolution, distribution and culture. Aristotle is supposed to have been the first to use the term. Magnus Hundt's (1449–1519) *Anthropologium de Hominis Diginate* (1501) deals with the anatomy and physiology of the human body. It was defined as 'a treatise on man' by Diderot and D'Alembert in 1772. The term was used in its present sense by Johan Friedrich Blumenbach (1752–1840), professor of medicine at Göttingen. Immanuel Kant (1724–1804), a German philosopher and professor of logic and metaphysics from Königsberg suggested an animal origin for man in *Anthropology* published in 1798. Physical evidence for the antiquity of man was unearthed by Johan Friedrich Esper (1732–1781) at Gailenreuth Cave in 1770. An attempt to trace man's ancestors was made by Heinrich Phillip August Ernest Haeckel (1834–1919) in his *Generelle Morphologiae* published in 1866. British surgeon, Edward Tyson (1649–1708) from Bristol published *The Anatomy of the Pigmy compared with that of a Monkey, an Ape and a Man* in 1698. It became a branch of science in the 18th century due to the work of Thomas Huxley, Charles Darwin (1809–1882), Sir Charles Lyell (1797–1875), Edward Tylor, Arthur Keith (1866–1955), Paul Broca (1824–1880), Rudolph Virchow (1821–1902) and Blumenbach. The first Anthropological Society was formed in Paris by Broca in 1859. The Anthropological Society in England was founded in 1863 with John Hunt. *Antiquity of Man* was published by Lyell in the same year. Pierre Marcellin Boule (1861–1942), professor at the Natural History Museum in Paris who made the first complete construction of Neanderthal skeleton, published *Les Hommes Fossiles* in 1921. *See evolution.*

Anthropometry [Greek: *anthrops*, man + *metron*, measure] The study of proportional measurement of organs and the body in humans and in their predecessors, particularly in relation to the skull and the brain. An early study was done by British surgeon, Charles White (1728–1813) around 1755. Paul Broca (1824–1880) founded the science of anthropometry with his invention of 27 craniometric and cranioscopic instruments. Belgian mathematician and statistician, Lambert Adolphe Jacques Quetelet (1796–1874) wrote *L'Anthropometri, ou measure des differentes facultes de l'homme* in 1871. The metafacial angle of anthropometry (Serres angle) was described in 1824 by Antoine Etienne Renaud Augustin Serres (1786–1868), professor of anatomy and natural history at the Jardin des Plantes, Paris. *See craniology.*

Antibiosis [Greek: *anti*, against or opposite + *bios*, life] Bacterium that produced a substance that killed another bacterium was observed by Louis Pasteur (1822–1895) and J. Joubert (1834–1910) in 1886. Inhibition by *Pseudomonas pyocyanae* of growth of anthrax was found by French bacteriologist, C.G. Bouchard, in the same year. It was named 'antibiosis' by P. Vuillemin in 1889, and was the first step towards the discovery of antibiotics.

Antibiotics [Greek: *anti*, against or opposite + *bios*, life] The term 'antibiosis' was introduced by P. Vuillemin as the opposite of 'symbiose'. It was later used to denote a substance produced by one organism that was capable of destroying another organism or inhibiting its growth. The introduction of the first antibacterial sulfonamide compound, Protonsil, revolutionized the treatment of bacterial disease. A report of a case of a 10-month-old infant dying of staphylococcal septicemia and saved by treatment with a drug, Streptozon, was given by O.H. Foerster of Germany in 1933. Clinical trials in Germany by Gerhard Domagk (1895–1964) and others established the successful treatment of conditions such as empyema, erysipelas and puerperal fever with Protonsil in 1935. Sulfanilamide was measured in blood by Eli Kennerly Marshall (1889–1966), professor of pharmacology at Johns Hopkins University in 1937. The importance of maintaining therapeutic blood levels of antibiotics in treatment was demonstrated by Perrin Hamilton Long (b 1899) and E.A. Bliss in 1939. Although Sir Alexander Fleming (1881–1955) discovered the antibacterial action of *Penicillium* mold while working at St Mary's Hospital in 1929, the difficulty of obtaining the antibiotic in a pure form prevented its therapeutic use. It was isolated in a pure form from *Penicillium notatum* later, in 1940. Streptomycin was isolated in 1944 by an American microbio-logist of Russian origin, Selman Abraham Waksman (1888–1973), and was used in the treatment of tuberculosis in 1948. He use the term 'antibiotic' in 1941 and received the Nobel Prize in Physiology or Medicine for his work in 1952. *See chemotherapy, sulfonamides, penicillin.*

Antibody [Greek: *anti*, against + *bodig*, body] An immunoglobulin that binds to a specific antigen. Their presence in blood of atopic or allergic individuals was demonstrated by a British immunologist of German origin, Otto Carl Willy Prausnitz (1876–1973) and Heinz Kustner in 1921. They were shown to be gamma globulins by Arne Wilhelm Kaurin Tiselius (1902–1971) and Elvin Abraham Kabat in 1939. Prausnitz transferred fish hypersensitivity of his partner Kustner to his own skin by a method of sensitization and the hypersensitive reaction of the skin was named the Prausnitz–Kustner reaction. His finding was subsequently used clinically to diagnose atopic hypersensitivity. Antibodies in the IgA globulin fraction of atopic individuals were discovered by J.F. Heremans and co-workers in Belgium. IgE antibodies were identified in serum by Kimishige Ishizaka and co-workers in Denver in 1970. The presence of a higher concentration of IgE antibodies in the serum of patients with hay fever and asthma was also demonstrated by Ishizaka and this contributed to further research in the pathogenesis of immediate hypersensitivity reactions. *See immunoglobulins, bacteriolysis.*

Anticardiolipin Antibodies [Greek: *anti*, against + *kardia*, heart + *lipos*, fat] Discovered in blood by August Paul Wasserman (1866–1925) who used liver extract as antigen in 1907. A pure form of cardiolipin antigen, or active phospholipid, was obtained from beef heart by Mary Candace Pangborn (b 1907) and was introduced as an agent for serological diagnosis of syphilis in 1942. *See antiphospholipid syndrome.*

Anticoagulants [Greek: *anti*, against or opposite + *coagulare*, to curdle] Swiss physiologist, Jean Louis Prevost (1790–1850), used defibrinated blood in Paris to prevent clotting during experimental blood transfusion on animals in 1821. Leeches were used to prevent the clotting of blood during treatment with an artificial kidney by John Jacob Abel (1857–1938) of Johns Hopkins University in 1910. The leech was used because it produces an anti-clotting factor, hirudin, but this method was abandoned as thousands of leeches had to be processed to produce a significant anticoagulant effect. Oxalates and citrate solutions were shown to be effective anticoagulants by Maurice Nicholas Arthus (1862–1945) and Calixte Pages in 1890 and their work was confirmed by C.A. Peckelharing in 1892. Heparin was discovered in 1918 by William Henry Howell (1860–1945) of Johns Hopkins University and became available after 22 years. The story of warfarin, one of the coumarin group of anticoagulants, began with a cattle disease that occurred around 1920 in the mid-western United States and Canada. This disease killed hundreds of thousands of cattle and all the affected animals bled excessively during their illness. A veterinary pathologist, Frank Schofield of Ontario, observed that these animals had all eaten moldy or spoilt clover. His observation went unheeded until a toxic substance, dicoumarol or coumadin, was isolated from clover by a biochemist, Karl Paul Link of Wisconsin, in 1940. This was later called 'warfarin' and is used to produce anticoagulation.

Anticonvulsants *See antiepileptic drugs.*

Antidepressants [Greek: *anti*, against + *deprimere*, to press down or to lower] Lithium was recommended as treatment for gout by Alfred Baring Garrod (1819–1907) of King's College, London in 1859 and became an over-the-counter treatment around 1867. As periodic depression was suspected to be due to uric acid diathesis, Alexander Haig in London tried lithium for depression in 1892. When the drug Iproniazid was used for the treatment of tuberculosis it was noted to produce an elevation of mood. This observation led to the search for similar compounds to treat depression – called 'psychic energizers' prior to use of the term 'antidepressants'. Iproniazid was noted to have monoamine oxidase inhibiting properties in 1952 and further research led to the discovery of other tricyclic and monoamine drugs as treatment for depression. Imipramine, the first tricyclic compound with antidepressant properties, was developed by Ronald Kuhn in 1956. However, its parent substance iminobenzyl was synthesized by Thiele and Holzinger in 1898. *See melancholy, lithium.*

Antidiptheria Serum Produced from the blood of infected horses by Emil Adolf von Behring (1854–1917) in 1891. The toxin–antitoxin substance produced by Behring was employed for active immunization against diphtheria by William Hallock Park (1863–1939) and colleagues in 1914.

Antidiuretic Hormone (vasopressin) A pituitary extract was shown in 1901 to produce diuresis by a German professor of pharmacology at Utrecht, Rudolf Magnus (1873–1927) and the British physiologist, Ernest Starling (1866–1927). The presence of colloid droplets in the posterior pituitary was described by Percy Theodore Herring (1872–1967) in 1908. The physiological effects of the extract was demonstrated by John Jacob Abel (1857–1938) of Johns Hopkins University. He mistakenly attributed the mixed action of the extract on the urine, uterus and blood pressure to a single hormone. British pharmacologist, Ernest Basil Verney (1894–1967) noted the association between polyuria of diabetes insipidus and the action of the posterior pituitary extract in 1929. The two closely related hormones, vasopressin or antidiuretic hormone and oxytocin, were identified and synthesized by an American biochemist and professor at Cornell University, Vincent du Vigneaud (1901–1978) in 1950. He was awarded the Nobel Prize in 1955. Inappropriate secretion of antidiuretic hormone in patients with bronchial carcinoma was described by W.B. Schwartz, W. Bennet, Frederic C. Bartter and co-workers in 1957.

Antidotarium A book of mainly herbal treatments written by Nicholas Praepositus of Salerno in the 12th century. It was translated into many languages and remained an apothecary's handbook for centuries.

Antidote [Greek: *anti*, against or opposite + *didonai*, to give] *See toxicology.*

Antidromic Stimulation Neurophysiological method to determine the refractory period of the motor neuron. Devised by New Zealand-born British neurologist, Derek Ernest Denny-Brown (1901–1980), in 1929.

Antiepileptic Drugs [Greek: *anti*, against + *lepsis*, seizing] Aulus Cornelius Celsus (25 BC–AD 50) mentioned that some people were cured of epilepsy after drinking the blood of a stabbed gladiator. Burnt human bones were suggested as a cure by Galen (129–200). The *Materia Medica* of Dioscorides in the middle of the first century mentions liver of ass, stomach of weasel and blood of turtle as antiepileptics and hoof of the elk was used by the Norwegians. Belladonna was used over 300 years ago and was followed by digitalis. Silver salts were used for hysteria and epilepsy in England in the 18th century. Drugs used in the 19th century include bromides of sodium, potassium and ammonium, borax and nitroglycerin. Bromide of potassium was recommended by Sir C. Locock (1799–1875) in 1853 and subsequently it became one of the most commonly used compounds for nearly a century. A major drawback of the drug was depression and drowsiness due to overdose. A synthetic camphor preparation, cardiazol or metrazol, was used as an injection in the early 1930s. Diphenyl hydantoin (epinutin) or hydantoin, were introduced by Hiram Houston Merrit (1902–1979) and Tracy J. Putnam in 1938. Secret remedies were common at the turn of the century. The role of flicker mechanisms in precipitating fits was recognized by G.H. Monrad-Krohn of America in 1936 and this led to a significant reduction in the number of attacks.

Antigens [Greek: *anti*, against + *genos*, birth] Substances capable of generating the production of antibodies. Observed by Edmund Weil (1800–1922) and Arthur Felix (1887–1856) in 1916. They found the 'O' and 'H' factors with specific antigenic properties in *Proteus* bacteria. Tissue-specific antigens were found by Paul Theodor Uhlenuth (b 1870) of Germany in 1903. Histocompatibility antigens were demonstrated on an experimental basis by American geneticist, Clarence Cook Little (1888–1971) in 1916. The importance of histocompatibility in organ transplantation was shown by French immunologist, Jean Dausset (b 1916) of Toulouse in 1958 and his contribution led to the procedure of tissue typing before transplantation.

Antihelmintics [Greek: *anti*, against + *helminth*, worm] Male fern was used against tapeworms and roundworms by Theophrastus (370–285 BC), Pliny (AD 28–79) and Galen (129–200). This was revived as treatment for hookworm by Edoardo Perronicito (1847–1936) in 1880 and thymol was recommended by Camillo Bozzolo (1845–1920) of Turin in 1881. *Chenopodium* was used as an antihelmintic by W. Schuffner and H. Vervoort in Sumatra, in 1913. A critical method of testing the efficacy of antihelmintics on animals was introduced by a veterinarian from the US Bureau of Animal Industry, Maurice Crowther Hall (1881–1938) and E.B. Cram in 1915. Carbon tetrachloride was introduced by Maurice C. Hall in 1921. However, the active ingredient of oil of *Chenopodium*, ascaridole, continued as the most commonly used drug for hookworm and roundworm. Tetrachloroethylene replaced carbon tetrachloride in 1925, owing to its lower toxicity. The curative effect of emetine against schistosomiasis was demonstrated by A.C. Hutcheson in 1913. *See Dryopteris felix mas.*

Antihemophilic Factor A globulin effective in promoting coagulation in hemophiliacs was isolated from normal human plasma by Francis Henry Laskey Taylor (1900–1959) and Jackson Arthur Patek (b 1904) in 1937. Despite this finding, the transfusion of blood or fresh frozen plasma remained the main treatment for hemophiliacs until 1954. Robert Gwyn Macfarlane (1907–1987) at Oxford obtained factor VIII from bovine blood in 1953. It was isolated in a purer form from human plasma and became the main treatment for hemophilia.

Antihistamine [Greek: *anti*, against + *histos*, tissue + *ammoniokon*, resinous gum] Research on drugs to combat rhinitis, urticaria, hay fever and pruritis began in France in 1937. Daniele Bovet (1907–1992) of the Pasteur Institute discovered the antihistamine properties of aminoethanol derivatives in 1936, but these were too toxic for therapeutic use. An effective antihistamine was introduced in 1939, followed by Antergan in 1942 which paved the way for the treatment of human allergic conditions. Research on similar compounds continued in America and diphenhydramine was prepared by Loewi in 1945.

Anti-Infective Vitamin *See vitamin A.*

Anti-Inflammatory Drugs *Salix alba*, the white willow, the source of salicylic acid was a folk remedy for fever and rheumatism for centuries. Its anti-inflammatory properties were demonstrated by Franz Striker of Germany in 1875. Acetanilide followed in 1875 and phenacetin was introduced in 1886. Use of salicylates in acute rheumatism was shown by Peter W. Latham, who wrote *On the Administration of Salicylates in Acute Rheumatism* in 1895. Phenylbutazone was introduced for rheumatoid arthritis by J.P. Currie, R.A. Brown and G. Will in 1953. The mechanism of anti-inflammatory action of aspirin and similar drugs through inhibition of prostaglandin formation was demonstrated by J.R. Vane and co-workers in 1970.

Anti-Lymphocyte Globulin An early substance similar to anti-lymphocyte globulin was observed by Elie Metchnikoff (1845–1916) in 1899. B.H. Waksman in 1961 showed that delayed hypersensitivity could be reduced using anti-lymphocyte globulin. It was used experimentally to prolong the survival of transplanted skin allografts by M.F.A. Woodruff and A. Anderson in 1963.

Antimalarials [Greek: *anti*, against + *mal*, bad + *aer*, air] *Cinchona* bark was used in treatment of malarial fever or ague prior to the isolation of quinine from it by Joseph Pelletier (1788–1842) in 1820. Mepacrine or atebrine was introduced in 1933 which drastically reduced the mortality of troops from malaria during World War ll. Development of resistance to mepacrine by *Plasmodium falciparum* was noted by N.H. Fairley in 1947. Chloroquine was tested by Robert Frederick Loeb in 1946. Paludrine or proguanil was synthesized in England in 1944 and tested against avian malaria by F.S.H. Curd and co-workers in 1945. Alfred Adams introduced paludrine as treatment of human malaria later in the same year. The effectiveness of paludrine on a large scale was demonstrated by N.H. Fairley from the Medical Research Unit of the Australian army in 1946. Primaquine, an 8–aminoquinoline derivative, was introduced as treatment by Harold John Edgcomb and co-workers in 1950. R.S. Hockwald, J. Arnold, J. Clayman and A.S. Alving noted that 5–10% of previously healthy African– American troops developed hemolytic anemia after treatment with primaquin in 1952. Subsequent studies by P.E. Carson, C.L. Flanagan, C.E. Ickes and A.S. Alving in 1956 showed that the hemolysis was due to genetically linked deficiency of glucose-6–phosphate dehydrogenase in the red blood cells. *See cinchona, Baike William Balfour, chloroquin, Peruvian bark.*

Antimony In Rome, wine allowed to stand in goblets made of antimony produced *Calices vomittori* or *Pocula emetica* as it absorbed the antimony and was then used to induce vomiting. The practice of making goblets out of antimony was revived during the Middle Ages. Basilius Valentinius, a Benedictine monk and alchemist, rediscovered antimony in the 15th century. It was known as *stibium* during the time of Paracelsus (1493–1541). In 1566 doctors in Paris opposed

the use of antimony and their lobbying produced a ban. When King Louis XIV had typhoid fever, antimony was used as treatment and, following his recovery, was restored to the pharmacopoeia. It was promoted as a medicine by Johan Tholde, an alchemist who wrote *The Triumphal Chariot of Antimony* in 1606. Tartar emetic or potassium antimony tartarate was introduced by Adrian van Mynsicht in 1631. Intravenous administration was given by A. Broden and J. Rodhain in 1906 and its effectiveness in treating trypanosomiasis in experimental animals (maladie du sommeil) was shown by Harry George Plimmer (1856– 1918) and John D. Thompson in 1908. J.E.R. McDonagh used it in treatment of vesical bilharziasis in 1915.

Antimony Poisoning The dangers of keeping vinegar and other acidic foods in antimony dishes were observed by Lehmann in 1902. Outbreaks of antimony poisoning due to lemonade made from lemon stored in enamelware occurred in Newcastle-upon-Tyne in 1928, Folkestone in 1929 and later in London. The outbreak in London occurred at a hospital Christmas party in 1932 and affected 65 persons who developed vomiting and collapsed. The Ministry of Health issued a warning in 1934 about the danger of drinking lemonade or similar products stored in enameled vessels.

Antineurasthin Sold as a nerve and brain food for neurasthenia in the early 20th century. Its analysis later showed that it was mainly composed of protein, lactose and potato starch.

Antiphlogistica [Greek: *anti*, against + *phlogist*, burn] Drugs used for inflammation, otherwise known as anti-inflammatory drugs. *See anti-inflammatory drugs.*

Antiphospholipid Syndrome (Syn. Hughes syndrome) Thrombosis, abortion and cerebral disease in the presence of lupus anticoagulant in the blood. Described by G.R.V. Hughes in the *British Medical Journal* in 1983. The presence of antiphospholipid antibodies that predispose patients to thrombotic events was pointed out by H. P. McNeil and co-workers in 1985.

Antipyretics [Greek: *anti*, against + *pyrexia*, fever] Ice, cold baths, diaphoretics, alcohol, quinine, aconite, purgatives and venesection formed the main treatment for fever until salicylic acid was introduced by Herman Kolbe (1818–1884) in 1874. The other antipyretics were: antipyrin (1884), phenazone (1884), acetanilide or antefebrin (1886), phenacetin (1887) and aspirin (1899).

Antipyrin [Greek: *anti*, against + *pyrexia*, fever] Derivative of phenyl hydrazine, synthesized by Ludwig Knorr at the

University of Würzburg in 1883. It was the first complete synthetic drug to be produced and was introduced into clinical practice as an antipyretic by Wilhelme Filehene in 1884. *See antipyretics.*

Antirabies Vaccine One of Louis Pasteur's (1822–1895) greatest achievements was the development of a rabies vaccine from the stored infected brains of animals. He used this for human inoculation on a young boy named Joseph Meister, who was bitten by a rabid dog, on 6 July, 1885. Further study and development of the vaccine was continued at the Pasteur Institute in Paris, founded with a public donation of 2.5 million francs in 1888. Rabies vaccine was also tried in shock treatment therapy for neurosyphilis by several workers including L. Tommasi and L. Cruveilhier (1933).

Antisepsis or asepsis [Greek: *anti*, against + *septikos*, that which causes putrefaction] The word 'antiseptic' was used by Sir John Pringle (1707–1782) in his essay *Experiments upon Septic and Antiseptic Substances* published in 1750. The concept was initiated on a scientific basis by Ignaz Semmelweiss (1818–1865) of Vienna. He demonstrated in 1847 that mortality due to puerperal fever could be reduced from 18% to less than 2% if students and doctors washed their hands before attending patients in the ward. However, his findings were ignored and he was ridiculed and persecuted. Louis Pasteur (1822–1895) in 1857 proved that microorganisms were the cause of fermentation, thus undermining the theory of spontaneous generation. Around the same time, in 1860, Joseph Lister (1827–1912) advocated use of carbolic acid for the prevention of infection during surgery, with remarkable effect. Destruction of microorganisms by heat was shown by Pasteur in 1868. Thomas Porter Blunt, while working with Sir Arthur Henry Downs (1851–1938), demonstrated the retarding effect of sunlight on putrefaction in 1877. Use of rubber gloves in surgery was introduced in the early 1900s by American surgeon, William Halstead (1852–1922).

Antiseptics Sir John Pringle, (1707–1782) investigated the effect of various substances on putrefaction in 1750. His work was not followed up for more than a century until H. Buchholtz used an infusion of tobacco leaves to investigate antiseptic effects in 1875. Sir Arthur Henry Downs (1851–1938) and Thomas Porter Blunt demonstrated the retarding effect of sunlight on putrefaction in 1877 and the resistance of bacterial spores to sunlight was demonstrated by E. Duclaux in the same year. Robert Koch (1843–1910) and Wolffhugel studied the effect of heat on bacteria in 1881 and later in the same year Koch introduced the method for comparing the germicidal effects of various substances. A quantitative study of disinfectants was introduced by Bernhard Theodor Ludwig Claus Kronig (1863–1918) and Theodore Paul (1862–1928), who also showed the disinfectant effects of acids and alkalis on bacteria in 1897. The antiseptic effect of alcohol was demonstrated by Epstein in the same year. Simon Flexner (1863–1946) showed that a 0.85% solution of sodium chloride caused the disintegration of meningococcal bacteria in 1907. Gentian violet was used by John Woolman Churchman (1877–1937) in 1912. The effect of ultraviolet light was studied by Laroquette and he also discovered, in 1918, that blue wavelengths were more effective as disinfectants.

Antistreptolysin Titer Hypersensitivity to streptococcal proteins in patients with rheumatic fever was demonstrated with skin tests by Birkhaug who published his findings in *Journal of Infectious Diseases* in 1929. Bernard Schlesinger (1896–1984) and Frederick John Poynton (1869–1943) in their contribution to *Recent Advances on Rheumatism* in 1931, pointed out that post-streptococcal arthritis following tonsillitis was due to allergy to bacterial products rather than to toxins from the bacteria. Their contribution led directly to the use of the antistreptolysin titer as a diagnostic marker in post-streptococcal rheumatic fever and nephritis.

Antithyroid Drugs The goitrogenic effects of cabbage were noted by Alan M. Chesney (b 1888) of Johns Hopkins Hospital while he was experimenting with syphilis in rabbits in 1928. Julia and Cosmo Mackenzie from the same hospital identified the antithyroid properties of thiourea while they were experimenting with other products to induce intestinal suppression of bacterial flora in 1930. Phenyl thiourea was discovered about the same time by Curt Richter. However, the effectiveness of thiourea on humans was established much later, in 1940, by Edwin B. Astwood (b 1909) of Boston who also introduced thiourea and thiouracil as treatments for hyperthyroidism in 1943. Radioactive iodine as a treatment for thyrotoxicosis was introduced by G.W. Blomfield and co-workers in 1951.

Antitoxins [Greek: *anti*, against + *toxicon*, poison] Antibody against a toxin. Two antitoxins successfully tried in animals were for diphtheria and tetanus. Their effectiveness in animals was demonstrated by Emil von Behring (1854–1917), an army surgeon from Western Prussia and Shibajaburo Kitazato ((1852–1931) of Tokyo in 1890. Successful clinical use of diphtheria antitoxin in a child suffering from diphtheria in Berlin was demonstrated by von Behring in 1891. The child recovered within a few days and he received the first Nobel Prize for Physiology or Medicine in 1901.

Antivenom Serum or antivenene [Greek: *anti*, against; Latin: *venenum*, poison] First prepared by Sir Richard Thomas Fraser (1841–1919) against cobra venom in 1895. *See ophidism.*

Antiviral Drugs *See Acyclovir.*

Antivivisectionists [Greek: *anti*, against; Latin: *vivus*, living + *secare*, to cut] The Society for the Prevention of Cruelty to Animals was founded in 1824, but use of living animals in experimentation was questioned in England by the *Medical Times and Gazette* only in 1858. Societies for preventing cruelty to animals were formed in Dresden and Paris in 1859. The antivivisectionist movement gained momentum and lobbying led to the appointment of a Royal Commission which recommended restriction of animal experiments. The National Antivivisectionist Society, the Antivivisectionist Association and the Church Antivivisection League were founded in 1875, 1876 and 1899, respectively.

Anton Syndrome Denial of visual disturbance or blindness. Described by an Austrian neurologist, G. Anton (1858–1933) in 1899. He graduated from the University of Prague in 1882 and succeeded Wernicke at Halle in 1905.

Antrum of Highmore [Latin: *antrum*, cave or hollow] Maxillary antrum. Illustrated by Leonardo Da Vinci (1452–1519) around 1500. Nathaniel Highmore (1613–1685) gave a description in 1651. Two cases of empyema of the antrum were described by M. Saint Hillaire in 1898.

Antyllus (AD 250) Greek surgeon who distinguished between a traumatic aneurysm and an aneurysm due to dilatation. He devised a method of tying the aneurysm at both ends, known as the Antyllus operation, which was in use until the end of the 19th century.

Anus [Latin: ring] First used in anatomy by Aulus Cornelius Celsus (25 BC–AD 50). The term was used during earlier Roman times to denote an old woman with wrinkled skin.

Aonian Christian physician commissioned by Al-Mansour, Caliph of Baghdad, in the 8th century to translate some of the Greek classics, including the aphorisms of Hippocrates (460–377 BC) and the works of Galen (129–200).

Aorta [Greek: *aeiro*, to lift, or *aorte*, the great artery] Term used by Hippocrates (460–377 BC) to refer to a branch of the windpipe. Aristotle used it around 350 BC to denote 'the large artery from which the heart was hung'. The expression 'arch of the aorta' was introduced by German surgeon, Lorenz Heister in 1732.

Aortic Aneurysm [Greek: *aneurysma*, dilatation; French: *eurys*, wide] An antemortem diagnosis was made by Andreas

Vesalius (1514–1564) in 1555 and was confirmed 2 years later at autopsy of the same patient. Another antemortem diagnosis was made by Raymond de Vieussens (1641–1715) around 1700. Phrenic nerve palsy as a sign of thoracic aortic aneurysm was described by Scottish surgeon and cardiologist, Allan Burns (1731–1813), in *Observations of Some of the Most Important and Frequent Diseases of the Heart* published in 1809. Tracheal tugging, as a physical sign of thoracic aneurysm (Porter sign), was described by William Henry Porter (1790–1861) in 1826. A case in the thorax which communicated with the pulmonary artery was described by physician, Sir Willoughby Francis Wade (1827–1906) of Bray, Wicklow in 1861. Visible pulsation of the arteries in the nostrils (Bozzolo sign) was described by Camilo Bozzolo (1845–1920) in 1880. A modern operative technique, Babcock operation, was designed by William Wayne Babcock (1872–1963), surgeon to the Samaritan and American Stomach Hospitals, Philadelphia, in 1926. An operative method for abdominal aneurysm was devised by Babcock in 1929. A description of the dissecting aneurysm of the aorta was given by Frank Nicholls (1699–1778), a physician to George II. He also described its pathogenesis. Resection of a saccular aneurysm of the thoracic aorta was performed by John Alexander and Francis Byron in 1944. Michael Ellis DeBakey (b 1908) and Arthur Denton Cooley (b 1920) resected a thoracic aneurysm and replaced it with a graft in 1953.

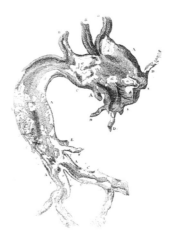

Aortic Aneurysm. Wepfer, J-J, *Observationes Medico-Practae de Affectibus Capitis.* Courtesy of the National Library of Medicine

Aortic Coarctation Described as an 'amazing narrowness of the aorta near the heart' by Giovanni Battista Morgagni (1682–1771) in 1761. M. Paris gave a classic description in 1791 and it is called 'maladie de Paris'. Erosion of the ribs in coarctation was observed by J.F. Meckel in 1827 and was radiologically detected by Hugo Roesler (b 1899) of

Germany in 1928. Infant and adult types were classified by L.M. Bonnet in 1903. Successful surgical resection and anastomosis of cut ends was performed by Clarence Crafoord (1899–1984) and Karl Gustav Wilhelm Nylin (1892–1961) of Sweden in 1944. Robert Edward Gross (1905–1988) operated on the second patient in the USA in 1945 and demonstrated the success of the procedure by operating on 60 patients in 1949. *See cardiac surgery.*

Aortic Depressor Nerve Thomas Willis (1621–1675) described a branch of the vagus supplying the aorta as a wandering nerve in 1664. Thiele (1824) and E. Cyon (1865) showed that the stimulation of this nerve caused a drop in blood pressure. Julius Bernstein (1864) and Carl Ludwig (1866) demonstrated slowing of the cardiac rate by stimulating it. N. Wooldridge identified it in the dog in 1883 and named it the aortic nerve. In humans this nerve was found to be represented by a branch of the superior laryngeal nerve.

Aortic Dissection *See dissecting aneurysm.*

Aortic Incompetence *See aortic insufficiency.*

Aortic Insufficiency The condition was noted by English physician William Cowper (1666–1709) of Hampshire in 1705. Thomas Hodgkin (1798–1866) gave a description in 1828 and a classic account with an illustrated plate was given by Sir Dominic John Corrigan (1802–1880) in 1832. Corrigan pulse or waterhammer pulse, characterized by a sudden impact and rapid fall in aortic insufficiency, was also described by him. The two separate murmurs heard over the femoral and solidus or brachial artery during the diastolic and systolic phases of the heart, were described by French physician, Louis Paul Duroziez (1826–1897) in 1861. The mechanism of production of these murmurs was explained by Herman Ludwig Blumgart (1895–1977) in 1933.

Aortic Stenosis Noted by Lazare Riviere (1589–1655) in 1674 and a postmortem description of calcific aortic stenosis was given by Theophile Bonet in 1679. An illustrated plate was drawn by an English physician, William Cowper (1666–1709), in 1705. The Austin Flint murmur, an apical mid-diastolic or presystolic functional murmur originating from the mitral valve, was described by Austin Flint (1812–1886) of New York in 1862. Johann Georg Monkeberg (1877–1925) of Bonn described two causes: one with inflammation and the other due to sclerosis, in 1904. Successful correction by surgery was done by Theodore Tuffier (1857–1929) in 1912. Charles Bailey became interested in the surgical treatment following the

death of a colleague, Horace Smithy, who had a critical aortic stenosis. Smithy had earlier worked on devising a successful surgical method but died before he could make further progress. Continuing the work started by Smithy, Bailey demonstrated a successful commissurotomy in 1950.

Aortic Valve An accurate illustration of the aortic valve and its root was given by Leonardo Da Vinci (1452–1519). Charles Anthony Hufnagel (1916–1989) was the first surgeon to explore the possibility of developing an artificial aortic valve. He commenced his research in 1940 and after 10 years he produced the first practical aortic valve prosthesis. An implant of this valve in a female patient was done at the Georgetown University Medical Center in 1952. Although the patient lived for several years, her case was further complicated by a coexisting coarctation of the aorta, and she succumbed to progressive cardiac failure. *See aortic stenosis, aortic insufficiency.*

Aortitis Syphilitic aortitis described by Arnold Ludwig Gotthilf Heller (1840–1913), professor of pathological anatomy at Kiel in 1900. *Treponema pallidum* was discovered in the syphilitic aorta by Karl Otto Reuter (b 1873) in 1906.

Aortocoronary Bypass *See coronary artery bypass graft.*

Aortopulmonary Defect or arterial septal defect A congenital malformation noted by John Elliotson (1791–1868) of University College, London in 1830. A series of cases was published by H. Perelman and co-workers in 1949.

Apepsia Hysterica *See anorexia nervosa.*

Aperient [Latin: *aperiens*, opening] Mild medicines which produce a gentle action on the bowel. Castor oil is mentioned as a purgative in the Ebers papyrus from 1550 BC. Leaves from the shrub *Senna* were used by Arabs in AD 750. Paul of Aegina (625–690) mentioned rhubarb, soft eggs, mallows and soup of shellfish as mild aperients. For a stronger laxative effect he recommended the leaves of the elder tree, *Sambucus*, the root of oak-fern, *Polypodium*, milk-whey with salt and dodder of thyme taken in wine after supper.

Aperitif Asafoetida gum was used by the Saracens to stimulate appetite and, owing to its aroma, it is still used in many food products and sauces. The French used mainly red wines as aperitifs with the addition of bitter ingredients. Wormwood has been known as an appetite stimulant for centuries and is still in use as a bitter ingredient in vermouth, which is sometimes taken to stimulate appetite.

Apert, Eugene (1868–1940) Parisian endocrinologist and pediatrician. In 1910 he classified manifestations of hypernephrosis or adrenal cortical hyperfunction on the basis of age of onset, from the embryo to old age. He also described the condition associated with syndactyly, mental retardation and visual loss (Apert syndrome) in 1906.

Apex Beat [Latin: *apex*, summit] Contraction of the heart in systole forcing the blood out of the ventricles. Described in the second chapter of William Harvey's (1578–1657) great work on the circulation of the blood, *Exercitatio anatomica de motu cordis, et sanguinis in animalibus* published in 1628. In the third chapter he stated 'At the moment when the heart contracts and when the breast is struck, when in short the organ is in a state of systole, the arteries are dilated, yield a pulse and are in a state of diastole'. Cardiac palpation as an aid to diagnosis was introduced by Hippolito Francisco Albertini (1662–1746) of Italy in 1728.

Apgar Score Proposed in an attempt to evaluate the state of newborn infants under different conditions of delivery and anesthesia by a graduate of Columbia University, Virginia Apgar (1909–1974) in *A Proposal for a New Method of Evaluation of New Born Infants* published in 1953.

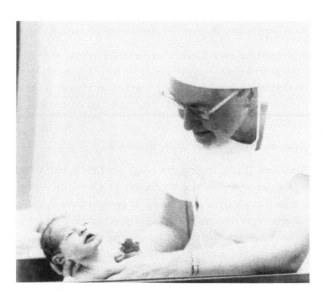

Virginia Apgar (1909–1974)

Aphakia [Greek: *a*, negative or without + *phakos*, lentil or lens] Absence of the lens in the eye.

Aphasia [Greek: *a*, negative + *phasia*, speech] Described by Carl Linnaeus (1707–1778) in 1745. The site of the lesion in the brain was suggested by Jean Baptiste Bouillaud (1796–1881) in 1825. It was called 'alalia' by J. Lordat in 1841. Paul Broca (1824–1880) re-named it, 'aphemia'. The current name was given by a Greek scholar, Chrysaphis. In 1869 a British neurologist, Henry Charlton Bastian (1837–1915),

described sensory aphasia, to which the word 'deafness' was assigned by Adolf Kussmaul (1822–1902). The site of the lesion in sensory aphasia was identified by Karl Wernicke (1848–1905) in 1874. *See speech disorders.*

Aphemia Defective articulation of speech or motor aphasia. *See aphasia.*

Aphorisms of Hippocrates (460–377 BC) [Greek: *aporismos*, definition] Contains 406 famous sayings, thought to be later works by his disciples. A translation into English was done in 1610, followed by others by: Sprengel (1707), Coar (1822) and Underwood (1828).

Aphrodisiac Love potion. Named after the Greek goddess of love, Aphrodite. Since ancient times thousands of substances have been suggested including: vaginal discharge from mares in heat, tongue of certain birds, roe mixed with wine and pigeon blood, and tiger testicles in arrak. Pliny the Elder (AD 23–79) recommended the feet of the hippopotamus and Dioscorides suggested aniseed. Rhinoceros horn is used in several parts of the world.

Aphthous Ulcers or apthae [Greek: *apto*, inflame] Hippocrates (460–377 BC) described apthae amongst the other diseases of dentition. Aretaeus the Cappadician (81–138) noted the abundance of these mouth ulcers amongst the Egyptians and attributed it to impurities in the water. Various recommendations such as honeyed water, juice of the pomegranate, vegetable acids and borate of soda were made by Paul of Aegina (625–690), Avicenna (980–1037) and Galen (129–200).

Apicolysis *See collapse therapy.*

Apnea [Greek: *a*, without + *pneuma*, breath or air] The earliest study on its physiology in humans was by Italian physiologist, Angelo Mosso (1846–1910), in 1903. *See cardiac resuscitation.*

Apollina Patron saint regarded as the guardian of teeth and patron of toothache, after she attained martyrdom in AD 250 at the hands of an anti-Christian mob in Alexandria, who broke all her teeth.

Apollo On the island of Delos he killed the great snake which symbolized disease and thereby became the Greek god of health. He also had the power to unleash pestilence and to confer health.

Apollonius of Citium Physician who lived around 100 BC. He wrote a commentary on the Hippocratic treatise on articulations, with a number of illustrations.

Apomorphine [Greek: *apo*, from + *morphia*, form] Organic base obtained by Matthieson and Wright by adding hydrochloric acid to morphine in 1869. It was used as an antiemetic in the same year by London physician, S. Gee.

Aponeurosis [Greek: *apo*, from + *neuron*, tendon] Term in anatomy refers to the insertion of a muscle that was not made of fleshy fibers.

Apophysis Term used by Galen (129–200) to refer to the blunt end of a bone.

Apoplectiform Cerebral Congestion Condition described by Armand Trousseau (1801–1867) of Paris around 1850, probably the syndrome now known as transient ischemic attack. He described transient acute neurological deficits such as loss of speech, loss of sight and staggering that lasts for a few seconds and related these to areas of internal carotid artery distribution in the brain. Despite the name, he believed that there was no congestion of the brain. In 1860 Lamare-Picquot thought that the presence of excess red globules in the blood predisposed the patient to it and prescribed arsenic. This was probably the first suggestion of increased risk of stroke in patients with an excess of red blood cells or polycythemia. A case of internal carotid artery reconstructive surgery in a patient with intermittent hemiplegia or transient ischemic attacks was reported by Regius professor of medicine, George White Pickering (1904–1980), H.H.G. Eastcott and C.G. Rob in *The Lancet* in 1954.

Apoplexy [Greek: *apo*, from + *plexein*, to strike] In ancient usage 'apoplexy' denotes a condition in which the individual suddenly falls, like an ox felled by the butcher. Paul of Aegina (625–690) stated that 'When the common origin of the nerves is affected and from it all other parts of the body have lost their motion and sensibility, the affection is called apoplexy'. He recommended use of clysters, bleeding and rubbing of oil as treatments. It is known to have had a poor prognosis, and this was reflected in the aphorism of Hippocrates (460–377 BC) that 'It is impossible to remove a strong attack of apoplexy and not easy to remove a weak attack'. Aretaeus of Cappadocia (81–138) and Caelius Aurelianus, a physician in the 5th century, observed that cold winter weather predisposed a person. A scientific study with associated changes in the brain was published by Johann Jacobus Wepfer (1620–1695) in 1648. The term was confused with epilepsy during these times. The occurrence of Cheyne–Stokes respiration in apoplexy was mentioned by John Cheyne (1771–1836) in 1818 and later by William Stokes (1801–1878) in 1854.

Apostasis [Greek: *apo*, away + *stasis*, standing] The end of an attack of a disease. A theory of pathogenesis proposed by Hippocrates (460–377 BC) states that if morbid residue fails to be evacuated by mouth, rectum, urethra or skin pore it will result in an eruption, tumor or gangrene.

Apothecaries Act Act of Parliament to regulate the practice of apothecaries in England and Wales. Passed in 1815 during the reign of King George III.

Apothecary The official name for the person in the royal palace or great household in England who administered drugs, spices, perfumes and sweetmeats. Previously known as spicers or pepperers. The office of Court Apothecary existed from the time of King John and one of the earliest mentions of the apothecary in England is found in Oxford records from 1277. Several references have been made to 'apothecaria' or 'ipotecaria' in deeds found at Oxford around 1320. Another early record shows them as court officials during the reign of King Edward II in 1313. Falcand de Luca was the first apothecary to sell medicine in England in 1357. In the 14th century they belonged to the Spicer's Guild or Guild of Grocers. They later joined the 'craft and mistery of the Company of Grocers' and remained members until the charter for the Society of Apothecaries was granted by James I of England in 1617.

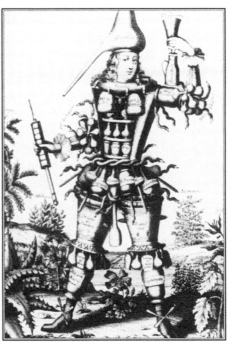

Fifteenth century depiction of the apothecary. P. Bousell and H. Bonnemain, *Histoire de la Pharmacie* (1977). Bibliothèque Nationale, Paris

Apothesis An ancient term for placing the fractured limb in a resting position.

Appendicitis [Latin: *appendix*, an addition or supplement; Greek: *itis*, inflammation] A description of the appendix vermiformis was given by Italian surgeon, Jacopo Berengario da Carpi (1470–1530) in 1521. An abscess of the vermiform process was described by German surgeon, Lorenz Heister (1683–1758) in 1711 and a case of inflamed appendix was recorded by Mestivier in 1759. His patient was a 45-year-old man who underwent drainage for appendicular abscess but failed to survive the operation. A rusty pin-like organ – the appendix – was found later during his postmortem examination. Successful drainage of an abscess was performed by Henry Hancock (1809–1880) of Charing Cross Hospital in 1848. John William Keys Parkinson (1785–1838), a London physician, described perforated appendix and recognized it as a cause of death in 1812. An operation in America was done by Willard Parker (1800–1884) in 1867 and the term was coined by Reginald Heber Fitz (1843–1913), a surgeon from Boston in 1886. Henry Barton Sands (1830–1888) of New York successfully removed an appendix before rupture in 1888. His assistant, Charles McBurney (1845–1913), described the site of maximal tenderness, the McBurney point. Sir Frederick Treves (1853–1923) was amongst the first to advocate the current practice of removal of the appendix during early stages of infection to prevent complications. He saved the life of King Edward VII by persuading him to postpone his coronation for 2 days and successfully removing his inflamed appendix in 1902.

Appendix Vermiformis [Latin: *appendix*, supplement + *vermis*, worm] Called the 'worm of the bowel' by ancient physicians in Egypt, and known as 'caecum intestinum' around 1600. A description was given by Jacopo Berengario da Carpi (1470–1530), an Italian surgeon, in 1521. *See appendicitis.*

Appert, Nicolas François (1749–1841) French confectioner who discovered a method of preserving meat and vegetables by excluding air from the containers. Joseph Gay-Lussac (1778–1850) examined Appert bottles and found that they were devoid of oxygen and concluded that oxygen caused putrefaction. Appert used the autoclave for sterilization in 1810 and he opened a canning factory in 1812. In 1795 he won a prize offered by Napoleon for finding a practical way of preserving food.

Appetite Regarded as an index of physical health and the loss of appetite as a symptom of physical disease since the time of Hippocrates (460–377 BC). The sensations of appetite and hunger were described by William Beaumont (1785–1853) in *Physiology of Digestion* (1845) and by Anton

Julius Carlson (1875) in *Control of Hunger in Health and Disease,* published in 1916. An early description of loss of appetite or anorexia in malignancy was given by William Brinton (1823–1867) of St Thomas' Hospital, London in *Diseases of the Stomach* published in 1859. *See hunger.*

Apprenticeship Part of every doctor's training until about 1870. During the 18th and 19th centuries each surgeon had one to four apprentices who paid large fees ranging from £250 to £1000 to their master. They were bound to him for 7 years at the Surgeon's Hall. One of the duties of the Barber–Surgeons Company was to supervise both master and apprentice during the apprenticeship. At the end the young surgeons took an examination and were granted three different levels of license depending on the examiners' perception of their capability and performance.

APUD Cells or concept An acronym for Amine Precursor Uptake and Decarboxylation. The concept of cells responsible for production of polypeptide hormones was proposed by A.G.E. Pearse in 1966 and extended to include endocrine, neural and neuroendocrine cells in 1975.

Aqua Regia Mixture of nitric and hydrochloric acids developed by Arab alchemist, Geber, during his search for potable gold or elixir of eternal youth.

Aqua Vitae [Latin: *aqua*, water + *vitae*, life] Term used for alcohol by Arab alchemist Geber who lived around the 8th century at Seville.

Aquae Sulis *See bath.*

Aqueduct of Fallopius [Latin: *aqua*, water + *ducere*, to lead] The canal for the facial nerve in the temporal bone was named after Italian anatomist Gabriele Falloppio (1523–1562).

Aqueduct of Sylvius [Latin: *aqua*, water + *ducere*, to lead] A channel that passes through the midbrain. Described by Franciscus Sylvius (1614–1672), also known as Sylvius de la Boë, of Leiden in 1660.

Aquilian Law of Rome Enacted to control surgery and healing in 300 BC.

Aquinas, Thomas (1225–1274) Pupil of Albertus Magnus (1192–1280). He separated the body from the soul and attributed sensory functions entirely to sensory organs and not the brain. He also sought to embrace all sciences into Christianity.

Aquino de Chateau, Lyon or Peter Louis (d 1797) French physician who published *Lettres sur le Hommes Celebres dans les Sciences.*

Arab Medicine A modification of Greek medicine translated and adapted to suit the religion, climate and race. The rulers of Baghdad from AD 750–1258 helped to preserve the Greek and Roman works on medicine and other sciences. Hippocrates (460–377 BC) was known as *Ibucrat* or *Bukrat* to the Arabs and his treatises were translated between AD 750–850. The works of Aristotle (384–322 BC) was translated by Sergius of Ras-al-'Ayn (AD 530) and Hunayn ibn Ishaq (AD 850). Some of the great Arab medical men during this period include, Rhazes (850–932) who described measles and smallpox in AD 900, Haly Abbas (930–994) who wrote the great medical book *Al-maleki*, Avicenna (980–1037) who wrote the *Canon* and Albucasis (d 1013) who wrote an illustrated surgical treatise around AD 1000. Arabic works in translation exercised a great influence on European medicine and astrology from the Middle Ages to the beginning of the 16th century. *See Abbasides, Cordova, Nestorian medicine.*

Arachnodactyly Term suggested by Charles Émile Achard (1860–1944) of Paris in 1902 to denote the spider-like appearance of fingers in patients with Marfan syndrome. The long, slender limb features of Marfan syndrome were described as 'dolicho-stenomelia' by French pediatrician, Bernard Antonin Jean Marfan (1858–1942) in 1896.

Arachnoid Layer [Greek: *arachne*, spider] The term 'arachnoeides' was first used by Hippocrates (460–377 BC) to refer to sediments in urine. Galen (129–200) used it to mean any plexus of veins or arteries. The present term for the cobweb-like membrane lying between the pia mater and dura mater was introduced by the Anatomical Society of Amsterdam in 1664.

Arachnoiditis [Greek: *arachne*, spider] Inflammation of the spinal canal. Described in a patient as 'meningitis circumscripta spinalis' by William Gibson Spiller (1863–1940), J.H. Musser and Edward Martin (1859–1938) in 1903. A description of a similar case as 'meningitis serosa spinalis' was given by K. Mendel and Saul Adler in 1908. Victor Horsley (1857–1916) described it as 'chronic spinal meningitis' in 1909. War injuries were thought to be responsible by T. Mauss and H. Krugger in 1918. Chronic arthritis of the spine was incriminated by C. Vincent in 1930. J.D. French in 1946 pointed out a protrusion of an intervertebral disc as a cause. A presently established cause, spinal anesthesia, was identified by W.G. Haynes and F.A. Smith in 1942. Lipiodol and other contrast media were noted as a cause by P. Bucy and I.J. Spigel in 1943.

Arantius (1530–1589) *See Aranzi, Giulio Cesare.*

Aranzi, Giulio Cesare or Arantius (1520–1589) Physician and anatomist who was professor of medicine and surgery at the University of Bologna. He named the hippocampus of the brain and described the choroid plexus, foramen ovale and ductus arteriosus. He wrote *De Humano Foeto* in 1564.

Aran–Duchenne Disease Progressive spinal muscular atrophy. Described by French neurologist Guillaume Benjamin Duchenne (1806–1875) in 1849. Another French physician, François Amilcar Aran (1817–1861) published his description in 1850. *See amylotrophic lateral sclerosis.*

Arber, Agnes, née Robertson (1879–1960) English botanist, born in London and educated at University College. She developed the technique of using serial sections for studying plant anatomy and studied early printed herbals. Her *Herbals, Their Origin and Evolution* was published in 1913.

Arbor Vitae Cerebelli [Latin: *arbor*, tree + *vitae*, life] Term used to denote a tree-like arrangement of the white fibers in the cerebella structure of the brain by Danish anatomist Begnigmus Winslow (1669–1760) in 1740.

Arbuthnot, John (1667–1735) Writer and physician, born at Arbuthnot near Montrose and educated at Aberdeen. He was appointed physician to Queen Anne in 1709. He became a fellow of the Royal College in 1714. His medical works include *Effect of Air on Human Bodies* and *Essay concerning Ailments*. *Miscellaneous Works of Dr Arbuthnot* was published in Glasgow in 1751.

Arbutin A hydroquinone glycoside. The leaves of *Arbutus* have been used as a remedy for urinary conditions since the time of Galen (129–200), and its chief constituent, arbutin, was isolated by Kawalier in 1852.

Archaeopteryx Almost the entire remains of a primitive bird from the Jurassic period were found in deposits of a quarry at Solenhoven in southwest Germany in 1861. Wagner named the bird 'Gryphosauraus' after the Greek mythical bird 'Gryphon'. Herman von Meyer renamed it 'Archaeopteryx' to denote a primordial bird. Sir Richard Owen (1804–1892), an opponent of Darwinian theory, published *On the Archaeopteryx von Meyer* in which he pointed out the existence of these birds prior to the Tertiary period. Darwin in *Origin of Species* has quoted this strange bird in support of his theory.

Archaeus [Greek: *archaios*, ancient] The principle of life, postulated by Paracelsus (1493–1541) of Switzerland. If activity of life takes place in a normal manner, unimpeded by any obstacle, the state is called health. If activity is impeded by some factor, it is called disease. It is an essence equally distributed in all parts of the body.

Archagathos of Peloponnesus Greek physician who practiced in Rome around 219 BC. He was initially a successful surgeon but, being too ready with the knife, he was nicknamed, Carnifex, the executioner.

Archelaus Greek philosopher before the time of Socrates. He was one of the first to propose that the Earth was not flat.

Archetype [Greek: *arche*, beginning + *typos*, type] Meaning original and adapted to psychiatry by Carl Gustav Jung (1875–1961).

Archezoic Period [Greek: *archaios*, ancient or primitive + *zoic*, life] Earliest geological era which started with unicellular life.

Archiatri Public physicians in ancient Rome who belonged to the Collegium Archiatrorum. The 'archiatri populares' were district physicians, 'archiatri palatini' were the court physicians, and 'archiatri municipali' were municipal physicians.

Archibald, Cameron (1707–1753) Scottish physician who studied for the bar before he took medicine. He was executed at Tyburn for participating in the Rebellion of 1745.

Archigenes Greek surgeon who lived around AD 100. He amputated limbs for indications such as gangrene and malignant tumors and suggested the use of ligature to stop bleeding during amputation. He listed several applications for toothache including: spirit of nitre, hot fermentation with vinegar and heated linseed. He recommended filling holes in teeth caused by caries.

Archimatthaeus A physician in Salerno in the early 12th century. He wrote *The Instructions of the Physicians* and *The Practice*.

Archimedes (287–212 BC) The father of hydrodynamics was born at Syracuse in Sicily. He discovered the principles of flotation while he was contemplating an experiment to determine the content of gold. He also discovered the lever and its mechanism and the Archimedian screw. He was killed by a Roman soldier during the capture of Syracuse by the Romans.

Architecture Its contribution to medicine and health has been significant by way of providing hospitals. The temples of Aesculapius were probably the first buildings devoted to healing and inpatient treatment. The Roman architect, Markus Vitruvius who lived around 50 BC pointed out the damage caused to health by lead pipes used for drainage in Rome. During Medieval times sick rooms became attached to churches and places of religious healing. This pattern of architecture led to later hospitals such as the Lazaretto near Milan (1488) and Hospital de Santa Cruz, Toledo (1505). Leone Battista Alberti (1404–1472) of Italy specified that hospitals for infectious diseases should be built away from towns and highways. In England Robert Hooke (1635–1703) designed the new Bethlem Hospital which opened at Moorfield in 1676. Sir Christopher Wren (1632–1723) designed several hospitals in London.

Architronics Subdivision of the brain into different regions of specific structure. Pioneered by Swedish histologist, Hammarberg in 1895. Knowledge was advanced in England by Alfred Walter Campbell (1868–1937) and in Germany by Cecile Vogt (1875–1962) and Oskar Vogt (1870–1959). Cytoarchitronics, dealing with cell structure and specific areas of the brain, was pioneered by Campbell in 1905 and later by Lewis Bevan in 1909.

Archives de Psychologie Founded by Swiss psychologist, Edouard Claparede (1873–1940) and his cousin Theodore Flournoy (1854–1920) in 1901.

Archusia Carcinogenic growth stimulator. *See Burrows, Montrose.*

Arculanus, Johanus or Giovanni d'Arcoli (1412–1484) French professor and surgeon at Bologna. He suggested the use of amber electrified by friction for extracting metal splinters from the eye. *See artificial teeth.*

Arcus Senilis [Latin: *arcus*, bow + *senilis*, aged] A circular opacity surrounding the cornea. Attributed in the past to various causes, such as deposition of hyaline bodies, lime particles, fatty degeneration and arrest of corneal development. In 1870 Jacob Mendes da Costa (1833–1900) associated corneal change seen in arcus senilis with fatty degeneration of the heart.

Ardent Fever or ardentes febres [Latin: *ardere*, to burn] Paul of Aegina (625–690), Areatus, Avicenna (980–1037) and Rhazes (850–932) described the symptomatology of ardent fever which occurred in several diseased states. Hippocrates (460–377 BC) referred to long walks, summer weather and protracted thirst as causes. A commonly practiced method of treating high temperature during ardent fever was by external cooling with cold sponges and oral intake of cold fluids. Hippocrates in *Epidemics* described the symptomatology which occurred with great heat, thirst, dry tongue and delirium. The mechanism was thought by Hippocrates to be the veins becoming dry and attracting bilious humors. He considered that cases which occurred with black or dark urine would often be fatal. These description were later found to be consistent with blackwater fever by John William Watson Stephens in 1937, although some authorities earlier (Fuchs, 1866) have attributed them to typhus. *See black water fever.*

Arderne, John (1307–1360) Warwickshire surgeon who practiced and wrote on surgery. He was mostly self-taught, although it is possible that he may have received some training in Montpellier, France. He specialized in proctology and his practice was initially at Mitcham, Surrey before he moved to Newark in Nottinghamshire. His fees were said to be enormous and sometimes consisted of ransoms meant for knights who were held by the Turks during the Crusades. *See anal fistula.*

Aretaeus of Cappadocia (81–138) From eastern Asia Minor who lived in Alexandria. He ranks beside Hippocrates (460–377 BC) in his study and description of disease. He gave the name 'diabetes', distinguished between spinal and cerebral paralysis and gave classic descriptions of angina, elephantiasis, dysentery, asthma and many other diseases. He observed mentally ill patients and established that manic and depressive states could occur in the same patient. This was probably the earliest recognition of bipolar illness. He described the prepsychotic personality. His only surviving work *De Cavesis et signis Acutorum Morborum* was published in 1552.

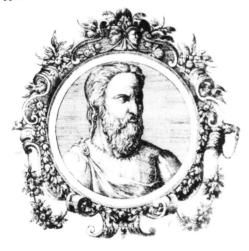

Aretaeus of Cappadocia (81–138). Courtesy of the National Library of Medicine

Argellata, Peter (d 1423) Physician in the 15th century who became professor of logic at Bologna. His work on surgery was printed posthumously in 1480 and it passed through several editions.

Argentaffinoma [Latin: *argentum*, silver + *affinitas*, affinity] (Syn. Carcinoid syndrome) The term *Karzinoide* (carcinoid) was introduced in 1907 by S. Obendorfer to describe a group of intestinal tumors. Carcinoid syndrome, consisting of flushing, wheezing, diarrhoea and valvular lesions was described by P. Masson in 1928. The suggestion that abdominal carcinomatosis may be associated with a direct release of hormones was made by Maurice A. Cassidy in 1931. A tumor with the classic symptoms and involvement of the valves of the right heart in a 19-year-old boy was described by G. Biorck, O. Axen and A.R. Thorson in the *American Heart Journal* in 1952. The same workers reported seven more patients who had excess 5-hydroxytryptamine or serotonin levels, thought to be responsible for their symptoms, in 1954. As the cells responsible for this tumor contained granules which showed an affinity for silver stain, the condition was named argentaffinoma. The high concentration of serotonin in the tumor, serum and urine was demonstrated by B. Pernow and J. Waldenstorm in 1954.

Argentier, John (1513–1572) Piedmont physician who opposed Galen's (129–200) views. Some of his works were printed in Venice in 1592.

Argentum [Greek: *argos*, shining] The chemical symbol Ag was assigned to silver by Berzelius (1779–1848). *See silver.*

Arginase A key enzyme in Krebs cycle was isolated by London chemist, Henry Drysdale Dakin (1880–1952) and Albrecht Kossel (1853–1827) at Marburg.

Arginine Amino acid isolated by Schulz from lupin seedlings in 1886. Its presence in the basic proteins of cell nuclei was demonstrated by a professor of physiology at Hamburg, Albrecht Kossel (1853–1927), in 1896.

Argon The English physicist John William Strutt Rayleigh (1842–1919), during his experiments, repeatedly noticed that nitrogen from air was heavier than nitrogen obtained otherwise. Scottish chemist, Sir William Ramsay (1852–1916) pointed out to him at a Royal Society meeting in 1894 that Henry Cavendish (1731–1810) had noted this finding a hundred years earlier. Ramsay and Rayleigh announced their discovery of argon, which had previously escaped detection due to its inertness, at the British Scientists Research Workers meeting on August 13, 1894.

Argyll Robertson Pupil Light rigidity of the pupil. Douglas Argyll Robertson (1837–1909), an ophthalmologist at Edinburgh Royal Infirmary, described four cases of spinal meiosis in his remarks on the action of light on the pupil in the *Edinburgh Medical Journal* in 1869. This condition associated with taboparesis was later named after him. *See Argyll Robertson, pupillary reaction.*

Argyll Robertson, Douglas Moray Cooper Lamb (1837–1909) Scottish ophthalmic surgeon who gave the first course in practical physiology at Edinburgh Royal Infirmary. He showed the constructive effect of eserine from

Calabar bean on the pupil and described the Argyll-Robertson pupil in 1869. *See Argyll Robertson pupil.*

Argyria Confusion with congenital heart disease, discovered in the latter half of the 19th century due to its association with skin discoloration. It was later found to occur as a result of using nose drops containing silver.

Ariboflavinosis The occurrence of a magenta-colored smooth tongue devoid of papillae in riboflavin deficiency was noted by Hugh Stannus (b 1877) in 1911. P.H. Bahr described the tongue lesions in *A Report on Researches in Sprue in Ceylon,* published in 1912. Additional features, such as neuritis and impairment of vision, were observed in Jamaicans by H.H. Scott in 1918. These signs and symptoms were produced experimentally in American prisoners by an Austrian-American physician, Joseph Goldberger (1874–1929) and Wilber Fred Tanner (1888) in 1925. Occurrence of retrobulbar neuritis was demonstrated by Fitzgerald Moore in 1930 and yeast extract was noted as a cure. A complete neurological picture was given by J.V. Landor and R.A. Pallister in 1935. It was shown to be due to riboflavin deficiency by W.H. Sebrell and R.E. Butler who named it ariboflavinosis in 1938.

Ariege Cave French cave in which paintings done by Cro-Magnon man, who lived 39,000 years ago, are found showing a human wearing a skin around the shoulders with deer's antlers on his head but naked from the waist down.

Aristotle (384–324 BC) Greek philosopher and scientist born in the province of Chalcidice next to Macedonia. His father was court physician to the King of Macedonia who was the grandfather of Alexander the Great. When he was 18 years he traveled to Athens to study under Plato (428–348 BC) and remained his pupil for 20 years. At 41 years he was appointed teacher to Alexander the Great who was 13 years old. When Alexander's father King Philip was assassinated in 336 BC Aristotle returned to Athens at the age of 53 years. His earliest and the greatest treatise on biology, *Historia Animalorum,* was written after his return to Athens. His other works include *De Anima , De Generatione Animalorum* and *De Partibus Animalorum.* Aristotle formed his Lyceum in Athens during the year 336 BC. A Latin translation of his three great biological treatises was published by Theodore Gaza (1400–1478) in Venice in 1476. Most of his teachings remained valid for 2000 years.

Arithmetic [Greek: *arithmos,* number] The earliest documentation is found in the papyrus written by an Egyptian priest named Ahmes in 1800 BC. It contains some common arithmetic operations and multiplications. Babylonian

numerals had bases of 10 and 60 and Egyptian numerals were based on symbols for 1 and multiples of ten. Hieroglyphic symbols were also allocated for numbers by the Egyptians. The oldest Greek numbering system consisted of assigned numbers to the 24 letters of the Greek alphabet. Ancient Roman numbers also had symbols for multiples of 5 as well as for powers of 10. We use the Arabic system of numbers.

Arkwright, Joseph Physician and great-grandson of industrialist Sir Richard Arkwright (1732–1792). He gave up medicine owing to ill health and joined the Lister Institute as a bacteriologist in 1906. He discovered the rickettsial bodies which were later identified as the cause of typhus fever. He also observed the rough and smooth colonies of dysentery bacilli and their relevance to antigenic properties.

Arloing, Saturnin (1846–1911) A physician who designed a seroagglutination test for the tubercle bacillus in 1898.

Arlt Sinus A dilatation of the lachrymal sac. Described by Carl Ferdinand Ritter von Arlt (1812–1887), professor of ophthalmology at Prague in 1855.

Armiger, Thomas Jeremiah (1782–1844) Demonstrator in anatomy at the London Hospital. He wrote *The Rudiments of the Anatomy and Physiology of the Human Body,* illustrated with plates, in 1816.

Armstrong, Charles (1886–1967) Microbiologist who identified the causative viruses of St Louis encephalitis and lymphocytic choriomeningitis in 1934.

Armstrong, George (1719–1789) He opened a dispensary for the poor in London in 1769, at Red Lion Square. He treated thousands of poor children at his own expense and started the movement to provide medical care for the poor. His *An Essay on the Diseases most Fatal to Infants* was published in 1767.

Armstrong, John (d 1779) Poet and physician from Castleton. He graduated from Edinburgh in 1732 with a thesis *De Tabe Purulente* dedicated to Sir Hans Sloane (1660–1753). He published an anonymous essay on the study of physick in 1735 and wrote *The History and Cure of Venereal Diseases* in 1737. A poetical work, *The Art of Preserving Health,* was published in 1744 and a collection of his medical essays appeared in 1773.

Army Medicine and Surgery Pythagorus is said to have served as an army physician. After being captured by the Persians in 500 BC he is supposed to have gained his freedom by successfully treating King Darius for a dislocated ankle and Queen Atossa for breast cancer. Field hospitals were established by the Byzantine Emperor, Leo VI, in the 9th century. He also had ambulance men known as *deputati* to carry the wounded men. Queen Isabella of Spain introduced one of the earliest systems of army medical services in the 15th century that provided a mobile unit of physicians and surgeons. Gunshot wounds were a major cause of morbidity and mortality and they were studied in detail by many surgeons such as Ambroise Paré (1510–1590) of France and Jerome of Brunswick. Harris von Gersdorf produced a field book of army surgery in 1517. Dominique Jean Larrey (1766–1842) of Paris was one of the greatest military surgeons in history. While working in the Hôtel Dieu in Paris in 1789 he introduced the 'flying ambulances' to provide first aid for the wounded. These ambulances were two- or four-wheeled carts drawn by horses. He later wrote five volumes of *Memoires de Chirurgie Militaire* in 1812. Army medical services in the British Isles remained a regimental system from 1660 to about 1873. James McGregor (1771–1858) was an army surgeon who served for nearly 50 years from 1815. George James Guthrie (1785–1856) from London was a surgeon in America and in the Peninsular War, was named the 'British Larrey'. He wrote *On Gunshot Wounds of the Extremities* in 1816 and *Commentaries on the Surgery of War* in 1855. Another two reformers of the British Army medical system were William Taylor and William Muir who brought an integrated hospital system to the military services in the 19th century. Nicolai Ivanovitch Pirogoff (1810–1881) from Moscow served in the Crimean War and advocated female nursing for the wounded. He published *Principles of General Military Surgery*, in 1854.

Arndt-Schultz Law Weak stimuli cause strong physiological responses and strong stimuli diminish or abolish physiological activity. Proposed by German psychiatrist, Rudolf Arndt (1835–1900).

Arneman, Justus (1763–1807) Professor of surgery at Göttingen who pioneered the study of diseases of the ear.

Arneth, Joseph (1873–1955) German physician who differentiated polymorphs into 5 groups according to their nuclear configuration, in 1904. He described a method of counting cells in each group to assess bone marrow response to toxemia and infection. His method, initially known as the Arneth count, was later renamed the polymorphonuclear count by William Edmond Cooke and Eric Ponder in 1914.

Arnisaeus, Kenningus (d 1635) German professor of physics at Helmstadt. He wrote several treatises on politics and was physician to the King of Denmark.

Arnold of Villanova (1234–1313) Italian physician from Valencia in Spain who also studied theology and law. He was professor at Montpellier for most of his career and was physician to Peter III (1285) and King Philip at Paris (1299). He also had three popes as his patients but came into conflict with the church owing to his unorthodox views on theology. This led to some of his work being publicly burnt. His voluminous work, amounting to about 138 treatises on medicine, astronomy and chemistry, *Opera Omnia*, was published in Lyons in 1532.

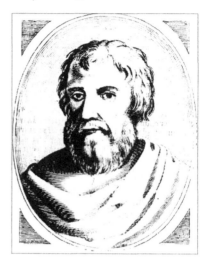

Arnold of Villanova (1234–1313). Courtesy of the National Library of Medicine

Arnold, Friedrich (1803–1890) Professor of anatomy from Heidelberg who described the otic ganglion of the 5th cranial nerve (Arnold ganglion) and several other structures which now bear his name.

Arnold, Joseph (1782–1818) Physician from Beccles, Suffolk who graduated from Edinburgh. His main interest was botany and he accompanied the British colonial administrator, Sir Thomas Raffles (1781–1826), on an expedition to Sumatra, where he died. He discovered the largest flower in the world, *Rafflesia arnoldi*, which measures over a meter in diameter.

Arnold, Julius (1835–1915) Succeeded his father, Friedrich Arnold (1803–1890) as professor of anatomy at the University of Heidelberg. He described fragments of red blood cells (Arnold granules) in 1897.

Arnold, Thomas (1742–1816) Physician from Leicester who devoted himself to mental disorders. He wrote *Observations on Insanity* (1782), *Dissertatio de Pluratide* (1766), *A case of Hydrophobia Successfully Treated* (1793) and *Observations on the Management of the Insane* in 1809.

Arnold–Chiari Syndrome A tongue-like abnormal protrusion of the cerebellum and medulla oblongata through the foramen magnum causing hydrocephalus and atrophy of brain tissue. Described by Austrian pathologist, Hans Chiari (1851–1916) in 1891 and further described by German pathologist, Julius Arnold (1835–1915), a professor at Heidelberg, in 1894.

Arnot, Henry (1843–1931) Surgeon and lecturer at St Thomas' Hospital, London, who wrote *Cancer, Its Varieties and Diagnosis* in 1874. He held several Church appointments and was made honorary canon of Rochester in 1905.

Arnott, James M. (1794–1885) Surgeon at Middlesex Hospital who founded the Middlesex Hospital Medical School.

Arnott, Neil (1788–1874) Scottish physician, inventor and philanthropist. In 1827 he published *Elements of Physics,* which was translated into several languages. In 1855 he gave up medicine to pursue research. He invented a smokeless grate known as Arnott Stove, a waterbed, a ventilator, a hydrostatic bed and other devices. His last invention was a chair bed to prevent seasickness. He also gave large sums of money to the University of London and Scottish universities. He never patented his inventions and did not seek to profit from them.

Aromatherapy The application of essential oils through baths, inhalation and massage has been practiced from ancient times to treat disease and revive health. Myrrh has been in use since biblical times and Egyptian priests used it to treat chronic diseases such as arthritis. Theophrastus, a botanist who lived around 300 BC, wrote a treatise on odors in which he described the effects of various scents on body and mind. The term 'aromatherapy' was coined by French chemist, René-Maurice Gattefosse in 1928. His interest began with the accidental discovery that lavender oil healed a severe burn on his hand and prevented scarring. He later established an oil-house and started demonstrating the benefits of essences on the body. Around the same time, French physician, Jean Valnet and skin-care specialist, Maguirete Maury, established aromatherapy.

Aromatics Burnt in large fires in an attempt to control plague in Athens in 429 BC and used during pestilence up to the Middle Ages.

Aronson Culture Medium For growing *Vibrio cholerae.* Devised by German bacteriologist, Hans Aronson (1865–1919).

Arrhenius, Svante August (1859–1927) Swedish chemist, born in Wijk near Uppsala. He moved to Stockholm in 1881 and became a student of Jacobus Henricus Van't Hoff (1852–1911). He advanced the theory of electrolyte dissociation, or the ionic theory, previously proposed by Van't Hoff and established the concept of the dissociation constant in 1883. He formulated the effect of temperature on the rate of chemical reaction in 1889 and was awarded the Nobel Prize for Chemistry in 1903.

Arrhenius, Olof Son of Swedish chemist, Svante Arrhenius. He applied pH measurement in determining the suitability of specific crops in relation to acid, alkaline or neutral soil.

Arrhenoblastoma [Greek: *arrhen,* male + *blastos,* bud] Tumor of the ovary consisting of convoluted tubules resembling the seminiferous tubules of the testis. Described by E.P. Pick of Berlin in 1905. G. Schikele described a second case with similar histology in 1906. The term was proposed in 1930 by Robert Meyer (1864–1947) to denote this group of masculinising tumors.

Arrhythmia [Greek: *a,* without + *rhythmos,* measured motion] The irregularities of the heart rate have been noted from ancient times from studying the pulse. The Chinese emperor and physician, Huang Ti Nei Ching Su Wen, who lived around 2000 BC, described the irregular rhythm and volume of the pulse. Paul of Aegina (625–690) described rhythmic and arrhythmic pulse. A description of paroxysmal tachycardia was given by Irish physician William Stokes (1807–1878) in 1854, but the term 'paroxysmal tachycardia' was coined by Leon Bouveret (1851–1925) of Paris in 1889. A report of syncope due to cardiac arrest or heart block was given by Marcus Gerbezius (1658–1818) in 1692. The same condition was described as 'epilepsy with slow pulse' by Giovanni Battista Morgagni (1682–1771) in 1761 and an account of 'a clear case of syncopal attacks with heart block' was given by Robert Adams (1791–1875) in 1827. Pulsus bigeminus was described by a professor of pathology at Berlin, Ludwig Traube (1818–1876) in 1872. An account of death due to ventricular fibrillation was given by Alexander John MacWilliam (1857–1937) in 1889. A graphic record of arrhythmia was achieved by Sir James MacKenzie (1853–1925) with his polygraph in 1897. The nature and ECG characteristics of atrial fibrillation were established around the same time by Sir Thomas Lewis (1881–1945) of University College, London. Lown–Ganong–Levine syndrome, a condition of shortened PR interval and normal QRS on ECG tracings associated with paroxysmal tachycardia, was described by Bernard Lown of Brigham Hospital, Boston, W.F. Ganong and Samuel Albert Levine (1891–1966) in 1952. *See Stokes–Adams, auricular flutter, heart block, paroxysmal atrial tachycardia, ventricular tachycardia, ventricular fibrillation, Wolf–Parkinson–White syndrome.*

Arrow Poison The South American arrow poison, curare, was described by Peter Martyr Angherius in 1516 and an account of its paralyzing effects was given by Charles Waterton (1782–1865) in *Wanderings in South America* published in 1825. Claude Bernard (1813–1878) demonstrated the neuromuscular blocking effect of curare in 1856. The search for the medicinal effects started around 1880, when it was noted that poison from *Antiaris toxicaria*, the upas tree from the Malay Archipelago had effects similar to digitalis in small doses. The explorer and doctor, David Livingstone (1813–1873), described the effects of an arrow poison called kombe obtained from the *Strophanthus* vine during his travels in southwestern Africa. A sample of this was analyzed by Sir Thomas Richard Fraser (1841–1919) of Edinburgh in 1885, who found it to be similar to digoxin and equally effective in the treatment of dropsy. Tetanus toxin in an unidentified crude form was used as an effective arrow poison by people of the South Pacific islands.

Arrowroot A starch prepared from *Maranta arundinacea*, and used in special diets. A reference to it as *Canna indica radice alba alexipharmica* was made by Sir Hans Sloane (1660–1753), a physician to the Governor of Barbados, in his catalogue of plants from Jamaica published in 1696.

Arrow Wound Theodoric of Cervia (1260) described a method of surgical removal of an arrow while chanting prayers. French surgeon, Guy de Chauliac (1300–1370) of Auvergne, wrote on instruments for withdrawing arrows embedded in the body. David Livingstone (1813–1873), the great African explorer and surgeon, described the surgical removal of arrowheads from wounded patients by African surgeons. On one occasion the surgeon successfully excised part of the lung in order to remove an arrow from the chest.

Arsenic [Greek: *arrenikon*, male] Compounds of arsenic were known in Egypt during the time of the 18th dynasty. The term 'arsenicon' was used by the Greek herbalist Dioscorides in AD 50 to denote a substance that was used as a cure for asthma. Early alchemists, including Roger Bacon (1214–1294) and Albertus Magnus (1192–1280), were also familiar with the properties of arsenic.

Arsenic Cancer Arsenic was suggested to be a carcinogen by John Ayerton Paris (1785–1856) in 1820. A case of cancer due to arsenic exposure in a 34-year-old clerk was recorded by Jonathan Hutchinson (1828–1913) in 1872.

Arsenic Poisoning Arsenic has been used as a poison as it is tasteless and odorless. Arsenic poisoning occurred in Vienna in the 1930s owing to an apple cake being mistakenly 'sugared' with arsenic. It also results from spraying fruit and vegetables with arsenic-containing insecticides. Traces of arsenic were found in common food products such as jams, marmalade, sweets, lemonade and liqueurs around 1910 and the practice of coloring food products with arsenical pigments also became a common problem in the 1920s until it was banned by the Public Health Act related to Preservatives in 1925.

Arsenic Preparations Found by A. Lingard, in 1899 to cure trypanosomal disease called 'Surra' in horses in India. The African explorer David Livingstone (1813–1873) was the first to use arsenic in treatment of the African horse disease or 'nagana' in 1857. An aromatic arsenical was prepared by Bechamp in 1860. Atoxl (*p*-amino phenyl arsenate) was identified as a cure for human African trypanosomiasis by Harold Wolferstan Thomas and Anton Breinl in England in 1904, but its toxic properties on the optic nerve limited its use. Paul Ehrlich (1854–1915) pursued the search for safer arsenic compounds and produced salvarsan (arsphenamine) which was found to cure relapsing fever, syphilis and trypanosomiasis, in 1911.

Arsphenamine Used in the treatment of Oroya fever by J. Arce in 1918. *See arsenic preparations.*

Artane or benzhexol Introduced as treatment for Parkinson disease by Kendall Brooks Corbin (b 1907) in 1949.

Artedi, Peter (d 1735) Swiss physician and friend of Carl Linnaeus (1707–1778) who wrote on fossils and quadrupeds. His work on ichthyology was completed and published after his death.

Artemisia absinthium Wormwood probably obtained its name from its paralyzing effect on intestinal worms. It is included in the *Materia Medica* of Dioscorides as a treatment for intestinal worms. It was an ingredient of absinthe which was a popular social drink amongst the elite in Paris around 1860. *See absinthe.*

Artemisia maritima A plant known to the ancient Greeks and Romans for its medicinal values. Dioscorides mentioned the seeds of the plant which he found growing in Cappodocia as treatment for Ascarides and Lumbrici around AD 60. Alexander of Tralles (525–605) advocated its use against intestinal worms. Kahler, an apothecary at Dusseldorf, extracted the active ingredient in 1830. Augustus Alms, a druggist's assistant at Penzilin in Mecklenburg-Schwerin, independently extracted the same substance and named it santonin, which was widely used as an antihelmintic in the 19th century.

Arterial Baroreflex The part played by the arterial baroreflex in control of circulation was demonstrated by German physiologist, Heinrich Ewald Hering (1866–1948) at Leipzig in 1923. The presence of sensors in or around the heart to detect variation in blood pressure in order to adjust the blood volume was suggested by John Peters in 1935.

Arterial Blood Gas Analysis *See blood gas analysis.*

Arterial Embolism François Quesnay, a surgeon in Paris, suggested an arterial cause for gangrene in *Traite de la Gangrene* published in 1739. Hebred in 1817 proposed that gangrene was caused by an obstacle in the interior of the blood vessels and embolism as a cause of gangrene was pointed out by H. Ball in *Thesis de Paris* published in 1862. A classical description of dislodged arterial emboli from the heart was given by William Senhouse Kirkes (1823–1864) in 1852. Hematuria with focal glomerular lesions in the kidney, due to minute bacterial emboli from endocardial vegetations in bacterial endocarditis, was observed by Max Hermann Friedrich Loehlein (1877–1921) of Leipzig in 1907. The method of arterial embolectomy through a balloon catheter was devised by Thomas J. Fogarty and colleagues in 1963. *See embolism.*

Arterial Encephalography or cerebral angiography Introduced by Antonio Caetanode Egas Moniz (1874–1955), clinical professor of neurology at the University of Lisbon. He demonstrated serial radiograms after injection of 25% sodium iodide into the carotid artery in 1931.

Arterial Pyemia Probably the first account of bacterial endocarditis, called 'arterial pyemia' was given by Sir Samuel Wilkes (1824–1911) in 1870. *See subacute bacterial endocarditis.*

Arterial Suture The end-to-end suture of the femoral artery was performed by John Benjamin Murphy (1857–1916) of America, in 1896. The modern technique was devised by Alexis Carrel (1873–1944) in 1902.

Arteriogram [Greek: *aer*, air + *tero*, I preserve + *graphein*, to write] A record of the impulse of the heart on the radial artery during the cardiac cycle was made on a smoke-covered drum by Etienne Jules Marey (1830–1904) in 1863. This was initially referred to as an arteriogram by several cardiologists, including Paul Wood (1907–1962) in the early 20th century. The term 'arteriogram' currently refers to radiological visualization of arteries after injection of radio-opaque dyes. *See angiography.*

Arterioles Although the capillaries were described by Marcello Malpighi (1628–1694) in 1661, a clear distinction between capillaries and arterioles was made much later by British physiologist, Marshall Hall (1790–1857) of Nottingham in 1831.

Arteriosclerosis [Greek: *aer*, air + *tero*, I preserve + *skeleros*; hard] Thickening of the arteries was described by Antonio Scarpa (1747–1832) of Italy in 1804. The term 'arteriosclerosis' was introduced by Frederic Martin Lobstein (1777–1835), professor of pathology at Strasburg in 1833. He used the term to refer to thickening and hardening of the arteries. It was later named atherosclerosis by Felix Jacob Marchand (1846–1928) of Leipzig in 1904. *See atherosclerosis.*

Arteritis [Greek: *aer*, air + *tero*, I preserve + *itis*, inflammation] *See temporal arteritis, polyarteritis nodosa, Takayasu syndrome, aortitis.*

Artery [Greek: *aer*, air + *tero*, I preserve or *terein*, to keep] The Greek physician Erasistratus, who lived around 300 BC, postulated that arteries contained air or the 'breath of life' and veins carried nutrients, and the word artery is derived from this. Galen (129–200) declared that arteries were full of blood. Thereafter no significant progress was made until William Harvey (1578–1657) discovered the role of arteries in the circulation of the blood in 1628. *See blood circulation.*

Artery Forceps Catch forceps were used to occlude blood vessels by producing a twist or torsion by Jean Zulema Ammusat (1796–1856) of France, Robert Liston (1794–1847) of London and others from 1830 to 1850. This replaced the previous practice of using the assistant's fingers to control bleeding. Spring clips or bulldog forceps were introduced to occlude veins in 1850. Thomas Spencer Wells (1818–1897) designed and advocated crushing vessels with the forceps, known as 'forci-pressure'. Serrated teeth on forceps were introduced by Webber in 1863. Eugene Koeberle (1828–1915) and Emile Jules Pean (1830–1898) in France modified them to include a locking device around 1865. In 1879 Spencer Wells (1818–1897) added variable pressure adjustment to the locking device, and this has changed very little up to the present.

Arthritis [Greek: *arthros*, joint or *arthrosia*, to articulate + *itis*, inflammation] Greek physicians used the term 'arthritis'. English medical writer in the 13th century, Gilbertus Anglicus, believed that it was caused by sexual excess. John of Gaddesden in the 14th century thought that overindulgence in food followed by sexual intercourse led to it. Rheumatoid arthritis was used to describe a form that differed from gout by Sir Alfred Baring Garrod (1819–1907) of King's College, London in 1858. *See rheumatoid arthritis, gout.*

Arthrodesis [Greek: *arthros*, joint + *desis*, binding] A method of surgical fixation of a joint by fusion of joint surfaces in cases of destructive joint disease. Performed by Henry Park (1744–1831) in 1733. Eduard Albert (1841–1900) of Vienna, who performed the procedure in the ankle of a paralytic foot in 1882, coined the term. Arthrodesis for deformities of the foot was pioneered in the USA by G. Davis (1913), M. Hoke (1921), E.S. Ryerson (1923). J.A. Key described positive-pressure arthrodesis or the compression method for tuberculosis of the knee joint in 1932. In England, Herbert Alfred Brittain (1904–1954) of Norwich performed subtrochanteric osteotomy and wrote *Architectural Principles of Arthrodesis* in 1941.

Arthrogryposis Multiplex Congenita [Greek: *arthros*, joint + *grypes*, hooked] A clinical description of the condition in infants was given by a professor of anatomy at Breslau, Wilhelm Adolf Otto (1786–1845).

Arthroplasty [Greek: *arthros*, joint + *plasmein*, to mold] First tried with success on a 21-year-old male named John Coyle with tuberculosis of the hip by J. Rhea Barton (1794–1871), a surgical graduate of the University of Pennsylvania, in 1818. Modern arthroplasty for ankylozed joints was pioneered by John B. Murphy (1857–1916), an American orthopedic surgeon of Irish origin at Appleton, Wisconsin, in 1913.

Arthroscopy [Greek: *arthros*, joint + *skopein*, to look] A modified form of a cystoscope was devised in 1918 by Kenji Takanagi (1888–1963), a professor at Tokyo University. An account of the procedure using a modified laparoscope in a series of 18 patients was published by Swiss surgeon, Eugen Bircher, in 1921. A description of the arthroscopic appearance of the joints on a cadaver was given by Michael S. Burmann in 1931. An atlas of arthroscopy was published by Masaki Watanabi of Japan in 1957. Arthroscopic surgery of the knee in the USA was mostly developed by Richard L. O'Connor (1933–1980), an orthopedic surgeon in California, and founding member of the International Arthroscopic Association. D.J. Dandy popularized the procedure in England.

Arthrosia Podagra [Greek: *arthorosia*, to articulate + *podos*, feet + *agra*, seizing] Radulphus, a Dominican doctor referred to gout as '*cum gutta quam podagram vel arthriticam*' in the 13th century. *See gout.*

Arthus Phenomenon A local skin reaction following the injection of antigen in experimental animals (rabbits) which were previously sensitized through repeated systemic injections of horse serum. Demonstrated by French physiologist, Maurice Nicholas Arthus (1862–1945) at the School of Medicine, Marseilles in 1903.

Artificial Anus An operation for congenital atresia of the anus was designed by Pierre Duret (1745–1851) in 1798. A more popular operation for treatment of anal atresia was described by Jean Zulema Amussat (1796–1856), a surgeon in Paris, around 1840. American surgeon, Phillip Syng Physick (1768–1837) devised another operation in 1821. *See Amussat operation, colostomy.*

Artificial Eye The French surgeon Ambroise Paré (1510–1590) designed artificial eyes, limbs and teeth. The eyelids were also sometimes made with gold and the eye was held in position by a large spring on the side of the head.

Artificial Feeding Extrabuccal feeding has existed as a therapeutic resource for over 1000 years. Rectal feeding was practiced by Spanish physician, Avenzoar (1113–1162). He also carried out nasogastric feeding through a metal tube in a patient with esophageal stricture. This method, by placing the food into the stomach through a tube, called 'gavage', was revived by Georges Maurice DeBove (1845–1920) in 1881. Other methods, such as rectal feeding through an enema and percutaneous feeding by rubbing nutrients into the skin, were in use in the 19th century. In 1927, Stejskal estimated from his experiments that 1350 calories could be supplied daily through the skin.

Artificial Fever W. Bierman in *History of Fever Therapy in Treatment of Disease* (1942) attributed the saying 'give me the power to produce fever and I will cure all disease' to Hippocrates (460–377 BC). Use as treatment for mental diseases was introduced by Austrian psychiatrist, Julius von Wagner-Jauregg (1857–1940) in *The Influence of Fever Producing Diseases on Mental Disorders* published in 1877. He won the Nobel Prize for Physiology or Medicine in 1917 for his discovery of malarial fever therapy for the late stage of syphilis. J.G. Kiernan, during his work on variola and insanity in 1883, observed that some patients with taboparesis improved after an attack of smallpox. A method of inducing hyperpyrexia up to 39.5 °C was introduced by K. Phillips in 1883. Wagner-Jauregg succeeded Robert Krafft-Ebing (1840–1902) as professor of psychiatry at Graz in 1889, and demonstrated the beneficial effects of treating general syphilitic paresis by inoculation with malaria in 1917. W. Kahler and F. Knollmeyer used a cabinet heated with electric light to induce pyrexia in 1929 and many other special means, such as diathermy, high-frequency currents and electromagnetic induction, were developed during this period. However, complications such as shock, coma and dehydration continued to be the main limitations. Most of the machines for producing pyrexia in

America received the approval of the Council on Physical Therapy of the American Medical Association. Such methods of producing artificial fever continued to be practiced for syphilis and other conditions until the advent of chemotherapy in the early 1940s. Another important monograph was written by Clarence Adolphe Neymann (b 1887) in 1938.

Artificial Heart A prototype was developed by Alexis Carrel (1873–1944) and A. Lindbergh in 1936. The first artificial heart was implanted into an animal by Soviet scientist Vladimir P. Demikhov in 1937. A 'heart' made of Silastic was later inserted successfully into a calf and maintained for 121 days, in 1969. Based on this finding, Michael De Bakey (b 1908) of Houston, Texas applied the procedure to humans and succeeded after three trials. Denton Cooley (b 1920) and Domingo Liotta kept a patient alive for over 2 days, while he awaited a living heart transplant in 1969. Willem Kolff of America implanted an artificial heart in a man and kept him alive for 112 hours in 1982. The heart used in this operation was devised by the American Robert Jarvick, and it was called Jarvick-7. *See cardiac transplant.*

Artificial Heart Valve American surgeon, Charles Anthony Hufnagel (1916–1989) explored the possibility of developing an artificial aortic valve. He commenced his research in 1940, and eventually produced the first practical aortic valve prosthesis. Implant of this in a patient was at the Georgetown University Medical Center in 1952. Cardiac valve surgery was revolutionized by the invention of several artificial valves which were mainly heterografts, in 1960. F.H. Ellis used the first flap valve in 1960. The ball-valve prosthesis developed by Albert Starr of the University of Oregon Medical School became popular during this time. J.P. Binet and A. Carpentier improved the valves and the latter introduced glutaraldehyde treatment in 1968 for the porcine valve prior to its insertion. The pig aortic valves fixed with glutaraldehyde were introduced by G.A. Kaiser and colleagues in 1969. *See aortic valve.*

Artificial Hip Joint The first recorded prosthetic replacement of a hip joint was performed by Themistocles Gluck (1853–1942) of Germany in 1890. Pierre Louis E. Delbet (1861–1925) replaced the femoral head with a prosthesis in 1903. Ernest Williams Hey-Groves (1872–1944) of England used an ivory ball and stem for hip arthroplasty in 1923. A total hip replacement with a joint made of steel was developed in 1938 by English surgeon, Phillip Wiles (1899–1967) at the Middlesex Hospital in London. G.R. Mckee of Norwich, England produced an entirely metal prosthesis

around 1951. English orthopedic professor at Manchester University, John Charnley (1911–1982), developed a prosthesis for total hip replacement around 1965.

Artificial Insemination Bartolommeo Eustachio (1524–1574) advised a husband to insert his finger into the vagina of his wife after intercourse in order to push the semen into the mouth of the uterus. The technique was performed on a dog by Lazzaro Spallanzani (1729–1799) in 1785. In 1790 John Hunter (1728–1793) performed it successfully in a woman whose husband had hypospadias. James Marion Sims (1813–1883) used it with success in 1866 in a patient with a history of 9 years of infertility. The first center for artificial insemination was founded by Russian biologist, Ilaya Ivanovich Shigry (b 1870) in 1901.

Artificial Kidney Extracorporeal hemodialysis. A dialyzing membrane was constructed for use in experimental animals by John Jacob Abel (1857–1938), Leonard George Rowentree (1883–1959) and Benjamin Bernard Turner (b 1871) who published *On the Removal of Diffusible Substances from the Circulating Blood by Means of Dialysis* in 1913. G. Hass treated a human with an artificial kidney using the type of membrane described by Abel. This method was inefficient as the area of the membrane used was small and nearly 24 hours were required to reduce blood nitrogen by 4 mg/100 ml. H. Necheles improved this method in 1923 using a peritoneal layer of ox cecum, known as 'gold beater's skin' since it was used to separate hammered gold leaf. W. Thalheimer in 1937 used cellophane as a dialyzing membrane and heparin as an anticoagulant. Dutch-born American physician, Willem Johan Kolff (b 1911) constructed the rotating-drum artificial kidney and treated his first patient in 1943. An artificial kidney of therapeutic significance was designed by H.T.J. Berk in 1944. Several workers, including N. Alwall (1946), L.T. Skeggs (1947) and J.R. Leonards (1949), continued to improve the design and function. Kolff and B. Watschinger reported two cases of uremia treated by hemodialysis and ultrafiltration with their twin-coil kidney in 1956. Their dialyzer and ultrafilter later came to be mass produced as a disposable unit. The shunted cannula, which made long term repetitive dialysis possible for patents with chronic renal failure, was developed by W. Quinton and colleagues in 1960.

Artificial Limb The earliest limb prosthesis, probably belonging to the Etruscans, was found in Capri. This was for use in amputation above the knee and was made of wood and bronze. A German pirate, Gotz von Berlichingen

(1480–1562), used an iron hand prosthesis in 1509. The Prince of Homberg (1633–1708) was fitted with an artificial leg, which he used for 50 years. French surgeon Ambroise Paré (1510–1590) designed and fitted ingenious artificial limbs on a larger scale. In England, Sir George Cayley (1771–1857) of Scarborough, a mechanical physicist and pioneer in aviation, designed artificial limbs in the early 19th century. The current internationally known artificial limb-fitting center at Queen Mary's Hospital in London was established in 1915.

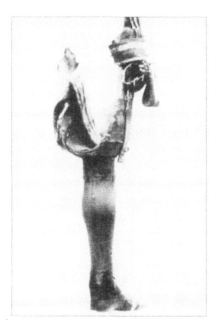

Artificial leg made for the Prince of Homberg (1633–1708)

Artificial Pacemaker *See cardiac pacing.*

Artificial Pneumothorax James Carson (1772–1843) of Liverpool advocated induction of a pneumothorax as treatment for patients with pulmonary tuberculosis, in 1821. James Houghton described a case in a bricklayer of advanced tuberculosis that improved after a spontaneous pneumothorax, in 1833. William Stokes (1804–1878) pointed out the beneficial effects in tuberculous patients in 1837. Pierre Carl Edouard Potain (1825–1901) treated a case of hydropneumothorax by withdrawing the fluid and replacing it with air in 1884. John Cayley treated several cases of hemoptysis by incising the chest wall and reported his study to the Clinical Society of London in 1885. Its induction was established as regular treatment for pulmonary tuberculosis by Italian surgeon, Carlo Forlanini (1847–1918) in 1888. In 1927 Clive Riviere, a London chest physician, wrote 'no more hopeful ray of sunshine has ever come to illuminate the dark kingdom of disease than that introduced into the path of the consumptive through the discovery of artificial pneumothorax'. Treatment for tuberculosis continued until the advent of chemotherapy in the early 1930s.

Artificial Respiration The first experiment on artificial respiration in animals was performed in 1667 by Robert Hooke (1635–1703), who kept the animals alive by blowing air through their lungs with bellows. Similar experiments were done by Robert Boyle (1627–1691) in the same year. John Fothergill (1712–1780), a physician from Yorkshire, in 1744 referred to the recovery of a man dead in appearance by distending his lungs with air. In 1855 Marshall Hall (1790–1857) of Nottingham, began his pioneering studies and introduced a method of artificial respiration. Theodore Tuffier (1857–1929) and Louis Hallion used the insufflation method in a patient during surgery for partial resection of his lung in 1896. This method was improved by Eugene Louis Doyen (1859–1916) and Rudolph Matas (1860– 1957), who were cardiothoracic surgeons. The negative-pressure chamber was developed by German surgeon, Ferdinand Sauerbruch in 1903, and was in use up to 1940. Endotracheal insufflation used on a wider basis in early 1900 made it practical and revolutionized surgery and anesthesia.

Artificial Silk As early as 1664, Robert Hooke (1635–1703) in his *Micrographia* suggested that it was possible to make an artificial glutinous compound resembling silk. The first of such filaments was produced by Sir Joseph Wilson Swan (1828–1914) of Sunderland in 1883 by squirting solutions of nitrocellulose. Artificial silk sutures with high tensile strength were developed around 1950.

Artificial Sweetener Saccharin (2–sulfobenzimide), the first artificial sweetener, was obtained from coal tar by two Americans, Constantin Fahlberg and Ira Remsen in 1879. It remained as a prescription product until the Food and Drug Administration allowed it to be used as an industrial food additive in 1938. Another sweetener, aspartamine, 200 times sweeter than sucrose, was prepared from two amino acids, phenylalanine and aspartic acid, in 1965.

Artificial Teeth Teeth made of ivory were used in ancient Rome. Fragments of an ancient skull with gold-inlaid teeth have been found at the Atacames site in Ecuador. Albucasis, the Arab surgeon in the 11th century, described replacement with ivory teeth. Guy de Chauliac (1300–1370) recommended replacing fallen teeth with those of another person or artificial teeth made of ox bone. Johannes Arculanus (1412–1484), a professor at Bologna, referred to gold leaf as a filling material and French surgeon Ambroise

Paré (1510–1590) designed artificial teeth, often made of gold. Peter Lowe (1560–1610) in his treatise on surgery written in 1654 mentioned artificial teeth made of whalebone and ivory fastened by wire. Parisian dentist, Nicholas Dubois de Chement, wrote a dissertation on artificial teeth in 1788. Porcelain teeth were introduced in France in 1774 and into America in 1814. The method of taking a plaster cast for replacement of teeth was invented in America in 1844. Use of atmospheric pressure to fix dentures to the jaw was discovered by James Gardette of Philadelphia in 1800. Sir John Tomes (1815–1895), a dental surgeon to the Middlesex Hospital, wrote a detailed book *The Management of Artificial Teeth,* in 1851. His name is also associated with the discovery of odontoblast processes which continue into the tubules of dentine. *See dental caries, dentistry.*

Artistic Anatomy Antonio Pollaiuolo (1428–1498) and Andrea del Verrocchio (1435–1499) of Italy applied accurate surface anatomy to their drawings. Michelangelo (1475–1554) and Raphael (1483–1520) did dissections in order to study and represent human forms with anatomical accuracy. Leonardo Da Vinci's drawings showed in great detail anatomic representations of human internal organs such as the heart, its valves and the aortic root. Albrecht Dürer (1471–1528) of Nuremberg was an artistic anatomist who made painstaking studies of the proportions of the human body which he represented in his drawings. *A Manual of Artistic Anatomy* was published by Robert Knox (1791–1862), a comparative anatomist at Edinburgh, in 1852. One of the revivers during modern times was Matthias Marie Duval (1844–1907), professor of anatomy at the National School of Fine Arts in Paris who published *Artistic Anatomy* in 1880. Max Brodel (1870–1941) was an artist from Leipzig who did medical illustrations. He traveled to America in 1893 and later came to be recognized as the founder of illustrative medical art there.

Arytenoid Cartilage [Greek: *aretaina*, ladle + *eidos*, form] The structure derives its name from its resemblance to the spout of a pitcher. Galen (129–200) used the term for the cartilage in the neck but believed that there was only one cartilage in humans. The existence of paired arytenoid cartilages was established in the 15th century.

Asafetida [Latin: *asa*, gum] A gum resin obtained from a perennial plant, *Ferula asafetida*. In the past considered to be an excellent remedy for hysterical disorders.

Asbestosis [Greek: *a*, not + *sbestos*, inextinguishable] The use of asbestos to make clothes was mentioned by the Greek historian, Herodotus (485–425 BC). A case of asbestosis was observed in a man who worked on a carding machine for 14

years whose autopsy at Charing Cross Hospital in 1900 revealed extensive pulmonary fibrosis. Ten others who worked with him died before the age of 30 years and these observations were reported by M. Murray in 1907. An unequivocal relationship between asbestos and pulmonary fibrosis was established by Edmund Henry Seiler (1891–1978) in 1928. The first recorded case of carcinoma of the lung in asbestosis was described by Kenneth Merrill Lynch (b 1887) and W.A. Smith in 1935 and the first case of mesothelioma in an asbestos worker in England was published by H. Wyers in 1946. A definite association between mesothelioma and exposure to asbestos was pointed out by I.C. Wagner, C.A. Sleggs and P. Marchand of South Africa in 1960.

Ascariasis Intestinal worms resembling earthworms were described by Paul of Aegina (625–690). An anatomical description of *Ascaris lumbricoides* or roundworms was given by Edward Tyson (1649–1708) in 1683. The egg and the reproductive process were described by Francesco Redi (1626–1697) of Italy in 1684. The migration of larvae through the lungs was discovered by F.H. Stewart in 1916, and the full life history was worked out by Brayton Howard Ransom (1879–1925) in 1917.

Ascaris lumbricoides *See ascariasis.*

Asch, Baron George Thomas de (1729–1807) Russian physician and pupil of Albrecht von Haller (1708–1777) at Göttingen. He made considerable donations to Göttingen University and also contributed to the Russian pharmacopoeia and wrote several treatises.

Ascham, Roger (1515–1568) British educational reformer from Kirkby Wiske. A book containing his views on education, *Scholemaster,* was published 2 years after his death.

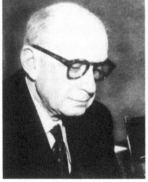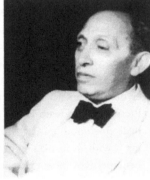

Selmar Ascheim and Bernhardt Zondek. Reproduced with permission from *Klin Wchschr.* 7, 8–9, 1928

Aschheim and Zondek Test for Pregnancy Two German gynecologists at Berlin, Selmar Aschheim (1878–1965) and

Bernhardt Zondek (1891–1966) while investigating the influence of the pituitary on sexual development, conceived the idea of concentrating the urine and injecting the concentrate into animals to study its effects. In 1927 they found marked devolvement of the ovaries in experimental animals. This enabled them to diagnose early pregnancy for the first time by a laboratory test. *See estrogen.*

Aschheim, Selmar (1878–1965) *See Aschheim and Zondek test for pregnancy.*

Aschoff Body A characteristic histological lesion found in rheumatic carditis. Described by Karl Albert Ludwig Aschoff (1866–1942) of Germany in 1904.

Aschoff Nodule *See Aschoff, Karl Albert Ludwig.*

Aschoff, Karl Albert Ludwig (1866–1942) German pathologist whose work on rheumatic myocarditis and the reticuloendothelial system has held its ground up to the present. He described the characteristic lesion called the Aschoff body, found in rheumatic carditis in 1904 and also coined the name 'endothelial system' in 1913.

Ascia A winding method of application of a bandage. Described by Hippocrates (460–377 BC).

Ascites [Greek: *askos*, leather bottle] Edema of the body was described by Paul of Aegina (625–690): 'the liver is greatly congealed, sometimes primarily, as when it has been inflamed, indurated or otherwise affected, or when from the sympathy of the other parts, the process of sanguification ceases and the affection is called dropsy'. He was probably referring to edema or dropsy from hepatic causes. He also accurately defined ascites as a great collection of fluid with a very small proportion of air between the peritoneum and the intestines. Hippocrates (460–377 BC) described the causes and treatment of dropsy due to disease of the spleen and the liver and advocated paracentesis abdominis as treatment.

Asclepiades of Bythnia (110–40 BC) *See Aesculapiades.*

Asclepios *See Aesculapius.*

Ascoli, Alberto (1877–1957) *See Bacillus anthracis.*

Ascorbic Acid [Greek: *askos*, bag + *karpos*, fruit] Vitamin C was isolated by S.S. Zilva in 1924 and later by Charles Glen King (1896–1988) and W.A. Waugh of Pittsburgh, in 1932. Its role in scurvy was identified by Albert Szent-Gryögyi (1893–1986) of Hungary in 1928. It was synthesized independently by Walter Norman Haworth (1833–1950) of England and Tadeus Richenstein (b 1897) of Switzerland in 1933 and Haworth named it ascorbic acid. A method of

determining small quantities in the blood was devised by Chester Jefferson Farmer and A. F. Abt in 1936. It was used to cure infantile scurvy by Leonard Gregory Parsons (1879–1950), a pediatrician at Birmingham Children's Hospital. *See scurvy.*

Aselius *See Aselli, Gaspar.*

Aselli, Gaspar (1581–1626) Italian physician and the discoverer of lacteals. He was born in Cremona and studied medicine at the University of Pavia where he was later professor of anatomy. While vivisecting a dog in 1622 he noticed milky filaments in its abdomen which he called white veins or 'lacteals'.

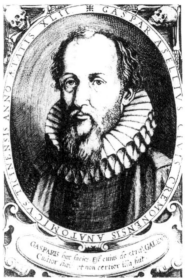

Gaspar Aselli (1581–1626). Courtesy of the National Library of Medicine

Asepsis *See antisepsis.*

Aseptic Meningitis Acute lymphocytic choriomeningitis. A clinical condition characterized by signs of meningeal irritation and sterile cerebrospinal fluid. Described by Arvid Johan Wallgren (1889–1973) of Stockholm in 1924. The causative virus was identified by Charles Armstrong (1886–1967) and Ralph Dougall Lillie (b 1896) in 1934. Several viruses including lymphocytic choreomeningitis virus, ECHO virus and coxsackie virus were later identified as causes.

Aseptic Necrosis Necrosis of the bone following fractures and other causes. Treated surgically by American orthopedic surgeon, Dallas Burton Phemister (1882–1951) of Pennsylvania in 1930.

Ashby, Henry (1846–1908) Born at Carlshalton, England and studied medicine at Guy's Hospital. He was physician to Manchester Children's Hospital and Victoria Hospital and contributed to the improvement of the health and living conditions of children in Manchester.

Ashby, Winifred (1879–1935) London-born American pathologist. She emigrated to the USA with her family in 1893 and graduated from Chicago University (1903) and Washington University, St Louis (1905). She later joined the Mayo Clinic and developed a special technique for estimating red cell survival and demonstrated for the first time the life span of the red blood cell.

Asherman Syndrome Intrauterine adhesions with amenorrhea. Described by a Czechoslovakian obstetrician, Joseph Asherman (1889–1968) in 1948. In 1844 James Young Simpson (1811–1870) observed a similar condition in which the uterine cavity was obliterated. Trauma due to curettage and cauterization was pointed out as a cause by Henry T. Ford in 1903.

Ashurbanipul King of Assyria (668–626 BC) Thousands of clay tablets related to the Assyrian culture were found in the remains of his royal library at Nineveh in the late 19th century. The cuneiform texts in these tablets were studied by Cambell Thompson in 1906 and they unlocked vast knowledge of historical, medical, astronomical, social, literary and religious aspects of ancient Assyria.

Ashwins Offspring of the sun and Hindu physicians of the god who united the 5th head of Brahma when it was severed by Bairava. According to Hindu mythology they also healed the paralyzed arm of the goddess Indra.

Asiatic Cholera *See comma bacillus, cholera.*

Askanazy, Max (1865–1940) German physician from Tübingen. The first to relate the findings of osteitis fibrosa cystica to parathyroid tumors in 1904.

Askew, Anthony (1722–1784) Westmoreland physician who graduated from Cambridge. He printed a small pamphlet which was meant to be a specimen of his intended book *Aeschylus,* which never materialized. He was also one of the holders of the famous gold headed cane and a great collector of books. He purchased many rare collections including the greater part of the collection of Richard Mead (1673–1754). After his death his collection was advertised as 'the best, rarest and most valuable collection of Latin and Greek books that were ever sold in England' and was auctioned. The Auction lasted for over 25 days in 1775 and realized a total of £4090 and 10 shillings.

Asklepios *See Aesculapius.*

Asoka (273–232 BC) Aryan king of India. A humanist who was initially a Hindu and converted to Buddhism. Records from rock inscriptions in Girnar, near Junagarh in India, show that he built many hospitals where people were given herbal treatment as well as physical therapy. He published 14 edicts, one setting out a system of medicine for humans and animals.

Asot *See antistreptolysin titer.*

Asparagine The first amino acid to be discovered. Obtained from asparagus by Louis Nicholas Vanquelin (1763–1829), a French analytical chemist, and Jean-Pierre Robiquet (1780–1840) in 1806.

Aspartamine A sweetener that is 200 times sweeter than sucrose. Prepared from phenylalanine and aspartic acid in 1965. It was approved as an artificial sweetener for soft drinks in 1983.

Aspartic Acid Prepared by Plisson in 1826 and isolated from a protein hydrosylate by H. Ritthausen in 1868.

Aspergilloma *See aspergillosis.*

Aspergillosis A description of human pulmonary aspergillosis was given by T. Sluyter in 1847 and this was followed by another by Rudolph Ludwig Carl Virchow (1821–1902) in 1856. The term was introduced by G. Fresenius in 1863. In 1894 G. Dieulafoy of France noted the increased incidence of pulmonary aspergillosis amongst French gaveurs de pigeons, or squab feeders, who acquired the disease from their habit of chewing nuts and forcing them down the gullet of the pigeons with their tongue. A differentiation between forms – allergic, saprophytic and septicemic – was made by Hinson and Plummer in 1952. Aspergilloma was differentiated from bronchopulmonary aspergillosis by F. Deve in 1938.

Asphyxia [Greek: *a*, without + *spuxis*, pulse] Pierre Flourens (1794–1867) produced asphyxia in experimental animals by identifying and inducing a lesion in the bilateral 'vital nodes' of the respiratory centers of the medulla oblongata in 1837. It was classified on the basis of its causes by Edmund Goodwin (1756–1829) as follows: asphyxia due to hanging or drowning as 'suffocationus'; asphyxia arising from inhalation of gases as 'metaphytica'; asphyxia caused by electricity and lightning as 'electrica'; and asphyxia from extreme cold as 'algida'. Local or regional asphyxia (ischemia) due to deprivation of blood was studied by Friedrich Julius Cohnheim (1839–1884) in 1872 and by Graham Brown in 1879.

Asplenium [Greek: *aspis*, shield] The fern was described as a destroyer of vermin by Dioscorides around AD 60. Since then its use as a worm treatment remained popular up to the 19th century.

Aspiration Biopsy The method was used for establishing the diagnosis of malignant infiltration of bone marrow by H.E. Martin and E.B. Ellis in 1930.

Aspirin *See acetyl salicylic acid.*

Aspirin Sensitivity Such sensitivity causing asthma, especially in patients with nasal polypi. Described by Frank Coke in *The Practitioner* in 1929. *See Francis triad.*

Assezat, Jules (1832–1876) French anthropologist who did pioneer studies on comparative craniology.

Assipu Priests Babylonian physicians around 2100 BC who later became lay physicians and were called 'Asu'. Their medicines or cures consisted of a mixture of animal sacrifice, attention to the influence of celestial bodies, demonology and drugs. Medical practice during their time was controlled by King Hammurabi's code. *See Hammurabi.*

Assman Sign 'Hilar dance' demonstrating the vigorous pulsation of the pulmonary arteries during fluoroscopic screening of patients with patent ductus arteriosus. Described by radiologist H. Assman of Leipzig in 1924.

Association of American Medical Colleges Founded in 1876, with 22 medical schools as members, to promote a high standard of medical school education. The association failed to exert its influence on many of the medical schools and had to suspend its activities from 1882 to 1889. In 1889 Sir William Osler (1849–1919), during his address at a meeting of the Medical and Chirurgical Faculty of the State of Maryland, made a strong appeal to correct the system of American medical education. Five medical schools, along with staff of the Johns Hopkins Hospital, issued a circular in 1890 appealing to all medical schools in the USA to send representatives to a conference for the purpose of organizing a unified curriculum for medical education. Following this meeting in 1890, a curriculum was introduced and the Association of American Medical Schools was reactivated to become the guardian of medical educational standards in America.

Astasia-abasia [Greek: *a*, without + *basis*, step] A fear of walking or standing, leading to a locomotor disturbance. Described by Paul Oscar Blocq (1860–1896) of Paris in 1888. *See Blocq disease.*

Astbury, William Thomas (1889–1961) Biochemist, born in Stoke-on-Trent, England, who studied at Cambridge with William Lawrence Bragg (1890–1971). He demonstrated the diffraction pattern of DNA in 1937, and used the method to classify proteins into different groups: keratin, myosin, elastin and collagen.

Asteroid Bodies Caused by precipitation of antigen–antibody complexes on the cell surface in sporotrichosis. First noted by Alfonso Splendore (1871–1953) in 1908.

Asthenia or aesthenia [Greek: *a*, without + *sthenos*, strength] Condition produced by lack of stimulation and nervous weakness, described by John Brown (1735–1788), a physician from Berwickshire, England. His system of medicine known as Brunonian theory, advocated the use of stimulants for treatment. The term was used to describe one of the delayed symptoms noted in animals after experimental removal of the cerebellum by Luigi Luciani (1840–1919), professor of physiology at Florence in 1891. Eugene Bouchat (1818–1891) recognized the clinical state of nervous exhaustion and asthenia, which he described as 'nervosisme' in 1860. The concept of asthenia was established by George Miller Beard (1839–1883) in 1869. *See chronic fatigue syndrome.*

Asthma Term is derived from the Greek for 'panting attack'. The symptoms were described in the Ebers papyrus from BC 1600. Aretaeus, a physician who lived around AD 100, gave a description in his work, translated into Latin in 1554. *Tractus contra Passionem Asmatis* was written by a Jewish physician, Maimonides, in the 12th century. English physician, John Floyer (1649–1734) wrote a treatise in 1698 in which he described perfumes or scents as precipitating causes. Henry Hyde Salter (1823–1871) in 1868 pointed out that contact with animals could cause it in *On Asthma, its Pathology and Treatment.* The hereditary predisposition was mentioned by William Cullen (1784), Thomas Ryan (1698), and William Davidson (1795). An important study of the mechanism was done by Franz Daniel Reissensen (1773–1828) of Strasbourg in 1808. He demonstrated contraction of the smooth muscles in the walls of the smallest bronchial tubes. The contractility of bronchial tubes under various stimuli was shown by Charles James Blasius Williams (1805–1889), who published his findings in *Diseases of the Chest* in 1840. John Elliotson (1791–1868), professor of medicine at University College, London described hay fever and asthma and suggested pollen as a precipitating cause in 1831. Skin reaction to grass pollen in hay fever patients was shown by Manchester physician, Charles Blackely (1820–1900) in 1873. The spirometer to measure lung functions was introduced by John Hutchison (1811–1861) in 1846 and the vitalograph came into use in 1954.The use of the peak flow meter for clinical monitoring started around 1960. Bronchoscopy was used in the management of asthma by Franz Nowotny (1872–1925) in 1907. The antispasmodic effect of theophylline on bronchial smooth muscles was demonstrated on by David Israel Macht (1882–1961) in 1921. Epinephrine (adrenaline) was used in asthma in the form of an inhaler by Percy William Leopold Camp (1877–1956) in 1929 and subcutaneous injections came into use later. Specific receptors in the bronchi were identified in 1948, and later led to the development of b² agonists. Sodium cromoglycate (Intal) was obtained from the plant *Ammi visnaga*, which had been used for centuries for the treatment of asthma, by British physician of Armenian origin, Roger Edward Collingwood Altounyan (1922–1987), in 1967. He also developed the spinhaler based on aerodynamic principles for delivery to the lungs. Up to 1950 some physicians used gold therapy for treatment. Steroids were commenced as standard treatment in 1954. *See bronchospasm, bronchial lavage.*

Astigmatism [Greek: *a*, without + *stigma*, point] Distortion of vision due to irregular refraction was described by English physician Thomas Young (1773–1829) in *On the Mechanism of Eye*, published in 1801. William Whewell of Trinity College, Cambridge named it 'astigmatism', since the retina was not able to identify a definite point or spot, but saw it as an oval or circle. Astronomer Sir George Biddle Airy (1801–1892), who himself suffered from astigmatism, corrected it using a lens in 1824. The cause due to the uneven nature of the lens of the eye was explained in 1864 by Dutch ophthalmologist, Franciscus Cornelis (1818–1889) of Utrecht. Modern spectacles to correct it were developed by Swedish professor and inventor of the slit lamp, Alvar Gullstrand (1862–1930) in the early 1900s.

Astigmometer Measures the degree of astigmatism. Invented by Louis Emile Javal (1839–1907) in 1867.

Aston, Francis William (1877–1945) English physicist who improved the apparatus to study isotopes in 1924. He also designed a mass spectrograph in 1919 with which he established the isotopic nature of neon and 21 other naturally occurring isotopes.

Astragalus [Greek: *astragalos*, a dye] Term used in Homer's *Iliad* to denote the cervical vertebrae which, with the arches removed, were used for playing dice.

Astrocytes [Greek: *astron*, star + *kytos*, hollow vessel] In nervous tissue, discovered by German physician, Otto Friedrich Carl Deiters (1834–1863) in 1863.

Astruc, Jean (1684–1766) French physician from Sauves in Languedoc who graduated from Montpellier. He had a successful practice in Paris and was later professor there. He wrote a systematic treatises on syphilis, *De Morbis Veneris libri sex* in 1736. He considered that it originated in America and spread to Europe in 1493. His other works include *On the Inoculation of Small Pox, Origine de la Peste, De Mortu musculare, A Treatise on Therapeutics* and *The Diseases of Women*. He was physician to the King of Poland in 1743.

Astrup Technique Micromethod of measuring acid–base status in the blood devised by Poulle Astroup (b 1915) in 1953.

Asturian Leprosy or pellagra *See Asturian rose.*

Asturian Rose or pellagra Noted in ancient Asturia and some other parts of Spain by Spanish physician Gasper Casal (1679–1759), who described it as *mal de la rosa* in 1735.

Astwood, Edwin Bennet (1909–1976) *See antithyroid drugs.*

Asylum The Arabs were the first to show a more humane approach to the mentally ill. They built asylums in Morocco, Damascus and Baghdad around AD 800. A European hospital devoted entirely to the care of the insane was built in Valencia, Spain, in 1409. One of the oldest hospitals in England, the Hospital of St Mary of Bethlehem, became an asylum for the mentally ill in 1402. During the Middle Ages patients were discharged to the community under the care of relatives and returned to the hospital when needed. Though the care of the mentally ill was sympathetic during this period, the attitude towards them changed during the 15th century and they were regarded as witches and devils. Their persecution continued up to the early 19th century. Overall care deteriorated across Europe in the 18th and 19th centuries. Bethlehem Hospital became a place to which the mentally ill were condemned, rather than a place of care. Patients were chained, held behind bars and exhibited to the public, often for a fee. The name of the hospital led to the expression 'bedlam'. Conditions were very much the same in France at Bicêtre and Salpêtrière Hospitals. Vincenzo Chiarugi (1739–1820) was one of the first in Europe to prescribe regulations for humane treatment in asylums in 1789. Around the same time, Phillipe Pinel (1745–1825), a neuropsychiatrist at the Bicêtre, unchained them. He proposed a treatable underlying physical cause for mental illness. The Retreat for Insane at York was founded by William Tuke (1732–1822), a British philanthropist and reformer of the care of the mentally ill in England. *See Holloway Sanatorium, Bethlehem Hospital, Aversa.*

Ataractic Modern tranquilizers to relieve emotional stress in humans. Term derived from the Greek *ataraxia*, which means lack of perturbation, or peace of mind. Ataraxia is the essential goal in the two Greek philosophical philosophies of Stoicism and Epicureanism. *See Stoics, Epicurean, tranquilizer.*

Ataralgesia Term proposed by J.T. Hayward-Butt in 1957 to denote a process of induction of general analgesia as opposed to general anesthesia.

Ataraxia *See ataractic.*

Atavism [Latin: *atavus*, ancestor] The apparent inheritance of a characteristic from a remote ancestor due to chance recombination of genes. Explained on Mendelian principles by American, Charles Benedict Davenport (1866–1944) in 1910. He also provided strong evidence for the hereditary nature of epilepsy, with David Fairchild Weeks (1874–1829) in 1911.

Ataxia [Greek: *a*, without + *taxis*, order] One of the delayed symptoms in animals after experimental removal of the cerebellum. Described by Luigi Luciani (1840–1919), professor of physiology at Florence in 1891. The first real advance was made by the neurologist Moritz Heinrich Romberg (1795–1873) of Berlin who published his treatise on nervous diseases in 1840. *See locomotor ataxia, Friedrich ataxia.*

Atebrine or mepacrine Acridine derivative produced by H. Mauss and F. Mietzsch of Germany in 1932. It was found to be superior to quinine in treatment and prevention of malaria, owing to its lower toxicity and was used extensively during World War ll. It was replaced by proguanil in 1945. *See antimalarials.*

Atelectasis [Greek: *ateles*, imperfect or unfinished] Partial collapse of the lung during the post-operative period. Described in detail by William Tennant Gairdner (1824–1907) of Glasgow in 1850.

Atharva-Veda One of the earliest systems of medicine practiced by the ancient Hindus of India. It contains spells, incantations and magic with reference to diseases and health. *See Ayurvedic medicine.*

Athenaeus A physician from Sicily and contemporary of Pliny (AD 23–79). He postulated that disease first attacked the animated spirit in the body. He wrote *The Deipnosophists* in 15 books, which contained a most exhaustive miscellany of anecdotes, quotations, customs and practice.

Atheroma [Greek: *athara*, porridge or groates] Term used by Galen (129–200) to denote a kind of fatty tumor, for which

he advocated surgery. Aulus Cornelius Celsus (25 BC– AD 50) and Paul of Aegina (625–690) also used the term to denote similar tumors. It was adopted to denote fatty degenerative lesions in the arteries by Albrecht von Haller (1708–1777), a Swiss physiologist, in 1755. *See atherosclerosis.*

Atherosclerosis Evidence has frequently been found in Egyptian mummies. The term 'atheroma' was adopted to denote fatty degenerative lesions in the arteries by Albrecht von Haller (1708–1777), a Swiss physiologist, in 1755. Jean George C.F. Martin Lobstein (1777–1835) used the term 'arteriosclerosis' in 1833. A classic description was given by Giovanni Battista Morgagni (1682–1771) on a 90-year-old woman in 1761. Felix Jacob Marchand (1846–1928) introduced the term in the modern sense in 1904. The key to its pathogenesis was provided by A.I. Ignatovski of the Russian Imperial Military Academy, who demonstrated in 1908 that rabbits, when fed with milk and egg yolk, developed it. The modern theory of pathogenesis was initiated in 1946 by J.B. Duguid who proposed that the atheromatous plaques were essentially mural thrombi that became incorporated into the vessel wall. His *Pathogenesis of Arteriosclerosis* was published in 1949. The stage of platelet deposition in atherogenesis was studied by L.A. Harker and colleagues in 1981. This later led to the use of antiplatelet agents. *See coronary artery disease.*

Athetosis [Greek: *athetos*, without fixed position] Hammond disease, associated with failure to maintain a fixed posture owing to abnormal involuntary movements. Described by American neurologist, William Alexander Hammond (1828–1900) in 1872. Victor Horsley (1857–1916), a neurosurgeon, abolished athetosis in a male patient in 1909 by removing a part of the precentral cortex. Athetosis arising out of basal ganglionic lesions of the brain was studied by Roy Richard Grinker of America in 1943 and by Samuel Alexander Kinnier Wilson (1878–1937) of King's College Hospital London, who proposed that the choreoathetoid movements originated from the cerebral cortex.

Athletics [Greek: *athleein*, to compete] Bronze statues and paintings of athletes by the Greeks dating back to around 1500 BC reveal their awareness of the importance of athletics in health. *See sports medicine.*

Athymia [Greek: *a*, negative or without + *thyreos*, shield] A term for dejection of the spirit, in psychiatry.

Atisar Term used in the Ayur-Veda of the Brahmins to refer to dysentery. *See dysentery.*

Atlas [Greek: *atlao*, I endure or sustain] In Greek mythology, a Titan who had the weight of the world on his shoulders.

The first vertebra, called rotos spondylos by Galen (129–200), was renamed the 'atlas' by Andreas Vesalius (1514–1564) in 1540. The word was used to describe a book of maps by Flemish geographer, Gerardus Mercator (1512–1594) in 1585. His book, which had a cover with a drawing of the Titan Atlas holding a globe on his shoulders, was completed by his son after his death. The name atlas for mainly illustrative medical books became popular in the latter half of the 19th century.

Atlee, Washington Lemuel (1808–1878) Surgeon in Pennsylvania who was a pioneer in the surgical treatment of uterine fibroids. He firmly established the place for ovariotomy by performing over 400 such operations.

Atmosphere The word is derived from the Greek term meaning a body of vapor in a spherical form. Air was regarded as an element until 1674, when English physician, John Mayhow (1641–1679) demonstrated that if a substance is burnt in an enclosed vessel the volume diminished and combustion stopped. Knowledge was advanced by Swedish apothecary and chemist, Carl Wilhelm Scheele (1742–1786). In the latter half of the 19th century experiments from balloons contributed significantly to its study.

Atmospheric Pressure Otto Guericke (1602–1686), the Mayor of Magdeburg in Germany and inventor of the air pump, demonstrated the effects of atmospheric pressure at the Court of the Emperor and devised a method of measuring it in 1657. The effect of atmospheric pressure on blood and circulation at high altitude was studied by Sommerbrodt in 1887. *See barometer.*

Atomic Disintegration A hypothesis that radioactive elements made of complex particles undergo spontaneous changes or disintegration and discharge high velocity negatively charged electrons or beta rays and positively charged particles or alpha rays. Suggested by Ernest Rutherford (1871–1937) and Frederick Soddy (1877–1965) in 1902.

Atomic Radiation The atomic bomb was as a result of chance discovery in 1938 by a group of Germans, Otto Hahn (1879–1968), Lise Meitner (1878–1968) and Fritz Strassman, that uranium when bombarded with neutrons was capable of breaking down into other elements with a release of energy. Meitner escaped from the Nazis and conveyed the possibility of the Germans making the bomb to the Danish physicist, Niels Bohr (1885–1962) who went to America to work on the atomic project at Princeton. A nuclear reactor was built by Italian scientist, Enrico Fermi (1901–1954) and Leo Szilard (1898–1964) of Chicago in 1942. The first trial of the bomb was carried out on 16th July 1945 in New Mexico. Twenty days later it was dropped on Hiroshima and it turned out to be 10 times more destructive than expected. A second bomb was dropped on Nagasaki on 6 August 1945. The devastating effect of atomic radiation became apparent to the world after these bombs. *See Chernobyl nuclear accident.*

Atomic Structure The Greek philosophers Democritus (460–360 BC) and his master Leucippus of the school of Abdera (500 BC) stated that all things in nature were made of small particles. These particles were named 'atoms' by Leucippus which means 'not to be cut'. The Roman poet, Lucretius (98–55 BC) stated 'matter does not cohere inseparably massed together, but is made of first beginning of things'. Ancient Sanskrit writings also describe atom as indivisible matter. Joseph Louis Proust (1754–1824) in 1794 proposed the Law of Multiple Proportions related to the combining properties of the atoms. John Dalton (1766–1844), the father of atomic theory, determined the atomic weight of various elements in 1808. J.W. Nicholson, professor of mathematics at King's College London calculated the wavelengths of spectral lines from a model of an emitting atom in 1911. The first constructive hypothesis that led to the modern theory of atomic structure was proposed by the English physicist Ernest Rutherford (1871–1937) in the same year. He conceived the idea of an atom as a miniature replica of our solar system with the sun as the positively charged central nucleus and the planets as the electrons. Henry Gwyn-Jeffreys Mosley (1887–1915), a student of Rutherford, showed that the number of positive charges on the nucleus is equal to its atomic number, in 1913. Two theories existed up to 1950 to explain the atomic nucleus: that the nuclear particles were arranged in concentric shells; and that the nucleus was analogous to a liquid drop. Both these theories were explained through the same model by American physicist James Leo Rainwater (b 1917) of Idaho in the early 1950s.

Atomic Theory The law of constant or definite proportions, fundamental to chemistry, states that different atoms always combined in definite proportions to form a compound. Proposed by John Dalton (1766–1844) in 1803 and published in 1807. The theory of atomic structure was proposed by Ernest Rutherford (1871–1937) at the Manchester Literary and Philosophical Society on May 7 1911. *See atomic structure.*

Atomic Weight English chemist, John Dalton (1766–1844) determined the atomic weight of many elements. Johann Wolfgang Dobereiner (1780–1849), a German professor of chemistry in Jena, established a relationship of atomic weights which later formed the basis for Menderleff periodic tables. Berzelius (1779–1848) determined atomic weights of many elements in 1826 and proposed the system of representing elements by the Latin letter(s) of their name. John Alexander Reina Newlands (1837–1898), a London chemist, arranged the elements in order of their atomic weights and recognized the similarity between every eighth element. A method of more accurately determining them was devised by American chemist and Harvard graduate, Theodore William Richards (1868–1928) of Pennsylvania around 1900. He was awarded the Nobel Prize for his work in 1914.

Atonia [Greek: *a*, without + tone] Term used in 1891 by Luigi Luciani (1840–1919), professor of physiology in Florence, to describe one of the delayed symptoms in animals noted after experimental removal of the cerebellum.

Atopy [Greek: *atopos*, out of place] Term coined by Arthur F. Coca of Cornell University to denote a form of hypersensitivity. He named antibodies in serum of atopic individuals as 'atopic reaginins'. The presence of antibodies in the blood of atopic or allergic individuals was shown by Otto Carl Willy Prausnitz (1876–1973), a British immunologist of German origin, and Heinz Küstner, in 1921. Prausnitz transferred the fish hypersensitivity experienced by his partner Küstner to his own skin by a method of sensitization. This hypersensitive skin reaction was named Prausnitz–Küstner reaction, and was used to diagnose atopic hypersensitivity.

ATP *See adenosine triphosphate.*

Atrial Fibrillation or auricular fibrillation [Latin: *atria*, antechambers + *fibrilla*, small fiber] Irregular pulse in mitral stenosis, observed by Robert Adams (1791–1875) in 1827 and by James Hope (1801–1841) in 1839. The first pulse tracing of atrial fibrillation was published by Etienne Jules Marey (1830–1904) in 1863. Fibrillar contractions of the atrium were noticed *in vivo* in a dog by A. Vulpian in 1873. The irregular contractions of the atria and ventricles of the heart were also noted by John Alexander MacWilliam (1857–1937) of London in 1887. Sir James Mackenzie (1853–1925), with the help of his polygraph, noted the disappearance of waves in veins produced by the contracting auricle in 1897. He named this auricular paralysis in 1902. He also studied the symptomatology and described the disappearance of the presystolic murmur, later named auricular fibrillation by Thomas Lewis (1881–1945), in 1909. In the same year, Carl Julius Rothberger (b-1871) of Germany and Heinrich Winterberg (1867–1929) of Austria, independently demonstrated atrial fibrillation in

humans. A series of investigations performed on normal hearts by Lewis from 1909 to 1916 led to the explanation of the QRST complexes as a sequential spread of electrical excitation over different parts of the atria and ventricles. He traced the excitation from the sinoauricular node down the bundle of His to the Purkinje fibers. On the basis of these findings, he studied the electrical and visible contractile changes that occurred in the auricle during electrically induced atrial fibrillation in animal hearts. Direct evidence in an exposed diseased heart of a horse was noted by him in 1912. He also recognized ventricular fibrillation and its incompatibility with life.

Atrial Flutter *See auricular flutter.*

Atrial Natriuretic Factor The presence of secretory granules in the atrium of the heart of guinea pigs was observed by B. Kisch in 1956. These were suggested to be associated with changes in the volume of body fluid by J.P. Marie, H. Guillemot and P.Y. Hatt in 1976. The potential natriuretic response to atrial myocardial extract in the rates was demon-strated by A.J. de Bold and co-workers in 1981.

Atrial Septal Defect The earliest mention of the foramen ovale was made by Galen (129–200), who noticed that the hole in the auricular septum contained a valve that closed at birth. Giulio Cesare Aranzi (1520–1589) described the foramen ovale in 1557 and Leonardo Bottallo (1530–1588) described it in 1564 and named it Bottallo foramen. An illustration was given by Andre du Laurens (1558–1609) in 1599. The passage of blood through it into the left ventricle in the fetus was noted by William Harvey (1578–1657) and John Baptiste Senac (1693–1770) recognized the persistence of it in adult life in 1745. An account of the different types of atrial septal defect was given by Karl Rokintansky (1804–1878) in 1875. The clinical picture was given by René Lutembacher (b 1884) in 1916, Maude Elizabeth Semour Abbot (1869–1940) of Canada in 1926 and Helen Brooke Taussig (1898–1986) of Johns Hopkins in 1938. An experimental attempt to repair an atrial septal defect in an animal was made by Roy Cohn of San Francisco Hospital in 1947 but, although his method was successful in dogs, he never tried it in humans. A year later, Gordon Murray of Toronto performed the correction in a 12-year-old girl, but unfortunately her prognosis was limited by a left-to-right shunt leading to pulmonary hypertension. Attempts at perfecting the method continued and several people, including Forest Dodrill (1949), P. Marion (1950) and Charles Bailey contributed towards improvement. Robert Edward Gross (1905–1988) of Boston later demonstrated some impressive results with his surgical technique for treating it in 1952.

Atrial Tachycardia Paroxysmal atrial tachycardia was noted by Leon Bouveret (1851–1929) in 1889 and named. Electrocardiographic changes were recognized by Sir Thomas Lewis (1881–1945) in 1909 and it was described in more detail by P.S. Barker and colleagues in 1943. Its occurrence in digitalis toxicity was pointed out by G.R. Herrmann in 1944 and his observation was confirmed by Bernard Lown and co-workers in 1958. Lown–Ganong–Levine syndrome, consisting of shortened PR interval and a normal QRS on ECG, associated with paroxysmal atrial tachycardia was described by Lown, W.F. Ganong and Samuel A. Levine in 1952. *See Wolf–Parkinson–White syndrome.*

Atrioventricular Anomalous Conduction An electrocardiogram showing a short PR interval and a prolonged QRS complex indicative of anomalous conduction. First published by Frank Norman Wilson (1890–1952) in 1915. Similar electrocardiographic changes were studied and explained by Louis Wolff (b 1898), Sir John Parkinson (1885– 1976) and Paul Dudley White (1886–1973) in 1930, and it was named Wolf–Parkinson–White syndrome. The existence of an abnormal pathway which explained the anomalous conduction was demonstrated by Francis Clark Wood (b 1901), Charles Christian Wolferth (1887–1965) and G.D. Geckler in 1943. The name 'Bundle of Kent' was given in honor of Albert Frank Stanley Kent (1863–1958) who described the anomalous tissue in an animal heart in 1893.

Atrioventricular Bundle (bundle of His) Bundle of the conducting system of the heart, independently described by Albert Frank Stanley Kent (1863–1958) of Wiltshire, England and Wilhelm His, Junior (1863–1934) of Germany, in 1893. The first recording of electrical activity of it in a dog was made by J. Alanis, H. Gonzalez and E. Lopez in 1958. Attempts to record this in humans were made by Brian Hoffmann in 1959. The catheter technique for recording electrical activity was developed by Benjamin Scherlag at Columbia University in 1969.

Atrioventricular Node Node of the conducting system of the heart discovered by a Japanese anatomist and pupil of Karl Albert Ludwig Aschoff (1866–1942), Sunao Tawara (1873–1952), while he was working in Germany in 1906.

Atriplicism A disease in North China and Beijing caused by poisoning from the plant *Atriplex littoralis*. Described by Matignon in 1898.

Atrium Latin term for the front hall of a Roman house. The atrial chamber of the heart derives its name from this.

Atromid or clofibrate One of the first cholesterol reducing drugs. Developed by Thorpe and Waring in 1962. An acute muscular syndrome associated with the intake of this drug was recognized by T. Langer and R.I. Levy in 1968.

Atropa belladonna (Syn. deadly nightshade) [Greek: *Atropos*, one of the Fates, who was supposed to cut the thread of life; Italian: *belladonna*, fair lady] Extracts of the leaves were used by a physician and naturalist at Zurich, Conrad Gesner (1516–1565), to relieve pain in 1540 and it was introduced into the London pharmacopoeia in 1809. It was employed in ophthalmic surgery by A.H. Reimarus (1729–1814) of Hamburg. An outbreak of belladonna poisoning occurred in London when its berries were sold as edible fruit by ignorant fruit dealers in 1846. *See Belladonna, atropine.*

Atrophy [Greek: *a*, without + *trophe*, to nourish] Wasting through lack of nourishment.

Atropine An alkaloid obtained from *Atropa belladonna*. Albert von Bezold (1836–1868) of Leipzig demonstrated that atropine in small doses blocked the vagal activity of the heart, thereby increasing heart rate. The antisalivary effects were demonstrated by Rudolf Peter Heinrich Heidenhain (1834–1897) in 1872. *See Atropa belladonna.*

Atwater, O. Wilber (1844–1907) American physicist who constructed a calorimeter to measure heat production, oxygen consumption and carbon dioxide elimination in 1892.

Atypical Pneumonia An 'unusual form of bronchopneumonia' or atypical pneumonia with cold agglutinins. Studied by Mildred Clark Clough (b 1888) and R.M. Richter of Johns Hopkins Hospital in 1918. Outbreaks of sporadic cases of pneumonia different from pneumococcal pneumonia or bronchopneumonia were noted in England by A.M. Gill in 1938. Monroe Davis Eaton (b 1904), G. Meiklejohn and W.J. van Henrick demonstrated the transferability of the agent causing atypical pneumonia in experimental animals in 1944. This was later named the Eaton agent. The mycoplasma which caused it was isolated by Louis Diennes and Geoffrey Edsall in 1937.

Aubert, Albert or James (d 1586) A physician at Lausanne who wrote *Libellus de Peste, Des Natures et Complexions des Hommes, De Metallorum ortu et causis* and other works.

Aubrey, John (1626–1697) Wiltshire physician and a contemporary of Oxford historian Anthony Wood. His fascination with his fellow men and their achievements prompted him to write several biographical works including one of William Harvey (1578–1657).

Aubry, John Francis French physician who wrote a book on ancient medical writers and their practice, *Les Oracles de Cos,* published in Paris in 1775.

Audiology [Latin: *audire*, to hear] A comparative study of the organs of hearing in humans and other animals was made by Antonio Scarpa (1747–1832) in 1789. The mechanism of hearing based on resonance, previously mentioned by Albrecht von Haller (1708–1777), was analyzed and explained by Hermann Ludwig F. von Helmholtz (1821–1894) in 1863. The Weber test for hearing was introduced by Ernest Heinrich Weber (1795–1878) in 1843 and its clinical significance was demonstrated by his pupil, Eduard Schmalz (1801–1871) in 1846. The Rinnie test, using a tuning fork to differentiate between sensorimotor deafness and conduction deafness, was devised by German otologist, Heinrich Adolf Rinnie (1819–1863) in 1855. The transmission of sound through the cranial bones was used in diagnosis of the diseases of the ear by August Lucae (1835–1911) in 1870. A modern study of the ear and the mechanisms by which it analyses and transmits sound to the brain was made in 1947 by Georg von Bekesy (1899–1972), Hungarian-born American physiologist. He published his *Hearing* in 1960. *See audiometer.*

Audiometer [Latin: *audire*, to hear; Greek: *metron*, measure] An oscillator with amplified connections to ear-phones constructed to measure the power of hearing in humans by David E. Hughes in 1879. An earlier version was devised by Arthur Hartmann (1849–1931) in 1878.

Audiometry *See audiology, audiometer.*

Audouin, Jean Victor (1797–1841) Entomologist and naturalist at Paris Natural History Museum who worked on silkworm disease. The fungus *Microsporum audouini* was named after him by another mycologist, David Gruby (1810–1898), in 1843.

Auenbrugger, Joseph Leopold (1722–1809) The son of an innkeeper in Vienna who learned the art of percussion by tapping wine in casks to detect the contents. He became physician in chief to the Hospital of Holy Trinity in Vienna and developed the clinical method of examination of the chest by percussion in 1751. He described it in *Inventum Novum* published in 1761. His findings were discarded by his contemporaries until Jean Nicolas Covisart (1755–1821) revived it and gave the credit to Auenbrugger in 1808.

Auerbach, Charlotte (b 1899) A pioneer and colleague of Hermann Müller (1890–1967) in the study of mutation. Born at Krefeld in Germany and educated in Berlin. In 1933 she emigrated to Edinburgh, where she worked with Müller and became a lecturer in genetics in 1947. She discovered chemical mutagenesis during her work on the effects of mustard gas on *Drosophila*.

Auerbach Plexus A network of autonomic nerve fibers in the intestinal wall. Described in 1862 by Leopold Auerbach (1828–1897), professor of neuropathology at Breslau. Histological changes of the plexus in achalasia were described by G. W. Rake in 1926.

Aufrecht Disease Infectious jaundice and changes in the parenchyma of the liver and kidneys. Described by German physician, Emmanuel Aufrecht (1844–1933).

Aujeszky Disease (Syn. pseudorabies, infectious bulbar palsy) An acute infection of the central nervous system of obscure etiology, affecting cats, horses, cattle, goats, pigs and sheep. Described by A. Aujeszky in 1902.

Aura Seminalis During the time of Galen (129–200) and Aristotle (384–322 BC) fertilization of the ovum was thought to take place by a mystic process called 'aura seminalis'. It was believed that the ovum was complete in itself and was capable of producing an embryo after a suitable stimulus was received.

Aura Warning signs before an attack of epilepsy. Term derived from the Greek word for 'breeze'. It was used by a Roman youth to explain his spreading sensation of epilepsy to the Roman physician Galen (129–200).

Aurelius, Anselmus A chief physician to the Duke of Mantua in the 16th century. He published a book on old age, *Gerocomice sive de fenum regimine,* in 1606.

Aurelius, Augustinius (354–430) Also known as St Augustine. Born in North Africa and studied rhetoric at Carthage and became a teacher in Milan. His *Confessions* was a brilliant work on introspective psychiatry and is considered one of the earliest contributions on self analysis based on psychological principles. He is regarded by some historians as the greatest introspective psychiatrist before Sigmund Freud (1856–1939). He became a priest and later a bishop in his home town of Tagaste.

Aurelius, Caelius *See Caelius Aurelianus.*

Aurelius, Markus Emperor of Rome and a victim of the plague in AD 180. Being a wise man and good father, he refused to see his son during his last 7 days of illness, lest he should transmit it to him.

Aureomycin [Latin: *aurum*, gold; Greek: *mykes*, fungus] Chlortetracycline, the first tetracycline antibiotic. Discovered in 1944 by Benjamin Minge Duggar (b 1872) of Wisconsin, in a fungal culture from a Missouri farmyard.

Auricle [Latin: *auricula*, little ear] Term used by Andreas Vesalius (1514–1564) to refer to the two small chambers of the heart.

Auricular Fibrillation *See atrial fibrillation.*

Auricular Flutter [Latin: *auricle*, ear flap] Noted and named by William Thomas Ritchie (1873–1945) of Edinburgh in 1905. Sir James Mackenzie (1853–1925) and Sir Thomas Lewis (1881–1945) advocated digoxin in treatment. The first electrocardiogram showing it was published by Willem Einthoven (1860–1927) in 1906. Ritchie later wrote a classic monograph on it in 1914.

Auricular Septal Defect *See atrial septal defect.*

Auriculoventricular Bundle *See atrioventricular bundle.*

Aurignac Caves Discovered in 1860 in the Haute Garonne in the Pyrenees by a French paleontologist, Edouard Armand Isidore Lartet (1801–1871) and Henry Christy. Several Neolithic skeletons from around 15,000 BC were found, along with evidence of their culture, the Aurignacian.

Aurignacian Man Early *Homo sapiens* around 15,000 to 20,000 BC. *See Aurignac caves.*

Aurum [Latin: gold] The chemical symbol for gold, Au, was proposed by Berzelius (1779–1848) in 1826. *See gold.*

Auscultation [Latin: *auris*, ear + *cult*, used or exercised] Method of examination of the chest discovered by René Theophile Laënnec (1781–1826) of Brittany, France in 1819. He studied medicine in Paris under Jean Nicholas Corvisart (1755–1821) and Guillaume Dupuytren (1777–1835). While working as a physician at the Necker Hospital, he was consulted by a young woman whose age and gender prevented him from putting his ear against her chest wall as a part of his clinical examination. However, his previous observation that a pin scratched at one end of a piece of wood could be heard at the other end by applying one's ear to it inspired him to roll a piece of paper and hold it against the chest wall of the patient and listen. He published his treatise on auscultation in 1819. His initial stethoscope was made out of wood, and paved the way for the flexible tube stethoscope invented by Caspar Wistar Pennock of America in 1839. Thomas Davies, a physician from Wales who studied under Laënnec at the Necker Hospital in Paris, introduced the method in England. His *Lectures on the Lungs and Diseases of the Heart* was published in 1835. An English physician who used the stethoscope in clinical medicine around the same time was John Elliotson (1791–1868), professor of surgery at the University of London. Its application to the brachial artery to determine diastolic pressure, with the help of the sphygmomanometer, was introduced by Russian physician, Nikolai Sergeievich Korotkov (1874–1920).

Austin Flint Murmur Apical mid-diastolic or presystolic functional murmur originating from the mitral valve in patients with aortic stenosis. Described by New York physician, Austin Flint (1812–1886), in 1862. He was born in Petersham, Massachusetts and graduated from Harvard in 1832. He helped to establish the Buffalo Medical College, where he later became professor of medicine.

Austin Moore Prosthesis Made of metal for hip arthroplasty. Devised by Austin T. Moore (1899–1963) of America in 1957.

Australasian Medical Gazette Published in Sydney as the official journal of the Australian branches of the British Medical Association in 1881. It merged with the *Australian Medical Journal* to become the *Medical Journal of Australia* in 1914.

Australia Antigen A previously unknown lipoprotein detected in 1964 in the serum of Australian Aborigines by New York biochemist, Baruch Bernard Samuel Blumberg (b 1925) during his search for genetic markers in the sera of people belonging to different races. Four years later, Alfred M. Prince of the New York Blood Center observed the same lipoprotein specifically in patients with hepatitis B and renamed it the hepatitis B surface antigen in 1968.

Australian Aborigines They were familiar with herbal remedies including purgatives, emetics, narcotics, aphrodisiacs and aromatics. They practiced cupping and blood letting, partly by mouth suction and partly using simple instruments such as bones and horns. They stitched small wounds with thorns and opened abscesses with sharp objects. The Aborigines of the Darling River in New South Wales believed that sickness was caused by an enemy who used a charm called *yountoo,* a piece of bone wrapped in dried flesh from a deceased friend, or *molee,* a piece of white quartz used in ceremonies. To effect a cure the doctor had to suck out the piece of bone or cast the *molee* into water. A tribe of Australian Aborigines known as Kalkadoona, adjoining the Mygoodano tribes, used flint knives to operate on the urethra.

Australian Medical Journal Published in 1846 in Sydney, discontinued and restarted in Melbourne in 1854. It continued under different titles for the next 54 years and merged into the *Medical Journal of Australia* in 1914.

Australopithecus afarensis Fossils of previously unknown hominid species, nearly 4 million years old, were found in the Afar Triangle in Ethiopia by an American anthropologist, Donald Carl Johanson (b 1943) in 1972. His findings included the remains of 13 individuals, a female was nicknamed Lucy. Another jaw bone of *Australopithecus afarensis* was found by Andrew Hill in Kenya in 1984 and this appears to be a part of one of the oldest skulls, dating back 5 million years.

Australopithecus africanus The suspected missing link in evolution of man was found by Arthur Dart (1893–1988) in the west of the Rift Valley in South Africa in 1925. The owner of the skull was nicknamed Abel. Since this finding, eight other *Australopithecus* remains have been found.

Autism [Greek: *autos*, by itself] Described as the mental life of a patient who is kept apart from the outside world, by Paul Eugene Bleuler (1857–1939) in his essay on *Schizophrenias*, in 1910. He explained it as a psychotic thought process that was not influenced by reality and did not follow normal logic. The term was used by American psychiatrist, Leo Kanner in *Autistic Disturbances of Affective Contact*, published in 1943. He also published a textbook, *Child Psychiatry* in 1935.

Autoclave [Greek: *autos*, by itself] Following Louis Pasteur's (1822–1895) research on methods of killing bacteria, his pupil Charles Chamberland (1851–1908) devised the pressure steam sterilizer or autoclave in 1880, based on the principle of Papin's steam digester . The method was included in the official *British Pharmacopoeia* in 1930.

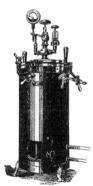

Autoclave using steam under pressure for sterilization. Albert Schneider, *Pharmaceutical Bacteriology* (1912). Blakiston, Philadelphia

Autoerasty [Greek: *autos*, by itself + *erastikos*, relating to love] Another term for narcissism or abnormal self love. *See narcissism.*

Autohemotherapy Practiced as treatment for a variety of ailments including blackwater fever, skin conditions and syphilis, until the early 20th century. It involves repeated withdrawal of 5–10 ml of blood and injecting it back subcutaneously or intramuscularly into the same patient for a few days. It was supposed to impart a form of protein shock to the patient.

Autoimmune Disease [Latin: *autos*, self + *immunis*, free] Paroxysmal hemoglobinuria was shown to be due to an autoimmune disease by the presence of autoantibodies by Julius Donath (1870–1950) and Carl Landsteiner (1868–1943) in 1903. An example of experimental induction of autoimmune disease was shown by Thomas Milton Rivers (1888–1962) and Francis F. Schwentker of the Rockefeller Institute in 1940. They produced autoimmune encephalitis in animals by injecting them with their own brain tissue. The concept was put forward by Ernest Witebsky (1901–1969) from Germany, who emigrated to America in 1934. He was chief of immunology at the New York State University, Buffalo, and proposed the *Postulate of Autoimmune Diseases* around 1942. Hemolytic anemia, one of the first observed autoimmune diseases in humans, was described by William Dameshek (1900–1969) in 1940. The autoimmune nature of glomerular nephritis was demonstrated by M. Masugi who produced changes in a rat kidney similar to those found in glomerular nephritis by injecting them with antiserum to rat kidney in 1933.

Autoimmune Thyroiditis [Greek: *autos*, self + *immunis*, free + *thyreon*, shield + *itis*, inflammation] *See Hashimoto thyroiditis.*

Autointoxication [Latin: *in*, within; Greek: *toxikon*, poison] Toxemia resulting from the absorption of food products in the intestines under the influence of bacterial action. Described by Charles Jacques Bouchard (1837–1915) in 1887. Until the early 20th century intestinal autointoxication was thought to be responsible for conditions such as anemia, neuralgia, neuritis, headaches, arteriosclerosis, rheumatism and many other diseases. The variety of symptoms was later explained by mechanical pressure of intestinal gases such as carbon dioxide and hydrogen sulfide.

Autonomic Nervous System Thomas Willis (1621–1675) introduced the concept of 'involuntary' and 'voluntary' or 'volitional' movements in 1664. The earliest theory of reflex action was put forward by Edinburgh physician Robert Whytt (1714–1766) in 1751. The concept of the action of spinal nerves independent of cerebral influence was introduced by French surgeon Pourfour du Petit in 1727. Evidence for the autonomic ganglionic chain was presented by Danish anatomist, James Benigmus Winslow (1669–1760) who gave the name *grand sympatheque* to it in 1732. Visceral and somatic functions were recognized by Marie François Xavier Bichat (1771–1802) in 1800 and an account of the unmyelinated fibers arising from the sympathetic ganglion was given by Robert Remak (1815–1865) in 1838. Differentiation between white and gray rami was established by Thomas Snow Beck (1814–1877) in 1846. Claude Bernard (1813–1878) in 1851 and Charles Brown-Séquard (1817–1894) in 1852, contributed to the discovery of vasomotor nerves. The inhibitory effects of the vagus nerve on the heart were demonstrated by Eduard Weber and Ernst Heinrich Weber in 1845. The 'preganglionic' and 'postganglionic nerves' were identified and named by British physiologist, John Newport Langley (1852–1925) in 1893. He also introduced the term 'autonomic' at the suggestion of Jebb in 1898. The anatomical arrangement of the autonomic system is given in the monographs of Walter Holbrook Gaskell (1847–1914) in 1916 and J. N. Langley in 1900. *See Bell–Magendie law.*

Autoplastic Adaptation *See alloplastic adaptation.*

Autopsy [Greek: *autos*, self + *opsis*, sight] A judicial postmortem was held by the famous French surgeon, Ambroise Paré (1510–1590), in 1562. Thereafter the practice became common and autopsies were done on many eminent personalities and royalty.

Autoscopy A method of directly examining the trachea and larynx without a laryngeal mirror. Devised by Alfred Kirstein (1863–1922) of Berlin in 1895. M. Thorner of Cincinnati later improved it and translated Kirstein's monograph on autoscopy into English.

Autosome A chromosome that does not take part in sex determination during meiosis. Described and named by American cytologist, T. H. Montgomery (1873–1912) in 1906.

Autumn Fever (Syn. Sakushu fever, nanukaymi, seven-day fever) An illness resembling Weil disease, occurring in some rural areas of Japan in 1900. Its causative agent, *Leptospira hebdomadis*, was identified by three Japanese workers Yutaka Ido (1881–1919), H. Ito and Hidetsune Wani in 1918.

Avebury, Lord *See Lubbock, John.*

Aveling, James Hobson (1828–1892) London obstetrician who designed a repositor (Aveling repositor) for reducing the inversion of the uterus.

Avellis Syndrome Unilateral paralysis of the larynx and soft palate with loss of sensation for pain and temperature on the contralateral side of the body due to a bulbar lesion. Described by German otorhinologist, Georg Avellis (1864–1916) in 1891.

Avenzoar (1113–1162) Abu Mervan Abdul-Malik ibn Zuhr, born in Seville to a noble Spanish family of Jewish origin. He learned medicine from his father and achieved fame as a physician in Spain and North Africa. In *Altersir* or *Theisir* he described the mite, *Ascaris scabei*, pericarditis, mediastinal abscess and many other conditions. He also did nasogastric feeding through a metal tube in a patient with esophageal stricture. His works were published in Venice as *Abumeron Avenzohar* in 1490.

Averrhoes (1126–1198) Abul Walid Muhammad ibn-Ahmed ibn-Mohammad ibn-Ruschid of Cordoba. A philosopher and physician who was a professor at the University of Morocco before succeeding his father as a judge in Cordoba. He wrote *Book of Universals*, based on Aristotle's philosophy and was persecuted for his free thinking on philosophy of the soul and the nature of man. He was tried by King Mansur of Morocco and was publicly disgraced by having his head shaved. He was later exonerated and reinstated by the king. His works were translated into Hebrew by Moses Ben Tibbon in 1260.

Aversa A leprosy hospital near Naples established in the 13th century. It was converted into a convent for the Order of St Mary Magdalene in the 15th century and became an asylum for the mentally ill in 1813.

Avertin Trade name for tribromoethyl alcohol. Synthesized in 1923 by Richard Willstaetter (b 1872) and Duisberg who used it as rectal treatment for whooping cough in 1926. Fritz Eicholtz and O. Butzengeiger of Germany independently discovered the anesthetic effects in 1927 and it was advocated as a basal anesthetic in 1927. It was used intravenously by Martin Kirschner (1879–1942) in 1929. It later came to be widely used as a basal anesthetic in England and for a short period in the treatment of chorea.

Avery, Theodore Oswald (1877–1955) Bacteriologist from Halifax, Nova Scotia, who spent most of his career at the Rockefeller Institute Hospital, New York. He pioneered immunochemistry and molecular biology. He discovered type III antigen of pneumococcus and demonstrated its antigenic functions in 1944.

Avesta Holy Iranian book which originated in 700 BC and is supposed to have been given by Ahuru-Mazda, the Persian god of goodness, to the prophet Zoroaster. It contains therapeutics such as herbal treatment, incantation and surgery.

Avian Sporotrichosis Essentially a fatal disease of geese found along certain stations of the Transcaucasian railway. Described by N. Sakharoff in 1891. Its causative agent was later identified as *Treponema anserinum*.

Avian Tubercle Bacillus [Latin: *avis*, bird] Discovered independently by several workers including Rivolta, Angelo Maffucci and W. K. Sibley in 1890. *See tubercle bacillus.*

Aviation Medicine The history of aviation began with a demonstration of an air balloon by Joseph Michael Montgolfier (1740–1810) and Jacques Etienne Montgolfier (1745–1799) in Annoay near Lyons in 1783. Later, Jacques

Alexander Charles, a French physicist, completed a manned balloon journey in December 1783, but was first casualty of aviation with aero-otitis media. The first fatality occurred in 1785 when Pilatre de Rozier and his companion Pierre Romane plunged to their death from a malfunctioning balloon. Scientific observations and physiological data were recorded during a balloon ascent by James Glashier and Coxwell at Wolverhampton in England in 1862. They observed diminution of visual and auditory acuity, paralysis and loss of consciousness at a height of 8700 m. The importance of oxygen at high altitude was shown by Paul Ebert and Tissandier in 1875. A liquid-hydrogen apparatus for high-altitude ascents was developed by Louis Paul Cailletet (1832–1913) of Paris, who installed a 300 m manometer on the Eiffel Tower. Paul Ebert, successor to Claude Bernard (1813–1878), was the father of aviation medicine owing to his outstanding work on high-altitude physiology between 1869 and 1878. With the development of airplanes, the problems of high altitude dictated the need for establishment of aviation medicine and the first school was formed in Mineola, Long Island in America in 1922. The Air Commerce Act, the first legislation to require fitness tests for airmen, was introduced in 1926 in the USA. A journal was published in 1930 and later became the *Journal of Aerospace Medicine*. The problems were mostly overcome with the introduction of pressurized aircrafts around the early 1940s. *Principles and Practice of Aviation Medicine* was published by H.G. Armstrong in 1939. *See air travel.*

Avicenna (980–1037) The greatest physician, after Rhazes (850–932) in the history of Arab medicine. He was born in Chorassan, Persia and followed his father to Bokhara. He mastered medicine, philosophy, astronomy, poetry and other subjects before the age of 16 years and he became chief physician to the Baghdad Hospital before the age of 18 years. His *Al-Qanun Fil Tibba*, consisting of five books, elaborated on every aspect of the medicine. The first two books dealt with physiology and hygiene, the third and fourth with treatment and the fifth with materia medica. He is said to have died under abject circumstances at Hamadhan in West Africa. His *Canon* remained a standard work for over 800 years and was used as a textbook in the University of Montpellier up to 1650.

Avogadro Law Equal volumes of gases at the same temperature and pressure contain equal numbers of molecules. Proposed in 1811 by Italian physicist, Amedeo Avogadro (1776–1856).

Avogadro, Amedeo (1776–1856) Italian physicist at the University of Turin, who proposed Avogadro Law in 1811.

He also used the name 'molecule' for the smallest possible quantity of water. *See Avogadro Law.*

Axel, Julius (b 1912) American pharmacologist, born in New York. After studying chemistry and biology, he joined the National Institutes of Health in 1949 and obtained his PhD in 1957. In 1960 he demonstrated, by radioactive means, that norepinephrine was taken up selectively and maintained in the sympathetic nerves. His discovery completed the final link between norepinephrine and the sympathetic nervous system. He also discovered catechol-o-methyl transferase which regulates the production of norepinephrine.

Axel, Richard (b 1946) A pioneer in the study of cloning and genetic engineering through induction of a specific mutation. Born in New York and graduated from Johns Hopkins University in 1970. In 1975 he showed that DNA in chromatin can be cleaved at specific points by staphylococcal nucleases. This was an essential step towards understanding genetic regulation.

Axenfeld, Karl Theodor Paul Polykarpos (1867–1930) Ophthalmologist at Freiburg who designed an operation for ptosis. The causative bacteria of angular conjunctivitis (Morax–Axenfeld bacillus) in man was described by him and French ophthalmologist, V. Morax (1866–1935) in 1896.

Axis [Greek: *axon*, axle] The second vertebra on which the atlas pivots was called *epistropheus* (to rotate upon) by Galen (129–200). The name 'axis' was given to it by Andreas Vesalius (1514–1564) in 1540.

Axis Traction Forceps For applying traction along the line of the pelvic axis during delivery. Designed by French obstetrician, Etienne Stéphene Tarnier (1828–1987). *See obstetric forceps.*

Axon Reflex Term used by British physiologists, John Newport Langley (1852–1925) and Hugh Kerr Anderson (1865–1928) in 1894 to denote the reflex response of the urinary bladder to nerve stimulation.

Axon Camillo Golgi (1844–1926), professor of histology at Pavia, identified and named the axon and dendrites of the nervous system, using his new staining method with metallic salts, around 1880.

Ayala, Gabriel Spanish physician who graduated from Louvaine in 1556 and practiced in Brussels. His publications around 1562 include *Popularia epigrammata Medica, Carman pro vera Medicina* and *De Lue Pestilenti*.

Ayerza Disease Associated with pulmonary hypertension and right heart failure, essentially corpulmonale. Described by Argentinean physician, Abel Ayerza (1861–1918) in 1901.

Ayleff, Sir John (1490–1556) Alderman to the City of London and surgeon to King Henry VIII.

Ayur-Veda *See Ayurvedic medicine.*

Ayurvedic Medicine [Sanskrit: *ayur*, life + *veda*, knowledge] The earliest records of Indian Ayurvedic medicine are to be found in Sanskrit documents from 1500 BC. It was probably practiced for a much longer period, from the time of the Indus Valley civilization around 2000 BC. Their early systems of medicine contained a mixture of incantations, herbs and witchcraft and the period of their maximal influence ended around 1000 BC. The medicine of the Brahmins gradually replaced the magical beliefs with more scientifically based medicine. Diseases were classified and described, methods of examination such as inspection and palpation were introduced, explanations of disease were proposed as a process of imbalance between air, bile and phlegm, and prognoses were gauged. The three great medical men of this era were Charaka (100 BC), Susruta (AD 500) and Vagbhata (AD 700). Of them, Susruta contributed most by describing hundreds of diseases and medicinal herbs in his *Charaka Samhita*. The remedies mentioned include dung from various animals including snakes, crocodile, horse, cow and elephant. It also contains an oath of a physician similar to that of Hippocrates (460–377 BC). His compendium of mainly surgical works contained a description of over 120 surgical instruments and operations such as amputation, cesarean section, rhinoplasty, lithotomy, excision of tumors and cataract extraction. The Vagbhata Samhita included midwifery. Medicine in South India relied less on surgery and the physicians there were called vaidyas and their system of Sitha medicine included magic, herbs and alchemy.

Azathioprine (Imuran) Drug synthesized by an American biochemist, George Herbert Hitchings in 1955. Its immunosuppressive properties of azathioprine were demonstrated by R. Schwartz and William Dameshek (1900–1969) in 1959. It was introduced as an immunosuppressive agent in organ transplantation in 1962.

Azilian Period A link between the later Paleolithic period and the Neolithic period. Named after the culture which existed during the Mesolithic stage at the site of Mas d'Azul, a small town at the foot of the Pyrenees. It was preceded by the Aurignacian culture.

Azo Dyes The red azo dye, Protonsil, was found by Gerhard Domagk (1895–1964) in 1935 to be the first antibacterial substance to give specific protection against streptoccocal infection. The active antibacterial component was found to be sulfanilamide. Domagk received the Nobel Prize for his discovery of Protonsil in 1939. *See antibiotics.*

Azoic Period [Greek: *a*, without + *zoe*, life] Precambrian period. The rocks which belonged to an age before the Cambrian period were observed to contain no fossils or any other evidence of life by Sir A.C. Ramsay around 1863. *See Cambrian period.*

Azoospermia [Greek: *a*, without + *sperma*, seed] Alexandre Donne (1801–1878) noted sperm in fluid recovered from the vagina in 1844. This contributed to the study of azoospermia which became important in the search for causes of sterility. Live spermatozoa were noted in the cervical mucus of a woman 8.5 days after coitus by S.R. Percy in 1861. The motility and the number of spermatozoa were estimated during postcoital examination by New York urologist, Max Huhner (1873–1947) in 1913. He performed testicular aspiration to study male infertility due to azoospermia.

Azote [Greek: *a*, without + *zoe*, life] Name given to nitrogen gas. *See nitrogen.*

Azotemia [Greek: *a*, without + *zoe*, life] Georges Fernand Isidore Widal (1862–1929) coined the term in 1905 to denote a syndrome that resulted from retention of nitrogenous materials which normally would have been eliminated by the kidneys. Jean Louis Prevost (1790–1850) and John Baptist Andrea Dumas (1800–1884) observed in 1821 that urea accumulated in the blood after extirpation of the kidneys. Large quantities were noted in the brain as well as the blood of patients who died with granular kidneys by Robert Christinson (1797–1882) of Edinburgh in 1829. The concentration of urea in the blood was estimated using the physicochemical method involving the freezing point by Sandor Koranyi (1866–1944) in 1897. In 1934 Donald Dexter Van Slyke (1883–1971) conducted experiments to demonstrate that urea clearance paralleled blood flow through the kidneys.

Azoth Universal remedy consisting of mercury, silver and gold. In use until the late 16th century.

Azoturia A morbid state in which an absolute and relative increase of urea in the urine occurs. Found by British biochemist, William Prout (1785–1850) in 1848. R. Willis named it.

Aztecs South American tribe which spread throughout Mexico around AD 1400. Tlazolteotl was their goddess for medicine men and Tzapotlatenan was the goddess of drugs. Their medicine man passed on his skill to his son, who was not allowed to practice until the death of his father. A high standard of medicine existed in the Aztec kingdom until the arrival of the Spanish conquest in the 16th century. The city of Tenochtitlan, now Mexico City, had pharmacies, steam baths for rheumatic diseases, hospitals and a higher standard of hygiene than was found in the Old World. Over 1000 herbal medicines were listed in their pharmacies.

Azygos or azygus vein [Greek: *a*, negative + *zygos*, pair] Greek term for the unpaired vein situated in the thorax. Introduced into anatomy by Galen (129–200).

B

B Hepatitis *See hepatitis B.*

B Virus Herpes simiae virus. Isolated by American bacteriologist, Albert Bruce Sabin (1906–1993) and Arthur M. Wright from the brain of a laboratory worker who died from the bite of an apparently normal monkey in 1934.

Baal or Balder God and source of fertility. In the form of a conical stone, worshipped by the Phoenicians. His wife, Baalat, was goddess of fertility. The festival of Baal, celebrated with a symbolic fire called 'baldersbal' in Scandinavia on midsummer night, has provided the evidence of Phoenician influence in Europe.

Baarsdorp, Cornelius Physician to Emperor Charles V in the 16th century. He wrote *Methodus Universe Artis Medicae* in 1538.

Babcock Operation *See Babcock, William Wayne.*

Babcock Test Test for estimating the fat content in milk using sulfuric acid as reagent. Devised by American agricultural chemist, Stephen Moulton Babcock (1843–1931) of Bridgewater, New York State. His work on the effect of a selective diet in cattle in 1907 led to the concept of accessory food factors by Frederick Gowland Hopkins (1861–1947).

Babcock, William Wayne (1872–1963) Surgeon to the Samaritan and American Stomach Hospitals, Philadelphia. He described a new operative technique, Babcock operation, for thoracic aneurysm in 1926. He designed a surgical method for abdominal aneurysm in 1929.

Babes, Victor (1854–1926) Rumanian bacteriologist who devised the mallein test for diagnosis of glanders in 1891. *See Babes–Ernest granules.*

Babes–Ernest Granules Intracellular bodies with a strong affinity for nuclear metachromatic stains, noted by Paul Ernest (1859–1937) a German pathologist, in 1888. Victor Babes (1854–1926), a Rumanian bacteriologist, observed the same granules independently in 1889. Their function was not known at the time, but they were thought to represent a part of the endoplasmic reticulum.

Babesiasis (Syn. Texas cattle fever, redwater fever, hemoglobinuric fever) The tick was shown to be a vector in babesiasis, essentially a disease of cattle and horses, by Theobald Smith (1859–1934), professor of microbiology at Harvard University, in 1888. Smith also demonstrated the presence of the causative protozoan in the red blood cells of affected animals in the same year, while he was working for the US Bureau of Animal Industry. It was called redwater fever as it causes hemoglobinuria. A pathologist at Johns Hopkins University, George Henry Faulkiner Nuttall (1862–1937) and S. Hadwen introduced trypan blue as treatment in 1909.

Babington, Guy Benjamin (1794–1866) English otologist and son of another physician, William Babington (1756–1833). He was educated at Charterhouse and studied medicine at Guy's Hospital. He designed a glottiscope (for visualizing the glottis), which he demonstrated to the Hunterian Society of London in 1827. He invented a laryngoscope in 1829, and described hereditary epistaxis in 1865. His glottiscope was later named after him.

Babington, William (1756–1833) Physician at Guy's Hospital who wrote *Outlines of Lectures on Medicine* with James Currie (1756–1805) in 1802. He was a founder of the Geological Society and the Hunterian Society. His son, Guy Benjamin Babington (1794–1866) was also a physician at Guy's Hospital.

Babington Glottiscope *See Babington, Guy Benjamin.*

Babinski Reflex An abnormal extensor plantar response in pyramidal lesions. Described by Jules François Babinski (1857–1932) of Paris in *Sur le Reflexe Cutane Plantaire dans Certaines Affections du Systeme Nervoux Central*, published in 1896.

Babinski Sign *See Babinski reflex.*

Babinski Syndrome Associated with cardioaortic syphilis and neurosyphilis, and described by Jules François Babinski (1857–1932) in 1896.

Babinski, Jules François Felix (1857–1932) A student of Jean Marie Charcot (1825–1893) in Paris. He described dystrophia adiposa genitalis in 1900, and is also known for his work on hysteria. *See Babinski Reflex, Babinski–Nageotte syndrome, anosognosia.*

Babinski–Nageotte Syndrome Associated with hemianesthesia and crossed hemiplegia. Described jointly by Jean Nageotte (1866–1948) and Jules François Babinski (1857–1932) in 1902. Babinski was a Polish political refugee in Paris in 1848, and graduated from the University of Paris with a thesis on multiple sclerosis in 1884. He worked under

Jean Marie Charcot (1825–1893) at the Salpêtrière from 1890 to 1927, and described dystrophia adiposa genitalis, a year before Alfred Fröhlich (1871–1953) in 1900. Nageotte was born in Dijon and graduated in medicine from Paris in 1893. He was physician to the Bicêtre in 1898 and also described the lateral medullary syndrome with Babinski.

Babylonian Medicine The Accadians (Akkadians) probably migrated from the Persian mountains around 4000 BC. They attributed a spirit to every object and disease, and each physician had his personal god for healing. Their chief god of healing was Ninurta, and they practiced exorcism to drive away demons and cure diseases. The idea of punishment of sins by way of disease was held by the Chaldeans, who belonged to a later civilization of Babylon. They had no doctors but had the wisdom to expose a patient publicly in the market so that anybody who had suffered from a similar disease was free to give the patient advice. Their goddess of fertility was Ishtar, and their king, Nebuchadnezzar II, built one of the eight monumental gates of Babylon and dedicated it to this goddess around 570 BC. The clay tablets of Ashurbanipal were dated around 600 BC and contain many incantations to drive away disease. When the physicians started practicing in Babylon, around 1700 BC, King Hammurabi introduced a code of laws that in part contained the rules and the fees for physicians' practice. It also prescribed punishment for their failure. *See Hammurabi, Nineveh.*

Baccio, Andreas (1550–1600) A native of Ancona and physician to Pope Sextus V. He wrote *De Thermis Libre Septem* in 1571 and *Tabula Simplicium Medicamentorum* in 1577.

Bache, Franklin (1799–1864) American physician and main contributor to *Dispensatory of the United States* published at Philadelphia in 1833.

Bache, William Earliest physiologist in the latter half of the 18th century to investigate the effect of carbon dioxide on higher animals. He published *On the Morbid Effect of Carbonic Acid Gas on Healthy Animals* in 1794.

Bachtisshua, George or Juris Bukht–Yishu Christian physician, in Jundishapur in southwestern Persia. He practiced at the Court of Caliph Al-Mansour around AD 500. His son Gabriel became physician to Harun-al-Rashid.

Bacillary Dysentery [Latin: *bacillus*, small staff or wand; Greek: *dys*, ill or out of order + *enteron*, bowel] Distinguished from amebic dysentery by George Balingall (1780–1855) in 1808. A monograph on it was published by Johann Georg Zimmermann (1728–1795) in 1771. The rough and smooth colonies of dysentery bacilli and their relevance to antigenic

properties were discovered by Joseph Arkwright, a physician and bacteriologist at the Lister Institute in 1906. *See dysentery, typhoid, enteric fever.*

Bacille Calmette–Guérin *See BCG.*

Bacilli [Latin: *bacillus*, staff or rod] The term was used before the advent of bacteriology to denote medicines prescribed by ancient Arab physicians. It was also used for scented candles used to overcome the smell of putrefying bodies. Bacillus was used to refer to microorganisms by Otto Muller (1730–1784) of Copenhagen.

Bacillus anthracis [Latin: *bacillus*, staff or rod; Greek: *anthrax*, coal] Name for bacterium causing anthrax given by Ferdinand Julius Cohen (1828–1898) in 1875. The genus was earlier called *Bacteridium* by French physician, Casimir Joseph Davaine (1812–1882), in 1864. Robert Koch (1843–1910) isolated it in 1876. *See anthrax.*

Bacillus botulinus [Latin: *bacillus*, staff or rod + *botulus*, sausage] Deadly bacteria which cause sausage poisoning. Described by Belgian bacteriologist, Emile Pierre Marie van Ermengem (1851–1932), in 1896. *See botulism.*

Bacitracin Antibiotic obtained from *Bacillus subtilis* and introduced by B. Johnson and co-workers in 1945.

Backhouse, William (1593–1662) Alchemist and astrologer from Berkshire who wrote *The Complaint of Nature*, and translated *The Pleasant Fountain of Knowledge* from French. He invented a 'way-wiser', an early form of odometer. Elias Ashmole (1617–1792), the founder of Ashmolean Museum, Oxford was a disciple.

Bacon, Francis (1561–1626) Lord Chancellor of England, philosopher and scientist. He introduced inductive reasoning in interpreting nature in *Novum Organum*, published in 1620. He died as a result of a chill contracted while he was experimenting with the refrigeration of a hen.

Bacon, Roger (1214–1298) English monk of the Franciscan order, scientist and alchemist. His search for the 'philosopher's stone' led to the development of the science of experimentation. He investigated refraction in raindrops, and suggested flying machines, camera obscura and mechanized ships. He wrote *Opus Majus* and was imprisoned for over 10 years for his ideas by Pope Nicholas IV in 1277. A medical work on therapeutics, *The Cure of Old Age* was printed in Oxford in 1590.

Bacquerre, Benedict de Physician in the 17th century who wrote *Senum Medicus* which was published in Cologne in 1673.

Bacteremia *See sepsis.*

Bacteria [Greek: *bakterion*, little rod or staff] *See bacterial culture, bacterial resistance, bacterial structure, bacteriology.*

Bacterial Culture Anton van Leeuwenhoek (1632–1723) found bacteria in a decoction of corn in 1683. A modern medium for bacterial culture was prepared by Louis Pasteur (1822–1895) in 1861. It contained sugar, ammonium tartrate and yeast, dissolved in water and sterilized. Theodore Albrecht Edwin Klebs (1834–1917) introduced the fractional method of obtaining pure cultures in 1873 and Joseph Lister (1827–1912) obtained a pure culture by an improved fractional method in 1877. Solid media, such as potato and gelatin, were introduced by Robert Koch (1843–1910) in 1881. The value of peptone and meat extract as culture media was discovered by Karl von Nageli (1817–1891) in the same year. Broth or bouillon containing meat infusion was introduced by August Johannes Löffler (1852–1915) and Julius Petri (1852–1921), an assistant to Koch, introduced Petri dishes for plating bacteria in 1887. *See agar.*

Bacterial Endocarditis *See subacute bacterial endocarditis.*

Bacterial Endotoxin *See endotoxin.*

Bacterial Filter Tiegel used a filter made of porous clay to separate anthrax bacteria from the medium in 1871. Another filtering device was designed by Charles Chamberland (1851–1908) of France in 1884 and was modified by Louis Pasteur (1822–1895) and named the Chamberland–Pasteur filter. Other filters were developed by H. Nordt-meyer and W. Pukall (1893).

Bacterial Resistance A demonstration using serial subculture in media containing antiseptics was given by M.G. Kossiakoff in 1887. In 1889 J. Massart of Paris showed that flagellate bacteria could be trained to survive in toxic concentrations of sodium chloride. A strain of *Staphylococcus aureus* which could withstand exposure to mercuric chloride was found by A.C. Abbott at Johns Hopkins in 1891. Charles Benedict Davenport (1866–1944) and H.V. Neal developed a resistant strain of protozoa by exposing them to sublethal concentrations of quinine and mercuric chloride in 1895. A variant of *Bacillus anthracis* capable of tolerating five times the normal inhibitory concentration of arsenic was grown by a Polish bacteriologist, J. Danysz (1861–1928) in 1900. The fundamental discovery that trypanosomes treated with suboptimal doses of trypanocidal drugs led to the development of drug resistance was made by Paul Ehrlich (1854–1915) in 1908. Cross resistance to drugs was demonstrated by Claus W. Jungeblut (b 1897) in 1923. The advent of clinical chemotherapy with sulfonamides increased resistant bacterial strains such as pneumococci, as

shown by I.H. Maclean, K.B. Rogers and Sir Alexander Fleming (1881–1955) of England in 1939. Further work by Edward Penley Abraham (b 1913), Ernest Boris Chain (1906–1979) and C.M. Fletcher led to recognition of bacterial resistance to penicillin and streptomycin in 1946.

Bacterial Structure Detailed examination was made possible by the introduction of ultraviolet light for microphotographic study by August Kohler in 1904. Joseph Edwin Barnard (1870–1949) further improved this method in 1919. Electron microscopic studies and high-speed centrifugation for organelles were developed by Albert Claude (1899–1983) of Luxembourg.

Bactericidal Substances [Greek: *bacterion*, rod + *caedere*, to kill] Danish physician, Niels Ryberg Finson (1861–1904) of Copenhagen demonstrated the bactericidal effect of sunlight. Similar properties in noncellular blood were found by American scientist, George Henry Falkiner Nuttall (1962–1937) while he was working towards his PhD at Göttingen in 1888. In 1895 Jules Jean Baptiste Vincent Bordet (1870–1961), a Belgian physiologist and authority on serology, showed that serum devoid of cells had bactericidal properties. *See antiseptics, antibiotics.*

Bacteriology [Greek: *bacterion*, rod + *logos*, discourse] The dogma of spontaneous generation existed up to the 16th century until Fracastorus (1478–1553), a physician in Vienna, proposed a possible cause for infectious diseases in *Contagium Vivum*, published in 1546. The earliest recorded attempt to view microscopic organisms was made by Athanasius Kircher (1601–1680), a Jesuit priest, in 1658. He examined the blood of a victim of plague with his primitive microscope and described what he saw as 'worms' of plague in *Scrutinium physico-medicim contagiosae luis quae pestis dicitur*. Anton van Leeuwenhoek (1632–1723), a Dutch lensmaker, described microscopic forms of 'animalcules', mostly protozoan organisms, in 1683. Nicholas Andry (1658–1742) proposed the possibility of infection by germs in 1701. Louis Pasteur (1822–1895) showed the presence of living cells in the fermentation process. Robert Koch (1843–1910), a German bacteriologist, isolated the first bacillus, causing anthrax, in 1876 and described a method of growing it in a culture. Since then, progress was sustained with a rapid succession of discoveries: mycobacterium causing leprosy by Gerhard Hansen (1841–1912) in 1874; gonococcal bacteria by Albert Neisser (1855–1916) in 1879; staphylococcus by Alexander Ogston (1844–1929) in 1881; and tubercle bacilli by Koch in 1882.

Bacteriolysis [Greek: *bakterion*, rod + *lysis*, loosing] From 1893 to 1895, a Polish bacteriologist, Johannes Richard

Friedrich Pfeiffer (1858–1945) and colleagues demonstrated granular degradation or bacteriolysis of cholera and other bacteria when injected into the peritoneal cavity of guinea pigs that had been previously inoculated with the same bacteria and that these substances were present in blood, serum and other body fluids. This was the first scientific evidence for the presence and effect of antibodies. Lysis of bacterial colonies in a culture was observed by Frederick William Twort (1877–1950) in 1915 and by Felix Hubert D'Herelle (1873–1949) in 1917.

Bacteriophage [Greek: *bakterion*, rod + *phagein*, to devour] Lysis of bacterial colonies in a culture was observed by Frederick William Twort (1877–1950) in 1915 and by Felix Hubert D'Herelle (1873–1949) in 1917. This was named the 'Twort–Herelle phenomenon', and Twort later isolated the agent responsible, *Bacteriophagum intestinale*, subsequently named bacteriophage. Electron micrographs were made by an American biologist of Italian origin, Salvador Edward Luria (1912–1981) in 1942. He studied medicine at Turin and emigrated to America and worked at the Indiana University. In 1951 he demonstrated that bacteria and phage genes can undergo mutation. A technique for preparing bacteriophage was developed by Swiss microbiologist, Werner Arber (b 1929) in 1953. A group using it as an experimental tool was established by Seymour Benzer, Max Delbruck (1906–1981), Alfred Day Hershey (b 1908) and Luria around 1960.

Bacteriotropins [Greek: *bakterion*, rod + *trope*, turn] Substances similar to opsonins in antistreptococcal and antipneumococcal sera. Discovered by Fred Neufield (1861– 1945) and William Rampau in 1904.

Bacterium [Greek: *bakterion*, rod] Christian Gottfried Ehrenberg (1795–1876) used the name *Bacterium triloculare* in his classification of microbes in 1838. It became a generic name given to most intestinal bacteria by Charles Edward Amory Winslow (1877–1957) and co-workers in reports of the American Committee in 1920. Four main types were assigned to this group: *Bacterium typhosum* (typhoid bacillus); *Bacterium coli* (coliforms); *Bacterium shigae* and *Bacterium flexner* (dysentery).

Bacteriuria Rod-shaped bacteria in the urine were observed by William Roberts (1830–1899) of Manchester in 1881. The reduction of nitrate to nitrite in the infected urine was noted by J. Cruikshank and J. Moyes of England in 1914. These workers used this to devise the diazotization test for detecting infection in urine. L.A. Rantz and C.S. Keefer in 1940, while assessing the value of sulfanilamide in treatment of urinary tract infection in 1940, noted that most patients with acute pyelonephritis had a growth of 100,000 or more organisms per milliliter of urine. This criterion is still being applied to the diagnosis of urinary tract infection. The value of 'clean catch' mid-stream urine for detecting urinary tract infection was demonstrated by E.H. Kass in 1955. *See pyelitis, pyuria.*

Bactishua, George *See Bachtisshua, George*

Badal Operation Partial section of the infratrochlear nerve as treatment for pain in glaucoma. Devised by French ophthalmologist, Antoine Jules Badal (1840–1929).

Baden A name given to different towns in Germany and Switzerland which provided therapeutic baths.

Badham, Charles (1780–1845) Physician from London and professor of physick at Glasgow in 1827. He published several treatises on lung diseases, including *Observations on the Inflammatory Affections of the Mucous Membrane of the Bronchiae* (1808) and *Essay on Bronchitis, with Remarks on Pulmonary Abscess* (1814). He also distinguished acute and chronic bronchitis from pleuropneumonia and pleurisy. *See bronchitis.*

Baelz Disease Painless papules on the mucous membrane of the lips. Described by German physician, Erwin von Baelz (1845–1913).

Baer, Carl Ernst von (1792–1876) Russian scientist from Estonia who founded embryology with his description of germ cell layers and the early processes of embryonic differentiation in 1769. He also described the structure of the mammalian ovum (1826), and the development of the spinal cord. He was professor of zoology at St Petersburg from 1834 to 1867.

Baer, William Stevenson (1872–1931) Baltimore orthopedic surgeon who suggested treatment of osteomyelitis with maggots in 1931. He also devised a method (Baer method) of injecting oil into joints to prevent adhesions. *See maggot.*

Baeyer, Johann Friedrich Wilhelm Adolf von (1835–1917) An organic chemist from Berlin and a student of Robert W.E. Bunsen (1811–1899) and Friedrich A. Kekule (1829– 1896). His research included the mechanism of photosynthesis, and the condensation of phenols and aldehydes. His work on the synthesis and study of the dye, indigo, in 1882 led to the recognition of the phenomenon currently known as tautomerism. He was awarded the Nobel Prize for Chemistry in 1905.

Bagard, Charles (1686–1772) French physician who wrote several medical treatises including *Histoire de Theriaque,*

Dissertation sur les Tremblemens de Terre, et les Epidemies and *Explication d'un Passage d'Hippocrate sur les Scythes qui Deviennent.*

Bagassosis [French: *bagasse*, cellulose fiber extract of sugar-cane] Respiratory disease caused by moldy overheated sugarcane. Found in Louisiana in 1937. An outbreak in workers on a cane shredder was reported in England in 1940. It was diagnosed using the precipitin reaction by Salvaggio and Seabury in 1966.

Baghdad Sore Cutaneous leishmaniasis (Syn. Oriental sore, Aleppo boil) Observed in Baghdad by an English physician Sturrock who practiced there for 4 years. A description was given by Jean Louis Alibert (1766–1837) in 1829. Antimony tartrate was used in treatment by L.B. Scott in 1917.

Baghdad Spring Anemia Acute form of hemolytic anemia due to inhalation of pollen by atopic individuals. Described by Max Lederer (1885–1952) in 1941.

Baglivi, Giorgio (George Baglivi) (1668–1707) A founder of the Iatrophysical School of Medicine, born to a poor family at Ragusa in Italy. He was educated in Naples and moved in 1692 to Rome, where he had a successful medical practice. He was a friend of Marcello Malpighi (1628–1694), on whom he attended following a stroke in 1694. He also conducted his postmortem. Baglivi was professor of anatomy at the Papal University in Sapienza, before he became the professor of practical medicine there in 1696. He distinguished between smooth and striped muscles. At the age of 28 he wrote *De Praxi Medica* and *De fibra motrice et morbosa.* He also published *Opera Omnia Medico Practica, et Anatomica* and several other works, which were collected and printed by Phillipe Pinel (1745–1825) in 1710. *See iatrophysics.*

Baier, John James (1677–1730) German physician from Jena, professor of physiology and director of the botanical gardens at Altorf. He wrote *Horti Medi Acad Altorf Historiae* (1727), *Orationes varii Argumenti* and several other works.

Baike, William Balfour He demonstrate the prophylactic effect of cinchona bark against malaria while traveling through malarious areas of the River Niger for 6 weeks in 1854. He and his crew took 6 grains of cinchona bark twice a day and thus escaped malaria. Unfortunately, he died from an attack of malaria as he discontinued taking cinchona prematurely after his return.

Bailey, Hamilton (1894–1961) London surgeon who design-ed a suprapubic trocar for puncturing the urinary bladder. He was a senior surgeon at the Royal Northern Hospital and he published *Noble Names in Medicine and Surgery* with William John Bishop (1903–1961) in 1944.

Baillarger, Jules Gabriel François (1809–1890) French psy-chiatrist who gave the name *folie a double forme* to the bipolar illness which had alternating states of depression and hyper-mania, currently known as manic depressive psychosis. He also noted white lines in the cerebral cortex which con-tained two bands separated by a thin dark line, later named 'internal and external bands of Baillarger' or 'Baillarger lines'.

Baillie, Matthew (1761–1823) A nephew of John Hunter (1728–1793) from Lanarkshire. He practiced at St George's Hospital and attended King George III during his last ill-ness. He wrote *Morbid Anatomy of Some of the Most Important Parts of the Human Body* (1793), the first book to treat pathol-ogy systematically. It contains illustrations of emphysema of the lungs, observed at the postmortem of Samuel Johnson (1709–1784). Baillie described dextrocardia with situs inver-sus viscerum in 1788, and associated rheumatic disease with valvular lesions in the heart in 1797. He left his collection of books, anatomy specimens and drawings to the Royal College of Physicians.

Baillou, Guillaume de (1538–1616) Physician to the Dauphin and first to describe whooping cough in 1578. His treatises including *Conciliorum Medicinalium Libri duo Paris* (1635), were printed posthumously in Geneva and Paris.

Bailly, Jean Sylvanus (1736–1793) French astronomer who made several important contributions to astronomy, includ-ing *History of Indian and Oriental Astronomy,* published in 1787. He was on the committee in Paris to inquire into animal magnetism in 1784. He was guillotined during the French Revolution in 1793.

Bailzie, William Scottish physician in the 15th century who became professor at Bologna in 1484. He wrote *Apologia pro Galeni Doctrina contra Empericos* in 1552.

Bain, Alexander (1808–1903) Considered a founder of mod-ern systematic psychology. He wrote *Senses and the Intellect* (1855) and *Emotions and the Will* (1859). He was professor of logic at Aberdeen in 1860.

Bainbridge Reflex Variable heart rate in response to pressor receptors in the right atrium and great veins. Described by English physiologist, Arthur Francis Bainbridge (1874–1921) in 1914.

Bainbridge, Arthur Francis (1874–1921) English physiolo-gist, born in Stockton-on-Tees, who graduated in natural sciences from Trinity College, Cambridge in 1897. He obtained his medical degree from St Bartholomew's Hos-pital in 1901, and became a lecturer in pathology at Guy's Hospital in 1905. He was appointed to the chair of physiology at St Bartholomew's Hospital in 1915 and remained in post until his death. He discovered that cardiac inhibition was produced by vagal tone, and that accelerator nerves caused cardiac excitation, in 1914. He was also a bacteriologist who classified various strains of Salmonella in 1909. *See Bainbridge reflex.*

Bainbridge, John (1582–1643) Astronomer and physician from Leicestershire who was appointed as the first Savilian professor of astronomy at Oxford by Sir Henry Saville (1549–1622) in 1619. He published several treatises including *An Astronomical Description of the Late Comet, Procli Sphaera, et Ptolomi de hypothesibus Planaterium liber Singularis* and *Canicularia.*

Bakehouses Welfare Order A law to ensure hygienic measures amongst bakehouse workers, passed in 1927.

Baker Cyst An affection of the knee joint, named after English surgeon, William Morrant Baker (1839–1896) of St Bartholomew's Hospital, who described it in 1877. He was born in Andover and graduated (1861) from St Bartholomew's Medical School where he became a surgeon in 1871.

Baker Itch Occupational disease affecting the hands and arms of bakers, known for centuries. Robert Willan (1757–1812) described it as psoriasis diffusa in 1798. The etiology was studied by R.P. White in the early 1900s. He demonstrated it to be an allergic reaction to one of the wet ingredients in baking.

Baker Lung Collection of starch granules in the lung and sputum of bakers. Observed by Carl J.C. Adolph Gerhardt (1833–1902) of Germany in 1896.

Baker, George (1540–1600) Elected Master of the Barber–Surgeon's Company in 1597 and had a successful practice in London. He wrote a testimonial verse as a foreword to Peter Lowe's book *The Whole Course of Chirugerie* in 1597.

Baker, George (1722–1809) Physician from Devonshire who was educated at Eton and King's College Cambridge. In his *An Essay Concerning the Causes of the Endemic Colic in Devonshire* he maintained that lead poisoning in Devonshire colic (colica Pictonum) was due to cider presses used in Devon. He practiced in London and was physician to the king and the queen. His other works include: *An Inquiry into a new Method of Inoculating the Small Pox* (1766), *De Catarrho et de Dysenteriae Londinis* (1763), *Oratio ex Harveii Instituto, Habita in Theatro Coll. Regi. Medicorum* (1761) and *De Affectibus animi et Morbis inde oriundis, dissertatio habita in Canterbrigiae in Scholis Publis* (1755).

Baker, Henry (1698–1774) English microscopist in London who improved the microscope. He recapitulated much of Anton Leeuwenhoek's (1632–1723) work in The *Microscope made Easy* in 1743. *See salmon disease.*

Baker, Robert Surgeon from Leeds who was appointed (1834) as medical supervisor for factory workers following industrial health reforms in 1830. He was promoted to medical inspector of factories in 1858.

Baker, William Morrant (1839–1896) Surgeon and lecturer at St Bartholomew's Hospital who gave a description of erythema serpens in 1873. He also described formation of the synovial cyst (Baker cyst) in diseased knee joint in 1877. He published a successful *Handbook of Physiology* with Vincent Dormer that ran to over 13 editions.

Bakerian Lecture Created at the Royal Institution in 1774 by an antique dealer and amateur scientist, Henry Baker, who left a sum of £100 for the purpose of granting a regular award to any person giving a lecture on an important scientific discovery. The first Bakerian Lecture was delivered by Peter Woulfe. Sir Humphry Davy (1778–1829) reported his experiment on electrolysis of water at the Bakerian Lecture held at the Royal Institution in 1806.

Bakey, Michael Ellis de (b 1908) American cardiovascular surgeon, born in Lake Charles in Louisiana. He graduated from Tulane University and was lecturer in surgery at the same institution until he moved to Baylor University College of Medicine in Houston, Texas in 1948. At Houston he joined with Arthur Denton Cooley (b 1920) and developed a surgical cardiovascular center of international repute.

BAL *See British Anti-Lewisite.*

Balamio, Ferdinand Physician to Pope Leo X. He translated several works of Galen (129–200) from Greek into Latin in the 15th century.

Balance, Torsion *See coulomb.*

Balaneology [Greek: *balanos*, bath + *logos*, discourse] Hydrotherapeutics, a science of treatment of diseases by baths, springs and mineral waters. *See baths.*

Balaneotherapeutics [Greek: *balanos*, bath + *therapeia*, healing] The study of application of baths in the treatment of diseases. *See baths.*

Balanitis [Greek: *balanos*, acorn, foreskin + *itis*, inflammation] Earlier known as bastard clap or blennorrhagia balnai.

Balantidium coli A protozoan parasite in the large intestine. Described by Swedish physician, Pehr Henrick Malmsten (1811–1883) in 1857. Fritz Schaudinn (1871–1906) from

Germany described several other species belonging to the genus in 1899.

Balard, Antoine Jerome (1802–1876) French chemist who started as an apothecary. He discovered that iodine turned blue in the presence of starch. This finding formed the basis for testing for starch, and also revealed the similarity between chlorine, bromine and iodine.

Balbiani, Eduard Gerard (1823–1899) From Santo Domingo, Haiti, he was professor of comparative embryology in France who described the yolk nucleus of the ovum in 1893.

Balbuties An ancient term for stuttering. *See stuttering.*

Bald *See Leech Book of Bald.*

Baldinger, Ernest Gottfried (1738–1804) German physician and professor of medicine at Marburg. He became an army physician and wrote *A Treatise on the Diseases of the Army* in 1775. His other publications include *Sylloge Opuluscurrorum Selectorum argument Medico Practica* and a journal for physicians.

Baldini, Bernadin Physician, mathematician and poet from Milan in the 15th century who wrote *De Multitudine Rerum* and *In Pestilentium Libellus.*

Baldwin, James Fairchild (1850–1936) American gynecologist from Ohio. He designed an operation for congenital absence of the vagina (Baldwin operation) in which a loop of ileum was transplanted between the bladder and the rectum.

Baldy Operation A procedure, now obsolete, in which the round ligaments were used to correct retroversion of the uterus. Designed by a gynecologist, John Montgomery Baldy (1860–1934) of Philadelphia.

Baley or Bailey, Walter (1529–1592) Physician from Dorset, educated at Winchester School. He became physician to the Queen and wrote a monograph on ophthalmology in England, *A briefe Treatise touching the preservation of eie sight.* His other works include *Directions for Health Natural and Artificial* and *Explicatio Galeni du Potu Convalesentium et Senum.*

Balfour Disease Associated with greenish nodular tumors of the periosteum and leukemic changes in the blood. Described by George William Balfour (1822–1903) of Edinburgh.

Balfour, Francis Maitland (1851–1882) Edinburgh lecturer on animal morphology at Cambridge. He was an embryologist and wrote *Treatise on Comparative Embryology* in 1880. He died in a mountaineering accident.

Balfour, George William (1823–1903) Cardiologist at Edinburgh who published *Hematophobia* (1858) on blood letting, *Introduction to the Study of Medicine, Clinical Lectures on the Diseases of the Heart and Aorta* (1876), *Senile Heart* and several other important treatises.

Balfour, John Hutton (1808–1884) Physician and botanist at Edinburgh whose efforts led to the establishment of the Botanical Society of Edinburgh, now known as the Botanical Society of Scotland. He wrote several botanical treatises and retired as professor of botany at Glasgow University in 1879.

Balfour, Sir Andrew (1873–1931) Physician who graduated from Edinburgh. One of his main interests in medicine was the study of tropical diseases and he founded the world famous Museum of Tropical Diseases while he was director of Wellcome Research Laboratories in 1918. He was the first director of the London School of Hygiene and Tropical Medicine in 1924. He was also a novelist and wrote *The Golden Kingdom* in 1903.

Balfour, Sir Andrew (1630–1694) Edinburgh physician and botanist, who studied under William Harvey (1578–1657) in London in 1650. He established the botanic garden in Edinburgh, which later became the Royal Botanic Gardens. He was the first president of the College of Physicians Edinburgh, and he bequeathed his private museum to Edinburgh University.

Ballance, Sir Charles Alfred (1865–1936) Neurosurgeon in London who graduated from St Thomas' Medical School in 1881. He researched nerve regeneration with James Purves-Stewart (1869–1949) and worked with Victor Horsley (1857–1916) in removing the first spinal tumor. He performed a mastoidectomy in England and wrote *Essays on the Surgery of Temporal Bone* in 1919. He introduced nerve grafting for facial palsy in 1932. He was the first president of the British Neurological Surgeons.

Ball Operation For radical cure of abdominal hernia. Described by an Irish surgeon, Charles Bent Ball (1851–1916) in 1887.

Ball, Charles Bent (1851–1916) Surgeon and proctologist at Dublin. He described the rectal valves (Ball valves), previously described by Morgagni, in *The Rectum and Anus, their diseases and treatment* published in 1887.

Ball-and-Tube Flow Meter Meter to measure the rate of flow of liquids, invented by Sir Alfred Ewing, in 1876. His principle was used to develop flow meters for anesthetic apparatus.

Ballantyne, John William (1861–1923) Born in Midlothian, he became a lecturer in midwifery and gynecology at Surgeons Hall Edinburgh, and published his first treatise *Deformities of Fetus* in 1895. His interest in teratology led directly to the campaign for improved antenatal care. He is regarded as the father of antenatal care in Britain. *See antenatal care.*

Ballantyne–Runge Syndrome Postmaturity syndrome. Prolonged gestation leading to postmaturity and overweight of the newborn infant. Described by John William Ballantyne (1861–1923) in 1902 and re-described by H. Runge of Germany in 1942.

Ballet, Gilbert (1853–1916) French physician in Paris who described paralysis of the extraocular muscles (Ballet disease) in cases of thyrotoxic exophthalmos.

Ballet, John English surgeon who traveled as third mate in Woodes Roger's pirate ship *Duke*, in 1708.

Ballingall, George (1778–1855) Professor of Military Surgery at the Royal Infirmary, Edinburgh, who wrote *Outlines of Military Surgery* in 1832. He also described Madura foot (Ballingall disease) in 1818 and differentiated between bacillary dysentery and amebic dysentery in the same year.

Ballistocardiograph [Greek: *ballein*, to throw + *kardia*, heart + *graphein*, to write] Instrument to measure cardiac output through detection of vibrations set up by the ejection of blood from the left ventricle into the aorta. The principle was demonstrated by J.W. Gordon in 1877. L. Landois devised a vertical model in 1880. The term was coined by Isaac Starr in 1939.

Balloon Angioplasty *See angioplasty.*

Balloon *See air balloon.*

Ballottement [French: *ballottement*, shaking about or tossing of a ship] A valuable sign for tumors of the kidney. Described by J.C.F. Guyon (1831–1920) at the Congres de Chirurgie in 1886.

Balsam Copaiba oil. Recommended as a remedy by a priest named Acugua in 1638.

Balsamo, Giuseppe or Count Alessandro di Cagliostro (1743–1795) A quack Italian physician who treated patients with magnets.

Balzar, M. Felix (1849–1929) *See bismuth.*

Bamberger Disease Jerky movements and acholalia seen in schizophrenia and hysteria. Described by a physician, Heinrich von Bamberger (1822–1888) of Vienna, in 1859.

Bamberger, Heinrich von (1822–1888) A physician in Würzburg and Vienna who differentiated pericardial pseudocirrhosis of the liver from cirrhosis in 1872. It was redescribed by Friedel Pick (1867–1926) in 1896, and is known as Bamberger disease as well as Pick disease.

Bamberger, Eugene (1858–1921) German physician who described progressive polyserositis, leading to ascites and pleural effusion, in 1881. It was later named Bamberger disease. *See clubbing.*

Bamberger–Marie Disease Hypertrophic pulmonary osteoarthropathy. Described by Eugene Bamberger (1858–1921) in 1881 and by Pierre Marie (1853–1940) of Paris in 1890.

Bancroft, Edward (1718–1787) A self-taught American physician who initially practiced as a medical attendant in Dutch Guyana. He published *Natural History of Guyana* in 1769. He came to England and studied for a short period at St Bartholomew's Hospital before he became a leading physician in London. He is mostly known for his extensive research on the application of dyes in industry. He also played a prominent political role, and in the process served as a British spy in America during the War of Independence.

Bancroft, Joseph (1872–1947) British physiologist who investigated the respiratory functions of the blood in 1925. He also published a work on maternal physiology, *Researches in Prenatal Life*, in 1946.

Bancroft, Sir Joseph (1836–1894) He was born at Stretford, Manchester and studied medicine at Manchester Royal School of Medicine and Surgery, before he graduated from St Andrew's in 1859. He emigrated to Australia as a ship's doctor in 1864, and practiced medicine in Brisbane. He discovered the adult worm *Wuchereria bancrofti* as a cause of filariasis, in the aspirate from a hydrocele in patients in Brisbane in 1876. As a public health officer he made significant contributions to the improvement of hygiene in Queensland.

Bandl, Ludwig (1842–1892) Professor of obstetrics and gynecology at the University of Vienna who pointed out in 1875 that rupture of the uterus in obstructed labor was nearly always confined to the lower segment of the uterus. In 1875 he described Bandl ring of the uterus which occurred during obstructed labor.

Bandl Ring A line of demarcation between the contracted upper segment and the thinned lower segment of the uterus which occurs during obstructed labor. Described by Viennese obstetrician, Ludwig Bandl (1842–1892) in 1875.

Bang Disease A widespread disease in cattle known as 'contagious abortion', named after Bernhard Laurits Frederik Bang (1848–1932), a Danish physician and veterinarian who discovered its causative organism, *Brucella* in 1897. *See brucellosis.*

Bang, Bernhard Laurits Frederick (1848–1932) Danish bacteriologist and veterinarian born at Soro and educated at Copenhagen, where he became director of the veterinary school. He discovered the causative bacterium of 'contagious abortion' in cattle in 1897. The same organism was discovered by Sir David Bruce (1855–1931) in the spleen of patients dying of Malta fever, in 1887, and he named it *Micrococcus melitensis*. This bacterium was later named *Brucella*. *See brucellosis, abortus fever, Mediterranean fever.*

Banister, John (d 1624) A physician and surgeon who graduated from Oxford in 1573. He published: *A Needful New and Necessary Treatise on Chirurugerie* in 1575 and *Historie of Man Sucked from the Sappe of Most Approved Anathomistes* in 1578.

Banister, Richard (1585–1633) A relative of the surgeon John Banister (d 1624), and an ophthalmologist. He wrote *A Treatise on One Hundred and Thirteen Diseases of the Eyes and Eye lids* and *Banister's Breviary of the Eyes.*

Bankart procedure Operative treatment for separation of anterior part of glenoid labrum in recurrent shoulder dislocation. Described by Arthur Sydney Blundell (1879–1951), the first orthopedic surgeon to Middlesex Hospital, London.

Banks, Sir Joseph (1743–1820) Naturalist from London who accompanied James Cook (1728–1779) on his voyage around the world. He bequeathed his botanical collection and books to the British Museum, of which Robert Brown (1773–1858) was appointed first curator.

Bannister Disease Angioneurotic edema previously described by John Laws Milton (1820–1898) and Heinrich Quincke (1842–1922). Re-described by Henry Martyn Bannister (1844–1920), a physician from Chicago, in 1894. *See angioneurotic edema.*

Banti Disease A syndrome of splenomegaly and anemia leading to cirrhosis and ascites. Described by an Italian physician Guido Banti (1852–1925) in Florence in 1894. He described its natural history in three stages in 1910. He suggested splenectomy as treatment of hemolytic anemia.

Banti, Guido (1852–1925) *See Banti disease.*

Banting, Sir Frederick Grant (1841–1941) Canadian orthopedic surgeon who later became an assistant in physiology at the Western Hospital in Ontario. In 1921 he set up a laboratory with the help of a British professor, John James Rickard Macleod (1876–1935) in Toronto and a first-year medical student, Charles Herbert Best (1899–1978) in search of a cure for diabetes. They discovered insulin in the islet cells of the pancreas in 1922. The Nobel Prize for Physiology or Medicine for the discovery of insulin was shared by Banting and Macleod in 1923 *See insulin.*

Banting, William (1797–1878) English coffin maker who proposed a diet devoid of saccharine or sweets and oily substances as treatment for corpulence in 1863.

Bantu *See African medicine.*

Barany Chair A chair that rotates for the purpose of studying nystagmus. Introduced by Robert Barany (1876–1936) of Vienna in 1906.

Barany Syndrome Unilateral deafness, vertigo and occipital headache. Described by Alfred Bing as cystic serous meningitis of the posterior fossa in 1911. Robert Barany (1876–1936) described several cases in detail in 1918. George John Jenkins (d 1939) in 1926 gave an account of two patients in whom a cure was achieved by opening and draining a collection of fluid in the precerebellar region, and he named it precerebellar cyst. These cysts were shown to be dilatations of the saccus endolymphaticus by J.S. Fraser and A.R. Tweedie in 1927.

Barany, Robert (1876–1936) An otologist, born in Vienna, and graduated from the university there in 1900. He joined the Ear Clinic of Adam Politzer (1835–1920) in Vienna in 1905, and studied the labyrinthine function of the ear. He devised the Barany caloric test for labyrinthine function in 1906 and was awarded the Nobel Prize for Physiology or Medicine while he was a Russian prisoner of war in Siberia in 1914. He was released in 1918 and was made the head of the otorhinology department at Uppsala in 1918. *See Barany chair, Barany syndrome.*

Barba Spanish physician who wrote on cinchona bark. His description was published in Seville in 1642. *See cinchona bark.*

Barbados Leg (Syn. Elephantiasis) *See Elephantiasis.*

Barber-Surgeons The barbers of England during the Middle Ages performed bloodletting, opened abscesses and extracted teeth. Gradually they took on more involved surgical procedures which brought them into conflict with surgeons. The various guilds of barbers and surgeons were mentioned in records as early as 1308, and the Company of Surgeons was mentioned around the mid-14th century. An act of Parliament during the reign of Henry VIII in 1540 united the two companies as 'Masters or Governors of the Mystery and Commonality of the Barbers and Surgeons of London'. The duties of each party was defined, and the barbers' practice was confined to minor surgery and dentistry. The company existed as the Barber–Surgeons Company until 1745, when the surgeons obtained their own charter and reverted to independent status. The College of Surgeons Museum started with the Hunterian collection in 1800 and its library was founded in 1801. The college building at Lincoln's Inn Fields was remodeled in 1836 and its interior was completed a year later. The Company of Surgeons continued in this form until 1840, when it be-came the Royal College of Surgeons London. It was again given a new charter as Royal College of Surgeons, England by Queen Victoria in 1843.

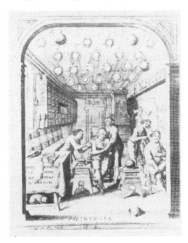

The Barber–Surgeons guild. Courtesy of the National Library of Medicine

Barber, A.H. Freeland Assistant professor of midwifery at the University of Edinburgh and president of the Royal Medical Society. He donated the first bed for antenatal care at Edinburgh in 1882. *See antenatal care.*

Barbeu, Duborg J. (1709–1779) French physician from Mayenne. He published *Code de la Raison Humaine* and *Eloge de Medecine Charles Gillet.*

Barbeyrac, Charles (d 1699) Physician from Provence who wrote *Traites de Medicine* (1654) and *Questiones Medicae Duodecim* in 1658. John Locke (1632–1704), his contemporary, compared him to Thomas Sydenham.

Barbiers *See Beriberi.*

Barbiturates The first, Veronal, named after the Italian city of Verona, was synthesized by Emil Fischer (1852–1919) and Josef von Mering (1849–1908) in 1902, and introduced into clinical practice in 1903. Its dependence property were pointed out by W. Willcox in 1913. Phenobarbitone was discovered in 1912. Somnifaine was the first barbiturate to be used intravenously on an operational basis, by G. Bardet in 1921. P. Fredet and R. Perks administered it intramuscularly in 1924. Hexabarbitone was synthesized by Kropp and Taub and introduced as an intravenous anesthetic by Helmut Weese and Walther Scharpff in 1932.

Barbon, Nicholas (1637–1698) Physician who played an important role in rebuilding London after the Great Fire in 1666. He also introduced insurance against fire.

Barclay, Alfred Ernest (1876–1949) A radiologist at Manchester who described the protrusion of barium into the duodenal ulcer crater (Barclay niche).

Barclay, John (1760–1826) From Cairn, Perthshire in Scotland. He became a lecturer of anatomy at Edinburgh in 1797 and wrote *A New Anatomical Nomenclature* in 1803 and *Muscular Motion* in 1808. He was a founder of the Dick Veterinary College of Edinburgh. The Barcleian Museum of the Edinburgh College of Surgeons was established on his anatomical collection.

Barcroft, Sir Joseph (1872–1947) Irish professor of physiology at Cambridge, known for his study of changes in hemoglobin during respiration. He devised an apparatus for blood gas analysis and published his work on respiratory physiology, *The Respiratory Function of the Blood*, in 1914. He pioneered studies on the physiology of the developing fetus and measured fetal blood volume, placental blood flow and transfer of gases across placental membranes. His *Researches on Pre-Natal Life* was published in 1946.

Bard Syndrome Pulmonary metastasis in cancer of the stomach. Described by Swiss physician, Louis Bard (1742–1821).

Bard, Louis (1857–1930) Swiss physician who described cancer of the pancreas while working with Adrien Pic (b 1862) in 1888. It is also known as Bard–Pic syndrome.

Bard, Samuel (1742–1821) French Huguenot from Philadelphia. He became professor of physick at the age of 28 years at King's College, New York, which later became Columbia College. He introduced the term 'angina suffocativa' for diphtheria in 1771.

Bardinet, Bartholemy Alphonse (1809–1874) Professor at the School of Medicine at Limoges who described the humero-olecranon ligament (Bardinet ligament) of the posterior part of the capsule of the elbow joint in 1869.

Bard–Pic Syndrome *See Bard, Louis.*

Bärensprung Disease A chronic contagious skin infection

mainly affecting the thigh, scrotum, perineum and axilla, due to microsporon species (*Tinea cruris*). Described by German physician, Friedrich Wilhelm Felix von Bärensprung (1822–1864).

Barfoed Test Test for monosaccharides using acetic acid as a reagent. Devised by Swedish physician, Christen Thomas Barfoed (1815–1899).

Barger, George (1878–1939) British chemist born at Manchester, educated at King's College Cambridge. He isolated histamine from ergot and studied norepinephrine action while working with Henry Hallet Dale (1875–1968) in 1910. He also determined the structure of thyroxine and achieved its chemical synthesis in 1927. He coined the term 'sympathomimetics' and published *Ergot and Ergotism* in 1931.

Baritosis A type of benign pneumoconiosis amongst baryta miners in Italy who worked with barium sulfate. Described by Arrigoni of Valsassina in Italy in 1933.

Barium [Greek: *baryata* or *barytes*, heavy] Barium was found by Carl Wilhelm Scheele (1742–1786) in 1774, and a process of mining it was suggested by Jakob Berzelius (1778–1848) and Pontin. Sir Humphry Davy (1778–1829) obtain-ed it by using their method in 1808.

Barium Enema Introduced as a diagnostic procedure for colonic diseases in 1914.

Barium Meal *See barium swallow and meal test.*

Barium Swallow and Meal Test Wolf Becher (1862–1906) of Germany demonstrated that the gastrointestinal tract can be outlined by X-rays using lead subacetate in animals in 1896. Walter Bradford Cannon (1871–1945) of Harvard University in 1898 demonstrated, by means of X-ray and fluorescent screens, the act of deglutition in animals, following a bolus of bismuth-impregnated food. He adapted this to study the alimentary tract of humans, and replaced bismuth with barium in 1924. Alfred Ernest Barclay (1876–1949), a radiologist at Manchester, described the protrusion of barium into an ulcer crater (Barclay niche) during a barium meal test.

Barker, Arthur Edward James (1850–1916) London surgeon who described a method of excision of the hip by an anterior approach (Barker operation).

Barker, John (d 1748) Physician to the Westminster Hospital from 1746 to 1748. He wrote, *Essay on the Agreement between Ancient and Modern Physicians on Acute Diseases* (1748) and *An Inquiry into the Nature Cause and Cure of the Epidemic Fever* in 1740, 1741 and 1742.

Barking Disease Mal de Laira, an epidemic of convulsive dancing and barking like dogs occurred amongst women in Ammou, near Aego in Hungary and some convents in Germany during 1613. It was first thought to be due to sorcery but was later attributed to hysteria.

Barkla, Charles Glover (1877–1944) Professor of physics at King's College London. He studied X-rays and established their wavelength. He correlated the position of an element in the periodic table with the number of electrons it contained. This was the first step towards the determination of atomic numbers. He became professor of natural philosophy at the University of Edinburgh in 1913, and was awarded the Nobel Prize for Physics in 1917.

Barkow, Hans Karl Leopold (1798–1873) Professor of anatomy at Breslau who described several ligaments attached to the carpels and tarsals (1841), some of which now bear his name.

Barlow Disease Infantile scurvy. *See Barlow, Thomas.*

Barlow, Thomas (1845–1882) The son of a cotton manufacturer at Edgeworth in Lancashire. He graduated in 1873 from University College London where he was professor of medicine from 1895 to 1907. In 1883 he described infantile scurvy (Barlow disease).

Barnard, Christiaan Neethling (b 1922) The son of an African missionary, Adam Barnard, he was born at Beaufort West, South Africa. He graduated from Cape Town Medical School and did postgraduate work in America before he returned home in 1958. He was the first to perform a human heart transplant. This took place at Groote Schuur Hospital in Cape Town in 1967. His patient, Louis Washkanski, survived for 17 days but died of pneumonia. *See cardiac transplant.*

Barnard, Joseph Edwin (1869–1949) English microscopist who improved microscopic study of bacterial structure through dark ground photography with ultraviolet light in 1919. *See bacterial structure.*

Barnardo, Thomas John (1845–1905) He suffered from poor health during his early childhood and at one time was given up for dead, until somebody noticed his feeble pulse when his coffin arrived. He came to London to train as a missionary to China. While in London, he volunteered to work during the cholera epidemic and encountered many homeless and destitute children. He became involved with missionary work with the children in England and founded the East End Juvenile Mission in 1867. At the request of Sir Anthony Ashley Cooper (1801–1885) he prepared statistics on the causes of destitution in England and was moved by the fact that more than 85% of the destitute children reached their plight because of the drinking habits of their parents and grandparents. He rescued over 60,000 children and the Custody of Children Act was passed mainly owing to his effort to protect children from parental abuse and neglect. The act was also known as 'Barnardo Act' and the homes for the children (Barnardo Homes) offered refuge to tens of thousands of children. He obtained the Licentiate of the Royal College of Surgeons in 1876 and was elected Fellow in 1879.

Barnardo Homes *See Barnardo, Thomas.*

Barnes Dilator A rubber bag for dilating the os and cervix uteri. Designed by English obstetrician, Robert Barnes (1817–1907).

Barnes, Robert (1817–1907) Norwich scientist and son of Phillip Barnes, the founder of the Royal Botanic Gardens, London. He became an assistant obstetric physician to the London Hospital in 1859 and was made full physician in 1863. He devised the Barnes dilator used in obstetrics.

Barometer [Greek: *baros*, weight + *metron*, measure] Italian, Evangelista Torricelli (1608–1647) from Faenza, a contemporary of Galileo (1564–1642), developed the theory of atmospheric pressure. He discovered that the unit in each column of water or mercury corresponded to a measure of pressure exerted by the atmosphere. On the basis of this, he worked with Vincenzo Vivianni (1622–1703) and constructed the first barometer in 1643. The fact that height of a fluid in a column depended on external pressure was proved by Robert Boyle (1627–1691) in 1659. Otto von Guericke (1602–1686) constructed a water barometer in 1672. The height of a mountain was recorded accurately using a barometer by Swiss geologist, Jean André Deluc (1727–1817), who came to England in 1774 as reader to Queen Charlotte.

Baron, Theodore Hyacinthe (1686–1758) Professor and dean of the Faculty of Medicine in Paris. The principal author of the Pharmacopoeia of Paris in 1732.

Baroreflex *See arterial baroreflex.*

Barotrauma [Greek: *baros*, weight + *trauma*, wound] (Syn. aero-otitis media) Damage to the middle ear due to sudden changes in pressure. *See aviation medicine.*

Barr Body *See Barr, Murray.*

Barr, Murray Llewellyn (b 1908) Canadian physician from Belmont, Ontario. He graduated from Western University,

Ontario in 1930. While working with George Bertram Ewart (b 1923) in 1949, he discovered that the extra X chromosome in the female formed a dark spot when stained. This extra chromatin material in the female was later named the 'Barr body' and is used as a marker for female tissues and cells.

Barraquer Reflex *See grasp reflex.*

Barré–Lieou Syndrome Occipital headache, vertigo, tinnitus and facial spasms due to involvement of the sympathetic plexus around the cervical vertebrae in cases of rheumatoid arthritis. Described by Jean Alexander Barré (1880–1967), professor of neurology at Strasbourg. Y.C. Lieou described it in 1928. He described Guillain–Barré syndrome in 1916.

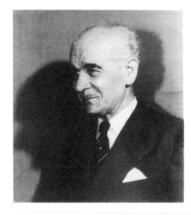

Jean Alexander Barré (1880–1967). Courtesy of the National Library of Medicine

Barrere, Peter (d 1765) Physician from Perpignan, France, who wrote *Dissertation sur la Couleur des Negris* in 1742.

Barrett Esophagus Transformation of the mucosa of the esophagus into columnar epithelium due to esophagitis, hiatus hernia or stricture. Described in 1950 by Australian-born British surgeon, Norman Rupert Barrett (1903–1979).

Barrett, Norman Rupert (1903–1979) Born in Adelaide, Australia and graduated from St Thomas' Hospital, London in 1928. He reported a case of successful surgical repair of a ruptured esophagus in 1947, and he named 'reflux esophagitis' in 1949. He wrote on diverticula of the esophagus in 1933 consisting of 113 cases. *See Barrett esophagus.*

Barrier Vacuoles Peribronchitic abscesses. Described by a French physician, François Magarite Barrier (1813–1870).

Barry, James (d 1865) Name taken by Miranda Stewart, an army surgeon who posed as a male student and obtained her MD from Edinburgh in 1812. She joined the army in 1813 and became a staff surgeon in 1819. She was Inspector-General of Hospitals to both lower and upper Canada in 1858, and kept her secret until her death in London at the age of 71 years.

Barry, Martin (1802–1855) Embryologist and surgeon from Edinburgh who observed the union of spermatozoon and ovum in the rabbit in 1843. He published it in *Researches in Embryology* in 1839.

Bart Hemoglobin Abnormal hemoglobin consisting of 4 alpha chains. Named for the place in which it was described, St Bartholomew's Hospital.

Barth Nitrous Oxide Cylinders Nitrous oxide for anesthesia was not readily available before 1868, and a cumbersome apparatus had to be used on site to produce it. Coxeter and Barth in Britain devised a method of liquefying the gas and supplied it in smaller cylinders on a commercial scale in 1868.

Bartholin Duct The sublingual gland and its duct (Bartholin duct). Described by Caspar Bartholin, the Younger (1655–1738), a Danish physician at Copenhagen, in 1684.

Bartholin Glands The vulvovaginal glands, described by Caspar Bartholin the Younger (1655–1738), professor of anatomy at Copenhagen in 1677. Also noted in the cow by French anatomist, Joseph Guichard Duverney (1648–1730) in 1683. Friedrich Tiedmann (1781–1861), an embryologist from Munich and professor at Heidelberg, described them in 1840.

Bartholin, Caspar, the Elder (1585–1629) Danish physician who described the functions of the olfactory nerve in 1611. He wrote *Controversiae Anatomicae* (1621), *Anatomicae Institutiones* (1611), *Enchyrdion Physicum* (1625), *Systema Physicum* and several other works.

Bartholin, Caspar, the Younger (1655–1738) Danish anatomist at Copenhagen and a son of Thomas Bartholin the Elder (1616–1680). He described the sublingual gland and its duct (Bartholin duct) in 1684. In 1677 he described the vestibular or vulvovaginal glands of the female reproductive system (Bartholin glands).

Bartholin, Erasmus (1625–1698) The son of Caspar Bartholin the Elder (1585–1629). He studied medicine at Leiden and was professor of mathematics and medicine at Copenhagen in 1669. He discovered the double refraction of light in Iceland feldspar, later explained by Christian Huygens (1629–1695) and Isaac Newton (1642–1727).

Bartholin, Thomas, the Elder (1616–1680) A son of Danish physician, Caspar Bartholin the Elder (1585–1629). He described the thoracic duct and the lymphatic vessels in 1652 and named the pancreas the 'biliary vesicle of the spleen' in 1666. He wrote: *Anatomia caspari Bartholini Parentis novis observersionibus Primum locupleta* (1641), *De Unicornis observertiones Novae* (1645) and *Antiquatatum Veteris Puperii Synopsis* (1646). He established the Danish pharmacopoeia and founded the first Danish scientific journal.

Bartholomew, Anglicus English Franciscan monk in the 12th century who wrote *De Proprietatibus Rerum* which included an account of medicine during medieval times.

Bartish, George (1536–1606) Oculist at Dresden who specialized in ophthalmology. He removed a bulbous cancer of the eye, and published a printed illustrated textbook of ophthalmology in 1583. *See eye.*

Bartlett, Sir Frederick Charles (1889–1969) Psychologist from Stow in Gloucestershire who pioneered a cognitive approach to understanding of human memory. He published *Psychology and Primitive Culture* in 1923, *Remembering* in 1932 and several other works.

Barton Fracture Fracture of the posterior articular margin of the lower end of the radius. Described by American surgeon, John Rhea Barton (1794–1871) in 1838.

Barton, John Rhea (1794–1871) Born in Lancaster, Pennsylvania. He performed osteotomy for ankylosis of the hip joint in 1826. He also described Barton fracture of the radius in 1838.

Bartonella bacciliformis The bacterium responsible for Peruvian Oroya fever. Found in red blood cells by Peruvian physician A.L. Barton (1871–1950) in 1909 and named in his honor by Richard Pearson Strong (1872–1948) in 1917. Arsphenamine was used in the treatment by J. Arce in 1918.

Bartram, George Ewart *See Barr, Murray.*

Bartram, John (1699–1777) A self-taught botanist and farmer from Pennsylvania. He had one of the largest collections of North American plants and Carl Linnaeus (1707–1778) considered him a great botanist.

Bartter Syndrome Diminished sodium resorption by the proximal tubule of the kidney leading to hypokalemic alkalosis. Described by American physician, Frederick C. Bartter (1914–1985) and colleagues in 1958. He was born in Manila in the Philippines and graduated from Harvard in 1940. Inappropriate secretion of antidiuretic hormone in patients with bronchial carcinoma was described by him and W.B. Schwartz in 1957.

Baruch Sign Resistance of high rectal temperature to cooling in a water bath. Described as a sign of typhoid fever by New York physician, Simon Baruch (1840–1921).

Barwell, Richard (1826–1916) London surgeon who described the correction of genu valgum by osteotomy of the tibia (Barwell operation).

Barwick, Peter (1619–1705) English physician who attended St John's College, Cambridge. He was appointed physician to the king. He supported William Harvey's (1578–1657) theory of blood circulation.

Bary, Heinrich Anton de (1831–1888) German botanist considered by some to be the founder of modern mycology. He studied the morphology and physiology of fungi and published *Comparative Anatomy of Ferns and Phanerogams* in 1877.

Baryphonia [Greek: *baros*, weight + *phone*, sound] Old term for difficulty in speaking. *See aphasia.*

Basal Ganglia [Latin: *basis*, base; Greek: *ganglion*, little tumor] Suggested to be internodes connecting the medulla oblongata and the cerebrum by Thomas Willis (1621–1675) in 1664. Marie Jean Pierre Flourens (1794–1867) in 1824, studied them by stimulating rabbits but failed to obtain a response. His studies were repeated in 1824 by François Magendie (1783–1855), who obtained jerks on both sides of the body on bilateral stimulation. Despite further research by William Hale White (1890), Sir David Ferrier (1897) and others, no specific function was identified. Samuel Alexander Kinnier Wilson (1878–1937) in 1912, recognized the related syndrome of chronic lenticular degeneration. Cecile Vogt (1875–1962) described a variety of motor disturbances associated with lesions of its striae complex. The interrelation between the lenticular structure and the substantia nigra was established in the 1940s. The clinical syndrome of basal ganglia associated with paralysis agitans and athetosis was described by Kinnier Wilson in 1946

Basal Metabolic Rate *See BMR.*

Basedow Disease (Syn. Graves disease, Parry disease) Exophthalmic goiter. Caleb Hillier Parry (1755–1822), a Bath physician, gave a detailed account of exophthalmic goiter in 1786. He did further studies and published 8 more cases in 1825. Robert James Graves (1796–1853), a Dublin physician, gave an account of three more cases in 1835. Carl Adolph Basedow (1799–1854) from Merseberg near Leipzig, described four more cases in 1840. *See antithyroid drugs, Merseberg triad.*

Basedow, Carl Adolph (1799–1854) German physician and general practitioner in Merseberg. He described the occurrence of exophthalmic goiter and palpitations in hyperthyroidism, and named these clinical symptoms the 'Merseberg Triad'. *See Basedow disease.*

Basel In Switzerland, an important center of printing and publishing during the Renaissance period. Many important early works including *De Fabrica* of Andreas Vesalius (1514–1564) in 1543, a collection of Archimedes' works (287–212 BC) in 1544 and Galen's (129–200) *Opera* in 1536 were printed in Basel. The University was founded in 1460.

Basel Nomina Anatomica or BNA The anatomical terminology accepted by the Anatomical Society at Basel in 1895.

Basham Mixture A popular remedy consisting of ferrous and ammonium acetate. Prepared by English physician, William Richard Basham (1804–1877).

Basil (d 1118) A physician during the 11th century in Constantinople. He belonged to a religious sect called the Bogomiles for which he was burnt alive.

Basilar Artery The term 'basilare' was used to denote the basilar artery by James Benigmus Winslow (1669–1760) in 1740.

Basilar Membrane The part played by the basilar membrane of the ear in hearing was explained by Hermann Ludwig Ferdinand von Helmholtz (1821–1894) in his 'resonance theory' in 1863.

Basilus Valentinius Benedictine monk and chemist who lived during the 15th century. He discovered antimony and wrote a treatise on it, *Triumphal Chariot Antimony.*

Baskerville, Sir Simon (1573–1641) Physician from Exeter who attended James and Charles I. He had a prosperous practice in London and was known as 'Baskerville the rich'.

Basophilic Adenoma [Latin: *basis*, base; Greek: *philein*, to love] A description of basophilic adenomata of the anterior pituitary in two patients was given by Jacob Erdheim (1874–1937) of Austria, in 1903. American neurosurgeon, William Harvey Cushing (1869–1939), recognized the clinical syndrome produced by basophilic tumors of the anterior pituitary, and named this 'pituitary basophilism' in 1932.

Bassen–Kornzweig Syndrome Ataxia, retinitis pigmentosa and abetalipoproteinemia. Described by Canadian-born American physician, F.A. Bassen (b 1903), and New York ophthalmologist, A.L. Kornzweig (b 1900) in 1950. *See abetalipoproteinemia.*

Basset Operation A form of radical vulvectomy as treatment of carcinoma of the vulva. Designed by French gynecologist, Antoine Basset (1882–1951) in 1912.

Bassi, Agostino (1773–1856) Italian lawyer who became a farmer. He demonstrated the fungal cause of muscardine disease of the silkworm in 1835. His work provided the evidence for pathogenesis caused by germs. The fungus he discovered was named *Beauveria bassiana*.

Bassini Operation *See Bassini, Edoardo.*

Bassini, Edoardo (1844–1924) Italian surgeon from Padua who designed an operative method for radical cure of inguinal hernia in 1887. He also described an operation for femoral hernia in 1893. Both these procedures bear his name.

Bassius, Henry (1690–1754) A surgeon and anatomist from Bremen who became professor of anatomy at Halle. He wrote: *Disputatio de Fistula Ani feliciter Curanda* (1718), *Observationes Anatomicae Chirurgicae Medicae* and *Tractatus de Morbis Veneris*.

Bassol, John (d 1347) Scottish physician who studied theology in the 14th century. He wrote several works on theology at Mechlin.

Bastian Law *See Bastian, Henry Charlton.*

Bastian, Adolf (1826–1905) Ethnologist from Bremen and a founder of comparative psychology. He studied in five universities across Europe before he became a ship's doctor. He studied the psychology of different races and proposed the theory that folk culture can be traced to geographical influence. He published the results of his first journey, which lasted for 8 years, in 1860.

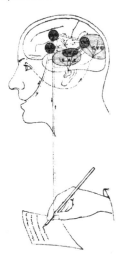

Word centers and commissures of the left cerebral hemisphere together with afferent and efferent paths. Henry Charlton Bastian, *A treatise on Aphasia and other Speech Defects* (1898). Lewis, London

Bastian, Henry Charlton (1837–1915) From Truro, Cornwall, a founder of British neurology. His work on aphasia in 1869 was based on his axiom 'we think in words', and he published a treatise on word blindness and word deafness, *A Treatise on Aphasia and Other Speech Defects,* in 1898. His description of the abolition of the tendon reflexes in the lower extremities associated with lesions above the lumbar segment of the spinal cord is called Bastian law. He also wrote *The Brain as an Organ of Mind* which had a biochemical approach to mental disorders. He also described the guinea worm, *Dracunculus,* in 1863.

Bastwick, John (1593–1650) Physician from Essex who graduated from Padua. He was imprisoned at St Mary's, Scilly for libel against the church and was released in 1640.

Bate, George (1608–1669) From Maid's Morton, Buckinghamshire, a physician to Charles I, Oliver Cromwell and Charles II.

Bateman, Thomas (1778–1821) Dermatologist from Whitby, Yorkshire, who described lichen urticatus, molluscum contagiosum and eczema in 1813. He also believed that ringworm disease of the scalp in children was due to poor nutrition, habits and living conditions. He described herpes praeputalis or herpes genitalis in *Practical Synopsis of Cutaneous Diseases,* in 1813.

Bates, Henry Walter (1825–1892) Leicestershire naturalist and colleague of Alfred Russel Wallace (1823–1913), with whom he traveled to South America in 1848. He collected over 8000 new species of insects.

Bateson, William (1861–1926) Yorkshire geneticist who popularized the work of Gregor Mendel (1822–1884) on peas in 1860. He wrote *Mendel's Principles of Heredity,* in 1902, *Materials for the study of Variation,* in 1894, and introduced the word 'genetics' in 1906. *Problems of Genetics* was published in 1913. He was the first director of the John Innes Horticultural Institution at Merton, Surrey and founded the Genetical Society in 1919.

Bath Salts Of various kinds, these were sold during the late 19th century as treatment for rheumatism and gout.

Bath English city located in Somerset, known to have had hot mineral springs for nearly 2000 years. The Romans built baths in the town and its bathing station was called *Aquae Sulis*. Several treatises have been written on the therapeutic effect of its waters. *See Baylis, William, baths.*

Bathmis Old term for the acetabular cavity of the shoulder joint.

Baths Probably used as a form of hydrotherapy since prehistoric times. Natural hot water baths with Bronze Age pipes have been found at St Moritz in Switzerland. They were also a popular remedy for various illnesses in ancient Greece and were introduced into Rome by Agrippa. Musa, a physician to Emperor Augustus around 20 BC, prescribed cold baths as specific treatment. Pliny (AD 23–79), Paul of Aegina (623–690) and others advocated them. In 600 BC the temples of Aesculapius used baths to heal patients. Galen (129–200), Aetius (AD 502–575), Avicenna (980–1037) and others said that a bath should not be taken after a meal. The Himalayan warm springs of Yeuntong have long been used therapeutically. The use of cold baths for fever was introduced in the 18th century and remained as a therapeutic option until the turn of the 19th century. Sir John Floyer advocated cold bathing in *Enquiry into the Right Use of Baths* published in 1697. The use of cold baths for fever in England was promoted by William Wright (1753–1819) and James Currie (1756–1805). An act to promote and establish public baths in England and Ireland was passed in 1846. The Jacuzzi was invented by an American of Italian origin, Candido Jacuzzi (1903–1986). He suffered from arthritis from infancy. *See Bath.*

Battey Operation *See Battey, Robert.*

Battey, Robert (1828–1895) A graduate of Jefferson Medical College from Georgia. He performed oophorectomy and excision of uterine appendages for non-uterine conditions such as painful menstruation and neurosis in 1872. His method (Battey operation) was adapted by Alfred Hegar (1830–1914) and others for treatment of other pelvic conditions.

Battie, William (1704–1776) Physician from Devon, educated at Eton and King's College Cambridge. He became the superintendent of St Luke's Hospital, and presented the Harveian Oration in 1746 and Lumleian Lecture in 1757 He published a *Treatise on Madness* in 1758.

Battle Sign Bluish discoloration of the skin over the mastoid process in cases of fracture of the base of the skull. Described by English surgeon, William Henry Battle (1855–1936), born in Lincoln and graduated (1877) from St Thomas' Medical School.

Battley Sedative A popular hypnotic remedy in the 19th century which contained extract of opium. Prepared by English chemist, Richard Battley (1770–1856).

Baudelocque Operation A method of removal of the ovum through an incision in the posterior vaginal cul-de-sac, as treatment for extrauterine pregnancy. Devised by French obstetrician, Jean Auguste Baudelocque (1800–1864), a nephew of Jean-Louis Baudelocque (1746–1810).

Baudelocque, Jean-Louis (1746–1810) Professor of gynecology in Paris. He defined the external conjugate diameter of the pelvis, Baudelocque line.

Bauderon, Brice (1542–1623) French physician who wrote *Paraphrase sur la Pharmacopi* (1588) and *Praxis Medica in duo Tractus Distincta* in 1620.

Bauer, George *See Agricola, George.*

Bauhin or Bauhinus of Amien (1511–1582) The first physician of the Bauhin family. His two sons, John and Gaspard were famous physicians and botanists.

Bauhin, Caspar (1560–1624) Professor of anatomy, medicine and Greek at Basel. He wrote an important treatise in gynecology, *Gynaecivorum sive de muliarium affectibus commentari*, and another on anatomy, *Theatrum Anatomicum*, in 1605. The iliocecal valve is named after him (Bauhin valve). He is better known for his works on botany, *Phytopinax*, published in 1596 and *Pinax Theatri Botanici*, containing a description of over 6000 plants. *See Bauhin.*

Bauhin, John (1541–1613) Elder brother of Caspar Bauhin (1560–1624). He was a botanist and physician. His wrote: *Historiae Plantarum Prodromus* (1619), *Historia Plantarum Universalis* (1651), *De Aqatis Mediactis Nova Methodus* (1655) and several other works on botany.

Baume Law A child who is affected with syphilis will not infect the mother if she has no signs of syphilis. Proposed by French physician, Pierre Prosper François Baume (1791–1871).

Baume Scale A scale in hydrometers for measurement of specific gravity of liquids. Proposed by French chemist, Antoine Baume (1728–1804) in 1768. He was a professor at the School of Pharmacy in 1752.

Baumgarten, Alexander Gottlieb (1714–1762) A philosopher from Berlin who wrote *Metaphysica* (1739) and *Aesthetica* (1758).

Bausch, John Lorenz (1605–1665) Physician from Schweinfort who wrote *Schediasmata Bina Curiosa de Lapide Hamatite et Oetite*.

Bausch, Leonard The father of physician, John Lorenz Bausch (1605–1665), himself a physician. He wrote two volumes on Hippocratic works.

Baxter, Andrew (1686–1750) Philosopher and physician from Aberdeen who wrote *An Inquiry into the nature of the Human Soul*.

Bayard Ecchymoses Capillary hemorrhages seen in the pleura and pericardium of infants who attempted to breathe prematurely *in utero*. Described by French physician, Henry Louis Bayard (1812–1852).

Bayer 205 (Suramin, Germanin) A synthetic remedy for try-panasomiasis, introduced in 1920. Tried for its clinical effectiveness by Ludwig Hadel and Wilhelm Jotten of Germany in the same year. The structure was not disclosed by the Germans, and Ernest Forneau, a French physician, in 1923 produced, Moranyl or Forneau 309, which had an identical structure. The discovery of Bayer 205 was achieved through research on a previous trypanocidal compound, afridol violet, discovered in 1906. The first trial of Bayer 205 on a case of human trypanosomiasis was done by P. Muhlens and W. Menk, on a German infected with *Trypanosoma gambiense*, in 1921. The second human trial was by British parasitologist, Warrington Yorke (1883–1943) on a patient infected with *Trypanosoma rhodesiense* in the same year. M. Mayer and Menk again demonstrated the effectiveness of the compound on a Belgian with *Trypanosoma gambiense* infection in 1922.

Bayer, Johann (1572–1625) Bavarian astronomer who designated the Greek letters of the alphabet to represent the brighter stars.

Bayes, Thomas (1702–1761) English mathematician and minister in Tunbridge Wells. He studied statistical inference and wrote *Essay Towards Solving a Problem in the Doctrine of Chances,* published posthumously in 1763.

Bayle Disease (Syn. dementia paralytica) General paresis. Described by Antoine Laurent Jesse Bayle (1799–1858) in 1822. *See Bayle, Antoine Laurent Jesse.*

Bayle Granulations The tubercular nodules of the lung that undergo fibroid degeneration. Described by French physician, Gaspard Laurent Bayle (1774–1861).

Bayle, Antoine Laurent Jessie (1799–1858) Physician from Paris who studied pathological lesions of the brain in psychiatric patients and described general paresis. Progressive paralysis of the insane is named Bayle disease.

Bayle, Gaspard Laurent (1774–1816) Physician from Provence who graduated from Paris in 1801. He made valuable contributions to understanding of the pathology of the lung in tuberculosis. An important works is *Recherches sur la Phthisie Pulmonaire,* published in 1810.

Baylis, William (d 1787) Scottish physician who practiced in Bath. He moved to Berlin and was appointed physician to Frederick the Great. He published *An Essay on Bath Waters* and *A Historical Account of the General Hospital at Bath.*

Bayliss, Sir William Maddock (1860–1924) Physiologist from Wolverhampton. He worked at University College London. He married the sister of Ernest Henry Starling

(1866–1927), with whom he conducted most of his experiments. The concept of the hormone and its feedback mechanism was developed by Bayliss and Starling during their pioneer work on secretin and other hormones. Bayliss' classic *Principles of General Physiology* was published in 1915.

Baynes, Sir Thomas (1622–1681) Physician and contemporary of politician and physician Sir John Finch (1626–1682). He was educated at Christ's College Cambridge and studied medicine at Padua. His later life was spent in Florence.

Bayro, Peter de (1478–1558) Italian physician who wrote *De Medendis Humani Corporis Malis Enchyridion* (1563), *De Pestelentia Ejusque Curatione per Preservationum et Curationum Regimen* and other treatises. He was physician to Charles II, Duke of Savoy.

Bazin Disease Erythema induratum scrophulosorum (shopgirls' disease) accompanied by a positive tuberculin test. Described by French dermatologist, Ernest Bazin (1807–1878) in 1861.

Bazin, Ernest Pierre Antoine (1807–1878) Early advocate of a parasitic cause for ringworm disease, opposed by some famous dermatologists including Erasmus Wilson (1809–1884). He was born in a village near Paris into a family of physicians. In 1847 he joined the Hôpital St Louis, where he remained for the rest of his career.

BCG or Bacille Calmette–Guérin vaccination L.C. Albert Calmette (1863–1933), a French bacteriologist from Nice, and Camille Guérin (1872–1961), of the Pasteur Institute Paris, started experiments in 1921 to produce acquired immunity by injecting attenuated tuberculous bacilli. Although their initial results in 1924 were successful with cattle, their large-scale trial on 251 children at Lübeck led to 72 deaths, mainly due to contamination by a virulent strain during preparation of the vaccine. Despite this setback, the vaccine was introduced in France and Norway around 1930. Britain was one of the last countries to accept routine immunization with BCG vaccine, after a memorandum by the Joint Committee of the Tuberculous Association of England led by W.H. Tyler in 1946.

Beach, Frank Ambrose (b 1911) American comparative psychologist and endocrinologist from Emporia, Kansas, who proposed the control of evolution through sexual behavior and hormones. He wrote *Hormones and Behavior* (1918), and *Sex and Behavior* (1965).

Beadle, George Wells (1903–1989) American geneticist from Wahoo, Nebraska. He worked with Edward Lawrie Tatum (1909–1975) at Stanford University and developed the concept that specific genes control specific enzymes. He shared the Nobel Prize for Medicine or Physiology with Tatum and Joshua Lederberg (b 1925) in 1958.

Beagle, HMS The English Naval ship that carried Charles Darwin (1809–1882) as its naturalist during its voyage of 1831–1836. Captained by a meteorologist, Robert Fitzroy (1805–1865) from Suffolk. The aim of the expedition was 'to complete the survey of Patagonia and Tierra del Fuego; to survey the shores of Chile, Peru and some islands in the Pacific; and to carry a chain of chronological measurements around the world'. Darwin spent 4 years on the ship without pay, studying the flora and fauna of South America and the Galapagos Islands. On his return, he worked on his theory of evolution for 20 years and published his *On the Origin of Species by Means of Natural Selection* in 1859. *See evolution theory, Darwin, Charles.*

Beale, Lionel Smith (1828–1906) Microscopist from Covent Garden, London who became professor of physiology and morbid anatomy at King's College London at the age of 24 years. He wrote his first book, *Microscope and its Application to Clinical Medicine* in 1854, and identified malignant cells in sputum in 1860. He also illustrated and described cells of the cardiac ganglion in 1863. When he died Sir William Osler (1849–1919) wrote 'His influence as a scientific investigator and a clinician was much more widespread than perhaps was recognized in London or Great Britain at large. Both in Canada and United States there are scores of men of my day, who like myself knew Dr Beale mainly through his writings, who will always be thankful for the stimulating work which he did in Medical Microscopy'.

Beard Disease *See Beard, George.*

Beard Regulator Pressure-reducing valves are necessary to regulate the flow of gases during anesthesia. An early regulator was devised by R.R. Beard in 1889. It continued to be used in anesthesia until the 1950s.

Beard, George Miller (1839–1883) American physician who introduced the concept of neurasthenia and nervous exhaustion in 1869. It was later named Beard disease. *See chronic fatigue syndrome.*

Beard, R.R. *See Beard regulator.*

Beatty, Sir William (d 1842) English naval physician during the battle of Trafalgar. He was knighted in 1831 and was physician to the Greenwich Hospital.

Beau Lines *See Beau, Simon Joseph Honore.*

Beau, Simon Joseph Honore (1806–1865) French cardiologist who described cardiac insufficiency and cardiac asystole.

He also described the Beau lines seen as transverse grooves on the fingernails in relation to previous episodes of serious illness.

Beaumont, William (1785–1853) Army surgeon from Connecticut, who in 1822, performed studies on the role of gastric secretion in humans. His subject was a French Canadian named Alexis St Martin who sustained a traumatic gastric fistula due to a gunshot wound. Beaumont appointed him as his personal servant and carried out a series of analyses of his gastric aspirate through this fistula. His *Experiments and Observations on the Gastric Juice and the Physiology of Digestion,* published in 1833, was a significant contribution to physiology in America.

Beauperthuy, Louis Daniel (1803–1871) A pioneer of tropical medicine from the West Indies. He studied medicine in Paris and investigated virulent epidemics of yellow fever in Venezuela and the West Indies. He pointed out the causal relationship of mosquitoes in marshes to these epidemics.

Beauvaria bassina See Bassi, Agostino.

Beauvis, Vincent (1190–1264) Medical encyclopaedist who transcribed from Averroes and Aristotle.

Beccari Membrane Hypothetical membrane of the nerve synapse. Described by Nello Beccari, professor of comparative anatomy at the University of Florence in 1907.

Beccaria, Cesare Marchese de (1738–1794) A philosopher of Milan who advocated a system of reform for criminals. He denounced capital punishment and sought to prevent crime through education. His work had a profound influence on the punishment and prevention of crime in Europe.

Beccaria, James Bartholomew (1682–1766) Physician from Bologna who was professor of chemistry. He wrote a treatise on the impurities of air and another on the motion of fluids.

Becher, Johann Jochium (1645–1685) Professor of medicine in Bavaria and an eminent chemist who wrote *Physica Subterranea, Institutiones Chymicae* and *Epistole Chymicae*. He invented a machine for spinning silk.

Bechia Old term for expectorating medicines used in the treatment of cough.

Bechterev, Vladimir (1857–1927) Contemporary of Karl Westphal (1833–1890), who founded the Psychoneurological Institute in St Petersburg in 1907. He was a neurologist and described the superior nucleus of the vestibular nerve in 1898. His last post was as professor of neuropsychiatry at the Military Medical Academy at St Petersburg.

Beck Syndrome *See anterior spinal artery syndrome.*

Beck Triad *See Beck, Claude Schaeffer.*

Beck, Claude Schaeffer (1894–1971) American surgeon born in Shamokia, Pennsylvania, who graduated from Johns Hopkins in 1921. He established collateral circulation for the heart by implanting the pectoral muscle to the pericardium in 1935. He was a pioneer in open cardiac massage in cases of cardiac asystole and described the Beck triad, consisting of low arterial pressure, high venous pressure and absent apex beat in cases of cardiac tamponade.

Becker Muscular Dystrophy A benign X-linked recessive form of muscular dystrophy involving pectoral and pelvic girdle muscles. Described by a German geneticist, P.E. Becker, professor of human genetics at the University of Göttingen in 1957.

Becker Phenomenon A pulsation of the retinal arteries in exophthalmic goiter. Observed and described by German oculist, Otto Heinrich Enoch Becker (1828–1890).

Becker, Daniel (1627–1683) Physician from Brandenburg who wrote *Medicus Microcosmus* (1660), *De ungumento Armario* and several other works. His treatise *De Cultivaro Prussiaco,* published in 1648, gives an account of a Prussian shoemaker who swallowed a knife which afterwards came out of his side.

Beckmann Thermometer *See Beckmann, Ernst Otto.*

Beckmann, Ernst Otto (1853–1923) German organic chemist at Leipzig. He devised apparatus for measuring freezing and boiling points, and discovered a mechanism of transformation of oximes into amides. He invented a sensitive thermometer, named after him.

Beckwith–Wiedemann Syndrome Exomphalos, macroglossia and gigantism, associated with hypoglycemia in infants. Described independently by American professor of pediatric pathology at Washington University, J.P. Beckwith (b 1933), and German pediatrician H.R. Wiedemann in 1964.

Beclard Triangle The area bounded by the posterior border of the hyoglossus, the posterior belly of the digastric and the greater cornu of the hyoid bone. Described in 1824 by Pierre Augustine Beclard (1785–1825), professor of anatomy in Paris.

Becquerel, Alexandre-Edmond (1820–1891) French physicist and assistant to his father, Antoine Cesare Becquerel (1788–1878). He succeeded him as director of the National History Museum at Paris in 1878, and made important contributions to the study of electricity and magnetic properties of solar radiation. He devised an actinometer to measure the intensity of sunlight.

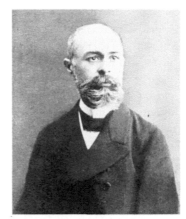

Antoine Henri Becquerel (1852–1908). F.J. Moore, *A History of Chemistry* (1918). McGraw-Hill Book Company, Inc. New York

Becquerel, Antoine Henri (1852–1908) French physicist from Paris, who discovered, in 1895, that certain substances emit radiation. This was the first recognition of radioactive substances and the phenomenon was named 'radioactivity' by him. He shared the Nobel Prize in Physics for his work with Marie and Pierre Curie in 1903.

Becquerel, Cesar Antoine (1788–1878) Chemist from Chatillon-sur-Loing in France who did research on electricity. He improved the electric magnet, invented several instruments for precise measurements of electromagnetic forces and wrote *Traite Experimental de l'electricite et du Magnetisme* (1834–1840).

Bed Bug *Cimex lectularius,* an insect belonging to the order Hemiptera, which has been known since ancient Roman times. It was noted in England mainly in seaports during the 16th century, and was thought to have arrived from the eastern Mediterranean. Asthma caused by its bites was described by Sternberg in the *Journal of Allergy* in 1929.

Bed Sore The warning signs of sacral sores in patients who had prolonged confinement to bed, and prevention of these by various applications, such as cabbage, knot grass, plantain and bread with nightshade, were described by Paul of Aegina (625–690). Aetius of Amida in AD 600 described the mechanism of development of pressure sores and prescribed various forms of treatment. Robert Graves (1796–1853) in *Clinical Lectures on the Practice of Medicine* published in 1848, described the causes and treatment. He referred to general measures such as nutrition, regular change of posture, judicious use of alcohol and use of the hydrostatic bed invented by a physician, Neil Arnott (1788–1874). Local or topical applications recommended by him include poultice of linseed oil, balsam of Peru and castor oil. Jean Martin Charcot (1825–1893) gave a classic account of bed sores in neurological disease.

Beddoes, Thomas (1760–1808) Son of a farmer at Shiffnal in Shropshire. He graduated as a physician from Edinburgh in 1786 and was professor of chemistry at Oxford. He gave up his position in 1892 to practice medicine in Bristol. He wrote *Translations of Schlee's Chemical Essays* in 1786 and *Chemical Experiments and Opinion.* He founded the Medical Pneumatic Institution to study the role of inhalation of gases in treatment of disease in 1799. Sir Humphry Davy (1778–1829) was his assistant. The poet and physician Lovell Beddoes was his son.

Beddoes, Thomas Lovell (1803–1849) A physician from Bristol and eldest son of Thomas Beddoes. He wrote several poems and plays including *The Bride's Tragedy* (1882) and the *Fool's Tragedy.* His last work, *Death's Jest-book,* was published a year after his suicide.

Bedlam Derived from the Bethlam Hospital and used by English clergyman, Thomas Adams in his book *Mystical Bedlam* or *World of Mad-Men* published in 1615. *See asylums.*

Bednar Aphthae *See Bednar, Alois.*

Bednar, Alois (1816–1888) Viennese pediatrician who wrote a treatise on diseases of infants in four volumes from 1850 to 1853. He described lesions of the palate in the newborn caused by the sucking of foreign objects, Bednar aphthae.

Beds The ancients slept on animal skins and feathers, and couch-like beds were used by the Roman upper classes. Air beds and water beds were introduced when the manufacture of india rubber cloth started in 1813, and Neil Arnott (1788–1874), an English inventor and physician, designed the hydrostatic bed in 1830. The term 'clinical' denoting the practice of medicine at the bedside is derived from the Greek word *kline* for bed.

Bedson, Sir Phillipe Samuel (1886–1969) Professor of bacteriology at the University of London. He devised a laboratory diagnosis for lymphogranuloma venereum through skin testing with an antigen in 1936. He produced conclusive evidence for the etiological agent of psittacosis.

Bee Sting Benson and Semenov attributed the effects of bee sting to allergy caused by contaminated pollen and other subtonics rather than to the venom itself, in the *Journal of Allergy* in 1929. English physician, Rupert Waterhouse (b 1873) in 1914 described a case of a bee keeper who gradually became sensitized to bee stings leading to an acute collapse. The effectiveness of epinephrine in treating it was shown by Braun in *South African Medical Records,* in 1925.

Beef Tapeworm *Taenia saginata,* described in 1782 by John Augustus Ephraim Goeze (1731–1786), a German clergyman and naturalist from Halle.

Beekman, John Anthony (1739–1811) Professor of philosophy at Göttingen who wrote a history of discoveries and inventions, and a treatise *De Mirabilis Auscultationibus* related to Aristotle's works.

Beer Drinker Disease Enlarged heart, tachycardia, hepatomegaly and marked edema in men who drink large amounts of beer, about 10 bottles per day. Described by an American, P.H. McDermott, in 1966. It became rare after the removal from the market of beer contaminated with cobalt.

Beer Law Transmission of light through a solution is a function of the concentration of the solution and the path length. Proposed by German physicist, A. Beer (1825–1863).

Beer *See addiction, alcohol.*

Beet Sugar Sugar was extracted from sugar beet by a German chemist, Sigismund Marggraf (1709–1782), in 1747. He demonstrated that the crystals in it were identical to glucose. This was probably the first instance of the use of the microscope in chemistry. German agricultural chemist, Franz Karl Achard (1753–1821), who succeeded Marggraf as director of the Royal Prussian Academy in 1799, established the first factory to make beet sugar on a commercial basis in Silesia in 1801.

Beetle Used as amulets in the past. Pliny (AD 23–79) stated that a beetle amulet worn in the left hand cures quartan fever. Amulets in the shape of beetles, made of various materials, were used in ancient Egypt. The beetle was also an emblem of Khepera, Egyptian sun god.

Beevor Sign Upward displacement of the umbilicus from paralysis of the lower rectus abdominal muscle. Described by English neurologist, Charles Edward Beevor (1854–1908) of the Brown Institute in London.

Begbie, James Warburton (1823–1876) Physician who graduated from Edinburgh. He wrote *Contributions to Practical Medicine,* and became Fellow of the Royal College of Physicians in 1852. He was a physician to the Royal Infirmary at Edinburgh, and president of the British Medical Association in 1875.

Behavior Therapy Therapy (through Pavlovian conditioning and learning) for the treatment of neurotic disorders named by H.J. Eysenck around 1960.

Behaviorism American psychologist, John Broadus Watson (1878–1958) from Greenville, South Carolina, proposed the theory that people and animals could be studied objectively through their behavior, in 1913. He wrote *Behavior: an*

Introduction to Comparative Psychology (1914), *Behaviorism* (1924) and several other works. He considered the concepts of consciousness and introspection to be of less importance in the study of human psychology. Anna Freud (1895–1982) also advocated the psychological study of children through their behavior and activities. The theory was further developed by Clark L. Hull (1884–1952), Edward Guthrie (1886– 1959) and B.F. Skinner (b 1904).

Behçet Syndrome Associated with orogenital ulceration. Described in three patients by Turkish dermatologist Halushi Behçet (1889–1948) in 1937. He was chief physician at Kirklareli Military Hospital (1914) and later worked in Budapest (1918) and Berlin, before he returned to Turkey (1919) as professor of dermatology and syphilis from 1933 to 1947. The eye changes of uveitis were described earlier by W. Gilbert in 1925. It is also known as Gilbert–Behçet syndrome.

Behr Disease Degeneration of the macula lutea and optic nerve, associated with ataxia. Described by C. Behr of Germany in 1909.

Behring, Emil von (1854–1917) Son of a schoolteacher and an army surgeon from western Prussia. He and Shibajaburo Kitazato (1852–1931) of Tokyo showed the effectiveness of antitoxins in animals in 1890. Behring demonstrated the first successful clinical use of diphtheria antitoxin in a child suffering in Berlin in 1891. The child became well within a few days and this achievement established the foundation for a new branch of medicine, immunology. He had the singular honor of receiving the first ever Nobel Prize in Physiology or Medicine in 1901 for his work on antitoxins.

Beijerinck, Martinus Willem (1851–1931) Microbiologist who, in 1901, described *Azotobacter,* a genus of free-living, nitrogen-fixing bacteria in soil. The diffusible property of the tobacco mosaic virus in agar was demonstrated by him in 1898.

Beilstein, Friedrich Konrad (1838–1906) *See organic chemistry.*

Bekesy, Georg von (1899–1972) *See cochlear implant.*

Bekhterev Disease *See ankylosing spondylitis.*

Belchier, John (1706–1785) Surgeon and pupil of William Cheselden (1688–1752). He was born in Kingston, Surrey and educated at Eton. He became a surgeon at Guy's Hospital in 1736. He attempted vital staining of bones by feeding animals with madder. His *An Account of the Bones of Animals being Changed to a Red Colour by Aliment Only* contributed to the study of osteology.

Belfield Operation Vasotomy. Described by American surgeon, William Thomas Belfield (1856–1929) of Chicago.

Bell Disease Mania resulting from acute periencephalitis. Described by American physician, Luther V. Bell (1806–1862).

Bell Fairy Cure A secret remedy for neuralgia and headache, sold by an English company during the late 19th century. On analysis it was found to contain a mixture of acetanilide and phenacetin.

Bell, Alexander Melville (1819–1905) The father of Alexander Graham Bell (1847–1922), inventor of the telephone. He published a system of visualizing speech in 1882, showing the position of the vocal cords for each sound.

Bell, Andrew (1753–1832) St Andrews educational reformist for poor adults in Britain. He founded the National Society for the Education of the Poor, which later set up over 12,000 schools. He established the principle and practice of day schools for adults. The Madras system, or monitoral system, of education in which pupils were encouraged to teach, was introduced by him in 1789 while he was in Madras. His pamphlet *Experiment in Education* was published in 1797.

Bell, Benjamin (1749–1806) Born in Dumfries, a student of John Hunter (1728–1793) and one of the first surgeons at the Edinburgh Royal Infirmary. He wrote *System of Surgery* in six volumes, which rivaled Heister's (1683–1758) *System of Surgery.* He differentiated between syphilis and gonorrhea in *Gonorrhoea Virulenta and Lues Venera* published in 1793. *See Bell, Joseph.*

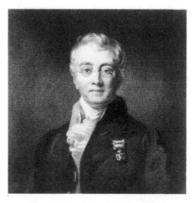

Sir Charles Bell (1774–1842). From Bell's *Institutes of Surgery* (1838). Adam and Black, Edinburgh

Bell, Sir Charles (1774–1842) A leading anatomist, physiologist and neurologist. He was the son of a Scottish clergyman at Edinburgh and brother of John Bell (1763–1820). He moved to London in 1804 and established his own school of anatomy. He was surgeon to the Middlesex Hospital in 1812, and a co-founder of the Middlesex Medical School in 1828. He recognized that lesions of the seventh nerve could give rise to facial palsy (Bell palsy). He wrote: *A System of Dissections* (1798), *Engravings of the Brain and Nervous System* (1802), *Essays on the Anatomy of Expression in Painting* (1806), *A System of Operative Surgery* (1809) and *Idea of a New Anatomy of the Brain* (1811). He also explained the part played by the dorsal nerve root in the sympathetic arc reflex in 1811. He returned to Edinburgh as professor of surgery in 1836 and remained in the post until his death. *See Bell–Magendie law.*

Bell, John (1691–1780) Physician from Stirling, Scotland, who traveled all over the world. He settled in Constantinople as a merchant in 1737, before he returned to Scotland in 1746. His *Travels* was published in 1763.

Bell, John (1763–1820) Brother of Charles Bell (1774–1842) and a lecturer in anatomy at Edinburgh. He established the first private anatomy school in Edinburgh, and published *Anatomy of Human Body* in 1783 and *The Principles of Surgery* in 1801.

Bell, Joseph (1837–1911) Surgeon in Edinburgh and grandson of Benjamin Bell (1749–1806). He showed shale oil to be a cause of scrotal cancer in 1876.

Bell, Thomas (1792–1800) Born in Poole, Dorset, he was a dental surgeon at Guy's Hospital. He was also a naturalist and wrote *British Stalk-eyed Crustacea* in 1853, and *Natural History of Selbourne* with Gilbert White in 1877. He was the first President of the Ray Society in 1844.

Bell–Magendie Law Law governing the part played by ventral (or motor) and dorsal (or sensory) nerve roots in reflex nerve conduction of the spinal cord. Formulated independently by Charles Bell (1774–1842) in 1811 and François Magendie (1783–1855) in 1822. *See autonomic nervous system.*

Bell Palsy Palsy arising from nuclear and infranuclear lesions of the facial nerve. Described by Sir Charles Bell (1774–1842) in 1821.

Belladonna [Italian: *bella*, beautiful + *donna*, lady] Deadly nightshade, the source of the alkaloid atropine. *See Atropa belladonna, Bailey, John.*

Bellini Ducts *See Bellini, Lorenz.*

Bellini, Lorenz (1643–1704) Physician of Florence, one of the greatest European medical man of his time. He introduced scientific thinking into medical practice, and explained fever through the physics of capillary circulation.

He was professor of philosophy at Padua and later professor of anatomy at the same institution. He described the anatomy of the kidney and discovered the renal excretory ducts, Bellini ducts. His work is considered to be on a par with that of Marcello Malpighi (1628–1694) and Giovanni Alphonso Borelli (1608–1679). He wrote: *Exercitatio Anatomica de Struc- tura et usu Renum* (1665), *Gustus Organum Novessimi deprehensum* (1665) and *De Urinis* (1683).

Bellocq Cannula A cannula for plugging the posterior nares. Designed by French surgeon, Jean Jacques Bellocq (1732–1807).

Belloste, Augustine (1654–1730) Army surgeon from Paris. He wrote *Chirurgian de l'Hospital* which was translated into many languages.

Bellows Invented for smelting metals, to keep the fire continuously burning. Anacharsis of Scythia, who lived around 569 BC, probably invented them, although studies suggest that they existed for manufacturing glass and smelting as early as 1600 BC in Mesopotamia. Wooden bellows were invented in 1669 by Martin and Nicholas Schelhorn from Schmalebuch in Germany. The principle of using bellows for artificial respiration was demonstrated on an experimental basis by Robert Hooke (1635–1703) in 1667.

Belon, Pierre or Bellonius (1517–1564) French physician from Le Mans. He was a great naturalist who wrote *History of the Nature of Birds* (1553), and *History of Fish* (1551). In his work on birds he compared the skeleton of the bird with that of man.

Benacerraf, Baruj (b 1920) Venezuelan-born American immunologist who did pioneering studies on immunological responses to diseased cells and in organ transplantation. He shared the Nobel Prize for Physiology or Medicine for his work on immunology with Jean Baptiste Gabriel Joachim Dausset (b 1916) and Georg Davis Snell (b 1903) in 1980.

Bence Jones Protein English physician, Henry Bence Jones (1814–1873), described the presence of albuminoid protein in 1847 in the urine of a patient who had two fractured ribs. He called it myelopathic albuminuria, later named Bence Jones proteinuria. He was born in Thorington Hall in Suf-folk and educated at Harrow and Trinity College, Cam-bridge before he entered St George's Hospital to study medicine. He became a physician there in 1845. The structure of Bence Jones protein or immunoglobulin 'light chains' was elucidated by German molecular biologist, Robert Huber (b 1937) in 1974.

Bence Jones, Henry (1814–1873) *See Bence Jones protein.*

Benda, Carl (1857–1933) Cellular biologist from Germany who identified and named mitochondria in cells. *See acromegaly.*

Bends *See caisson disease.*

Beneden, Edouard Joseph Louis Marie (1845–1910) Belgian cytologist and embryologist from Liège. In 1887 he discovered that the number of chromosomes was constant for each cell in a given body, and was characteristic of each species. He proposed the phylum Mesozoa to include organisms of a transition state between unicellular and multicellular.

Benedict Test Copper sulfate solution used in detection of sugar in the blood and urine. Devised in 1931 by Stanley Rossiter Benedict (1884–1936), an American physiological chemist and professor at Cornell University.

Benedict, Stanley Rossiter (1884–1936) American professor of pathology at Cornell University Medical College, New York. He used copper sulfate solution for detecting sugar in the blood while he was a second-year medical student. *See creatinine, phosphate.*

Benedictine Order Established by a physician, Saint Benedict (AD 480–543) from Nursia near Spoleto in Italy. The first monastery was at Mountcassino, between Rome and Naples. A hospital was erected later at this site by Abbot Desiderius in 1050. Their monastic medicine transformed the previous system of ancient medicine which consisted of prayers and incantations, into that of Galen (129–200) and Hippocrates (460–377 BC). *See monastic medicine.*

Benedictus or Benedetti, Alexander Physician from Verona during the 15th century who was professor of medicine at Padua until 1495. He wrote: *Collectiones Medicinae sive Aphoriseme de Medici et Aegri Officio* (1506), *Anatomis sive de Historia Corporis Humani di Lib V* (1493), *De Obsevatione Pestilentia* and *De Omnium Capite ad Calcum Morborum Causis* (1500).

Benedikt Syndrome *See Benedikt, Moritz.*

Benedikt, Moritz (1835–1920) Hungarian-born Austrian physician who modernized the use of electricity for treatment of diseases between 1868 and 1875. He described paralysis of the oculomotor nerve associated with tremors and ataxia on the contralateral side, due to a lesion in the midbrain involving the third nerve (Benedikt syndrome) in 1889.

Beneke, Friedrich Eduard (1824–1825) A founder of systematic psychology. His *Lehrbuch Der Psychologie als Naturwissenschaft* was published in 1832.

Benevieni, Antonio *See Benivieni, Antonio.*

Benevoli, Anthony (1685–1756) Chief surgeon at the Hospital of St Mary in Florence. He published works on the eye and general surgery including *Lettera Sopra Catarrata Gleucomatosa* and *Nuova Propozitoniae Intorna alla Caruncula dell Uretera della Carnosita.*

Benger Food Digestive enzyme products developed by William Roberts of Manchester Royal Infirmary and a pharmaceutical chemist, Benger, in 1912.

Bengue Balsam A secret remedy for rheumatism, neuralgia and gout at the turn of the century. It was a mixture of menthol and methyl salicylate and was prepared and sold in England and Paris.

Benham, W. Rhoda (1894–1957) Microbiologist who founded the first scientific laboratory for mycology in America. She established a comprehensive postgraduate course in the Medical School of Columbia University, NY for medical mycology where Chester Emmons (1900–1985) and Arturo L. Carrion worked.

Benign Albuminuria March albuminuria. The earliest description was given in 1841 by Becquerel in a man with albuminuria who was otherwise healthy. In 1877 von Leube reported that 4% of 110 healthy soldiers in his study had albumin in their urine and 16% developed albuminuria after a march. Frederick William Pavy (1829–1911) in 1885 noted that the albumin in similar patients was absent in the early morning urine sample but appeared later in the day, and named the condition 'cyclic albuminuria'. Benign albuminuria was shown in 5.62% of healthy soldiers in England by Hugh Maclean (1879-1957) in 1919.

Benignus Morbus Old term for a benign disease with a favorable prognosis.

Benini, Vincent (1773–1764) Physician from Cologne who had his own printing press on which he published several commentaries on the works of Aulus Cornelius Celsus (25 BC–AD 50), Fracastorius and others.

Benivieni, Antonio (1443–1502) Surgeon from Florence who pioneered pathology from autopsies and founder of pathological anatomy. His *De Aditis Causis Morborum* published in 1507 contains classic descriptions of diseases such as fibrinous pericariditis, biliary calculi, diseases of the hip joint and ruptured intestines.

Bennet, Alexander Hughes (1848–1901) English neurologist who described the diagnosis and operative removal of a brain tumor in 1884. He also gave a definition of 'muscular tonicity'.

Bennet, Christopher (1618–1655) Physician from Somerset who published *Exercitationes Diagnosticae* (1654) and several other treatises under the name of Benedictis.

Bennet, James Henry (1816–1891) English obstetrician who differentiated between benign and malignant tumors of the uterus in 1845.

Bennet, Sir Norman Godfrey (1870–1947) Dental surgeon in London who proposed a classification (Bennet classification) for occlusion and malocclusion of teeth.

Bennett Fracture Fracture involving the first metacarpal bone and the carpometacarpal joint, complicated by subluxation. Described by Edward Hallaran Bennett (1837–1907), professor of surgery at Dublin in 1882.

Bennett, George (1804–1893) Born in Plymouth and became a Fellow of the Royal College of Surgeons in 1859. He was a naturalist who traveled to New Zealand, and many zoological and paleontological specimens have been named after him. He wrote *Wanderings of a Naturalist* (1834) and *Gatherings of a Naturalist* in 1860.

Bennett, John Hughes (1812–1875) Professor of physiology at Edinburgh. He recognized the importance of the microscope in investigation of disease, and lectured on histology in 1841. In the same year he published *Cod-Liver Oil as a Therapeutic Agent*. He described leukocythemia in 1845, in which illustrated the microscopic blood picture in leukemia. He also studied the pathogenesis of pulmonary tubercle in a series of patients in 1845, and published *The Restorative Treatment of Pneumonia* in 1865. His other publications include: *Outlines of Physiology* (1855) and *Clinical Lectures in Medicine* (1856).

Benson Disease Small degenerative white spherical bodies in the vitreous of the eye, seen in advanced age. Described by Dublin ophthalmologist, Arthur Henry Benson (1852–1912).

Bentham, Jeremy (1748–1832) English social reformer, born in London, and founder of University College. His brother George Bentham (1800–1884) was a biologist who published a number of books on botany.

Benzene Observed by Michael Faraday (1791–1867) in whale gas prepared by the Portable Gas Company in 1825. Hofmann discovered it in coal tar around 1840, and Friedrich August Kekule (1829–1896) discovered the six carbon ring structure in 1865. It became a major cause of industrial poisoning owing to its wide use in manufacture of rubber and coal tar products. Its leukotoxic action was demonstrated by L. Selling of Johns Hopkins Hospital in 1910, and this led to its use in treatment of leukemia. The dangers and side-effects of benzene therapy were demonstrated by Alex von Korany of Budapest, who effectively halted its therapeutic use at the 17th International Congress of Medicine held in London in 1913.

Benzhexol *See artane.*

Benzodiazepines Chlordiazepoxide was synthesized by Sternbach of Cracow, Poland in 1955, following his investigation into similar drugs over 20 years. Its pharmacological properties were investigated in 1957, and its anxiety-relieving properties became clear only around 1960. Sternbach synthesized diazepam (Valium) in 1959. Nitrazepam and Oxazepam soon followed.

Benzoin Resin from the tree *Styrax benzoin,* indigenous to Southeast Asia. The first mention appears amongst the commodities of Arab traders in the 10th century. It was a precious commodity in the 15th century and was included amongst the gifts sent by the Sultan of Egypt to the governors of Venice. An accurate account of it as a drug was given by Garcia de Orta, a physician from Salamanca, while he was stationed at Goa in 1563. It was known in England as Gum Benjamin and was imported in the 17th century.

Benzyl Benzoate Treatment of scabies introduced by A. Kissmeyer in his article in *The Lancet* in 1937.

Berard, Auguste (1802–1846) A surgeon in Paris who described the suspensory ligament of the pericardium (Berard ligament) in 1836.

Beraud, Bruno Jacques (1823–1865) A surgeon in Paris who described the valve (Beraud valve) located at the junction of the lachrymal duct and its sac, in 1854.

Beraud, Laurence (1703–1771) Mathematician, astronomer and philosopher from Lyons who was professor of humanity in Vienna. He wrote *La Physiques des corps Animes.*

Berchillet-Jourdain, Anselme Louis Bernard (1734–1816) French surgeon in Paris. He described chronic suppurative peridonditis, Jourdain disease.

Berdmore, Thomas (1740–1785) English dental pioneer and dentist to George III. He wrote *A Treatise on the Disorders of the Teeth and Gums* in 1768.

Bereavement Noted as a cause of melancholy by Robert Burton (1576–1640) in *Anatomy of Melancholy* in 1621. Sigmund Freud (1856–1939) studied the association between grief reaction and bereavement in 1917. A more detailed study of the symptomatology and treatment of the grief reaction was done by American psychiatrist, Eric Linde-mann in 1944.

Berengario da Carpi, Jacopo (1470–1530) Also known as Berengarius, he was an Italian surgeon from Pavia who gave a clear description of the appendix vermiformis and the thymus in 1521. He dissected over 100 bodies and gave a description of valvular heart disease and dilated heart. He produced accurate drawings of his human dissections. He and his father, who was also a surgeon, performed vaginal hysterectomy.

Berg, Fredrik Theodor (1806–1887) A mycologist who discovered the causative fungus of thrush in 1841. *See candidiasis, thrush.*

Bergen, Charles Augustus (1704–1760) Anatomist and physician who wrote *Elementa Physioligae* (1749), *Anatomes experi- mentalis* (1755) and works on botany.

Berger Disease Immunoglobulin A gammaglobulinopathy associated with glomerular nephritis due to mesangial deposition of IgA. Described by French pathologist, E.J. Berger in 1968.

Berger, Emil (1855–1926) Austrian ophthalmologist who described irregular pupils (Berger sign) seen in cases of early neurosyphilis.

Berger, Johannes (1873–1941) German professor of psychiatry at the University of Jena. He invented the electroencephalogram during his studies to correlate psychological states with various physiological parameters in 1929. *See Berger rhythm.*

Berger, Paul (1845–1908) A surgeon who, in 1887, wrote an extensive monograph on the interscapulothoracic amputation, known as the Berger operation.

Berger Operation *See Berger, Paul.*

Berger Rhythm Alpha rhythm found in the electroencephalogram. Named after German neuropsychiatrist, Johannes Berger (1873–1941), who gave the first description in 1924. He was a pioneer in psychophysiology and committed suicide.

Bergeron Disease Hysterical chorea. Described by French physician, Etienne Jules Bergeron (1817–1900).

Bergius, Peter Jonas (d 1791) Physician and botanist at Stockholm who published *Flora Capensis* and a materia medica just before his death.

Bergman, Torbern Olof (1735–1784) *See mineral waters.*

Bergmann Incision An incision for exposing the kidney through the outer border of the erector spinae muscle at the level of the 12th rib towards the junction of the outer and middle third of the Poupart ligament. Described by German surgeon, Ernest von Bergmann (1836–1907).

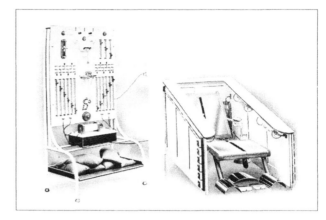

Bergonie switchboard and chair. Percy Hall Browne, *Ultra-Violet Rays in the Treatment and Cure of Disease* (1924). Heinemann, London

Bergonie Chair Designed by French physicist and radiologist, Jean Alban Bergonie (1857–1925), for reducing weight. It was connected to electricity to give regulated electric impulses to treat flabby muscles and obesity.

Bergson, Henri (1859–1941) Professor of philosophy at the College de France, born in Paris. He proposed the theory of creative evolution in *l'Evolution Creatice* published in 1907. He considered the mind as the center and architect of all living things. His book was translated into English as *Creative Evolution* in 1911.

Beriberi (Syn. kakke, barbiers) The origin of the word is obscure. Some historians suggest that it is derived from the Hindi word *bheree* a sheep, as the patients affected showed a gait similar to that of the sheep. Others believe that it is from the Hindi word *bher-bheri* for a sore or a swelling. *Bhari* also means a sailor in Arabic and the disease may have received its name from its occurrence amongst sailors. It was called *kakke* in China and is described in a Chinese pamphlet dating from the 2nd century. A similar illness was described amongst the Roman soldiers in the Red Sea region in 24 BC. It was noted in Sri Lanka in the 17th century, and the Sinhalese words *bari-bari,* meaning 'I can't, I can't' denoting a state of neurasthenia or nervous exhaustion. Jacobus Bontius (1592–1631) gave a description of dry beriberi in *De Medicina Indorum* published in 1642. C. Rogers gave an account of wet beriberi in *De Hydrope Asmatico Ceylonia* in 1808. John Grant Malcomson (d 1844) recognized that both dry and wet beriberi were manifestations of the same disease in his *Practical Essay on the History of Beri Beri Madras* published in 1835. The infantile form was described by Z. Hirota in 1897. Erwin Otto Eduard von Baelz (1849–1933) described the peripheral neuritis of beriberi in 1880. It was eradicated in the Japanese navy by the Director General of the Medical Department, Admiral Kanehiro Takaki (1849–

1915), by supplementing fresh food into the diet of polished rice in 1882. It was conclusively established as a deficiency disease by a Dutchman, Christian Eijkman (1858– 1930) in 1890. The anti-beriberi factor was isolated in 1911 by a Polish chemist, Casimir Funk (1884–1967) who named it *vitamine*. *See thiamin.*

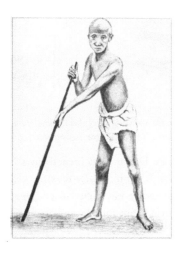

Paraplegic beriberi. Sir Patrick Manson, *Tropical Diseases* (1914). Cassell and Company Limited, London

Berkeley, George (1685–1753) Irish philosopher and clergyman from Kilkenny who wrote *Essay Towards a New Theory of Vision* (1709), *A Treatise Concerning the Principles of Human Knowledge* (1710) and several other works. He was Bishop of Cloyne in 1734.

Berkenhout, John (1730–1791) Physician from Leeds who wrote *On the Bite of a Mad Dog* (1788), *Pharmacopoeia Medici* (1766) and *First Lines of the Theory and Practice of Philosophical Chemistry* (1788).

Berkfeld Filter A bacterial filter made of compressed earth, known as Kieselguhr, in Hannover, Germany. Introduced by H. Nordtmeyer in 1891. The owner of the mine was Wilhelm Berkefeld (1836–1937) a German manufacturer of the filters.

Berkow Table Table for estimating surface burn lesions. Proposed by New Jersey surgeon, Samuel Gordon Berkow (b 1899).

Berlin Academy Joachim Jung (1587–1657), a physician and botanist from Lübeck, founded one of the earliest scientific societies, Societas Ereneutica, in Berlin in 1622, which lasted for only 2 years. A brotherhood of physicians, Collegium Naturae Curiosum, was established in 1655, followed by Collegium Curiosum sive Experimentale in 1672. The Berlin Academy was formed in 1700 by the mathematical genius Gottfried Wilhelm Leibniz (1646–1716).

Berlin Disease A condition of traumatic edema of the retina. Described by German oculist, Rudolf Berlin (1833–1897).

Berlin Psychoanalytic Society Founded by Viennese psychiatrist, Karl Abraham (1877–1925) in 1908.

Bernard of Menthon (923–1008) A monk from Annecy, France who built two hospitals, the Great and Little St Bernard Hospitals for travelers at the summit of the Alps.

Bernard, Claude (1813–1878) Outstanding French physiologist from Villefranche, where his parents were winemakers. He entered the University of Paris as a medical student in 1835 and worked with François Magendie (1783–1855) from 1839 to 1844, before he succeeded him as professor of physiology in 1855. He discovered glycogen and described its metabolism in 1853. He established the mechanism of vasomotor reflex responses in 1851. The concept of the cell in relation to the internal environment of the body was introduced by him in his *Introduction to the Study of Experimental Medicine*, published in 1865. His *Leçons sur la Chaleur Animale et sur les effets de la Chaleur et sur la Fievre* (1876), dealing with temperature, blood pressure measurement and experimental methods, is a classic in experimental physiology.

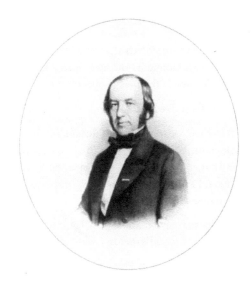

Claude Bernard (1813–1878). Courtesy of the National Library of Medicine

Bernard, John Stephen (1718–1793) Born in Berlin, he graduated in medicine from Holland. His work *De curatione morborum* was published in 1794. He wrote several other essays on Greek medical works.

Bernard–Soulier Syndrome An autosomal recessive trait causing prolonged bleeding time and thombocytopenia with abnormal platelets. Described by French physician J. Bernard (b 1907) and a hematologist, J.P. Soulier (b 1915) of Paris, in 1948. Soulier obtained the blood fraction for treating factor IX deficiency.

Bernhardt Disease Meralgia paresthetica of the external cutaneous nerve of the thigh. Described by Martin Max Bernhardt (1844–1915), a German neurologist at Berlin, in 1878. It was also described by Russian neurologist, V.K. Rot (1848–1916).

Bernheim Syndrome Right heart failure due to bulging of hypertrophied interventricular septum in hypertension. Described by Hippolyte Bernheim (1837–1919), professor of clinical medicine at the University of Nancy, in 1910. He was a pioneer in the study of hypnotism and hysteria and wrote *Hypnotism, Suggestion, Psychotherapy with New Considerations in Hysteria* in 1903.

Bernheimer, Stephan (1861–1918) Professor of ophthalmology in Vienna who described the fibers of the optic tract (Bernheimer fibers) in 1889.

Bernier, F. (1625–1688) Frenchman who classified the human race. He published an anonymous essay *Journal des Scavans* (1684), in which he distinguished the human race into five species on the basis of physical features and geographical distribution.

Bernoulli, Daniel (1700–1782) Second son of Jean Bernoulli (1667–1748). Swiss mathematician and physician at Basel. After becoming professor of mathematics at St Petersburg in 1725, he returned to Basel as professor of anatomy in 1732. He wrote several treatises on science and astronomy although his main interest was differential equations. His *Hydrodynamica,* which explored the relationship between pressure, velocity and density in flowing fluids, was published in 1738. He formulated the laws for the flow of liquids through pipes of various diameter and explained the Boyle law of gases.

Bernoulli, Jacques (1654–1705) Swiss mathematician and brother of Jean Bernoulli. He was a professor at Basel in 1687 and introduced the term 'integral' in differential calculus in 1690. He published an edition of Descartes geometry in 1695.

Bernoulli, Jean (1667–1748) Graduated in medicine from Basel in 1694 and studied mathematics. He was professor of mathematics at Gröningen in 1695, and at Basel in 1705. He founded the dynasty of Bernoullis who excelled in mathematics.

Bernoulli, Nicholas (1695–1726) Eldest son of Jean

Bernoulli of Gröningen. He died by drowning while he was mathematical professor at St Petersburg.

Bernstein, Julius (1839–1917) German professor of physiology at Halle. He invented a differential rheotome in 1890 to record voluntary contractions of muscle on a time-related basis. He proposed the cell membrane theory to explain electrical properties of the muscle, in 1912.

Bernstein, Nicholas (1896–1966) Moscow-born Russian physiologist who made a lifetime study of the physiological mechanisms involved in human locomotion. This led to the concept of self-regulated motor systems and cybernetics. His *On the Construction of Movements* was published in 1947.

Berry Aneurysm Aneurysm of the circle of Willis. Described by Canadian surgeon, Sir James Berry (1860–1946). *See intracranial aneurysm.*

Berry Circles Stereoscopic charts inscribed in circles. Devised by Sir George Andreas Berry (1853–1940), an ophthalmologist at Edinburgh.

Berry Ligament *See Berry, Sir James.*

Berry, Sir James (1860–1946) Canadian-born British surgeon at the Royal Free Hospital who specialized in surgery of the cleft palate and thyroid gland. The lateral fascial ligament of the thyroid gland is named after him.

Berryat, John (d 1794) French physician and superintendent of mineral waters in France. He wrote a treatise on mineral waters and published a compilation, *Collectiones Acedemique.*

Bert, Paul (1833–1886) French physiologist and student of Claude Bernard (1813–1878), whom he succeeded as professor of physiology at the Sorbonne in 1869. He experimented on the effect of anoxemia on blood and the circulation using pressure chambers. He proved in 1878 that symptoms at high altitude were due to anoxemia, and his *La Pression Barometrique* was published in the same year. He was the minister of education in France and founded the universities at Lyon and Lille. *See aviation medicine.*

Bertapaglia, Leonardo (d 1460) Professor at Padua who practiced dissections. He wrote on surgery with a strong influence of Arabic medicine and surgery.

Berthelot, Marcellin Pierre Eugene (1827–1907) Physician who studied medicine at Turin and Paris and obtained his medical degree from the College de France, where he was professor of pharmacy in 1860. He produced benzene and naphthalene in 1851. His *Organic Chemistry founded on Synthesis* was published in 1860. He discovered 'invertin' in yeast, responsible for hydrolysis of sugar. He named 'acetylene' and introduced a standard method of determining the latent heat of steam. He succeeded Louis Pasteur (1822– 1895) as Secretary of the French Academy of Sciences in 1889.

Berthold, Arnold Adolph (1803–1861) German physiologist who proved the existence of internal secretions, hormones. In 1849 he transplanted a cock's comb to another bird that had been castrated, thereby preventing the sequelae of castration and maintaining the growth of the comb.

Berthollet, Louis Claude (1748–1822) Born in Talloires in France. He graduated as a physician from Turin at the age of 19 years. His passion was chemistry and he revolutionized the process of bleaching. He made significant contributions to bread and beer making and manufacture of explosives. He suggested the relationship between the rate of a chemical reaction and the mass of the reagents which led to the formulation of the law of definite proportions by Joseph Louis Proust.

Bertillon, Alphonse (1853–1914) French criminologist who proposed a system for identification of criminals through measurement of their physical characteristics.

Bertin, Experius Joseph (1712–1781) Anatomist from Brittany who published several works on anatomy, including *Traite de Osteologie* in four volumes in 1784.

Bertin, René Joseph Hyacinthe (1767–1828) The son of French anatomist, Joseph E. Bertin (1712–1781). He was medical officer to the French prisoners in Plymouth. His most important contribution to medicine was a treatise on the heart *Traite des Maladies du Coeur et des gros Vaisseaux,* published in 1824.

Bertini, Anthony Francis (1658–1726) Italian physician who wrote *la Medicina Diffsa Contra la Calumini Degli Nomini Volgare* in several volumes from 1699 to 1709.

Bertrand, John Baptist (1670–1752) French physician who wrote an account of the plague at Marseilles and two other treatises, one on muscular motion and the other on sea air.

Berylliosis *See beryllium.*

Beryllium Element discovered by French chemist, Vanquelin (1763–1829), in 1798 and isolated by Friedrich Wohler (1800–1882) in 1828. In 1935 M.S. Fabroni of Milan exposed experimental animals to beryllium carbonate and named the resulting condition 'berylliosis'. Occupational disease due to beryllium oxyfluoride was demonstrated by I. Gelman of Moscow in 1936.

Berzelius, Jöns Jacob (1779–1848) Born in Sweden, he studied medicine in Uppsala but his main interest was chemistry. He calculated the atomic weight of many metals and proposed the system of representing elements by the first Latin letter of their name. He made many other important contributions to chemistry including a description of isomeric bodies, later known as isomers. He used the term 'organic chemistry' and defined it as 'the part of physiology which describes the composition of living bodies, and the chemical processes which occur in them' in *Lectures in Animal Chemistry* published in 1806. He coined the word 'protein' from the Greek word *proteios* which means 'primary'. *See bile, proteins.*

Besler, Basil (1561–1629) Botanist and apothecary from Nuremberg who wrote *Hortus Eystettensis* and *Icones Florum et Herbarum*.

Besler, Michael Robert (?–1661) Anatomist and the son of a botanist, Basil Besler of Nuremberg, who wrote *Observatio anatomica-medica* and *Admirande Fabricae Humanae mulirius partium*.

Besnier Prurigo *See Besnier, Ernest.*

Besnier, Ernest (1831–1909) French dermatologist from Honfleur who described flexural pruritis amongst infants in 1892. This was later named Besnier prurigo. He graduated in 1857 and became a physician at the St Louis Hospital in 1872, where he developed an interest in dermatology. He wrote a treatise on rheumatism in 1876 in which he described chronic synovitis. *See Boek sarcoidosis.*

Best Disease A hereditary form of childhood macular degeneration transmitted through an irregular dominant trait. Described by German physician, Franz Best in 1905.

Best Operation Subcutaneous suture of the abdominal ring as treatment for hernia. Devised by Scottish surgeon, Van Best (1836–1875).

Best, Charles Herbert (1899–1978) Canadian physician from West Pembroke, Maine. In 1922, while a first-year medical research student in Toronto, he assisted Frederick Banting (1891–1941) in isolating insulin from the islet cells of the pancreas. He subsequently obtained his medical degree in 1929 and succeeded John James Rickard Macleod (1876–1935) as professor of physiology at Toronto. He introduced heparin as an anticoagulant and demonstrated the long-acting property of insulin when combined with zinc in 1936. *See insulin.*

Bestiality [Latin: *bestia*, beast] Copulation with birds and beasts is an ancient practice. Different names were given to those who practiced sex with different animals. In ancient

Egypt an infertile woman had symbolic intercourse with a bull to open the pathway for conception. Havelock Ellis (1859–1939) quoted instances of bestiality in his studies.

Beta Blockers Term introduced by an American pharmacologist from Montana, Raymond Perry Ahlquist (1914–1983), who identified the two important groups of alpha and beta adrenergic receptors in 1948. The terms beta-1 and beta-2, to denote the further selective properties of the beta receptors were introduced by A. Lands in 1968. Dichloroisoproterenol or DCI was the first drug belonging to the class of beta blockers to be produced, but the sympathomimetic action due to its isoprenaline group limited its therapeutic value. Pronethalol was introduced by Sir James Black but was withdrawn as it induced tumors in animals.

Beta Cells of the Pancreas The alpha and the beta cells in the islets of Langerhans of the pancreas were identified independently by M.A. Lane (1907) and R.R. Bensley (1911) of America.

Beta Hemolytic Streptococci Since the introduction of the name 'streptococcus' by Anton Julius Friedrich Rosenbach (1842–1923) in 1884, a controversy has continued regarding their classification. Classification into alpha, beta, and gamma, based on the type and degree of hemolysis produced on the blood agar plate, was introduced by J.H. Brown (b 1884) in his monograph in the medical researches of the Rockefeller Institute in 1920. Those bacteria producing greenish discoloration or partial hemolysis were designated to the alpha group and those showing a greater degree of hemolysis were named beta.

Beta Oxidation Theory *See Knoop, Franz.*

Beta Rays *See atomic disintegration.*

Beta Thalassemia A condition associated with bone changes, splenomegaly and severe anemia in infancy and early childhood. Described by Thomas Benton Cooley (1871–1945) and P. Lee in 1925.

Bethencourt, Jacques de French physician who described syphilis as a new disease as 'Morbus venereus' in 1527.

Bethesda A pool in Jerusalem where diseases were cured during the time of St John the Baptist.

Bethlehem Hospital Established as the Priory of St Mary of Bethlehem under the leadership of a monk and Sheriff of London, Simon Fitzmary, during the reign of King Henry III in 1247. The monks ran a 20-bed hospital which was taken under the administration of the Mayor of London in 1340. It was used as a hospital for the insane around 1403,

and moved to Moorfields in 1675, and to St George's Field in 1814. Care at the hospital deteriorated in the 18th and 19th centuries. Patients were chained, held behind bars and exhibited to the public. The name 'bedlam' became synonymous with wild tumult. It remained the only asylum for the insane in England until Bethel Hospital was established in 1724. St Lukes asylum for the insane in London followed in 1751.

Betts, John A physician who took his doctor's degree from Christ Church, Oxford in 1654 and became physician to King Charles II. He wrote *De Ortu et Natura Sanguinis* (1669) and *Anatomae Thomae Parr.*

Betz Cells Giant motor cells in the fifth layer of the cerebral cortex. Described by Vladimir Betz (1834–1894), a Russian professor of anatomy at Kiev in 1874. A later description were given by a Leeds physiologist, William Bevan-Lewis (1847–1929).

Bevan, Aneurin (1897–1960) From Tredigar, Monmouthshire, he was one of 13 children born to a poor miner. He worked in the pits and became a politician through trade unionism. He was the Minister of Health for the Labour Government in 1945 and founded the National Health Service in Britain in 1946.

Bevan, Arthur Dean (1860–1943) American surgeon in Chicago who described the 'Bevan method' for the operation of undescended testis in 1899.

Bevan, John *See Bevis.*

Bevan-Lewis, William (1847–1929) Professor of mental diseases at Leeds who described the large cells of the motor cortex (Bevan-Lewis cells) in 1879.

Beverwick, John de or Beverovicious (1594–1647) Physician from Dort who published several works in Amsterdam, including *De termino Vitae Fatali an Mobili* (1644), *De Excellencia Sexus Foeminei* (1639) and *Introductio ad Medicinum Indegenam* (1663).

Beveridge, Sir William Henry (1879–1963) British civil servant and economist, born in Rangpur, India. He paved the way for the provision of social security in England through his report *Social Insurance and Allied Services* in 1942.

Beveridge, William Ian Beadmore Professor of anatomy and pathology at the University of Cambridge who wrote *Influenza: The Last Great Plague* in 1977 and *The Art of Scientific Investigation* in 1950.

Beverovicious *See Beverwick, John de.*

Bevis or Bevan, John (1693–1771) A physician from

Pembrokeshire, Wales. He made lenses by adding borax to improve the refractive power. He wrote several treatises and also published Halley astronomical tables.

Bewick, Thomas (1753–1828) Artist from Northumberland and an engraver on wood who wrote *A General History of Quadrupeds* in 1785.

Bezoar [Arabic: *bazahr*, counter-poison] Concretions of high-phosphate stones found in certain ruminant animals, such as the goat. They were used as medicines and amulets to treat a wide variety of maladies since ancient times. The Arabs used a special species of goat, *Capra aegagus,* to obtain their bezoars. They also introduced their use as medicine and amulets into Europe around the 9th century.

Bezoar Animale A 17th-century remedy which consisted of the dried powdered liver and heart of vipers.

Bezold Disease Otitis media complicated by the release of pus into adjacent structures such as the sternomastoid muscle, mastoid bone, back of the neck and thoracic cavity, often leading to a fatal outcome. Described by an otologist, Friedrich von Bezold (1842–1908) of Germany, in 1881.

Bezold, Albert von (1836–1868) German physiologist who demonstrated the accelerator nerve fibers of the heart and their origin in the spinal cord in 1862. He described the nerve ganglia in the interauricular septum (Bezold ganglia) in 1863. He was professor of physiology at Würzberg at the age of 23 years, but died 10 years later from rheumatic heart disease.

Bezold, Friedrich von (1842–1908) *See Bezold disease.*

Bial Test Test for detection of pentose sugar in the urine, using hydrochloric acid as one of the reagents. Devised by German physician, Manfred Bial (1870–1908).

Bianchi Syndrome Sensory aphasia accompanied by apraxia and alexia, seen in lesions of the left parietal lobe. Described by Italian neuropsychiatrist, Leonardo Bianchi (1848–1927). He established the teaching of psychiatry in Naples in 1890 and was Minister of Public education.

Bianchi, Giovanni Battista (1681–1761) Anatomist from Turin who wrote *Historia Hepatica* (1710), *Ductus Lachrymalis Anatome* in 1715 and other works on anatomy.

Bianchi, John (1693–1775) Also known as Janus Plankus. A physician at Rimini who wrote *Lettere Interno alla Cataratta* (1720), *De Monstris et Rebus Monstrosis* (1749) and a number of other treatises.

Bianconi, John Lewis (1717–1781) Physician at Bologna

who translated Benignus Winslow's book, *Anatomy* into Italian in six volumes.

Bibliography in Medicine The first known was by an Arab, Abi'Usabi'a (1203–1269), who wrote *Lives of the Physicians* (*Uyunu l'Anba fi Tabaqati'l Attiba*) in 1245. It was translated into Latin as *Fontes Relationum de Classibus Medicorum.* A bibliography of 52,000 scientific works was produced by Swiss physician, Albrecht von Haller (1708–1777) of Bern in 1776. *A Catalogue of Medical Books* (1812) was published by Robert Watt (1774–1819), a physician from Ayrshire, Scotland, and President of the Faculty of Physicians and Surgeons at Glasgow. He also compiled *Bibliotheca Britannica.* An American biography was compiled by James Thacher (1754–1844) in 1828. An exhaustive medical bibliography with a catalogue of authors and subjects was produced by John Shaw Billings (1838–1913) in 1876. *Garrison and Morton's Medical Bibliography* was compiled by Leslie T. Morton, who incorporated Fielding Garrison's previous work, which provided over 4200 items, and added over 1600 before he published the first edition of the Garrison–Morton bibliography in 1949.

Bichat, Maria Francis Xavier (1771–1802) Physician from Thoitette, France who worked at the Hôtel Dieu in Paris. A founder of microscopic anatomy, a field later known as histology. He advocated the study of anatomy on the basis of different tissues in the body. He wrote *Recherches Physiologiques sur la vie et la Mort, Anatomie Generale Applique a la physiologie* (1801) and *Traites des membranes.*

Bicuspid Valves [Latin: *bis*, twice + *cuspis*, point] *See mitral valve.*

Bidder Ganglion *See Bidder, Friedrich.*

Bidder, Friedrich Heinrich Wilhelm (1810–1894) Professor of anatomy at Dorpat who investigated the autonomic nervous system in 1842, and showed that it was made up of small medullated fibers from the sympathetic and spinal ganglia. He discovered the ganglionic cells (Bidder ganglion) at the junction of the auricles and ventricles in 1852. He demonstrated the reflexive copious production of acid gastric juice at the sight of food in gastrostomized dogs in 1852.

Bidloo, Godfrey (1649–1713) Anatomist and poet from Amsterdam. His chief work, *Anatomia Humani Corporis,* consisting of 105 beautifully engraved plates, was published in 1685.

Biedl, Arthur (1869–1933) German physician worked on the neural control of the viscera through splanchnic centers in 1895. He demonstrated the importance of adrenal glands in the role of internal secretions in 1910, and Lawrence–Moon–Biedl syndrome was described in 1922.

Bier, August Karl Gustav (1861–1949) Pioneer from Kiel in studying the tissue response to local asphyxia produced by deprivation of blood in 1887. He discovered the action of cocaine as a spinal anesthetic in 1889.

Biermer Disease Progressive pernicious anemia. It showed no response to any therapeutic measures. Described by Swiss professor of medicine, Anton Biermer (1827–1892) in Zurich in 1872.

Biermer, Anton (1827–1892) *See Biermer disease.*

Biernacki Syndrome Analgesia of the ulnar nerve seen in dementia paralytica and tabes dorsalis. Described by Polish physician, Edmund Biernacki (1867–1912) from Lemberg, Austria.

Biesiadecki Fossa A recess of the peritoneum over the psoas muscle. Described by Polish physician, Alfred von Biesiadecki (1839–1888).

Biett Disease *See systemic lupus erythematosus.*

Biett, Laurent Theodore (1781–1840) A physician from Paris who gave an early description of lupus erythematosus.

Bifilar Magnetometer A bar magnet suspended by two vertical wires constructed by Sir W. Snow Harris in 1836, and improved by Wilhelm Weber (1804–1891) and Karl Friedrich Gauss (1777–1855).

Bigelow, Erastus Bigham (1814–1879) American inventor, from West Boylston, Massachusetts who invented looms in the textile industry. He founded the Massachusetts Institute of Technology (MIT) in 1861.

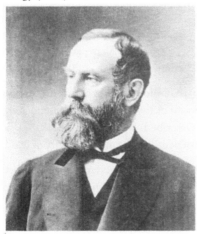

Henry Jacob Bigelow (1816–1890). Courtesy of the National Library of Medicine

Bigelow, Henry Jacob (1816–1890) Surgeon in Boston who described the Y-shaped iliofemoral ligament of the hip joint (Bigelow ligament) in 1869. He also adopted the single-word nomenclature in compilation of the American Pharmacopoeia in 1820. He assisted the surgeon John Warren (1778–1856) in a demonstration of ether as a surgical anesthetic at Massachusetts General Hospital in 1846. The success of this procedure was announced in his article in the *Boston Surgical and Medical Journal* of 18 November, 1846.

Bigelow, Jacob (1787–1879) A visiting physician to the Massachusetts General Hospital and professor of materia medica and surgery at Harvard. He was also a botanist and wrote *American Medical Botany* in three volumes from 1817–1820 which had 60 plates and 6000 colored engravings.

Bigeminy [Latin: *bigemina*, twin] Pulses bigeminius, in which two pulses occur in rapid succession. Described by Ludwig Traube (1818–1876) in 1872.

Bignami, Amico (1862–1929) While working with Ettore Marchiafava (1847–1935) in Rome, he identified the role of the *Anopheles* mosquito as a vector in transmission of malaria. A neurological disorder consisting of tremor, convulsions and coma related to alcohol intake (Marchiafava–Bignami syndrome) was described by them in 1903.

Bile [Latin: *bilis*, bile] Considered to be an important factor in production of disease during ancient times by Hippocrates (460–377 BC) as well as the Hindu Brahmins. A study of the composition of the bile was done by Louis Jacques Thenard (1777–1857), a contemporary of Joseph Gay-Lussac (1778–1850) in 1803. He called it *picromel* to denote the sweetish bitter substance in it. Jöns Jacob Berzelius (1779–1848) also investigated it and thought that it contained resin. A test for bile was devised by German chemist, Max von Pettenkoffer (1818–1901) in 1844, and Paul Ehrlich (1854–1915) devised further tests in 1883. Bile acids were shown to be steroids based on the structure of cholesterol by German organic chemist, Heinrich Otto Wieland (1877–1957) in 1912. The Nobel Prize in Chemistry was awarded to Wieland for his work on bile acids while he was a professor at Munich in 1927. Synthesis of the bile acid ester, taurocholic acid, from cholesterol was done by a Swedish biochemist from Stockholm, Sune Karl Bergstrom (b 1916) in 1952.

Bile Acids *See bile.*

Bile Stones Gallstones observed by Gentile da Foligno, a professor at Padua in 1340. Bernard Naunyn (1839–1925) of Berlin did important clinical studies on gallstones in 1898, and advocated drainage of the bile duct in cases of cholestasis due to gallstones.

Bilguer, John Ulric de (1720–1796) Swiss army surgeon. His chief work *Dissertatio Inauguralis Medico-Chirugica de Membrorum Amputatione rarissime adminstranda aur quasi Abroganda* was published in 1761, and later translated into English and French.

Bilharzia *See bilharziasis.*

Bilharziasis The eggs of *Schistosoma haematobium* have been found in the dry tissues of 3000-year-old mummies in Egypt, indicating the antiquity of the disease. Theodor Maximilian Bilharz (1825–1862), a German professor of zoology at Cairo, discovered the parasite in the portal system of the blood of patients in 1851, and it was named after him by Thomas Spencer Cobbold (1828–1886). Wilhelm Griesinger (1817–1868) demonstrated the fluke in the mesenteric veins of the bladder and other organs in 1854. The endemic status of bilharziasis in the South Africa was shown by John Harley (1883–1921) in 1864.

Biliary Atresia *See congenital biliary atresia.*

Biliary Cirrhosis *See primary biliary cirrhosis.*

Biligrafin *See cholecystography.*

Bilirubin [Latin: *bilis*, bile or green + *rubin*, red] Isolated by W. Heintz (1817–1880) in 1857. A method of estimating it in biological fluid, based on Paul Ehrlich's diazo reaction, was devised by a physician at Utrecht, Albert Abraham H. van den Berg (1869–1943) and P. Muller in 1916. *See bile.*

Bilis Atra Another term for melancholy.

Biliverdin Obtained by Jöns Jacob Berzelius (1779–1848) in 1840. Basilius Valentinus prepared a crystalline form in 1859.

Bill of Health Originally a document issued by the consul to the master of a vessel before he was allowed to sail.

Billing, Archibald (b 1791) Born in Cromlyn, he graduated from Trinity College, Dublin in 1818, and was physician to the London Hospital, where he organized practical teaching at the bedside. He wrote *The First Principles of Medicine* (1831), *Practical Observations on Diseases of Lungs and Heart* (1852), *The Treatment of Asiatic Cholera* (1848) and *The Science of Gems, Jewels, Coils and Medals, Ancient and Modern* (1867).

Billings, John Shaw (1838–1913) Born in Indiana, he was an army surgeon during the Civil War. He founded the library of the Surgeon General in Washington DC, one of the largest libraries in the world. In 1876 he published a catalog of authors and subjects and in 1880 he produced the first volume of the Index catalog of the library, the most exhaustive bibliography ever. He planned and built the Johns Hopkins Hospital, which took him over 14 years.

Billroth Operation II (Syn. Billroth II anastomosis) Resection of the pylorus with the greater part of the lesser curvature of the stomach, closure of the cut ends of the duodenum and stomach, followed by a gastrojejunostomy.

Billroth Operation Excision of the pyloric end of the stomach followed by axial anastomosis with the duodenum. Described by Emile Jules Pean (1830–1898) of Paris in 1879. Theodor Billroth (1829–1894) used this method and it was named the Billroth I operation. The Billroth II operation, in which the stomach is excised with closure of the duodenum, followed by anastomosis with the jejunum, was also devised by Billroth. It was modified by Eugene Alexander Pólya (1875–1944) of Germany in 1911. *See gastrectomy.*

Billroth, Theodor (1829–1894) Professor of surgery in Zurich and Vienna. He performed experimental resections of the cervical esophagus in animals in 1871. His work was followed up by his assistant Vincenz Czerny (1842–1916) who did the first successful resection of the esophagus in a human in 1877. Billroth performed a distal partial gastrectomy in 1881 and resection of the larynx in 1883. *See Billroth operation.*

Biloptin *See cholecystography.*

Binet, Alfred (1857–1911) French experimental psychologist from Nice who graduated in medicine from the Sorbonne, where he became the Director of the Department of Psychology in 1892. He published *L'Etude Experimentale de l'Intelligence* in 1903. He also wrote a book on the psychology of reasoning in 1886. He initiated the intelligence quotient (IQ). *See intelligence quotient.*

Binet–Simon Test A test for intelligence devised by Alfred Binet (1878–1956), a French experimental psychologist and Theodore Simon (1873–1961) of Paris in 1911.

Bing Sign Extension of the great toe following stimulation of the dorsum of the foot or toe, in cases of pyramidal tract lesions. Described by R. Bing (1878–1956), French professor of neurology at the University of Basel.

Bing Tuning Fork Test A test to differentiate between middle and inner ear lesions. Devised by Austrian otologist, Alfred Bing (1844–1922).

Binocular Vision [Greek: *binus*, two + *ocular*, eye] Le Pere Cherubin, a French philosopher, viewed small objects under the microscope conjointly with both eyes in 1677.

Sir Charles Wheatstone (1802–1875) investigated binocular vision and constructed the stereoscope based on this principle. The binocular technique later became a permanent feature of the microscope.

Binswanger Disease A progressive subcortical encephalopathy leading to a classic picture of dementia, which occurs mostly in the fifth and sixth decades of life. Described by a professor of psychiatry at Jena, Otto Ludwig Binswanger (1852–1929) in 1894. *See subcortical dementia.*

Binz, Carl (1832–1912) A pupil of Rudolph Virchow (1821–1902). He founded the Pharmacological Institute of the University of Bonn in 1869, and was its first director. He published a book on the history of anesthesia in 1896, and a textbook of materia medica in 1866. His work was translated by Peter W. Latham, professor of medicine at the University of Cambridge, and published in two volumes by the New Sydenham Society in 1897.

Biochemistry [Greek: *bios*, life + *chemia*, mutation] The application of chemistry to medicine started with Theophrastus Bombastus von Hohenheim (1493–1541). The union of chemistry with medicine was named iatrochemistry and was studied by Johannes Baptista van Helmont (1577–1644), Johann Rudolph Glauber (1604–1670) and Robert Boyle (1627–1691). Antoine Lavoisier (1743–1794) stated that 'life is a chemical function'. Important works that contributed to early biochemistry were: *Chemistry in its Application to Agriculture and Physiology* (1840) and *Organic Chemistry in its Application to Physiology and Pathology* (1842), both by Justus von Liebig (1803–1873) of Germany and *Chemical and Physiological Balance of Organic Nature* (1844) by Jean Baptiste Dumas (1800–1884) and Jean Baptiste Joseph Dieudonne Boussingault (1802–1887). Much is founded on the pioneering works of Josiah Willard Gibbs (1839–1903) on chemical thermodynamics, Jacobus Henricus Van't Hoff (1852–1911) on chemical kinetics and Svante Arrhenius (1859–1927) on electrolytic dissociation. William Dobinson Halliburton (1860–1931), professor of physiology at King's College London, was an English pioneer in biochemistry who wrote *The Essentials of Chemical Physiology* in 1892. The first of the amino acids, tryptophane, was discovered by Sir Frederick Gowland Hopkins (1861–1947) in 1901. The study of the amino acids and their sequence in proteins and research on enzymes occupied most of the early period. A significant advance was made by the introduction of electrophoresis, a method of analysis based on the different mobility of substances in an electric field by Arne Wilhelm Kaurin Tiselius (1902–1971) in 1930. His technique was simplified in 1944 by A.H. Gordon and John Porter Archer

Martin who used water on cellulose (filter paper) as a medium for analysis. Their technique was used by Charles Dent to identify 60 different amino acids in 1948. The biochemical processes of the body were shown to be regulated by genes by Edward Laurie Tatum (1909–1975) at the Rockefeller Institute. A turning point in the study of structural biochemistry came with Emil Fischer's (1852–1919) research on the principal components of living matter such as fats, proteins and sugars. A valuable account of the early development of biochemistry is given in F. Leben's *Geschichte der Physiologischen Chemie* published in 1935.

Biofeedback *See feedback mechanism.*

Biogenesis [Greek: *bios*, life + *genesis*, origin] The theory that living matter always arises by the agency of pre-existing living matter. Term coined by Thomas Henry Huxley (1825–1895) in 1870.

Biological Clock Proposed as a biological mechanism to determine the period during which one species has been separated from another species by Linus Pauling (1901–1994).

Biology [Greek: *bios*, life + *logos*, discourse] Term introduced in 1802 by Gottfried Reinhold Treviranus (1776–1837) of Bremen to denote the science of life. Jean Baptiste de Monet Lamarck (1744–1829) independently used it in the same year. Aristotle (384–322 BC), the father of biology, wrote *De Anima* which dealt with the essence of life or psyche, and distinguished living from non-living things. His second book, *Historia Animalium*, contained observations, investigations and descriptions of several forms of animal life. His other extant works are *De Generatione Animalium* on the generation of animals and *De Partibus Animalium* on the parts of animals. Theophrastus (380–287 BC), the founder of botany, wrote *Historia Plantarum*. Some notable biologists include: Herbert Spencer (1820?–1903), John Ray (1627–1705), Carl Linnaeus (1707–1778) and Charles Darwin (1809–1882).

Biopsy [Greek: *bios*, life + *opsis*, sight] *See liver biopsy, rectal biopsy, bone marrow biopsy.*

Boisbaudran, Paul Emile Lecoq de (1838–1912) *See gallium.*

Biot Sign A variant of Cheyne–Stokes respiration seen in medullary compression of the brain. Described by French physician, Camille Biot (b 1878).

Biotin A coenzyme necessary for the growth of bacteria. Found in high concentration in egg white by W.G. Bateman in 1916. It was named 'vitamin H' by Paul Gyorgy (1893–1976) in 1931, and was renamed 'coenzyme R' by F.E. Allison in 1933. The composition was established by American biochemist and professor at Cornell University, Vincent du Vigneaud (1901–1978) in 1941. Synthesis was achieved by Stanton Avery Harris (b 1902) and co-workers in 1943.

Bipolar Illness [Latin: *bis*, twice + *polos*, pivot] *See manic-depressive psychosis.*

Birch-Hirschfield, Felix Victor (1842–1899) German pathologist who devised a method of staining amyloid tissues with gentian violet and Bismarck brown.

Bird, Golding (1814–1854) London physician who described oxaluria (Bird disease) and treated bedsores by galvanism.

Bird-Breeders' Lung A disease with symptoms resembling farmers' lung, described amongst bird breeders around the 1950s. It was shown to be due to antigenic properties of the excreta of budgerigars and pigeons by F.E. Hargreave, J. Pepys and others in 1966.

Bird-Fanciers' Lung Bird-breeders' lung in patients who plucked geese or chicken feathers. Described by M.M. Plessener of Germany in 1960.

Birds Eye Inclusion bodies in cancer cells described by Rudolph Virchow (1821–1902).

Birkbeck, George (1776–1841) Born in Settle, Yorkshire, he graduated as a physician from Edinburgh when he was 21 years old and became professor of natural history at the Andersonian Institution in Glasgow soon after his graduation. After practicing as a physician in London, he took up engineering and founded the London Mechanics Institution in 1822. This became Birkbeck College in 1907 and was later incorporated into London University.

Birley Anti-Catarrh A secret remedy in the form of a liquid, advertised as a 'special remedy for catarrh for cold and influenza' by a London company at the turn of the 19th century. On analysis it was found to contain mainly sugar and traces of tartaric acid.

Birmingham, Ambrose (1864–1905) Irish professor of anatomy who described the stomach bed, the organs on which the posterior part of the stomach rested in 1896.

Birth Control The first suggestion of contraception is found in Aristotle's *Historia Animalium* in which he recommends covering the cervix with a mixture of the oils of cedar and olive. Violent body movements by women after intercourse as a method of preventing conception was mentioned by Greek and Roman medical men, including Galen (129–200). During Egyptian times, around 1800 BC, pessaries made of crocodile dung, vaginal irrigation with honey and sponges soaked in gum were used to prevent pregnancy. Various herbal abortifacients, such as jugri from molasses and leadwort, were also used in India. Dioscorides in the 2nd century described several methods of contraception, including magical prescriptions or amulets, potions, pessaries and the local application of contraceptive materials. The most scientific treatise on contraception during the Roman period was written by Soranus of Ephesus in the 1st century. He specialized in gynecology and distinguished abortifacients and contraceptives. Aetius of Amida, around the 6th century, described pessaries in his encyclopedic work on medicine. Contraceptive recipes are described in the Chinese medical texts written by Sun Ssu-Mo, in AD 695. Condoms were introduced into Europe during the 17th century, supposedly by a Colonel Cundum. They were made of the dried gut of the sheep. Practical birth control in England was introduced by Francis Place (1771–1854) who wrote a treatise in 1822, *Illustrations and Proofs of the Principles of Population*. He and his assistants organized distribution of handbills on birth control in London and across the north of England in 1823. His disciples included Richard Carlile, Richard Hassel and William Campion. The economic, medical and social aspects of birth control were discussed by Carlile in *Every Woman's Book or What is Love*, published in 1826. Other forms of contraception using vaginal metal caps and diaphragms were used during this period. The birth control movement in America was initiated by Robert Dale Owen (1801–1877) in 1828. He published the first book on birth control in America in 1830, *Moral Physiology* in which he recommended coitus interruptus. A physician from New York, Charles Knowlton (1800–1850), advocated douching in *Fruits of Philosophy*, published anonymously in 1832. The douche and vaginal sponges were advocated by a physician, George Drysdale in his treatise *Elements of Social Science* published in 1854. Charles Brandlaugh, Annie Bessant and Edward Truelove were prosecuted in England on grounds of obscenity because of their attempts to promote public education on contraception during the years 1878 and 1879. A scientific forum for birth control was created in England by Sir Clifford Allibut (1836–1925) and William Bateson (1861–1926) in 1912. In the same year Sir James Barr, President of the British Medical Association, endorsed birth control, and he was joined by Abraham Jacobi (1830–1919), the first President of the American Medical Association. A year later the Malthusian League printed a pamphlet with advice on birth control and distributed it on a large scale free of charge. *See condom, contraceptive devices, coitus interruptus, coitus reservatus, Sanger, Margaret.*

Births and Deaths Registration Act Originally enacted in 1836 and followed in 1874 by an Act which specified the statutory duty of the doctor to issue a certificate for a patient on whom he attended during his or her last illness in England.

Bischoff, Theodor Ludwig Wilhelm (1807–1882) Professor of anatomy and embryologist at Heidelberg who described the zona radiata of the mammalian ovum in 1884.

Bishop, John Michael (b 1936) *See oncogenes.*

Bishop Licenses To allow physicians to practice in England, instituted by an act of Parliament in 1511. Bishops were empowered to hold an *ad hoc* examination by a panel of physicians before allowing a physician to practice. One of the earliest licenses to practice psychiatry (for the melancholy and mad) as a specialty is found in Archbishop Whitgift's *Register* in 1600. Although the right to grant Bishop's licenses ceased after the Medical Act of 1858, it remained on the statute book until 1948.

Bismuth Discovered by the German physician, George Agricola (1494–1555) in 1520. It was prepared by French chemist, Nicholas Lemery (1645–1715) from Rouen, who sold it as a secret remedy for spasms of the stomach and migraine. It was suggested as a treatment for syphilis by Felix Balzar (1849–1929) of Paris in 1889. It came into general use following publication of a treatise by a physician L. Odier of Geneva, who recommended it as an antispasmodic in 1786. Bismuth subnitrate was used in treatment of amebic dysentery in Panama by W.E. Deeks in 1908. Its curative action on spirochaetosis of fowls was shown by A.E. Robert and B. Saunton in 1916, and in 1921 Robert Sazerac (b 1875) and Constantin Levaditi (1874–1953) used it effectively in treatment of syphilis. Thereafter, about 200 bismuth compounds appeared within a short period, as treatment for rheumatoid arthritis, syphilis and other conditions.

Bismuth Meal Walter Bradford Cannon (1871–1945) from Harvard University demonstrated by means of a X-ray tube and fluorescent screens the act of deglutition in animals, following a bolus of bismuth-impregnated food, in 1898. He adapted this to study the alimentary tract of humans and replaced bismuth with barium as a purer and cheaper contrast medium in 1924.

Bisset, Charles (1717–1791) Scottish physician from Glenalbert, Perthshire. He wrote *Treatise on Scurvy* (1755), *An Essay on the Medical Constitution of Great Britain* and *Medical Essays and Observations.* He later studied engineering in Europe and wrote *A Treatise on Fortification.*

He subsequently served as a military surgeon in Jamaica for a short period before he returned to settle in Skelton, Yorkshire.

Bistoury French term for a small surgical knife. The bistoury cache used in surgery was invented by French surgeon, Bienaise (1601–1631).

Bistoury Laser Used in surgery. Developed by the Americans, D.R. Herriott, E.I. Gorden, H.A.S. Hale and W. Gromnos in 1967. *See laser.*

Bistovol (bismuth stovarsol) Prepared by C. Levadetti in 1925. It was used as treatment for syphilis by L. Fourinier and A. Schwartz in the same year.

Bitot Spots Cheese-like patches on the cornea due to vitamin A deficiency, leading to keratomalacia. Described by French anatomist and surgeon, Pierre A. Bitot (1822–1888) in 1863. He was born in Pondesac and studied medicine at Bordeaux before he graduated from the Faculty of Paris in 1848. He was professor of surgery for sick children at Bordeaux in 1878.

Bittorf Sign In which referred pain occurs in the distribution of the genitofemoral nerve because of lesions of the testis or ovary. Described by Alexander Bittorf (1876–1949), a pathologist in Leipzig.

Bizzozero, Giulio Cesare (1846–1901) Italian physician who described the platelets as the third elementary constituent of blood in 1882. In a later treatise in 1887 he gave more details of platelets, including their size and other properties. *See sideroblasts.*

Bjerrum Chart For testing vision. Devised by Danish professor of ophthalmology, J.P. Bjerrum (1851–1920) from Copenhagen.

Black Bile Thought to be the cause of melancholia by Hippocrates (460–377 BC), who proposed purgatives as treatment. Several centuries later, Cicero disputed this idea and attributed melancholia to psychological difficulties.

Black Crown A porcelain-faced crown for the anterior tooth, fastened by a screw into a gold-lined tooth canal. Devised by Greene Vardiman Black (1836–1915), a dentist from Chicago.

Black Death A terrible pestilence that swept England in 1348. Referred to as the Great Pestilence or the Great Mortality. It was probably bubonic plague and it ravaged England for 2 years, reducing the population from about 4 million to a million. *See bubonic plague.*

Black Fever *See Rocky mountain spotted fever.*

Black Leg (Syn. blackquarter, charbon symtomatique) A fatal disease, mainly of sheep and cattle. Described by Saturnin Arloing (1846–1911) in 1881. The causative agent was identified by several workers and named *Clostridium chauvoei*.

Black, Joseph (1728–1799) Scottish chemist, educated at Belfast and studied medicine at Glasgow and Edinburgh. He succeeded William Cullen (1710–1790) as professor of chemistry and anatomy at Glasgow in 1756. He became a lecturer in chemistry at Edinburgh in 1766. He developed the theory of latent heat, disproved the theory that when a substance is burnt it gives off a substance called phlogeston, and rediscovered carbon dioxide. He presented his thesis *De Humore acido a cibis orto, et Magnesia Alba,* for his doctorate degree in 1754.

Black, Sir James Whyte (b 1924) A physician whose major interest was cardiovascular medicine. He graduated from St Andrews, Scotland in 1946. He discovered prothenolol, the first betablocker which led to the development of propranolol. He was a major contributor to the development of burinamide which was a prototype of the H2 antagonist, cimetidine. He was knighted in 1981 and awarded the Nobel Prize for Medicine or Physiology in 1988.

Black, William (1750–1829) A physician from Ireland who was educated at Leiden. He wrote: *A Dissertation on Insanity Extracted from Between Two and Three Thousand Cases in Bedlam* (1810), *A Historical Sketch of Medicine and Surgery from their Origin to the Present Time* (1782), *A Comparative View on the Mortality of the Human at All Ages* (1788) and other treatises.

Blackall, John (1771–1860) English physician and one of the earliest workers to demonstrate albuminuria in dropsy. He wrote *Observations on the Nature and Cure of Dropsies* in 1813.

Blackley, Charles Harrison (1820–1900) Manchester physician who demonstrated that hay fever can be produced by applying pollen to the eyes. He published his work on hay-asthma, *Experimental Researches on the Causes and Nature of Catarrhus Aestivus* in 1873.

Blackman, Frederick Frost (1866–1947) Botanist born in Lambeth, London and graduated in medicine from St Bartholomew's Hospital in 1885. He researched respiration of plants and factors limiting plant growth.

Blackmore, Sir Richard (1650–1729) Born in Wiltshire, he was physician to King William and Queen Anne. He was also a poet and his philosophical poem *Creation* ran into several editions. *Satyr against Wit* was another successful work in 1700. He wrote treatises on medical subjects including smallpox, consumption, spleen, gout and dropsy.

Blackwater Fever Hippocrates (460–377 BC) gave a description which has puzzled physicians as regards to its etiology for nearly 2000 years. Quinine was considered to be the cause by Veretas, a Greek physician in 1858 and by Salvatore Tommasi (1813–1888) of Italy in 1874. Robert Koch (1843– 1910) also supported this theory. Sambon in 1898 thought that it was a disease similar to babesiasis or Texan fever of cattle. In the early 1940s it was established to be a malignant form of falciparum malaria infection. Primaquin, an 8-aminoquinoline derivative, was noted to induce signs similar to those of blackwater fever in healthy African– American troops by R.S. Hockwald, J. Arnold, J. Clayman and Alving in 1952.

Blackwell, Alexander (d 1748) A physician from Aberdeen who studied under Herman Boerhaave (1668–1738) at Leiden. He went to Sweden in 1740 and practiced as a public health engineer. He was later suspected of having taken part in Count Tessin's plot and was beheaded.

Blackwell, Elizabeth (1821–1910) Born in Bristol, she emigrated to New York with her father in 1832. She obtained her MD from New York in 1849 to become the first woman graduate of medicine in America. She returned to England in 1879 and became the first woman to be licensed to practice medicine in England. She later became professor of obstetrics and gynecology at the London School of Medicine, and pioneered medical education for women.

Blackwell, Elizabeth Wife of Alexander Blackwell, the physician executed for treason in 1747. She wrote *The Curious Herbal; containing 500 of the most useful plants which are now used in the Practice of Physic* in 1737. A second volume appeared in 1739.

Blackwell, Emily (1826–1910) Sister of Elizabeth Blackwell, the first woman to graduate in medicine in America. She was a surgeon and assistant to James Simpson. She established the New York Infirmary for Indigent Women and Children with her sister in 1856, and became professor of obstetrics at the Women's Medical College attached to the Infirmary in 1869.

Bladder Ammonius, a surgeon of Alexandria, described a method of extraction of stones from the bladder in 240 BC. Rhazes (850–932) of Persia found that hematuria was a symptom of bladder disease. Albucasis (936–1013) in his surgical book *Altasrif* written in the eleventh century, described a surgical operation for bladder stones. Benjamin Bell (1749–1806) suggested suture of the bladder for rupture in 1789 and it was used by Willet of St Bartholomew's Hospital. Bladder stones in patients with cystinuria were noted by William Hyde Wollaston (1766–1828) in 1810. A cystine stone from the bladder of a boy of six years was removed by Julius Muller in 1852. The external sphincter of the bladder was discovered by German histologist, Friedrich Gustav Jakob Henle (1809–1885). The Mercer bar, a transverse curved ridge joining the internal openings of the ureter within the bladder, was described in 1848 by Louis Auguste Mercier (1811–1882) of Paris. London surgeon, George James Guthrie (1785–1856) published a monograph, *On the Anatomy and Diseases of the Neck of the Bladder* in 1834. Cancer of the bladder due to aniline in the dye industry was shown by: Ludwig Rehn (1849–1930) of Germany (1895), Leuenberger of Basle (1912), Heinrich Curshmann (1846–1910) of Germany (1920) and Oppenheimer. A cystoscope was invented by Philipp Bozzini (1773–1809) of Mainz in 1804 and a lens system was added by Max Nitz (1848–1906) in 1879. Practical visualization of the interior was made possible by Hartwig of Berlin who placed a light in a cystoscope in 1887. The Brown-Buerger cystoscope to irrigate as well as observe the bladder was devised by Leo Buerger (1879–1943) in 1909. A catheter, manometer and a moving strip of bromide paper to measure and record bladder and sphincter behavior was designed by Derek Ernest Denny-Brown (1901–1981) and Robertson in 1933. They used this to study the bladder and sphincters following complete transection of the spinal cord and Stewart developed their method into a cystometer in 1942.

Bladder Cancer This was first ascribed to a chemical compound involved in fuchsin manufacture. Described by a German surgeon, Ludwig Rehn (1849–1930) in 1892. The association of bladder cancer with the dye industry was demonstrated by S.G. Leuenberger of Basel in 1912. F. Curshmann of Germany (1920), R. Oppenheimer (1926) and M.W. Goldblatt (1949) demonstrated the carcinogenic properties of aniline and its related compounds on the bladder.

Bladder Carcinoma *See bladder cancer.*

Blair, William Bell (1871–1936) Liverpool obstetrician who used oxytocin in labor in 1909. He was a founder of the Royal College of Obstetricians and Gynaecologists.

Blair, Patrick (1666–1728) A surgeon and botanist from Dundee, who practiced medicine in Boston, Lincolnshire. He published *Anatomy of Elephant* after dissecting an elephant in 1710, *Miscellaneous Observations on Physic Anatomy Surgery and Botany* (1718) and *New Dispensatory of*

Pharmaco-Botanalogia (1728). His *An Account of the Dissection of a Child in 1717* contained a description of congenital hypertrophic pyloric stenosis.

Blair, Vitray Papin (1871–1955) A plastic surgeon who, with James Barrett Brown (1899–1971), introduced split skin grafts in 1929. He was a pioneer in modern maxello-facial surgery.

Blak Thyrol Female Pills A secret remedy for amenorrhea in the early 1900s. Prepared from the moon plant of South Virginia.

Blake, Clarence John (1843–1919) Otologist in Boston who devised a paper prosthesis for repairing a hole in the eardrum.

Blakemore–Sengstaken Tube A triple-lumen tube with two inflatable balloons for applying esophageal tamponade to stop bleeding from esophageal varices. Devised by an American surgeon from New Jersey Robert William Sengstaken (b 1923) and Arthur Hendley Blakemore of New York in 1950.

Blakeslee, Albert Francis (1874–1954) Geneticist from Genesco, New York who worked on plants. He demonstrated in 1937 that polyploidy could be induced in plants by treating them with colchicine.

Blalock, Alfred (1899–1964) American pioneer in cardiac surgery for congenital heart diseases, born at Culloden in Georgia. He graduated from Johns Hopkins University and did his postgraduate studies at Vanderbilt University Hospital. He was the chair of surgery at the Johns Hopkins Hospital in 1942, where he worked with Helen Taussig (1898–1986). They designed the Blalock–Taussig shunt in 1945. He pioneered surgery of patent ductus arteriosus in children. He treated myasthenia gravis by performing thymectomy. His collected papers were published by one of his pupils in 1966.

Blalock–Taussig Shunt Surgical treatment for Fallot tetralogy, performed by Alfred Blalock (1899–1964) and Helen Taussig (1898–1986) of Johns Hopkins Hospital in 1945.

Blancard or Blanchard, Stephen (1625–1703) Professor of history at Middelburg before he became a physician at Franeker, The Netherlands. He produced a dictionary of medicine, surgery and anatomy in 1684. He wrote *Lexicon Medicum Gracio Latinum*.

Blanchard Apiol and Steel Pills Secret remedy for treatment of amenorrhea during the late 19th century. It contained Barbados aloes and iron.

Blanchard, Elston Charles (b 1868) A proctologist who wrote: *The Romance of Proctology* (1938), *Epitome of Ambulant Proctology* (1924), *Textbook of ambulant Proctology* (1928) and *Ambulant Proctology Clinics* (1925).

Blandrata, George (d 1690) Physician from Saluzzo, Italy who had a stormy life because of his politics. He escaped from prison in Pavia and lived in various parts of Europe. He wrote *Brevis Enaratio disputationis Albanae de Deo trine et Christio Duplici* in 1658. He was murdered by his nephew over a monetary disagreement.

Bland-Sutton, Sir John (1855–1936) Surgical pathologist and gynecologist. In 1889 he demonstrated that animals with rickets could be cured by treatment with crushed bones and cod liver oil. He was a pioneer in the study of cancer and wrote *Cancer Clinically Considered* (1909) and *Tumors, Innocent and Malignant* in 1922. The Bland-Sutton Institute of Pathology was established at the Middlesex Hospital in London. *See rickets.*

Bland–White–Garland Syndrome In young children, anomalous origin of the left coronary artery from the pulmonary artery, leading to angina and myocardial infarction. Described by American physician, E.F. Bland (b 1901), a Boston cardiologist, Paul Dudley White (1886–1973) and J. Garland (1893–1973) of Gloucester, Massachusetts. H.S. Brooks gave a description in two cases in 1886.

Blane, Sir Gilbert (1749–1834) Born in Blanefield, Ayrshire, he first went to Edinburgh to train as a clergyman, but later took medicine at the inspiration of William Cullen (1710–1790). He accompanied Admiral Rodney as his physician during an expedition to the West Indies in 1780, and used lime juice in treatment of scurvy amongst seamen. He was a physician at St Thomas' Hospital, where he wrote several treatises on medicine.

Blasius, Gerhard (1626–1682) Professor of anatomy at Amsterdam. He discovered the duct of the parotid gland in 1662.

Blassig, Robert (1830–1878) The director of the Ophthalmic Hospital at St Petersburg. He described the spaces in the anterior part of the retina near the ora serrata in 1863.

Blastema Theory [Greek: *blastema*, bud] The original theory of cancer, which stated that it arose from a fluid 'blastema' released by the tissues owing to pathogenic changes induced by adverse conditions. This was accepted by medical men such as Rudolph Virchow (1821–1902), Karl von Rokintansky (1804–1878) and others until 1860.

Blastoderm [Greek: *blastos*, bud + *derma*, skin] The three germ cell layers in the chick embryo were discovered by an embryologist and paleontologist, Heinrich Christian von Pander (1794–1865) of St Petersburg in 1817. *See Pander cells.*

Blastomycetes [Greek: *blastos*, bud + *mykes*, fungus] A carcinogenic agent, suggested by William Russell in 1890 in the *British Medical Journal*. His theory led to a search for other biological agents with carcinogenic properties.

Blastomycosis Thomas Casper Gilchrist (1862–1927) of Johns Hopkins described chronic granulomatous lesions of the skin associated with bony lesions, caused by a fungus (*Blastomyces dermatidis*) in 1897. This was first thought to be exclusive to North America and was named American blastomycosis. It was described in South America by Lutz Alolfo in 1908.

Bleaching Powder Charles Tennant (1768–1838), a Scottish industrial chemist from Ochiltree, patented the manufacture of bleaching powder from chlorine and slaked lime in 1799. Louis Claude Bertholot (1748–1811), a physician and chemist from Talloires in France, manufactured it with his new method.

Bleeding Time *See Duke, William Waddell.*

Blegny, Nicholas de (1652–1722) French surgeon who established the Academy of New Discoveries at his house in Paris, where he edited a journal in which he announced various discoveries in medicine. He was considered a quack by some and was imprisoned in the castle of Angers for 8 years. One of his famous works *Maladies Veneriens* was published in three volumes in 1683.

Blepharoxyston (Syn. speculum oculi) An ancient instrument for examining the eye.

Bleuler, Eugene (1857–1939) Professor of psychiatry at Burgholzli Hospital in Vienna, where Carl Jung (1587–1657) was one of his students. He coined the term 'schizophrenia' to include dementia praecox in 1911 and established concepts such as autism and ambivalence.

Blind Person Act Passed in 1920 in England. It specified the criteria needed for a person to register as blind. Amongst the other benefits conferred on the blind, the act reduced the retirement age for a pension for a blind person from 70 to 50 years.

Blind Schools The first public school for the blind was established in Paris in 1784 by Valentine Hauy (1746–1822), who also printed raised or embossed letters to help the blind to read. The first blind school in England was founded in Liverpool in 1791. Edinburgh and London followed, with the establishment of their blind schools in 1799. Louis

Braille (1809–1852) devised an alphabet for the blind with varying combinations of six dots in 1834. An embossed system based on Roman capitals was devised in 1845 by William Moon (1818–1894), an English inventor from Kent, who himself became partially blind at the age of 4 years. Education for blind and mute children was made compulsory in Scotland through an Act of Parliament in 1890. The optophone, a device with which blind people could read by ear, was invented by Edmund Edward Fournier D'Albe, a physicist from London, in 1923. The Talking Book Service, mainly for the elderly blind, was introduced in 1935.

Blind Spot Of the retina, discovered in 1668 by Edeme Mariotte (1620–1684), a prior at the Cloister of Saint Martin in France.

Blizard, Sir William (1743–1835) Qualified from St Bartholomew's Hospital and became a surgeon at the London Hospital in 1780. He tied the superior thyroid artery for goiter, and was a founder of the London Hospital Medical School in 1785. He cultivated his poetic talents during his spare time.

Blizard, Thomas (1788–1838) A cousin and pupil of Sir William Blizard (1743–1835). He was surgeon to the London Hospital.

Bloch, Konrad Emil (b 1912) German-born American biochemist who was appointed to the first chair of biochemistry at Harvard University in 1954. His work on fatty acids and cholesterol led to the understanding of the formation of ketones and cholesterol, for which he was awarded the Nobel Prize for Physiology or Medicine in 1964.

Bloch, Oscar Thorvald (1847–1926) A surgeon who devised the two-stage operation for carcinoma of the colon in 1892. His method was modified by Johann von Mikulicz-Radecki (1850–1905) in 1903, and is known as the Mikulicz operation.

Block *See heart block.*

Block, Brachial Plexus *See brachial plexus block.*

Block, Extradural Sacral *See caudal anesthesia.*

Block, Extradural *See extradural block.*

Block, Paravertebral Somatic *See paravertebral somatic block.*

Block, Thoracic Sympathetic *See thoracic sympathetic block.*

Block, Trans-Sacral *See transsacral block.*

Blockly Hospital Now known as Philadelphia General Hospital. It began as an almshouse in 1720. It is probably the

oldest hospital in America to have functioned continuously since its formation.

Blocq Disease The inability either to stand or to walk in a normal manner. Named after Paul O. Blocq (1860-1896), French physician. *See astasia-abasia.*

Blondel, James Augustus English physician of French origin who became involved in the controversy over Mary Tofts, the 'rabbit woman of Godalming', who claimed to have given birth to a rabbit in 1727. He wrote *The Strength of Imagination in the Pregnant Women Examined,* and *The Power of Mother's imagination Over the Fetus Examined.*

Blood [Anglo-Saxon: *blod*, blood] Ancient Sumerians who lived around 4000 BC knew that the blood was the essence of all vital activities. They also considered the liver to be an important organ, as it was known to store blood. Empedocles (500–430 BC) of Agrigentum in Sicily upheld the view that 'the blood is the life' and he identified the innate heat of the blood with the soul. *See anemia, blood circulation, blood letting, blood transfusion, ABO blood group, blood analysis, blood coagulation, hematology.*

Blood Analysis The difference between arterial and venous blood was demonstrated in 1668 by John Mayow (1643–1679). Chemical analysis was done by Robert Boyle (1627–1691) in 1684. A series of clinical blood analyses was performed by Alfred Baring Garrod (1819–1907) during his work on uric acid in the blood of a number of patients in 1848. Carl Schmidt (1822–1894) published his researches on blood analysis in patients with fatal cholera in 1850. Microchemical methods of estimating blood glucose were introduced by Ivor Christian Bang in 1913. Otto Knut Olof Folin (1876–1934) and Hsien Wu devised colorimetric methods to estimate blood glucose, blood nitrogen and uric acid around 1919. *See blood gas analysis, chemical pathology.*

Blood Bank Term first used by Bernard Fantus (1874–1940) in 1937, when he started a center for preserving blood at the Cook County Hospital in Chicago. A major initial problem in storing blood was coagulation. Albert Hustin (b 1882) of Belgium in 1914 added small quantities of citrate to prevent coagulation in stored blood. In 1915 Richard Weil (1876–1917) of New York showed that blood could be safely stored for 3.5 days using sodium citrate. Francis Peyton Rous (b 1879) and J.R. Turner of the Rockefeller Institute in 1916 stored blood for several weeks by adding dextrose. The concept of storing human blood under special conditions for transfusion during emergencies was proposed by Sergei S. Yudin (b 1891) of the Moscow Skilifosovsky Institute in 1931.

Blood Circulation Empedocles (500–430 BC) of Agrigentum in Sicily considered the heart to be the center of the system of blood vessels through which the blood (life) distributed innate heat to other parts of the body. His view was upheld by Aristotle. The term 'circulation' in relation to the movement of blood in the veins and arteries was coined by Andrea Caesalpino (1525–1603) of Italy in 1559. Erasistratus, who lived around 300 BC, postulated that the arteries contained bloodless spirit or air and the veins carried the nutrients. He also believed that the valves of the heart directed the blood towards the veins. Galen (129–200) proposed that blood from the left ventricle reached the right side of the heart via pores in the interventricular septum. He also knew that the pulmonary artery carried blood to the lungs. His teaching was accepted for over 1000 years until William Harvey (1578–1657) announced the discovery of the circulatory system in *Excercitatio Anatomica du Motu Cordis et Sanguinis in Animalibus* published in 1628. In 1608, Harvey's teacher Fabricius Hildanus (1560–1634) had noted that the valves in the veins opened towards the heart, but he offered no explanation for this. Harvey pointed out in his work that these valves prevented venous reflux. Capillary circulation was discovered by Marcello Malpighi (1628–1694) in 1661 and John Hunter (1728–1793) in 1785 demonstrated the presence of a collateral circulation of the arteries. Ernst Heinrich Weber (1795–1878) in 1827 showed that the motion of the blood through the vessels was similar to the progression of waves. The cardiac ganglia, which exert nervous control on the muscular activity of the heart, were discovered by Robert Remak (1815–1865) in 1844. Carl Friedrich Wilhelm Ludwig (1816–1895) located the center in the brain that acted as a 'master switchboard' to control and regulate the circulatory system, around 1854. *See fetal circulation, heart.*

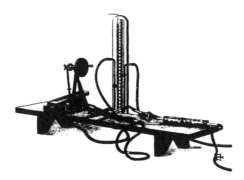

A laboratory model used for demonstrating blood circulation. G.V. Anrep and D.T. Harris, *Practical Physiology* (1923). Churchill, London

Blood Coagulation One of the first to investigate the subject of coagulation of blood was Andrew Buchanan (1798–1882), a physician who graduated from Glasgow in 1822. The classical theory of clotting is derived from the work of Olof Hammarsten (1841–1932) of Uppsala in 1875, Alexander Schmidt (1831–1894) of Leipzig in 1892 and Paul Oskar Morawitz (1879–1936) of Germany in 1903. Hammarsten demonstrated the splitting of fibrinogen into fibrin and other products during the process of clotting. The enzymatic nature of the process was suggested by Morawitz, who also introduced the term 'thrombokinase'. Morawitz's enzymatic theory was verified by F. R. Bettelheim and K. Bailey in 1952. Until 1903, only four factors – thrombokinase, prothrombin, fibrinogen and calcium – were known to be involved in clotting. A fifth factor, factor V, was announced by Paul Arnor Owren (b 1905) of Scandinavia in 1947. Factor VI was used to denote a hypothetical derivative of factor V proposed by Owren. Factor VII was discovered and named by F. Koller and co-workers in 1951. The system of numerical terms was applied to several subsequently discovered factors in 1953.

Blood Count The method of estimating the number of cells in the blood was invented by Karl Vierordt (1818–1884) of Germany in 1852. He used a capillary tube to collect his own blood and counted the number of cells in a cubic millimeter. White cells were counted by Hermann Welcher (1822–1897) in 1853. The pipette for dilution before counting was invented by Pierre Carl Edouard Potain (1825–1901) in 1867, and a modern counting chamber was devised by William Richard Gowers (1845–1915) in 1877. The discovery of staining methods for blood cells by Paul Ehrlich (1854–1915) of Germany was an important contribution to the field of hematology. He used aniline dyes to stain and identify white blood cells in 1877, and introduced the differential blood cell count in 1879. *See leukocyte count.*

Blood Depots or reservoirs Lungs as a storehouse for blood were mentioned by Marcello Malpighi (1628–1694). John Hunter (1728–1793) noted that the veins accommodated the excess blood when the arteries contracted. Several organs of the body, used as reservoirs for blood that was not needed immediately for metabolism, were mentioned by Thomas Hodgkin (1798–1866) in 1822. Joseph Barcroft (1872–1947) in 1934 estimated the reserve blood capacity of the organs as follows: liver 20%, spleen 16% and skin 10%.

Blood Gas Analysis Italian anatomist, Matteo Realdo Colombo (1516–1559), while vivisecting a dog, made an incision into the pulmonary vein and found that the blood in it was bright red, unlike other blood. This led him to suggest that the lungs had rendered the blood 'spirituous'.

His observation was the first on oxygenated blood. Chemical differences between arterial and venous blood were shown in 1668 by John Mayow (1643–1679). A micrometer, was devised by Hans Winterstein in 1905. British physiologist John Scott Haldane (1860–1936) analyzed respiratory gases in 1898. An improved apparatus was invented by Donald Dexter Van Slyke (1883–1971) in 1924.

Blood Glucose The microchemical method of estimation of blood glucose was devised by Ivor Christian Bang of Germany in 1913 and improved by Otto Folin and Hsien Wu in 1919. A method of preparing blood filtrates for determination of sugar content was devised by Michael Somogyi (1883–1971), professor of biochemistry at St Louis, Missouri in 1930. Analysis of whole blood for sugar, Benedict test, was devised by Stanley Rossiter Benedict (1884–1936) of Cornell University, New York in 1931.

Blood Groups *See ABO blood groups.*

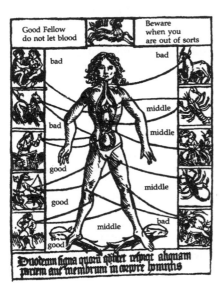

Sites of blood letting in relation to the zodiac, 15th century

Blood Letting Hippocrates (460–377 BC) practiced venesection but did not leave any treatise on the subject. Galen (129–200) wrote three treatises on venesection. Aulus Cornelius Celsus (25 BC–AD 50) described the technique in his *De Re Medicina*, and the Talmud, the Hebrew book written in AD 500, also mentions the practice. Islamic teaching that the blood should be let from the opposite side to the disease or lesion was refuted by Pierre Brissot (1478–1522) of Paris, who venesected on the same side and also as close to the lesion as possible. Exotic anatomical charts were issued to illustrate the various sites in the human body for blood letting during this period. The practice was popular in Italy in the time of Leonardo Botallo

(1519–1587), and costly Venetian bleeding cups were treated as family heirlooms. Thomas Sydenham (1624–1689) practiced blood letting in England, but with clinical prudence. Matthew Baillie (1761–1823), a physician and nephew of John Hunter (1728–1793), criticized and denounced the practice in 1817. *See cupping.*

Blood Meal The Aborigines from the River Darling in New South Wales fed their sick and debilitated patients on the blood drawn from male friends. The donors often willingly bled themselves to the point of fainting in order to provide blood for the sick.

Blood Pressure Stephen Hales (1677–1761) of Hertfordshire, was the first person to measure blood pressure. He inserted a copper tube into the femoral artery of a horse and connected it to a glass tube, and recorded the rise of the column. He published his findings in *Hemastatiks* in 1733. Jean Leonard Marie Poiseuille (1799–1869) constructed a mercury manometer in 1828, the Poiseuille Hemodynometer. A practical method of frequently measuring blood pressure in humans, by applying counter-pressure to the artery, was devised by Karl Vierordt (1818–1884) of Germany in 1854. His method was cumbersome, owing to the attachment of weights, and further improved models of the sphygmomanometer using a pneumatic cuff were produced by Samuel Ritter von Basch (1837–1905) in 1881, and Riva Rocci (1863–1937) in 1896. A pioneer in the study of blood pressure in clinical medicine was Henry Horatio Akbar Mahomed (1849–1884), a physician at Guy's Hospital. He used his own modified sphygmograph. Blood pressure measurements became a part of routine clinical examination in the 1920s. *See diastolic blood pressure, diurnal blood pressure, essential hypertension.*

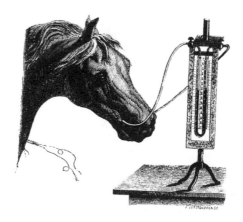

Differential manometer. Claude Bernard, *Leçons sur la chaleur animale* (1876). Bailliere, Paris

Blood Root Or pacoon, an ancient North American medicine. The active ingredient in the root was isolated and named sanguirina.

Blood Transfusion The idea was suggested as early as 1628 by Johannes Colle (1558–1631) who recommended that the blood from the vein of a young man should be transmitted per fistulum into the vein of an old man. Richard Lower (1631–1691) of Cornwall, and Edmund King (1629–1701) physician to Charles II, performed the first blood transfusion from one animal to another in 1665. Jean Baptist Denys (1625–1704), professor of surgery in Paris, transfused 12 ounces (336 g) of blood from a lamb to a dying man in 1667. In the same year Lower and King demonstrated a similar transfusion in a volunteer named Arthur Coga. James Blundell (1790–1877) gave the first transfusion of human blood to a bleeding woman in childbirth in 1824. In 1839 Samuel Armstrong Lane (1802–1892), surgeon at St George's Hospital, gave an account of successful transfusion to an 11-year-old boy who had a bleeding diathesis. He was advised by Blundell on the procedure. This was probably the first record of blood transfusion to a hemophiliac and the article was published in *The Lancet* of 1840. The first transfusion in Ireland was given at Jervis Street Hospital by an Irish surgeon R.M. Donnell, on 28 April 1865. They were made relatively safe in the early 1900s by the discovery of ABO groups by Karl Landsteiner (1868–1943). Ronald Arthur Kimpton (b 1881) and James Howard Brown (b 1884) introduced containers lined with paraffin wax to prevent clotting during transfusion, in 1913. In 1914 Louis Agote (1868– 1854) and Albert Hustin (1882–1967) of Belgium independently added sodium citrate to donor blood to prevent coagulation. J. Nurnberger increased the storage time by preserving it in ice in 1922. *See ABO blood groups.*

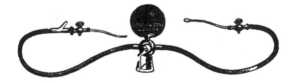

Early apparatus for blood transfusion. W. Braithewaite, *The Retrospect of Medicine* (1883). Simpkin, Marshall & Co., London

Blood Viscosity The physical properties of fluids in relation to their flow through a tube was studied by Jean Leonard Marie Poiseuille (1799–1869) in 1840. Early work was published by A. du Pre Denning and John H. Watson in the *Proceedings of the Royal Society* in 1906. Russell Burton-Opitz then published *The Viscosity of Blood* in the *Journal of the American Medical Association* in 1911. An apparatus to measure the viscosity of fluids was designed by Emil Hatschek in 1913. The viscosity of blood related to pathological states was studied by J. Nurnberger in 1942.

Blood Volume A method of estimation was proposed by Gabriel Valentin in 1838 which involved drawing a sample of blood from an individual, evaporating it to dryness and weighing it before and after injection of water, but this was unreliable. Another method, by calculating the circulation time, was proposed by Karl Vierordt (1818–1884) in 1842, but its clinical value was uncertain. The first estimation of total blood volume and the volume of red blood cells was by Hermann Welcker (1822–1897) of Germany, in 1863. A method of estimating plasma and blood volume by injecting a dye was introduced by Norman Macdonnell Keith (1885–1976) and co-workers in 1915.

Blood–Brain Barrier This barrier that prevented many of the substances dissolved in blood from reaching the brain was discovered by Paul Ehrlich (1854–1915) in 1885.

Bloom Syndrome An autosomal recessive condition, consisting of photosensitivity, skin changes and short stature with increased risk of leukemia. Described by a Warsaw-born American dermatologist, D. Bloom (b 1892) in 1954.

Blue Baby Fallot tetralogy.

Blue Disease *See Rocky mountain spotted fever.*

Blue Nevus Mongolian spot. Noted amongst infants of the Mongolian race by Ferdinand Jean Darier (1856–1938) in 1913.

Blue Ointment A mixture of fat and metallic mercury, and a common remedy in the treatment of syphilis in the 18th and 19th centuries.

Blue Pus *See Pseudomonas pyocyanea.*

Blumberg Sign Rebound tenderness in cases of peritoneal inflammation. Described by a German surgeon and gynecologist, J.M. Blumberg (1873–1955). He established the X-ray and Radium Institute in Berlin, and emigrated to England during the Nazi regime.

Blumberg, Baruch Samuel (b 1925) American biochemist who studied at Columbia University and Oxford. He was professor of biochemistry at Pennsylvania University in 1964, and in the same year discovered a previously unknown lipoprotein (Australia antigen) detected in the serum of Australian Aborigines, while he was looking for genetic markers in sera of people of different races. This lipoprotein was later found to be associated with hepatitis

B, and was renamed hepatitis B antigen. He introduced a vaccine for hepatitis B in 1969.

Blume, Karel Lodewijk (1796–1862) German physician and botanist who was the head of the vaccination program at Java in 1818. He returned to The Netherlands in 1828 and spent the rest of his career on botanical studies. He wrote *Flora Javae* (1828), *Rumphia* (1835–1845) and other works.

Blumenau, Leonid Wassiljewitsch (1862–1932) A neuroanatomist from St Petersburg who described the lateral nucleus of the cuneatus in 1907.

Blumenbach, Johann Friedrich (1752– 1840) Professor at Göttingen and pioneer in craniology. In his treatise *De Generis Humanis Varietate Nativa* published in 1776, he dealt with the variation of skull, face and skin in different races.

Blumer Sign Hard tissue is felt on rectal examination, due to metastasis in the rectovesical pouch or pouch of Douglas. Described by a physician at San Francisco, George Albert Blumer (1858–1940).

Blumgart, Herman Ludwig (1895–1977) A pioneer in the use of isotopes in diagnostic medicine. He introduced the use of radioactive substances in the evaluation of cardiac functions and velocity of blood flow, along with Soma Weiss (1898–1942) in 1927. *See nuclear medicine, isotopes.*

BMA *See British Medical Association.*

BMR or basal metabolic rate [Greek: *metabole*, change] A study on the metabolism of the human body was done by Sanctorio Sanctorius (1561–1636), a physician at Padua. He designed a balance to calculate the weight of invisible perspiration, respiration and excretion. He also invented the first clinical thermometer, which was fundamental to the study of metabolism. His work on metabolism lasting over 30 years was published as *Ars de statica medicina* in 1614, and later translated into English by John Quincy (d 1723). The relationship of the thyroid to basal metabolic rate was studied by Adolf Magnus-Levy (1869–1955), a German-born physiologist in America. In 1895 he administered thyroid extracts from animals to normal men and found that their basal metabolic rate became elevated. Levy's extensive work was published in 1899. The correlation of pulse and pulse pressure with BMR was demonstrated by Jay Marion Read (b-1889) in 1922. *See metabolism.*

Boas Sign Hyperaesthesia below the right scapula posteriorly, and the ninth and 11th ribs, in acute cholecystitis. Described by German gastroenterologist, Ismar Isidor Boas (1858–1938).

Boas, Franz (1858–1942) Anthropologist from Minden, Germany, who emigrated to America in 1886, and became a professor at Columbia in 1889. He wrote *The Mind of Primitive Man* (1911), *Anthropology and Modern Life* (1928) and other works.

Boate, Gerard A Dutch physician who settled in Ireland. He wrote *Ireland's Natural History* in 1652.

Bobb Operation Cholecystotomy for removal of gallstones. Described by American surgeon, John Stough Bobb (1809–1870).

Bochdalek Duct A lateral duct of the salivary gland opening into the lower remnant of the thyroglossal duct. Described by Vincenz Alexander Bochdalek (1801–1883), professor of anatomy at Prague. He also discovered puncta lachrymalia of the lachrymal ducts in 1866.

Bochdalek Hernia A congenital hernia through the remnant of the pleuroperitoneal canal in the left posterolateral part of the diaphragm. Described by Vincent Alexander Bochdalek (1801–1883), professor of anatomy at Prague, in 1848.

Bocium *See bronchocele.*

Bock, August Carl (1782–1833) A surgeon and anatomist from Magdeburg, Russia. He described the cavernous ganglion around the portion of the carotid artery within the cavernous sinus in 1817.

Bock, Carl Ernest (1809–1874) The son of the surgeon, August Carl Bock (1782–1833), and an anatomist who wrote *Atlas and Handbook of Human Anatomy.*

Bockhart Impetigo A form of superficial staphylococcal folliculitis occurring as a complication of various skin conditions including scabies and eczema. Described by a German physician, Max Bockhart in 1887.

Bodansky Unit A unit for measuring alkaline phosphatase in the serum, named after an American biochemist of Russian origin, A. Bodansky (1896–1941), in 1933. He graduated in medicine from the University of Chicago in 1935, and was professor of pathology at the University of Texas.

Bodenstein, Ernst August Max (1871–1942) German physical chemist who was professor in several universities (Leipzig, Hannover) before he was appointed to the chair of chemistry at Berlin in 1923. His research on halogens – chlorine, bromine and iodine – formed the basis for the kinetic theory of gases.

Bodington, George (1799–1882) English physician from Sutton Coldfield. He pointed out the value of fresh air in pulmonary complaints.

Bodleian Library Founded at Oxford by Sir Thomas Bodley (1545–1613) from Exeter. He was a diplomat in Denmark, Holland and France, and returned to Oxford and married a wealthy widow. He offered his magnificent collection of books to the library through Ravis, Dean of Christ Church in 1597. The library at Oxford, originally established by Humphrey, the Duke of Gloucester, was extended to receive his books. It was named the Bodleian Library and opened in 1602.

Bodmer, Sir Walter Fred (b 1936) German-born English geneticist who pioneered the study of the human leukocyte antigen (HLA) histocompatibility system which later proved to be vital in transplantation medicine. He graduated from Clare College, Cambridge and was a lecturer there before he moved to Stanford University. He returned as professor of genetics at Oxford University in 1970, and became the Director of Research at the Imperial Cancer Research Fund in 1979.

Body Snatchers *See Anatomy Act, Burke and Hare murders, resurrectionists.*

Boeck Sarcoidosis (Syn. Besnier–Boeck–Schaumann disease, osteitis tuberculosa multiplex cystoides) A syndrome of benign sarcoid described by a Norwegian dermatologist, Peter Caesar Moeller Boeck (1845–1915) in 1899. French dermatologist, Ernest Besnier (1831–1909) of Honfleur, gave an account of lupus pernio and other features of sarcoidosis in 1889. The systemic nature was described by Jorgen Nilson Schumann (1879–1953).

Boeck, Peter Caesar Moeller (1845–1917) In 1896 he was the first dermatologist in Norway to be appointed professor of medicine at the University of Oslo. *See Boeck sarcoidosis.*

Boehmer, George Ralph (1723–1803) Professor of anatomy and botany at Wittemberg who published several works on botany.

Boerhaave Syndrome Herman Boerhaave (1668–1758) described the spontaneous rupture of the esophagus in Baron de Wassenaer, Grand Admiral of Holland, in 1723. Norman Rupert Barrett (b 1903) of England described three cases in 1946.

Boerhaave, Abraham Kaan (1715–1753) Nephew of Herman Boerhaave (1668–1738). Professor of medicine at St Petersburg. He wrote *Perspiratio Dicta Hippocrate* and *Impentum Faciens Hippocrate per corpus consentiens Physiologice et Physiologice illustratum.*

Boerhaave, Herman (1668–1738) Eminent physician of Leiden, the son of a clergyman. After an attempt at studying theology, he developed his interest in science and obtained his medical degree at Haderwijk in 1693. In 1709 he was made professor of botany and director of the university botanic garden at Leiden, where he became renowned for his knowledge of languages, mathematics, botany, chemistry, classics and medicine. He taught medicine and chemistry to famous medical men including William Cullen (1710–1790), Albrecht von Haller (1708–1777), John Pringle (1707–1782), David Pitcairn (1749–1809) and several hundred others across Europe. He described rupture of the esophagus and established the site and nature of pleurisy. His publications include *Institutiones medicae* (1708), *Aphorismi de cognoscendis et curandis Morbis* (1709) and *Elementa Chemiae* (1724).

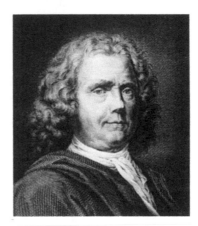

Herman Boerhaave (1668–1738). Courtesy of the National Library of Medicine

Bogden or Bogdanus, Martin Born in Dresden, he was a pupil of Tommaso Bartholini (1616–1680). He defended his teacher's claim to the discovery of the thoracic duct and lymphatics against the claims of Olof Rudbeck (1630–1702) in 1652

Bogros, Annet-Jean (1786–1823) Anatomist from the Faculty of Medicine, Paris, who described the retroperitoneal passage of the external iliac artery in 1823.

Bogrow Fibers Fibers running from the optic tract to the thalamus. Described by Russian anatomist, Sergei Livovich Bogrow (1878–1923).

Bohn, John **or Bohinius** (1640–1718) A physician at Leipzig whose main interest was chemistry. He wrote: *Dissertationes Chemici-Physicae* (1685), *Medicationes Chemico-physicae* (1689) and *De Alkalie et acidi insufficienta pro principorum corporum Naturelium Munere Gerondo* (1675).

Bohr Effect The effect of carbon dioxide on the dissociation of oxygen from hemoglobin. Named after Danish physician, Christian Bohr (1855–1911), father of the eminent physicist Niels Bohr. He described the S-shaped oxygen dissociation curve of hemoglobin in 1904.

Bohr, Aage Niels (b 1922) The son of Niels Bohr (1885–1962). A physicist at his father's Institute of Theoretical Physics in Copenhagen. He developed the collective model theory for the atomic nucleus and was awarded the Nobel Prize for Physics in 1975.

Bohr, Niels Henrick David (1885–1962) Danish physicist who proposed the dynamic theory of the structure of the atom in 1926. In America, he worked with John Archibald Wheeler (b 1911), an American physicist, at the Princeton laboratory on the atomic project. During their work they established that the atomic bomb could be produced with uranium-235. In his work on hydrogen, he postulated that a massive, charged central nucleus was surrounded by a single electron traveling around it. He worked in England for a brief period with Joseph John Thomson (1856–1940) and Ernest Rutherford (1871–1937).

Bois-Reymond, Emil du (1818–1896) Professor of physiology at the University of Berlin who first described the injury potential of the muscle, in 1840. *See action potential.*

Boll, Franz Christian (1849–1879) Professor of anatomy in Genoa who described the basal cells of the lachrymal glands in 1869. He discovered the photosensitive pigment in the retina in 1877.

Bologna The first scientific school of medicine and surgery in Europe was established in Bologna in 1260. This later became a leading center of learning where eminent men such as Alexander Achillini (1463–1512), Julius Arantius (1530–1589), Pietro Argillata (d 1423) and others studied during the Renaissance period.

Bolometer A sensitive instrument for measuring changes up to one millionth of a degree centigrade. Devised by Samuel Pierrepont Langley (1834–1906), a pioneer in aeronautics and secretary of the Smithsonian Institute in 1881.

Boltwood, Bertram Borden (1870–1927) American chemist from Amherst, Massachusetts. He was a pioneer in the study of isotopes. He discovered ionium, later known as thorium-203. He invented a radioactive method of dating rocks.

Boltzmann, Ludwig (1844–1906) Austrian physicist from Vienna who was professor of physics at several universities, including Graz, Vienna, Munich and Leipzig. He proposed the law of equipartition of energy, known as Boltzmann law.

Bolus [Greek: *bolus,* lump] Term originally used to denote the maximum convenient oral dose of any medicine that is thicker than honey. In present practice it usually means a loading dose of an intravenous drug.

Bonaventura, Giovanni (1221–1274) Leading French philosopher who based his philosophy on the scientific study of nature and the human mind.

Bonds The concept of bonds in chemistry was introduced by Scottish chemist, Archibald Scott Couper (1831–1892). In his *On a New Chemical Theory* to be presented to the French Academy in 1858 by his teacher Charles Adolphe Wurtz (1817–1884), Couper explained the formation of links between atoms which formed the basis of organic chemistry. Wurtz delayed the presentation of Couper's paper and the credit for the discovery of bonds was claimed by Friedrich August Kekulé (1829–1896).

Bone Graft Fred Houdlett Albee (1876–1945) of Philadelphia grafted living bone tissue for internal splints. He transplanted tissue from a tibia into a diseased spine of a patient with Pott disease. Bone grafts were also used for non-union of a fractured neck of the femur by Melvin Anderson and co-workers at the Mayo Clinic in the 1940s. The use of ceramic plaster material as a substitute for bone in surgery was pioneered by an orthopedic surgeon, Lyman W. Smith (1912–1991) of Cleveland, Ohio, in 1963.

Bone Marrow Aspiration [Anglo-Saxon: *ban*, bone + *mearg*, pith] Sternal needle puncture for the study of bone marrow was described by Carley Paul Seyfarth (b 1890) of Germany in 1923. The use of the needle puncture technique in the study of hemopoietic diseases was popularized in 1927, by Mikhail J. Arinkin (1876–1948) of Germany. Bone marrow aspiration was developed and promoted as a diagnostic procedure by Richard Phillip Custer (b 1903) in 1933.

Bone Marrow Biopsy [Anglo-Saxon: *ban*, bone + *mearg*, pith] A microscopic examination of bone tissue in a blood disorder was done in 1846 by John Dalrymple (1804–1852) of Dublin on William Macintyre's patient with multiple myeloma. Diagnostic bone marrow biopsy on a femur with the use of a trocar was performed by G. Pianese in 1903. He also described anemia in children owing to bone marrow infiltration by leishmania as *Leishmania infantum* in 1905. Study of the bone marrow by trephining the upper half of the tibia was carried out by Giovanni Ghedini of Genoa in 1908. *See bone marrow aspiration.*

Bone Marrow Infusion [Anglo-Saxon: *ban*, bone + *mearg*, pith] The administration of fluids into the bone marrow cavity in patients with no accessible veins, because of shock or other causes, was advocated by N. Henning in 1940. He used the sternum in adults and the tibia in newborn babies and infants for his procedure. J.D. Gimson continuously infused an infant through the tibia for 6 days in 1944.

Bone Marrow Transplantation [Anglo-Saxon: *ban*, bone + *mearg*, pith] Early animal experiments on bone marrow transplantation in animals were conducted by D.W.H. Barnes, M.J. Corp and co-workers in 1955. They gave sufficient X-ray doses to leukemic mice to destroy the bone marrow, followed by injection of normal marrow from mice of the same strain. Entire body irradiation of leukemia patients, followed by marrow transfusion was carried out by Edward Donnell Thomas (b 1936) and colleagues, in 1959. Of the 11 patients who underwent this treatment, three were successful and the other eight died of sepsis. He became professor at Washington University School of Medi-cine at Seattle in 1963 and continued his research into the use of bone marrow transplantation for genetic diseases and aplastic anemia, for which he was awarded the Nobel Prize for Physiology or Medicine (with Joseph Edward Murray) in 1990. In France, the application of bone marrow transplantation for leukemia was pioneered by George Mathe at the cancer and immunogenetic research institute at Ville-juif, Paris in 1960.

Bone Necrosis An early English treatise, *A Practical Essay on Certain Disease of the Bones Termed Necrosis* was written by James Russell (1755–1836), professor of clinical surgery at Edinburgh in 1794. *See osteomyelitis.*

Bone Scan [Anglo-Saxon: *ban*, bone] The technique of radionuclide scintigraphy of the skeleton, known as bone scanning, was pioneered in orthopedics by C.H. Baur of Stockholm while he was professor of orthopedics at Cornell University in 1962.

Bone Setters In the past they were the equivalent of modern-day osteopaths and chiropractors. A celebrated bone setter in England was Sara Mapp at Epsom. She was the daughter of a Wiltshire bone setter and she started her practice at Epsom in 1830, becoming an important social figure in London through her prosperous practice. Queen Victoria consulted her and Hans Sloane (1660–1753), the President of the Royal College and a notable medical personality, also sought her to treat his niece who had a spinal deformity. Despite her success, she died in abject poverty and was buried with parish funds. Hugh Owen Thomas (1834–1891), the father of modern orthopedic surgery in England, developed his knowledge and practice from the experience of his ancestors who were bone setters through seven

generations. A treatise on bone setting was written by Wharton Peter Hood (1833–1916) of London in 1871.

Bone, William Arthur (b 1871) Born at Stockton-on-Tees, he was a chemist and head of the chemical department at the Battersea Polytechnic in London in 1896. In 1911 he invented the system of flameless combustion using a mixture of coal gas and air, and projecting it on to porous material.

Bonet, Juan Pablo (1579–1633) Devised a new system of communication for the deaf and dumb in 1620. He probably learnt the system from another Spaniard, Pedro Ponce de Leon (1510–1584), a pioneer in the field.

Bonet, Theophile (1620–1689) Born in Geneva, he published an extensive treatise on pathology *Sepulchretum* following postmortem findings from nearly 3000 cases in 1679. One of his reports includes the first postmortem description of calcific aortic stenosis. His other publications include: *Labrinthi Medici* (1675), *Pharos Medicorum* (1668), *Prodromus anatomiae Practicae* and *Course de Medicine et de la Chirugie.*

Bonifacio Hospital Founded in Italy for the mentally ill by Grand Duke Pietro Leopoldo of Tuscany in 1788.

Bonnaire, Erasme (1858–1918) An obstetrician in Paris who described a method of dilatation of the cervix by the fingers of one hand while pressing above the pubic symphysis with the other hand.

Bonnet, Amedée (1802–1858) A surgeon from the Hôtel Dieu, Lyons. The posterior part of the sheath of the eyeball described by him bears his name.

Bonnet, Charles (1720–1793) Born in Copenhagen. In 1769 he described visual hallucinations in old age not associated with any mental disorder (Bonnet syndrome).

Bonnevie-Ullrich Syndrome Lymphedema of the extremities, nail dystrophy, webbed neck, short stature, and lax skin. Independently described by American geneticist, K. Bonnevie (1872–1950) in 1934 and German pediatrician Otto Ullrich (1894–1957) in 1930.

Bonnier, Pierre (1861–1918) A physician in Paris who described a syndrome of vertigo, trigeminal neuralgia and locomotor weakness due to lesions of the vestibular apparatus and fifth nerve nucleus (Bonnier syndrome), in 1903.

Bontius or Gerard de Bont (1536–1599) A physician and first professor of medicine at Leiden University.

Bontius, Jacobius or Jacob de Bondt (1592–1631) A physician at Leiden who recognized tropical medicine as a distinct branch. He described beriberi. He wrote: *Medicina*

Indorum (1642), *De Medicina Egyptorum* (1718) and *Historia Naturiae et Med Indiae Orientalis* (1658).

Bonwill Triangle Formed by both heads of the mandible and the center of the alveolar margin. Described by American dentist, William Gibson Arlington Bonwill (1833–1899).

Books on Medicine The oldest known medical handbook, in the form of a cuneiform tablet, belongs to Sumerian physicians around 2200 BC. The Kahun papyrus is the oldest extant Egyptian medical papyrus, written around 2150–1900 BC. Consilia were early medical books in the 14th and 15th centuries in Europe which contained experience and case records of famous physicians from the past. One such was written by a Paduan professor, Gentile da Foligno, around 1340. The first medical work to be printed in Latin was that of Aulus Cornelius Celsus (25 BC–AD 50), which appeared in 1478. The first important printed scientific book (*Buch der Natur*) in Germany with illustrations of animals and discussions on medical subjects such as plague, physiology and anatomy was by Conrad von Megenberg (1308–1374) and published in 1475. A medical book to appear in England was *A Passing Gode Lityll Boke Necessarye and Behoveful agenst Pestilence* published around 1480. It was a translation of a work written by the Papal physician Johannes Jacobe of Montpellier in 1374. The second English book, *The Governayle of Helthe,* was published in 1491. Printed illustrations of the viscera were given by Magnus Hundt (1449–1519) in his *Anthropologium de Homis Dignitate, natura, et Propriatatibus* published in 1501. An anatomy book in English was written by Davis Edwardes (1502–1542), who performed dissection in England in 1531. A book on anatomy, *A Treasure for Englishmen, containing the Anatomie of Man's Body* was written by Thomas Vicary, a surgeon from London, in 1548. A book devoted to the anatomy of the head, *Anatomia Capitis Humani,* with 11 woodcuts, was written by Johan Dryander (1500–1560) in 1536. A book on surgical anatomy, *Anatomia Chirugica,* was written by an Italian, Bernardino Genga (1665–1734) in 1672. *See American medical books.*

Boole, George (1816–1864) A self-taught mathematician and son of a cobbler from Lincoln. He became professor of mathematics at Cork, and did important work on differential equations. He wrote *Mathematical Analysis of Logic* (1847) and *Laws of Thought* in 1854.

Boorde, Andrew (1490–1549) Carthusian monk from Sussex who became Bishop of Chichester. He later left the order and traveled to the Continent to study medicine. On his return he settled in Glasgow to practice medicine. He was a friend of Thomas Cromwell (d 1540) and Latinized his name to Andreas Perforatus. He wrote *The Breviary of Healthe* and *The Fyrst Boke of the Introduction of Knowledge* which reflected his wide traveling experience. The story of 'Tom Thumb' is said to have been written by him. Towards the last stages of his life he was imprisoned for some obscure reason and died in Fleet prison.

Boothby, William Meredith (1880–1953) Physician at the Mayo Clinic, who recommended preoperative intravenous iodine administration in exophthalmic goiter, and glycine for treatment of myasthenia gravis. He perfected the nitrous oxide–ether–oxygen apparatus for anesthesia in 1912, the Boothby–Coton Flow Meter. *See Boothby–Lovelace–Bulbian mask.*

Boothby–Coton Flow Meter *See Boothby, William Meredith.*

Boothby–Lovelace–Bulbulian Mask For delivery of oxygen, developed by William Meredith Boothby (1880–1953), Randolph William Lovelace (1907–1965) and Arthur H. Bulbulian (b 1900) in 1938.

Borax Name derived from the Arabic term *booruk*. Pliny referred to it as *chrysocollo*. The main source in the past was Tibet. It was also called chrysocolla [Greek: *krusos*, gold] by the German physician, George Agricola (1494–1555) in 1530. William Homberg (1652–1715) of Batavia prepared sal sedativum, a free acid of borax, in 1702, and it was found to be a compound of soda in 1747. The antiseptic properties of boric acid were discovered by French chemist Jean Baptiste Dumas (1800–1884) in 1872.

Borborygmi A medical term to denote loud intestinal sounds produced by contractions. Derived from the Greek term for 'rumbling'.

Borde, Andrew *See Boorde.*

Bordenave, Toussaint (1728–1782) Professor of surgery in Paris who wrote *Dissertations sue les Antiseptiques* and translated Haller's work on physiology into French.

Bordet, Jules Jean Baptiste Vincent (1870–1961) Belgian physiologist and authority on serology, born in Soignies. He graduated from the University of Brussels in 1895 and did extensive research on antigen–antibody agglutination reactions and proposed several theories related to their mechanism of interaction. In 1895 he showed that serum devoid of cells had the same bactericidal property as peritoneal fluid, one of the most significant findings in the field of immunology. In 1900 he described 'complement', previously called 'alexin' by Eduard Buchner (1860–1907). While working with his brother-in-law, Octave Gengou

(1875–1957) in 1906, he extracted the endotoxin from whooping cough bacillus and prepared a vaccine for this disease. He was awarded the Nobel Prize for Medicine or Physiology in 1919.

Bordet–Gengou Bacillus (Syn. pertussis bacillus) The causative agent of whooping cough, isolated by Jules Vincent Bordet (1870–1961) and Octave Gengou (1875–1957) in 1906.

Bordeu, Theophile de (1722–1776) Physician from Bern who wrote *Recherches sur Glandes* (1746), *Recherches anatomiques sur la Position de Glandes et sur leur Action* (1756) and other works. He suggested that the internal secretions of the testis and ovary had remote and overall effects on the organism. This was the first suggestion of the concept of hormones.

Borel, Peter (1620–1689) A physician from Languedoc who wrote: *Historiae et Observationum Medico-Physicarum Centuria Prima et Seconda* (1653), *Bibliotheca Chymeca* (1656), *De Vero Teloscopie Inventore* (1655) and other works.

Borelli, Giovanni Alphonso (1608–1679) A mathematician and philosopher in Naples who established the iatrophysical school of medicine which explained bodily functions on the basis of physical laws. He wrote *Theoria Medicorum Planaterium et Causis Deductae* (1666), and his *De Motu Animalium* was published posthumously in 1681. *See iatrophysics.*

Boric Acid Discovered by chemist and physician, William Homberg (1652–1715) of Batavia, in 1702. He practiced as a physician in Rome before his appointment as physician to the Duke of Orleans in Paris.

Borlace, Edmund (d 1682) A physician and son of Sir John Borlace, Lord Justice of Ireland. He qualified from Leiden in 1650. His publications were mainly non-medical related to topography and history.

Born, Max (1882–1970) A German physicist from Breslau. In 1936 he became the professor of natural philosophy at Edinburgh, where he pursued his research on quantum theory based on matrix mechanics which led to a statistical approach to the subject. He was awarded the Nobel Prize for Physics with Walter Wilhelm G. Bothe (1891–1957) in 1954.

Bornholm Disease (Syn. pleurodynia) An epidemic myositis which occurred in the Danish island of Bornholm in the Baltic Sea. Described by Ejner Oluf Sylvest Sorenson (1880–1931) in 1930.

Boron A non-metallic element discovered by Joseph Louis Gay-Lussac (1778–1850) and Louis Jacques Thenard (1777–1857) in 1808. *See borax.*

Borovskii, Peter Fokiah (1863–1932) A bacteriologist from Russia who gave a description of *Leishmania tropica,* in 1898.

Borozail A type of venereal disease noted in Ethiopia around 1500, found to be different from French pox.

Borrelia duttonii (Syn. *Spironema duttonii*) A spirochete transmitted by a tick, causing African relapsing fever. Identified by Joseph Everett Dutton (1876–1905) and John Lancelot Todd (1876–1949) in 1905. It was named after French bacteriologist, A. Borrel and Joseph Dutton. *See relapsing fever.*

Borrelia recurrentis The causative organism of relapsing fever, a spirochete, was discovered by Otto Hugo Franz Obermeier (1843–1873) in 1873. *See relapsing fever.*

Borrichius or Borch (1626–1690) A physician in Denmark who wrote *Hermetes Aegyptorum et Chemicorum Sapentia* in 1674 and other treatises.

Bosch, Carl (1874–1940) German chemist from Cologne who invented the Bosch process by which hydrogen is obtained from superheated steam through high pressure.

Bose, Sir Jagadis Chandra (1858–1937) A physicist and botanist from Calcutta who did research on electric waves and the growth of plants. He demonstrated the process of wireless telegraphy and became the first Indian physicist to be elected as a Fellow of the Royal Society in 1920.

Bosquillon, Marie Edouard François (1744–1814) Professor of medicine at the Faculty of Medicine Paris, and professor of languages at the College Royal France. He became an honorary associate of the Society of Medicine Edinburgh and wrote *Aphorismes et Prognostics D'Hippocrate* in 1814.

Bostock Botanic Eye Ointment A secret remedy advocated for all kinds of eye diseases by a London company during the late 19th century. It contained traces of ammoniac mercury, paraffin and lard.

Bostock Catarrh (Syn. catarrhus aestivus, allergic rhinitis, vasomotor rhinitis) Hay fever, described by John Bostock (1773–1846) of Guy's Hospital in 1817. *See allergy, Bostock, John, hay fever.*

Bostock, John (1773–1846) A physician at Guy's Hospital gave a detailed description of hay fever in 1819. *See hay fever, asthma, allergy.*

Boston Sign A sign in exophthlamic goiter where jerky arrest of the descent of the eyelid occurs when the eyeball is turned downwards. Described by a Philadelphia physician, L. Napoleon Boston (1871–1931). He was professor of clinical medicine at the Women's Medical College of Pennsylvania in 1928, and wrote *Clinical Diagnosis by Laboratory Methods.*

Bostroem, Eugen (1850–1928) A mycologist who devised a staining method for actinomyces in 1890. *See Actinomyces graminis.*

Bosworth, Francke Huntington (1843–1925) A pioneer of American rhinology who described purulent rhinitis, dislocation of the columnar cartilage of the nasal septum and diseases involving the ethmoid cells.

Botallo, Leonardo or Botallus (1519–1587) Italian physician who, while working in France in 1530, gave a description of the ductus arteriosus and foramen ovale. These were later named Botallo duct and Botallo foramen, respectively. He also described 'summer catarrh' or hay fever in 1564. His publications include *De Curandis Vulneribus Sclopitorum* (1560) and *De Curatione per Sanguis Missionem* (1583).

Botallus *See Botallo, Leonardo.*

Botanical Gardens or physick gardens The cultivation of medicinal herbs in special gardens has been practiced since ancient times. Such gardens existed in Europe in Salerno and Venice in the 14th century. The first botanical gardens without special attention to medicinal herbs were established at the universities of Padua and Pisa. The physick garden at Oxford was established by Henry Danvers, Earl of Danby, in 1632. He presented Oxford University with £250 with which a piece of land near East Gate was bought Its plants were cataloged by Jacob Bobart, professor of botany, in 1675. Many eminent physicians, such as William Withering (1741–1799) in England and Hermann Boerhaave (1668–1738) in Germany, had their own herbal gardens.

Botany [Greek: *botane*, pasture or herb] Aristotle initiated the scientific study of plants. Theophrastus followed with his treatise *Historia Plantarum* in 320 BC. Interest in plants was sustained by Galen (129–200) who listed over 300 herbal medicines and Dioscorides who described over 600 plants around AD 600. An early printed book containing realistic plant illustrations was produced by Otto Brunfels (1489–1534) of Mainz in 1530. Clusius (1525–1609) of Antwerp published several illustrative works on the plants of India and Europe. Matthias de l'Obel (1538–1616) of The Netherlands was an eminent botanist and director of the botanical garden of Queen Elizabeth I in England. He used the morphology of leaves as the basis of his classification of plants, and the genus Lobeliaceae was named after him.

Caspar Bauhin (1560–1624) helped to clear the confusion on the names of plants with his work on botanical synonyms *Pinax Theatri botanici* published in 1623. One of the first English books on the subject, *Anatomy of the Plants,* was published by Nehemiah Grew (1641–1712) in 1682. He described different tissues in plants and identified the male and female parts of flowering plants. A system of classification to include the genus and species was introduced by Carl Linnaeus (1707–1778) in 1750, in his description of 11,800 species of plants. Larger botanic gardens with an interest in medicine were established in the 1600s in various places including Leiden, Padua and Chelsea. *See Biology.*

Bothor An ancient Arabic term for measles or smallpox.

Böttcher, Arthur (1831–1889) Professor at the University of Dorpat who described the ganglion around the cochlear nerve within the internal auditory meatus, in 1856.

Bottger, Johan Friedrich (1642–1715) An apothecary and alchemist in Berlin. His claim to the discovery of transmutation of metals into gold brought him into favor with Frederick I and the King of Poland. He was later exposed as a fraud but continued his experiments on porcelain and invented Meissen pottery. He was imprisoned by Augustus the Strong, King of Poland, at Meissen, where he manufactured his porcelain until his death. The secret of Meissen porcelain was kept for over a century after his death.

Bottini Operation The use of galvanocautery to make a channel through an enlarged prostate. Designed by Italian surgeon, Enrico Bottini (1837–1903).

Bottoni, Albertino A physician in Padua in the 16th century who wrote *De Morbis Mulibribus* (1585) and *De Vita Conservanda* (1582).

Bottoni, Domini (1641–1731) A physician from Sicily who wrote, *Febris Rheumaticae Malignae Historia Medica,* in 1712.

Botulism [Latin: *botulus*, sausage] Described by a German poet and physician Justinus Kerner in 1820. It was called 'sausage poisoning' in Germany and was thought to be due to contamination of sausages by copper and lead vessels during cooking. In 1822 Kerner published two monographs on epidemics of botulism in Germany. A series of 29 cases was presented by Weiss in 1824, and a larger series of 62 cases was presented by Muller in 1863. The etiological agent, *Clostridium botulinum,* was isolated by Emile Pierre Marie van Ermengem (1851–1932), during his investigation of a small outbreak in the village of Ellezeles, Belgium in 1896. The first recorded outbreak in Britain occurred in Gairloch, Scotland in 1922. It claimed the lives of eight people who ate sandwiches made from potted wild duck paste at a hotel at Loch Maree.

Bou Bou *See dengue fever.*

Bouchard Nodes Found in the second interphalangeal joints of the hands, initially thought to be due to gastrectasis. Described by French physician, Charles Jacques Bouchard (1837–1915) of Paris.

Bouchard, Abel Henry (1833–1899) French physician who described the shooting pains of tabes dorsalis while working with Jean Marie Charcot (1825–1893) in Paris in 1866. He also described miliary aneurysms and associated them with cerebral hemorrhage.

Bouchard, Charles Jacques (1837–1915) French physician and dean of the Faculty of Medicine at Paris who studied nutrition. He described acute gastric dilatation in 1884 and autointoxication in 1887. He described the spider nevi seen in liver disease. He wrote *Maladies par Raletissement de la Nutrition* in 1882. *See Bouchard nodes.*

Boucher de Perthes, Jacques (1788–1868) French archeologist from Rethel. He found evidence of early Stone Age or Paleolithic culture in Abbeville, France in 1805. Stone instruments and the remains of extinct animals provided evidence that humans existed over 20,000 years ago. He presented his findings to the Society of Emulation of Abbeville in 1838 and it was published in 1847.

Bouchut, Jean Antoine Eugene (1818–1891) Paris physician who recognized the state of nervous exhaustion and asthenia, which he called 'nervosisme' in 1860. It was described by Miller George Beard (Beard disease) in 1869. *See chronic fatigue syndrome.*

Boudewins, Michael (d 1681) A physician from Antwerp who wrote *Ventilabrum Medico Theologicum* in 1666.

Bougie [French: candle] Metal bourgies for relief of obstruction of the urethra were introduced by Scultetus of Ulm, Germany in the mid-17th century.

Bouillaud Syndrome Acute rheumatic carditis. *See Bouillaud, Jean.*

Bouillaud, Jean Baptiste (1796–1881) Physician from Angoulême, France who located the site of the lesion in the brain which causes aphasia in 1825. He also correlated carditis with acute rheumatic fever, Bouillaud syndrome. He described acute rheumatic polyarthritis in 1832.

Bouillet, John (1690–1770) French medical historian who wrote *Avis et Remedes Contre la Peste* (1721), *Recueil des Lettres et Autres Pieces pour Servir l'historiae de l'Acedemie de*

Beziers in 1736 and a treatise on dropsy, *Observationes sur l'anafarque.*

Boule, Pierre Marcellin (1861–1942) Professor at the Natural History Museum in Paris. He made the first complete construction of a Neanderthal skeleton and wrote *Les Hommes Fossiles* in 1921.

Boullion A culture medium for bacteria containing beef in a suspension of water and peptones. Devised by the discoverer of the tubercle bacillus, Robert Koch (1843–1910).

Bourgeous, Louise (1563–1636) Parisian midwife and pupil of Ambroise Paré (1510–1590). She wrote an important treatise in midwifery in 1609 which was translated into English as *The Compleat Midwife's Practice,* in 1659.

Bourgery, Marc Jean (1797–1869) Surgeon in Paris who described the posterior ligament of the knee joint in 1837.

Bourneville, Désiré Magloire (1840–1909) French neurologist in Paris who described adenoma sebaceum associated with mental deficiency and epilepsy (epiloia) in 1880. He founded the *Progres Medicale* in 1873 and established the first school for mentally defective children in France.

Bourneville Disease (Syn. Pringle disease) *See adenoma sebaceum, Bourneville, Désiré Magloire.*

Boussingault, Jean Baptiste Joseph Dieudonné (1802–1887) French agricultural chemist from Paris. He demonstrated the ability of legumes to increase nitrogen in the soil by fixing it from the atmosphere.

Bouvart, Michael Philip (1717–1787) French physician who opposed inoculation.

Bouveret, Leon (1851–1925) *See Bouvert syndrome.*

Bouvert Syndrome Paroxysmal atrial tachycardia. Described by Leon Bouveret (1851–1925) of Paris in 1889. *See atrial tachycardia.*

Boveri, Theodor (1862–1915) German biologist and pioneer in cytology. He graduated in medicine in 1885 and studied the changes of chromosomes in cell division in *Ascaris.* The centrosome was named by him in 1888. He also drew up a general scheme for spermatogenesis and oogenesis in 1892.

Bovet, Daniel (1907–1992) Italian pharmacologist who studied chemistry at Geneva before he joined the Department of Chemical Therapeutics at the Pasteur Institute in Paris in 1929. He established a laboratory for chemotherapeutics in Rome, and discovered the first antihistamine compound in 1936 and developed the drug, Antergan, from it. He pioneered the study of drugs that blocked the action of epinephrine and norepinephrine. He made synthetic analogs of succinyl choline used in anesthesia and was awarded the Nobel Prize in Physiology or Medicine in 1957.

Bovine Spongiform Encephalopathy *See scrapie, Kuru, prion, prion disease.*

Bovine Tuberculosis A clear distinction between bovine and human tubercle bacilli was made by Theobald Smith (1859–1934), professor of microbiology at Harvard University in 1898. The transmission of the bovine tubercle bacillus to humans through milk and meat was demonstrated by French biologist, Edmond Isidore Etienne Nocard (1850–1903).

Bowden Indian Balm A secret remedy prepared in the west of England at the turn of the century. It was used as a topical application for skin inflammation, and contained mainly lard and coconut oil.

Bowditch, Henry Pickering (1840–1911) American physiologist at Boston who established a physiology laboratory in America, at Harvard in 1871 where he did important studies on the physiology of the heart muscles and nerves. His experiments on nerve block contributed to the development of local anesthesia. He founded the American Physiological Society in 1887 and was dean of the Harvard Medical School from 1883 to 1893.

Bowdler, Thomas (1754–1825) Studied at St Andrews University and obtained his MD from Edinburgh in 1770. He was known for *The Family Shakespeare* in ten volumes, published in 1818, in which certain words and phrases were removed, making it suitable for family reading, and which led to the expression 'to Bowdlerize'.

Bowen Disease *See Bowen, John Templeton.*

Bowen, John Templeton (1857–1941) American dermatologist, born in Boston. He graduated from Harvard where he was professor of dermatology in 1907. He described a variant of basal cell epithelioma which occurred as a precancerous lesion of the skin, Bowen disease, in 1912.

Bowlby, Sir Anthony Alfred (1855–1929) Surgeon at St Bartholomew's Hospital.

Bowlby, Edward John (1907–1990) The son of the surgeon Anthony Bowlby. He is known for his pioneering work on the effects of maternal deprivation on mental health and development of children.

Bowman Capsule *See Bowman, William, glomerular filtration.*

Bowman Membrane *See Bowman, William.*

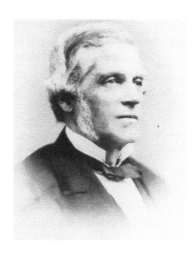

Sir William Bowman (1816-1892). Courtesy of the National Library of Medicine

Bowman, Sir William (1816–1892) English physician and demonstrator in anatomy at King's College London. Born in Nantwich, Cheshire and graduated from King's College. He developed the concept of glomerular filtration and tubular secretion in 1842. He described the capsule of the glomerular apparatus, Bowman capsule. He later (1846) practiced ophthalmology at the Royal Ophthalmic Hospital, Moorfields and perfected irridectomy and removal of cataracts. The basement membrane of the cornea (Bowman membrane) was described by him, and he wrote *Lectures on the Operations of the Eye* in 1849.

Bowman–Heidenhain Theory A modification of Sir William Bowman's (1816–1892) theory on glomerular filtration and secretion, proposed by German physician, Rudolph Peter Heinrich Heidenhaim (1834–1897) in 1874.

Box Golden Pills A wonder cure for various diseases in the early 1900s. It was found to contain mainly capsicum and gentian. The golden fluid, another version from the same makers, contained a decoction of lobelia and products injurious to health.

Boyd, William Clouse (1903–1983) American biochemist and immunologist, born at Dearborn, Mississippi and graduated from Harvard. He was professor of biochemistry at Boston University School of Medicine, where he trained, in 1938. He was a pioneer in immunochemistry and studied blood groups in relation to race. He wrote: *Fundamentals of Immunology* (1943), *Genetics and the Races of Man* (1950), *Biochemistry and Human Metabolism* (1952) and *Introduction to Immunochemical Specificity* (1968).

Boyer Cyst *See Boyer, Alexis.*

Boyer, Alexis (1757–1833) A tailor's son from Limousin who rose to be imperial surgeon to Napoleon. He was professor of anatomy in Paris and wrote *Du Corps Humain* in four volumes in 1802. His surgical works, which contained a description of subhyoid bursa (Boyer cyst), were published later in eleven volumes. *See anal fissure.*

Boyer, Herbert Wayne (b 1936) American biochemist and pioneer in genetic engineering, born in Pittsburgh, Pennsylvania. He was professor of biochemistry at the University of San Francisco in 1976, and demonstrated how DNA of a plasmid could be joined to bacterial DNA or DNA from a toad. He used his methods for commercial production of insulin, and formed Genentech in 1976.

Boyer, John Nicholas (1693–1768) A physician from Marseilles who wrote several treatises on epidemics.

Boyle Apparatus For use in anesthesia, devised by Henry Edmund Gaskin Boyle (1875–1941), an anesthetist at St Bartholomew's Hospital in 1917. It was improved over the next 20 years by: addition of vaporizing bottle to flow meters (1920); addition of second vaporizing bottle and bypass controls (1927); addition of a plunger device (1930); and replacement of water sight-feed by a dry-bobbin flow meter (1937). *See Boyle, Henry Edmund Gaskin.*

Boyle Law Related to volume and pressure of gases. Proposed by eminent British chemist, Robert Boyle (1626–1691) in 1662.

Boyle, Henry Edmund Gaskin (1875–1941) An anesthetist at St Bartholomew's Hospital, who wrote *Practical Anaesthetics* in 1907. He was one of the first members of the Association of Anesthetists of Great Britain and Ireland, and he was awarded an OBE for his wartime service as an anesthetist. He introduced the Boyle apparatus for anesthesia in 1917. *See Boyle apparatus.*

Boyle, Robert (1626–1691) Father of modern chemistry. He was the seventh son of the Lord High Chancellor of Ireland, from Lismore. He improved Guericke's air pump in 1659, and used it for studying the properties of air. This led to the discovery of the fundamental law of gases related to pressure and volume in 1662. His other contributions include: the relationship between boiling point and atmospheric pressure; preparation of acetone from lead acetate and lime; the concept of elements; demonstration of the necessity of air for life; discovery of the expansive power of freezing water; and production of methyl alcohol from wood. While he was in Oxford he founded the Invisible College with Christopher Wren (1632–1723), Thomas Willis (1621–1675)

and Seth Ward (1617–1689) in 1655. It promoted the science of experimentation and observation, and later became the Royal Society with a charter from King Charles in 1668. *See gas laws.*

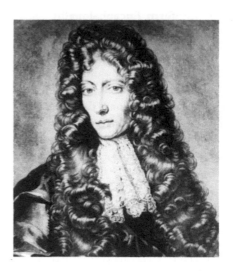

Robert Boyle (1626–1691). Courtesy of the National Library of Medicine

Boyle–Van't Hoff Law Derived from Robert Boyle (1626–1691) and Jacobus Henricus Van't Hoff's (1852–1911) theories of the relationship of pressure to temperature. *See Boyle, Robert, Van't Hoff.*

Boys, Sir Charles Vernon (1855–1944) English physicist and inventor from Wing in Rutland. He invented: an improved torsion balance with fused quartz fibers; an extremely sensitive radiometer capable of detecting the heat from a candle several hundreds yards away; a calorimeter for use with coal gas; and a camera with a moving lens.

Bozemann Catheter A double-channeled urethral catheter. Designed by American surgeon, Nathan Bozemann (1825–1905).

Bozzolo Sign *See Bozzolo, Camilo.*

Bozzolo, Camilo (1845–1920) A physician who introduced thymol as treatment for ankylostomiasis in 1880. He also described the visible pulsation of the arteries in the nostrils as a sign of thoracic aortic aneurysm (Bozzolo sign).

BR Compounds (BR 68,34) The prototype arsenic compounds linked to heterocyclic rings, introduced by A. Binz and C. Rath as treatment of trypanosomiasis in 1927.

Brachial Neuritis [Latin: *brachium*, arm; Greek: *neuron*, nerve + *itis*, inflammation] Neuritis due to lateral herniation of the cervical intervertebral disc was described by B. Stooky in 1940 and by R. Semmes in 1943.

Brachial Plexus Block [Latin: *brachium*, arm; *plexus*, braid] Achieved by injecting the plexus with an anesthetic under direct vision by American surgeon, George Washington Crile (1864–1943) of Cleveland in 1897. Hirschel performed the block by injecting the anesthetic blindly through the axilla in 1911. A supraclavicular technique was devised by Kulenkampf, who experimented with the method on himself in 1912. It was modified by J. Patrick of England in 1940. A monograph, *Local Anaesthesia: Brachial Plexus* was written by Robert Reynolds Macintosh and W.W. Mushin in 1946.

Brachial Plexus Injuries [Latin: *brachium*, arm + *plexus*, braid] Studied and explained by James H. Stevens (1871–1932), a surgeon from Rochester, New Hampshire. A syndrome of lower brachial palsy, consisting of enophthalmos, ptosis and paralysis of the area of the ulnar nerve following injury to the 8th cervical nerve and first thoracic root was described by Joseph Jules Dejerine (1849–1917) and Augusta Klumpke (1859–1927) of Paris in 1885.

Bracht Maneuver A maneuver for breech delivery that permitted spontaneous delivery of the infant. Described by Berlin gynecologist, Erich Franz Eugen Bracht (1882–1969) in 1935.

Bracht-Wachter Bodies Perivascular microabscesses seen in the myocardium in acute bacterial endocarditis. Described by Berlin pathologist, Eric Franz Eugen Bracht (b 1882) and German physician, H.J.G. Wachter (b 1878).

Bradford Frame A rectangular frame made of pipework, to which a heavy sheet of canvas was attached. Designed and used as a bed frame for patients with tuberculosis of the spine and fractures of the thigh by a Boston orthopedic surgeon, Edward Hickling Bradford (1848–1926).

Bradinham, Robert (c 1596) A surgeon on board Captain Kidd's ship *Adventure Galley*. He later gave evidence which led to Kidd's conviction for piracy and murder. Kidd was executed by hanging at Wapping.

Brady, Robert (d 1700) A physician from Denver, Norfolk. He was Regius professor of medicine at Cambridge, and a friend of Thomas Sydenham (1624–1689). He was also physician to King Charles II and King James II.

Bradycardia [Greek: *brados*, slow + *kardia*, heart] The first report of syncope due to cardiac arrest or heart block was given by Marcus Gerbezius (1658–1718), a Slovenic physician in 1692. The same condition was described as 'epilepsy with slow pulse' by Giovanni Battista Morgagni (1682–1771) in 1761. Dublin physician, Robert Adams (1791–1875) presented *A Clear Case of Syncopal Attacks with Heart*

Block in 1827. Allan Burns (1731–1813), a Scottish surgeon and cardiologist, described the occurrence of neurological symptoms in extreme bradycardia.

Bragg, Sir William Henry (1862–1942) English physicist from Westward, Cumbria, educated at Trinity College, Cambridge. He became professor of mathematics at Adelaide, Australia in 1886. He returned to England as professor at Leeds in 1909, and worked with his Australian-born son Sir William Lawrence Bragg (1890–1971) in 1912. Together they constructed the first X-ray spectrometer and discovered X-ray diffraction, a key technique in analysis of proteins. They won the Nobel Prize for Physics in 1915, and he moved to University College London in the same year. His published works include *Studies on Radioactivity* (1912), *X-rays and Crystal Structure* with his son in 1915 and *Universe of Light* (1933). *See X-ray crystallography.*

Brahe, Tycho (1546–1601) One of the greatest astronomers. He was born at Knudstrup in the south of Sweden, at that time a province of Denmark. He began his career in astronomy with his observation on the eclipse of the sun which occurred in August 1560. He made several discoveries and contributions in astronomy and wrote *Astronomiae Insaturate Mechanica* (1598) and *Astronomia Nova* in 1609. *See astronomy.*

Brahmins Hindu priests who were descendants of Indo-European or Aryan people, according to Max Muller (1823–1900). They wrote the four immortal Vedas – Rig, Yajur, Sama and Athara. The subcaste of Brahmins, 'Vaidya', became physicians and practiced incantations, surgery and herbal medicine. Charaka (100 BC), Susruta (AD 500) and Vagbhata (AD 700) were three of their greatest medical men.

Braid, James (1808–1860) A Manchester surgeon, born in Fife. He rediscovered hypnotic phenomena and earned the title 'the initiator of the scientific study of animal magnetism'. He was interested in the application of mesmerism to induce anesthesia, and substituted the word 'hypnotism' in place of 'mesmerism'. He wrote *Neurohypnology or Rationale of Nervous Sleep* in 1843. He also devised an operation for club foot. *See hypnosis, animal magnetism.*

Braidism (Syn. hypnotism) *See Braid, James.*

Braidwood, Thomas (1715–1806) Scottish teacher who studied at Edinburgh. He founded the first British school for the deaf and dumb in Edinburgh in 1760. This was transferred to Hackney, London in 1783.

Braille, Louis (1809–1852) He was blind, and attended the first blind school at Paris, founded by Valentine Hauy (1746–1822). In 1834, he devised an alphabet for the blind with varying combinations of six dots. This is still in use after further modifications. He also improved the method of embossed printing for the blind.

Brain [Anglo-Saxon: *braegen*] Recognized as the center of the nervous system and seat of intelligence by Herophilus of Chalcedon in 300 BC. A monograph was written by Jason Pratensis (1486–1588) in 1549. Thomas Willis (1621–1675) gave a modern description of the nervous system in 1664 and identified the cerebrum as the seat of intelligence. Pierre Flourens (1794–1867), a French physiologist in Paris, conducted animal experiments to study the functions of different parts of the brain, in 1824. Robert Remak (1815–1865) observed that the gray matter of the brain contained cellular tissue in 1825, and Gottfried Ehrenberg (1795–1876) noted that the white matter consisted of conduction fibers. Gustav Theodor Fritsch (1838–1891) and Eduard Hittig (1838–1907) demonstrated that stimulation of certain areas produced localized motor movements and convulsions in the body, in 1870. Their finding was a landmark in the study of localization of brain lesions in motor disorders. The distribution of blood vessels within the substance of the brain was described by Henry Duret (1849–1921) and Johann Otto Leonhard Heubner (1843–1926) of Germany in 1872. *See cerebral circulation, cerebral cortex, cerebellum, motor cortex.*

Brain Death Inactivity of the brain, rather than stoppage of the heart, as a sign of death. Adopted by the French Academy of Medicine in 1966.

Brain Injury *See concussion.*

Brain Tumor One of the earliest surgical removals of a brain tumor arising from the dura mater was performed by Sir William Macewen (1848–1924), professor of surgery at the Glasgow Royal Infirmary in 1879. The next successful diagnosis and removal during life was achieved by Alexander Hughes Bennett (1848–1901) and Sir Rickman Godlee (1849–1925). Bennett diagnosed and localized the tumor in a 23-year-old patient at the Hospital for Epilepsy and Paralysis at Regent's Park, London and Godlee successfully operated on the patient in 1884. Eugene Hahn of Germany is also credited with having removed a brain tumor in 1881. The gamma helmet, a device for delivering precise radiation to brain tumors using cobalt-60, was invented by Swedish physicists, Lars Leksell and Borje Larsson in 1968. *See neurosurgery.*

Brain, Walter Russel (1895–1966) The Baron of Eynsham, neurologist and a medical statesman. He was the Chairman of the Royal Commission on Marriage and Divorce, a member of the Standing Committee on Drug Addiction and held several other positions in important committees.

Brambell, Francis William Rogers (1901–1970) Irish zoologist educated at Trinity College, Dublin. His work on reproductive cycles of mammals while he was professor of zoology at the University College of North Wales, Bangor, led to the discovery of the route of transmission of maternal antibodies to the fetus.

Branchiogenic Carcinoma A primary epithelioma of the neck arising from branchiogenic cysts. Described by Richard von Volkman of Germany in 1882.

Brande, William Thomas (1788–1866) He succeeded Sir Humphry Davy (1778–1829) as professor of chemistry at the Royal Institution of Great Britain in 1813, and delivered a series of celebrated chemical lectures to students from 1816 to 1850. He devised the Brande test for quinine, using chlorine, water and ammonia as reagents.

Brandt Method Deep massage of the Fallopian tubes, employed for expressing pus out of a pyosalpinx. Devised by Swedish physician, Thure Brandt (1819–1895).

Brandt, Georg (1694–1768) Swedish chemist who studied medicine and chemistry at Leiden under Hermann Boerhaave (1668–1738). He investigated arsenic and its compounds and published a systematic treatise on it in 1733. He also discovered cobalt in 1730 and distinguished between potash and soda. He was the first chemist to condemn alchemy and promote chemistry as a science.

Brandt, Hennig Sebastian (1458–1521) German alchemist and merchant who discovered a waxy substance in the urine, which glowed in the dark. He named it phosphorus.

Brandy [German: *branntwein*, burnt wine] Distilled from wine by the Italians in 1100. It was called the elixir of life by Arnold of Villanova who introduced it in the pharmacopoeia in the 13th century.

Brasavalo, Antonius Musa (1500–1555) A physician of Ferrara who wrote several commentaries on the Aphorisms of Hippocrates (460–377 BC), and a complete index to Galen's (129–200) works.

Brasbridge, Thomas A physician from Northamptonshire. He wrote *The Poor Man's Jewel; viz. A Treatise of the Pestilence; to which is annexed a Declaration of Herbs* in 1578.

Brasdor Operation A distal ligation applied to an aneurysm. Devised by French surgeon Pierre Brasdor (1721–1798).

Brashear, Walter (1776–1860) A surgeon from Maryland who performed amputation at the hip joint in 1806.

Brass Founders' Ague The ill effects of inhalation of metal fumes by workers in brass were described by Potissier in 1822. Charles Turner Thackrah (1795–1833), a pioneer of industrial medicine in England, described intermittent fever in brass workers in 1831 without identifying its cause. E.H. Greenhow established that it was caused by zinc fumes in 1862.

Brauer, Ludolph (1865–1951) Described thoracoplasty for the treatment of tuberculosis in 1908. He also pioneered the use of nitrogen instead of air in the production of artificial pneumothorax.

Braun, Ferdinand (1850–1918) German physicist from Fulda who constructed the first cathode-ray oscilloscope (Braun tube) in 1897. He shared the Nobel Prize with Guglielmo Marchese Marconi (1874–1937) in 1909.

Braun, Friedrich Wilhelm (1862–1934) Leipzig physician who introduced novocaine as a local anesthetic and discovered a method of prolonging its effect by adding epinephrine.

Braun, Max (1850–1930) A physician who later became professor of zoology at Dorpat, in 1884. Most of his contributions were on parasitology.

Braune, Christian Wilhelm (1831–1892) German who studied and described locomotion on a mathematical basis in 1891. He pioneered the use of frozen sections for studying fetal abnormalities in 1872.

Braun-Fernwald Sign Asymmetrical enlargement of the uterus with the appearance of a longitudinal furrow. Described by Viennese obstetrician, Carl Braun von Fernwald (1823–1891).

Braxton Hicks Sign Intermittent contraction occurring after the 3rd month of pregnancy. Described by English obstetrician, John Braxton Hicks (1825–1897) of Lymington. He studied medicine at Guy's Hospital and graduated from the University of London in 1847. He was obstetric physician to Guy's Hospital from 1868 to 1893.

Braxy (Syn. bradsot, quick plague) A fatal disease of sheep in Norway, Scotland, Germany and Australia. It was found to be caused by *Clostridium septique* by Nielson in 1888.

Brazier Disease (Syn. zinc chills, brass chills, foundry fever, welder's ague) Disease due to inhalation of zinc and metal dust in industry. Recognized by Potissier in 1822.

Break Bone Fever *See dengue fever.*

Breakfast Cereal The first breakfast cereal was made from shredded wheat by Henry Perky of Denver, Colorado in 1893. He was given the idea by a person with indigestion who described to Perky how he took boiled wheat soaked in milk every morning to sooth his stomach. William Kellogg (1852–1943), a physician from Tyrone in Michigan, introduced the method of flaking the grains into crispy flakes in 1894.

Breast Cancer Aulus Cornelius Celsus (25 BC–50 AD), a Roman physician, practiced excision of the breast for cancer and kept the pectoralis major intact. In AD 180 Leonidas of Alexandria excised breast cancer with the removal of surrounding healthy tissues, a method that is similar to modern radical mastectomy. According to Paul of Aegina (625–690), cancer arises out of thick, over-heated bile. He stated that 'it can occur in any part of the body, but the breasts of women were commonly affected due to its laxity which admitted humors, that caused it'. Hippocrates (460–377 BC) described a fatal case. Rhazes (850–932) was wary of removing cancers of the breast and described a case of cancer which occurred in the breast of the other side after its removal from the one side. Antyllus, in AD 300, recommended that advanced cancers should be left, as they were inoperable. An important early treatise on the breast was written by Alfred Armand Louis Marie Velpeau (1795–1867) of Paris in 1854. Andre Victor Cornil (1837–1908), a histopathologist from Paris, gave a description of the malignant transformation of the acinar epithelium of the breast in 1865. Sir James Paget (1814–1899) gave an original description of eczema of the nipple and mammary cancer in 1875. The supraclavicular operation was designed by the American surgeon William Halstead (1852–1922) in 1889. English surgeon, Charles Hewitt Moore (1821–1870), a pioneer in the treatment of cancer, was one of the first to insist on the entire removal of the breast. Oophorectomy was performed as treatment by Sir George Thomas Beatson (1848–1933) in 1896. The embolic theory for its spread was elaborated by Roger Williams in *Diseases of the Breast,* published in 1894, and his theory was advocated by Marmaduke Shield in 1898. Stephen Paget wrote in *The Lancet* opposing the embolic theory in 1889. Radium was introduced as treatment by Sir Geoffrey Langdon Keynes (1887–1982) in 1932. Androgens were used in treatment by Alfred A. Loeser in 1938, and estrogens were tried by Sir Alexander Haddow (1907–1976) in 1944. Charles Brenton Huggins (b 1901) and Dao in 1951 successfully performed adrenalectomy for the condition, and ablation or removal of the pituitary was pioneered by Rolf Luft and Herbert Olivecrona (1891–1980) in 1952.

Breastfeeding Aristotle forbade wine for nursing women in his statement 'it is the same whether the nurse or the child, drink it'. Galen (129–200) in his treatise on infancy, stated that infants should be fed with the milk of their mother as this was more natural to them than that of a stranger. Chinese women breastfed their aged grandfathers before feeding their own hungry children. Jews breastfed their infants for the first 2 years, and Aetius of Amida (AD 600) recommended breastfeeding for 20 months. Up to the 15th century in England, suckling was continued for 2–3 years, and by the end of the 17th century the suckling period was reduced to about 24 months. Artificial feeding was introduced in England around the 18th century, and the suckling period was reduced to about 9 months in the 19th century.

Breathalyzer The first to detect the amount of alcohol in the breath was devised by Lallamand, Perrin and Duroy of Paris in 1860.

Breech Delivery *See Bracht maneuver, Wigand maneuver.*

Bregma [Greek: *brechein*, to moisten + *bregma*, forepart of the head] Ancient Greek physicians used the term to refer to the most humid – and delicate – part of the infant's skull. Aristotle used it for the bone in the anterior part of the skull that was the last to fuse after birth. It was renamed the vertex by Galen (129–200).

Breisky Disease Kraurosis vulvae, described by German gynecologist, August Breisky (1832–1889).

Bremer Test Test for detecting sugar in the blood, using methylene and eosin as reagents. Devised by American physician, Ludwig Bremer (1844–1914).

Brenda Disease Brazilian yaws, described by Italian dermatologist, Achilles Brenda towards the end of the 19th century.

Brennemann Syndrome Abdominal pain and fever due to mesenteric lymphadenitis in children following a throat infection. Described by Joseph Brennemann (1872–1944) in 1927.

Brenner Tumor A peculiar neoplasm of the ovary, described as 'oophoroma folliculare' by German physician, Fritz Brenner (1877–1969) in 1907. He graduated from Heidelberg in 1904 and, after working with Eugen Albrecht at his pathology institute, he emigrated to South Africa in 1910. A similar neoplasm of the ovary was described by Ernst Gottlob Orthmann (1858–1922) in 1899.

Brenner, Sydney (b 1927) South African-born British biologist who was Director of the Medical Research Council Molecular Biology Laboratory in Cambridge. He worked with Francis Harry Compton Crick (b 1916) to unravel the genetic code, and together they worked out the nucleotide code for 20 amino acids in 1961. He introduced the term 'codon' for the unit of three nucleotides that coded for one amino acid.

Breschet, Gilbert He succeeded Jean Cruveilheir (1791–1874) as professor at the University of Paris in 1818. He described the diploic venous spaces within the cranial bones in 1819.

Bretonneau, Pierre (1771–1862) A physician in France who performed tracheotomy in croup. He gave the present name diphtheria to the disease in 1826. He also gave a classic pathological description of typhoid in 120 patients at autopsy and demonstrated the characteristic features of Peyer patches which occurred in the intestines of typhoid patients.

Bretylium Tosylate A ganglion-blocking drug, introduced as treatment for hypertension by A.L.A. Boura and A.F. Green in 1959.

Breuer, Josef (1842–1925) A contemporary of Sigmund Freud (1856–1939). In his initial interviews with a patient Anna O (pseudonym), he used hypnosis to bring out her experiences. He called this 'talking cure', and Freud conceived his idea of psychoanalysis from this. He also described the Hering–Breuer reflex in 1868.

Brewer Kidney Hematogenous abscesses following septicemia. Described by American surgeon, G.E. Brewer (1861–1939) of Westfield, New York. He graduated from Harvard in 1885 and established himself in general practice at New York in 1887. He continued to develop his surgical skills and traveled to Britain to study anatomy under Sir William Turner (1832–1916) of Edinburgh. He was elected President of the American Surgical Association in 1920.

Brewster, Sir David (1781–1868) Scottish physicist, born in Jedburgh. He obtained his LLD from Aberdeen and commenced the *Edinburgh Encyclopaedia* in 1808 which he completed in 1830. He invented the polyzonal lenses for lighthouses (1811), the kaleidoscope and the lenticular stereoscope. He wrote *Depolarisation of Light* (1813), *Optics* (1831), *Letters on Natural Magic* (1831) and *More Worlds than One* (1854). He was awarded the Rumford Gold Medal in 1818 for his work on polarization of light.

Bridewell Hospital A royal palace built for Henry VIII by the Knights Hospitallers and presented by Edward IV, 22 years later, to the City for beneficial uses. The hospital initially functioned as a reform house for vagrants and prostitutes in 1553.

Bridges, Robert (1844–1930) A student of St Bartholomew's Hospital who later became a physician to the Royal Northern Hospital and Great Ormond Street Hospital. When he retired he wrote several poems, the last of which, *The Testament of Beauty* was published on his 85th birthday.

In 1913 he was appointed Poet Laureate.

Bridgewater Treatises Francis Henry Egerton, Earl of Bridgewater, (1756–1829) left a sum of £8000 to be given to eight persons appointed by the President of the Royal Society to write essays 'on the power, wisdom, and goodness of God, as manifested in his creation'. These were written by: the surgeon Sir Charles Bell, Scottish theologian, Thomas Chalmers, John Kidd, William Buckland, William Prout, Peter M. Roget, Whewell and William Kirby from 1833–1835.

Bridgman, Percy Williams (1882–1961) A physicist at Cambridge, Massachusetts who was awarded the Nobel Prize for his work on high-pressure physics and thermodynamics in 1946. He proved that viscosity increases with pressure.

Briggs, William (1556–1630) A physician from Norwich, at St Thomas' Hospital, whose *Theory of Vision* was published by Hooke. He also wrote *Ophthalmographia* in 1687.

Brigham Hospital In Boston, Massachusetts, the first hospital to do a renal transplant. Although its first transplant was not successful, it was followed by a second successful kidney transplant from an identical twin by Joseph E. Murray in 1954. *See renal transplant.*

Bright Disease Richard Bright (1789–1858), an eminent physician at Guy's Hospital, was the first to associate the symptoms and signs in nephritis with the peculiar inflammation found in the kidneys on postmortem. His classic description was published in the *Reports of Medical Cases* published in 1827.

Bright, Richard (1789–1858) An eminent physician at Guy's Hospital, born in Bristol and studied medicine at Edinburgh, London, Berlin and Vienna. One of his first publications was *Travels from Vienna through Lower Hungary* (1818). He joined Guy's Hospital in 1820 and was instrumental in founding the *Guy s Hospital Reports*. He differentiated renal dropsy from cardiac dropsy, and gave a classic description of chronic non-suppurative nephritis (Bright disease) in 1827. He continued to work at Guy's Hospital for 20 years and became one of its most distinguished physicians. He also gave an original description of acute yellow atrophy of the liver, and unilateral epilepsy.

Brill Disease An illness resembling typhus, described amongst immigrants from Europe by New York physician, Nathan Edwin Brill (1860–1925), a graduate of University Medical College, New York in 1880. He was professor of clinical medicine at the College of Physicians and Surgeons, Columbia in 1910. The above illness was shown to be a true recrudescence of typhus by American immunologist and professor at Stanford and Harvard Universities, Hans Zinsser (1878–1940), in 1934.

Brill, Nathan Edwin (1860–1925) *See Brill Disease.*

Brillat Savarin, Anthelme (1755–1826) A lawyer from Jura who became his city's mayor. He fled to Switzerland during the French Revolution and published *Physiology du Gout* (1825) in which he treated gastronomy as a fine art based on psychological principles. This is considered a classic on obesity and diet.

Brill–Symmers Disease Follicular lymphadenopathy and splenomegaly. Described by Nathan Edwin Brill (1860–1925) in 1925. Douglas Symmers (1879–1952), an associate professor of pathology at the Bellevue Hospital, described it in 1928.

Brill–Zinsser Disease *See Brill disease.*

Brimstone *See sulfur.*

Brinster, Ralph Lawrence (b 1932) *See genetic engineering.*

Brinton Disease Linus plastica. *See Brinton, William.*

Brinton, William (1823–1867) A physician from St Thomas' Hospital who described peptic ulcer disease with over 7000 postmortem findings in 1857. His *Diseases of the Stomach* published in 1859 contains an original description of linus plastica (Brinton disease) of the stomach.

Briquet Syndrome Hysteria, named after French physician, Paul Briquet (1786–1881), who wrote a monograph on it in 1859.

Briquet, Paul (1786–1881) A physician in Paris who described pulmonary gangrene in bronchiectasis in 1841. *See Briquet syndrome.*

Brissaud, Edouard (1852–1909) A pediatrician and neurologist who trained under Jean Marie Charcot (1825–1893) at the Salpêtrière in Paris. He outlined a condition of uncontrolled tic spasms in children in 1896, and described infantile myxedema in 1907. He was operated on for a brain tumor by Victor Horsley (1857–1916) in Paris, but died. *See Brissaud–Siccard syndrome.*

Brissaud–Siccard Syndrome Facial spasm and contralateral paralysis of the limbs. Described by French neurologist, Edouard Brissaud (1852–1909), and French physician and radiologist, Jean A. Siccard (1872–1929) of Paris, in 1908.

Brissot, Pierre (1478–1522) Professor from Poitou at the Paris faculty who opposed the Islamic method of blood letting and promoted the Greek and Roman methods. He also wrote a treatise in defense of phlebotomy. *See blood letting.*

Bristowe Syndrome An insidious onset of hemiparesis on one side, with frank onset of hemiplegia on the contralateral side, accompanied by dysphasia and coma, due to tumor of the corpus callosum. Described by London physician, John Syer Bristowe (1827–1895) in 1884.

Britannica A name given to a herb noted to cure scurvy during late Anglo-Saxon times.

British Anti-Lewisite (BAL) 2-3 dimercaptopropanol was discovered as an antidote to the chemical war gas lewisite by London biochemist, Sir Rudolph Albert Peters (1889–1982) and co-workers during World War ll. It was later found to be effective as a chelating agent in treatment of poisoning by heavy metals. Its most frequent use in the late 19th century was in treatment of toxic side-effects resulting from arsenotherapy. *See Lewisite.*

British Association for the Advancement of Science (BAAS) Sir David Brewster (1781–1868) was a founder member in 1831. British chemist and clergyman, William Venables Vernon Harcourt (1789–1871) of Sudbury, Derbyshire was another and was its president in 1839. Its first annual meeting was held in the same year at York, and Queen Victoria presented the Kew Observatory to the Association in 1842.

British Journal of Anesthesia First published in 1923.

British Journal of Surgery Founded in 1913 by orthopedic surgeon, Ernest Williams Hey Groves (1872–1944).

British Medical Association (BMA) Founded at a meeting of 50 medical practitioners convened by Sir Charles Hastings (1794–1866) at the Worcester Royal Infirmary in 1832. It was initially named 'Provincial and Surgical Association' and its transactions were published in *The Provincial Medical and Surgical Journal.* By 1848 it had eight branches extending from Yorkshire to southwestern and southeastern regions and by 1853 its membership had increased to nearly 2000 from an initial 70. The first overseas branch was formed in Jamaica in 1877, and the first branch in the Indian subcontinent was established in Sri Lanka in 1887. The name was changed to the British Medical Association in 1855, taking the same name of a previously known association in London which had ceased to exist. Its journal was renamed *British Medical Journal* in 1857. Christine Murrell, the first woman member on the council of the BMA, was elected in 1924.

***British Medical Journal* (BMJ)** The forerunner, the *Midland Surgical and Medical Reporter,* was commenced by Charles Hastings (1794–1866) in 1828. It was revived and renamed, *The Provincial Medical and Surgical Journal* then became *British Medical Journal* in 1857.

British National Formulary (BNF) Developed from the national (war) formulary, first published in 1949. It was designed to serve as a handbook for prescribers in the late 1970s, and its present style appeared in 1981.

British Nurses Association Established with a view to regulating nursing and registering all nurses, by Mrs Bedford Fenwick in 1886. *See nursing.*

British Orthopaedic Association Founded by the English orthopedic surgeons, Robert Jones (1858–1933), Harry Platt (1886–1986), Ernest Muirhead Little (1854–1935), T.H. Openshaw (1856–1929) and Boston surgeon, Robert Osgood (1873–1956) in 1917. Muirhead Little was its first President, and Harry Platt was its first Secretary.

British Orthopaedic Society Founded by Robert Jones (1858–1933), Noble Smith and several other orthopedic surgeons in 1894. It ceased to exist in 1900.

British Pharmaceutical Codex (BPC) First published as a complementary volume to the *British Pharmacopoeia* in 1907. It was the first publication to specify standards for surgical dressings, vaccines, antisera and other blood products.

British Pharmacopoeia Developed from the pharmacopoeias of London, Edinburgh and Dublin, first published in 1864. *The Edinburgh Pharmacopoeia* was first published in 1699, followed by the *Dublin Pharmacopoeia* in 1793. *See London Pharmacopoeia.*

British Red Cross The forerunner of the establishment was founded as the National Society for Aid to the Sick and Wounded in 1870, and it became the British Red Cross in 1905. Sir Frederick Treves (1853–1923), a surgeon from Dorchester, played an important role its establishment.

British Society for Prevention of Cruelty to Animals Founded in an attempt to prevent vivisection in 1824, and it led to the Cruelty to Animals Act in 1876.

Brittain, Herbert Alfred (1904–1954) *See arthrodesis.*

Britton, Nathaniel (1859–1934) A botanist from Staten Island, New York. He established the New York Botanic Garden in 1896 and was its first director. He wrote several treatises on botany.

Broadbent Sign *See adherent pericardium.*

Broadbent, Sir William Henry (1835–1907) Born in Huddersfield, Yorkshire, he was a member of the Royal College of Physicians in 1857 and worked in France with Armand Trousseau (1801–1867) and Phillipe Ricord (1799–1889). On his return, he joined St Mary's Hospital as an obstetric officer and he later became physician to the Queen and the president of the Harvean, Medical, Clinical and Neurological Societies. He was an eminent cardiologist and a neurologist who described 'adherent pericardium' and proposed the 'Broadbent's hypothesis' for recovery of motor power of the muscles in paralysis. He described apoplexy due to cerebral hemorrhage into the ventricles in 1876. *See adherent pericardium.*

Broca Area Named after French surgeon Paul Broca (1824–1880) who located the motor area of speech in the brain of a 21-year-old man in 1861. *See Broca, Paul.*

Broca, Paul (1824–1880) French surgeon and anthropologist, born at Saint-Foyla-Grande, Gironde. He obtained his medical degree from the University of Paris in 1849. He identified the motor speech center in the third frontal convolution of the brain in a 21-year-old patient with aphasia who died in 1861. He was appointed to a commission to report on excavations in the cemetery of the Celestines in 1847, and became interested in craniology. He invented a series of instruments to measure the skull and founded anthropometry.

Brock Syndrome Atelectasis and chronic pneumonitis of the middle lobe due to compression of the middle lobe bronchus (middle lobe syndrome). Described by Russel Claude Brock, Baron Brock of Wimbledon (1903–1980), of Guy's Hospital, in 1937.

Brock, Sir Russell Claude (1903–1980) A pioneer of thoracic surgery in England, who graduated from Guy's Hospital in 1927, and started his career in thoracic surgery as a Rockefeller Traveling Fellow in St Louis in 1929. He was surgeon at Guy's and Brompton Hospitals in 1936 and performed the first cardioesophageal resection for carcinoma of the cardia in 1942. He reported three cases of pulmonary stenosis treated by valvulotomy in 1948, and recognized hypertrophic cardiomyopathy at an operation in 1957. *See Brock syndrome.*

Brockbank, E.M. (1866–1959) Dean of medical studies at Manchester Royal Infirmary and author of: *Foundation of Provincial Medical Education in England* and *Diagnosis and Treatment of Heart Disease.*

Brocklesby, Richard (1722–1797) Physician from Somerset who qualified in Leiden and established a practice in London. He was a friend of Samuel Johnson (1709–1784) and his published works include: *Account of a Poisonous Root Found Mixed with Gentian, Dissertatio et Saliva Sana et Morbosa* and *Essay Concerning the Mortality of Horned Cattle.*

Brocq Disease A condition similar to psoriasis and lichen planus with lichenification. Described by Anne Jean Louis Brocq (1856–1928), a dermatologist in Paris in 1902.

Brodel, Max (1870–1941) An artist from Leipzig who did medical illustrations. In 1893 he traveled to America and became the founder of illustrative medical art.

Broden, A. *See antimony.*

Brodie Abscess An abscess of long bones due to *Staphylococcus aureus*. Described in 1828 by Sir Benjamin Collins Brodie (1783–1862), an eminent surgeon at St George's Hospital.

Brodie Tumor (Syn. cystosarcoma phyllodes, giant fibroadenoma) An essentially benign serocystic tumor of the breast, sometimes reaching a large size. Described by Sir Benjamin Collins Brodie (1783–1862) of St George's Hospital in 1840.

Brodie, Charles Gordon (1860–1933) A demonstrator in anatomy at the Middlesex Hospital, who wrote *Dissections Illustrated* in 1895. The transverse humeral ligament (Brodie ligament) is named after him.

Brodie, Sir Benjamin Collins (1783–1862) A surgeon from Wiltshire, who worked at St George's Hospital from 1808 to 1840. One of his interests was physiology and he wrote: *The Effect of Influence of the Brain on the Action of the Heart* (1810), *Effect of Certain Vegetable Poisons* (1811), *The Influence of the Nervous System on the Production of the Animal Heat* (1812) and *The Influence of the Pneumogastric on the Secretions of the Stomach,* in 1814. He perfected many surgical instruments and performed the first operation for varicose veins, in 1814. His most important work, *On the Pathology and Surgery of the Diseases of the Joints,* was published in 1819.

Brodmann, Korbinian (1868–1918) German neuropsychiatrist at Jena who classified the cortical areas (Brodmann areas) of the brain in terms of numbers, on the basis of the structure and morphology of cell layers.

Brodum, William A successful quack practitioner in the 18th century in England. He practiced at Blackfriars and then moved to the West End of London, where he established a prosperous practice with 'cure-all' remedies. He wrote an unscientific treatise: *Guide to Old Age and Cure for Indiscretions of Youth* in 1795. When he was challenged by the Royal College of Physicians regarding his qualifications, he produced a duly signed certificate which he had obtained for a fee from Marischal College, Aberdeen in 1791. Although Marischal College later accepted that the issue of Bro-drum's certificate was due to an oversight, the Royal College of Physicians could not curb his practice since he had a legally valid certificate. *See quackery.*

Bromfield, William (1712–1792) London surgeon who founded the Lock Hospital. He became a surgeon to St George's Hospital and wrote: *An Account of the English Night Shades, Thoughts Containing the Present Mood of Inoculating for the Small Pox, Chirurgical Cases and Observations* and *Narrative of a Physical Transaction with Mr. Aylet, Surgeon of Windsor.*

Bromide Used in the 19th century for sedation and other conditions such as epilepsy, climacteric symptoms and hypertension. *See antiepileptic drugs.*

Bromidrosis [Greek: *bromos,* stench + *hidros,* sweat] Fetid perspiration.

Bromine [Greek: *bromos,* stink] Discovered in salt water by Antoine Jèrome Balard (1802–1876), an apothecary at Montpellier, who called it 'muride' in 1826. Its potassium salts were used in treatment by French physicians. Bromide of potassium was recommended as treatment for epilepsy by Sir C. Locock (1799–1875) in 1853. Ten years later it became one of the most commonly used compounds in treatment of epilepsy.

Bromism *See antiepileptic drugs.*

Brompton Cocktail Analgesic mixture containing morphine, cocaine, heroin and alcohol, for use in terminal cancer. Introduced at the Brompton Hospital by H. Snow in 1896.

Brompton Consumption and Cough Specific A secret remedy sold in the late 19th century by a London company with no relation to the Brompton Hospital. It contained ipecacuanha and tincture of opium.

Bronchial Arteries [Greek: *brongchos,* windpipe] The term 'bronchial' was used in 1665 by Frederick Ruysch, professor of anatomy at Amsterdam, to describe the arteries and veins around the bronchi.

Bronchial Asthma *See asthma.*

Bronchial Carcinoma *See carcinoma of the lung.*

Bronchial Cast Found in a patient with chronic pulmonary disease. Described by Nicholas Tulp (1593–1674) in his *Observationes Medicae* first published in 1641. Richard Warren (1731–1797) of Cavendish in Suffolk and physician

to George III, illustrated them in 1772.

Bronchial Lavage The bronchoscope was used in the treatment of asthma to clear the secretions and exudates of the mucosal epithelium of the bronchi by an American pioneer in laryngology, Horace Green (1802–1866), in 1838. His *Treatise on the Diseases of the Air Passages* was published in 1846.

Bronchial Spasm *See bronchospasm.*

Bronchiectasis [Greek: *bronchus,* windpipe + *ektasis,* extension] First noted by René Laënnec's (1781–1826) assistant, Jean Bruno Cayol, in 1808. Laënnec later described it and differentiated it from conditions such as emphysema and pleurisy. Paul Briquet (1796–1881) of Paris described pulmonary gangrene in bronchiectasis in 1841. Successful removal of bronchiectatic lobes of the lung was performed by Werner Korte (1853–1937) of Berlin in 1909.

Bronchiolitis [Greek: *bronchus,* windpipe + *itis,* inflammation] Acute inflammatory condition of the finer bronchioles causing asthma. Described by Ludwig Traube (1818–1876), professor of medicine at Berlin, in 1847.

Bronchitis [Greek: *bronchus,* windpipe + *itis,* inflammation] Described in detail by English physician Charles Badham (1780–1845) who named in 1808.

Bronchocele [Greek: *bronchus,* windpipe + *cele,* tumor] Goiter or tumor in the top or middle part of the windpipe. Also known as bocium.

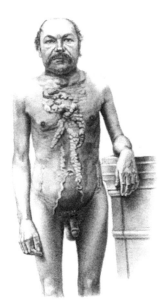

Malignant bronchocele. Theodor Billroth, *Clinical Surgery* (1881). New Sydenham Society, London

Bronchogram [Greek: *bronchus*, windpipe + *graphein*, to write] A radiological method of studying bronchiectasis by injecting bismuth through the bronchoscope was used by Henry Lowndes Lynah (1879–1922) and William Holmes Stewart (b 1868) in 1921. A method of outlining the bronchial tree using an oil containing radio-opaque iodine compound, lipiodol, was devised by Jean Athanase Sicard (1872–1929) and Jacques Forrestier (b 1890) in 1922.

Bronchophony [Greek: *bronchus*, windpipe + *phone*, voice] (Syn. bronchial breathing).

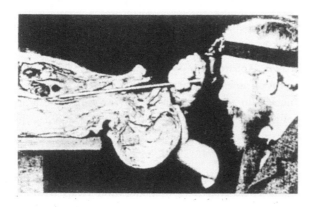

Bronchoscopy. Demonstration by Gustav Killian. Courtesy of *Ann. Thorac. Surg*, 22,310, (1976)

Bronchoscopy [Greek: *bronchus*, windpipe + *scopos*, a watcher] The earliest attempt to view the larynx and trachea directly was made by Alfred Kirstein (1863–1922) of Berlin in 1895, and direct bronchoscopy was performed by Gustav Killian (1860–1921) in 1898. It was used in the management of asthma by Franz Novotny (1872–1925) in 1907, and a book on intestinal endoscopy, which included tracheobronchoscopy, was written by American laryngologist Jackson Chevalier (1865–1958) of Pittsburgh in the same year. He also performed the first removal of an endobronchial tumor through a bronchoscope in 1917 and was the first professor of bronchoscopy at the University of Pennsylvania in 1920.

Bronchospasm [Greek: *bronchus*, windpipe + *spasmos*, tension] William Cullen (1710–1790) suggested spasm of bronchial muscles as a cause of asthma in 1778. An important study of the mechanism of asthma was done by Franz D. Reissensen (1773–1828) of Strasbourg in 1808. He showed the contraction of muscles in the bronchial wall during an asthmatic attack. Alfred Wilhelm Volkmann (1800–1877) of Dorpat produced bronchospasm by stimulation of the vagus nerve in 1844, and Sandleman induced it by irritation of the nasal mucosa in 1890. The auscultatory signs were described by René Laënnec (1781–1826) following

his invention of the stethoscope in 1819.

Bronchotomy [Greek: *bronchus*, windpipe + *tome*, cutting] Described by Fabricius ab Aquapendente (1533–1619), Hermann Boerhaave (1668–1738) and others. In 1759 M. Louis, a French surgeon, gave a tragic account of a 7-year-old girl who had a bean seed stuck in her windpipe. Despite his attempts to save the child by performing a bronchotomy, he was prevented by other physicians who advised the child's parents against it. After the death of the child, he demonstrated on the child's body how easy it was to remove the foreign body, much to the sorrow of the parents and physicians.

Bronchus [Greek: *bronchus*, windpipe] Derives its name from the belief by the Greek philosopher Plato (428–348 BC) that fluids, when drunk, passed down the trachea, creating its moistness [Greek: *brechein* + to moisten].

Bronk, Detlev Wulf (1887–1975) American neurophysiologist from New York who worked with Lord Edgar Douglas Adrian (1889–1977) on the biophysical properties of motor nerve fibers at Cambridge, in 1927. They recorded the activity of single motor units by introducing concentric needle electrodes in 1928.

Brønsted Theory Acid gives off a proton in solution and bases accept the proton. Proposed by Danish physical chemist, Johannes Nicolaus Brønsted (1879–1947) in 1928. A similar definition was also put forward by Martin Thomas Lowry (1874–1936), professor of chemistry at Guy's Hospital Medical School in 1923.

Bronze Age Started in Western Asia around 2000 BC and in Western Europe around 1500 BC. Bronze implements from 1500 BC unearthed from the graves of Mycenae show an alloy content of 88% copper and 12% tin. It came to China at the time of Emperor Ta-Yu in 2200 BC and ended around 600 BC.

Bronze Diabetes Iron is deposited in the liver, skin and other organs leading to pigmentation, cirrhosis and diabetes. Described by Armand Trousseau (1801–1867) as 'glycosurie, diabete-sucre' in 1865 and by Charles Emile Troisier (1848–1919) in 1871. Two workers from Paris, Victor Charles Hanot (1844–1896) and Antole Marie Emile Chauffard (1855–1932), described it in 1882. It was named hemochromatosis by Friedrich Daniel von Recklinghausen (1833–1910) in 1889. J.H. Sheldon postulated in 1927 that it was an inborn error of metabolism.

Bronzerio, John Jerome (1577–1630) Italian physician who wrote *Disputatio de Principatu Hepatis ex Anatomie Lampetrae,*

De Principio Effectivo semini Insito and other works.

Brooke Disease Acanthoma adenoides cystecum. A familial skin disease of dominant inheritance, described by English dermatologist, Henry Ambrose Grundy Brooke (1854–1919) of Manchester in 1892.

Brooks, Keith William (1848–1908) Born in Cleveland, Ohio, he was a professor at Johns Hopkins University who contributed to the knowledge of embryology with his work on the oyster.

Broom, Robert (1866–1951) South African paleontologist, originally from Paisley, Scotland. He graduated in medicine from Glasgow and practiced in South Africa. He found a partial skeleton of *Australopithecus*, the ancestor of humans, in 1947 and wrote *The Coming of Man* in 1933.

Brophy Operation Operation for cleft palate designed by American oral surgeon, Truman William Brophy (1848–1928).

Brosse, Guy de la (d 1641) Physician to Louis XIII in Paris who published several works on plants.

Brothel Parliament sanctioned establishment of brothels in 1161 and they were known as 'stews'. Bernard Mandeville advocated regular medical inspection of prostitutes in *A Modest Defence of Public Stews* published in 1724. *See prostitution.*

Broussais, François Victor Joseph (1772–1838) Son of a physician at St Malo, France. He graduated in medicine in 1803 and was a physician in the navy and army, before he became a professor at Val-de-Grace. He considered gastroenteritis or irritability of the mucous membrane of the alimentary canal, as a basis for most diseases and advocated deprivation of food and extensive use of leeches. His views were opposed by René Laënnec (1781–1826) but Broussais' popularity overcame his critics.

Brown, James (1854–1895) Surgeon as the Johns Hopkins Hospital. In 1893, he catheterized male urethras.

Brown, James Howard *See blood transfusion.*

Brown, James William (1897–1958) A member of the editorial board of the *British Heart Journal* in the 1920s. In 1930 he joined D.C. Muir in establishing heart clinics for school children and became consultant to Grimsby and neighboring hospitals in 1938. His *Congenital Heart Disease,* published in 1939, was of great importance in establishing cardiac surgery in England.

Brown, John (1735–1788) A physician from Berwickshire, Scotland, and an assistant to William Cullen (1710–1790). He was a clergyman and a school teacher before studying medicine. He proposed the Brunonian theory which classified diseases into: 'asthenic' or debilitated, and 'sthenic' or excitable. He prescribed stimulants for treatment of asthenia. He was a heavy drinker and was imprisoned for improper behavior.

Brown, John (1810–1882) A physician from Edinburgh who was apprenticed to James Syme (1799–1870). He wrote a novel, *Rab and his Friends* (1859), a narrative of the surgical tragedies and difficulties caused by sepsis and lack of anesthesia. He also wrote *Horae Subsecivae* in three volumes and was known as the 'Charles Lamb' of Scottish literature.

Brown, Phillip King (1869–1940) Gave a description of fatal leukopenia in 1901.

Brown, Robert (1773–1858) A physician and botanist who went on an expedition to Tasmania. He described the cell nucleus in 1831 and named it. He explained the process of generation in plants by means of pollen, and described the movements of fine particles of fluid in 1827. *See Brownian movement.*

Brown, Sir Dennis (1892–1967) English anesthetist who designed the ether inhaler (Dennis Brown Inhaler) in 1928.

Brown, Sir George Lindor (1903–1971) English physiologist who studied the effects of acetylcholine on muscles with Sir Henry Hallet Dale (1875–1968) in 1929. *See acetylcholine.*

Brown, Thomas (1778–1820) Scottish physician who received his education at Edinburgh. After qualifying as a lawyer, he studied medicine from 1798 to 1803. He lived in Kew for a short period before returning to Edinburgh. His main interest was philosophy and he wrote *Lectures on Philosophy of Human Mind* in 1820, and was regarded as the founder of systematic psychology. He also published some poetry.

Brown, Thompson Richardson (1872–1950) English physician who, in 1898, described the occurrence of eosinophilia and its diagnostic importance in trichinosis.

Brown, William (1752–1792) Editor of the first pharmacopoeia of America in 1778.

Browne, Edward (1642–1708) Son of Sir Thomas Browne (1605–1682) and a physician. He obtained his degree from Oxford in 1667 and became physician to Charles II.

Browne, Edward Granville (1862–1926) A graduate of St Bartholomew's Hospital who gave up medicine to become professor of Arabic and Persian languages. Most of his contributions were on oriental history, literature and religion.

Browne, John (1642–1700) English surgeon from Norwich who studied at St Thomas' Hospital, London where he became a surgeon. He was also surgeon to William III. He gave a description of cirrhosis of the liver in the *Philosophical Transactions of the Royal Society* in 1685.

Browne, Patrick (1720–1790) Physician from Ireland. He qualified from Leiden and practiced for a short time in Paris and London before he settled in Jamaica. He wrote *Civil and Natural History of Jamaica*.

Browne, Sir Thomas (1605–1682) The son of a London merchant from Upton in Cheshire. He was born in Cheapside and entered Pembroke College, Oxford. After studying medicine he practiced for a short while in Oxfordshire. He pursued his medical studies at Montpellier, Leiden and Padua before settling in Halifax. In 1635 he wrote *Religio Medici,* an expression of religious faith and spiritual life with medical scepticism. His other works include: *Urn Burial* (1658) on mortality and immortality and burial customs, *Pseudodoxia* (1646) on the vulgarity of mankind, and *Christian Morals* (1716), incomplete but meant to be a continuation of *Religio Medici*. He became a general practitioner in Norwich in 1636. He was buried at St Peter's Mancroft in Norwich.

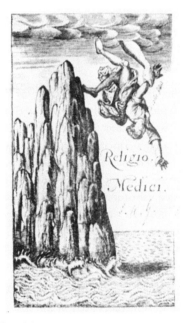

Religio Medici (1642) by Sir Thomas Browne

Browne, William (1692–1774) He obtained his medical degree from Cambridge in 1792, and practiced at Norfolk before he moved to Great Ormond Street in London. He published several pieces of orations, prose and poetry. He awarded three gold medals to scholars of Latin and Greek at Cambridge and founded a scholarship at Peterhouse.

Brownian Movement Robert Brown (1773–1858) observed the movements of pollen grains suspended in water using a crude microscope in 1827. He described the movements as the 'dance of the elements' in the *Philosophical Magazine* in 1828. They were suggested to be due to temperature irregularities by Victor Regnault (1810–1871) in 1858. The collision between the pollen grains and the molecules of the liquid was proposed as the cause of the movements by Christian Wierner (1826–1896) in 1863. His view was shared by Sir William Ramsay (1852–1916) in 1879. It was elucidated by M. Smoluchowski (1872–1917) and experimentally demonstrated by Jean Perrin (b 1870).

Browning, Carl Hamilton (1881–1792) He studied the property of resistance of parasites to therapeutic agents and showed a species of trypanosome resistant to Atoxyl in 1908. He introduced acriflavin as an antiseptic in 1917. In 1922 he demonstrated the 'interference phenomenon' of chemotherapeutic agents which was probably the first scientific recognition of drug interaction. He published an essay entitled *Biological Principles in Immunity* in the *British Medical Journal* of 1927.

Brown–Buerger Cystoscope *See Buerger, Leo.*

Brown–Séquard Syndrome *See Brown-Séquard, Charles Edouard.*

Brown-Séquard, Charles Edouard (1817–1894) French neurophysiologist. His father was a sea captain from Philadelphia, and he was born in Mauritius. He was educated in Paris and became professor of physiology at the medical faculties of Harvard (1864) and Paris (1869). He described hemiplegia associated with crossed anesthesia (Brown-Séquard syndrome) in 1850. He demonstrated the importance of the suprarenal capsule by producing adrenal insufficiency in dogs by removing their adrenal glands in 1856.

Brucaeus, Henry (1531–1593) A physician from Flanders who wrote *De Primu Mortu* (1580), *Propositiones de Morbo Gallico* and other treatises.

Bruce, Alexander (1854–1911) Scottish neurologist at Edinburgh who described the descending posteriomedial part of the spinal tract in 1901.

Bruce, Sir David (1855–1931) A physician and microbiologist of Scottish origin who was born in Melbourne, Australia and studied medicine in Edinburgh. He identified the causative agent of nagna disease of African horses, a trypanosome, in the blood of diseased animals in 1894. In 1887, while he was in Malta as an army doctor, he discovered the cause of the mysterious disease later known as Malta fever. The organism responsible was named *Brucella* and the disease was called brucellosis.

Brucella abortus *See brucellosis.*

Brucellosis (Syn. Bang disease, Mediterranean fever, undulant fever, Rock fever of Gibraltar. First named Malta fever) Sir David Bruce (1855–1931) isolated the bacterium responsible in the spleen of patients dying of the disease in Malta in 1887 and named it *Micrococcus melitensis*. The same organism, causing a widespread disease in cattle called 'contagious abortion', was discovered by Bernhard Bang (1848–1932) in 1897. The genus of bacteria was later named *Brucella*, by Karl Friedrich Meyer (b 1884) and E. Shaw of America in 1920. *Brucella suis*, the natural host of which is the pig, was described by J.E. Traum of America in 1914.

Bruch Membrane A transparent membrane adjoining the retina, separating it from the capillaries of the choroid. Described in 1844 by Karl Wilhelm Ludwig Bruch (1819–1884), a German professor of anatomy at Basel and Giessen.

Bruck Disease Bone deformities, multiple fractures and ankylosis of the joints, described by Alfred Bruck of Germany in 1897.

Brucke, Ernest Wilhelm von Ritter (1819–1892) A leading physiologist of Europe who visualized the fundus of the eye with artificial light in 1822. He also described the radial fibers of the ciliary muscles in 1844.

Brudzinski Sign A diagnostic test for meningitis in which flexion of the ankle, knee and hip occurs when the neck is bent. Described by Polish physician, J. Brudzinski (1874–1917) in 1909.

Brugsch Papyrus *See papyri.*

Bruit *See murmur.*

Brumpt, Alexandre Joseph Emile (1877–1951) French parasitologist who described the life cycle of *Trypanosoma cruzi* in 1912. He also discovered the parasitic nematode of humans, *Oesophagostomium brumpti* in 1902. *See piedra.*

Brunn, Albert von (1849–1895) A student of Waldeyer who later became professor of anatomy at Göttingen in 1872. He described the cell mass found in the male urethra in 1893.

Brunner Glands Glands in the duodenum of dogs and humans, described by Swiss anatomist, Johan Brunner (1653–1727) in 1687. These glands were first observed by Jacobus Wepfer (1620–1695) of Schaffhausen,

who was his father-in-law.

Brunner, Johan Conrad (1653–1727) Swiss anatomist from Diessenhofen who studied under Joseph Guichard Duverney (1648–1730) at Paris. He conducted the first experiments on endocrinology. He demonstrated the symptoms of thirst and polyuria of diabetes in dogs by surgical excision of their pancreas. He wrote *Glandula Pituitaria* (1688) and *Glandula Duodeni seu Pancreas Secundum Detectum* (1715).

Bruno the Calabrian A surgeon at Padua in the 13th century. He completed his *Chirurgia Magna* in 1252 and also wrote, *Chirurgia Parva,* which had a strong Islamic influence.

Bruno, Giordano (1548–1600) Astronomer of Naples who suggested that the universe was infinite in terms of both time and space. He was burnt at the stake for his heretical theories.

Brunonian Theory *See Brown, John.*

Bruns Syndrome Vertigo caused by sudden movements of the head, due to cysticercosis of the fourth ventricle in the brain. Described by German neurologist, Ludwig Bruns (1858–1916) in Hannover.

Brunsfels, Otho (d 1534) A public physician in Bern who published *Catalogus Illustrium Medicorum, Herbarium Viva Icones* and other treatises.

Brunton, Sir Thomas Lauder (1844–1916) Born in Roxburghshire and graduated in medicine from Edinburgh in 1866. He was a lecturer at the Middlesex Hospital before he became a physician at St Bartholomew's Hospital. He introduced amyl nitrite in treatment for angina in 1867. He classified albuminuria into two categories – true and false – and suggested valvotomy for relief of symptoms in mitral stenosis in 1902. His well known *Textbook of Pharmacology and Therapeutics* was published in 1885. It was one of the first complete textbooks on the subject and it was translated into several languages. *See angina pectoris, amyl nitrite.*

Brushfield Spots (Syn. Mongolian spots) Whitish yellow pinpoint spots sometimes seen in the iris of infants with Down syndrome. Described by London physician, Thomas Brushfield (1858–1937) in 1924.

Bruton, C. Ogden (b 1908) *See combined immunodeficiency.*

Bryant Triangle *See Bryant, Thomas.*

Bryant, Thomas (1828–1914) Surgeon from Kennington who worked at Guy's Hospital and described the iliofemoral triangle (Bryant triangle) in 1861. This is used for surface marking in the diagnosis of fracture of the neck of the femur. He was surgeon to Queen Victoria in 1896.

Bryce, Thomas Hastie (1862–1946) Anatomist in Glasgow who carried out one of the earliest studies on human embryos.

Bryson Sign Reduced expansion of thoracic movement seen in exophthalmic goiter. Described by English physician, Alexander Bryson (1802–1860).

Bubo [Greek: *bubon*, groin] An ancient term used by Galen (129–200), Aulus Cornelius Celsus (25 BC–AD 50), Paul of Aegina (625–690) and other physicians for tumor or inflammation of the glands in the groin. *See climatic bubo.*

Bubonic Plague One of the earliest recorded epidemics, probably due to bubonic plague, occurred amongst the Philistines in 1000 BC. The first mention of the disease, according to Rufus of Ephesus, was made by Dionysios as *pestilentes bubones* in 277 BC. It was also mentioned by Dioscorides and Poseidonios around AD 100. It appeared again in Lower Egypt around AD 540 and reached Byzantium within 2 years, killing over 10,000 people each day. The pandemic Black Death in the 14th century occurred first in a Crimean port in 1347, and was carried to Genoa by Italian merchants. From Genoa it swept the whole of Europe, killing over 24 million people, until it reached Moscow in 1352. It is said to have reached England via a ship that arrived at Weymouth, Dorset, in 1348, and from the west of England it spread to the whole country in 1350. The disease remained endemic for a further 300 years and another epidemic, the Great Plague of London, occurred in 1665. It was only in the late 18th century that England became free of the threat of plague. In 1864 Pringle in India was told that people of the Shurwal district of the Himalayas knew that an exodus of rats always occurred just before the plague arrived, and they then left the district whenever this occurred. The causative organism was isolated independently by Alexander Emile Jean Yersin (1863–1943) and Shibasaburo Kitasato (1852–1931) in Hong Kong in 1894.

Bubonocele Protrusion of the bowel occasioned by a rupture of the peritoneum, or relaxation of the muscle, described by Paul of Aegina (625–690). When the intestines remained in the groin he called the condition bubonocele, and when they fell into the scrotum he named it enterocele. He recommended pomegranate, gall-nuts and diluted wine. He also advocated bandages to retain the intestines within the abdomen. Herniorrhaphy was practiced earlier by Aulus Cornelius Celsus (25 BC–AD 50). Alsaharavius or Albucasis (936–1013) found none of these measures helpful,

unless the protruded parts were returned (reduced) and secured by bandages.

Buchan, William (1729–1805) Born in Roxburghshire, Scotland in 1729 and practiced medicine in London. He wrote a popular book, *Domestic Medicine* in 1769, which went to 19 editions during his lifetime. He also wrote *Advice to Mothers* and *Treatise on Venereal Disease.*

Buchanan, Francis Hamilton (1762–1829) Born in Callander, Scotland and was a surgeon to the East India Company. He wrote *A Journey from Madras* (1807) and *Account of Nepal* in 1819.

Buchheim, Rudolf (1820–1879) Professor at Leipzig and a leading pharmacologist in Germany who investigated the action of potassium salts, ergot and cod-liver oil. He published a textbook of materia medica in 1856.

Büchner, Eduard (1860–1917) Professor of chemistry at Munich and brother of the German bacteriologist, Hans Büchner (1850–1902). He extracted the enzyme 'zymase' from yeast in 1897, and demonstrated its capability of fermenting sugar in the absence of yeast, for which he was awarded the Nobel Prize for Chemistry in 1907.

Büchner, Hans (1850–1902) German bacteriologist and brother of Eduard Büchner. He graduated in medicine from Leipzig in 1874 and was a professor at Munich in 1880. He did pioneering work on proteins in the blood that combined with invading microorganisms and protected against infection. These proteins were later named gammaglobulins.

Buck, Gurdon (1807–1877) Surgeon in New York who established the method of treating fractures of the thigh by applying traction through weights and pulleys. The fascial sheath of the penis was described by him in 1848.

Buckland, Francis Trevelyan (1826–1880) A surgeon from Oxford whose admiration for John Hunter (1728–1793) motivated him to search for his coffin. After examining over 3000 coffins, he succeeded and transferred it to Westminster Abbey in 1859. His best known works are: *Curiosities of Natural History* in four volumes (1857–1872), the *Log Book of a Fisherman and a Zoologist* (1875) and *Natural History of Fishes* (1881).

Buckland, William (1784–1856) Professor of geology and clergyman at the University of Oxford and one of the greatest authorities on geology in the first half of the 19th century. He discovered several fossil remains of animals extinct in Britain, such as the hippopotamus, rhinoceros and elephant, in a cave near Kirkdale in Yorkshire. His work, *Reliquiae Diluvianiae ,* was published in 1823.

Budd Disease *See Fasciolopsis buski, Budd, George.*

Budd, George (1808–1882) Professor of medicine at King's College London who described Budd–Chiari syndrome and cirrhosis of the liver due to the nematode *Fasciolopsis* (Budd disease) in 1845.

Budd, William (1811–1880) English physician and brother of George Budd (1808–1882). He proposed excreta as a source of typhoid and he wrote *Typhoid Fever: Its Nature Mode of Spreading and Prevention* in 1873.

Budd–Chiari Syndrome Occlusion of the hepatic veins leading to cirrhosis and portal hypertension. Observed by Karl Rokitansky (1804–1878) in 1842. It was described by an English physician, George Budd (1808–1882) in 1845 and by an Austrian pathologist, Hans Chiari (1851–1916) in Vienna in 1898.

Buddha, Gautama Siddartha (568–488 BC) A Hindu prince from the Sakaya tribe at Kapilavastu situated about 100 miles north of Benares. He founded Buddhism which proposed the concept of nirvana and transmigration of souls. *See Buddhist, nirvana.*

Buddhadasa King of Ceylon, who lived around AD 341. He is supposed to have been a skilled surgeon, and he built several asylums and hospitals.

Buddhist Follower of Gautama Buddha, whose concept of nirvana emphasized complete withdrawal of interest from the external world to the innerself. It is a tranquil state devoid of passion attained through four stages of meditation. These appear to be the earliest form of psychotherapy.

Budge, Julius Ludwig (1811–1884) Professor of physiology at Bonn who described the ciliospinal and genitospinal centers of the spinal cord in 1841.

Budin, Pierre (1846–1907) The originator of infant welfare services. He became the Chief of Staff at the Maternity Hospital in Paris in 1895 and organized the first clinic, Consultation de Nourrisons, where mothers brought their babies for health screening, a month after delivery.

Buerger Disease Obliteration of most of the arteries of the leg by a chronic proliferative process. Described by Felix von Winiwarter (1852–1931) in 1879. He observed a new growth of intima in the blood vessel and named it 'endarteritis obliterans'. The same condition was observed to be caused by occlusion of the blood vessels secondary to thrombosis by Leo Buerger (1879–1943) of New York who named it 'thromboangiitis obliterans' in 1908. His further work on the subject confirmed the disease to be due to arteriosclerosis in 1926.

Buerger, Leo (1879–1943) American urologist of Viennese origin who graduated from the College of Physicians and Surgeons in 1901. He designed the Brown–Buerger cystoscope in 1909 which helped to irrigate the bladder during cystoscopy. *See Buerger disease.*

Bufalini, Marizio (1787–1875) Italian physician from Florence who wrote *Essay of the Doctrine of Life* while he was a student in 1813. He pointed out the importance of observations in medicine in *Fondamenti della Patolia Analitica* published in 1819.

Buffer The term 'puffer' in German describes the ability of certain substances to resist any change in pH. It was introduced by Danish physicist, Sören Peter Lauritz Sörensen (1868–1939) of Copenhagen. It was later corrupted to 'buffer' in English.

Buffon, George Louis Leclerc, Compte de (1707–1788) French naturalist, son of a wealthy lawyer in Montbard, Burgundy. After graduating in science and law, he took natural science and wrote *Histoire Naturelle* in 44 volumes while he was director of the king's garden (Jardin du Roi) in Paris from 1749–1767. He was one of the earliest to propose the idea of evolution when he agreed that life forms in the animal kingdom were successively derived from one another. He suggested that the earliest life forms originated from polar regions and the ocean. He translated Isaac Newton's *Fluxions* while he was on a visit to England in 1733.

Buhl Disease Icterus neonatorum, described by German pathologist, Ludwig von Buhl (1816–1880).

Buist, John Brown (1846–1915) Appointed as a pathologist at the Edinburgh Medical School in 1880. He described the elementary body in the skin lesions (Buist–Paschen body) seen in smallpox and vaccinia.

Buist, Robert Cochrane (1860–1939) Born in Dundee, he was a lecturer in midwifery and gynecology at St Andrews. He described a method (Buist method) of resuscitating an asphyxiated newborn infant by alternately holding the child on the stomach and the back.

Bulbar Palsy or pseudobulbar palsy Described as 'primary labioglossolaryngeal paralysis' by Benjamin Amand Duchenne (1806–1875) and attributed to bulbar nuclei in 1861. Wachsmuth described it in more detail and named it 'progressive bulbar palsy' in 1864. Jean Martin Charcot (1825–1893) established the nuclear origin of the disease in 1870. Its association with amyotrophic lateral sclerosis was pointed out by Joseph Jules Dejerne (1849–1917) in 1883.

Bulimia [Greek: *bous*, ox + *limos*, hunger] Insatiable desire for food, named by Erasistratus in 300 BC. An identical condition was observed in some patients with accidental traumatic lesions of the brain by Stephen Paget in 1897 and a Russian physician, Vladimir Michailovich Bechterev (1857–1927) in 1901.

Bulleyn, William (d 1576) A physician of Ely who wrote *The Government of Health* (1558) and *Regimen against Pleurisy* (1562). He was accused of having murdered Sir Thomas Hilton, who in fact died of malignant fever. He wrote most of his treatises while he was serving a prison sentence for non-payment of debts.

Bulwer, John English physician in the 17th century who wrote: *Chirologia or the Natural Language of the Hand* (1644), *Man Transformed or the Artificial Changeling* and *Pathomyotomia or a Dissection of the Significative Muscles of the Affection of the mind* (1649).

Bundle Branch Block Hans Eppinger (1879–1946) and Carl Julius Rothberger (b 1871) described changes of the bundle branch block seen in the electrocardiogram in 1910. P.S. Barker of America described it in 1930 and R.H. Bayley specified the changes in the electrocardiogram due to right bundle branch block in 1934.

Bundle of His *See atrioventricular bundle.*

Bundle of Kent *See atrioventricular anomalous conduction, Kent, Albert Frank.*

Bunge Spoon An instrument for eviscerating the eyeball designed by German ophthalmologist, Paul Bunge (1844–1920).

Bunge Theory A causal relationship proposed between alcoholism in the father and inability to suckle a child in his daughter. Suggested by a Swiss physiologist, Gustav von Bunge (1844–1920) of Basel.

Bunsen Burner The principle of mixing air with coal gas to bring about complete combustion and increase the heating efficiency of the flame was devised by Robert Bunsen (1811–1899) of Germany in 1854. A similar type of burner is supposed to have been used in England by Michael Faraday (1791–1867).

Bunsen, Robert (1811–1899) Eminent German physicist, born in Göttingen. He received his doctorate of science from the University of Göttingen at the age of 20 years in 1831. While working with G.R. Kirchhoff (1764–1833) in 1829, he detected dark lines in the solar spectrum due to the absorption of certain wavelengths by the atmosphere. While working on spectroscopy, they discovered the elements cesium and rubidium. In 1841 Bunsen invented the carbon–zinc battery which became known as Bunsen battery. His most famous invention was the 'Bunsen burner' in 1854, which came to be used in most chemical laboratories. His other inventions include a grease-spot photometer, an ice calorimeter and an actinometer. *See Bunsen burner.*

Burdach, Charles Frederick (1776–1847) Professor of medicine at Dorpat who described the posterior column of the spinal cord (Burdach column) in 1819.

Burdwan Fever Similar to kala azar, first observed in lower Bengal in 1850.

Burials *See burying alive, coffin.*

Burinamide *See Black, Sir James.*

Burke and Hare Murders Two Irishmen, William Hare, a lodge keeper in Edinburgh and William Burke were partners in performing 16 murders in Edinburgh to supply bodies to Surgeon's Square for profit. In 1827 an old army pensioner in their lodge died without paying his rent of £4 and Burke and Hare supplied his body for dissection to Robert Knox's assistant in return for money. *See Burke, William, Knox, Robert.*

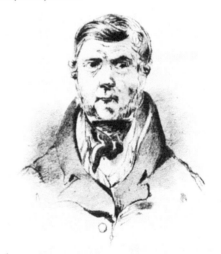

A sketch of William Burke taken in court. George MacGregor, *The History of Burke and Hare* (1884). Morison, London

Burke, William (1792–1829) Notorious murderer, born in Orrey, County Tyrone in Ireland. He deserted his wife and seven children and emigrated to Scotland in 1813. He met Helen McDougal and moved with her to Edinburgh around 1827. The couple moved into William Hare's lodgings where Burke and Hare teamed up to perform 16 murders to supply bodies to Surgeon's Square for profit. Hare turned Crown witness, and Burke was found guilty and hanged.

Burkitt Lymphoma Multiple tumors in African children were observed by Sir Albert Cook, a medical missionary, who described the tumor as a sarcoma in his report to the *Journal of Tropical Medicine* in 1902. African children with the tumor usually underwent mutilating surgery in an attempt to cure them. Denis Parsons Burkitt (1911–1993) established the place of chemotherapy in its treatment in 1960, and it was named Burkitt lymphoma.

Burkitt, Denis Parsons (1911–1993) Pioneer of chemotherapy for cancer. He was born in Enniskillen, Northern Ireland. He first studied engineering at Dublin University and later switched to medicine and qualified as a doctor in 1935. He became a member of the Royal College of Surgeons in 1938 and proceeded to work in Somalia, Kenya, Sri Lanka and Uganda. He first noticed multiple tumors of the jaw in African children while he was working at the Mulago Hospital in Kampala. He traveled extensively in Africa in order to study the incidence and geographical distribution of the tumor before describing it in detail. He found it to be different from a sarcoma. He used methotrexate and cyclophosphamide for treatment in 1960. It was later named Burkitt lymphoma. *See Burkitt lymphoma.*

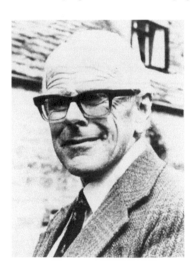

Denis Parsons Burkitt (1911–1993)

Burman, John (d 1779) Physician and pupil of Hermann Boerhaave (1668–1738) in Leiden. He was professor of botany at the Botanic Gardens, Amsterdam in 1738. He published several works on botany, the last of which was on American plants, illustrated with plates.

Burn Space *See Burns, Allan.*

Burnet, Sir Frank Macfarlane (1899–1985) Australian immunologist. He worked at the National Institute for Medical Research under Sir Henry Hallet Dale (1875–1968) for 3 years, starting in 1931, and perfected the technique of growing viruses in living chick embryos. He predicted the phenomenon of immunological tolerance and was awarded the Nobel Prize for his work on immunology which he shared with Peter Brian Medawar (1915–1987) in 1960.

Burnet, Thomas Scottish physician during the 17th century who wrote *Thesaurus Medicinae Practicae* (1673) which went to 12 editions and *Hippocrates Contractus* in 1685.

Burnett Syndrome Milk–alkali syndrome. Alkalosis and hypercalcemia as result of excessive intake of milk was described by American physician, Charles H. Burnett (1913–1967) of Colorado in 1949.

Burnett, William English physician who described a case of epilepsy associated with a remarkable slowness of pulse in 1820. This was one of the first descriptions of heart block.

Burning Glass A name given to lenses used for creating fire. Archimedes (287–212 BC) used a lens to focus light rays and burn an enemy fleet during the siege of Syracuse in 214 BC. The largest ever lens or burning mirror was made by Parker in 1800 in England and was exported to China.

Burning the Dead Practiced amongst ancient Greeks, Romans and Brahmins. Heraclitus (c 500 BC) of Greece thought that the soul was purified by burning, and the practice became common to most parts of ancient Greece. Sir Thomas Brown (1605–1682) in his *Hydriotaphia* mentioned the ancient custom of burning the dead. The practice of burning the dead and collecting the ashes is thought to have originated in Asia and been brought to the West during the Greek and Roman period. *See cremation.*

Burns Ancient physicians were familiar with the treatment of burns, and Paul of Aegina (625–690) recommended vinegar, pickled olives, raw egg and light earth as applications. He also advised the use of fig leaves for stimulating hair growth in the affected parts of the skin or scalp. Galen (129–200) and Avicenna (980–1037) recommended cimolian earth as an application. A modern monograph was published by Fabricus Hildanus (1560–1634) in 1607. Benjamin Bell (1749–1806) advocated emollients and astringents around 1790. London physician, George Cleghorn (1716–1789) applied vinegar, Sir James Earl used cold water and ice and Dominique Jean Larrey (1766–1842), the French army surgeon, applied linen bandages including alcohol and opium. Contractures following burns were first treated with skin grafts by George David Pollock in 1871. A modern classification of burns is included in the monograph by David Goldblatt in 1927.

Burns, Allan (1731–1813) Scottish surgeon and cardiologist who suggested that angina was due to coronary artery obstruction in *Observations of Some of the Most Important and Frequent Diseases of the Heart*, in 1809. Phrenic nerve palsy due to thoracic aneurysm is also described in his treatise. He correlated neurological symptoms with extreme bradycardia. He suggested ligation of the innominate artery and the fascial space above the suprasternal notch was described by him in *Observations on the Surgical Anatomy of the Head and Neck* published in 1812. This space was later named 'Burns space'.

Burns, John (1775–1850) The first professor of surgery at the Andersonian School of Medicine in Glasgow. He attained a worldwide reputation with his *The Principles of Midwifery* and *The Principles of Surgery*.

Burrowes, George London physician who did research on cerebral circulation, and published *On the Disorders of the Cerebral Circulation and the Connections between the Affections of the Brain and Diseases of the Heart* in 1846. He considered the flow of blood in the brain to be fixed but influenced by posture.

Burrows, Montrose Thomas (1884–1947) While working with Alexis Carrel (1873–1944) he demonstrated the method of growing tumor tissue *in vitro*. He also postulated the theory of origin of cancer in which he described a substance called 'archusia' which stimulated abnormal growth in cells when exposed to adverse conditions.

Burton Line Bluish discoloration of the gums seen in lead toxicity. Described by London physician, Henry Burton (1799–1849) of St Thomas' Hospital in 1840.

Burton, Henry (1799–1849) Physician at St Thomas' Hospital who described a line seen on the gums due to lead poisoning in 1840.

Burton, Robert (1576–1640) Born at Lindley in Leicestershire, he received his primary education at Sutton Coldfield. In 1599 he became a student at Christ Church Oxford and wrote one of the greatest books on psychiatry *The Anatomy of Melancholy*, which was published in 1621. He is said to have suffered from melancholic depression, which gave him insight into this problem and contributed to the success of his work.

Burton, William (1697–1759) A physician from Ripon in Yorkshire who was educated at Christ Church Oxford. He wrote a history of Yorkshire.

Burying Alive The first story of burying a live person was in 1225 BC, in Boetia, Greece, when Creon ordered Antignone, sister of Polynices to be buried alive. Roman vestals, virgins consecrated to the goddess Vesta, were buried on suspicion of immorality.

Buss, Carl Emil *See salicylic acid.*

Busulphan *See chronic myeloid leukemia.*

Butazolidine Phenylbutazone, introduced as treatment in rheumatoid arthritis by J. P. Currie, R. A. Brown and G. Will in 1953.

Butenandt, Adolf Friedrich Johann (b 1903) German biochemist and pioneer in the study of sex hormones. Born at Bremerhaven and educated at Marburg and Göttingen. He isolated the first steroid hormone, estrone, from urine obtained during pregnancy, in 1929. He obtained a crystalline form of a male hormone in 1931 and named it androsterone. He was awarded the Nobel Prize for Chemistry with Leopold Ruzicka (1887–1976) in 1939, but was forbidden to accept it by the Nazi regime.

Butlin, Sir Henry Trentham Bart (1845–1912) A surgeon at St Bartholomew's Hospital who obtained the Jacksonian Prize for his work on ununited fractures in 1873. He was a member of many medical societies and associations and was President of the British Medical Association in 1911 and 1912.

Butter Known to the ancient Romans as *butyrum*, and as medicine and not food. Aristotle called butter the fat of milk with the consistency of oil. Methods of preparing curd and butter were mentioned by Pliny in the 1st century. Mostly Christians of Egypt used butter instead of oil for their lamps in the 3rd century.

Butter, William (1726–1805) Physician from Derbyshire who graduated from Edinburgh and practiced in London. He wrote: *A Method of Cure for the Stone, An Account of Puerperal Fever as it Appeared in Derbyshire in 1782, An Improved Method of Opening the Temporal Artery, A Treatise on Angina Pectoris, A Treatise on the Worm Fever* and *A Treatise on the Venereal Rose*.

Buzzi, Francesco (1751–1805) An optic surgeon in Milan who identified the most important part of the retina, the 'yellow spot' or macula lutea and the central fovea in 1782.

Byrthe of Mankynde An English translation of a manual for midwives *Rosengarten*, published by a German physician, Eucharius Rosslin (d 1526) in 1513. The translation of the book was done by Thomas Raynalde of London in 1540, and it remained popular for over a century until its final edition in 1676. The first book contained a description of the genitourinary system of the female, and the second was concerned with obstetrics. The third book dealt with infant feeding and care, and the final book was on household remedies.

Byssinosis [Greek: *byssos*, fine flax] A condition affecting workers involved in the cotton, jute or hemp fiber industries, described by J. Leach in 1863. The symptoms presenting as 'Monday tightness' (after a weekend break), or 'return to work tightness' (after a holiday) were known amongst the cotton workers a century earlier. The condition was studied in more detail by J. T. Arlidge in 1892.

Byzantium Founded by Byzas in 667 BC, it was taken over by the Romans in AD 73. The first Christian Emperor, Constantine, moved his capital from Rome to Byzantium in AD 330, mostly because of recurrent epidemics of malaria and plague in Rome. It was later named Constantinople and is now known as Istanbul. A notable early Byzantine physician was Oribasius, who compiled Greek and Roman medical works around AD 360. The Byzantine period, since the formation of its empire, lasted for nearly 2000 years until about AD 1400.

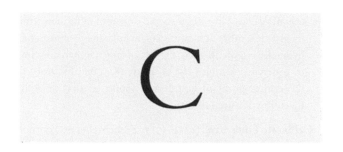

Cabanis, Peter John George (1756–1803) French physician from Cognac who was one of 500 members in the Council during the Revolution. His works include: *Observationes sur les Hospitaux, Melanges de Litterature Allemande, Journal de la Maladie et de la Mort de Mirabeau,* and *Rapports du Physique et du Moral de l'homme.*

CABG *See coronary artery bypass graft.*

Cabot Splint A posterior wire splint for immobilizing the lower limb. Designed by a Boston surgeon, Arthur Tracy Cabot (1852–1912).

Cabot, Hugh (1872–1945) American urologist from Rochester, Minnesota who specialized in the treatment of hypospadias. He devised an operation for undescended testis in 1936.

Cabot, Richard Clark (1868–1939) Born in Brooklin, Massachusetts, he graduated in 1892 from Harvard Medical School, where he spent the rest of his career. He was professor of medicine at Harvard in 1918 and became professor emeritus in 1933. In 1897 he described the cytoplasmic ring arrangement within red blood cells (Cabot rings) sometimes seen in megaloblastic anemia.

Cacatoria Febris Term used for intermittent fever by Sylvius de la Böe (1614–1672).

Cachexia [Greek: *kakos*, bad + *hexis*, habit] Described in the third group of diseases in William Cullen's (1710–1790) nosology (1769), which classified diseases into neurosis, fevers, local disorders and cachexias. Aretaeus (81–138) gave an accurate description of the features of cachexia and stated that it terminated in dropsy, phthisis or wasting. Aetius of Amida, a physician in the 6th century, identified scirrhus of the spleen and the liver as occasional causes. The word has been added to a variety of related conditions such as anemia of young women or chlorosis (cachexia virginium), myxedema following thyroidectomy (cachexia strumpriva) and Simmond disease (pituitary cachexia).

Cachexia Strumpriva Term used by Swiss surgeon, Emil Theodor Kocher (1841–1917) in 1883 to denote myxedema after total removal of the thyroid gland.

Cachexia Virginium *See cachexia.*

Cacophony [Greek: *kakos*, bad + *phone*, sound] A disorder of the voice leading to aphony or dysphony, described by Galen (129–200) and Theophrastus (BC 300).

Cadaveric Sex *See necrophilia.*

Cadaveric Transplant *See cadaver.*

Cadaver [Latin: *cadaver*, dead body] Herophilus and Erasistratus were the first to do dissections on human cadavers around 250 BC. Human dissections were banned in the Roman Empire, and from this period up to the time of Andreas Vesalius (1514–1564) knowledge of anatomy remained patchy and inaccurate. The official source of cadavers in England and other places for five centuries was official executions of criminals. The need for cadavers outstripped the supply, especially in the 18th and 19th centuries, and the resurrectionist movement appeared, supplying stolen bodies from graves in return for money. Some of the earliest experiments of human organ transplantation and other fields were carried out on cadavers. In 1888 John Cummings Munroe (1858–1910) used an infant cadaver to demonstrate that patent ductus arteriosus could be ligated. In 1887 A. Eugen Fick, a physician in Zurich and a pioneer of the contact lens, tried his device first on animals and then on cadavers. Corneas from cadavers were shown to be effective in corneal transplants by a Russian surgeon, Petrovich Filatov (1875–1956). Knee and other joint transplants from cadavers as treatment for advanced joint disease were used by German surgeon, Erich Lexer (1867–1937) at Freiburg in 1908. Sergei S. Yudin (b 1891) of the Moscow Skilifosovsky Institute was the first to use cadaver blood successfully, in 1930. Renal transplantation from cadavers was introduced in the early 1950s, and the first series of nine patients was reported by David Milford Hume (1917–1973), J.P. Merrill and G.W. Thorn in 1955. Following the establishment of transplantation medicine, the Human Tissue Act of England was passed in 1961 to regulate the procedure for obtaining tissues from cadavers for transplantation. The act specified that consent must be obtained from the next of kin, or from a coroner in other circumstances, before the tissue was removed. The Eurotransplant organization to tissue-type all potential donors and cadavers, in order to computer-match them to recipients was established in Stockholm in 1966.

Cadmium Element discovered by Friedrich Stromeyer (1776–1835) of Göttingen in 1817. Its most common compound, cadmium oxide, was described by Joseph Louis Gay-Lussac (1778–1850). Three cases of cadmium poisoning in the paint industry were described by Thomas Legge

(1863–1932) in 1924, and mass poisoning due to cadmium oxide fumes was reported by P. Ross in 1944. An account of an outbreak of chronic cadmium poisoning in workers in factories producing alkaline storage batteries was given by L. Frieberg from Sweden in 1945.

Cadogan, William (1711–1797) English pediatrician who wrote an early English treatise on the care and feeding of infants, published in 1748. He wrote a book on gout in 1771.

Caduceus The wand of Hermes or Mercury, used as a symbol of the medical profession and an emblem of the Medical Corps of the United States Army. The emblem carries two serpents under a pair of wings.

Caducus Morphus (Syn. falling sickness or epilepsy).

Cadwalader, Thomas (1708–1779) A physician from Philadelphia and a founder of the Pennsylvania Hospital and the Philadelphia Medical Society. He gave the first description of osteomalacia as *An Extraordinary Case in Physic* in 1744.

Caelius, Aurelianus A physician of African origin and pupil of the Roman physician, Soranus, around the 4th century. He wrote *On Acute Diseases and Chronic Diseases* and other works, which were printed in Amsterdam in 1722.

Caesalpinus, Andreas (1519–1603) A physician from Arezzo who wrote *Libri XVI de Plantis X* and other medical works. He had some insight and knowledge of the circulation of blood prior to William Harvey (1578–1657) that was reflected in his *Questiones Peripateicae* published in 1571.

Caffeine An alkaloid obtained from the seeds of *Coffea arabica* by a German chemist, Friedlieb Ferdinand Runge (1795–1867), in 1820. It was later obtained in a pure form in 1822 by Joseph Caventou (1795–1878), professor of pharmacy in Paris. Another chemically identical substance, theine, was discovered in the leaves of Chinese tea by C. Jobst in 1838. The action of caffeine on animals was studied by Carl Binz (1832–1912) in 1878 and, owing to its effect on the heart, it came to be used in place of digitalis for a brief period. The signs and symptoms after caffeine withdrawal, which include headache, were studied by C. Pfeiffer in 1943.

Caffey Disease Infantile cortical hyperostosis consisting of periodic painful swelling of the mandible during infancy. Described by American professor of pediatric radiology at the College of Physicians and Surgeons, Columbia University, New York, J. Caffey (b 1895), in 1945.

Cagniard de La Tour, Baron Charles (1777–1859) French physical chemist and engineer, born in Paris and educated at the École Polytechnique. He gave a demonstration of the

role of yeast as a live microscopic organism in fermentation in 1838. His other achievements include: the invention of a hydraulic engine in 1809; the use of an Archimedian screw to generate a strong blast of air in 1815; the discovery of the critical point of liquids and vapors in 1823; and the invention of a siren in 1819.

Cailletet, Louis Paul (1832–1913) French chemist, born at Chatillon-sur-Seine and educated at the École des Mines at Paris. He commenced his work on gases in 1870 and liquefied hydrogen, nitrogen and oxygen, through a process of compression, cooling and sudden expansion, in 1877. He studied the application of liquid hydrogen apparatus in high altitude ascents by installing a 300-meter manometer on the Eiffel Tower.

Cainotophobia [Greek: *kainos*, new + *phobos*, fear] Morbid aversion to anything novel.

Cairns, Hugh John Foster (b 1922) A molecular biologist and virologist who graduated from Oxford University and trained at the Radcliffe Infirmary. He was professor at several universities including the State University of New York at Stony Brook and the Harvard School of Public Health. He was a pioneer in the study of causes of cancer and demonstrated that it develops from a single cell by mutation of the DNA.

Cairns, Sir Hugh William Bell (1896–1952) An eminent Australian neurologist and surgeon who became the Nuffield professor of surgery at Oxford in 1937. He described hydrocephalus following obstruction of the flow of cerebrospinal fluid secondary to tuberculous meningitis in 1949. He specialized in neurosurgery with Harvey Williams Cushing (1869–1939) for a year and was an advisor for head injuries to the Ministry of Health in England during World War ll.

Cairo Built on the site of the ancient capital Fostath in AD 968 by Giavahar, the first Caliph of the Fatimites. Al-Mansur Hospital was one of the earliest hospitals, established in Cairo in 1276.

Caisson Disease Diver's disease, occurring in men who worked in caisson chambers used for laying foundations under water. Described by Benjamin Babington of England in 1863. The first caisson was used in England to build a bridge over the River Thames in 1738. The physiological explanation for caisson disease was given in 1878 by the French physician, Paul Bert (1833–1886), who did extensive research on respiratory physiology. His work was advanced by British respiratory physiologist, John Scott Haldane (1860–1936) in 1895. He devised a safe method for deep-sea divers to rise to the surface in 1907. Further work was done by English physician, Sir Erskin Leonard Hill (b 1866) in 1915.

Caius College *See Caius, John.*

Caius, John (1510–1573) Born in Norwich and educated at Gonville Hall, Cambridge. He studied under Andreas Vesalius (1514–1564) at Padua and obtained his MD in 1541. He returned to England to become the royal physician, and obtained royal authority to refound Gonville Hall. He used his own wealth to achieve this in 1557, and it was later named after him. He was elected President of the Royal College of Physicians nine times. *A Bok or Counseille Against Disease Commonly called Sweate or Sweatying Sicknesse* is considered to be a classic description of epidemic disease.

Cajal, Santiago Ramón y (1852–1934) Spanish professor of histology and morbid anatomy at Madrid (1892–1922) who graduated from Zaragoza University in 1873. He described the horizontally placed multipolar nerve cells of the cerebral cortex in 1899, and the structure of the synapse in detail in 1903. He shared the Nobel Prize for Physiology or Medicine with Camillo Golgi (1843–1926) in 1906.

Calabar Bean Faba Calabaria, the seed of *Physostigma venenosum*. The plant was first found to grow in the mouths of the Niger and Old Calabar rivers in the Gulf of Guinea in Africa. West African tribes used the seeds as an ordeal poison for trying those accused of witchcraft. English physician W.F. Daniell first made the plant known in England in 1840, and subsequently presented a paper to the Ethnological Society in 1846. W.C. Thompson, a missionary in West Africa, forwarded the plant to John Hutton Balfour (1808–1884) of Edinburgh in 1859 who described it as a new genus. The poisonous effects of the seed were studied by Sir Robert Christison (1797–1882) who self-experimented in 1876. He found the seed to be intensely poisonous and recommended it for official executions in Britain. Physostigmine, a poisonous alkaloid present in it, was identified and named by C. Jobst and Hesse in 1863. Another active substance was isolated by Vee and Levin in 1865 and named eserine. Another alkaloid, calabarine, was detected by Harnack and Witkowski in 1876.

Calamus The angle in the floor of the fourth ventricle between the inferior cerebella peduncles. Named by Herophilus in 320 BC.

Calcar A friend of Andreas Vesalius (1514–1564) who prepared the 300 illustrations for *De Humani Corporis Fabrica* in 1543.

Calciferol A more potent antirachitic substance than cod-liver oil, obtained through irradiating ergosterol by Robert Benedict Bourdillion (1889–1971) and co-workers in 1931.

Calcification [Latin: *calx*, lime + *facere*, to make] A description of calcified coronary arteries was given by Giovanni Battista Morgagni (1682–1771) in 1761. The ectopic calcifications in the tissues known as Rainey corpuscles were described by George Rainey (1801–1844), a demonstrator at St Thomas' Hospital. Mönckeberg arteriosclerosis caused by calcification of the medial layer of the arteries was described by a pathologist, Johann Georg Mönckeberg (1877–1925) of Bonn in 1903. Hypervitaminosis D associated with metastatic calcification and renal calculi following high intake of irradiated ergosterol in experimental animals was shown independently by Pfannensteil and Kreitmer in 1928. Further studies on metastatic calcification due to vitamin D excess were carried out by I.E. Steck in 1937.

Calcitonin The C cells, or parafollicular cells, in the thyroid gland noted in 1876, were shown to be of an endocrine nature by J.F. Nonidez, in 1932. A hormone from these cells was extracted by Douglas Harold Copp (b 1915) and E.C. Cameron in 1961 and named 'calcitonin'. Around 1961, P.F. Sanderson and F. Marshall, independently demonstrated the presence of calcitonin. It was introduced in treatment of Paget disease by O.L.M. Bijvoet and co-workers in 1967.

Calcium [Latin: *calx*, lime] Element discovered by Sir Humphry Davy (1778–1829) in 1808. Use of calcium in treatment of tetany following parathyroidectomy was shown by a Canadian-born pathologist, William George MacCallum (1874–1944) of Johns Hopkins University. Elevation of serum calcium in sarcoidosis was observed by G.T. Harrell and S. Fisher in 1939. A demonstration of its role in blood coagulation was given by Maurice Nicholas Arthus (1862–1945) and Calixte Pages in 1890. The need for calcium and its daily requirement in humans was established by American biochemist, Henry Clapp Sherman (1875–1955) of Columbia University in 1931.

Calcium Antagonists A family of vasodilators which mimic the cardiac effects of calcium withdrawal was named by A. Fleckenstein in 1963. He observed this property in verapamil or isoptin. The antiarrhythmic effects of verapamil were demonstrated by F. Bender and co-workers in 1966.

Calcium Channel The influence of calcium on excitability and contraction of heart muscle was described by the English physiologist, Sydney Ringer (1834–1910) in 1883. Calcium as a link between excitation and contraction was shown by L.V. Heilbrunn and F.J. Wiercinski in 1947. The existence of calcium channels in cells was suggested by Robert Michael in 1975. Verapamil was the first calcium channel blocker and its antiarrhythmic effects were studied by L. Schamroth and co-workers in 1972. A protein that regulated the passage of calcium ions in and out of muscle cells during contraction and relaxation was identified by Kevin P. Campbell and Roberto Coronado in 1987.

Caldani, Leopold Marco Antonio (1725–1813) Professor of anatomy at Padua who succeeded Giovanni Battista Morgagni (1682–1771) to the chair in 1771. He described the coracoclavicular ligament in 1721 which bears his name.

Caldwell–Luc Operation A radical antrostomy described by American otorhinologist, George Walter Caldwell (1834–1918) of New York in 1893. Henry Luc (1855–1925) of Paris described the procedure in 1889.

Caledonian Asylum An asylum for the indigent children of Scottish parents, founded in 1813 at Islington, London.

Caliphates The Eastern caliphate was controlled by Baghdad, where eminent Islamic physicians such as Mesu Senior (777–857), Johannitus Onan (809–873), Rhazes (850–932) and Haly Abbas (930–994) practiced. Ruled by the dynasty of Abbasides, it was an important center for translating Greek manuscripts into Arabic. Other important towns of the Eastern caliphate included Alexandria, Damascus and Basra. The Western caliphate, situated in Spain, had Toledo and Cordova as its educational centers. Some eminent physicians of the western caliphate include Avenzoar (1113–1162), Albucasis (936–1013), Avicenna (978–1036) and Maimonides (1135–1208).

Callaway, Thomas (1791–1848) London orthopedic surgeon. He devised a test (Callaway test) for dislocation of the shoulder in which the vertical measurement round the axilla and the outer part of the clavicle is greater on the dislocated side.

Calleja, Sanchez Camillo (d 1913) Professor of anatomy at Madrid who described the islets of the olfactory cells in the hippocampal cortex in 1893. These now bear his name.

Callandar, C. Latimer (1892–1947) American surgeon from San Francisco who designed an operation for amputation at the lower third of the thigh, in 1935.

Callendar, Hugh Longbourne (1863–1930) English physicist from Gloucestershire who became a professor at McGill University in Montreal in 1893. He was appointed to the chair of physics at University College London in 1898. His contributions include: invention of a constant pressure air thermometer capable of measuring up to 450°C in 1891; construction of a platinum resistance thermometer in 1886; and invention of a continuous flow calorimeter to measure the specific heat of liquids.

Callender, George William (1830–1875) London surgeon who devised maxillary clips (Callender maxillary clips) for treating overgrowth of the incisor process of the maxilla.

Calisthenics [Greek: *kayos*, beautiful + *thenos*, strength] A system of light gymnastics to promote strength and grace of carriage. Practiced by the ancient Greeks, who also established gymnasiums for this purpose. The revival of gymnastics in the 19th century was brought about by a Swede, Per Henrick Ling (1776–1839), who established an institute for training teachers of gymnastics in Stockholm in 1813. An early 20th century book on calisthenics, *Eurhythm, Thought and Action,* was written by H.H. Hubert of St Thomas' Hospital, London in 1921.

Callus [Greek: *calco*, to tread] In the 16th century, the French physician Ambroise Paré (1510–1590) compared the process of callus formation in a fracture to the gluing of two pieces of wood. Other surgeons around this time described it as an exudation of the bony juice.

Call–Exner Bodies Minute degenerative cysts in ovarian granulosa cells. Described by Emma Call and Siegmund Exner (1846–1926) of Vienna in 1875. Some historians have mistakenly credited Friedrich von Call (1844–1917), a physician in Vienna, with this discovery.

Calmette, Leon Charles Albert (1863–1931) French bacteriologist, born in Nice. He founded the Pasteur Institute at Lille in 1895 and was its director from 1895 to 1919. He developed the bacille Calmette–Guerin vaccine (BCG vaccine) for tuberculosis with Alphonse Guérin (1872–1961) in 1908. Calmette also developed antiserum for *Amanita phylloides* poisoning in 1897 and discovered an antiserum for snakebite while he was stationed in Saigon.

Calmiel, Louis Florentine (1798–1895) French physician in Paris who showed pathological lesions in the brain of patients with general paresis at a time when the cause of syphilis was not known.

Calomel [Greek: *kalos*, beautiful + *melas*, black] Hydrogyrum chloratum, a compound of mercury prepared by French chemist, Jean Beguin (1550–1620) from Lorraine in 1608. It became a general remedy in Europe in the 16th century, and Crollius or Osualdus in the 17th century used it as treatment for many ailments, including dropsy. J. Casper in his treatise published in Tübingen in 1760, mentioned it as a panacea. By end of the 18th century it was used internally and topically by almost every physician. The main constituents were organic mercurial compounds and mercurous chloride, responsible for its diuretic effect. It continued to be used as a diuretic until the 1950s.

Calorescence John Tyndall (1820–1893), an Irish physicist and professor at the Royal Institution in England, heated metals to incandescence or until they emitted visible light. He named this process 'calorescence'.

Calorie, Luigi (1807–1896) Professor of descriptive anatomy at the University of Bologna. He described the serous space (Calorie bursa), which is inconsistently found between the trachea and the arch of the aorta, in 1874.

Calorimeter [Latin: *calor*, heat; Greek: *metreon*, measure] The heat changes in the body were studied in 1780 by Antoine Laurent Lavoisier (1743–1794) and Pierre Simon de Laplace (1749–1827) using ice and water. Scharling in 1849 used an air calorimeter to study energy changes in the body. In 1870, Robert Bunsen (1811–1899) devised an ingenious calorimeter in which the quantity of ice melted and its contraction in volume were used as a measure of heat. Carl von Voit (1831–1908) of Munich and German chemist, Max von Pettenkofer (1818–1901) developed the differential calorimeter in 1886. Metabolic changes in the body were measured with the use of an animal's body as a calorimeter by Max Rubner (1854–1932), a physiologist in Munich in 1891. A modern calorimeter capable of measuring heat production, oxygen consumption and carbon dioxide elimination was devised by an American, Wilber Olin Atwater (1844–1907) in 1892. A continuous flow type was introduced by H. Callendar in 1902 and a special form for measuring specific heat at low temperatures was designed by German physicist, Hermann Walther Nernst (1864–1941) and English physicist, Frederick Alexander Lindemann Cherwell (1886–1957) in 1911.

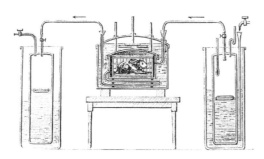

A modified calorimeter by P.L. Dulong (1785–1838). J G M'Kendrick, *A Textook of Physiology* (1889). James Maclehose & Sons, Glasgow

Calorimetry [Latin: *calor*, heat; Greek: *metron*, measure] *See calorimeter.*

Calvé Disease Osteochondrosis of the vertebra. Described by French orthopedic surgeon, J. Calvé (1875–1954). An orthopedic surgeon at Harvard Medical School, Arthur Thornton Legg (1874-1939) and Geog Clemens Perthes (1869-1927) of Tübingen described it independently in 1910.

Calvé –Legg–Perthes Disease *See Calvé disease.*

Calvities [Greek: *calvus*, baldness] (Syn. baldness)

Cambrian Period [Latin: *Cambria*, Wales] The rocks found below those of the Silurian period in the Lake District were studied by Adam Sedgewick (1785–1873), a geologist from Yorkshire, who named it in 1834. *See Azoic period.*

Cambridge Philosophical Society Formed in 1819. It received the Royal Charter in 1832.

Cambridge University [Latin: *Cantabrigia*] Said to have been founded by King Sigebert of East Anglia in AD 630. It was neglected during the Danish invasion and was restored by Edward the Elder in 915. The Royal Charter was granted by Henry III in 1231. Most of the records of the University were burnt in 1381 during Wat Tyler's rebellion. Queen Victoria conferred a new charter on the university in 1857.

Camerarius, Joachium or Camerer (1534–1598) German botanist and physician, who wrote *Hortus Medicus et Philosophicus* (1588) and other works. He provided proof for sexuality in plants in *De Sexu Plantarum Epistola,* published in 1694.

Camerarius, Rudolph Jacob (1665–1721) German physician and botanist who studied sexuality in plants.

Camerer Law Children of the same weight had the same food requirements, regardless of age. Proposed by German pediatrician, Wilhelm Camerer (1842–1910).

Cameron, Archibald (1707–1753) A medical practitioner from Lochaber, Scotland. He became a medical officer in the army raised by his brother, head of the Cameron Clan, in support of the Young Pretender's rebellion of 1745. Cameron was captured in Scotland and executed at Tyburn.

Cammann Stethoscope One of the first binaural models, devised by New York physician, George Philip Cammann (1804–1863).

Camp Fever (Syn. typhus fever) *See typhus fever.*

Campbell Area *See Campbell, Alfred.*

Campbell De Morgan Spots Small benign telangiectatic spots appearing increasingly with age. Described in 1872 by English surgeon, Campbell de Morgan (1811–1876) at the Middlesex Hospital, London.

Campbell, Alfred Walter (1868–1938) Australian pathologist, who graduated in medicine from Edinburgh in 1892 with a gold medal for his thesis, *Pathology of Alcoholic Insanity*. He did histological studies related to localization of function in the cerebral cortex in 1905 and defined the precentral area of the cerebral cortex (Campbell area).

Campbell, William Francis (1867–1926) Brooklyn professor of surgery at Long Island College Hospital. He described the suspensory ligament of the axilla (Campbell ligament) in 1908 in his textbook on surgery.

Campbell, Willis Cohoon (1880–1941) Orthopedic surgeon from Memphis, Tennessee. He devised the Campbell bone-block operation for paralytic pes calcaneocavus, in which a block of bone is used to maintain the normal position of the foot. He published one of the most important textbooks on orthopedics, *Operative Orthopedics*, in 1939.

Camper, Peter (1722–1789) Dutch surgeon at Leiden who wrote *Demonstrationum Anatomico-Pathologicarum Liber Primus* in 1760. Another of his books was translated into English as *The Works of the late Professor Camper on the connections between Science and Anatomy* by Thomas Cogan in 1794. Camper described the superficial layer in the fascia of the abdomen (Camper fascia). He attempted to measure the skull from an anthropological point of view. He was a talented artist who provided the illustrations for William Smellie's famous textbook on midwifery.

Camphor Introduced to the west by Arabs and Avicenna (978–1036) popularized it. Hermann Boerhaave (1668–1738) considered it to be a volatile resin. A report in England on its efficacy was published by a physician, David Bayne Kinnier of Edinburgh in 1727. The regular use of it in medicine was established by Leopold von Auenbrugger (1722–1809) in 1761. As it has a distinct aroma it was used as an ingredient in various medicinal preparations. A synthetic camphor preparation, Cardiazol or Metrazol, was used in injections to control epileptic fits in the early 1930s.

Campion, Thomas (1567–1620) Born in Witham in Essex, he first practiced as a lawyer and later qualified in medicine in 1602. He wrote poems in English and Latin.

Campylobacter jejuni [Greek: *campylos*, curved or bent; Latin: *jejunos*, empty] Identified as a cause of intestinal illness by David A. Robinson of the Public Health Laboratory at Withington Hospital, Manchester in 1980.

Campylobacter pylori [Greek: *campylos*, curved or bent + *pylorus*, gatekeeper] Identified as the cause of gastritis and probably duodenal ulcers by an Australian, Barry J. Marshall, in 1984. It was later renamed *Helicobacter pylori*.

Camus, Anthony (1722–1782) French physician in Paris who published several medical works including *Physic for the Mind* and *Abdeker or Art of Preserving Beauty*.

Canadian Medical Association Formed in 1867 at a meeting at Laval University presided over by James A. Sewell from Edinburgh. Its first president, Charles Tupper (1821–1915), a physician, and two of its first vice-presidents Hector Peltier and R.S. Black, were also graduates of Edinburgh.

Canal of Schlemm Canal at the junction of the cornea and sclera. Described by a professor of anatomy, Friedrich Schlemm (1795–1858) of Berlin, in 1830.

Canal Rays Positively charged particles of atomic mass, described by a German physicist, Eugen Goldstein (1850–1930) from Silesia, in 1886.

Canavan Disease (Syn. spongy degeneration of infancy) A form of familial degenerative disease of the white matter of the central nervous system, seen in certain Jewish families. Observed by American pathologist, M.M. Canavan (1879–1953) in 1931.

Cancer [Latin: *cancer*, crab] Mentioned in the Ebers papyrus, written around 1500 BC. Greeks used the term 'gangrene' and Romans called it 'lupus' because it consumed like a wolf. Galen (129–200) thought that the puffed-up veins looked like a crab. Ancient Egyptians treated cancer with excision, cautery and astringents. According to Paul of Aegina (625–690), it is produced by thick overheated bile. He stated that 'it can occur in any part of the body, but the breasts of women were commonly affected, due to its laxity which admitted humors, that caused it'. Hippocrates (460–377 BC) also described a fatal case of cancer of breast. Aulus Cornelius Celsus (25 BC–AD 50) observed that they became unequal and immovable, which is equivalent to the presently established signs of irregularity and fixation of malignant cancers. Rhazes (850–932) was wary of removing cancers of the breast and described a case which occurred on the other side after the removal of one breast. Antyllus, in AD 300 recommended that advanced cancers should be left as they were inoperable. Alexander Monroe (1697–1767) of Edinburgh discouraged surgery for all forms of cancer. The first American book on tumors was published by an American surgeon, John Collins Warren (1778–1856) in 1837. Edwin Klebs (1834–1913), an American scientist born in Vienna, noted an abnormality of chromosomes in cancer cells in 1889. One of the earliest workers on cancer statistics was an American, Frederick Ludwig Hoffman (b 1865), who wrote *The Mortality from Cancer Throughout the World* in 1915. He also pointed out the possible harm from asbestos dust. An English pioneer was Sir John Bland-Sutton (1855–1936), who wrote *Cancer Clinically Considered* (1909) and *Tumors, Innocent and Malignant* in 1922. The etiology remained unclear until the 1940s, and several agents were tried for the treatment on an empirical basis. *See cancer therapy, carcinoma, carcinogenesis, P53 gene.*

Cancer Act Introduced in England in 1939 to facilitate early diagnosis and prompt treatment of cancer.

Cancer Surgery *See cancer, mastectomy, hysterectomy, esophageal carcinoma, carcinoma of cervix.*

Cancer Therapy Several agents were tried as treatment on an empirical basis until the 1940s. Lead was used as a local applicant to tumors by French surgeon, Thomas Goulard (d 1784) in 1760. Selenium was tried by M. Wasserman and later by F. Keysser of Germany in 1911. Blair Bell (1871–1936) used injections of colloidal lead in 1922 and A. T. Todd used selenium colloids in 1928. Castration as treatment of advanced breast cancer in women was performed by a Scottish surgeon, Sir Thomas George Beatson (1848–1933) in 1896. Similar treatment was suggested independently by German surgeon, A. Schinzinger in 1889. The beneficial effects of it and estrogens in the treatment of prostatic carcinoma were demonstrated by Charles Brenton Huggins (b 1901) in 1941. A landmark in the development of therapy was the discovery by Alfred Gilman (b 1908) and Frederick Stanley Phillips (b 1916) in 1946 that nitrogen mustards could bring about regression of certain lymphomas and leukemias. Methotrexate was introduced by Sidney Farber (1903–1973) in 1949, who also introduced actinomycin D in 1956. Denis Parsons Burkitt (1911–1993) was a pioneer of modern chemotherapy. He first used methotrexate and cyclophosphamide for Burkitt lymphoma in 1960. The cytotoxicity of *cis*-platinum was serendipitously discovered in 1965, when an electric current was passed between platinum electrodes through a nutrient medium in which bacteria were growing. B. Rosenberg and colleagues further investigated the matter and noted that bacterial growth was inhibited by chlorides of *cis*-platinum formed during electrolysis, and their work led to the introduction of *cis*-platinum for cancer therapy. Fungi are also an important source for several anti-cancer agents such as mitomycin (introduced by J. Colsky in 1960), adriamycin and daunomycin.

Candida albicans Name given to the fungus causing thrush by Christine Berkhout from Delft at the University of Utrecht in 1923. *See candidosis.*

Candidosis Described (with illustrations) by Bernard Rudolph Conrad von Langenbeck (1810–1887) in 1839.

Frederick Theodor Berg (1806–1887) discovered the fungus in lesions seen in thrush in 1841, and around the same time David Gruby (1810–1898) independently identified the same organism as a cause of thrush. The fungus was first named *Oidium albicans* by Charles P. Robin (1821–1885) in 1853 and was initially classified under a new genus, *Syringospora* by M. Quinquad in 1868. W. Zopf of Breslau later included it in the *Monilia* genus in 1890. It was named *Candida albicans* by Christine Berkhout from Delft in 1923. *See thrush.*

Candolle, Augustine Pyrame de (1778–1841) Swiss botanist from Geneva and professor of botany at Montpellier, who introduced the term 'taxonomy' to botany in his *Theorie Elementaire de la Botanique* published in 1813. His son Alphonse Louis Pierre Pyrame de Candolle (1806–1893) was also an eminent botanist who published several important books.

Cannabis indica (Syn. Ganja, herba cannabis, hashish, Indian hemp) Referred to as *Rh-ya*, in the Chinese herbals of the 5th century. The Hindu medical works of Susruta and Charaka mention it as a remedy. It was brought to Europe sporadically from the East around 1563, and the bulk of it was brought by Napoleon's returning army in the 19th century. It later became a fashionable drug amongst the elite, and in Paris intellectuals and poets such as Theophile Gautier (1811–1872) and Charles Pierre Baudelaire (1821–1867) used (or abused) it. An important treatises on cannabis intoxication was published by Jacques Joseph Moreau (1804–1884) of Paris in 1845. *See hashish.*

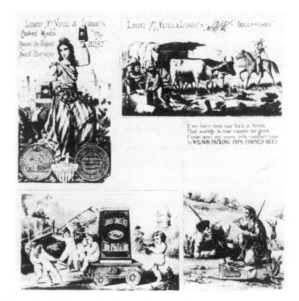

Canned Food. Picture taken from card given with canned corned beef in the USA early this century

Canned Food Italian biologist, Lazzaro Spallanzani (1729–1799), suggested in 1765 that food could be preserved by being sealed in containers which did not allow air to penetrate. French confectioner, Nicolas François Appert (1749–1841), used the autoclave for sterilization of food in 1810 and opened the first canning factory in the world in 1812. *See food industry.*

Cannibalism An account amongst Paedian Indians was given by the Greek historian Herodotus around 400 BC. The people of Papua New Guinea practiced it for centuries and were prone to a viral disease called kuru. The origin and method of transmission of this disease were first studied by American virologist, Daniel Carleton Gajdusek (b 1923) in 1957. He demonstrated the transmission via the central nervous system of humans to another species.

Cannizaro Reaction The formation of benzoic acid and benzyl alcohol by treating benzaldehyde with potassium hydroxide. Discovered by Italian chemist, Stanislao Cannizaro (1826–1910) of Rome.

Cannizaro, Stanislao (1826–1910) Italian organic chemist and statesman born in Palmero. He was professor of chemistry at Genoa, Palmero and Rome. He distinguished between atomic weight and molecular weight and introduced the term 'hydroxyl' for the OH radical. He was made a Senator in 1871 and died in Rome.

Cannon Syndrome An increase in adrenal output due to emotional stress which prepared the animal for 'fight or flight'. Described by American physiologist, Walter Bradford Cannon (1871–1945) in 1911.

Cannon, Walter Bradford (1871–1945) An eminent American physiologist, born at Praire du Chien in Wisconsin, and educated at Harvard, where he was head of the Physiology Department from 1906 to 1942. He introduced the concept of the influence of the emotions on involuntary reactions of the body in situations such as rage and fear. He also coined the word 'homeostasis' to denote the internal physiological balance of the body and published *Wisdom of the Body* in 1932. He died of cancer due to exposure to X-rays during his research on intestinal motility. *See Barium swallow and meal test, Cannon syndrome.*

Cannstadt Skull One of the earliest discoveries of a skull of primitive man, in 1700.

Cannula [Latin: *canna*, reed] A modern cannula for draining a liver abscess was devised by an English surgeon, Joseph Fayrer (1824–1907). This was adapted to drain a lung abscess by John Rickman Godlee (1849–1925) in 1884.

Canon of Avicenna *See Avicenna.*

Canstatt, Carl Friedrich (1807–1850) German physician who wrote a book on geriatrics in 1839.

Cantlie, Sir James (1851–1926) London surgeon who designed a cannula (Cantlie cannula) for draining amebic abscesses of the liver.

Cantwell, Andrew Irish physician in the 18th century who wrote *History of a Remedy for Weakness of the Eyes, Account of Small Pox* and other treatises.

Capelluti, Rolando Italian surgeon from Palma in the 13th century. He was a pupil of Roger Frugard (b 1170) and re-edited *Practica Chirurgiae.*

Capgras Syndrome A rare psychological disorder in which the patient believes that familiar persons have been replaced by impostors. Described by J.M.J. Capgras (1873–1950) in 1923. He named it 'L'illusion des Sosies' after Socias, a servant of Amphitryon in the play on Greek mythology written by Moliere. Zeus seduced Amphitryon's wife by impersonating him, and arranged for Mercury to take the form of Socias to complete his deception. The syndrome was named after Capgras by a French neurologist, J. Levy-Valensi in 1929.

Capillarity The ascent of liquid in small tubes was noted by Leonardo Da Vinci (1452–1519) in 1490. The capillary ascent of sap in plants was observed by Niccolo Agiunti of Pisa in 1630. The theory behind it was studied by Isaac Newton (1642–1727), Pierre-Simon Laplace (1749–1827) and others in the 17th century. The modern capillary theory was proposed by English physician, Thomas Young (1773–1829) in 1803.

Capillary Basement Membrane Demonstrated in the glomerulus by D. Ohmori of Germany in 1921. It was described in detail by Canadian physician, Leone McGregor (b 1900) in 1929.

Capillary Circulation [Latin: *capillus*, hair] William Harvey (1578–1657) in his work on the circulation of the blood *Exercitatio Anatomica de Motu Cordis, et Sanguinis in Animalibus* in 1628 failed to establish the connection between arteries and veins. This gap was remedied by Marcello Malpighi (1628–1694) with his description in *De Pulmonibus* published in 1661. Dutch microscopist, Antoni van Leeuwenhoek (1632–1723), also wrote a letter on it to the Royal Society but it was not published. Regulation of the mechanism of the capillaries was discovered by a Danish physiologist, Schack August Steenberg Krogh (1874–1946) of Copenhagen, around 1915. He won the Nobel Prize in 1920. *See blood circulation.*

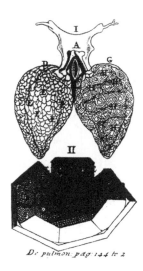

Sketch by Malpighi of the lungs and capillary circulation of a frog. Courtesy of the National Library of Medicine

Capillary Electrometer An instrument that magnifies minute fluctuations of electrical potential. Invented by French physicist, Gabriel Jonas Lippmann (1845–1921) in 1875. It was adopted by Augustus Waller (1856–1922) of St Mary's Hospital to record electrical potential in the human heart in 1887. *See electrocardiograph.*

Capital Punishment [Latin: *caput*, head] The Amherst papyri give an account of Egyptian state trials around 1500 BC where condemned persons were asked to choose their mode of death. Impalement was a method of execution of criminals in ancient Rome during the time of Nero. The first execution by hanging in England was carried out for piracy in 1241. During the reign of King Henry VIII, over 72,000 alleged criminals were executed over a period of 38 years. Sir Samuel Romilly (1757–1818) of Soho advocated the abolition of capital punishment for stealing, and through his efforts managed to have an Elizabethan statute repealed. Punishment by death was abolished for most crimes by Sir Robert Peel's (1788–1850) Acts. The electric chair for official executions was invented by two Americans, Harold P. Brown and E.A. Kennealley, in 1888.

Caplan Syndrome A combination of pneumoconiosis and rheumatoid arthritis which caused well defined X-ray opacities in the lungs of miners. Described by Anthony Caplan a member of the Pneumoconiosis Panel in Cardiff in 1953. He graduated from the University of London in 1931 and studied medicine at St Bartholomew's Hospital, before becoming a member of the Royal College of Physicians in 1935.

Capon-Comb Test *See androgen.*

Cappadocia In Asia Minor, the birth place of the great physician Aretaeus (81–138). Founded by Pharnaces in 744 BC. It became a Roman province in AD 15. It was captured by the Saracens in 717 and annexed to the Turkish empire in 1360.

Captopril (ACE Inhibitor) *See angiotensin converting enzyme inhibitors.*

Caput Medusae Where subcutaneous distension of veins over the abdomen becomes visible owing to cirrhosis. Named by a Roman state physician, Marcus Aurelius, in AD 160 It takes its origin from Medusa, the Greek mythical queen of the Gorgons whose head was covered with snakes. George Budd (1808–1882) of King's College, London stated that 'these veins answer a good purpose' in 1845, implying that they served as collaterals. Marie Philibert Constant Sappey (1810–1896) of Paris demonstrated the collateral flow with illustrations in 1883.

Carabelli Tubercle A small tubercle occasionally seen on the lingular surface of the molar tooth. Described by a Viennese dental surgeon, Georg Carabelli (1787–1842).

Carat [Greek: *keration*, horn-like pods] Unit of weight for measurement gold, originally related to the average weight of the seeds of the carob, a native tree of Africa. When diamonds were discovered in India, the seeds were transported there to be used as weights. The English carat was fixed at 3.1683 grains by the Board of Trade in 1888 and this was replaced by the metric carat in 1914.

Carbimazole A currently used antithyroid drug, synthesized by Alexander Lawson, C. Rimington and C.E. Searle in 1951.

Carbinoxolone Introduced as a treatment of gastric ulcer by F. Avery Jones in 1965.

Carbohydrates [Latin: *carbo*, coal; Greek: *hydor*, water] Glycogen and its metabolism were discovered and explained by Claude Bernard (1813–1878) in 1853, and an early treatise on carbohydrate metabolism was written by Frederick William Pavy (1829–1911) of England in 1862. The role of the citric acid cycle in the aerobic metabolism of carbohydrates was described by Sir Hans Adolf Krebs (1900–1982) in 1937, who shared the Nobel Prize for his work with Fritz Lipmann (1899–1986) in 1953. *See glucose.*

Carbolic Acid Phenol, a product of distillation of coal tar discovered by a chemist, Friedlieb Runge (1795–1867) at Hamburg in 1834. It was studied by Augustin Laurent

(1808–1853) and Charles Frederic Gerhardt (1816–1856) who named it phenol. It was used for the deodorization of sewage and employed as a disinfectant during the cholera epidemic in London in 1866. It was first used as an antiseptic spray by Paris chemist, François Jules Lemaire (1814–1886), who wrote an exhaustive treatise on it in 1864. Joseph Lister (1827–1912) experimented on the antiseptic properties in 1866 and devised a hand-driven spray for its use during surgery. The spray was later made steam driven and remained in use for the next two decades.

Carbon Identified as a distinct element by Antoine Lavoisier (1743–1794) in 1788. He demonstrated that it existed as a pure form in diamond by burning diamond to yield carbon dioxide.

Carbon Dating Use of radioactive carbon-14 in dating ancient objects was introduced by Williard Frank Libby (b 1908) of Connecticut in 1946.

Carbon Dioxide [Latin: *carbo*, coal + *di*, two; Greek: *oxys*, sharp] First obtained in the 16th century through burning charcoal by Jean Baptiste van Helmont (1580–1644), who named it 'gas'. Joseph Black (1728–1799), professor of chemistry at Glasgow University, rediscovered it 100 years later and named it 'fixed air'. William Bache published *On the Morbid Effect of Carbonic Acid Gas on Healthy Animals* in 1794. Michael Faraday (1791–1867) liquefied it by using atmospheric pressure in 1823. Henry Hill Hickman (1800–1830) studied its inhalational effects for inducing anesthesia, in 1824. The anesthetic effects of excess inhalation of carbon dioxide were shown by Alberico Benedecenti in 1896. Evidence that it produced vasodilatation was presented by L. Severini in 1888. Ludwig Traube (1818–1876) noted a rise in blood pressure due to carbon dioxide in asphyxia in 1863, and Belgian physician, Jean Hubert Thiry (1817–1897) proposed the theory that it acted via the medullary center in controlling respiration in 1864.

Carbon Disulfide Discovered by W.A. Lampadius of Freiburg in 1796. It was used as treatment for a variety of diseases and was tried as an anesthetic agent before the use of chloroform. Symptoms and signs of carbon disulfide poisoning were described by A. Payen (1851), A. Delpech (1856) and H.C. Charcot in 1889.

Carbon Monoxide In 1896 several deaths in a colliery explosion in south Wales attracted the attention of the British physiologist John Scott Haldane (1860–1936), who conducted investigations and found that the men had succumbed to carbon monoxide poisoning. Subsequently,

he did extensive research using animals and sometimes trying out the effect of the gas on himself. It was mainly though his work that the physiological mechanism and toxic effects were made known.

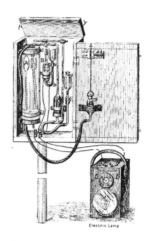

Portable apparatus for underground air analysis. Sir Clement le Neve Forster and John Scott Haldane (1860–1936), *The Investigation of Mine Air* (1905). Charles Griffin, London

Carbon Tetrachloride Introduced as a treatment for hookworm by H.C. Hall of the United States Bureau of Animal Industry in 1921. Its toxicity was shown by J.F. Docherty and E. Burgess. Three prisoners were cured of ascaris and ankylostoma but developed fatty changes and necrosis of the liver. A report was published in the *British Medical Journal* of 1922. *See antihelminthics.*

Carbonate of Soda Known as *neter* to the Hebrews, and the ancient Hindus called it *sajji noon*. It was obtained by burning algae and seaweed and used mainly as medicine.

Carbonic Anhydrase Isolated from tissues by Francis John Worsley Roughton (1899–1972) and Norman Urquhart Meldrum (1907–1933) in 1933. A crystalline form of the enzyme was obtained from beef erythrocytes by D.A. Scott of Toronto and A.M. Fisher in 1942.

Carboniferous Period [Latin: *carbo*, coal + *ferre*, to carry] Geological era identified by William Daniel Conybeare and William Phillips in 1822.

Carbuncle [Latin: *carbunculus*, little coal] Described as 'anthrax' by Paul of Aegina (AD 625–690) and other ancient authors. Aulus Cornelius Celsus (25 BC–AD 50) gave an accurate description and recommended burning the part affected, in the belief that it made the part insensible to heat and pain. *See anthrax.*

Carcassone, Maurice Professor of anatomy at Montpellier who described the 'triangular ligament' or the fascia of origin of the penile musculature in 1821. The ligament now bears his name.

Carcinoembryonic Antigen The presence of tumor-specific antigens in human colonic cancer was demonstrated through immunological and absorption techniques by P. Gold and S.O. Freedman in 1965. A laboratory method of assaying it in the management of cancer was described by H.J. Hansen and co-workers in 1974.

Carcinogenesis [Greek: *karkinos*, crab + *genesis*, descent] One of the first suggestions associating tobacco with cancer was made by a London apothecary, John Hill (1716–1775) in 1761. He cautioned against its use because of the formation of nasal polyps. Scrotal cancer in chimney sweeps due to chronic exposure to soot was described by Percivall Pott (1714–1788) in 1770. The association between pipe smoking and cancer of the lip was observed by Samuel Thomas Sommering (1755–1830) in 1795. A description of cancer caused by industrial tar and paraffin was given by Richard von Volkmann (1830–1889) in 1875. The carcinogenic effects of X-rays in humans was reported by a German physician, Ernst August Franz Albert Frieben (b 1875) in 1902. Carcinoma was experimentally transmitted through several generations in animals by Marau in 1894 and Leo Loeb (1869–1959) in 1900. Loeb managed to transmit cystic sarcoma of white mice though 40 generations, and Carl Oluf Jensen (1864–1934) in 1902 inoculated rats with tumor tissue and transmitted the tumor through 40 generations. Experimental production of malignant tumors using X-rays was demonstrated by Jean Clunet (1878–1917) of France in 1911 and the experimental production of cancer by injection of tar was demonstrated by Henry Peter George Bayon (1876–1952) in 1912. Johanes Andreas Fibiger (b 1867) identified nematodes as carcinogenic agents in rats in 1913, a finding which was later disproved. The carcinogenic property of tar was also demonstrated by Katsulsaburo Yamagiva (1863–1930) and Koichi Itchkawa (1888–1948) in 1915. Leukemia due to radium exposure was observed by Prosper Emile Weil (b 1873) and Antoine Marcellin Lacasagne (b 1884), in 1925. In 1927, 20 deaths occurred in painters of luminous dials in a company based at New Jersey owing to blood dyscrasia caused by radium. Several other irritants or agents were proved to be carcinogenic in the early 20th century. Cancer of the bladder due to aniline in the dye industry was demonstrated by several workers including Ludwig Rehn of Germany (1895), S.G. Lueunberger of Basel (1912), F. Curshmann of Germany (1920) and R. Oppenheimer (1926). Andrew Moynihan

described chronic gastric ulcer as a precancerous condition in 1923. Radium was noted to produce osteogenic sarcoma in young women who worked in American watch factories by H.S. Martland in 1929. Cigarette smoking as a cause of carcinoma of the lung was demonstrated by Richard William Shaboe Doll (b 1912) and Austin Bradford Hill (b 1897) in 1950. Cancer was shown to develop from a single cell initiated by mutation of DNA by Hugh John Foster Cairns (b 1922) who was head of the Imperial Cancer Research Laboratory (1973–1980) at Mill Hill in London. The capability of certain viruses to transform cells into a cancerous state was demonstrated by an Italian virologist, Renato Dulbecco (b 1914) while he was at the Imperial Cancer Research Laboratory in London. He was awarded the Nobel Prize in Physiology or Medicine in 1975. A great advance in the study of carcinogenesis was made with the discovery and isolation of the embryonal carcinoma cell as an experimental tool by a British geneticist from the University of Oxford, Anne Laura McLaren (b 1927) in the early 1970s. The tumor suppresser gene, *Rb1*, associated with rare childhood cancer of the retina was discovered by an American biochemist, Robert Allen Weinberg (b 1942) of Pittsburgh. *See P53 gene.*

Carcinogens *See carcinogenesis.*

Carcinoid Syndrome *See argentaffinoma.*

Carcinoma of the Breast *See breast cancer.*

Carcinoma of the Cervix The most useful contribution towards the diagnosis of cervical cancer was made by an American cytologist of Greek origin, George Nicholas Papanicolaou (1883–1962), who demonstrated that cytology could be used to diagnose it before the disease became clinically overt. He investigated the normal cyclical changes of the vaginal epithelium with Charles Rupert Stockard (1879–1939), a New York biochemist, in 1917 and described the use of the vaginal smear in diagnosis in 1928. Papanicolaou and Herbert Frederick Traut (b 1894) published their paper, *The Diagnosis of Uterine Cancer by Vaginal Smear* in 1943. The Schiller test, which permitted visualization of the suspected area of the cervix after staining with iodine, was devised by a Viennese gynecologist in America, Walter Schiller (1887–1960) in 1927. Important cytological studies were also carried out in England by Leonard Stan-ley Dudgeon (1876–1938) and C.V. Patrick in 1927, and Norman Rupert Barrett (b 1903) in 1934.

Carcinoma of the Gallbladder Mentioned in the medical literature by Maximillian Stoll of Swabia in 1777. The association between gallstones and cancer was suggested by

Friedrich Theodor von Frerichs (1819–1885) of Aurich in *Clinical Treatise on Diseases of the Liver* in 1861. Other early papers on the subject were published by J. Ludwig Courvoisier (1843–1918) of Basel in 1890 and D. Ames in 1894. A modern review of the subject was presented by C.F.W. Illingworth of England in 1935.

Carcinoma of the Lung Isaac Adler's (1849–1918) monograph on *Primary Malignant Growths of the Lungs and Bronchi* published in 1912 evoked vast interest and initiated further study on the subject in the early 20th century. The suggestion of the lung as a seat of carcinoma was made by Giovanni Battista Morgagni (1682–1771) in *De Sedibus et Causis Morborum per Antomen Indagatis* (1761). He described a hard adherent lung with a cancerous ulcer in a 60-year-old man with hemoptysis. Gaspard Laurent Bayle (1774–1816) of Paris mentioned some forms in *Recherches sur la Phtisie Pulmonaire* published in 1810. Further observations and studies were made by William Stokes (1842) and Walter Hayle Walshe (1871). Fragments of malignant tissue in the sputum were recognized by Walshe of London in 1843. The malignant cells were also identified in the sputum by Lionel Smith Beale (1828–1906) of King's College, London in 1860 and in gastric washings by Ottomar Rosenbach (1851–1907) of Germany in 1882. R. Huguenin of Paris gave a historical account of pulmonary cancer in *Cancer Primitif du Poumon* in 1928. A metastatic tumor of the mediastinum, from oat cell carcinoma of the lung, was described by George William Barnard (1892–1956) in 1926. Evarts Ambrose Graham (1883–1957), professor of surgery at Washington University, St Louis, was the first to remove a lung in a case of lung cancer. Pioneer work on sputum analysis for malignant cells for diagnosis was done by Leonard Stanley Dudgeon (1876–1938) and C.H.J. Wrigley in 1935. Graham was one of the first to associate tobacco smoking with lung cancer. Cigarette smoking as a cause was demonstrated by Richard William Shaboe Doll (b 1912) and Austin Bradford Hill (b 1897) in 1950.

Carcinoma of the Prostate *See prostatic carcinoma.*

Carcinoma of the Rectum *See rectal carcinoma.*

Carcinoma of the Stomach *See gastrectomy, gastric carcinoma.*

Carcinoma of the Uterus The modern surgical treatment for cancer of the uterus through the vaginal route was introduced by Vincenz Czerny (1842–1916), professor of surgery at Heidelberg, in 1878. Wilhelm Alexander Freund (1833–1918) introduced the abdominal operation in the same year, and his method was improved by Austrian gynecologist, Ernest Wertheim (1864–1920) in 1898.

Radical vaginal hysterectomy was introduced by Friedrich Schauta (1849–1919) in 1902. The development of cancer in the cervical stump following subtotal hysterectomy was described as a clinical entity by German gynecologist Rudolf Chrobak (1843–1910) in 1896. Other workers including Charles Horace Mayo (1865–1939) and John O. Polak recognized this risk in the early 1930s and advocated panhysterectomy to avoid its recurrence. Radiation treatment was introduced into Europe around 1908. *See carcinoma of the cervix.*

Cardanus, Hieronimus Girolomo (1501–1576) A physician born to a noble family in Milan, who was professor of medicine at Pavia (1543) and Bologna (1562). In 1551 he traveled to Scotland to cure John Hamilton, the archbishop of St Andrews, of a dangerous illness, and cast a horoscope for Edward VI. Cardanus was also a prodigious writer on subjects such as algebra and health. He described the characteristics or indicators of long life which, according to him, were: a family history of long life in at least of one of the parents; a cheerful easy disposition; and the ability to sleep long and soundly. He died a few weeks after publishing his autobiography, *De propria vita*. He had a tragic life, as one of his two sons was executed for murdering his wife, and the other son became a reprobate.

Cardiac Aneurysm *De Motu Cordis et Aneuriysmatibus* was written by Giovanni Maria Lancisi (1654–1720), professor of anatomy at the Collegio de Sapienza. A specific account of a case was published by Domenico Maria Gusmano Galeati (1686–1775) of Bologna in 1757. It was described in England by Thomas Bevill Peacock (1812–1882), a physician at St Thomas' Hospital in 1858. A detailed review was given by M. Pelvet of Paris in *Des Aneurysmes du Coeur* published in 1868. The first successful surgical operation was performed by a German surgeon, Ferdinand Sauerbruch (1875–1951) in 1903.

Cardiac Arrest The first report of syncope due to cardiac arrest or heart block was given by Marcus Gerbezius (1658–1718), a Slovenian physician in 1692. An identical condition was described as 'epilepsy with slow pulse' by Giovanni Battista Morgagni (1682–1771) in 1761. A successful cardiac resuscitation using electrostimulation to the thorax in a patient without a pulse in 1774 is found in the *Register of the Royal Humane Society of London*. Robert Adams (1791–1875) presented *A Clear Case of Syncopal Attacks with Heart Block* in 1827. Walter Hayle Walshe (1812–1892) of London suggested the use of electrostimulation in 1862. The first account of death due to ventricular fibrillation was given by a Scottish physiologist, Alexander John MacWilliam

(1857–1937) while at the University of Aberdeen in 1887. *See cardiac resuscitation, ventricular fibrillation.*

Cardiac Asthma Repiratory distress due to cardiac failure. One of the earliest descriptions was given by Leon Rostan (1790–1866) of France in 1817.

Cardiac Catheterization Claude Bernard (1813–1878), during his experiments on respiration in animals, passed a mercury catheter through the carotid artery of the horse into its left ventricle. Similar experiments were performed to study intracardiac pressure by French physiologists, Etienne Jules Marey (1830–1904) and Jean Baptiste Auguste Chauveau (1827–1917) in 1861. The first human cardiac catheterization using a ureteric catheter was performed by Fritz Bleichroder in 1912. The method was revived by Werner Forssmann (1868–1941) of Germany who performed it on animals in 1929. He later catheterized himself through a vein, using a ureteral catheter, and confirmed its position in the right atrium by X-ray. Studies of congenital heart diseases by venous catheterization were undertaken by Lewis Dexter in 1947. His work was followed by further pioneering work in 1949 by Andre Cournand (1895–1988) and Dickenson Woodruff Richards (1895–1973). A valuable modification of the percutaneous technique, which allowed the introduction of a catheter that had a larger diameter than the needle used for the initial puncture, was devised by Sven Ivar Seldinger in 1953. *See angiocardiography, left ventriculography.*

Cardiac Electrophysiology *See electrophysiology.*

Cardiac Enzymes *See diagnostic enzymology.*

Cardiac Massage *See cardiac resuscitation.*

Cardiac Murmurs *See murmur.*

Cardiac Neurosis *See effort syndrome.*

Cardiac Output William Harvey (1578–1657) estimated, from the number of heart beats and change in volume of the left ventricle, that about 500 ounces of blood were forced into the arteries by the heart in about 30 minutes. Although this was later proved to be low, it was probably the first attempt to quantify cardiac output. He also pointed out variation according to physiological and physical needs. In 1870 the German physiologist Adolf Fick (1829–1901) calculated it by estimating the difference of the oxygen content between the arterial and venous blood. In 1894 a Canadian-American physiologist, George Neil Stewart (1860–1930) discovered that it was possible to measure it in animals by injecting a dye into the vein and analyzing the amount of dye that appeared in arterial blood. This method

was later adapted for humans by an American physiologist, William Ferguson Hamilton (b 1893) and co-workers in 1932. The dye dilution curves obtained later became useful in diagnosis of congenital heart disease. A more complex method called 'foreign gas sampling' was introduced by A. Bornstein (who used nitrogen) in 1910, and A. Krogh (who used nitrous oxide) in 1912. X-ray comparison of cardiac volume at systole and diastole was proposed by W. Meek and J. Eyster in 1920. Ballistocardiography was also used to estimate it in the 1920s. Various experimental methods were discussed by the Finnish physiologist, Robert Adolf Armand Tigerstedt (1853–1923) in his work published in 1921. *See ballistocardiograph.*

Cardiac Pacing Luigi Galvani's (1737–1798) nephew, Giovanni Aldini (1762–1834) conducted experiments on cardiac electrostimulation using his uncle's invention, on the body of a criminal executed at Newgate, London in 1802. The effect of electrical stimulation of human tissues was studied by Guillaume Benjamin Amand Duchenne (1806–1875), a neurologist from Boulogne, in 1855. A description of an artificial pacemaker in experimental studies on cardiac resuscitation in animals was given by Solomon Albert Hymen (b 1893), a physician at the Beth David Hospital, New York, in 1932. Paul Maurice Zoll (b 1911) applied external cardiac pacing in ventricular standstill in two patients in 1932. Implantable artificial pacemaker was made possible with the invention of semiconductor tran-sistor by American scientists, William Bradford Shockley (1910–1989), John Bardeen (b 1908) and Walter Houser Brattain (1902–1987) who won the Nobel Prize for Physics in 1956. Endocardial electrodes for pacing were used in animals by John C. Callaghan and Wilfred G. Bigelow, in 1951. F. Furman and G. Robinson introduced intracardiac right ventricular pacing for heart block in 1958, and the first generator implant for cardiac pacing was applied at the Karolinska Hospital in Sweden in 1958.

Cardiac Resuscitation Cardiac arrest and apnea in patients have been treated with the application of galvanism since the mid-19th century. J. C. S. Jennings in 1861 recommended the application of one wire to the neck and another to the heart in order to deliver galvanism to patients with apnea. The basic principles of resuscitation: artificial respiration, galvanism (electric shock), injection into blood vessels and artificial circulation (external cardiac massage), were proposed by Benjamin Ward Richardson (1828–1896) in *Paper on Resuscitation* presented to the British Medical Association meeting at Manchester in 1861. Cardiac massage was given by Carl Johan August Langenbuch (1864– 1901) in 1887 but his attempts were unsuccessful.

Ernest Starling and William Arbuthnot Lane (1856–1943) performed the first successful transdiaphragmatic cardiac massage combined with artificial respiration following cardiac arrest during surgery in 1902. Intracardiac injection of epinephrine was introduced in the early 1920s. Solomon Albert Hymen (b 1893), a physician at the Beth David Hospital, New York in 1929 postulated that the benefit of the injection was mainly due to the effect of the needle piercing the heart and not due to epinephrine. M.C. Lidwell used this method in 1930 and made attempts to resuscitate stillborn infants by thrusting a needle into their ventricles. A description of the artificial pacemaker was given by Hyman in 1932. No further significant advances were made until 1947 when W.H. Sweet applied direct stimulation to the sinoatrial node in two patients who developed cardiac arrest during surgery. Arrest due to ventricular fibrillation during surgery was treated with electric countershock and direct cardiac massage to the exposed heart by Claude Schaeffer Beck (1894–1971) of Cleveland in 1947. A further advance was made by C.E. Herrod and co-workers who announced a combined pacemaker device and defibrillator in 1952. Wilfred G. Bigelow and Jack A. Hopps applied a similar device to clinical use in 1953. *See cardioversion, cardiac arrest, cardiac pacing.*

Cardiac Sounds Heart sounds were suggested as a key to the motion of the internal parts of the body by Robert Hooke (1635–1703). These were first interpreted for clinical purposes by René Laënnec (1781–1826) in 1819. Jean Baptiste Bouillaud (1796–1881) of Angoulême, France diagnosed heart diseases on the basis of cardiac sounds and murmurs in 1824. J. Rouanet of Paris also undertook clinical study in 1832. Arthur Leared (1822–1879), in his MD thesis at the University of Dublin, explained the mechanism of production of the first and second heart sounds. He also devised a biaural stethoscope in 1851. The mechanism and physiology of the second heart sound was explained in 1866 by a French cardiologist, Pierre Carl Edouard Potain (1825–1901) who also studied the mechanism of production of gallop rhythm, in 1875. Phonocardiography for recording them was introduced by Wilhelm Einthoven (1860–1927) and M.A.J. Geluk of Germany in 1890. The first heart sound was explained by William Dock of King's County Hospital, Brooklyn, New York in 1933. Asynchronous contractions of the left and right ventricles contributing to the components of the second heart sound were investigated by Carl John Wiggers (1883–1962), professor of physiology at the Western Reserve University, Cleveland in 1949. The third heart sound was studied and described by an American physician, William Sydney Thayer (1864–1932) of Johns Hopkins Hospital. *See murmurs.*

Cardiac Surgery The first series of cardiac operations to be performed were for stab wounds of the heart. Henry C. Dalton (b 1847) of Washington University sutured the torn pericardium from a stab wound in 1891 and Daniel Hale Williams (1858–1931) performed a similar operation at the Provident Hospital in Chicago's South Side in 1893. The first recorded successful cardiac surgery was performed on a 22-year-old man with a stab wound through the heart by Ludwig Rehn (1849–1930) of Frankfurt in 1896. The first successful surgical operation for cardiac aneurysm was performed by a German surgeon, Ferdinand Sauerbruch (1875–1951) in 1903. This was followed by a valvotomy for stenosis of the pulmonary valve by a Paris surgeon, Eugene Louis Doyen (1859–1916) in 1913, but his procedure was unsuccessful. Elliot Carr Cutler (b 1888) of the Western Reserve University of Cleveland, Ohio performed valvotomy for severe mitral stenosis through the transventricular approach in 1923. London surgeon, Sir Henry Sessions Souttar (b 1875) pioneered a valvulotomy procedure by introducing his fingers through the left atrium and splitting the mitral commisures in a case of mitral stenosis in 1925. An operation for an intracardiac congenital anomaly was carried out by Alfred Blalock (1899–1964) in 1944. Successful open heart surgery was performed (1953) by an American cardiovascular surgeon, John Heysham Gibbon (1903–1973) who used the heart–lung bypass machine on animals in 1939, and employed the first pump oxygenator on humans in 1954. He used his machine successfully to close an atrial septal defect in a 19-year-old woman in 1953. This was followed by a series of operations by Clarence Walton Lillehei (b 1918) who used human volunteers for cross circulation during his cardiac procedures. A modified heart–lung machine was introduced by J.W. Kirklin at the Mayo Clinic, and a successful operation for truncus arteriosus was performed by D.C. McGoon and G.C. Rastelli in 1967. Modern cardiac surgery in the 20th century was pioneered by Denton Arthur Cooley (b 1920) of Houston; he excised a ventricular cardiac aneurysm under cardiopulmonary by-pass in 1959. *See cardiac transplant, coronary artery bypass, pediatric cardiology, cardiology.*

Cardiac Thrombus An account of emboli from intramural thrombus of the heart was given by William Senhouse Kirkes (1823–1864) of Holker, Lancashire in *The Detachment of Fibrinous Deposits of the Heart* in 1852.

Cardiac Transplant First performed in animals by Alexis Carrel (1873–1944) and Charles Claude Guthrie (1880–1963) in 1905. Their technique was developed by Frank Charles Mann (b 1887) of Minnesota, who transplanted heterotrophic mammalian hearts by anastomosing the heart to the vessels in the recipient animal's neck in 1933. Successful canine orthotopic cardiac transplant was carried out by Richard Rowland Lower (b 1929) and Norman Edward Shumway (b 1923), an American cardiac surgeon of Michigan in 1960. James Daniel Hardy (b 1918) and colleagues carried out the first cardiac transplant with a xeno-graft (from a chimpanzee) in 1964, but it was a failure. The first cardiac transplant was performed by Christiaan Neethling Barnard (b 1922) at the Groote Schuur Hospital in Cape Town in 1967. His patient, Louis Washkanski, survived for 17 days, but succumbed to pneumonia. His second heart transplant patient, Philip Blaiberg, lived for 74 days in 1968. In the following ten years about 500 cardiac transplants were performed throughout the world.

Cardiac Valves *See artificial heart valve, aortic valve, mitral valve, tricuspid valve.*

Cardialgia [Greek: *cardia*, heart + *algos*, pain] An old term and synonym for heartburn or dyspepsia.

Cardiazol Metrazol, a synthetic camphor preparation used as injections to control epileptic fits in the early 1930s.

Cardica Passio Cardiac passion, an ancient Greek term for syncope.

Cardiff Medical Society Founded with 19 members at the Cardiff Royal Infirmary with Thomas Evans as its first president in 1870.

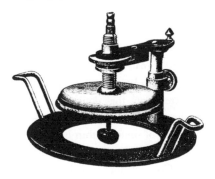

Improved design of Etienne Jules Marey's cardiograph. G V. Anrep and D T Harris, *Practical Physiology* (1923). Churchill, London

Cardiography [Greek: *kardia*, heart + *graphein*, to write] A method of recording cardiac impulses on a smoked paper drum devised by French physiologists, Etienne Jules Marey (1830–1904) and Jean Baptiste Auguste Chauveau (1827–1917) in 1863.

Cardiolipin Antigen A phospholipid obtained from beef by Candace Mary Pangborn (b 1907) in 1941. It was used in the serological test for diagnosis of syphilis by A. Harris, A. A. Rosenberg and L. M. Riedel in 1946.

Cardiology [Greek: *kardia*, heart + *logos*, discourse] Erasistratus who lived around 300 BC, believed that the valves of the heart directed the blood towards the veins. The ancient Chinese lacked precise anatomical knowledge of the heart and they believed that the trachea opened into the heart. The Roman physician Galen (129–200) proposed that blood from the left ventricle reached the right side of the heart via pores in the interventricular septum. His teaching was accepted for over 1000 years until William Harvey (1578–1657) announced his discovery of the circulatory system in 1628. David Dundas, a British physician in the late 17th century who did pioneer work on rheumatic diseases, was one of the first to concentrate on the heart and he published *An Account of Peculiar Diseases of the Heart* in 1808. The 'peculiar disease' described by him was later recognized as rheumatic heart disease. A description of coronary circulation was given by Raymond Vieussens (1641–1715) of France in his *Traite du Coeur* in 1715. The calcification of the coronary arteries was described by Giovanni Battista Morgagni (1682–1771) in 1761. David Pitcairn (1749–1809), a physician at St Bartholomew's Hospital, was one of the first to concentrate on the pathology of the heart. He noted the lesions in the heart valves following rheumatic fever and introduced the term 'rheumatic' in the description of heart disease in 1788. Jean Nicholas Corvisart (1755–1821) wrote an important treatise on the diseases of the heart in 1814. English cardiologist, Sir James Mackenzie (1853–1925), developed his own ink polygraph by which he simultaneously recorded arterial and venous pulsations during his study on arrhythmias. He was the first to note the loss of effective atrial contraction or 'atrial paralysis' which was later named 'atrial fibrillation' by Sir Thomas Lewis (1881–1945). Mackenzie also described the functional pathology of cardiac tissue in 1907 and established the place of digitalis in the treatment of auricular fibrillation. The first electrocardiogram of a man was recorded by August Desire Waller (1856–1922), a physiologist at St Mary's Hospital in London, in 1887. Dutch physiologist, Willem Einthoven (1860–1927), simplified the method with his invention in 1903 of the string galvanometer, which developed into the electrocardiograph. His apparatus was improved by Lewis who added two strings instead of a conventional single string, making it possible to record different leads. The first recording of a fetal electrocardiogram was reported by M. Cremer of Germany in 1906. Alexis Carrel (1884–1947), a French-born American biologist, reported the first heart transplantation in a dog in 1905, and the first human heart transplantation was achieved by Christian Neethling Barnard (b-1922) at Groote Schuur Hospital in Cape Town in 1967. Cardiac catheterization was performed by Werner Forssmann (1868–1941) of Germany on himself in 1929. A practical electrical defibrillator to treat the irregularity of the heart was constructed by an American professor of electrical engineering, William Bennett Kouwenhoven (1886–1975) of Johns Hopkins University, in 1936. An attempt at bypassing diseased coronary arteries by implanting pectoral muscles onto the pericardium was made by Claude Schaeffer Beck (1894–1971) of America in 1935. Other advances in cardiac surgery made in the United States were by: William Wayne Babcock (1872–1963), Claude Beck (1894–1971), Alfred Blalock (1899–1964), Robert Edward Gross (1905–1988), Michael Ellis DeBakey (b 1980) and Arthur Denton Cooley (b 1920). Rene G. Favaloro, a rural physician from La Plata, Argentina performed the first successful coronary artery bypass graft using the saphenous vein, on a woman who had an obstructed right coronary artery, at the Cleveland Clinic in 1967.

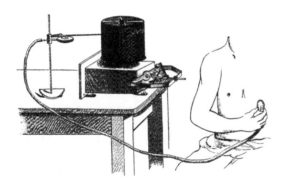

A cardiograph to measure the impulse of the heart. Augustus Waller, *An Introduction to Human Physiology* (1893). Longmans, London

Cardiomyopathy [Greek: *kardia*, heart + *myos*, muscle + *pathos*, suffering] Defined by the World Health Organisation in 1968 as a condition involving the heart muscle, of usually unknown etiology, with cardiomegaly and heart failure. The first mention of a dilated heart was made by Jacopo Berengario da Carpi (1470–1530) of Italy in 1521. Jean Nicholas Corvisart (1755–1821) differentiated between active and passive dilatation of the heart and Theophile René Laënnec (1781–1826) made a classification of the diseases of the myocardium. French pathologists, H. Liouville and L. Hallopeau, observed the anatomical features of hypertrophic cardiomyopathy in 1869. William Evans of the National Heart Hospital, London was the first to describe familial cardiomegaly in 1949. Henry Christian pointed out the condition as a separate entity from hypertension or coronary heart disease in 1950. Hypertrophic

cardiomyopathy was recognized at an operation by a surgeon from Guy's Hospital, Russell Claude Brock (1903–1980), in 1957.

Cardiopulmonary Bypass The concept of maintaining life without the action of the heart, by regular injection or supply of blood was proposed by a French physiologist, Caesar Julian Jean La Gallois or Lagallois (1770–1814) in 1812. C. Ludwig and A. Schmidt demonstrated artificial oxygenation of blood in 1869. An artificial lung for oxygenation was devised by W. von Schoeder in 1882. The first film oxygenator where the blood flowed on a thin film over the surface of a cylinder was devised by Max von Frey and M. Gruber in 1885. A prototype heart–lung machine was built by an American cardiovascular surgeon, John Heysham Gibbon (1903–1973) and his wife in 1935; they tried it experimentally on animals in 1939. A pump oxygenator was used during cardiac surgery on a patient named Cecelia Bovolek by Gibbon in 1953. *See cardiac surgery.*

Cardiothoracic Surgery *See cardiac surgery, cardiac transplant, coronary artery bypass, cardiopulmonary bypass aortic aneurysm, pneumonectomy, cardiology, pediatric cardiology.*

Cardiotomy Syndrome [Greek: *kardia*, heart + *tome*, to cut] *See Dressler syndrome.*

Cardiovascular System *See blood circulation, capillary circulation, heart, cardiology.*

Cardioversion [Greek: *kardia*, heart; Latin: *versio*, translation + *uertere*, to turn] In 1899 Jean Louis Prevost (1790–1850) and F. Battelli induced ventricular fibrillation in a dog's heart by applying a small current, and later terminated the arrhythmia by giving a larger dose of current. The effect of alternating current on the dog's heart was done by W.B. Kouwenhouven, D.R. Hooker and O.R. Langworthy in 1932. Induction of sinus rhythm by applying countershock to an intact animal was demonstrated by the same workers in 1933. Countershock to a fibrillating human heart leading to recovery was performed by Claude Schaeffer Beck (1894–1971) and colleagues of America, in 1945. Following their success, Paul Maurice Zoll (b 1911) and co-workers terminated ventricular fibrillation in four patients by applying alternating countershock current in 1956. Direct current capacitor discharge capable of depolarizing the myocardium transthoracically was developed B. Lowen and R. Amarasingham in 1962.

Cardon, Jerome (1501–1576) *See Cardanus.*

Carey, Matthew (1760–1839) The son of a baker in Dublin who emigrated to America in 1793. He founded the

Philadelphia Journal of the Medical and Physical Sciences in 1820 which was renamed *American Journal of Medical Sciences* in 1824. He gave one of the best accounts of the epidemic of yellow fever of Philadelphia in 1793.

Carey–Coombs Murmur A short mid-diastolic murmur heard during acute rheumatic carditis. Described by an English physician from Somerset, Franklin Carey Coombs (1879–1932). He was trained at St Mary's Hospital and graduated in 1903 before he moved to Bristol General Hospital, where he spent most of his career.

Caries of the Spine Described by Hippocrates (460–377 BC). The lumbar vertebrae from the mummy of an Egyptian priest of Ammon during the 21st dynasty (1100 BC) shows definite evidence of this disease. The first observation related to the tuberculous nature was made by French surgeon, Jacques Mathieu Delpech (1777–1832) in 1828. Percivall Pott (1714–1788) described the deformity and sequelae due to spinal caries (Pott disease) in 1779 but failed to describe the tuberculous nature. Modern orthopedic treatment, combined with advocation of a horizontal posture, were introduced by Thomas Baynton (1761–1820) of London in 1813. The method of wiring the spine in Pott disease was introduced by Berthhold Ernst Hadra (1842–1903) of America in 1891. The diseased spine of patients with Pott disease was treated with a bone transplant from the tibia by Houdlett Fred Albee (1876–1945) of Harvard in 1915.

Caries *See dental caries.*

Carlisle, Sir Anthony (1768–1840) Anatomist and physiologist from Willington, Durham. He moved to London and was a pupil of H. Watson at the Westminster Hospital, and succeeded him as senior surgeon in 1793.

Carlson, Chester Floyd (1906–1968)

Carmot A hypothetical constituent of the philosopher's stone in alchemy. *See alchemy.*

Carnochan, John Murray (1817–1887) New York surgeon who designed an operation for trigeminal neuralgia. It involved the removal of the semilunar ganglion and part of the trigeminal nerve through the maxillary antrum.

Carnot, Sadi (1796–1831) Scientist from Paris, considered a founder of thermodynamics. He defined work and postulated the second law of thermodynamics. His only published work, *Reflexions sur la Puissance Motrice du feu et sur les Machines propre a Developer cette Puisance,* appeared in 1824. He died of cholera. *See thermodynamics.*

Carophobia [Latin: *caro,* flesh; Greek: *phobia,* fear] An old term for abnormal aversion to meat.

Carotene *See vitamin A.*

Carotid Angiography Visualization of the carotid artery in patients presenting with cerebral symptoms was suggested by a New York neurologist, James Ramsay Hunt (1872–1937) in 1914. The method of radiologically visualizing the cerebral circulation by injecting radio-opaque sodium iodide into the carotid artery was introduced by Antonio Caetanode de Abreu Egas Moniz (1874–1955) of Portugal in 1927. Sodium iodide was later noted to give rise to fits and was replaced by another dye, thorotrast. Four cases of thrombosis of the internal carotid artery were diagnosed by Moniz and Almeida Lima in 1937 using angiography.

Carotid Arteriography *See carotid angiography.*

Carotid Artery [Greek: *karos,* deep sleep or stupefaction] Name derived from the belief by Aristotle that compression of the carotid artery resulted in a deep sleep or coma. Andreas Vesalius (1514–1564) referred to it as arteriae sopariae in 1550. Curtius in 1551 ligated both carotid arteries in a living animal and showed that it did not produce coma.

Carotid Artery Ligation Jean Louis Petit (1674–1750) observed that the brain could survive without one carotid artery in a case of carotid thrombosis. Ligation of the common carotid artery for cerebral hemorrhage was performed by John Abernethy (1764–1831) in 1798, but his patient died within 30 hours. Successful ligation following trauma was performed in 1803 by David Fleming, a British naval surgeon. Sir Astley Paston Cooper (1768–1841) ligated the artery for treatment of carotid aneurysm in 1805, but was not successful. On his second attempt in 1808, he succeeded and the patient lived for 13 years. Another operation for berry aneurysm was performed by Benjamin Travers (1783–1838), a surgeon at St Thomas' Hospital, in 1811. The first American to perform the procedure was William D. Macgill (1802–1833), who successfully tied both carotid arteries in 1823. Victor Horsley (1857–1916) used the operation for intracranial aneurysm outside the cavernous sinus in 1885. C. Pilz in 1863 presented a series of 600 ligations, of which 43% were fatal.

Carotid Artery Thrombectomy Surgical removal of a thrombus in the internal carotid artery to re-establish patency in the vessel during acute cerebral insufficiency was carried out by C. G. Rob and E. B. Wheeler in 1957.

Carotid Body A body in the artery, described as 'ganglion minutum' by Hartwig Wilhelm Ludwig Taube (b 1706) in 1743. A pathological account of carotid body tumors was given by Felix Jacob Marchand (1846–1928) in 1891. Reports of carotid body tumors secreting catecholamines were given independently by G.G. Glenner and P. Berdal in 1962.

Carotid Body Tumors *See carotid body.*

Carotid Endarterectomy The first case of internal carotid artery reconstructive surgery in a patient with intermittent hemiplegia or transient ischemic attacks was reported by Regius professor of medicine George White Pickering (1904–1980), H.H.G. Eastcott and C.G. Rob in *The Lancet* in 1954.

Carotid Sinus Depressor Reflex Described by Edgar Dewight Brown (b 1869) and Torald Hermann Sollmann (1874–1965) of Minnesota in 1912. The function and structure of the carotid nerve and the reflex effect of pressure on the carotid sinus were shown by Heinrich Ewald Hering (1866–1948) in 1924.

Carotid Sinus Syndrome Fainting and fits occurring due to an overactive carotid sinus reflex, following minimal stimulation of the carotid sinus. Described by Jean Marie Charcot (1825–1893) in 1872. It was described again and explained by American physician, Soma Weiss (1898–1942) in 1929 and by James Porter Baker (b 1913) in 1933.

Carpenter, William Benjamin (1813–1885) British physiologist, born in Bristol and graduated in medicine from Edinburgh in 1839. He proposed the concept of the subconscious mind. He was professor of forensic medicine at University College in 1849, and later took part in marine expeditions (1868–1871). He wrote: *Principles of General and Comparative Physiology* (1838), *Principles of Human Physiology* (1846), *The Microscope and its Revelations* (1856), *Principles of Mental Physiology* (1874) and *Nature and Man* (1888).

Carpue Operation Revival of the Indian method of rhinoplasty, described by English surgeon, Joseph C. Carpue (1764–1846).

Carpus [Greek: *karpos*, wrist] Galen (129–200) used the term collectively to mean the eight carpal bones of the hands. The carpus was described by Andreas Vesalius (1514–1564) in 1550.

Carrel, Alexis (1884–1947) French-born American biologist from Lyons, considered as the father of organ transplantation, owing to his pioneering work in the field. He obtained his medical degree in 1900, and perfected end-to-end arterial anastomosis by using triple thread sutures in 1902. He joined the University of Chicago as an assistant in physiology in 1904, and reported the first heart transplantation in a dog in

1905, before he moved to the Rockefeller Institute in 1906. He introduced the method of maintaining excised animal organs alive by providing physiological surroundings in 1911, and was also the first to grow tumor tissue. He received the Nobel Prize for his work on extra-vital cultivation of tissues. His *Man and the Unknown*, gave a technocratic vision of a world led by the intellectual elite and was published in 1935.

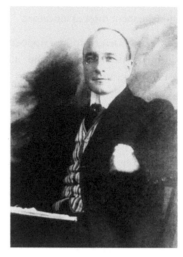

Alexis Carrel (1884–1947). Courtesy of the National Library of Medicine

Carrion Disease (Syn. verruga peruviana, Oroya fever) Named after a medical student, Daniel Carrion (1859–1885) of Lima, who died after self-experimenting by inoculating both his arms with matter from the lesion of a patient with the disease. After incubating the disease for 23 days, he died within 15 days of developing symptoms. *Bartonella bacilliformis,* the bacterium responsible, was found in red blood cells by A.L. Barton in 1915, and Richard Pearson Strong (1872–1948) and co-workers named the organism *Bartonella.* Arsphenamine was used in the treatment by J. Arce in 1918.

Carroll, James (1854–1907) English-born physician and director of the laboratory of the Army Medical School in America. He was a pioneer in the study of yellow fever and typhoid bacteria. He occasionally conducted experiments on himself and in 1898, during the process of developing a typhoid vaccine, he took an oral dose of typhoid bacteria. He also infected himself with yellow fever in 1900, and accompanied Walter Reed (1851–1902) on an expedition to Cuba to investigate yellow fever in 1901. William Osler (1849–1919) later suggested that Carroll died of chronic bacterial endocarditis as a result of self-experimentation on typhoid.

Carson, James (1772–1843) Physician in Liverpool who performed open pneumothorax as treatment for tuberculosis in 1820. He also studied the effect of the venous return of the blood of the heart and the property of elastic recoil of the lung by creating a negative pressure in the pleura.

Carswell, Sir Robert (1793–1857) Born in Paisley, a Scottish professor of pathological anatomy at University College London. He wrote *Illustrations of the Elementary Forms of Disease* in 1837. He was later the royal physician in Belgium, where he spent the rest of his life.

Carter, Henry Vandyke (1831–1907) Physician in the Indian Medical Service. He described madura foot, scrotal elephantiasis and several other diseases.

Cartilage [Latin: *cartilago*, gristle] Word used by Pliny the Elder (AD 28–79) to refer to the center of roots. It was introduced into anatomy by Aulus Cornelius Celsus (25 BC–AD 50).

Carus An ancient term for profound sleep from which the patient cannot be aroused by any external stimuli, including pain.

Carus, Carl Gustav (1789–1868) Professor of anatomy and an obstetrician at Montpellier. He studied pelvimetry in 1820, and defined the circle of Carus, which has its center at the pubis symphysis and pelvic outlet at its periphery. He later proposed the concept of psychosomatic disease.

Carvallo Sign *See tricuspid incompetence.*

Carver, Jonathan (1732–1780) A physician from Connecticut who gave up his profession to become an explorer. He wrote a work on his travels in 1778.

Casal Necklace Pattern of dermatitis involving the neck in pellagra, named after Gaspar Casal (1691–1759), a Spanish physician from Oviedo who first made a comprehensive study of pellagra in 1730.

Casal, Gaspar (1691–1759) Spanish physician who described *mal de rosa*, presently known as pellagra, in 1730. He practiced for over 30 years in Oviedo in Asturia and gave classic descriptions of several diseases which earned him the title of the Spanish Hippocrates. He later moved to Madrid and was appointed physician to King Ferdinand. *See pellagra.*

Casanova, (De Seingalt) Girolomo (1725–1798) An Italian wanderer and adventurer. His travels and sexual exploits in an edited form under the title *Memoires Ecrits par Lui-meme* were published in (1828–1838) in 12 volumes. He described the use of several contraceptive devices such as balls soaked in alkaline solution, half a small lemon as a cervical cap and the sheath.

Cascade Process Method used for liquefying oxygen, invented in 1877 by Raoul Pierre Pictet (1846–1929), a chemist from Geneva. His method involved the application of pressure at a relatively high critical temperature.

Casoni Test *See Casoni, Tomaso.*

Casoni, Tomaso (1850–1925) Italian physician at the Victor Emmanuel Hospital at Tripoli. He devised the skin sensitivity test (Casoni test) for the diagnosis of hydatid disease in 1912.

Casselberry, William Evans (1859–1916) Laryngologist in Chicago. He described the Casselberry position following intubation, which allowed the patient while lying prone to swallow without the fluid entering the tube.

Casserius, Giulio (1561–1616) Professor at Padua and a teacher of William Harvey (1578–1657). He described the muscles of the ossicles of the ear, the musculocutaneous nerve and the larynx. He practiced bronchotomy which he learnt from Fabricius, his assistant.

Cassiodorus (AD 468–560) A founder of monastic medicine, from a Syrian family who settled in Italy. He was a follower of St Benedict in caring for the sick and established a monastery at Scillace in Calabria. He also collected valuable ancient manuscripts and had them copied.

Castellani, Sir Aldo (1877–1971) Famous Italian bacteriologist, born in Florence, he identified the trypanosome as the cause of sleeping sickness in Uganda. In 1903 he went as a bacteriologist to Sri Lanka, where he described tea taster's lung due to moniliasis in 1905, and gave an account of yaws in 1906. He also identified and named the fungus *Tinea rubrum* in 1910 while he was there. On returning to Britain he established an internationally recognized practice in Harley Street and was physician to many royal families. He was later called to Italy to attend the Italian dictator, Benito Mussolini (1883–1945) and became Surgeon General to the Italian forces. He published over 200 papers on medical mycology and wrote his autobiography, *Microbes Man and Monarchs* in 1960.

Castelli, Bartholomew (d 1607) Italian physician who published *Lexicon Medicum Graeco-Latinum* in 1598.

Castle, William Bosworth (b 1899) *See pernicious anemia.*

Castration [Latin: *castrare*, to geld] The benefits of therapeutic surgical castration in treatment of advanced breast cancer were reported by Scottish surgeon Sir George Thomas Beatson (1848–1933) in 1896. Radical surgical treatment combined with prophylactic castration for primary breast cancer suggested by A. Schinzinger in 1889. The value of the procedure was clearly established by A. Siegert in 1952. *See eunuchs.*

Casts *See urinary casts.*

Casualty *See accident services.*

CAT Scanner Computerized axial tomography (CAT) was developed independently by a British scientist Godfrey Newbold Hounsfield (b 1919) and a South African-born American medical physicist, Allan Macleod Cormack (b 1924) around 1973. Hounsfield was born in Newark, and educated at the City and Guilds College, London. After serving as a radar engineer during World War II, he joined Thorn-EMI in 1952 and became director of its medical research department in 1972. Cormack and Hounsfield shared the Nobel Prize in 1979.

Cat Scratch Fever Characterized by lymphadenopathy and fever, following a cat scratch. Described in 1950 by Robert Debre (b 1882), a pediatrician and bacteriologist in Paris, and by William Edward Greer (b 1918) and Scott Chester Keefer (1897–1972) in 1951.

Catabolism [Greek: *kata*, down + *bolos*, throw] *See metabolism.*

Catacombs Depositories of the dead, used by the first Christians of Rome. Catacombs were also used by the Egyptians around BC 1500.

Catalysis [Greek: *kata*, down + *lusis*, loosening] Kirchhoff (1764–1833) in 1812 observed that starch was converted to glucose by the action of dilute acid but the acid itself remained unchanged. During the period 1817–1823 several workers, including Johann Wolfgang Dobereiner (1780–1849), Eilhardt Mitscherlich (1794–1863) and Louis Thenard (1777–1857), found that some metals accelerated chemical reactions without any change in the metal itself. Thenard also noted that fibrin in the blood accelerated the decomposition of hydrogen peroxide, an effect that was later explained to be due to methemoglobin. Following these observations, the concept of catalytic substances was introduced in 1837 by Jöns Jacob Berzelius (1779–1848). The mechanism of action of a catalyst was explained by Alexander William Williamson (1824–1904), professor of chemistry at University College, London (1849–1887) in 1854. In 1888, Friedrich Wilhelm Ostwald (1853–1932) discovered that a catalyst affects only the speed and not the equilibrium of a reaction.

Catalyst *See catalysis.*

Cataplasm [Greek: *kata*, down + *plasmein*, to mold] Poultice made of a variety of substances. A cataplasm of bread with nightshade was described by Paul of Aegina (625–690) for treatment of bedsores. Galen (AD 129–200) also described several poultices. Substances used have varied from herbal medicines to dung.

Cataplexis [Greek: *kata*, down + *lepsis*, seizing] Defined by Hippocrates (460–377 BC) as a sudden stupefaction of an organ or body.

Cataract Name derived from a Greek term which means 'to confound' or disturb. A similar word in Greek means waterfall [*kata*, down + *rhatoks*, precipice]. Islamic physicians called it 'gutta opaca' and Aulus Cornelius Celsus (25 BC–AD 50) named it 'suffusio'. It has also been described by Hippocrates (460–377 BC). Galen (AD 129–200) proposed the lens as the immediate organ of sight. Paul of Aegina (625–690) described a detailed operation as treatment. Freytag was the first surgeon to attempt the extraction of cataract in the 17th century. The nature of the cataract was pointed out by French ophthalmologist, Antoine Maitre-Jean (1650–1730) in 1706. Lotterius of Turin performed a successful operation, and Baron Wenzel from Vienna designed a knife for the purpose and improved the method in 1782. Ware later practiced Wenzel's method and published *Wenzel's Treatise on the Cataract*. Cataract due to the effect of lightning was described in an 18-year-old woman by Edwin Theodor Saemisch (1833–1909), an ophthalmologist in Bonn in 1864, and C. Hess induced cataract in animals by exposing them to electric current from a Leiden jar in 1888. 27 cases of cataract due to electricity were described by A. Gabriéldés in 1935. *See glass blowers' cataract, cataract extraction.*

Cataract Extraction Cataract operations were performed by the Brahmin surgeon, Susruta around 500 BC. Extraction of the lens by suction was known to the Arabs around AD 700. Surgical treatment of cataract by excision of the lens was performed in 1749 by French oculist, Jacques Daviel (1692–1762). Iridectomy was added to the procedure in 1854 by Albrecht von Graefe (1828–1870) who also introduced the method of linear extraction of a cataract in 1868. The suction method of extraction was promoted by Stowers in 1906 and Vard Houghton Hulen (1865–1939) in 1910. In 1917 Jose Ignacio Barraquer (1884–1965) designed an instrument called the 'erisiphake' which created a controlled vacuum by means of an air pump for suction of the lens. This method of operation, called 'phacoerisis', was widely in use until the 1930s. *See cataract.*

Catarrh [Greek: *kata*, down + *rhoia*, to flow] According to Hippocrates (460–377 BC) it was caused by the flow of fluid from the head to the mouth and then to the lungs.

Catatonia [Greek: *kata*, down or against + *tonus*, stretched] A condition in which a psychotic individual maintains peculiar rigid postures and remains mute. Described and named 'catatonia' by Karl Kahlbaum of Germany around 1860. *See Kahlbaum, Karl.*

Catecholamine *See epinephrine, norepinephrine, pheochromocytoma.*

Catgut [Latin: *catta*, gut] Made from animal intestines and used to make the strings of musical instruments such as harps and violins. It was used in surgery by Sir Astley Cooper (1768–1841) in 1817. Catgut treated with carbolic acid to promote asepsis was introduced by Joseph Lister (1827–1912) in 1869. Robert Abbe (1851–1928), a New York surgeon, used it for suturing intestines in 1889.

Catharsis A term given by Josef Breuer (1842–1925) to the therapeutic technique which he used on a female patient to bring out her repressed memories under hypnosis.

Catharetic Caustic substance used by ancient Greek and Roman physicians to treat superfluous growth or lesions.

Catheter [Greek: *kata*, down + *heimi*, to thrust into] The first urethral catheters during ancient times were made of silver and bronze tubes. Rhazes (850–932) a Persian physician, devised catheters with lateral holes to drain pus. He also used a lead catheter instead of bronze whenever flexibility was needed. Experiments in Europe on catheterization were conducted by J.Z. Amussat (1850–1932) in 1918. Flexible catheters made of woven silk cylinders covered with a coating of elastic gum were devised by M. Bernard, a silversmith in Paris, in the second half of the 18th century, and these were later manufactured by Walsh of London. Rubber urethral catheters were used by Auguste Nelaton (1807–1873). James Brown (1854–1895) of Johns Hopkins Hospital was the first to catheterize male ureters in 1893. The Charriere Scale used for grading the size of urethral and ureteric catheters was introduced by a Paris instrument maker, Joseph François Bernard (1803–1876). The Bozemann catheter, a double-channeled urethral catheter, was des-igned by an American surgeon, Nathan Bozemann (1825– 1905). A large bore suprapubic urinary catheter (Malecot catheter) was designed by a French surgeon in Paris, Achille Etienne Malecot (b 1852).

Cathode Ray Observed by a German physicist, Julius Plucker (1801–1868) in 1859. Emissions from the cathode during the passage of current were noticed by Hittorf (1824–1914) in 1869 and named cathode ray by Eugen Goldstein (1850–1930) a German physicist, in 1880. The theory that they consisted of a stream of negatively charged particles was proved by Jean Baptiste Perrin (1870–1942) in 1895. The ratio of the charge on a cathode to its mass was determined by Sir Joseph John Thomson (1856–1940) in 1897. He called these particles 'corpuscles' and they were later named 'electrons'.

Catomismus Term used by Paul Aegina (625–690) for reduction of a dislocated humerus.

Caton, Richard (1842–1926) English physician who identified electrical activity in the brain of living animals. *See electroencephalography.*

Cattalin, Alfred William Newman (1814–1886) A surgeon and dentist from Brighton, and a founder of the Odontological Society in England. He invented the 'Cattalin bag', a reservoir for re-breathing in anesthesia.

Cattle Disease Prevention Act Enacted in Britain in 1866 following a cattle plague which killed over half a million cattle in 1865. It restricted the movement of livestock and enforced the slaughter of affected animals, and had a dramatic effect in bringing the epidemic under control.

Caucasian Supposed to have descended from people who lived in the Caucasus. Term is now used to represent fair-skinned people.

Caudal Anesthesia Caudal block was described by a French surgeon, Fernand Cathelin (b 1873) in 1901 and was used clinically by H. Schlimpert in 1911. The procedure was introduced into obstetrics by W. von Stoeckel in 1909. The epidural space, which lies within the boundaries of the sacrum, was termed the caudal space by Mildred Trotter in 1947. A paper on continuous caudal block in labor was published by Robert Andrew Hingson (b 1913) and Waldo Berry Edward (b 1905) of America in 1942. They found that labor could be made entirely painless without inhibiting uterine contractions or harming the fetus. A.H. Galley and J.H. Peel were amongst the first to use the method in England in 1944. *See epidural anesthesia.*

Caudate Lobe of the Liver [Latin: *cauda*, tail] The Spieghel lobe, described in 1627 by Andrein van der Spieghel (1578–1625), professor of anatomy in Venice and Padua.

Cautery Ancient Egyptians treated cancer with excision, cautery and astringents. Cautery, or burning of the chest wall, was recommended as a treatment for empyema by Galen (AD 129–200) and Paul of Aegina (625–690).

Hippocrates (460–377 BC) recommended cautery for glaucoma and conditions such as liver abscess and other infections. The fontanelle [French: *fontanelle*, little fountain], a point where sagittal and frontal sutures join, was used during the Middle Ages to apply cautery to cure cerebral and ocular diseases. Cautery with a hot iron was used to control bleeding in Europe up to the 16th century, when Ambroise Paré (1510–1590) replaced it with ligature. Auguste Nelaton (1807–1873), an eminent French surgeon in Paris, was the first to use electrocautery in surgery. Modern galvanocautery was invented by another French surgeon, Charles Gabriel Pravaz (1791–1853) in 1853. French physician, Claude Andre Paquelin (1836–1905) published a work on cautery in 1877. Italian surgeon, Enrico Bottini (1837–1903), described the use of galvanocautery in surgery in 1873. A new form of cautery, consisting of a battery, a single cell with platinum with a large surface area for applying heat, was devised by Robert Ellis of England in 1861.

Cave Drawings One of the earliest records available to study prehistoric cultures. The pictures of mammoths, such as those found in the La Madeleine caves in France, have rendered support for the theory that early humans coexisted with such species during prehistoric times. The drawing of a witch doctor wearing a deer mask over his face, found in a cave at Les Trois Freres in France, is estimated to have been drawn about 39,000 years ago by Cro-Magnon man, the first modern humans of Europe. *See Altamira cave paintings.*

Cavendish Society For the publication of research in chemistry, established in 1846.

Cavendish, Charles (1703–1783) English physicist who constructed a maximum/minimum thermometer in 1757.

Cavendish, Henry (1731–1810) Nephew of the third Duke of Devonshire and a son of Charles Cavendish. He studied hydrogen and gave it the name 'inflammable air' in 1766. He combined hydrogen and oxygen by means of an electric arc in 1783, and demonstrated that water is a compound and not an element. His accuracy in measuring the gravitation and density of the Earth has not been surpassed by modern methods.

Cavendish, Margaret Duchess of Newcastle She fought against prejudice and became the first woman member of the Royal Society in 1667. No other woman was admitted to the Royal Society until 1945.

Caventou, Joseph Bienaime (1795–1877) Professor at the École de Pharmacie in Paris. He isolated the alkaloid emetine from ipecacuanha. While working with Pierre

Joseph Pelletier (1788–1842) he obtained strychnine and brucine from the plant *Strychnos*. His other achievements include the isolation of quinine and cinchonine from cinchona bark in 1820; caffeine from coffee beans in 1822; and veratrine in 1818. He also isolated chlorophyll and gave it its present name. *See cinchona.*

Cavernous Sinus Syndrome [Latin: *cavernosus*, chambered + *sinus*, curve or gulf] Thrombosis of the cavernous sinus with involvement of its lateral wall leading to paralysis of the third, fourth, fifth and sixth cranial nerves. Described by Charles Foix (1882–1927) of Paris in 1922.

Cecostomy H. Pillore of Rouen was the first to open the cecum onto the right iliac region through a peritoneal incision in a patient with carcinoma of the rectum, in 1776.

Cecum [Latin: *caecus*, blind] 'Blind gut' was first called the 'appendicula caeci' by Rufus of Ephesus in the 1st century. Paracelsus (1493–1541) named the structure the monocolon.

Celiac Disease Non-tropical sprue due to gluten-induced enteropathy. Described by Samuel Jones Gee (1839–1911) of St Bartholomew's Hospital, in 1888. It was redescribed by Christian Archibald Herter (1865–1910) in 1908 and Thorald Einar Hess Thayssen (1883–1986) in 1929.

Cell Division Studied by Matthias Jacob Schleiden (1804–1881) in 1838. A pioneer German botanist and professor at Bonn, Eduard Adolf Strasburger (1844–1912) published *Cell Formation and Cell Division* in 1875. Mitosis, the process of nuclear division involving the chromosomes in the cell, was described by Walther Flemming (1843–1905) in his classical account in 1882. The term 'anaphase' was introduced by Flemming in 1882. It was also described by German cytologist, Friedrich Anton Schneider (1831–1890).

Cell Nucleus [Latin: *cella*, compartment + *nucleus*, little nut] Described by Robert Brown (1773–1858) in 1831.

Cell Receptors The cell receptors embedded in the cell membrane of an egg cell were found by Thomas F. Roth and Keith R. Porter in 1964.

Cell Theory *See cell.*

Cell [Latin: *cella* or *celo*, to conceal] Robert Hook (1635–1703) adopted the term in biology to refer to the compartments that he noted in cork under the microscope in 1665. The structure of plants was observed two decades later by Marcello Malpighi (1628–1694) and Nehemiah Grew (1641–1712). The nucleus was described by Robert Brown (1773–1858) in 1831, and the nucleolus by Gabriel Gustav

Valentine (1810–1883) in 1836. The role of the nucleus in cell division and the formation of tissues was studied by a German botanist, Matthias Jacob Schleiden (1804–1881) in 1838. His *Grundzuge der Wissenschaftlichen Botanik* published in 1842 was one of the first books on plant cytology. The structure of specialized cells, such as nerve cells and smooth muscle cells, was examined by Theodor Schwann (1821–1902) in 1839. He coined the famous phrase *Omnis cellula e cellula* (every cell from a cell). Analysis of diseased tissue on the basis of cell formation and structure was done by Rudolph Virchow (1821–1902) in his *Cellular Pathology,* published in 1858. The first electron-microscopic study, showing structures such as the endoplasmic reticulum and mitochondria, was performed by an American cytologist of Belgian origin, Albert Claude (1899–1983), in 1945.

Cellier, Elizabeth English midwife in the 17th century who went to prison for her political involvement. She was largely instrumental in licensing midwives.

Cellular Respiration French chemist, Antoine Lavoisier (1743–1794), in his treatise on heat in 1780, stated that 'respiration is therefore a combustion, slow it is true, but otherwise perfectly similar to that of charcoal'. He thought that combustion of foodstuff occurred in the lung, and Justus von Liebig (1803–1873) believed that it took place in the blood. Eduard Pfluger (1829–1910) was the first to point out that tissues were the site of respiration. Cytochromes, hydrogen acceptors in cellular respiration, were discovered by C.A. MacMunn in 1886. Glutathione, a hydrogen carrier in cellular respiration, was isolated by Frederick Gowland Hopkins (1861–1947) of Cambridge University in 1921.

Cellulose *See nitrocellulose.*

Celom Theory [Greek: *koiloma,* hollow] *See gastraea theory.*

Celsius, Anders (1704–1744) Swedish astronomer who was appointed to the Chair of Astronomy at Uppsala in 1730. He defined the boiling point of water as 100° and the freezing point as 0° in his *Observationer om Tvenne Bestandiga Grader par en Thermometer* in 1742. The temperature scale he defined was later named Celsius. *See thermometer.*

Celsus, Aulus Cornelius (25 BC–AD 50) Roman physician who lived during the reign of Tiberius Caesar (42 BC–AD 37). His manuscripts on veterinary medicine, agriculture and medicine were lost for several centuries until they were discovered by Thomas of Sarzana who later became Pope Nicholas V in 1443. Celsus' greatest work *De Re Medicina* (eight books), the first classical treatise on medicine to be printed, in 1478. The four cardinal signs of inflammation: rubor, dolor, color and tumor, are found in his fourth book.

His other contributions include treatises on the use of antiseptic substances, plastic surgery to the face and skin grafting.

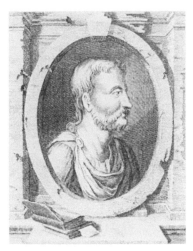

Aulus Cornelius Celsus. Courtesy of the National Library of Medicine

Census The first census was taken by Moses – of the Israelites. King David carried out a census in 1017 BC. The census became a regular feature in the Roman Empire. The first census in Ireland was taken by Sir William Petty (1623–1687) of Hampshire, in 1687.

Centrifuge A machine to increase the force of gravity and speed up the rate of sedimentation to measure the size of small particles. Used by Swedish physical chemist, Theodor Svedberg (1884–1971) and J.B. Nichols in 1923. It was used for separation of isotopes by mass by Jesse W. Beams in 1935.

Centriole Minute particles within the centrosome were described by German cytologist, Theodore Boveri (1862–1915) in 1888.

Centromere [Greek: *kentron,* center + *meros,* part] A self-propagating particle in the chromosome described by D.H. Wenrich. *See chromosomes.*

Centrosome [Greek: *kentron,* center + *soma,* body] A minute paired body in the ovum, lying outside the nucleus, was observed independently by Belgian cytologist, Edouard Joseph Louis Marie van Beneden (1845–1910) and Walther Flemming (1843–1905) of Germany in 1875. It was named by German biologist, Theodor Boveri (1862–1915) in 1888. It was later found in all cells and is regarded as the 'dynamic center' of cell division.

Cephalin [Greek: *kephale,* head] Cephalin and myelin in brain tissue were discovered by a German chemist, John Ludwig Wilhelm Thudichum (1829–1901), who worked as the director of the Chemical and Pathological Laboratory at St Thomas' Hospital, London.

Cerebellar Ataxia *See cerebellum.*

Cerebellum [Latin: *cerebellum*, small brain] Sometimes called the lesser brain, first distinguished from the main brain or cerebrum by Erasistratus of Chios (310–250 BC). Thomas Willis (1621–1675) in 1664 suggested that the cerebrum presided over voluntary motions, and the cerebellum controlled involuntary movements. No further study was made until Luigi Rolando (1773–1831) at Sassari in Sardinia published a series of observations on the effects of experimental removal in animals. He noted that ablation of the cerebellum did not affect mental characters or sensation. Luigi Luiciani (1840–1919) studied the consequence of removal of the cerebellum in higher mammals in 1891. The gang-lion cells in the cerebellum were observed by Johannes Evangelista Purkinje (1787–1869).

Cerebral Abscess One of the earliest operative treatments, by opening the lateral ventricles, was performed by William Detmold (1808–1897) of America in 1850.

Cerebral Angiography The method of radiologically visualizing the cerebral circulation by injecting radio-opaque sodium iodide into the carotid artery was introduced by Antonio Egaz Moniz (1874–1955) of Portugal in 1927. He and his assistant, Almeida Lima, injected sodium iodide into an exposed internal carotid artery. This substance was later noted to give rise to fits and was replaced with thorotrast, which itself was substituted with diodrast, used as a contrast material for many decades. Angiography was employed to differentiate between hemorrhage, thrombosis and em-bolism by I.S. Wechsler and S.W. Gross in 1949. *See cerebral circulation.*

Cerebral Circulation [Latin: *cerebrum*, brain] Ancient Egyptians thought that good pulsation of the brain at birth predicted will power, and this belief was also mentioned by Pliny, the Elder (AD 28–79). Thomas Willis (1621–1675) discovered the arterial supply of the brain by injecting the artery with 'aqua crocata' in 1664, and the network of arteries described by him was named the circle of Willis. Gabriele Falloppio (1523–1562) described the pulsation of the dural vessels in 1561 and cerebral vessels were mentioned by Humphrey Ridley (1653–1708), a London anatomist, in 1695. Alexander Monro (1733–1817) in 1793 believed that the arterial supply was fixed or limited as it was enclosed in a fixed cavity. London physician, George Burrowes, did research on cerebral circulation and published *On the Disorders of the Cerebral Circulation and the*

Connections between the Affections of the Brain and Diseases of the Heart in 1846. He considered the flow of blood in the brain to be fixed but influenced by posture. The circulation of blood within the brain was also described by Henri Duret (1849–1921) of Paris in 1873. Sir Leonard Erskine Hill (1866–1952) postulated the scientific theory that changes in the cerebral circulation were secondary to alterations in general circulation, in 1896.

Cerebral Cortex [Latin: *cerebrum*, brain + *cortex*, bark] The structural organization was observed in 1776 by an Italian anatomist Francesco Gennari (1750–1797) of Parma, while he was a medical student. He also made a special note of the white line in the cortex which was most prominent in the occipital area. This was identified as the primary visual cortex and named the 'Line of Gennari'. In 1840, the French psychiatrist Jules Gabriel François Baillarger (1809–1890) noted that these lines consisted of two bands separated by a thin dark line. They were traced throughout the cortex and named 'internal and external bands of Baillarger'. Theodore Herman Meynert (1833–1892) of Vienna systematically studied cortical cells and identified five horizontal layers in 1867. Knowledge on the different layers of the cortex was advanced by Russian neurologist, Vladimir Aleksandrovich Betz (1834–1894) in 1874, and by an English neuropsychiatrist, William Bevan Lewis (1847–1929) in 1878. The Italian neurologist Camillo Golgi (1844–1926) of Pavia discovered in 1886 that the cells with short axons ramified in the cortex. Elliot Smith (1871–1937) in 1907 divided the brain into 50 zones on the basis of Baillarger bands. *See brain, motor cortex, architronics.*

Cerebral Hemorrhage [Latin: *cerebrum*, brain + *haima*, blood] Shown to be the cause of apoplexy (stroke) in four cases at postmortem, by Johann Jacobus Wepfer (1620–1695) of Schaffhausen in 1658. Henry Bouchard, while working with Jean Martin Charcot (1825–1893) in Paris, described miliary aneurysms and associated these with cerebral hemorrhage in 1866. Apoplexy due to cerebral hemorrhage into the ventricles was described by Sir William Henry Broadbent (1835–1907) in 1876.

Cerebral Palsy *See spastic diplegia.*

Cerebrospinal Fever Meningitis. A report in England was given by Thomas Willis (1621–1675) in 1661, and in France by Gaspard Vieusseux (1746–1814) in 1805. A description in America was given 200 years later by Elisha North (1771–1843), a physician from Connecticut, in *A Treatise on Malignant Epidemic, Commonly called Spotted Fever* published in 1811. Intracranial infection as a result of head injury was recognized by Astley Paston Cooper (1768–1841) in 1824, but he did not differentiate between meningitis and encephalitis. The causative organism, the *Meningococcus* or *Diplococcus intercellularis meningitidis* was isolated from cerebrospinal fluid of patients with meningitis by Austrian pathologist, Anton Weichselbaum (1845–1920) in 1887. The symptoms of fever, vomiting, headache and irritability were described by William Richard Gowers (1845–1915) in 1888. Kernig sign in diagnosis was described by Russian neurologist, Michalovich Vladimir Kernig (1840–1917). Brudzinski sign as a diagnostic test, in which flexion of the ankle, knee and hip occurs when the neck is bent, was described by a Polish physician, J. Brudzinski (1874–1917). Simon Flexner (1863–1946), an American bacteriologist, prepared an antiserum for the treatment of cerebrospinal meningitis in 1908. Death due to circulatory disturbance and neural damage resulting from fulminating meningococcal septicemia was described by H. Worster, C. Drought and A.M. Kennedy in 1919.

Cerebrospinal Fluid (CSF) Hippocrates (460–377 BC) thought that the brain was a gland. The ancients believed that the secretions of the brain poured directly into the pharynx. Erasistratus, around the same time, described the four ventricles of the brain but did not mention any fluid in them. Galen (129–200) mentioned a fluid in the fourth ventricle which purged through the ethmoid into the nose. Andreas Vesalius (1514–1564) mentioned a 'watery humor of the brain' but without any description. The first definite mention was made by Italian anatomist, Costanzo Varoli (1545–1575) in 1573. It was observed and described in fish and turtles by Dominico Cotugno (1736–1822) in 1784, but he failed to detect it in humans. Antonio Maria Valsalva (1666–1723) mentioned a liquid similar to that found in joints when he cut open the brain of a dog in 1692. CSF rhinorrhea after trauma to the head was described by Stalpartius van der Wal in 1727. A clear-cut scientific description was given by Albrecht von Haller (1708–1777) in 1766. François Magendie (1783–1855) in 1825 described the functions, and Karl Friedrich August Lange (b 1883) in 1842 devoted nine pages to the fluid in his work on anatomy. The cell elements were studied by Jean Nageotte (1866–1948) and G.F. Isidore Widal (1862–1929) in 1901. The globulin content was precipitated with magnesium sulfate by French neurologist, Georges Guillain (1876–1971). William Dobinson Halliburton (1860–1931), professor of physiology at King's College London, studied the chemical composition, and the physics of cerebrospinal fluid pressure was studied by Bernard Naunym (1839–1925) of Berlin. The pathway and circulation of the fluid was elucidated by Lewis Hall in 1915. Analysis of proteins in the CSF, by precipitation with sodium chloride and gold solution, was developed from the findings of Richard Adolf Zsigmondy (1866–1930) by Lange in 1912. A method of detecting an increase in globulin in the CSF using carbolic acid was devised by a Budapest psychiatrist, Kalman Pandy (b 1868) in 1910. *See lumbar puncture.*

Cerebrovascular Accident Syn. stroke. *See apoplexy.*

Cervical Disc Prolapse [Latin: *cervix*, neck; Greek: *diskos*, disc; Latin: *prolapsus*, fallen or slid down] *See brachial neuritis.*

Cervical Rib Syndrome (Syn. thoracic inlet syndrome, thoracic outlet syndrome, scalenus anterior syndrome) E. Bramwell in 1903 pointed out the first cervical rib as a cause of pressure symptoms, and a classic treatise was written by William Williams Keen (1837–1932) of America in 1907. The division of the first rib as treatment was performed by T. Murphy in 1910. Other symptoms due to compression of the brachial plexus and blood vessels were recognized by Alfred Washington Adson (1887–1951) of Rochester, Minnesota and I. Caffey. Adson, a graduate of the University of Nebraska (1912), was a pioneer in neurosurgery at the Mayo Clinic, and described the sign (Adson sign) in which the radial pulse became obliterated when the head was turned to the affected side. He also recommended the division of the scelenus anterior muscle for relief of symptoms in 1947. The name 'scalenus syndrome' was given to the condition by an American surgeon, Howard Christian Naffziger (b 1884) of San Francisco in 1937.

Cervical Smear The use of cytology in a clinical setting was introduced by George Nicholas Papanicolaou (1883–1962), who commenced his work in 1917. He investigated the normal cyclical changes of the vaginal epithelium with Charles Rupert Stockard (1879–1939) and described the role of the vaginal smear in the diagnosis of cancer in 1928. Papanicolaou and Herbert Frederick Traut (b 1894) later published *The Diagnosis of Uterine Cancer by Vaginal Smear* in 1943. Important cytological studies were also done in England by Leonard Stanley Dudgeon (1876–1938) and colleagues in 1927 and 1934. The use of routine cytological examination for early detection of cervical carcinoma and preinvasive lesions was intensified by G.H. Green in 1965 and D.J.B. Ashley in 1966. Their value as a routine screen was established by T.N. Roman and J.P.A. Latour in 1967.

Cervix [Latin: *cervix*, neck] *See carcinoma of the cervix, cervical smear.*

Cesarean Hysterectomy The removal of a pregnant uterus was demonstrated in dogs and sheep by Joseph Cavallini in 1768. The procedure following delivery was performed by

Boston obstetrician, Horatio Robinson Storer (1830–1922) in 1868. Eduoardo Porro (1842–1902) of Padua Italy performed the operation on a 25-year-old primigravid dwarf in 1876.

Cesarean Section Numa Pompilius, the ruler of Rome around 700 BC, made a declaration that if any pregnant woman died without delivering her child her abdomen should be cut open to deliver it. This decree or Lex Regia later became known as Lex Caesare under subsequent emperors. The practice is mentioned by Pliny (AD 28–79) as a very ancient procedure, although no mention of it was made by Hippocrates (460–377 BC). It is next in *Chirugia Guidonis de Cauliaco* published around 1350 which recommended the practice only on a dead mother who had not delivered. Ambroise Paré (1510–1590) advocated the procedure in France in the same circumstances. Caspar Bauhin (1560–1624) gave an account of a Swiss sow-gelder, Jacob Nufer, who performed a Cesarean section on his wife in 1500. Nufer's wife is recorded to have had several other children and lived to 77 years. This is the first record of success of the procedure on a live mother. François Rousset (1535–1590), a contemporary of Paré, wrote the first complete treatise with case histories and illustrations in 1586. Hieronymus Mercurialis (1550–1616), the author of the first Italian book on obstetrics, advocated Cesarean section in cases of contracted pelvis in 1585. Modern Cesarean section on live mothers was pioneered by Raphael B. Sabatier (1732–1811) and Jean Louis Baudlocque (1746–1810) of France. A successful operation in England was reported by James Barlow of Lancashire in 1798. The first for childbirth in America was performed by John Lambert Richmond (1785–1855), a former coal miner who was a pastor as well as a physician in a small community outside Cincinnati in 1827. The chief causes of death following Cesarean operations in the 19th century were hemorrhage, nervous shock and peritonitis. In a set of statistics published by Pihan-Dueffilay in Germany in 1861, 38 patients out of 88 who underwent the procedure died.

Cesium Element discovered through spectrum analysis by G.R. Kirchhoff (1824–1887) and Robert Bunsen (1811–1899) in 1860.

Cestan–Chenais Syndrome Ipsilateral paralysis of the vocal cords and soft palate, with contralateral hemiplegia and sensory loss due to pontobulbar lesions caused by the occlusion of the vertebral artery below the level of the posterior inferior cerebella artery, or a tumor. Described by French neurologist, R. Cestan (1872–1934) and French physician, L.J. Chenais (1872–1950) in 1903.

Cetrimide Introduced as an antiseptic in 1947.

Ceylon (Sri Lanka) Eratosthenes (274–194 BC) of Alexandria estimated the distance from the Atlantic to the Eastern Ocean to be 7800 miles, and the distance of the Cinnamon Land or Tabrobane (Ceylon) from Thule to be 3800 miles. It was ruled in 160 BC by King Dutta Gemunu or Dutha Gamani, who is credited with having built 18 hospitals to which he formally appointed physicians. Buddhadasa, a king of Ceylon who lived around AD 341, is supposed to have been a skilled surgeon who built several asylums and hospitals. Herman Paul, a physician to Dutch settlers in Ceylon in the 17th century, published a description of several natural elements and plants from Ceylon in *Museum Zeylanicum* before he returned to Holland as the professor of botany at Leiden in 1685. The first overseas branch of the British Medical Association in the Indian subcontinent was established in Ceylon in 1887. Aldo Castellini (1877–1971) elucidated the etiology of yaws in 1906 and described pulmonary moniliasis (tea taster's lung) in 1905 while he was working as a bacteriologist in Ceylon from 1903 to 1915. The British surgeon, Sir Frederick Treves (1853–1923) in his *The Other side of Lantern*, described scenic beauty of Ceylon. *See Vedas.*

Chaddock Sign In which an extensor plantar response is obtained by stroking the skin in the area of the external malleolus in cases of pyramidal tract lesions. Described by a neurologist in St Louis, Charles Gilbert Chaddock (1861–1936).

Chadwick Sign Blue coloration of the vaginal mucosa in early pregnancy. Described by Boston gynecologist, James Read Chadwick (1844–1905), in 1887.

Chadwick, Edwin (1800–1890) Lawyer and sanitary reformer from Manchester, England. As a secretary to the Poor Law Commission set up by Lord Henry Grey (1802–1894) in 1834, he aroused public awareness of poor sanitation in England. His *Report on the Sanitary Conditions of the Labouring Population* was released in 1842. *See sewers.*

Chadwick, Sir James (1891–1974) English physicist, born near Macclesfield. He studied at Manchester, Berlin and Cambridge, and worked with Ernest Rutherford (1871–1937) on atoms. He discovered the particle almost exactly like a proton but with no charge on it, previously proposed by Rutherford (1920) in 1932. Chadwick named it 'neutron' and was awarded the Nobel Prize in 1935. He wrote *Radiation from Radioactive Substances* with Rutherford in 1930, and built the first cyclotron in England at Liverpool in 1935.

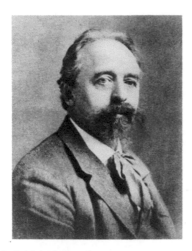

James Read Chadwick (1789–1869)

Chagas Disease South American trypanosomiasis due to *Trypanosoma cruzi*, first described in Lasance, a village in the state of Minas Geras in Brazil by a Brazilian physician, Carlos Chagas (1879–1974), in 1909. Some medical historians believe that Charles Darwin's symptoms during the latter part of his life were due to Chagas disease.

Chagas, Carlos (1879–1974) Brazilian physician from Oliveira who graduated from the medical school at Rio de Janeiro in 1903. In 1909, during one of his field missions to the village of Lasance situated in the interior of Brazil, he discovered the protozoan, *Trypanosoma* and its insect vector that caused South American trypanosomiasis. This disease was later named after him.

Chain, Sir Ernest Boris (1906–1979) German-born British biochemist of Jewish origin. He escaped from Nazi Germany and came to work in Cambridge and Oxford. At the Dunn School of Pathology, Oxford, he worked with Howard Walter Florey (1895–1968) and produced a pure extract of penicillin from *Penicillium notatum* in 1940. The chemotherapeutic effect of penicillin was also demonstrated by Chain and co-workers in the same year.

Chalazion Described as a concretion of inert fluid in the eye by Paul of Aegina (625–690). Aetius of Amida recommended incision as treatment in AD 600.

Chalcolithic Period An era of human culture during which time copper remained as the predominant metal.

Chaldea An ancient name for Babylon.

Chaldeans *See Babylonian medicine.*

Chamberlain Family Obstetricians, whose family arrived in England as Huguenot refugees from France. William

Chamberlain along with his wife and children, Peter, Simon and Jane, reached England in 1569. He understood the use of obstetric forceps and this was guarded as a family secret. His son, Peter Chamberlain, the elder practiced obstetrics in Southampton for some time, while his father and younger brother practiced in London. After the death of his father, Peter moved to London. He had two sons: Hugh Chamberlain, the elder (1632–1720) and Paul Chamberlain (1635–1717) who were also obstetricians. Hugh had a son of the same name (1664–1728) who was also an obstetrician in London. *See Chamberlain, Hugh, the elder.*

Chamberlain, Hugh, the Elder (1632–1720?) Grandson of Peter Chamberlain, the elder. Hugh graduated from Trinity College Cambridge in 1664 and became a male midwife and attended the wife of James II. He tried to sell the secret of the obstetric forceps, invented by his grandfather Peter, to the French obstetrician, François Mauriceau (1637–1709) on a visit to Paris, but Mauriceau set an almost impossible task to the overconfident Chamberlain by asking him to deliver the baby of a 30-year-old rachitic dwarf with a deformed pelvis who had been in labor for 8 days. Chamberlain, who claimed to be able to do it in quarter of an hour, gave up after trying for 4 hours. On his return from Paris, he brought a copy of Mauriceau's *Des Maladies des Femmes Grosses et Accouchees* which he translated into English. It remained a bestseller for the next century. Chamberlain later sold the forceps to a Dutch obstetrician, Rogier van Roonhuyze in 1692.

Chamberland, Charles (1851–1908) A pioneer in methods of sterilizing medical equipment who invented the autoclave. *See bacterial filters.*

Chamberland–Pasteur Filter *See bacterial filters.*

Chamberlayne, William (1619–1689) Medical poet who practiced in Shaftsbury, Dorset. His poems include *Love's Victory, a Tragy-Comedy* (1659) and *Pharonnida, a Heroick Poem.*

Chambre, John (1470–1549) English physician in Northumberland who studied medicine in Oxford and Padua. He became physician to King Henry VIII and the warden of Merton College, Oxford.

Chancroid Sexually transmitted infection characterized by ulceration of the male and female external genitalia. Studied by Leon Bassereau (1811–1888) of Paris, a pupil of Phillipe Ricord (1800–1889), in 1852. The causative organism was discovered by Augusto Ducrey (1860–1940) in 1889. It was later named *Haemophilus ducreyi*, in honor of its discoverer.

Chandos Professorship In medicine and anatomy at St

Andrew's Medical School in Scotland. Created by the Duke of Chandos (1673–1744) with a donation of £1000 through his son's tutor and physician, Charles Stuart, in 1722.

Chantemmesse, Andre (1851–1919) A bacteriologist from Paris who worked with Isidor Widal (1862–1929) on typhoid toxin and antityphoid serum. He isolated the dysentery bacillus in 1888.

Chapple Sign Limitation of abduction, occurring in congenital dislocation of the hip. Described by Charles Culloden Chapple in 1935.

Chaput, Henri (1857–1919) French surgeon who performed ureterosigmoidostomy for urinary diversion. He designed an operation for artificial anus in 1896.

Charaka A Hindu Brahman physician around 100 BC. His most important work on medicine, *Charaka Samhita,* displayed medical knowledge in the form of a dialogue between master and student. *See Ayurvedic medicine.*

Charas, Moses (1618–1698) Apothecary from Languedoc in France who wrote a pharmacopoeia in two volumes in 1673. This was translated into Chinese for the use of the Emperor. Charas was also known for his work on poisons.

Charcot Joints Progressive joint damage caused by excessive range of movement due to loss of pain sensation secondary to neuropathy or other neurological disease was described by Jean Martin Charcot (1825–1893) in 1868.

Charcot Triad Intention tremor, nystagmus and scanning speech, seen in multiple sclerosis is named after the French neurologist, Jean Martin Charcot (1825–1893).

Charcot, Jean-Martin (1825–1893) The greatest of French neurologists, born in Paris. He graduated in 1853, and became a physician to the great hospital of Salpêtrière in 1862. Apart from his vast contributions to neurology, he also did work on biliary passages, the liver and kidneys. His contributions to neurology include: *Localization and Functions of Cerebral Diseases* (1876), *Cortical Motor Centers in Man* (1895), *Lesions in Muscular Atrophy* (1886), *Peroneal Muscular Atrophy* (1886) with Pierre Marie (1853–1940), and *Miliary Aneurysms* with Abel Bouchard (1833–1899). In the last two decades of his career he started using hypnosis in diagnosis and treatment. This had a profound influence on one of his pupils, Sigmund Freud (1856–1939). Charcot's *Leçons sur les Maladies due Systeme Nerveux* was published in five volumes in 1872–1893. Sir William Osler (1848–1919) stated that 'no writer has more graphically described the trophic troubles following spinal and cerebral disorders particularly the acute bed sore than Charcot'. The

lenticulostriate artery described by Charcot is named after him. *See Charcot joints.*

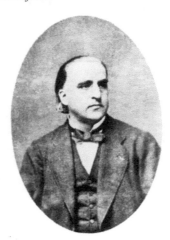

Jean-Martin Charcot (1825–1893). Courtesy of the National Library of Medicine

Charcot–Leyden Crystals Seen in the sputum of patients with bronchial asthma, named after the French neurologist, Jean Martin Charcot (1825–1893) and German physician, E.V. von Leyden (1832–1910).

Charcot–Marie–Tooth–Hoffmann Syndrome (Syn. peroneal muscular atrophy, familial atrophy) An autosomal dominant inherited muscular atrophy due to neurological changes in the nerves and the spinal cord. Described by Jean Martin Charcot (1825–1893) and Pierre Marie (1853–1940) in 1886. Howard Henry Tooth (1856–1926), an English physician, described it independently in the same year, and the German physician, Johan Hoffmann (1857–1919) gave a description in 1897.

Chardonnet, Comte Hilaire de (1839–1924) Pupil of Louis Pasteur (1822–1895) during the time that he was investigating silkworm disease. Inspired by the work of Pasteur on the subject, he invented the process of making artificial silk in 1884. He also experimented on the effect of ultraviolet light on organisms and invented an actinograph which was used to measure solar radiation in aviation.

Charing Cross Hospital Hospital and its medical school founded by Benjamin Golding in 1818. Its original site was in the Strand in central London. It moved to its present site on Fulham Palace Road in Hammersmith in 1973.

Charles Law The volume of a gas is proportional to its absolute temperature at constant pressure. Law proposed by Jacques Alexander Cesar Charles (1746–1823), professor of physics in Paris in 1787.

Charles, Jacques Alexander Cesar (1746–1823) Professor of physics in Paris who preceded Joseph Louis Gay-Lussac (1778–1850) in proposing the law of expansion of gases in 1787, but failed to publish his findings. Charles successfully flew along the Champs de Mars in a hydrogen balloon in 1783.

Charleton, Walter (1619–1707) Physician from Shepton Mallet in Somerset, who was attending physician to Charles I in 1641. He later accompanied Charles II abroad as his physician during his exile. He published *Chorea Gigantum or the most famous Antiquity of Great Britain, vulgarly called Stonehenge standing on Salisbury Plains, restored to the Danes,* in which he suggested a Danish origin for Stonehenge, in 1663. He was elected President of the Royal College of Physicians in 1689. He wrote the first English book on modern physiology based on experimentation in 1659.

Charmis Physician in Rome during the time of Nero, who mostly practiced quack medicine and charged extravagant fees.

Charnley Prosthesis Prosthesis for the hip joint devised around 1961 by Sir John Charnley (1911–1982) professor of orthopedics at Manchester University. *See Charnley, Sir John.*

Charnley, Sir John (1911–1982) Eminent British orthopedic surgeon, born in Bury, Lancashire and educated at Manchester University. After serving as an orthopedic surgeon during World War II, he returned to Manchester Royal Infirmary where he pioneered artificial hip joints in 1961. The long-term results of a series of Charnley's artificial joints made of Teflon were unsatisfactory. He started using polythene from 1962 and this gave better results. He was knighted in 1977.

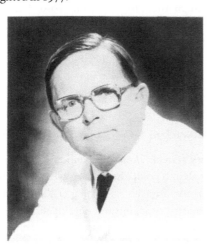

Sir John Charnley (1911–1982). Courtesy of the National Library of Medicine

Charriere Scale Scale for grading the size of urethral and ureteric catheters. Introduced by a Paris instrument maker, Joseph François Bernard (1803–1876).

Chartist Movement Movement to represent the problems of the working classes in London, activated from 1834 to 1848 on the basis of reforms preached by the English inventor and clergyman, Edmund Cartwright (1743–1823). This led to the formation of the London Work Men's Association in 1836 and the People's Charter in 1838.

Chassaignac, Marie Edouard (1805–1879) Surgeon in Paris who described the space between the pectoralis major and the mammary gland (Chassaignac space) in 1836. The carotid tubercle on the transverse process of the sixth vertebra (Chassaignac tubercle) is also named after him.

Chastity Belt Known in Europe during the second half of the 12th century. It is illustrated in one of the Göttingen manuscripts of Kyeser published in 1405. Although it is thought to have come from the East, the origin of the device is not certain. The girdle was known in Germany during the 16th century. John Moodie, a practitioner from Edinburgh, wrote a treatise on it in the 17th century in which he explained how to make chastity belts for girls who indulged in self abuse.

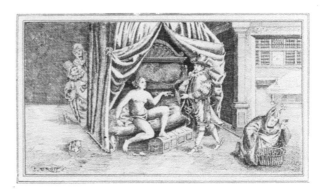

Chastity belt. Lucien Nass, *Curiosités Médico-Artistiques* (1907). Albin Michel, Paris

Chatelier, Henry le (1850–1936) Chemist from Paris. He discovered the law of equilibrium in a reaction, related to temperature and pressure in 1888.

Chaucer, Geoffrey (1340–1400) English poet, supposed to have written the earliest treatise on science in England, *Tractus Conclusonibus Astralabi* on his presentation of an astrolabe to his 10-year-old son. The influence of Aristotle during the Middle Ages in England is revealed by his phrase 'of Aristotle and his philosophye' in the Prologue of the *Canterbury Tales*. The English surgeon John of Arderne

(1307–1360) was probably the model chosen for Chaucer's Doctor of Physik, who had a love for gold. Some other medical historians believe that John of Gaddesden (1280–1361) was the Doctor of Physik in Chaucer's Tales.

Chauffard, Anatole Marie Emile (1855–1932) Physician in Paris. The point of tenderness below the right clavicle (Chauffard point) in cases of cholecystitis is named after him. He described rheumatoid arthritis in children between first and second dentition (Still–Chauffard syndrome), and pseudoxanthoma elasticum in 1889, He described Acholuric familial jaundice (Minkowski–Chauffard syndrome) in 1907.

Chauliac, Guy de (1300–1370) Born in Auvergne, France, the most celebrated surgeon in the 14th century. He was a student of the Italian anatomist Mundinus (1270–1326), who eliminated astrology and mysticism from surgery. He extracted cataracts, resected tumors and performed other operations which are described in his *Chirugia Magna* written in 1363.

Chaulmoogra Oil Obtained from the seed of the kalaw tree (*Gynocardia odorata*), it was already known to the Hindus as a cure for leprosy in India thousands of years ago. A Burmese legend states that Rama, the king of Benares, when he contacted leprosy, retired to the jungle and cured himself by taking the leaves and fruits of the kalaw or chaulmoogra tree. The AyurVeda of the Brahmins also refers to the value of chaulmoogra or *tuvarka*, the Chinese called it Ta-Fung-Tsze. The oil was introduced to the West by Frederick John Mourat (1816–1897) in 1854, and continued to be used as a treatment for leprosy until the 1920s. The contents of the oil were analyzed by Fredrick Belding Power (1853–1927) in 1902.

Chaussier, François (1746–1828) Anatomist and surgeon in Paris who discovered the external circumflex branch of the deep femoral artery which supplied the quadriceps muscle, in 1789.

Chavasse Operation Myomectomy of the inferior oblique muscle, devised by an ophthalmologist from Liverpool, Bernard Chavasse (1889–1941).

Cheadle Disease Infantile scurvy, named after London pediatrician, Walter Butler Cheadle (1836–1910), who differentiated between scurvy and rickets in 1877.

Cheatle Forceps For removal of instruments from a steam sterilizer. Devised by London surgeon, Sir George Lenthal Cheatle (1865–1951).

Chediak–Higashi Syndrome An autosomal recessive condition, in which vacuolated neutrophils and eosinophils occur in association with albinism, photophobia, nystagmus and recurrent infection. Independently described by a Cuban physician, M. Chediak (b 1903) in 1952 and a Japanese pediatrician, O. Higashi in 1954.

Cheese Hippocrates (460–377 BC) described cheese as indigestible and flatulent, and mentioned a special kind of cheese, hippace, made from mare's milk by the Scythians. Aulus Cornelius Celsus (25 BC–AD 50) also considered it as flatulent, and ranked it amongst other unwholesome articles of food. Galen (AD 129–200), in *De Alimente*, gave an ample description of the nature and properties of cheese. Pliny (AD 28–79) described several kinds of cheese and discussed the merit of each. He stated that salted cheese caused wasting and that soft cheese was nutritious.

Cheese Washer Lung Allergic condition due to *Penicillium caesi* spores in workers who removed mold from the surface of mature cheese. Described in Switzerland by Schlueter in 1973.

Chelsea Garden of Physick Garden of medical herbs established by the Apothecary's Society of London in 1676.

Chemical Pathology The first chemical investigation of blood was done by French physician and chemist, Hilaire Marin Rouelle (1718–1779), who found sodium carbonate, potassium chloride and sodium chloride in vertebrate blood in 1773. He also isolated urea from urine and demonstrated its high nitrogen content. Chemical pathology was established as a branch of medicine by Swedish professor of biochemistry at Harvard University, Otto Knut Olof Folin (1867–1934) with his microchemical method of estimation of blood glucose and other blood constituents, around 1915. His colorimetric method was later developed to measure microquantities of constituents such as urea nitrogen and uric acid in the blood, around 1919. The method of radioimmunoassay for measuring minute amounts of biologically active substances such as hormones and enzymes in the blood was introduced by Solomon A. Berson (1918–1972), Rosalyn Sussman Yalow (b 1921) a New York physiologist and colleagues in 1956. *See chromatography, diagnostic enzymology.*

Chemical Warfare *See gas warfare.*

Chemistry [Greek: *chemia*, alchemists' art of transmutating base metals into gold] The first person to apply chemistry to medicine was Paracelsus (1493–1541). This field, known as iatrochemistry, was further developed by Baptiste van Helmont (1577–1644). The first book of chemistry that was separated from the beliefs of alchemy was published by a German physician and chemist, Andreas Libavius or Libau

(1540–1616) of Halle. His book, *Alchemia* in 1597 described: stannic chloride as *spiritus fumans libavi*; the preparation of hydrated crystals of sugar; and the production of wine by fermentation. Another important book dissociated from alchemy, *Tyrocinium chymicum*, was published by Jean Beguin (1550–1620) of France in 1610. This was followed by that of van Helmont who described the properties of a gas and gave it the present name. Iatrochemistry was further developed by a German chemist and physician, Johann Rudolph Glauber (1604–1668). He refined the method of distillation and studied the reactions of the three main mineral acids. He is better known for his various secret remedies including Glauber salt. The calcination of metals on exposure to air was shown by Jean Rey, a physician from Paris in the early 16th century. The principles of physics were applied to gases by Robert Boyle (1627–1691) around 1662. Joseph Priestley (1733–1804), a clergyman and chemist from Leeds, made several discoveries in the field of chemistry and established it as a science in England. He helped to disprove the phlogiston theory, which had been held for over 100 years, by obtaining pure oxygen through heating a metal oxide. The compound of chlorine and hydrogen, muriatic acid, was also discovered by Priestley in 1772. A clear account of chemistry, *Cours de Chemie*, was written by French physician and chemist, Nicolas Lemery (1645–1715). A systematic chemical dictionary, *Dictionaire de Chyme*, was published by French chemist, Pierre Joseph Macquer (1718–1784) in 1766. Antoine Laurent Lavoisier (1743–1794) of Paris defined an element as 'a substance that cannot be split into a simpler form by any means', and investigated 'dephlogisticated air' which had previously been described by Priestley in 1774. He also proved that 'dephlogisticated air' was responsible for combustion and called it the 'acidifying principle', from which the present name oxygen [Greek: *oxys*, sharp + *gen*, to produce] is derived. The use of chemical symbols to denote the elements in chemistry was introduced by Berzelius (1779–1848) in 1811. Colloid chemistry was established by Thomas Graham (1805–1869) around 1857. Michael Faraday (1791–1867) was the first to liquefy carbon dioxide by applying pressure and he condensed chlorine into liquid in 1823. Industrial chemistry was established by Justus von Liebig (1803–1873) of Germany. A method of determining vapor density was discovered by John Baptiste Andre Dumas (1800–1884), an apothecary at Geneva, in 1823. A major advance in organic chemistry was made by Friedrich Wöhler (1800–1882) who synthesized urea from potassium cyanate and ammonium sulfate in 1829. Liebig and Wöhler published their work on the oil of bitter almonds, which essentially contained benzaldehyde, in 1831. Pierre Eugene Marcelin Berthelot (1827–1907) of

Paris produced benzene and naphthalene in 1851, and the six-carbon ring structure for benzene was proposed by Friedrich August Kekulé (1829–1896) in 1865.

Chemotherapy [Greek: *chemia*, mutation + *therapio*, to take care of] Term coined by Paul Ehrlich (1854–1915) to denote 'the use of drugs to injure an invading organism without injury to the host'. Only a few chemotherapeutic agents such as mercury were known before 1898. In 1904 he produced the first man-made chemotherapeutic agent, trypan red, which cured mice infected with trypanosomiasis. Harold Wolferston Thomas and Anton Breinl from the School of Tropical Medicine at Liverpool developed the second most effective drug 'atoxyl' against trypanosomes in 1905. This was followed by the discovery of arsphenamine, also known as salvarsan, by Ehrlich in 1910. The concept of a 'chemotherapeutic index', the ratio of minimal curative dose to maximal tolerated dose, was also developed by Ehrlich. Acriflavin was introduced as an antibacterial substance by Carl Hamilton Browning (1881–1972), a pupil of Ehrlich, in 1913. The phenomenon of drug interaction or therapeutic interference was discovered by Browning and R. Gulbransen in 1922. A major breakthrough in the fight against bacteria was achieved by the discovery of the first antibacterial sulfonamide, Protonsil, by Gerhard Domagk (1895–1964) in 1935. The science of analytical control of the blood level of therapeutic agents during therapy was established by Eli Kennerley Marshall (1889–1966) in 1937. *See antibiotics, cancer therapy.*

Chenopodium *See antihelmintics.*

Chernobyl Nuclear Accident Catastrophic accidental release of radioactivity at Chernobyl near Kiev in Russia on 26 April 1986. The incident, which led to dozens of deaths, was initially thought to be localized. Subsequent studies have revealed that the radioactivity from the reactor was found in many areas of Europe.

Cherubin, Le Pere A French friar, mathematician and philosopher of Orleans who applied binocular lenses to the microscope in 1677. He wrote *Dioptrique Oculaire* and *La Vision Parfaite*.

Cherwell, Frederick Alexander Lindemann (1886–1957). *See calorimeter.*

Cheselden, William (1688–1752) Born in Burrow-on-the-Hill, Leicestershire, he studied surgery at St Thomas' Hospital, London. He was a pupil of the famous anatomist William Cowper (1666–1709) and began to deliver lectures at the age of 22. He published a syllabus in 1711, and *Anatomy of the Human Body* in 1713. He became chief surgeon at St Thomas' Hospital and visiting surgeon at St George's Hospital and the Westminster Infirmary. He was famous as a lithotomist and wrote *Treatise on the High Operation for Stone* in 1723, and another treatise on anatomy of the bones in 1733. Architecture was one of his leisure interests and he designed the Old Surgeon's Hall at the Old Bailey. At the time of his death he was chief surgeon to the Chelsea Hospital.

Chevreul, Michel Eugene (1786–1889) French chemist and gerontologist from Angers. He is known as the 'father of fatty acids' because of his research on margarine, olein, stearin and other fatty acids. In 1823 he discovered that fat was composed of fatty acids and glycerol. Cholesterol, one of the earliest known sterols, was described by him in 1815. Towards the end of his career he studied the psychiatric effects of old age, which made him a pioneer in psychogeriatrics.

Chewing Platina Cremonensis, an Italian medical writer in the 16th century wrote specifically on the act of chewing. He advised tender people of small frame to chew their food well if they expected their stomach to digest it in his treatise on health addressed to Cardinal Roverella in 1529.

Cheyne Disease A morbid anxiety about health leading to hypochondriasis was described by George Cheyne (1671–1743) in 1733.

Cheyne, George (1671–1743) Scottish physician who completed his medical studies under Archibald Pitcairn (1652–1713) in Edinburgh. He later moved to London, where his change of eating habits caused him to reach a weight of over 32 stones (448 lb or 201 kg). He embarked on a successful reducing diet of vegetables and published his experience in *An Essay on Health and Long Life*. He also wrote *A New Theory of Fevers, Philosophical Principles of Natural Religion, An Essay on Method of Treating the Gout, The English Malady or Treatise of Nervous Diseases* and *The Natural Method of Curing the Diseases of the Body*.

Cheyne, John (1777–1836) Physician from Dublin and the son of a surgeon, who entered Edinburgh University at the age of 15 years. He studied anatomy with Charles Bell (1774–1842), and wrote his first book *Essays on the Diseases of Children* in 1801. He wrote an early monograph on laryngology, *Pathology of the Membrane of the Larynx and Bronchia* in 1809. He described acute hydrocephalus in 1808, and Cheyne-Stokes breathing, which occurred in apoplexy or stroke, in 1818. *See Cheyne–Stokes breathing.*

Cheyne–Stokes Breathing A poor prognostic sign in apoplexy, described by John Cheyne (1777–1836) of Dublin

in 1818 and by Irish physician William Stokes (1804–1878) in 1854.

Chiari, Hans (1851–1916) Austrian pathologist, who described Budd–Chiari syndrome in 1898. He also did extensive work on syphilis and wrote a history of pathology in 1903. *See Arnold–Chiari syndrome, Budd–Chiari syndrome.*

Chiari–Frommel Syndrome Galactorrhea and atrophy of the uterus associated with low levels of follicle stimulating hormone. Described by Austrian gynecologist, Johann Baptiste Chiari (1817–1854) in 1855, and German gynecologist, Richard Julius Ernst Frommel (1854–1912) in 1882.

Chiasma [Greek: *chiasmos*, cross] The crossing fibers of the two optic nerves in the brain. Described by Dutch professor of anatomy, Samuel Thomas Sommering (1755–1830) of Kassel in 1786.

Chicken Pox *See varicella, herpes zoster.*

Chicoyneau, Aime Francis (1702–1740) Son of Francis Chicoyneau (1672–1752), who studied anatomy under James Benignus Winslow (1669–1760). He was also an eminent botanist and Chancellor of the University of Montpellier.

Chicoyneau, Francis (1672–1752) Physician to the King of France and a Counselor of State. He served at Marseilles during the epidemic of plague, on which he later wrote a treatise. He advocated the theory that plague was not contagious.

Chiene, John (1843–1923) Professor of surgery in Edinburgh who established several surface markings (Chiene lines) of the head and neck in surgery.

Child Abuse The abuse of children (neglect, physical, psychological and sexual abuse) by parents and carers has probably been in existence for thousands of years. The present awareness was initiated by C. Henry Kempe and colleagues who published *The Battered Child* in 1962. Roberta Kalma gave a perspective on the diagnosis, treatment and prevention of child abuse in 1977. A review, *Child Abuse and Neglect*, was published by N.S. Ellerstein in 1981. *See child care, child labor, chimney sweeps.*

Child Care During the 19th century, poverty and pregnancies of unmarried mothers contributed to a surge in abandoned children in the streets of London. During the 4 years from 1819 to 1823, 150 children were found abandoned. This figure rose sharply, and in 1870 alone 276 babies were found dead in London. Child abuse, exploitation of children and child labor also flourished during this period causing great concern. *See adoption, adoption act, Barnardo, Thomas, child labor, chimney sweeps, infant mortality rates.*

Child Labor Exploitation of children in industry reached beyond humanitarian principles at the turn of the 17th century. Children were sold to mill and factory owners. Mentally handicapped children were also included in the deals. Later, owing to the efforts of men such as Jeremy Bentham (1748–1832), Michael Sadler (1861–1943), Sir Anthony Ashley Cooper (1801–1885) and Robert Owen (1771–18580), reforms were introduced to improve the condition of factory workers including children. The first infant schools in Britain were founded by the Welsh social and educational reformer, Robert Owen, and a select committee under Michael Sadler was appointed to inquire into the condition of children in 1831. The Factory Act of 1833 regulated the labor of children in mills and factories in the United Kingdom, and a Royal Commission was appointed to address the situation in 1840. The pitiful working conditions for children continued in the mines where they labored from the early hours of the morning to the late evening, some not seeing daylight except on a Sunday. The Coal Miner's Act of 1842 forbade the underground employment of children under the age of 13 years. The Ten-Hours Act, limiting the hours of work in factories, was passed in 1847, mainly owing to the efforts of the factory reformer, Richard Oastler (1789–1861) of Leeds.

Child Psychiatry Adult psychiatric illnesses were noted in children by Jean Étienne Dominique Esquirol (1838), Wilhelm Griesinger (1845) and Henry Maudsley in 1867. One of the earliest monographs, *Psychic Disturbances of Childhood*, was published by Herman Emminghaus in 1887. Another treatise, *Biographical Sketch of an Infant*, dealing with child behavior was written by Charles Darwin (1809–1882) in 1876. A comprehensive work, *The Studies in Childhood* was published by the psychologist James Scully in 1895. *The Pedagogical Seminary*, a journal for publication of studies in children, was founded in 1891 by Granville Stanley Hall, an American pioneer in child psychology. Extensive work on normal development in various stages of childhood was done by Arnold Lucius Gesell (1880–1961) from Alma, Wisconsin, professor of child hygiene at the Yale School of Medicine. He published several works on the subject, including *An Atlas of Infant Behavior* (1934), *Infant and Child in the Culture of Today* (1943) and *Child Development* (1945). Viennese psychoanalyst, August Aichhorn (1878–1949), in 1918 organized a system of reform for delinquents, and his methods were later adopted by many other institutions. The American Orthopsychiatric Association, consisting of psychiatrists, psychologists, criminologists, sociologists and

pediatricians, was formed in 1924 in order to adopt a multi-disciplinary approach to delinquency. Sir Cyril Ludowic Burt (1883–1971), a London psychologist, is considered as the first applied psychologist and pioneer in vocational guidance and child guidance in Britain. He published *Young Delinquent* (1925) and *The Backward Child* (1937).

Child Technique One-stage pancreatoduodenectomy with preservation of external pancreatic secretion, for carcinoma of the duodenum. Described by New York surgeon, Charles Gardner Child (b 1908) in 1948.

Childs, Borlase George (1816–1888) Born in Cornwall, and surgeon to the City of London police for 40 years. He invented the modern police helmet in 1861.

Chimney Sweeps After the Great Fire of London in 1666 tortuous chimneys were built for most dwellings and children were cruelly exploited to clean these. This practice continued into the 18th century, when the plight of juvenile chimney sweeps became acute. The English essayist, Charles Lamb (1775–1834) wrote *The Praise of Chimney Sweepers* in 1823, and the English author, Charles Kingsley (1819–1875) in 1863 described the story of 'Tom' the little chimney sweep. Lord Shaftbury's act in 1875 stipulated that all chimney sweeps should have a license from the police. Scrotal cancer in chimney sweeps due to chronic exposure to soot was described by the London surgeon, Percivall Pott (1714–1788) in 1770. The same cancer, due to chronic contact with tar and mineral oil was observed by H. T. Butlin in 1892.

Chimney Sweep's Cancer Cancer of the scrotum, the first occupational cancer, described by Percivall Pott (1714–1788) in 1770.

China Root Rhizome of *Smilax chinae* found in China, Formosa and Japan, used for centuries as a general remedy. Its medicinal value was also mentioned by Andreas Vesalius (1514–1564) in 1546.

Chinese Medicine It was governed for thousands years by the philosophy of the legendary Fu Hsi, Huang Ti and Shen Nung. Fu Hsi is said to have ruled around 3000 BC and is credited with many inventions, such as hierographics, numbers and basic trigonometry. Shen Nung, or the Red Emperor who lived around 2800 BC, organized a system of agriculture, experimented on plants and discovered their medicinal value. The great herbal, *Pen Tsoa*, describes over 365 drugs, and is attributed to Shen Nung. Huang Ti Nei Ching, the Yellow Emperor who lived around 2700 BC, revolutionized China with a public system of roads and industry under an organized government. His *Canon of*

Medicine was probably compiled around the 7th century, and is said to convey the system of medicine he practiced. Huang Ti is credited with the invention of acupuncture. He described the irregular rhythm and volume of the pulse in disease. Hua Tu (AD 115–205), a famous Chinese surgeon, used cannabis and other narcotics as anesthetics during his operations, which included laparotomy and excision of the spleen. The herbal drug, *Ma Hung,* used by the ancient Chinese for treatment of anaphylaxis over 2000 years ago, has been found to contain the alkaloid ephedrine as its active ingredient. The ancient Chinese also knew of the abortifeciant effect of rye contaminated with the ergot fungus, *Claviceps purpurea. Cannabis indica* or Indian hemp was known to the Chinese as *Rh-ya* in the 5th century. However, the Chinese lacked precise knowledge of anatomy, and they believed that the trachea opened into the heart and the spinal cord into the testicles. Li Shih-Chen (1518–1593), a physician to the Imperial Medical Academy, is considered the father of modern Chinese herbal medicine. His *Pen Tshao Kang Mu* (Great Pharmacopoeia), a product of 30 years of work, contains more than 11000 prescriptions. It also describes the use of silver and mercury before their introduction into European medicine. *See acupuncture, yang and yin.*

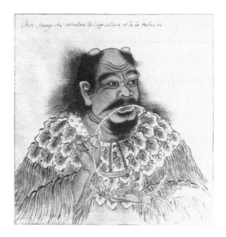

Shen Nung, author of the *Pen Tsoa.* P. Bousell and H. Bonnenmain, *Histoire de la Pharmacie* (1977). Bibliothèque Nationale, Paris

Chinese Restaurant Syndrome Dizziness and a burning sensation in the face and the chest, due to monosodium glutamate used in food. Described by R.H.M. Kwok in the *New England Journal of Medicine* in 1968.

Chirac, Peter (1650–1732) Born in Languedoc, he was professor of medicine at Montpellier and an army physician at Roussillon in 1692. He was physician to the French king in 1730. He wrote several medical treatises on wounds, fevers and the use of iron rust in incubus.

Chiromancy *See palmistry.*

Chironomia [Greek: *cheros,* hand + *nomia,* to judge or know] The art of expression through hand movements, probably originating at the time of the first dumb and/or deaf person. Giovanni Bonifacio wrote on sign language for the deaf and dumb in 1616, and a physician, John Bulwer, was the first English person to publish a treatise on chironomia in 1644. John Wallis (1616–1703), one of the founders of the Royal Society, was also a pioneer in teaching deaf-mutes through gestures and writing.

Chiropody [Greek: *cheir,* hand + *podes,* feet] A book on the subject was written by Rousselot (d 1772) of Paris in 1762. An early English treatise, *A Treatise on Corns, Bunions, the Diseases of the Nails and the General Management of the Feet,* was published by Lewis Durlacher (1792–1864), surgeon chiropodist to Queen Victoria, in 1845.

Chiropractic Medicine A form of bone setting, founded in 1895 by a storekeeper from Toronto, David Daniel Palmer (1845–1913), who practiced at Davenport, Iowa. He proposed that diseases could be treated by manipulation of the spine, and founded the Palmer School of Chiropractic in 1898 and the College of Chiropractic in Portland, Oregon. *See Abrams, Albert, spondylotherapy, bone setters.*

Chirurgische Bibliothek The first German journal in surgery commenced in 1771 and continued until 1797.

Chi-Square Test A statistical test for significance of the difference between a series of proportions, introduced by a mathematician Karl Pearson (1857–1936) of University College, London in 1900.

Chittenden, Russel Henry (1856–1943) American physiologist, born in New Haven, Connecticut, considered to be the founder of physiological chemistry and nutrition in America. His works include *Physiological Economy in Nutrition* (1905) and *Nutrition of Man* (1907).

Chloral Hydrate Discovered in 1832 by a German chemist, Justus von Liebig (1803–1873), by passing chlorine through alcohol. Its molecular formula was published by Jean Dumas (1800–1884) in 1834, and it was introduced into medicine by Rudolf Bucheim (1820–1879), who first tried it on himself in 1861. Oscar Liebreich (1839–1908) of the Charité Hospital, introduced chloral hydrate as a remedy for general use in 1869, and it was employed as an intravenous anesthetic by Oré of Lyons in 1872. It was used as a premedication before giving chloroform by a French surgeon, Forne, in 1877.

Chlorambucil First used for treatment of chronic lymphatic leukemia by David Abraham D. Galton and co-workers in 1951.

Chlorine [Greek: *chloros*, green] First obtained by Karl Wilhelm Scheele in 1774, and its bleaching action was discovered by Claude Louis Berthollet (1748–1822) in 1785. It was named by Sir Humphry Davy (1778–1829) in 1810, and Michael Faraday (1791–1861) later condensed the gas into liquid in 1823. It was used to purify water by William Cruikshank (1745–1800) of England in 1800. A method of obtaining it (Deacon process) by passing a mixture of hydrogen chloride and air through cuprous chloride was invented by H.W. Deacon (1822–1877) in 1868. It was used in Reading during an epidemic in 1910 to sterilize the water, and since then its use in water purification has become standard. Chlorine was the first gas to be used as a poison gas in chemical warfare by the Germans in 1914.

Chloroamphenicol *See chloromycetin.*

Chloroform Discovered by French chemist, Eugene Soubeiran, in 1831. Around the same time Justus von Liebig (1803–1873) of Germany and a physician, Samuel Guthrie (1782–1848) from Bloomfield, Massachusetts, announced their independent discovery of chloroform. Its composition was determined by Alexander Dumas (1800–1884) who gave it its present name in 1834. Its anesthetic properties were demonstrated on animals by French physiologist, Jean Pierre Marie Flourens (1794–1867) in 1847. Liverpool chemist, David Waldie (1813–1899), suggested trying the inhalational effects of chloroform to relieve labor pains to James Y. Simpson, (1811–1870) who used it with success in 1847. The first death due to chloroform in anesthesia occurred in a woman named Hannah Greener, near Newcastle upon Tyne in 1848. This and a few other deaths from chloroform raised widespread concern about its safety. John Snow (1813–1858) of Soho, London, who specialized in anesthesia, started conducting experiments on the compound and published *On Chloroform and other Anaesthetics* in 1858. The debate on the use of chloroform virtually came to an end when Snow successfully administered it to Queen Victoria during the delivery of Prince Leopold in 1853. A portable model of a chloroform inhaler was introduced by Joseph Thomas Clover (1825–1882) in 1862. In 1879 the British Medical Association, at a committee meeting, concluded that chloroform caused a depressor effect on the cardiovascular system. In 1889, the Nizam of Hyderabad granted a sum of money to Surgeon Major

Lawrie to investigate the effects of chloroform. The Hyderabad commission found that respiration always failed before the heart failed, and a second Hyderabad commission confirmed these findings. In 1900, the Anesthetics Committee of the British Medical Association, after analyzing the notes on 25,920 chloroform administrations, concluded that the most im-portant factor in the safety of the drug was the experience of the administrator. *See anesthesia.*

Chloromycetin Chloramphenicol was prepared from *Streptomyces venezuelae* from soil by John Ehrlich (b 1907), P.R. Burkholder and co-workers in 1947. Its effectiveness against rickettsial infections was demonstrated by Joseph Edwin Smadel (1907–1963) and Elizabeth B. Jackson in 1948.

Chlorophyll [Greek: *chloros*, green + *phyll*, leaf] Joseph Priestley (1733–1804) in 1774 and Jean Ingenhouez (1730–1799) around 1779 independently noted that plants which contain the pigment gave off oxygen when exposed to sunlight. Two French botanical chemists, Joseph Bienaime Caventou (1795–1878) and Pierre Joseph Pelletier (1788–1842) named the green substance chlorophyll in 1817. The importance of sunlight for the activity of chloroplasts was pointed out by Julius Sachs (1832–1897) in 1865. The structure of chlorophyll was discovered by Richard Wilstatter (b 1872) of Germany in 1905. Nobel Prize-winning work on the role of chlorophyll in photosynthesis was carried out in 1961 by an American chemist, Melvin Calvin (b 1911).

Chloropicrin English chemist, Stenhouse, prepared it by mixing bleach with picric acid in 1848. It was used in gas warfare by the Germans in 1917. *See gas warfare.*

Chloroquin When Allied troops occupied Tunis in 1943 they came across supplies of a German antimalarial drug called sontoquin. Chloroquin was developed later as a result of the search for other antimalarial compounds similar to sontoquin. Its activity was tested by Robert Frederick Loeb in 1946. In 1955, R.B. Arora and colleagues demonstrated that it exerted more antifibrillatory effect on the animal heart than did quinidine. Three years later, M.E. Hess and Schmidt showed that intravenous chloroquin terminated aconitine-induced atrial fibrillation in dogs. Following these findings it was used as treatment for atrial fibrillation until the early 1960s. It has also been in continuous use as an antimalarial agent since 1946. *See antimalarials.*

Chlorosis [Greek: *chloros*, green] (Syn. green sickness, icterrius amanterium, morbus virginius and cachexia .virginium) Anemia in young women for which no cause was found. Noted during puberty, and described by Johanes Lange in 1554. Hippocrates (460–377 BC) described a similar condition in his book on diseases of virgins. Robert Pierce (1620–1710), an English physician from Bath, gave an account under the title Green Sickness in 1697. The cause remained obscure, although oligocythemia was thought to be due to deficient red cell production. This is now known to be due to iron deficiency.

Chlorothiazide Synthesized by F.C. Novello and J.M. Sprague during their search for a carbonic acid inhibitor for treatment of hypertension in 1957. Initial studies on chlorothiazide as a diuretic were carried out by K.H. Beyer in 1958.

Chlorpromazine In 1947 French surgeon H. Laborit at the Military Hospital at Val de Grace in Paris started investigating the use of antihistamines to inhibit the reaction of the autonomic nervous system to physical stress in surgery. He was impressed by the effect of promethazine in making the patient calm and relaxed, and started investigating this group of drugs with the help of Parisian anesthetist, P. Huguenard, in 1949. Charpentier produced a phenothiazine, code named RP 4560, in 1950. Laborit found that this induced tranquillity without clouding consciousness and persuaded a group of psychiatrists, Hamon, Paraire and Velluz at Val de Grace Hospital, to try it on their patients. The news of their success spread and the drug was evaluated by French psychiatrists, Jean Delay (b 1907) and Pierre Deniker (b 1917) at the nearby St Anne's Hospital in 1952. It was then introduced under the name chlorpromazine in most mental hospitals in France in the same year and reached England in 1953.

Chlortetracycline Aureomycin, obtained from *Streptomyces aureofaciens* by Benjamin M. Dugger, a retired botany professor from Wisconsin, in 1948. It became the most commonly prescribed antibiotic over the next few decades.

Chnum Ram-headed god of Egypt, also regarded as the god of cataracts.

Cholagogues [Greek: *cholo*, bile + *agogos*, leading] Substances that lessen the amount of bile. Calomel, rhubarb, podophyllin and mercury preparations have been used for this purpose.

Choleangitis Bernard Naunyn (1839–1925) of Berlin in 1892 used the term to denote inflammation of the lining membrane of the smallest bile ducts which caused jaundice.

Cholecystectomy [Greek: *chole*, bile + *kystis*, bladder + *ek*, out + *temno*, to cut] Successful removal of a gallbladder was performed by Carl Johan August Langenbuch (1846–1901) in 1882.

Cholecystenterostomy The creation of a surgical fistula between the gallbladder and intestines, suggested by a Munich surgeon, Johann Nepomuk von Nussbaum (1829–1890), and performed by Alexander Winiwarter in 1882. French surgeon, Paul Jules Tillaux, later performed it in a case of cancer of the head of the pancreas invading the bile duct.

Cholecystography [Greek: *chole*, bile + *graphein*, to write] A contrast method in radiology with tetrabromophenolphthalein as an intravenous agent, to visualize the biliary tract. Invented by American surgeon, Evarts Ambrose Graham (1883–1957) of St Louis and Warren Henry Cole (b 1898) in 1924. It was used for nearly 30 years until it was replaced by intravenous iodipamide (Biligrafin) in 1953, which had the advantage of making the common bile duct visible. Oral cholecystography was made possible with the introduction of calcium or sodium ipodate (Biloptin).

Cholecystokinin [Greek: *chole*, bile + *kystis*, bladder + *kinein*, to move] In 1928 a Chicago physiologist, Andrew Conway Ivy (1893–1977) and Erie Oldberg found that when acid was injected into the duodenum a substance was released into the blood which caused the gallbladder to contract. This substance was named 'cholecystokinin' by Ivy. A preparation of cholecystokinin which produced contraction of the gallbladder after intravenous administration was made by J.E. Jorpes and V. Mutt in 1959.

Cholecystostomy [Greek: *chole*, bile + *kystis*, bladder + *tome*, cutting] The first suggestion that a distended gallbladder could be relieved by a puncture was made in 1743 by Jean-Louis Petit (1674–1750), a leading surgeon in Paris. It was performed by John Stough Bobbs (1809–1870), an American surgeon from Indianapolis, in 1867. The second recorded procedure was by James Marion Sims (1813–1863) of New York in 1878, but his patient died. The method described by Sims, was successfully used on a patient by Lawson Tait (1845–1899) in 1879.

Choledochal Cyst [Greek: *chole*, bile + *docoz*, containing or receiving] The anatomical abnormality in this condition was described by a German anatomist, Abraham Vater (1684–1751) in 1720, and the pathology and symptomatology were described by an English surgeon, John Douglas (d 1759) in 1752.

Cholelithiasis [Greek: *chole*, bile + *lithos*, stone] *See gallstones.*

Cholera (Syn. cholera morbus) Described by the ancient Hindu Brahmins in 400 BC. Hippocrates (460–377 BC) gave a description of several well detailed cases of cholera resulting from unwholesome food and unboiled pork. The symptoms arising from the stomach and intestines were vividly described by Aretaeus (81–138). Garcia del Huerto, a physician at Goa, described it in 1560. The more recent history of cholera dates back to 1817 when it occurred at Benares in India. The epidemic reached Hamburg via the Middle East and then spread to Sunderland in 1831. Several epidemics occurred in England during the periods 1831–1832, 1848–1849, 1853–1854 and 1865–1866, claiming over 25,000 lives. The bacillus responsible was identified by Robert Koch (1843–1910) in 1883. *See comma bacillus.*

Cholera Morbus [Greek: *cholera*, water gutter from the roof of a house] *See Asiatic cholera.*

Cholera Vaccine The first attempt at immunization against cholera on a large scale was made by a Spanish bacteriologist, J. Ferran in 1885, during an outbreak of cholera in Spain. He developed his own vaccine and submitted himself to be inoculated to study the effects. Owing to reactions caused by uncontrolled doses of vaccine, Ferran's campaign was stopped by the government. It was continued by Waldemar Haffkine (1860–1930) from Russia, who later became a pupil of Elie Metchnikoff (1845–1916). Haffkine also inoculated himself with virulent strains of cholera in 1892, and traveled to India, where he inoculated over 40,000 people over 29 months.

Cholesterol [Greek: *chole*, bile + *stereos*, solid] One of the earliest known sterols, described by Michael Eugene Chevril (1786–1889) in 1815. The presence of high levels in the diet as a cause of atherosclerosis was emphasized by S. Saltykow in 1908. The method of estimating serum cholesterol was devised by C.S. Myers and Wardell in 1918, and another simple method was described by S.L. Leiboff in 1924. The Nobel Prize in Chemistry for work on the structure was awarded to Adolf Otto Reinhold Windaus (1876–1959) of Germany in 1928. Timothy Leary of America made a microscopic study of coronary artery lesions in 1934 and concluded that the pathogenesis of atherosclerotic lesions was related to disturbance of lipid metabolism. Around the same time, Frederick Arthur Willius at the Mayo Clinic commenced extensive studies on lipids and demonstrated that high total lipid and cholesterol levels positively correlated with coronary artery disease. The statistical significance of a high cholesterol level in heart disease was demonstrated by C.A. Poindexter and M. Bruger in 1938. The mechanism of production of cholesterol in animals was worked out by Konrad Emil Bloch (b 1912) of Harvard University and Feodor Felix Konrad Lynen (1911–1979) of Munich who jointly received the Nobel Prize for their work in 1964. Further research was carried out by Michael Stuart Brown of the South Western Medical School in Texas in 1971 and his work, along with that of Leonard Joseph Goldstein, led to the discovery of low-density lipoprotein cholesterol (LDL) receptors. Synthesis of cholesterol in the living cell was elucidated by Sir John Warcup Cornforth, an organic chemist from Sydney, while he was in England at Sussex and Oxford Universities. He received the Nobel Prize for Chemistry in 1975. *See lipids.*

Cholesterolemia, Familial The familial clustering of patients with xanthomas, hypercholesterolemia and premature heart disease was noted independently by C. Muller and Siegfried Josef Thannhauser (b 1885) in 1938. The lack of receptor sites for low-density lipoprotein cholesterol (LDL receptors) in the liver of patients with familial hypercholesterolemia, leading to a rise in serum cholesterol, was shown by Joseph Leonhard Goldstein (b 1940), a molecular biologist and professor of medical genetics at the University of Texas. He was awarded the Nobel Prize for Physiology or Medicine for his work in 1985.

Chomel, James Francis A physician from Paris, and brother of another physician, John Chomel. He wrote *Universae Medicinae Theoricae pars Prima* in 1709.

Chomel, John Baptiste Lewis (d 1765) A physician and the son of Peter John Baptiste Chomel (d 1740). He published a work on the history of medicine in France.

Chomel, Peter John Baptist (d 1740) Paris physician to the king. He wrote a history of common plants.

Chopart Joints Astragaloscaphoid and calcaneocuboid articulations, described by François Chopart (1743–1795), professor of surgery in Paris, in 1792.

Chordata [Greek: *chorde*, cord] Animals with a notochord [Greek: *noton*, back] were classified in the phylum Chordata by a lecturer on animal morphology, Francis Maitland Balfour (1851–1882) of Edinburgh in *Treatise on Comparative Embryology* published in 1880.

Chordee [Greek: *chordee*, harpstring] An early term for painful erection of the penis during an attack of gonorrhea.

Chorea [Greek: *chorea*, dance] *See Sydenham chorea, Huntington chorea.*

Choreoathetosis [Greek: *chorea*, dance + *athetos*, lawless] *See Sydenham chorea, Huntington chorea.*

Choriocarcinoma [Greek: *chorion*, skin + *karkinos*, crab] The first case report was provided by Hans Chiari (1851–1916) of Germany in 1877. John Whitridge Williams (1866–1931) of Johns Hopkins Hospital gave the first case report in America in 1895.

Christ Referred to as a healer in many instances in the New Testament of the Bible. Touching has been observed as an important part of his healing. The calendar based on the birth of Jesus Christ was introduced by a monk, Dionysious Exiguus, in AD 525.

Christian, Asbury Henry (1876–1951) Boston physician who described Weber–Christian Syndrome with Frederick Parkes Weber (1863–1962) in 1925. Hand–Schuller–Christian syndrome, consisting of defective membranous bones, diabetes insipidus, pituitary dysfunction, and exopthalmos, was described by him in 1919.

Christiansen, Johanne Ostenfeld (1882–1968) Copenhagen physician and respiratory physiologist who discovered the part played by hemoglobin in the transport of carbon dioxide. He devised a method of preparing coagulated egg albumin for determining peptic activity.

Christison, Sir Robert (1797–1882) Physician from Edinburgh. He was appointed professor of jurisprudence at Edinburgh in 1822 and became physician to Queen Victoria in Scotland in 1849. He experimented on himself to study the poisonous effects of the calabar bean from tropical Africa in 1876. On finding it to be intensely poisonous he recommended it for official executions. His *On the Poisonous Properties of Hemlock and its Alkaloid Conia* was published in the *Transactions of the Royal Society of Edinburgh* in 1836.

Christmas Disease Hemophilia B due to lack of factor IX. Described by Rosemary Peyton Biggs in 1952. The disease is named after the patient (S. Christmas) in whom it was first described.

Chrobak, Rudolf (1843–1910) *See carcinoma of the uterus.*

Chromatid A half chromosome between early prophase and metaphase, described and named by American zoologist Clarence Ervin McClung (1870–1946) of Philadelphia in 1900.

Chromatin [Greek: *chroma*, color] Nuclear material of the chromosome was described by a German anatomist, Walther Flemming (1843–1905) in 1879. He also showed that nuclear division involves a longitudinal splitting of the chromosome and a migration of the daughter halves to the daughter nuclei.

Chromatography [Greek: *chroma*, color + *graphein*, to write] Studied by Christian Friedrich Schoenbein (1799–1868) in 1861. It was developed by a Russian botanist and organic chemist, Mikhail Semenovich Tswett (1872–1919) in 1906. He named the method 'chromatography' and used it to

identify the family of yellow plant pigments called carotenoids. It was revived for separating amino acids with the use of filter paper by British biochemists, John Porter Martin Archer and Richard Laurence Millington Synge (b 1914) in 1942. A book on chromatography designed for students, *An Introduction to Chromatography*, was published by Trevor Illtyd Williams at the Sir William Dunn School of Pathology, Oxford in 1946. It proved to be very valuable in studying the structure of proteins, and the Nobel Prize for Chemistry was awarded to its pioneers, Synge and Martin, in 1952. Column chromatography for identification and quantification of amino acids from the hydrolysates of proteins and physiological tissues was developed by Stanford Moore (1913–1982), an American biochemist, and William Howard Stein (1911–1980), at the Rockefeller Institute in 1950.

Chromium [Greek: *chroma*, color] Element described by Johann Lehmann, a German physician and metallurgist in the Berezov mine at Ekaterinberg in 1762. It was isolated by French analytical chemist, Louis Nicholas Vanquelin (1763–1829) in 1797. Cumming described 'chrome holes' occurring in the hands of workers who handled bichromate in Glasgow in the *Edinburgh Medical Journal* in 1827. Similar lesions were found in factory workers in Germany by Wutzdorf in 1897. The first case of adenocarcinoma due to chronic chromate exposure was described in a worker in Scotland by D. A. Newman in 1890. Further cases of cancer induced by chromium were noted in Germany by E. Pfeil in 1912.

Chromomere [Greek: *chroma*, color] The smallest particles in the chromosome, identified by their characteristic size and position, described by Edmund Beecher Wilson (1856–1939) of America in *The Cell in Development and Inheritance*, published in 1896.

Chromosomes [Greek: *chroma*, color + *soma*, body] Discovered and studied in 1875 by Walther Flemming (1843–1905), a German histologist of Sachsenberg. Their role as carriers of heredity was recognized by German physiologist Wilhelm Roux (1850–1924) of Halle in 1883. W. Waldeyer (1836–1921) named them chromosomes in 1888. Theodor Boveri (1862–1915) and Walter Stanborough Sutton (1877–1916) separately pointed out the individuality of the chromosomes in 1890s. The modern theory of chromosomes was initiated by D.H. Wenrich who provided anatomical evidence for their individuality. He observed the paired occurrence of maternal and paternal chromosomes and the linear arrangement of centromeres within the chromosome. In 1902, Clarence Erwin McClung (1870–1946), an American cytologist, suggested that the X or accessory chromosome was associated with sex characteristics. A chromosome map of sex-linked genes was produced by American geneticist, Alfred Henry Sturtevant (1891–1970) of Jacksonville, Illinois in 1911. He published *History of Genetics* in 1965. The number of chromosomes in humans was found to be 46, by Joe Hin Tjio and Albert Levan (b 1905) in 1956. *See genetics.*

Chronaxia The period of excitation of animal tissue. Defined by Louis Lapicque (1866–1952) of France in 1909. It denotes the shortest time that a current twice the strength of the rheobase must be applied to stimulate a response.

Chronic Active Hepatitis *See active chronic hepatitis.*

Chronic Fatigue Syndrome A state of nervous exhaustion and asthenia, first recognized by Eugene Bouchut (1818–1891) of Paris who called it *nervosisme* in 1860. American physician, George Miller Beard (1839–1883), introduced the term 'neurasthenia' for a similar condition in 1869, and it was named Beard disease. A state of neurocirculatory asthenia or cardiovascular neurosis amongst soldiers was noted by Arthur Bowen Richards Myers (1838–1921) in 1869. The presence of the same condition amongst soldiers during the American Civil War was described by Jacob Mendes Da Costa (1833–1900) of Jefferson Medical College, Philadelphia in 1871. Sir Thomas Lewis (1881–1945) described it as 'effort syndrome' in 1917, and Paul Wood (1907–1962), an eminent English cardiologist, attributed the somatic symptoms to psychoneurosis arising out of fear, in 1941. The concept of 'psychoasthenia', in which psychological weakness or asthenia followed shock, fatigue, or constitutional weakness, was proposed by Pierre Janet (1859–1947), professor of psychiatry at the College de France, and a contemporary of Jean Martin Charcot (1825–1893). The term 'fibrositis' was coined in 1894 by the London neurologist, Sir William Gowers (1845–1915) to denote an unexplained state of diffuse muscle aches and body pains. An outbreak of a paralytic illness amongst the staff of the Los Angeles County General Hospital occurred in 1934 and this, and epidemics elsewhere, were referred to as 'epidemic neuromyasthenia'. A similar outbreak at the Royal Free Hospital in London in 1955 suggested that it was a conversion hysteria possibly triggered by a viral illness, and it was named 'benign myalgic encephalomyelitis'. The term 'myalgic encephalitis' (ME) was later applied to the same condition. An attempt to apply specific criteria and define the illness was made by G.P. Holmes and co-workers in 1988. The symptoms were shown to be due to general fatigue rather than a myalgic disorder by R.H.T. Edwards and colleagues in 1993.

Chronic Myeloid Leukemia (CML) Busulphan (Myleran) as treatment for CML was suggested by Sir Alexander Haddow (1907–1976) in 1953, and was introduced as an effective treatment by David Abraham Goiten Galton and M. Till in 1955. *See Philadelphia chromosome.*

Chronic Subdural Hematoma Although the condition was observed at postmortem over several centuries, the first clear account was given only in 1817 by M. Houssard of Paris. Rudolph Virchow (1821–1902) used the term 'pachymeningitis hemorrhagica' for it and gave a histological description in 1857. It was described in detail by Sir Charles Alfred Ballance (1865–1936), a neurosurgeon in London, in 1907. Trauma as an important cause was pointed out by F. Robertson (1900), Wilfred Trotter (1914) and Tracy J. Putnam and Harvey Williams Cushing (1869–1939) (1925). A classic treatise, *Chronic Subdural Hematoma* was published in the *Bulletin of the Neurological Institute of New York* by a New York neurologist, Leo Max Davidoff (1898–1975) and Cornelius G. Dyke, in 1938.

Chronoscope [Greek: *chronos*, time + *skopein*, to look] Instrument to measure small intervals of time, invented by Charles Wheatstone (1802–1875) in 1840. His principle was later applied to the calculation of the velocity of projectiles. An improved chronoscope was constructed by Pouillet in 1844.

Chronothermalism [Greek: *chronos*, time + *therme*, heat] Disease concept proposed by London physician, Samuel Dickson around 1850. In his vague treatise he proposed that all diseases could be resolved by paying attention to time and temperature. However, he sensibly discarded blood letting, purging and starvation as treatments for all diseases except apoplexy and inflammation of the chest.

Chrysocolla [Greek: *krusos*, gold] Name given to borax by the German physician, George Agricola (1494–1555) in 1530, since borax was used for soldering gold.

Churchman, John Woolman (1877–1937) He demonstrated the effect of gentian violet as an antiseptic in 1912. He showed the selective bactericidal action of intravenous gentian violet against staphylococci in 1924.

Churg–Strauss Syndrome Allergic granulomatosis, described by J. Churg (b 1910), and New York pathologist, L. Strauss in the *American Journal of Pathology* in 1951. Churg was born in Poland, where he graduated in medicine before he emigrated to America in 1936. He was clinical professor of pathology at the Mt Sinai Hospital in 1966.

Chvostek Sign Facial muscles spasms on tapping the facial nerve, a diagnostic sign in cases of tetany. Described by Austrian surgeon, Frantisek Chvostek (1835–1884) in 1876.

Chyli Receptaculum of the Thoracic Duct Described by Jean Pecquet (1622–1674), a French anatomist, while he was a student in 1647.

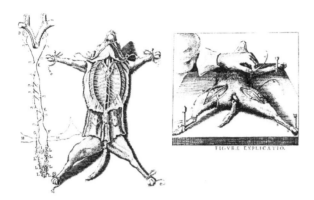

Chyli receptaculum. Jean Pecquet's figure of the thoracic duct in a dog. William Stirling, *Some Apostles in Physiology* (1902). Waterlow & Sons, London

Chylomicrons An anatomist, Simon Henry Gage (1851–1944), and Pierre Auguste Fish (b 1865) of Washington, DC observed and named the fine particles of fat seen in the blood during the transport of fat, in 1924.

Chymopapain First used to dissolve the nucleus pulposus of the intervertebral disc by Lyman W. Smith of North Western Medical School, Chicago, in 1963.

Chymotrypsin Enzyme produced in a crystalline form by an American biochemist, John Howard Northrop (1891–1987) of New York in 1935. His *Crystalline Enzymes* was published in 1939.

Ciaccio, Guiseppe Vincenzo (1824–1901) Professor of comparative anatomy at Bologna, who described the conjunctival glands (Ciaccio glands) in 1874.

Cicero (106–143 BC) Roman philosopher and orator who suggested that body ailments could result from emotional factors. He proposed several concepts which are fundamental to psychiatry and psychotherapy. He also disputed the idea of Hippocrates (460–377 BC) on black bile as a cause of melancholia and attributed it to psychological difficulties.

Cicuta A plant genus including the water hemlock, *Cicuta maculatum*. A preparation from this poisonous plant was used for centuries as treatment in conditions such as cancer and syphilis. William Withering (1741–1799) described its medicinal uses around 1792.

Cigarette Smoking *See smoking.*

Ciliary Ganglion [Latin: *cilium*, eyelid] Schacher ganglion, described by Polycarp Gottlieb Schacher (1674–1737), professor of pathology and surgery at the University of Leipzig, in 1737.

Ciliary Glands [Latin: *cilium*, eyelid] Described in detail in 1857 by Jacob Antonius Möll (1832–1914), an ophthalmologist at the Hague.

Ciliary Motion [Latin: *cilium*, eyelid] Motion of the epithelial tissues was described by Jan Evangelista Purkinje (1787–1869) and Gabriel Gustav Valentine (1810–1883) in 1835.

Ciliary Muscles [Latin: *cilium*, eyelid] Sir Philip Crampton (1777–1858), a surgeon from the Meath Hospital Dublin, described the radial fibers of the ciliary muscles, in 1805. The circular fibers were described by a French professor of physiology at Montpellier, Charles Rouget (1824–1904) in 1856. The mechanism of accommodation of the eye, which is brought about by the contraction of ciliary muscles effecting a change in curvature of the anterior surface of the lens, was shown by Herman Helmholtz (1821–1894).

Cimento [Italian: *cimento*, experiment] The Accademia del Cimento was one of the first important scientific academies since the establishment of the museum at Alexandria in AD 641. It was founded by Duke Leopold of Tuscany in Florence in 1657. *See Academy.*

Cinchona Bark Peruvian bark, known for its antipyretic properties by the people of South America before the Spanish conquest. In 1628 King Philip IV of Spain appointed Bobadilla Mendoz, the Count of Chinchon, as the Spanish Viceroy to Peru. While he was living in Lima his wife contracted malaria and was dying of it. Her physician, Juan del Vego, on the advice and experience of a local magistrate, prescribed cinchona or Peruvian bark. She made a remarkable recovery and del Vego, on his return to Spain in 1639, introduced the bark. A massive trade in cinchona from the New World to Spain followed, and from there it reached other parts of Europe. It was prescribed by Jesuit priests in England in 1655 and came to be known as Jesuit's powder or Jesuit's bark. The name 'cinchona' was given to the plant in honor of the Countess of Chinchon, by Carl Linnaeus in 1742. The alkaloid quinine was extracted by Pierre Joseph Pelletier (1788–1842) and J.B. Caventou (1795–1877) of Paris in 1820. Cinchona cultivation was introduced to Sri Lanka, Jamaica and Java in 1860, but it became established only in Java. The cinchona preparation ('febrifuge powder') was introduced as a treatment for malaria in India by J.E. de Vrij in 1874. *See quinine, Markham, Sir Robert.*

Cinelli, John (1625–1706) Italian physician who went to prison for criticizing the Royal Physician to Cosmo III. He published *Bibliotheca Volante,* which was reprinted in Venice in 1734.

Cinematography A camera that could take rapid pictures of the same scene was developed by the French physiologist, Etienne Jules Marey (1830–1904), who used it to study locomotion in animals in 1881. The production of rapid serial roentgenograms from the screen image was introduced into radiology in England by R.J. Reynolds in 1927. Cinematography was used to investigate stomach lesions by Walter Clements Alvarez (b 1884) of the Mayo Clinic in Rochester, Minnesota, in 1934. London zoologist, Sir James Gray (1891–1975), was one of the first to use it to study ciliary movement in cytology and he wrote *Textbook of Experimental Cytology* in 1928.

Circle of Willis *See cerebral circulation.*

Circumcision [Latin: *circum,* round + *caedere,* to cut] (Syn. Acrobystia) Circumcision of the male is the only surgical procedure mentioned in the Bible. It was also common amongst the ancient Egyptians. Cancer of the penis was almost unknown amongst circumcised Jews. Circumcision of females was practiced by ancient Egyptians according to the study of papyri by V.O. Peyron (1785–1870). The practice of female circumcision was also common in certain other Arab tribes, and in some parts of Africa and Asia.

Cirillo, Dominic (1730–1799) Professor of botany in Naples who was persuaded by Lady Walpole to come to London, where he attended the lectures of William Hunter (1718–1783). On his return to France in 1780 he published *Nosologiae Methodica Rudimenta.* When the French took over administration in Naples he accepted a position, but was executed when the government was restored in Naples.

Cirrhosis [Greek: *kirros,* yellow or tawny colored] Condition of a hard, shrunken liver was named by René Laënnec (1781–1826) of Paris.

Cis-**Platinum** The cytotoxicity was accidentally discovered when an electric current was passed between platinum electrodes through a nutrient medium in which bacteria were growing, by B. Rosenberg and colleagues during their experiments in 1965. They noted that bacterial growth was inhibited by chlorides of *cis*-platinum which formed during electrolysis, and further investigations enabled it to become an important drug in cancer therapy.

Cisternal Puncture *See occipital puncture.*

Citois, François (1572–1652) Born in Poitiers, he qualified from Montpellier and had a successful medical practice in Paris. He gave an account of Poitou colic in his treatise *Colica Pictonum* published in 1616.

Citric Acid Cycle The first important study on the complete oxidation of pyruvic acid was performed by Albert von Szent-Györgyi (1893–1986) in 1935. He used minced pigeon breast muscle known for its high rate of respiration and demonstrated the role of succinic, fumaric, malic and oxaloacetic acids in the respiratory cycle. The role of the other compounds – pyruvic acid, citric acid and alphaketoglutaric acid – in the aerobic metabolism of carbohydrates was described by Sir Hans Adolf Krebs (1900–1982) who published his work in *Role of Citric Acid in Intermediate Metabolism of Animal Tissues* with W.A. Johnson in 1937. Krebs was awarded the Nobel Prize in 1953.

Cladius, Deotatus Physician to the Bishop of Basel in the early 17th century. He published a book on preserving health, *Pantheon Hygiasticon Hippocraticum Hermenticum, de hominis vita ad centum ed viginte anos salubriter producenda* in 1628.

Cladius, Friedrich Matthias (1822–1869) Professor of anatomy at Kiel who described the supporting cells on the floor of the cochlear canal in 1858.

Clap *See gonorrhea.*

Clapeyron, Benoit Paul Emile (1799–1864) French physicist, born in Paris and educated at the École Polytechnique. He advanced Sadi Carnot's (1796–1832) work on thermodynamics, dealing with efficiency of heat engines. The concept of thermodynamics later became important in biological metabolic studies and physical chemistry.

Clapton Line Green line seen at the base of the teeth in cases of poisoning due to copper. Described by London physician, Edward Clapton (1830–1909).

Clark Operation Radical form of hysterectomy for cancer of the uterus. Described by American gynecologist, John Goodrich Clark (1867–1927) of Baltimore, in 1895.

Clark Sign Obliteration of liver dullness due to distension in peritonitis. Described by New York physician, Alonzo Clark (1807–1887). He also advocated the use of opium in peritonitis.

Clark, Alonzo (1807–1887) Physician at the Medical Department of Syracuse University, New York who introduced the use of large doses of opium in cases of peritonitis in 1855. He monitored the respiratory rate as an indicator of opium level.

Clark, Thomas (1801–1867) Physician from Ayr in Scotland, who held the chair of chemistry at Marischal College, Aberdeen in 1833. He devised the soap test for testing hard water, developed a process for softening hard water and discovered the pyrophosphate of soda.

Clark, William Mansfield (1884–1964) American chemist and physiologist in New York, whose study on the acidity of milk led to the discovery of a range of titration indicators. His *The Determination of Hydrogen Ions* was published in 1920.

Clarke Column *See Clarke, Jacob.*

Clarke, Jacob Augustus (1817–1880) Born in Pimlico in London, he was an eminent neurologist who described the nucleus dorsalis of the spinal cord (Clarke column) and the pigmented cells of the nucleus dorsalis (Clarke cells) in 1851.

Clarke, John (1761–1815) A graduate of St George's Hospital and leading obstetrician in London. He gave the earliest account of tetany in his *Commentaries on some of the Most Important Diseases of the Children* which was published in the year of his death.

Clarke, Sir Charles Manfield (1782–1857) English physician who described ulcer at the neck of the uterus as a cause of vaginal discharge in 1814.

Clarkson, Thomas (1760–1846) The son of a clergyman, born in Wisbech, England, and educated at St Paul's School. He devoted his life to the abolition of slavery, and was one of the founders of the Antislavery Society. He wrote *History of the Abolition of the African Slave-trade* in two volumes in 1808.

Claude Syndrome Ipsilateral paralysis of the third and fourth nerves with contralateral hemianesthesia, due to compression of the arterial supply to the inferior nucleus ruber (red nucleus) by mesencephalic lesions. First described by French neurologist, Henri C.J. Claude (1869–1945) of Paris in 1912.

Claude, Albert (1899–1983) Belgian-born American biologist who obtained his doctorate in medicine from the University of Liège in 1928. He joined the Rockefeller Institute for Medical Research in New York in 1928 and made major contributions to the study of the cell and its organelles. He pioneered electron microscopy of cells, and high-speed centrifugation for separating nucleus, mitochondria and microsomes. He showed that mitochondria are the site of respiration, and shared the Nobel Prize for Physiology or Medicine with George Emil Palade (b 1912) and Christian René De Duve (b 1917) in 1974.

Clausius, Rudolf J.E. (1822–1888) Professor of physics at Bonn, and contemporary of James Prescott Joule (1818–1889). He proposed the second law of thermodynamics which established that energy has a constant tendency to move in the direction of dissipation. The concept of thermodynamics was later applied to biological metabolic studies and physical chemistry.

Claviceps purpurea [Latin: *clavus*, club + *purpureus*, purple] Species of fungus in rye which causes ergotism. *See ergotism.*

Clavicle [Latin: *clavicula*, small key] Collar bone, which derives its name from its resemblance to an ancient key. American surgeon, Charles McCrearry (1785–1826) from Kentucky excised it in 1811. A bandage for fractured clavicle was described by French surgeon, Pierre Joseph Desault (1744–1795). Thomas Callaway (1791–1848), an English physician, wrote a treatise on fractures of the clavicle and shoulder joint in 1846. A method of strapping for fracture was described by American surgeon, H. Earle Conwell (b 1893) of Alabama in 1928.

Clayton, John Yorkshire clergyman and scientist in the middle of the 17th century. He showed that combustible gases could be produced by heating coal in airtight vessels, in 1688.

Cleft Palate The procedure of staphylorraphy was performed on a child by M. le Monnier, a Parisian dentist, around 1750. Uranoplasty, the operative treatment, was attempted by John Mattauer of America in 1837. Operative surgery was further advanced by American surgeon, Mason Warren in 1848. Avery of Charing Cross Hospital was the first surgeon in England to close a cleft in the hard palate successfully. The Diffenbach–Fergusson method originally designed by Johann Friedrich Diffenbach (1792–1856), professor of surgery in Berlin, was introduced into England by Sir William Fergusson (1808–1877) in 1874.

Cleland, John (1835–1925) Born in Perth, Scotland he was professor of anatomy at Glasgow who wrote *Scala Naturae and other Poems* in 1887. He was the co-author of *Cleland's and Mackay's Textbook of Anatomy* (1896), one of the earliest books on anatomy to contain photographic illustrations.

Cleopatra (68–30 BC) Queen of Egypt, and the last of the dynasty of the Ptolemies. She also practiced medicine and obstetrics and wrote a treatise on medicine. An inscription at the Temple of Esneh is believed to show Cleopatra in labor. Some historians believe that the medical works attri-buted to her were written by a contemporary, also named Cleopatra.

Clerc, Daniel le (1652–1728) Physician in Geneva who published *Historie de la Medicine* in 1696 and *Bibliotheca Anatomica*.

Cleveland, Emiline Horton (1829–1878) Graduate of the Female Medical College of Pennsylvania in 1855. After doing postgraduate work in Paris she returned to America, where she was appointed professor of obstetrics at the Woman's Hospital, opened by Ann Preston in Philadelphia, in 1861. In 1875 she became the first woman in America to perform major abdominal surgery and ovariotomy.

Clevenger Fissure Inferior sulcus of the temporal lobe, named after a psychiatrist, Shobal Vail Clevenger (1843–1920) of Chicago.

Climacteric [Greek: *klimakter*, step of staircase] Ancient Greek term for certain periods of life in an individual. Greek physiologists recognized five climacterics at the following years of life: the 7th, the 21st, the 49th, the 63rd and the 81st. The 63rd year was considered as the grand climacteric.

Climatic Bubo The first series on the disease involving 38 patients on the Zanzibar coast was described by Reinhold Ruge in 1896. As no cause, such as injury or sexual contact could be identified, Ruge named it climatic bubo. It was common in the 19th century in the English navy. Sailors contracted it from the East Indies. *See lymphogranuloma venereum.*

Climatology Hippocrates (460–377 BC) in one of his treatises said 'on arrival at a town with which he is unfamiliar, a physician should examine its position with respect to the winds and the sun'. In another place he wrote 'the contribution of astronomy to medicine is not a very small one but a very great one indeed. For with the seasons men's diseases, like their digestive organs suffer change'. In *On Airs, Waters and Places* he stated 'whoever wishes to investigate medicine probably should consider the seasons of the year and what effect it produces on them'. Italian physician and pioneer of occupational medicine, Bernadini Ramazzini (1633–1714), also stressed the effects of annual change of seasons and environment on health.

Clinical Medicine [Greek: *kline*, bed] Practice of medicine by the bedside. The system of case histories in teaching clinical medicine was introduced by Italian physician, Alderotti Taddeo (1223–1303) in Florence. Archibald Billing (b 1791) of Cromlyn, Dublin was the first in London to organize practical teaching by the bedside at the London Hospital in 1822. He continued to teach there until 1836. Dutch physician, Anton de Haen (1704–1776), was a pioneer in promoting bedside teaching in Europe. After presentation of clinical cases his students individually whispered the diagnosis in his ear so that they would not lose face in case their diagnosis was wrong.

Clinical Pathological Conferences The concept of presenting clinical cases followed by discussion and finally disclosure of the correct diagnosis by the pathologist was initiated by Richard Clark Cabot (1868–1939) of the Massachusetts General Hospital in 1895. He introduced it into the Harvard Medical School in 1900, and weekly clinical pathological conferences were started at the Massachusetts General Hospital by Cabot and James Homer Wright (1871–1928) in 1910. These were published in the *Boston Medical and Surgical Journal,* which became the *New England Journal of Medicine.*

Clinical Thermometry The significance of temperature as a sign of disease was recognized in ancient times, when warmth signified life and coldness meant death. Sanctorio Sanctorius (1561–1636) was the first use a thermometer, which he designed to record the temperature of the human body in 1614. It consisted of a convoluted capillary glass tube with a bulb at the end which was placed in the patient's mouth. The other end of the tube was dipped in water and the temperature was estimated from the amount of warm air that was expired. Herman Boerhaave (1668–1738) recommended its use in clinical medicine and his pupils, Gerard van Swieten (1700–1772) and Anton de Haen (1704–1776) made a number of temperature recordings in healthy people and compared these with recordings taken in disease around 1740. The ability of the body to maintain its temperature despite high room temperatures was demonstrated by Sir Charles Blagden (1748–1820) in 1774. Clinical thermometry was also advocated by George Martini (1702–1741) in his *Essays and Observations.* Diurnal variation in body temperature was observed by Chossat of France in 1838. George Zimmerman, an army surgeon at Hamm, did extensive experiments on thermometry and demonstrated the elevation of temperature secondary to the process of inflammation in 1850. Ludwig Traube (1818–1876) professor of medicine at Berlin, was one of the first to use the thermometer in clinical medicine, in 1850. A treatise on its application to clinical medicine was published by Carl Reinhold August Wunderlich (1815–1877), professor of medicine at Leipzig, in 1860. The effect of cold water on fever was extensively studied by James Currie (1756–1805) in England. The clinical thermometer remained a curiosity in medicine until around 1864. John Simon Bartlett, and another British physiologist, Sydney Ringer (1835–1910), independently published a series of temperature observations in England. Ringer's *On the Temperature of the Body as a means of Diagnosis in Phthisis and Tuberculosis*, published in 1865, remains a classic on the subject. Thermometers used up to this time were long and inconvenient and took about 20 minutes to record temperature. A more convenient form, a short-stemmed clinical thermometer, was invented by Sir Thomas Clifford Alibutt (1836–1925) of Dewsbury in 1866. The temperature curve in typhus, typhoid and pneumonia was described by T.J. Maclagan in 1868. It came into general use in England around 1873, following the publication of temperature charts in surgical patients by English surgeon, Joseph Bell (1837–1911).

Clippingdale, Samuel Dodd (1853–1925) London physician who graduated from Aberdeen in 1876. He later established a practice in Kensington and wrote several articles on the medical profession and its members.

Clitoris Female sex organ which takes its name from the Greek meaning 'to be enclosed or hidden', owing to its position in the external female genitalia.

Clomiphene Orally active non-steroidal compound chemically related to estrogen. Shown to inhibit the secretion of pituitary gonadotrophins and suppress ovulation by D.E. Holtkamp and co-workers of Cincinnati in 1960. It was found to induce ovulation in anovulatory women by D. Charles in England (1962) and R.B. Goldblatt (1961) in America. The first large trial in 102 anovulatory women was carried out by Peter M.F. Bishop (1905–1979) of London in 1965. It was used in treatment of infertility by C.J. Collins of Illinois in 1966.

Clonorchis sinensis [Greek: *clon*, branch + *orchis*, testis] Chinese liver fluke. In 1910 Harujiro R. Kobayashi (b 1887) of Japan discovered that cyprinoid fish acted as secondary intermediate hosts to *Clonorchis sinensis*. The complete life cycle was elucidated by Muto in 1917.

Cloquet, Hippolyte (1787–1840) Professor of anatomy at Paris who described the nasopalatine ganglion in 1816.

Cloquet, Jules Germain (1790–1883) Younger brother of Hippolyte Cloquet (1787–1840) and professor of anatomy at Paris. He described the lymphatic gland (Cloquet gland) in the femoral canal in 1817. Several other anatomical structures are named after him.

Closed-Circuit Anesthesia Based on the principle that if sufficient oxygen is added to supply the basal needs of the body and the resulting carbon dioxide is absorbed, the same mixture of gases can be used repeatedly for maintaining

anesthesia. Introduced by John Snow (1813–1858) in 1850. It was revived by Dennis Emerson Jackson (b 1878) during his work on animals in 1915, and American anesthetist, Ralph Milton Waters (b 1883) of Madison, Wisconsin used it for clinical anesthesia in 1920. The first clinical reports appeared in 1920 and a two-phase system was devised by Brian Sword (b 1889), an anesthetist from New Haven in 1926. A new closed circuit apparatus was patented by Drager in 1926, and caustic soda was used as an adsorber by W.B. Primrose of Glasgow in 1931. A closed circuit method for cyclopropane anesthesia was devised by American anesthetists, Ralph Milton Waters (b 1883) of Madison and Erwin Rudolf Schmidt (b 1890) in 1934.

Clostridium Etiological agent of botulism, isolated by Belgian bacteriologist, Emile Pierre Marie van Ermengen (1851–1932) during his investigation of a small outbreak in the village of Ellezeles in Belgium in 1896. *See botulism.*

Clotting *See blood coagulation, prothrombin time.*

Clouston, Sir Thomas (1840–1915) British psychiatrist, born in the Orkney Islands. He graduated from Edinburgh, where he became the superintendent of the Royal Morningside Asylum and lectured on mental diseases. He focused on mental aspects of adolescence and published *The Hygiene of the Mind* and *Clinical Lectures on Mental Diseases*. He was the first to associate juvenile paresis with congenital syphilis.

Clover, Thomas Joseph (1825–1882) Born in Aylesham, Norfolk, he was a leading anesthetist and lecturer at University College Hospital who made several contributions to anesthesia. He invented a quantitative chloroform inhaler in 1862, and devised a small portable apparatus, Clover inhaler, in 1876 which continued to be used for the next 75 years.

Clowes, William Surgeon to St Bartholomew's and Christ Church Hospitals during the 16th century. He also served in the army and was surgeon to Queen Elizabeth I. He published *Practice for all young Chirurgions* in 1591.

Club Foot Congenital disease of great antiquity. The mummy of Pharaoh Siphtah (1300 BC), now preserved at the Cairo Museum, shows evidence of this disease. The first surgical attempt to correct club foot or talipes was made by the German surgeon, Lorenz Heister (1683–1758) in 1784. G.M. Thilenius treated it by dividing the tendo achilles in the same year. The first accurate description was given by Antonio Scarpa (1747–1832) in 1803. A new method of subcutaneous section of the tendo achilles as treatment was introduced by Jacques Mathieu Delpech (1777–1832), professor of surgery at Montpellier, in 1816. His method was later employed by George Friedrich Ludwig Stromeyer

(1804–1876) in 1821. A classic English description was given by William John Little (1810–1894), a London surgeon who himself suffered from it, in 1839. He was operated on by Stromeyer.

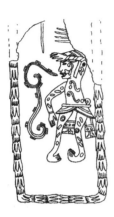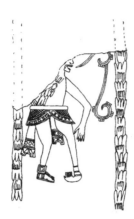

Drawing from frescoes of excavations at Teotihuacán, Mexico showing a boy (left) with bilateral club-foot and (right) an older person with unilateral club-foot. Le Vay, D, *The History of Orthopaedics*. Parthenon, London

Clubbing The first description of clubbing of the fingers was given by Hippocrates (460–377 BC) in his book of prognostics. Amongst the other symptoms, such as fever, sweats and dry cough in cases of empyema, he also noted that the nails in the hands of these patients were bent. A modern description of clubbing of the fingers and toes associated with arthritis and periostitis of the distal end of the long bones (pulmonary osteoarthropathy) secondary to anoxemia in chronic pulmonary disease or carcinoma of the lung was given by Pierre Marie (1853–1940) of Paris in 1890. It was also described by Viennese physician, Eugen Bamberger (1858–1921) in 1889.

Clutton Joints Form of chronic synovitis of the knee joint seen in congenital syphilis. Described by an English surgeon, Henry Hugh Clutton (1850–1909) from Sutton Walden, in 1886. He graduated from St Thomas' Hospital, London where he spent most of his career, and was made full surgeon there in 1892.

CMV *See cytomegalovirus.*

Cnidos Greek peninsula where one of the most famous ancient medical schools existed in 600 BC. At the school, each disease was studied and a specific remedy was sought. Famous physicians and scientists, including Democedes (600 BC) and Ctesius (500 BC) were from Cnidos, and their school ranked second only to the School of Cos attended by Hippocrates (460–377 BC).

Cnidus *See cnidos.*

Coagulase Test A test for pathogenicity of staphylococcal bacteria, introduced by H. Much (1880–1932) of Germany in 1908. *Staphylococcus pyogenes* was linked to coagulase-producing staphylococci by R. Cruickshank in 1937. The coagulase test was standardized by E.H. Gillespie in 1943.

Coagulation [Latin: *coagulum*, rennet] *See blood coagulation.*

Coal Miners' Disease A description of it in England is found in the *Saxon Chronicle* of Peterborough from AD 852. It was later referred to in Bishop Pudsey's *Bolden Book* in 1180. Chest disease was described by John Evelyn (1620–1706) of London in 1661. The disease known as 'black spit' amongst coal miners was correlated with autopsy findings in their lungs by W. Marshall of Glasgow in 1833.

Coarctation [Latin: *coarctare*, to press together] *See aortic coarctation.*

Coats, G. (1876–1915) Scottish ophthalmologist, born in Paisley, and graduated from Glasgow University in 1897. He studied ophthalmology in Vienna and many other centers in Europe before joining the Royal Ophthalmic Hospital in London in 1902. He wrote a classic treatise on thrombosis of the central vein of the retina, and described retinitis exudativa (Coats disease).

Coats, Joseph (1846–1899) A grand-uncle of the founder of the famous firm of cotton spinners, J & P Coats at Paisley. He was the first chair of pathology at Glasgow University in 1894. He pioneered pathology and started the first course for students in 1877. His *Manual of Pathology* was published in 1883.

Cobalt The name is derived from *kobold* which the miners of Saxony used to mean 'goblin'. The fumes of cobalt arsenite or smaltite were observed by miners in the 16th century. It was also known as 'mundic' in Cornwall. It was isolated by Swedish chemist Georg Brandt (1694–1768) in 1733. Tungsten carbide, a commonly used compound in the metal industry, was prepared from cobalt by Krupps of Essen, Germany in 1926. Pulmonary disease due to exposure to cobalt or tungsten was described by A.O. Bech and M.D. Kipling in 1962.

Cobbold, Thomas Spencer (1828–1886) London helminthologist who named the parasites, *Filaria bancrofti* and *Bilharzia hematobia* after their discoverers.

Cocaine The effects of the coca plant (*Erythroxylon coca*) in Peru were well known to the Incas. The Spanish explorer Augostin de Zarate was the first to focus attention of the rest of the world on coca plants from Peru in 1555. He pointed out that leaves, when chewed, produced a numbing effect. Nearly two centuries later a French chemist Angelo Mariani imported it to France and sold its products as 'Mariani wine', 'Mariani elixir', 'Mariani tea' and 'Mariani lozenges'. It was obtained from the plant by Gaedicke of Germany in 1855. Its active principle was obtained by Albert Niemann (1806–1877) of Germany, a pupil of Friedrich Wohler (1800–1882) in 1859. Niemann also named it cocaine. Pure cocaine was produced by Niemann and Sossen at Wohler's laboratory in Göttingen. A few years later Thomas Moreno y Maize, a surgeon in the Peruvian army, studied the effects and suggested that it could be used as a local anesthetic. These properties were described by Konstantinovich Vasili Anrep (1852–1915) in 1878. The addictive properties were first realized by Josef Breuer (1842–1925), a colleague of Sigmund Freud (1856–1939) in Vienna in 1884. Karl Koller (1857–1944) introduced it as a local anesthetic in eye surgery at the suggestion of Freud in the same year. C.L. Schleich (1859–1922) proposed its use for infiltration anesthesia in 1894. William S. Halstead (1852–1922) of Johns Hopkins University demonstrated the method of producing local anesthetia by injecting cocaine into the nerves in 1885. It was used as a spinal anesthetic in the same year by J.L. Corning (1885–1923). *See local anesthetic.*

Cocchi, Anthony (1693–1758) Professor of anatomy in Florence. He visited England to meet Isaac Newton (1642–1727), Richard Mead (1674–1754) and other important medical men and scientists. He published several medical treatises, some of which were translated into English.

Cocci [Greek: *kokos*, seed] *See Staphylococcus, Streptococcus.*

Coccidiomycosis [Greek: *kokos*, berry + *mykes*, fungus + *osis*, condition] A description of the causative organism was given by an undergraduate student of Robert Johan Wernicke (b 1873), Alejandro Posadas (1870–1902) of Buenos Aires, in 1892. American surgeon, Emmet Rixford (b 1865) of California and Thomas Caspar Gilchrist (1862–1927) of Baltimore named the fungus *Coccidioides immitis*, after consultation with the eminent American parasitologist Charles Wardell Stiles (1867–1941) in 1896. The mycelial nature of the fungus was demonstrated by William Ophuls (1871–1933) and Herbert C. Moffit in 1900. E.C. Dickson in 1915 studied the condition and thought that it was a mild form of tuberculosis due to the healed pulmonary lesions. The 'San Joaquin Valley Fever' of California was identified to be a milder form of coccidiomycosis by Myrnie Gifford in 1936.

Cochlear Implant [Latin: *cochlea*, snail shell; Greek: *koklias*,

snail] The idea of implanting a miniature prosthesis in the inner ear or cochlea to overcome deafness was first suggested by a Hungarian physiologist and physicist, Georg von Bekesy (1899–1972) in 1960. He also designed an audiometer which is still in use and published *Experiments in Hearing* in 1962. He was awarded the Nobel Prize for Physiology or Medicine in 1961. The first cochlear implant was made by the American firm 3M and it was implanted in 1973.

Cock, Edward (1805–1892) Surgeon at Guy's Hospital, London, and nephew of Sir Astley Cooper (1768–1841). He performed the first pharyngectomy in England, and described a method of urethrotomy in 1866.

Cock Peculiar Tumor Ulceration of a sebaceous cyst giving it an appearance of epithelioma. It is named after a surgeon at Guy's Hospital, Edward Cock (1805–1892).

Cockayne Syndrome Dwarfism, microcephaly, retinal atrophy, mental retardation and progressive upper motor neuron dysfunction with autosomal recessive inheritance. Described by English physician, Edward Alfred Cockayne (1880–1956) from Sheffield. He described epidermolysis bullosa in 1938.

Cod-Liver Oil Employed for centuries in Northern Europe as a treatment for rheumatic disorders. It was used for chronic rheumatism in England by Robert Darley who conveyed his findings to Thomas Percival (1740–1804) of Manchester in 1782. An early treatise *Experiences of the Great Curative Powers of Cod-liver Oil* was published by Johann Heinrich Schenckl, a physician from Siegen, in 1822. Another was published by Sir John Hughes Bennet (1812–1875) of Edinburgh in 1841. In 1855, Dutch physician, D.J. DeJongh, wrote a treatise in which he listed a variety of illnesses that benefited from treatment with it. Armand Trousseau (1801–1867) in France used it as a treatment for rickets in 1865. Its efficacy in treatment of rickets was experimentally demonstrated in 1889 in England by Sir John Bland-Sutton (1855–1936) who fed crushed bone and cod-liver oil to lion cubs with rickets. It came to be used as a treatment for most joint and bone diseases in the last part of the 19th century. The active substance that prevented rickets was detected by Elmer Verner McCollum (1879–1967) and colleagues at the Johns Hopkins School of Hygiene in 1922.

Codeine A base alkaloid of opium, isolated by Jean-Pierre Robiquet (1780–1840) in 1832.

Codman, Ernest Amory (1869-1940) Surgeon to Massachusetts General Hospital who devised the first anesthetic chart (with Harvey Cushing). He coined the term frozen shoulder in 1934.

Codronchi, Giovanni Battista (1547–1628) Italian physician who wrote on forensic medicine in 1597. He also published a monograph on diseases of the larynx in 1597.

Coenzyme [Latin: *cum*, with; Greek: *en*, in + *zyme*, leaven] A dialysable non-protein compound essential for enzymatic activity named by Bertrand in 1897. The first was discovered by an English chemist, Sir Arthur Harden (1865–1940) of Manchester in 1904. He shared the Nobel Prize for Chemistry with Swedish biochemist Hans Karl von Euler-Chelpin (1873–1964) in 1929. Coenzyme A, which takes part in the respiratory cycle, was discovered by American biochemist, Fritz Albert Lipmann (1899–1986) in 1951, and it was isolated from yeast by German biochemist, Feodor Felix Konrad Lynen (1911–1979) in the same year.

Coffee *See caffeine.*

Coffey, Robert Calvin (1869–1933) Surgeon from Portland, Oregon. In 1911 he designed the operation (Coffey operation) in which ureters are transplanted into the colon.

Coffey, Walter Bernard (1868–1944) Surgeon in San Francisco who treated cancer by injecting an extract from the suprarenal cortex of the sheep.

Coffin Elaborate coffins made during early times reflected the prosperity and status of the deceased. Athenians were buried in coffins made of cedar wood, and the Romans used marble and stone. Egyptian coffins made of wood had inlaid enamel hieroglyphics with the dead person's name. Alexander the Great is said to have been buried in a gold coffin.

Cogan, Thomas (1736–1818) Born in Northamptonshire, he qualified as a physician in Leiden in 1767, and founded the Royal Humane Society with another physician William Hawes. He translated the works of Dutch physician, Peter Camper (1722–1789), and published *A Philosophical Treatise on Passions, Ethical Questions or Speculations in Moral Philosophy* and *Theological Disquisitions.*

Cogan, Thomas (d 1607) Physician from Somerset, educated at Oriel College, Oxford. He was elected master of Manchester School in 1575 and wrote *Haven of Health* (1586) and *A Preservation from Pestilence.*

Cohausen, John Henry (d 1750) Physician from Lower Saxony who wrote several medical treatises, some of which were later translated into English by a medical writer named Campbell.

Cohen, Stanley (b 1922) American biochemist, born in Brooklyn, New York and educated at Brooklyn College and the University of Michigan. He was professor of chemistry at Vanderbilt University in 1959. He isolated nerve growth factor and epidermal growth factor.

Cohn, Ferdinand Julius (1828–1898) German bacteriologist and botanist who was born in Breslau and obtained his degree in botany from Berlin at the age of 19 years. He returned to Breslau as a professor in 1859 and established the world's first institute for plant physiology. He demonstrated the existence of bacterial spores while working with Robert Koch (1843–1910), and was one of the first to refute the theory of spontaneous generation.

Cohnheim, Julius Friedrich (1839–1884) German pathologist from Pomerania in Poland. After serving as an army surgeon in the Austrian war, he became professor of pathology at Kiel in 1868, and later was professor at Breslau until 1878. He made a series of important contributions and discoveries throughout his career. His achievements include: pioneer experiments on histology and pathology in his dissertation on inflammation of the serous membranes in 1861; introduction of the freezing method for fresh microscopic slide preparations; and silver staining for the study of nerve endings in muscles in 1863. His most important work was on inflammation and suppuration. He described diapedesis in 1867. His *Lectures on General Pathology* was published in 1877.

Coindet, Jean François (1774–1834) Physician at Geneva who initiated the treatment of goiter with iodine in 1820. *See iodine.*

Coiter, Volchard (1534–1576) Dutch anatomist at Gröningen who published *De Cartlagenibus Tabulae* and several other works on anatomy. He was one of the first to note the automaticity of the heart beat in an excised heart of a kitten.

Coitus Interruptus A method of contraception known since Biblical times. Many African tribes have practiced the method for centuries.

Coitus Reservatus Male continence, a method of contraception by avoiding climax during intercourse. Proposed by John Humphrey Noyes (1811–1866) of America in 1866. His *Male Continence* was published in 1872.

Colchicum Meadow saffron, known as 'ephemerum' to the ancients, who considered it to be very poisonous. It derives its name from Colchis on the Black Sea, one of the places where the plant grows. Dioscorides described its poisonous properties in the 1st century. Alexander of Tralles, around

AD 550, recommended it for gout. Its use in the treatment of gout was revived by the Arabs around AD 900. It was denounced as a medicine by several physicians including Jacques Grevin of Paris in 1568 and Wedel of Jena in 1718. It was first included in the *London Pharmacopoeia* in 1618. It was introduced into medicine in England by W.H. Williams, a physician at Ipswich in 1820, and it was entered into the *London Pharmacopoeia* in 1824.

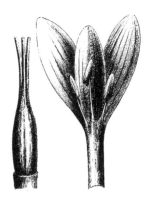

Ovary and perianth of *Colchicum autumnale*. Henry G. Greenish, *Materia Medica* (1899). Churchill, London

Cold [Anglo-Saxon: *ceald*] Described by Giovanni Baptista Della Porta (1543–1615) in his book of *Natural Magic* around 1600, to be similar to heat in that it could be reflected from a polished surface. His theory was proved with the use of a concave mirror at the Accademia del Cimento in 1684. Swiss physicist, Pierre Prevost (1751–1839) of Geneva defined cold as 'absence of heat' in 1791.

Cold Agglutinins First observed and described in the serum of patients suffering from 'an unusual form of bronchopneumonia' by Baltimore physician, Mildred Clark Clough (b 1888) and R.M. Richter of Johns Hopkins Hospital in 1918. *See atypical pneumonia.*

Cold Baths *See baths.*

Cole, William (1626–1662) A herbalist from Oxfordshire who wrote *The Art of Simpling* (1656) and *Adam in Eden or Nature's Paradise* in 1657.

Cole, William Sydney (1877–1952) Biochemist at Trinity College, Cambridge, he was the first to isolate tryptophan with Frederick Gowland Hopkins (1861–1947) in 1901. He published *Exercises in Practical Physiological Chemistry* in 1904.

Colet, John (1466–1569) Son of Sir Henry Colet, Lord Mayor of London. He was educated at Magdalen College, Oxford and later attended several colleges in Paris and Italy.

On his return to England in 1497 he took holy orders and was made the Dean of St Paul's. He pioneered grammar schools for studies in Latin and Greek, the first of which was St Paul's School, which he established with the proceeds from his own estate in Buckinghamshire in 1512.

Coley, William Bradley (1862–1936) American surgeon who graduated from Harvard in 1888, and was professor of clinical surgery at Cornell University. He induced erysipelas in patients to bring about tumor regression and prepared a streptococcal toxin (Coley toxin) to treat malignancies, but side-effects limited its use.

Colica Pictonum (Syn. Poitou colic, Devonshire colic, lead colic, colica vegetabilis, endemic colic) The earliest description of lead colic, from drinking artificially treated and stored strong wine, was given by Aethaeus in the 16th century. Citesius or François Citois (1572–1652) gave an account of colic of Poitou. George Baker (1722–1809), a physician in Devonshire, published *An Essay Concerning the Causes of the Endemic Colic in Devonshire*, in which he maintained that lead poisoning in Devonshire colic was due to cider presses used in Devon. It was also studied by James Hardy of Barnstaple, who wrote another treatise on the colic of Somerset and Poitou in which he attributed the cause to lead coating in drinking vessels. An epidemic in Devon in 1724 was described by John Huxam (1692–1768) in 1759. Lead colic in America (West India dry-gripes) was described by American physician, Thomas Cadwalander (1708–1779) in 1745.

Collagen Disease [Greek: *kolla*, glue + *genos*, descent] The first group of diseases called diffuse collagen disease was described by Paul Klemperer (1887–1964) and colleagues in 1942. Their description included disseminated lupus erythematosus and diffuse scleroderma. *See periarteritis nodosa, rheumatoid arthritis, connective tissue disease.*

Collapse Therapy Tuberculosis therapy, popular in the early 1900s. The principle is to rest the lungs and the methods employed included artificial pneumothorax, phrenic crush, apicolysis and thoracoplasty. Liverpool physician, James Carson (1772–1843), performed an open pneumothorax as treatment for tuberculosis in 1820. Phrenic crush, together with induction of pneumoperitoneum, to reduce the volume of the affected lung and raise the diaphragm, was introduced by Andrew Ladislaus Banyani (b 1893) in 1934. Apicolysis, a method of collapsing the affected apical lobe of the lung by removal of the adjacent bony structure of the chest wall, was originally suggested by Carl Boye Semb (b 1895) of Scandinavia in 1935. Thoracoplasty was introduced a few years later by several workers, including P.D. Crimm. The method of extrapleural pneumolysis was introduced in 1935, but it was abandoned because of the high rate of infection in the extrapleural space. *See artificial pneumothorax.*

Colles, Abraham (1773–1843) Irish surgeon, born near Kilkenny. He obtained the diploma of the College of Surgeons in 1795. After obtaining his MB from Edinburgh in 1797 he returned to Dublin, where he became a leading surgeon and professor of anatomy and surgery at the College of Surgeons, Ireland, in 1804. He was one of the first to tie the subclavian artery, in 1811, and is also thought to have been the first to tie the innominate artery successfully. He wrote a treatise on syphilis, *Practical Observation on the Venereal Disease,* in which he referred to immunity acquired to syphilis by a healthy mother in bearing a syphilitic child (Colles Law) in 1835. *See Colles fracture.*

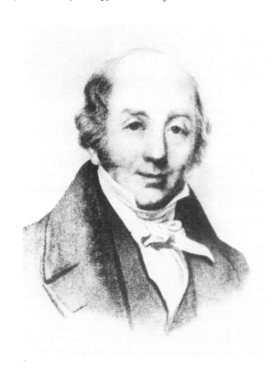

Abraham Colles (1773–1843). Courtesy of the National Library of Medicine

Colles Fracture Fracture of the distal radius of the forearm, described by Abraham Colles (1773–1843), professor of surgery at Dublin in 1814. Partial excision of the lower end of the ulna in cases of wrist deformity following Colles fracture was first carried out by an orthopedic surgeon, William Darrach (1876–1948) of Columbia University, in 1913.

Collet–Sicard Syndrome Palsy of the 9th, 10th, 11th and 12th cranial nerve as a result of fracture of the posterior cranial fossa. Described by French otorhinologist, Frederic

Justin Collet (b 1870) in 1915 and French radiologist, Jean Athanase Sicard (1872–1979) of Paris in 1917.

Collier, James Stanfield (1870–1935) London neurologist who described that part of the medial longitudinal bundle within the tegmentum of the midbrain (Collier bundle). He also gave a detailed description of subacute combined degeneration of the cord with James Samuel Riesien Russell (1863–1939) and others, in 1900.

Collier, Jeremy (1650–1726) Clergyman from Cambridge-shire, who served at a rectory in Suffolk. He later became a lecturer at Gray's Inn. He published *Essays Upon Several Moral Subjects* in three volumes in 1697, which dealt with pain, revenge, drunkenness, whoring, infancy and youth. The second edition was printed in 1707.

Collinson, Peter (1694–1768) Botanist from Kendal, West-morland and a contemporary of Carl Linnaeus (1707–1778) and Benjamin Franklin (1706–1790). Linnaeus named an American plant after Collinson, and Franklin conveyed his essays on electricity to him first.

Collip, James Bertram (1892–1965) Canadian chemist, born in Belleville, Ontario, who received his degree from Toronto University. He isolated a practical form of insulin for clinical use in 1923. He also extracted parathormone from the parathyroid glands in 1925, and identified hormones from the placenta. He was appointed professor of biochemistry at McGill University in 1928. He transferred to the chair of endocrinology in 1941. *See insulin.*

Collins, Samuel English physician who studied at Padua and took his degree at Oxford in 1659. He published a work on anatomy, and was made a censor of the College of Physicians in 1707.

Colloid Chemistry [Greek: *kolla*, glue + *oeidos*, form] Thomas Graham (1805–1869), the founder of colloid chemistry, distinguished crystalloid from colloid, on the basis of diffusion, in 1857. He called substances that passed through parchment paper crystalloids, and those that did not colloids. Further progress on the study of colloids was made by William B. Hardy (1864–1934) in 1900. Colloids were divided into 'hydrophile' and 'hydrophobe', depending on their affinity for water in a dispersed phase by Jean Perrin (1870–1942) of France in 1904. Clear proof that colloidal solutions had measurable osmotic pressure was provided by English physiologist, Ernest Henry Starling (1866–1927) in 1896. The Nobel Prize in Chemistry for work on colloidal solutions was awarded to an Austrian chemist Richard Zsigmondy (1865–1929) at Göttingen in 1925.

Colombo, Matteo Realdo (1516–1559) Italian anatomist and pupil of Andreas Vesalius (1514–1564), whom he succeeded at Padua in 1544. While vivisecting a dog he made an incision into the pulmonary vein and found that the blood in it was a brighter red. This led him to suggest that the lungs had rendered the blood 'spirituous'. His observation was the first on oxygenated blood. He described pulmonary circulation in 1559.

Color Blindness The first mention of the condition is found in a letter written by Joseph Huddart (1741–1816) to Joseph Priestley (1733–1804) in 1777. John Dalton (1766–1844), an English chemist from Eaglesfield, Cumberland, who himself suffered from it, was one of the first to investigate it in 1794. Some of the disasters on the railroads in England were recognized (in 1855) as due to colorblindness in drivers. Alarik Frithjof Holmgren (1831–1897) of Sweden introduced a test for color blindness in 1876. Thereafter, testing was obligatory in the railway services. The standard test was designed by a Japanese ophthalmologist, Shinobu Isihara (1879–1959) of Tokyo in 1917. The mechanisms involved in color discrimination were first explained by a Finnish-born Swedish physiologist, Ragner Arthur Granit (b 1900), who used microelectrodes to study the response of retinal cells to light of different wavelength and intensity. The 'retinex' theory, which led to further understanding of color vision, was developed by an American, Edwin Herbert Land (1910–1991) of Bridgeport, Connecticut, who also invented the Polaroid camera in 1947.

Color Vision *See color blindness.*

Colostomy or colotomy [Greek: *kolon*, great gut + *tome*, to cut] A method of establishing an artificial anus in the colon was proposed by Alexis Littre (1658–1726) of Paris in 1710. He advised the opening of the sigmoid flexure in the iliac region in certain cases of imperforate anus, and this was performed successfully by Dinet in 1793. H. Pillore from Rouen opened the cecum onto the right iliac region through a peritoneal incision for a patient with carcinoma of the rectum, in 1776. The first recorded colostomy for intestinal obstruction was performed by Pierre Fine (1760–1814) in 1805. Colostomies in England were performed independently by Freer and Pringle in 1821 for stricture of the rectum. Freer's patient died on the 10th day, but Pringle's patient survived. Lumbar colostomy through a vertical incision in the loin was performed by Danish surgeon, Adolph Callisen (1740–1824) of Copenhagen in 1817. Jean Zulema Amussat (1796–1856) carried out lumbar colostomy successfully in 1839. The earliest lumbar colostomy in England was performed by John Hilton (1804–1878) in 1857, and the second was by Thomas Bryant in 1859.

Colotomy *See colostomy.*

Colston, Edward (1636–1721) Philanthropist from Bristol who established several almshouses and schools. He made generous contributions to St Bartholomew's Hospital and Christ's Hospital in London.

Columbia University Founded as King's College, New York, in 1754. It reopened after the American Revolution as Columbia College in 1784. It was made Columbia University in 1912.

Coma Derived from the Greek term *koma*, to 'lie down' or 'deep sleep'.

Coma Vigil (Syn. agrypnia, typhomania) Lying awake in coma. Early physicians around the 17th century attributed it to diminished influx of nervous fluid into the medulla oblongata.

Combe, Charles (1743–1817) Physician and son of an apothecary from Bloomsbury, London. He studied at Harrow School and graduated in medicine from Glasgow in 1783. His main interests were antiquities and classical literature.

Combe, George (1788–1858) Edinburgh physician, brother of Scottish physician, Andrew Combe (1797–1847). He first practiced as a lawyer before taking to phrenology in 1837. He published *Essay on the Constitution of Man in Relation to External Objects, Essays on Phrenology* and several other works on education and phrenology. *See phrenology.*

Combe, James Scarth (1796–1883) Scottish physician who practiced at Leith and Edinburgh. His account, *A Case of Anaemia* presented before the Medico-Chirurgical Society of Edinburgh in 1822 was later recognized as the first on pernicious anemia.

Combined Immunodeficiency Swiss-type agammaglobulinemia. The first few cases of severe lymphopenia with extensive candida infection in infancy were described in Switzerland in 1950. A sex-linked familial condition of agammaglobulinemia was reported in an 8-year-old boy with recurrent infection by Ogden C. Bruton (b 1908), an American pediatrician, in 1952. Both were later classified as 'severe combined immunodeficiency'.

Comby Sign Whitish yellow patches seen in the inflamed buccal mucosa, before the onset of Koplik spots in measles. Described by French pediatrician, J. Comby (1853–1947).

Comenius, John Amos (1592–1671) Born in Moravia, a pioneer in educational reforms in Europe. He advocated education from infancy to adulthood, and wrote several works, including the first book on the Kindergarten, *School of Infancy.*

Comma Bacillus [Greek: *comma*, short clause; Latin: *bacillus*, small rod] The causative organism of cholera, *Vibrio cholerae*, was discovered by Robert Koch (1843–1910) in Egypt in 1883. Having realized the significance of his findings, Koch traveled to India on a special mission and isolated the bacterium from the intestinal contents of 42 people who had died of cholera, in 1884. *See Asiatic cholera.*

Commerson, Philibert (1727–1773) French physician who practiced in Montpellier. He was recommended by Carl Linnaeus (1707–1778) to the Queen of Sweden to assist in her collection of rare fish. He dedicated his life to botany and, following his voyage around the world in 1773, published several works. He wrote a dictionary and bibliography on the writers of natural history.

Committee on Safety of Medicines Appointed by the Department of Health in England in 1972.

Common Cold The viral etiology of the illness was demonstrated by a bacteriologist, Walther Kruse (1864–1943) of Bonn, in 1914. He also described bacillary dysentery in 1900.

Community Health Awareness of health in the community was stimulated by the poor sanitary conditions that prevailed during the early 19th century. The great sanitary reformer Edwin Chadwick (1801–1890) gave his report in 1842. The City Sewage Act was passed in 1848, and the first post of Medical Officer in London was created, to which a surgeon from St Thomas' Hospital, John Simon (1816–1904), was appointed. Sir Henry Duncan Littlejohn (1826–1914) was appointed Medical Officer of Health in Edinburgh in 1862 and presented his report on the sanitary conditions in the town in 1865. This led to significant improvement in the state of hygiene and a fall in the death rate. Another pioneer was Sir George Newman (1870–1948) of Leominster, a civil servant and physician. He was Chief Medical Officer to the Ministry of Health in 1919, and published *Hygiene and Public Health* (1917), *Outline of the Practice of Preventive Medicine* (1917), and *Building of a Nation's Health* (1939). *See sewers, public health.*

Comparative Anatomy Aristotle described parts of animals in his *De Partibus Animalium* and *Historia Animalium.* He compared organs such as the liver, spleen and kidneys of animals to those of humans. During early Roman times dissections on animals, animal sacrifices and slaughterhouses for animals were an important source for the study of anatomy. A modern work was written by Pierre Belon

(1517–1564) in 1553. The term was first introduced by a celebrated English botanist, physician and anatomist, Nehemiah Grew (1641–1712) of Coventry, in 1672. Use of the microscope was initiated by Marcus Aurelius Severinus (1580–1656) in his *Zootomia Democritaea* published in 1645. Other important comparative anatomists include: Johan Friedrich Meckel (1781–1833), professor of anatomy at Halle; Georges Leopold Cuvier (1769–1832) of Paris; Johan Muller (1821–1897) of Bonn; Robert Knox (1791–1862) from Edinburgh University; and Sir Richard Owen (1804–1892) from Lancaster. *See dissection.*

Comparative Psychology A book entitled *Animal Intelligence* was published by John George Romanes (1848–1894) in 1883. He was a naturalist and a friend of Charles Darwin (1809–1882) and did pioneering work on invertebrate animals and compared the mental development of animals and humans in *Mental Evolution in Animals* published in 1888.

Complement [Latin: *complere*, to fill up] *See alexin.*

Complexion Thought to be produced by four humors and hot and cold, moist and dry characteristics of the body and skin. An early treatise was written by Levinus Lemnius (1505–1568), a physician and monk in The Netherlands in 1561. It was translated into English by a school master and physician, Thomas Newton (d 1607) in 1576.

Compound F *See corticosteroids.*

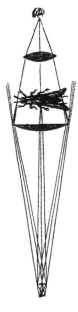

Earliest form of compound microscope with object glass and eye glass. Jabez Hogg, *Microscope, its History, Construction, and Teachings* (1854). Illustrated London Library, London

Compound Microscope Several convergent lenses with one having a short focal length. The first was probably invented by Zacharias Janssen who was a spectacle maker from Middelburg in Holland around 1590. It consisted of a double convex lens as an objective and a concave eyepiece. Dutch lens maker, Hans Lippershey (1571–1619), independently devised a compound microscope in 1609. Galileo (1664–1642) was one of the first to apply it to scientific studies. A description was given by Robert Hooke (1635–1703) who constructed his special microscope in 1665. His instrument had a single hemispheric lens as an objective and a plane convex lens as eyepiece. Eustachio Divini gave an account of his compound microscope to the Royal Society in 1666, and Phillip Bonnai published an account of two others in 1698. *See microscope.*

Computerized Axial Tomography CAT was developed independently by a British scientist, Godfrey N. Hounsfield (b 1919), and a South African-born American medical physicist, Allan Cormack (b 1924), around 1973.

Comrie, D. John (1875–1939) Physician at the Royal Infirmary of Edinburgh, and President to the History of Medicine section of the British Medical Association in 1927. He published a *History of Scottish Medicine* in two volumes in 1932.

Concato Disease Polyserositis due to tuberculous inflammation of serous membranes. Described by Italian physician, Luigi Maria Concato (1825–1882) in 1881.

Concave Lenses These came into use about two centuries after the introduction of convex lenses, in the mid-15th century. They were used in spectacle making in 1500.

Conchology [Greek: *kongche*, shell + *logos*, discourse] Study of shells, known to Pliny and Aristotle. A treatise was published by John Daniel of Kiel in 1675, and other important treatises were published by: Martin Lister (1685), James de Carle Sowerby (1842) and Edward Forbes (1848).

Concussion Described by Lanfranc (1290–1296) of Milan in *Chirurgia Magna* published in 1295. It was defined as 'an essentially transient state due to head injury which is of instantaneous onset, manifests widespread symptoms of purely paralytic kind, does not as such comprise any evidence of structural cerebral injury, and always followed by amnesia for the actual moment of accident' by Wilfred Trotter (1872–1939) in 1924. *See head injury.*

Condillac, Etienne de Bonnet (1715–1780) Born in Grenoble, he was a contemporary of the French political philosopher, Jean Jacques Rousseau (1712–1778) and disciple of John Locke (1632–1704). He proposed the theory that all knowledge comes from the senses. He published *Traite des Systemes* (1746) and *Traites des Sensations.*

Conditioned Reflex [Latin: *reflectere*, to turn back] The concept of a physiological basis for all psychological reactions to external stimuli was put forward by the great Russian physiologist Ivan Mikhailovich Sechinov (1829–1905) around 1860. Ivan Petrovich Pavlov (1849–1936) based his meticulous scientific investigation of reflexes on Sechinov's theory and established the theory of conditioned reflexes in the 1920s.

Condom Several suggestions have been made regarding the invention of the condom. Some historians believe that it was invented by Condom or Conton, a court physician to Charles II in the 17th century; others attribute the invention to a Major Condom of the Royal Guards. The first appearance of the word is found in a work on syphilis published by English physician Daniel Turner (1666–1741) in 1717. It is also mentioned in the *Classical Dictionary of the Vulgar Tongue* published in 1785. A description is found in *De Morbo Gallico* written by the Italian anatomist, Gabriele Falloppio (1523–1562). He pointed out its advantage, that it could be carried in a pocket, and recommended it for protection from syphilis, without any mention of its use for birth control. Handbills advertising condoms appeared in the last half of the 18th century. A particularly interesting handbill offering the sheaths [Anglo-Saxon: *sceth*, shell or pod] for sale was produced by a Mrs Phillips of the Strand in London in 1776. The first condoms were made of the dried gut of the sheep, and came into large-scale use only following the vulcanization of rubber, independently by Charles Goodyear (1800–1860) in America, and Thomas Hancock (1786–1865) in England, in 1844.

Conductor The term was first used in his *Dissertation on Electricity* by John Theophile Desaguliers (1683–1749) of La Rochelle, France. He was brought to London by his father, a clergyman, and became professor of philosophy at Oxford in 1710. He published several treatises including *A Course of Experimental Philosophy* and a treatise on building chimneys that prevented smoke.

Condylomata Accuminata [Greek: *kondylos*, knuckle] Genital warts have been known for over 2000 years and their occurrence following sodomy was mentioned by the Roman poet Juvenal in the 1st century. Aetius of Amida (AD 502–575) defined condylomata as tubercles which form in the soft wrinkled skin around the anus, and recommended their removal with forceps. Gabriele Falloppio (1523–1562) differentiated condylomata lata or syphilitic warts from genital warts.

Confessions A book of brilliance on self analysis, unprecedented in its time, was written by St Augustine in AD 386. It is considered to be one of the earliest significant works on self analysis based on psychological principles.

Congenital Agammaglobulinemia A sex-linked familial condition, reported in an 8-year-old boy with recurrent infection by American pediatrician, Ogden C. Bruton (b 1908) in 1952.

Congenital Atresia of the Esophagus Described in a 2-year-old child by Thomas Gibson, grandson of Oliver Cromwell and Physician General to the army in 1697. William Durston has been sometimes credited with first description in 1670 although the case that he described was that of conjoined females with many organs in common. After nearly 250 years, Martin published a case report in 1821 which was followed by a series of 43 cases by Morell Mackenzie (1837–1892), a British laryngologist in 1884. Gastrostomy as treatment was introduced in England by Steele in 1888. Sir Arthur Keith (1866–1955) traced 14 cases in the museums of London and gave an accurate description in 1910. Primary anastomosis of the esophagus was suggested as treatment by H.M. Richter in 1913. This operation was performed by Cameron Haight (1901–1970) and Harry A. Towsley in 1943.

Congenital Biliary Atresia First reviewed by J. Thompson of Edinburgh who presented a series of 50 cases in 1891. A collection of 120 cases from the literature was described by J.B. Holmes in 1916. Successful treatment by anastomosis was performed by W.E. Ladd in 1928. Up to 1960 only four cases were successfully treated by surgery in England, and the first success was achieved by T.E.D. Bevan and G.W. Duncan in 1946. Another large series of 146 cases was presented by Robert Edward Gross (1905–1988) in 1953.

Congenital Dislocation of the Hip Ambroise Paré (1510–1590) considered injury to be the cause of the disease in the 16th century. One of the earliest accounts was given by Guillaume Dupuytren (1777–1835) in 1826. In 1835 Charles Gabriel Pravaz (1791–1853) attributed it to inflammation. Aristide Auguste Vernuil (1866) and Edme Felix Alfred Vulpian (1871) considered it to be caused by a neuromuscular condition. German surgeon, Albert Hoffa (1859–1908) designed the Hoffa method of operative treatment in 1890. The Trendelenburg sign in CDH was described by Friedrich Trendelenburg (1844–1924) of Germany, in 1895. Pierre Germain Marie Damany (1870–1963) postulated that it was the consequence of bipedal gait. Tibial tripometry, a measure of the angle between the tibiae, was used as a diagnostic criterion by Damany in 1912. Clinical signs for diagnosis were described by George Perkins (1872–1979), professor of surgery from St Thomas' Hospital, in his *Signs by which to Diagnose Congenital Dislocation of Hip* published in *The Lancet* in 1928. A method of conservative treatment with the use of a harness with stirrups was introduced by a Czechoslovakian surgeon, Arnold Pavlik (1902–1965), in 1957.

Congenital Heart Disease One of the earliest accounts was given by Michael Underwood (1737–1820), a London pediatrician, in his treatise on children's diseases in 1789. A monograph was written by London physician, John Richard Farre (1775–1862) in 1814, and another on the malformations of the human heart was published by English physician, Thomas Bevill Peacock (1812–1882) in 1854. The method of measuring cardiac output in animals by injecting a dye into the vein and analyzing the amount of dye in the arterial blood was introduced by Canadian-American scientist, George Neil Stewart (1860–1930) in 1894. His method was used in clinical medicine by an American physiologist, William Ferguson Hamilton (b 1893) and co-workers in 1932, and the dye dilution curves obtained became a cornerstone for diagnosis. A modern clinical approach to congenital anatomical lesions of the heart was introduced by Maude Elizabeth Seymour Abbott, (1869–1940) of Canada in *Congenital Heart Diseases* published in 1927. She pointed out that it was associated with an 18% risk of other malformations. Study was further advanced by the introduction of venous catheterization by Lewis Dexter in 1947. James William Brown (1897–1958), a member of the editorial board of the *British Heart Journal* and a consultant to Grimsby Hospital, published *Congenital Heart Disease* in 1939, which was of great importance in establishing pediatric cardiac surgery in England. The increased risk of congenital heart disease and congenital cataracts in patients who contracted maternal rubella during their first trimester of pregnancy was pointed out by Sir Norman McAlister Gregg (1892–1966) in 1941. *See atrial septal defect, pediatric cardiology, Fallot tetralogy.*

Congenital Hypoplastic Anemia Erythrogenesis imperfecta. Condition in early infancy owing to bone marrow depression. Described by Kenneth Daniel Blackfan (b 1883) and Louis Klein Diamond in 1944.

Congenital Megacolon *See Hirschsprung disease.*

Congenital Spherocytosis (Syn. acholuric jaundice) Increased osmotic fragility of red cells, noted by Oskar Minkowski (1858–1931) in 1900. The connection between increased fragility of red cells and their spherical shape was pointed out by Max Gansslen (1859–1969) in his article

Uber Hemolytischen Ikterus published in 1922. The fragility of spherical red cells in hypotonic solution was studied in detail by a Kansas physician, Russell Landram Haden (b 1888) in 1934, by another American physician William Bosworth Castle (b 1899) of Boston and by G.A. Dalland in 1937.

Conical Refraction Phenomenon correctly predicted by Irish mathematician, Sir William Rowan Hamilton (1805–1865) of Dublin in his work on optics in 1827.

Conine Active alkaloid from the seeds of the deadly plant, hemlock (*Conium maculatum*), obtained in a pure form by P.L. Geiger (1785–1836) in 1831. *See hemlock.*

Coningham, John (d 1749) Born in Cumberland, he graduated from Rheims in 1719 and served as physician at the London Hospital.

Conjugal Sex [Latin: *conjugare*, to join together] The first royal decree to control conjugal sex was issued by Queen Joanna I (1326–1882) of Naples. Her decree stated 'Ne quis uxorum suam cogeat plus quam sexies pro die coire' (that no man must force his wife to have sexual intercourse more than six times a day). A book dealing with personal health, prevention of conception, hereditary well-being or health, physical excess and infanticide, *The Conjugal Relationship,* was published by Augustus K. Gardner a professor of midwifery at the New York Medical College in 1910.

Conn Syndrome Excessive secretion of aldosterone leading to hypernatremia, hypertension and hypokalemic alkalosis. Described by American physician, Jerome William Conn (b 1907) of the University of Michigan in 1955.

Connective Tissue [Latin: *cum*, together + *nectere*, to bind; French: *tissue*] Its nature and origin was explained by French neurologist, Jean Nageotte (1866–1945) in 1916.

Connective Tissue Stains Various stains were developed by J.H. Buzzaglo of Amsterdam (1934), Germain Crossman of Rochester, New York (1937), Franklin Burr Mallory of Boston (1897), and Robert Kingsbury Lee-Brown of Syd-ney (1929).

Connective Tissue Disease [Latin: *cum*, together + *nectere*, to bind; French: *tissue*] An early description was that of scleroderma by Carlo Crisio of Italy in 1754, and it was given its present name by E. Gintrac in 1844. Dermatomyositis, which is another form of connective tissue disease, was described by Ernest Leberecht Wagner (1829–1888) in 1863. *See periarteritis nodosa, rheumatoid arthritis, collagen disease.*

Connell, Karl (1878–1941) New York physician who designed a band with two hooks (Connell harness) for fixing the face-piece of anesthetic apparatus to the head during anesthesia.

Connor, Bernard (1666–1698) Irish physician who settled in Oxford in 1695. He published *Dissertationes Medico-Physicae* and *Evangilium Medici* in 1697.

Conolly, John (1794–1866) A resident physician at the Middlesex Asylum in Hanwell who was the first in England to advocate the removal of all forms of mechanical restraints for mental patients.

Conradi Line Drawn from the base of the xiphisternum to the cardiac apex, to denote the upper limit of normal dullness of the left lobe of the liver. Defined by Norwegian physician, Andrew Christian Conradi (1809–1869).

Consilia Medical books during the 14th and 15th centuries in Europe which contained experience and case records of famous physicians from the past. An important consilia was written by a Paduan professor, Gentile da Foligno around 1340. Another, containing 305 cases, was written by Bartolommeo Montagnana in 1470.

Constantin, Robert (1502–1605) A physician and professor at Caen. He published a lexicon in Greek and Latin in 1562.

Constantine The Great (AD 272–337) The Emperor of Rome who embraced Christianity and founded the Byzantine Empire. He was also a great humanist, who prevented the murder of unwanted children and offered them protection. *See Byzantium.*

Constantinus, Africanus (1020–1087) He gave a decisive impetus to medieval medicine. He was born in Carthage and traveled extensively in India, Babylon, Egypt and other places. He retired to the Montecasino Monastery in Salerno in 1070 and wrote several medical treatises. He translated important Arabic and Greek medical works into Latin, and was also the first to use the term 'variola' for smallpox. His work earned him the title of *Orientis et occidentis doctor.*

Constantinople *See Byzantium.*

Constipation Hippocrates (460–377 BC) recognized the importance of regular evacuation of normal stools in maintaining health. Paul of Aegina (625–690) stated that 'when the digestive faculty is in an atonic state, we must give food and applications of an astringent nature' and he recommended pomegranates, apples, pears and fragrant wines of astringent quality. Aulus Cornelius Celsus (25 BC–AD 50) recommended laxatives and diuretics. Haly Abbas (AD 930–994) treated it with prunes, tamarinds and clysters. Chronic intestinal stasis or chronic constipation was well recognized as a cause of cancer by several workers, including the surgeon E.G. Slesinger (1922), during the early 20th century. *See aperient, laxative, suppository.*

Constrictive Pericarditis Pericardiectomy as treatment was performed by French surgeon, Paul Hallopeau (1876–1924) in 1921. *See adherent pericardium.*

Consumption Cures Various quack medicines sold in the form of secret remedies for tuberculosis during the 19th and early 20th centuries. Some of these were Tuberculozyme, Brompton Consumption Mixture (which had no relation to the Brompton Consumption Hospital) and Steven's Consumption Cure, which was claimed by Dr Steven to contain a herbal medicine called *umckaloaba* from Africa. *See umckaloaba, Brompton consumption and cough specific.*

Consumption *See tuberculosis.*

Contact Lenses The original idea of covering the cornea with a protective shell was suggested by Leonardo da Vinci (1452–1519) in the 15th century. René Descartes (1596–1650) and Thomas Young (1773–1829) also made similar suggestions in the 17th and 18th centuries. The English astronomer Sir John Herschel (1792–1871) investigated the possibility of using a gelatinous transparent shell over the cornea to protect it from disease of the eyelids in 1827. Saemisch of Germany approached F.E. Muller of Wiesbaden, a glass blower and maker of artificial eyes, to make a thin glass shell suitable to be placed over the cornea for his own use. Saemisch used it for the next 20 years. In 1892, Muller made another lens for Fraenkel, a physician who had an entropion as a result of trachoma. The term 'contact lens' (*Kontakbrille*) was introduced by A. Eugen Fick, a physician in Zurich, who started investigating it as a refractive device in 1887. He conducted his experiments on animals and then cadavers and himself, before he tried them on his patients. Fick also obtained several contact lenses through the German physicist, Ernest Abbe (1840–1908) of Eisenach, an associate of Carl Zeiss (1816–1888). In 1889 August Muller, a medical student in Germany started his experiments which he presented for his doctorate thesis. He corrected his own myopia and proceeded to develop the technique. Lohnstein of Berlin (1896) and Siegrist of Switzerland made significant contributions to their development and Siegrist developed another parallel method, called the hydrodiascope in 1897. Leopold Heine (b 1870), an ophthalmologist in Kiel in Germany, demonstrated their practical value in correcting myopia, hyperopia and astigmatism in 1929. His work created worldwide interest and 4 years later a Hungarian ophthalmologist, Josef Dallos at the Carl Zeiss Institute, devised a technique for adding high correcting

power. The plastic contact lens was introduced in 1938 by Theodore E. Obrig, the founder of the Obrig Laboratories, which made them at Worcester, Massachusetts. Some of the early publications on the subject include *Contact Lenses* by Obrig in 1942 and a book on the contact lens technique by L. Lester Beacher of New York in 1941. *See hydrodiascope, Zeiss, Carl.*

Contagion [Latin: *contagio*, touch] Described as infection passing from one individual to another by Girolamo Fracastoro of Verona (1478–1553) in 1546. This was one of the earliest propositions on the contagion theory of infection. The existence of an infectious germ of disease was proposed by Armand Trousseau (1801–1867) of Paris in his *On Contagion* published in 1860. The germ theory of disease was proved by Louis Pasteur (1822–1895) in 1865. *See germ theory of disease.*

Contagious Diseases Act Act of Parliament to combat the spread of venereal diseases, passed in England in 1864. It was amended in 1867 to make medical examination compulsory for prostitutes who lived in areas that had naval and military bases. This act was repealed in 1886.

Contraception [Latin: *contra*, opposite or against + *captor*, receiver] *See birth control, contraceptive devices.*

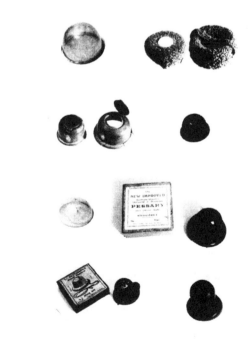

Early contraceptive devices. Courtesy of the IPPF

Contraceptive Devices During ancient Egyptian times, around 1800 BC, pessaries made of crocodile dung, vaginal irrigation with honey and various other methods were used to prevent pregnancy. Herbal abortifacients such as jugri from molasses and leadwort from Sri Lanka were known to the Indians. Sponges soaked in contraceptive materials such as gum were used in ancient times and mentioned in the Talmud. Condoms were introduced into Europe during the 18th century, supposedly by a Colonel Condom. The first condom was made of the dried gut of the sheep. After the discovery of vulcanization in 1840, condoms were made of rubber. Francis Place (1771-1854) wrote a treatise in 1822, *Principles of Population*, in which he suggested several measures for the prevention of conception. Other forms of contraception – vaginal metal caps and diaphragms – were used during this period. Latex condoms were introduced in 1930. The contraceptive pill was developed from studies on the ovary by an Austrian, Ludwig Haberlandt in 1921, and the work on progesterone as a contraceptive was pioneered by Willard Myron Allen (1904–1993) and George Wash-ington Corner (1889–1981) of America in 1929. Further development of the contraceptive pill was brought about by an American endocrinologist, Gregory Goodwin Pincus (1903–1967), who determined the correct amounts of progesterone to be used in it in the 1950s. An inert intra-uterine device was introduced as a method of contraception by Jack Lippes in 1961. *See birth control, condoms.*

Contraceptive Pill *See contraceptive devices.*

Contrast Media A mixture of bicarbonate and tartaric acid was one of the earliest contrast agents in radiology used for visualizing the lining of the stomach. It was later replaced by bismuth nitrate, bismuth sulfate and barium sulfate. Iodized oil was introduced by Athanase Siccard (1872–1929) in 1921. Gallbladder visualization was made possible by Evarts Ambrose Graham (1883–1957), professor of surgery at Washington University, St Louis, and Warren Henry Cole (b 1898) who used chlorinated and brominated phenolphthalein capable of being excreted by the liver, in 1929. Iodophthalein, which is less toxic, was introduced as an oral as well as an intravenous contrast medium by Whitaker and Miliken in 1929. Pheniodol replaced iodophthalein as a better contrast medium in 1940.

Convalescence Methods to treat those who were reduced in flesh and cachectic were described by Paul of Aegina (625–690). He mentioned the use of thick wine, and food with thick juices, along with slow exercise as a method of revival after an illness. Aetius of Amida (AD 502–575) recommended the rubbing of various herbal oils onto the skin, and Haly Abbas (AD 930–994) advocated the same, but with plenty of sleep. Rhazes (850–932) recommended food with plenty of meat and sleep.

Convalescent Institution The first in England was established at Walton-on-Thames in 1840, and later had branches for children in Mitcham and Hendon. Another was opened at Snaresbrook, East London, in 1866.

Convex Lens The evidence that the ancients had a knowledge of optics is provided by the discovery of a convex lens made of rock crystal in the ruins of Nimrud by Sir Austen Henry Layard (1817–1894). The oldest convex lens in existence today is from the island of Crete and dates to the Minoan civilization around 1000 BC. A polished crystal found in Nineveh, which may have been used as a lens, is in the British Museum. The magnifying power of convex lenses and concave mirrors was described by Seneca in AD 50. He also used them to aid his defective sight. A scientific study was done by Alhazen or Ibn Al-Haitham (AD 965–1038) of Basra. Convex spectacles were invented around 1270 in France, and convex lenses started to be produced industrially in Venice in 1300.

Convulsion [Latin: *con*, together + *vulsum*, tear away] *See epilepsy.*

Cook, Fredrick Albert (1865–1940) An explorer and physician from Calicoon, New York State. He graduated in medicine from Columbia University and joined the Arctic ex-pedition as a surgeon in 1891. Thereafter, he made several expeditions to the Antarctic and other places. He made his controversial claim to be the first man to reach the North Pole in 1908. His claim was challenged by Robert Peary, and Cook was discredited by an investigating committee in Copenhagen. He was imprisoned for another alleged fraud in 1923 but was subsequently pardoned.

Cooke, John (1756–1838) Born in Lancashire, he studied medicine at Guy's Hospital, London, and was elected in 1784 as physician to the London Hospital, where he served for the next 20 years. He published a *Treatise on Nervous Diseases* (1820–1823), which became a standard work.

Cooke, William Edmund (1881–1939) Born in Wigan, he was an English pathologist who modified Arneth's count for white blood cells and renamed it the polymorphonuclear count.

Cooley Anemia Thalassemia major, a hereditary hemolytic anemia associated with bone changes in children. Described by an American physician, Thomas Benton Cooley (1871–1945) of Michigan in 1925. He became the head of pediatric services at the Children's Hospital, Michigan in 1921 and was professor of pediatrics at the Wayne University from 1936 to 1941.

Cooley, Arthur Denton (b 1920) American cardiac surgeon, born in Houston, Texas. He graduated from Johns Hopkins and joined the Texas Heart Institution in Houston in 1962. Here he became a pioneer in open-heart and vascular surgery.

Coolridge, William David (1873–1975) American physicist, born in Hudson, Massachusetts, who received his degree from the Massachusetts Institute of Technology. He invented the prototype of the modern X-ray vacuum tube (Coolridge tube) in 1916. His other achievements include: a method of rendering tungsten ductile in 1908; a successful submarine detection system for use in World War II; and the development of radar.

Coombs Test Used to detect antigens in the blood. Devised by Amos Royston Robin Coombs (b 1921), Arthur Ernest Mourant and Robert Russell Race (1904–1984) in 1945.

Cooper, Samuel (1780–1848) A famous surgeon who served at the Battle of Waterloo and was later appointed to the chair of surgery at University College London. He published *A Dictionary of Surgery* in 1809, which became a popular book and underwent seven editions. This was later translated into German, French and Italian.

Cooper, Sir Astley Paston (1768–1841) Born in Brookhall, near Norwich and was induced by his uncle, William Cooper, a surgeon at Guy's Hospital, to come to London to study surgery. In London, Cooper studied under John Hunter (1728–1793) and attended Guy's Hospital where he later became a surgeon and eminent teacher of anatomy. He successfully ligated the external iliac artery for femoral aneurysm, and the common carotid artery for carotid aneurysm in 1808. He was also one of the first to perform an amputation at the hip joint.

Cope, Edward Drinker (1840–1897) American paleontologist from a Quaker family in Philadelphia. He wrote over 1400 articles and books on fossils and made several contributions to the theory of evolution. Because of financial difficulties, he sold his lifelong collection of fossils to the American Museum of Natural History.

Cope, Sir Vincent Zachary (1881–1974) A surgeon at St Mary's Hospital Paddington and Bolingbrook Hospital, Hunterian Professor, and Arris and Gale Lecturer of the Royal College of Surgeons. He wrote several books on surgery for diseases of the abdomen, including one on its history.

Copernicus, Nicolas (1473–1543) One of the greatest astronomers, who revolutionized the field. He was born in Thorn on the Vistula in Prussia. He studied astronomy at the universities of Cracow, Bologna, Rome and Padua and devised methods of accurately predicting the positions of the sun, moon and planets and increased the accuracy of calculations and tables. He also studied medicine at Padua from 1501 to 1505. One of his main contributions was on the movements of the planets, including the Earth, around the sun. His legendary *Nicolai Copernici Torinencis de Revolutionibus Orbium Coelistium Libri VI* was completed in 1530 and published in 1543. Copernicus received the first printed copy of it on the day of his death, on 24 May.

Copper Known to the ancient Egyptians, who used it to make utensils 15,000 years ago. It was probably the first metal known to the Egyptians during predynastic times. Copper mines existed in Sinai around 5000 BC and its use came into Europe around 4000 BC. It was employed as a medicine in the form of sulfate or 'blue stone' by Hindus and Arabs. During Roman times it was known as *cyprium* as it was abundantly found in Cyprus. Prehistoric relics made of copper, dating back to 2000 BC, have also been found in Ireland. The term 'cyprium' was later corrupted to the Latin word *cuprum* and is denoted by the symbol 'Cu' in chemistry.

Coprolalia [Greek: *kopros*, dung] Person uses spontaneous and involuntary obscene expressions. *See Gilles de la Tourette, Latah disease.*

Coproporphyrin [Greek: *kopros*, dung + *porphyros*, purple] *See porphyrin.*

Coram, Thomas (1668–1751) Born in Lyme Regis, Dorset, he was a philanthropist who established the first Foundling Hospital in England in 1739. The hospital opened at Hatton Garden in 1741 and gave medical care to infants who were brought from all over England. It moved to new premises in 1754.

Coramine Pyridine betacarbonic acid diethylamide, used as a coronary vasodilator in the 1930s and 1940s.

Cordotomy [Greek: *chorde*, cord + *tome*, to cut] The division of the anterolateral column of the spinal cord as treatment for intractable pain was performed by Gibson William Spiller (1863–1940) and Edward Martin (1859–1938) in 1912.

Cordova The birthplace of the great physician, Averrhoes (1126–1198), was founded in the south of Spain in 152 BC. It was taken by Goths in AD 572 and was later captured by Abderahman, who erected a great mosque there in 786. It became the most enlightened center of learning and a well planned city with libraries, a mosque-university, schools and industries during the Muhammedan era around AD 900. At the height of its glory it had one million inhabitants, 200,000 houses and 50 hospitals. The library of Cordova contained over 225,000 volumes. The Caliphs of Cordova also established libraries at Toledo, Seville and Muricia in AD 1000–1200. With the fall of Cordova in 1235 to the Christians, Arab medicine declined and lost its influence.

Cordus, Euricius (d 1538) Botanist, poet and physician whose real name was Henry Urban. He wrote several botanical and medical treatises including one on English sweating sickness in 1529.

Cordus, Valerius (1515–1544) The son of Euricius Cordus (d 1538) and a botanist. He was born at Simsthausen in Hesse and became a teacher of materia medica at Wittenberg at the age of 25 years. He wrote several works including the first German materia medica or pharmacopoeia, *Dispen-satorium*, in 1535. He prepared ether by treating oil of vitriol (sulfuric acid) with distilled sprits (alcohol) in 1549. He called this *Oleum Vitriole Dulce*. He died at the age of 29 in Rome.

Cori, Carl Ferdinand (1896–1984) He and his wife Gerty Theresa Radnitz Cori (1896–1957), were the third couple to receive the Nobel Prize after the Curies (1903) and the Jolliot-Curies (1935). They were born in Prague, graduated from Trieste and emigrated to America in 1922, where they both became professors at the Washington University Medical School at St Louis. They were amongst the first to demonstrate that defects in enzymes could be inherited, and won the Nobel Prize in Physiology or Medicine for their work on carbohydrates and enzymes.

Coringius, Hermanus (1606–1681) A physician at Leiden who wrote a philosophical treatise on the Aristotelian system.

Cormack, Allan Macleod (b 1924) South African-born American medical physicist who worked at Groote Schuur Hospital in Cape Town before he became professor at Massachusetts in 1964. He developed CAT scanning or computerized axial tomography, independently of Sir Godfrey Newbold Hounsfield (b 1919). The Nobel Prize for Physiology or Medicine was shared by Hounsfield and Cormack in 1979.

Cornarius, John (1500–1558) Born in Saxony, he practiced medicine in Germany and wrote several translations of Latin and Greek medical classics.

Cornaro, Luigi (1467–1566) Architect from Venice who wrote one of the earliest treatises on preservation of health in old age in 1550. He was 83 years old when he wrote the first book and it contained many sensible suggestions for living healthily in old age. His third book on the joys of old age was written at the age of 95 years. He died in his 99th year. A translation into English was published in 1753.

Corneal Graft [Latin: *cornu*, horn] The first attempt to use human donors for corneal transplants was made by Heinrich Sellerbeck (b 1842) of Germany in 1878. The procedure was described by Arthur von Hippel (1841–1917) of Germany in 1888. A successful corneal transplantation was by Eduard Conrad Zirm (1863–1944) in 1906. The procedure was initially found to be difficult to perform owing to the belief that the grafts had to be obtained from the living eye within a few minutes. New York ophthalmologist, Ramon Castroviejo (1904–1987), and Vladimir Petrovich Filatov (1875–1956) of Odessa, a Russian surgeon, demonstrated that the cornea from a cadaver was equally effective. J. W. Tudor Thomas (1893–1976) of Cardiff after extensive trials on animals, improved the rate of success of corneal transplantation with the use of small grafts.

Corneal Opacity [Latin: *cornu*, horn] Paul of Aegina (AD 625–690) in his treatise on ophthalmology, recommended crocodile dung as treatment. He also distinguished between cataract and amaurosis. A modern description was given by German ophthalmologist, Phillip Franz von Walther (1782–1849).

Corneal Transplant *See corneal grafts.*

Corner, Edmund Moss (1873–1950) London surgeon who devised a plug (Corner plug) for closing a perforated peptic ulcer.

Corner, George Washington (1889–1981) Anatomist from Rochester, New York, who published an anatomical text on the Middle Ages in 1924. He discovered progesterone in the corpus luteum with American physician, Willard Myson Allen (b 1904) of Rochester, Minnesota in 1929. *See oral contraceptives.*

Cornet Forceps Forceps for holding litmus paper while testing urine, devised by Berlin physician, George Cornet (1858–1915).

Cornil, Victor Andre (1837–1908) Histopathologist in Paris. He described malignant transformation of the acinar epithelium of the breast in 1865. *See breast.*

Corning, James Leonard (1855–1923) Born in New York, he introduced spinal anesthesia in 1885. He was also one of the earliest workers in America to recognize the dangers of cocaine addiction.

Coronary Angiogram *See coronary arteriogram.*

Coronary Arteriogram The coronary arteries in a human during life were outlined by S. Radner of Lund, Sweden in 1945. He used the ascending aorta through a sternal puncture for his procedure. J.A. Helmsworh and colleagues used the newly invented polythene catheter through the brachial artery for catheterization in 1950. The method of selectively visualizing coronary arteries by inserting a catheter into a major artery and passing it in a retrograde fashion into the mouth of the coronary artery, before injecting a radio-opaque dye, was devised by F. Mason Sones of the Cleveland Clinic and Charles T. Dotter of the University of Oregon Medical School in 1959.

Coronary Artery Aneurysm A major review in 31 patients was performed by N. Packard and H.F. Weschsler in 1939. The next important series consisting of 89 cases was presented by A.S. Dauod in 1963.

Coronary Artery Bypass Graft (CABG) An attempt at bypassing diseased coronary arteries by implanting pectoral muscles onto the pericardium, was made by Claude Schaeffer Beck (1894–1971) in America in 1935, in a 48-year-old coal miner. The first CABG was performed in 1962 but the patient died of a cerebrovascular accident. A rural physician from La Plata, Argentina, Rene G. Favaloro, who studied surgery at the Cleveland Clinic, performed the first successful bypass using the saphenous vein in 1967. By 1970 Favaloro and colleagues had performed over 2200 CABGs with an operative mortality of only 3%. Their successful results established the procedure as a standard treatment for coronary artery disease.

Coronary Artery Disease A description of coronary circulation was given by Raymond de Vieussens (1641–1715) of France in *Traite du Coeur* in 1715, and calcification of the coronary arteries was described by Giovanni Battista Morgagni (1682–1771) in 1761. Allan Burns (1731–1813), a Scottish surgeon and cardiologist, made the first suggestion that angina was due to coronary artery obstruction in his *Observations of Some of the Most Important and Frequent Diseases of the Heart,* published in 1809. The first case of correctly diagnosed coronary artery occlusion in life was reported by Adam Hammer (1818-1878) in 1876. George Dock of Pennsylvania diagnosed a case and later confirmed it at autopsy in 1896. Timothy Leary of America made a microscopic study of coronary artery lesions in 1934 and came to the important conclusion that the pathogenesis of the atherosclerotic lesions was related to disturbance of lipid metabolism. Around the same time Frederick Arthur Willius (1888–1972) at the Mayo Clinic commenced extensive studies on lipids and demonstrated that high total lipid and cholesterol levels positively correlated with coronary artery disease. The modern theory of atherosclerosis was initiated in 1946 by J.B. Duguid, who proposed that the atheromatous plaques were essentially mural thrombi that had become incorporated into the vessel wall. The stage of platelet deposition in atherogenesis was studied by L.A. Harker and colleagues in 1981. This led to the use of anti-platelet agents. *See angina pectoris, coronary artery bypass graft.*

Coronary Artery, Anomalous The anomalous origin of the coronary artery from the pulmonary artery was described by H. Brooks in 1885.

Coronary Atherosclerosis *See coronary artery disease.*

Coronary Care Unit (CCU) The concept of intensively monitoring the patient during the early stages of myocardial infarction was introduced around 1960 in both America and England. The first 11-bedded unit was established in America through the efforts of Hughes Day at the Bethany Medical Center in Kansas City in 1962. The early results of the unit were presented at a meeting of the American College of Chest Physicians later in the same year. The second CCU was opened at the Presbyterian Hospital in Philadelphia. In England, K.W.G. Brown and H.W. Day proposed the concept independently in 1963.

Coronary Thrombosis *See coronary artery disease, myocardial infarction.*

Corpora Quadrigemina Andreas Vesalius (1514–1564) was one of the first to give a clear account of the structure. Robert Whytt (1714–1766) of Edinburgh in 1768 demonstrated that the destruction of the anterior corpora quadrigemina resulted in the abolition of the pupillary contraction in reaction to light.

Corpulence [Latin: *corpus*, body + *lentus*, thick] Undue accumulation of fat in the body. *See obesity.*

Cor-Pulmonale *See Ayerza disease.*

Corpus Luteum [Latin: *corpus*, body + *luteus*, orange yellow] Described by Gabriele Falloppio (1523–1562). A more detailed account was given by the Dutch physician, Regnier de Graaf (1641–1673) in his work published in 1672. John Beard (1858–1924) of Edinburgh suggested that it may be an inhibitor of ovulation during pregnancy in 1897 and his views were confirmed by Auguste Prenant (1861–1927) in 1898. In 1901 Ludwig Frankel (1870–1951) and Franz Cohn (b 1880) demonstrated that the extirpation of corpora lutea from pregnant rabbits before the implantation of embryos, and at certain other times during pregnancy, resulted in termination. In 1911 Leo Loeb (1869–1959) of Germany demonstrated that extirpation in guinea pigs accelerated the next ovulation, whereas extirpation of other parts of the ovary had no such effect. W.L. Williams of America found that estrus and ovulation could be induced within 48 h in cows by squeezing it out by rectal manipulation in 1921. The hormone progesterone from corpus luteum was discovered by George Washington Corner (1889–1981) and Willard Myron Allen (b 1904) in 1929.

Corrected Transposition of the Great Arteries The pathological features of congenital corrected transposition of the aorta and pulmonary artery were described by Karl Rokitansky (1804–1878) in 1875. A clinical description, adequate to establish a diagnosis, was given by R.C. Anderson and colleagues in 1957.

Corrigan Button An instrument used to apply counter-irritation to the skin, first described by Sir Dominic Corrigan (1802–1880) in 1841. The button or rod measured about 6 inches (15 cm) and was made of iron. The second portion of the apparatus was a small spirit lamp used for heating one end of the rod before applying it to the skin. Corrigan stated that the heated button should be only lightly applied, so as to make only a slight brownish discoloration of the skin.

Corrigan Pulse Waterhammer pulse, characterized by a sudden impact and rapid fall in aortic insufficiency. Described by Dublin physician, Sir Dominic John Corrigan (1802–1880) in 1832. *See waterhammer pulse.*

Corrigan, Sir Dominic John (1802–1880) Physician in Dublin who described famine fever in 1847, and also wrote a treatise on the heart in 1832. *See Corrigan pulse, Corrigan button.*

Cortex, Adrenal *See corticosteroids, cortisone.*

Cortex John Hughlings Jackson (1834-1911), a British neurologist from Yorkshire, proposed in 1864 that areas in the cortex responsible for specific isolated movements existed. Theodor Fritsch (1838–1897), a military surgeon during the Prussian–Danish war in 1867, while attending on soldiers suffering from brain injury, noted that stimulation of one side of the brain caused the opposite side to twitch. He later joined with Eduard Hitzig (1838–1907), another brilliant neurologist, and did experiments on the stimulation of the brain in dogs. They established that the different compartments of the cerebral cortex had different functions. The localization of electrical activity in relation to the functions was further studied by Francis Gotch (1853–1913) and the

British neurosurgeon, Victor Alexander Haden Horsley (1857–1916), in 1892. Further knowledge was advanced by Swiss physiologist, Walter Rudolph Hess (1881–1973) through his technique of applying small electrodes to various parts of the brain in order to study its functions. Several specific areas in the prefrontal cortex, now known as Pitres areas, were described by Jean Albert Pitres (1848–1927) from Bordeaux. He was a contemporary of Jean Martin Charcot (1825–1893) in Paris in 1880. Jules Gabriel François Baillarger (1809–1890), a French psychiatrist, noted that the white lines in the cerebral cortex consisted of two bands separated by a thin dark line. These lines were found to be present throughout the cortex and were named the 'internal and external bands of Baillarger'. Betz cells, giant motor cells in the cerebral cortex, were described by Vladimir Betz (1834–1894), professor of anatomy in Kiev in 1874. *See cerebral cortex, brain, motor cortex, architronics.*

Corti, Bonaventura (1720–1813) Italian anatomist who described the receptor organ for sound, which consisted of a complex structure of basilar membrane, cochlea, hair cells and other structures. This was later collectively named the 'organ of Corti'.

Corti, Marquis Alfonso (1822–1888) Physician from Sardinia, who worked as a histologist in Berlin, Vienna and Turin. He discovered the spiral structure in the cochlea of the inner ear (organ of Corti) in 1851.

Corti, Matthew (1475–1544) Italian physician and professor at Pisa, who wrote *De Curandis Febris* and other works.

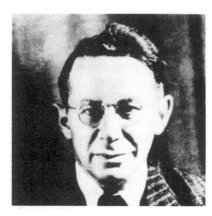

Tadeus Reichstein (b 1897). Courtesy of the National Library of Medicine

Corticosteroids [Latin: *cortex*, bark; Greek: *stereos*, solid] The first active cortical extract from the adrenal glands was prepared by Wilber Willis Swingle (b 1891) and Joseph John Pfiffner (1903–1975) in 1930. He demonstrated its remarkable effect on adrenalectomized animals. Cortisone was isolated independently by Tadeus Reichstein (b 1897),

Edward Calvin Kendall (1886–1972) and Oskar Paul Wintersteiner (1898–1971) in 1936. Reichstein also elucidated its structure and named it 'compound F'. Following the research on oxysteroids in America, dedydrocortisone was synthesized in 1945. Cortisone was first tried for rheumatoid arthritis in 1948 by Kendall, with remarkable beneficial effects. *See rheumatoid arthritis, adrenal insufficiency.*

Cortisone The first active extract of the adrenal cortex, later known as cortisone, was obtained by Edward Calvin Kendall (1886–1972) in 1935. It was isolated by Tadeus Reichstein (b 1897), who also demonstrated its structure in 1936. The compound was synthesized by Robert Burns Woodward (1917–1979) of Boston in 1951. *See corticosteroids.*

Corvisart, Jean Nicolas (1755–1821) Napoleon's favorite physician, who revived the clinical sign of percussion described by Leopold Auenbrugger (1722–1809) in 1751. He wrote an important treatise *Diseases of the Heart* in 1814. He was also the teacher to Guillaume Dupuytren (1777–1835), René Laënnec (1781–1826) and Georges Cuvier (1769–1832).

Corynebacterium diphtheriae Discovered by Theodor Albrecht Edwin Klebs (1834–1913) in 1883. The causal relationship between the organism and diphtheria was established by German microbiologist, Friedrich Loeffler (1852–1915) in 1884. The effects of diphtheria toxin in the disease were demonstrated by Pierre Paul Emile Roux (1853–1933) and Alexandre Emil Yersin (1863–1940) in 1889. The antitoxin was developed by Emil von Behring (1854–1915) and Shibasaburo Kitasato (1852–1931) in 1891. It was tried successfully for the first time on a child with diphtheria on the Christmas night of 1891.

Cos Greek island where one of the leading schools of the Aesculapiades existed from 600 BC. Hippocrates (460–377 BC) was born at Cos and he studied, practiced and taught at the school.

Cosme, John Bascllac (1703–1781) Franciscan lithotomist who wrote treatises on his subject.

Cosmogeny [Greek: *cosmos*, universe or world + *genos*, descent] *See geogeny, Earth.*

Costochondral Junction Syndrome (Syn. Tietze syndrome) A painful swelling at the costochondral junction of the sternum, of unknown etiology. Described by Alexander Tietze (1864–1927) a surgeon at Breslau, in 1921.

Cot Death Sudden death in apparently healthy infants, studied by A. Goldbloom and F.W. Wigglesworth of Canada in 1938. By 1954 at least 600 babies per annum were dying. Various theories, ranging from infection to suffocation or asphyxia, have been put forward over the past decades to explain these deaths.

Cotton, Nathaniel (1707–1788) English physician who qualified from Leiden. On returning to England he established an asylum for the insane at St Albans, which he named the Collegium Insanorum. He published *Observations on a Particular Kind of Scarlet Fever that Prevailed in and about St Albans* (1749) and a poem, *Visions, in Verse,* in 1751.

Cotton, Richard Payne (1820–1877) A successful practitioner in Kensington in London. His main interest was tuberculosis and he published *Phthiasis and the Stethoscope* in 1852. He also gave a description of paroxysmal tachycardia in 1869.

Cotton–Boothby Apparatus Used for nitrous oxide-oxygen–ether anesthesia. Devised by William Meredith Boothby (1880–1953) of Mayo Clinic and Boston surgeon, Frederic Jay Cotton (1869–1938), in 1912.

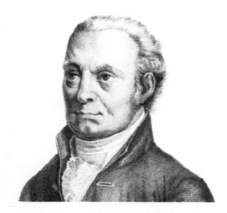

Dominico Cotugno (1736–1822). Courtesy of the National Library of Medicine

Cotugno, Dominico (1736–1822) Born in Bari, near the Adriatic coast of Italy, he was professor of anatomy at Naples. He observed the fluid in the brain of fish and turtles in 1784, although he could not detect it in humans. He described several structures of the labyrinthine apparatus in 1760 and gave a classic description of sciatica.

Couching [French: *coucher*, to lie down] A method of treating cataract by displacing the opaque lens of the eye by pushing it down into the vitreous body. *See cataract extraction.*

Coulomb A measure of electric charge proposed by Charles Augustus Coulomb (1736–1806), a French physicist who lived during the French Revolution. It is the charge produced by a steady current of one ampere in one second.

He invented the torsion balance (1785) named after him. He postulated the law governing the attractive or repulsive forces between two charged particles in relation to their distance.

Coumadin *See anticoagulants.*

Coumarin Plant-based flavoring for foods, synthesized by English chemist, William Perkin (1838–1907), in 1868. Its use was abandoned in 1954, following the discovery that it was hepatotoxic.

Councilman, William Thomas (1854–1933) Born in Baltimore, he graduated from the University of Maryland in 1878. He was Shattuck professor of pathology at Harvard University in 1892. He introduced the term 'amebic dysentery' in 1890.

Countertransference Term was used by Sigmund Freud (1856–1939) in 1910 to denote the psychotherapist's own emotional involvement with a patient during therapy.

Coupling The presence of two genes in the same chromosome in a double heterozygote. Described by William Bateson (1861–1926) in 1906.

Courmont, Jules (1865–1917) French pathologist who designed an agglutination test, now obsolete, for *Mycobacterium tuberculosis.*

Cournand Catheter With a unipolar electrode at the tip of the catheter for intracardiac pacing, manufactured by Unites States Catheter Company. It was named after André Frédéric Cournand (1895–1988). *See cardiac catheterization.*

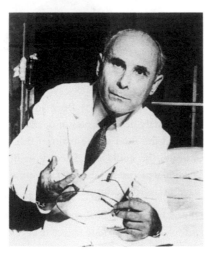

André Frédéric Cournand (1895–1988). Courtesy of the National Library of Medicine

Cournand, André Frédéric (1895–1988) Inventor of the cardiac catheter. He was born in Paris and emigrated to America in 1930. He commenced his pioneer work on cardiac catheterization in 1949 and was awarded the Nobel Prize, which he shared with Werner Forssmann (1904–1979) of Germany and Dickenson Woodruff Richards (1895–1973) of Columbia. Cournand was professor Emeritus of medicine at Columbia University in 1960.

Courtois, Bernard (1777–1838) French chemist from Dijon who studied pharmacy at Auxerre. He isolated the alkaloid, morphine, with Guyton de Morveau. He took over his father's factory for manufacturing saltpeter in 1804, and serendipitously discovered iodine when he added sulfuric acid to ash of seaweed in 1811.

Courvoisier Sign Localized tenderness in the right hypochondrium over the inflamed gallbladder in cholecystitis. Described by Ludwig Georg Courvoisier (1843–1918), professor of surgery at Basel, in 1890. He worked with Sir William Fergusson (1808–1877) and Sir Spencer Wells (1818–1897) in London and was one of the first to remove stones from the common bile duct.

Couvade [French: *couver*, to brood upon] Ancient custom amongst some tribes of Africa, the Balearic Islands and Turkestan. In this practice during pregnancy and childbirth the father confines himself for some time before and immediately after delivery, as if he also were giving birth to the child.

Couvelaire Syndrome Premature separation of a normally implanted placenta, accompanied by albuminuria, azotemia and shock. Described by French obstetrician Alexandre Couvelaire (1873–1948) from Bourg in 1911. He was professor at the University of Paris in 1914 and was later elected president of the Sociètè d'Obstètrique et de Gynècologie.

Coward, William (1656–1725) English physician of Winchester, also a poet who wrote *Second Thoughts Concerning the Human Soul* (1702), *Licentia Poetica; or the true test of Poetry* and *Ophthalmiatria.*

Cowley, Abraham (1618–1687) Physician who obtained his MD from Oxford in 1657. He devoted most of his time to publishing poetry.

Cowper Glands Glands of the male urethra, named after William Cowper (1666–1709), who described them in 1700. They were observed by Jean Mery (1645–1722), the first surgeon to Hôtel Dieu at Paris, in 1684.

Cowper, William (1666–1709) Surgeon from Hampshire who wrote *Myotomia Reformata* (1694) and *Anatomy of Human Bodies* in 1697. He described the pair of glands (Cowper glands) close to the male urethra in 1700. *See aortic insufficiency.*

Cowper, William (d 1767) Physician at Chester who published *A Summary of the Life of St Wyburgh* and a history of Chester.

Cox, Harold Rae (b 1907) American bacteriologist from Montana who prepared a typhus vaccine (Cox vaccine) from yolk-sac culture of rickettsial species in 1940.

Cox, Wilhelm Hendrix (1861–1933) Dutch bacteriologist who introduced a process of impregnating nerve cells and neuroglia with potassium salts, mercuric chloride and ammonia for histological studies.

Coxiella burnetii The causative organism of Q fever, observed during an outbreak of febrile illness amongst meat and cattle workers in Brisbane by Edward Holbrook Derrick (1898–1976) in 1937. The disease was named Q fever, (Q denoting query) before its causative organism was identified by Sir Frank Macfarlane Burnett (1899–1985) and Mavis Freeman in the same year. The organism was recovered from ticks during an outbreak in Montana by Herald Rea Cox (b 1907) and G.E. Davis in 1938 and named *Coxiella burnetti*, in honor of its discoverers.

Coxsackie Virus Isolated from the feces of two children during their acute phase of poliomyelitis in Coxsackie, New York by American pathologist, G. Dalldorf (b 1900) and Grace Mary Sickles (1898–1959) in 1948. Dalldorf was born in Iowa and graduated from New York University in 1924. He was professor of pathology at Cornell University in 1960. Cardiac involvement by coxsackie B virus was recognized in newborn infants in Johannesburg by S.N. Javett and colleagues in 1956.

CPK *See creatinine phosphokinase.*

Crabbe, George (1754–1832) Physician from Suffolk who published several poetical works including *The Library* (1781), *The Village* and *The Parish Register.*

Crafoord, Clarence (1899–1984) Stockholm surgeon who performed the first successful surgical resection of coarctation and anastomosis of its cut ends, with Carl Gustav Wilhelm Nylin (1892–1961) in 1945.

Crafts Test or reflex Dorsiflexion of the great toe occurring when the anterior surface of the ankle is stroked in cases of pyramidal tract lesions. Described by American neurologist, Leo M. Crafts (1863–1938) of Minneapolis.

Cramer, William (1878–1945) London pathologist who prepared a solution (Cramer–Bannerman solution) for indirectly enumerating platelets, with another London

pathologist, Robert George Bannerman (1891–1947).

Crampton, Sir Philip (1777–1858) Surgeon from Meath Hospital Dublin who graduated in medicine from Glasgow at the age of 23 years. He described the radial fibers of the ciliary muscles in 1805. He was President of the Dublin College of Surgeons for three years and was appointed surgeon to the Queen.

Cranial Arteritis *See temporal arteritis.*

Cranial Bruit A bruit on auscultation of the cranium in a case of caroticocavernous fistula. Described in 1809 by Benjamin Travers (1783–1838), a surgeon at St Thomas' Hospital. Its pathological significance, called 'cephalic bellows sound', was explained by J.D. Fisher in 1838. S.O. Steinheil observed this sign in a case of intracranial angioma in 1895, and Johan Hoffmann (1857–1919) diagnosed a case of angioma after hearing it in 1898.

Cranial Nerves *See abducent nerve, olfactory nerve, optic nerve, patheticus oculorum, facial nerve, trigeminal neuralgia, vagus, spinal accessory nerve.*

Craniology [Greek: *kranion*, skull + *logos*, discourse] Established by Johann Friedrich Blumenbach (1752–1940) of Göttingen who studied the variation of the skull in relation to race in 1775. He published *Decas Collectiones suae Cranorium diverasrum Gentium Illustrata* with 70 plates.

Craniometry [Greek: *kranion*, skull + *metron*, measure] *See anthropometry.*

Crawfurd, Andrew (1786–1854) Physician from Lochwinnoch, Scotland, who qualified from Glasgow. He published several poems including *A Glance Ayont the Grave, The Laird of Logan* and *Whistlebinkie.*

Cream, Neill Thomas (1850–1892) Graduated from Montreal in 1876 and later settled in England. He obtained his membership of the Royal College of Physicians and fellowship of the Royal College of Surgeons in 1878 and lived on Lambeth Palace Road, London. He pursued a career of blackmail, murder and abortion, and poisoned the husband of one of his mistresses with strychnine. He was sentenced to life imprisonment for his crime but was pardoned and released in 1891. However, he was arrested within a year of his release, for more blackmail and murders. This time he was found guilty and was executed at Newgate in November 1892.

Creatinine [Greek: *kreatos*, of flesh] A method of estimating it in blood was devised by Max Jaffe (1841–1911) in 1886, and its presence in urine was detected by Max von Pettenkofer

(1818–1901). *See creatinine estimation, creatinine clearance test.*

Creatinine Clearance Test Danish physician, Poul Brandt Rehberg of Copenhagen assumed that creatinine is solely excreted through the glomeruli, and used its clearance rate to measure glomerular filtration, as a test for renal function, in 1926.

Creatinine Estimation Max Jaffe (1841–1911) devised a method of estimating creatinine in the blood in 1886. He mixed blood with picric acid and sodium hydroxide and found that it gave a red color in combination with creatinine (Jaffe method) in the blood. This method was improved by Stanley Rossiter Benedict (1884–1936) in 1929. The prognostic value of the rise in blood creatinine in urological disorders was demonstrated by Frank Stewart Patch (b 1878) and I.M. Rabinowitch in 1928.

Creatinine Phosphokinase (CPK) Reported to be elevated in myocardial infarction by J.C. Dreyfus in 1960. The isoenzymes of CPK were recognized by S.B. Rosalki in 1965, and several isoenzymes were isolated by other workers in 1972 and 1973. Heart muscle was found to contain about 30% of one of the isoenzymes, MB-CPK (M, for muscle and B, for brain) which became substantially elevated in myocardial infarction. The test for the MB-CPK fraction was later used to differentiate myocardial infraction from other conditions that led to a rise of CPK activity.

Credè, Carl Sigmund Franz (1819–1892) Professor of obstetrics and gynecology in Leipzig who described a method of expulsion of the placenta (Credè maneuver) by applying pressure on the uterine fundus through the abdominal wall. He wrote on the prevention of ophthalmia neonatorum using silver nitrate in 1884.

Cremation Burning a body, practiced by the ancient Hindus who worshipped the fire god Agni. Romans and Greeks burnt their dead around 1225 BC. Brunetti of Italy performed the first modern cremation using an open outdoor furnace in 1869, and he later presented his experience on three cremations to the Vienna Exhibition in 1873. The advantages were pointed out in England by Sir Henry Thompson (18201–1904) in his *The Cremation: Treatment of Body after Death* published in 1874. The English Cremation Society was formed in the same year, and Thompson was elected as its first president. The first site for cremation in England was located at Woking, and its furnace was designed and supervised by Gorini of Italy. The next cremation society to be formed was in Milan, in 1876. The practice in England was opposed by the Home Office in 1879, and Sir Spencer Wells (1818–1897) made a plea to allow it at the British Medical Association meeting held at Cambridge in August 1880. A memorandum signed by the members at the meeting was sent to the Secretary of State asking for permission to use the crematoriums under supervision. The Cremation Act, which set the procedure for cremation, was passed in 1902.

Cremation Society of England *See cremation.*

Creosote [Greek: *creos*, flesh + *sote*, to preserve] Active ingredient of wood vinegar, obtained from the tar of beech wood by Justinius Kerner (1786–1862) in 1820. It was isolated and named by Karl Reichenbach in 1832. It became a popular remedy for consumption and other diseases for the next 50 years. It was revived as a specific remedy against pulmonary tuberculosis by Apollinaire Bouchardat (1806–1886) and Gimbert in 1877.

Cretaceous Period Period in Earth history identified and named by Jean Baptiste Julien Omalius d'Halloy of France in 1822.

Cretinism [Swiss French: *creitin*, human being (as Christian)] Felix Platter (1536-1614) of Basel gave one of the earliest descriptions in his *Praxeos Medicae* in 1602. An important work on cretinism and goiter was done by Italian physician, Michele Vincenzo Giacinto Malacarne (1744–1816) in 1789. François Emmanuel Fodere (1764–1835) of Italy studied it and considered it to be due to air in the valleys rather than water. Jean François Coindet (1774–1834), a physician in Geneva, administered iodine to patients with goiter and obtain a beneficial response. An accurate clinical description was given by Thomas Blizard Curling (1811–1888) of the London Hospital in 1850. Charles Hilton Fagge (1838–1833), a physician at Guy's Hospital, described sporadic cretinism in 1871, and Sir William Withey Gull (1816–1890) also from Guy's Hospital, gave a classical description and identified its cause in 1873. The term 'myxedema', for the condition in adults, was coined by William Miller Ord (1834–1902) in 1878.

Creutzfeldt–Jakob Disease A syndrome of dementia accompanied by pyramidal and extrapyramidal signs which usually occur after middle age. Described by Hans Gerhard Creutzfeldt (1885–1964) in 1920. Five patients with a similar condition between the ages of 30 and 50 years were described by Bavarian physician, Alfons Maria Jakob (1884–1931) in 1921. Jakob, the son of a shoemaker, graduated from Strasburg in 1909 and worked with two other eminent neurologists, Franz Nissl (1860–1919) of Heidelberg and Alois Alzheimer (1864–1915) of Breslau. The first possible transmission of the disease from human to human was noted in

1974, when a patient who received a corneal transplant from a known case died of the disease within 18 months after the procedure.

Cri du Chat Syndrome The chromosome abnormalities of babies with a mewing cry, mental and physical retardation, hypertelorism, low-set ears and microcephaly were studied by Jerome Lejeune and colleagues in 1963. They noted that part or all of one of the pair of chromosome 5 was deleted in this condition.

Crichett, George (1818–1882) Appointed in 1876 as ophthalmic surgeon to the Middlesex Hospital, where he became renowned for his invention of iridesis, a subcutaneous operation for squint and other ophthalmic procedures. His son, Sir Anderson Crichett, was also an eminent eye surgeon.

Crichton-Browne, Sir James (1840–1938) Born in Edinburgh and graduated in medicine from Edinburgh University, where he was a pupil of Joseph Lister (1827–1912). His father was a physician and commissioner on lunacy in Scotland, and he developed an interest in psychiatry as a student. He presented a paper, *Psychical Diseases of Early Life.* He was a founder of the journal *Brain* with Hughlings Jackson (1835–1911) and Sir David Ferrier (1843–1928), and was its co-editor. He started the first British journal of neuropathology, *West Riding Asylum Reports,* while he was director of West Riding Asylum, Wakefield in 1871. He was the Lord Chancellor's visitor in lunacy in reforms from 1875 to 1922. He published *Stray Leaves from Physician's Portfolio,* which contains a variety of interesting articles.

Crick, Francis Harry Compton (b 1916) British biologist, born near Northampton, who received his degree from University College, London. He later joined Cambridge University and worked with James Dewey Watson (b 1928) from America in elucidating the structure of DNA in 1953. Crick shared the Nobel Prize for Medicine or Physiology with Watson and Maurice Hugh Wilkins (b 1916) in 1962. His autobiography *What Mad Pursuit* was published in 1988.

Criggler–Najjar Syndrome Seven cases of infants with jaundice from the day of their birth were described by two American pediatricians, John F. Criggler (b 1919) and V.A. Najjar (b 1914) in 1952. Najjar was born in the Lebanon and graduated from the University of Beirut in 1935, before he came to America (1938) and joined the pediatric department at Johns Hopkins in 1949. Criggler graduated from Johns Hopkins and was a pediatrician at Harvard Medical School. None of the seven infants they described showed any evidence of hemolysis, infection or liver disease. Most died during the first year and kernicterus was found in one who came to autopsy. Two survivors were followed up by Najjar, and in 1956 their liver functions were found to be normal apart from jaundice, which was identified to be due to an inability to convert bilirubin to diglucuronide.

Crile, George Washington (1864–1943) American surgeon and physiologist, born in Chile, Ohio, and received his MD from the University of Wooster in 1887. He developed an interest in the study of surgical shock following the death of his friend, and became a pioneer in the field. He was one of the first to use blood transfusion and epinephrine in its treatment, and published a monograph on the subject in 1899. He was made professor of surgery at the Western Reserve School of Medicine in 1911, and founded the Cleveland Clinic Foundation in which he was the first director from 1920 to 1940. He devised the brachial plexus block by injecting the plexus with an anesthetic under direct vision in 1897. His other published works include *Blood Pressure in Surgery* (1903) and *Anemia and Resuscitation* (1914).

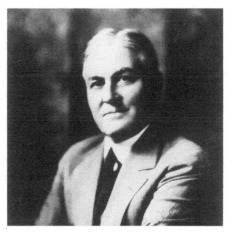

George Washington Crile (1864–1943). Courtesy of the National Library of Medicine

Criminal Responsibility One of the first to state that an insane person was not responsible for a criminal act was a Roman jurist, Domitius Ulpianus (AD 170–224). It is only in the past two centuries that insanity has been accepted as an excusable reason for crime. The first account of a trial in England where insanity was raised as defense was given by Richard Cosin (1549–1597) in 1592. In 1723 Justice Tracey stated that the person pleading insanity 'should know no more than an infant, a brute or a wild beast'. In one of the most important insanity pleas of the 19th century, in a trial of John Bellingham, a bankrupt Liverpool broker, for shooting the English lawyer and statesman Spencer Percival (1762–1812) in 1812, the accused was sentenced to death by Chief Justice Mansfield on the grounds that, if he could distinguish between right and wrong on other matters, he was responsible for his act of shooting. A debate continued for nearly a century with prominent psychiatrists, including Henry Maudsley (1835–1918), and forensic experts such as Alfred Swaine Taylor (1806–1880) contributing. One of the earliest works in America on medical jurisprudence regarding insanity was published by Isaac Ray (1807–1881) in 1838. *See McNaughten rule.*

Criminology [Latin: *crimen*, accusation; Greek: *logos*, discourse] One of the first studies on the subject describing how factors such as age, sex, education, climate and season affected the crime rate in France was published by Lambert Adolphe Quetelet (1796–1874) in 1831. A system of recorded measurement and description of criminals was devised by French criminologist, Alphonse Bertillon (1853–1914) in 1886. A system of criminal typing was proposed by Italian, Cesare Lombroso (1836–1909) in 1876.

Crippen, Harvey Hawley (1862–1910) Physician turned murderer. He was born in Michigan, and obtained a diploma as an ear and eye specialist in 1886. He came to London in 1900 as a manager to a drug-patenting company. He lived in Camden Hill with his wife, whom he married in America. Crippen poisoned her with hyoscine in 1910. He dissected the body and tried to destroy the remains by burning, but some were buried under the cellar. He tried to escape with his secretary and lover, Ethel, to America, but was recognized by the captain of the Atlantic liner, who made use of the newly invented teleradiography to inform Scotland Yard. This was the first time telegraphy was used in crime work. Crippen was tried for his crime and the forensic pathologist, Sir Bernard Henry Spilsbury (1877–1947), of St Mary's Hospital, London gave evidence as an expert witness during the trial. The trial resulted in Crippen's conviction and he was executed at Pentonville.

Cripps Operation A method of colotomy in the iliac region. Described by English surgeon, William Harrison Cripps (1850–1923) in 1880.

Critchett, George (1817–1882) London ophthalmologist who described several operations for the eyes, including one for squint.

Critical Temperature of Gases *See Thomas Andrews.*

Crocodile Pessaries made of crocodile dung were used to prevent pregnancy by the Egyptians around 1800 BC. In

300 BC Serapion of Alexandria, an opponent of Hippocratic medicine, also promoted crocodile dung for many diseases. As a result, these excreta became very costly to obtain. Galen (129–200) prescribed crocodile bile as treatment for wounds resulting from a crocodile bite. Crocodile dung was also used as a cure for consumption for centuries. A fossil crocodile was found in Doddridge, Gloucestershire in 1806, although it was not known to be indigenous to Britain.

Crocq Disease Acrocyanosis, named after Belgian physician, Jean B. Crocq (1868–1925) who described it in 1896.

Crohn Disease Regional ileitis, was described by an American physician, Burril Bernard Crohn (b 1884), L. Ginzberg and G.D. Oppenheimer in 1932. Crohn worked at Mt Sinai Hospital, New York and was President of the American Gastroenterology Society. Two important early pathological accounts of the disease were given by G. Hadfield in 1939 and G.W.H. Schepers in 1945.

Cro-Magnon Man Modern European man belonging to the species *Homo sapiens* appeared after Neanderthal man. He is supposed to have lived about 35,000 years ago in Europe during the Aurignacian phase of culture, and used flint implements. The name takes its origin from the cave in France where French workmen found five skeletons. The earliest discovery of Cro-Magnon remains in Britain were found by William Buckland (1784–1856) in 1823, at an ancient cave dwelling of Paviland known as Goat's Hole, in South Wales.

Cronkhite–Canada Syndrome Characterized by gastrointestinal polyposis and ectodermal changes including alopecia and nail and skin changes. Described by an American physician, Leonard W. Cronkhite of Massachusetts General Hospital, and an American radiologist, W.J. Canada, from St Luke's Hospital, Massachusetts, in 1955.

Crookes Tube German scientist Johann Wilhelm Hittorf (1824–1914) first noticed the glowing effect that occurred when electricity was passed through a vacuum tube. In 1869, Sir William Crookes (1832–1919) of London improved the degree of the vacuum achieved, and studied this phenomenon in greater detail. He observed the various effects of passing a current through the tube, and named the fluorescent phenomenon 'radiant matter'. His tube was later developed into the cathode ray tube which was a precursor of the tube used in the production of X-rays.

Crookes, Sir William (1832–1919) Molecular physicist and chemist in London who discovered thallium in 1861. He founded the *Chemical News* in 1859 and was its editor. He developed the Crookes tube, a forerunner of Röntgen's cathode or X-ray tube, in 1878. Joseph John Thomson (1856–1940) used it for his discovery of the electron in 1897. Crookes also invented the spinthariscope to demonstrate the fluorescence produced by X-rays. The *Select Methods of Chemical Analysis* was published by him in 1881. *See Crookes tube.*

Croone or Croune, William (1633–1684) Physician in London who qualified from Emmanuel College Cambridge. He became a traveling tutor to Howard, son of the Duke of Norfolk, and was appointed professor of anatomy at the Company of Surgeons in 1670. He published a treatise on muscle physiology, *De Ratione Motus Musculorum* in 1667. The Croonian Anatomical Lectures at the Royal Society and several regular lectures in algebra at Cambridge were founded by his widow. *See fixatives.*

Croonian Lectures *See Croone.*

Cross Resistance *See bacterial resistance.*

Cross, Philip Army surgeon from County Cork, who poisoned his wife with arsenic in order to marry his children's governess. He was found guilty in 1887 and hanged in January 1888.

Crossing-Over A process of exchange of corresponding segments between chromatids of homologous chromosomes, by breakage or reunion during pairing. Described by a geneticist from Kentucky, Thomas Hunt Morgan (1866–1945) in 1911.

Croup Term coined from the Scottish vernacular [*roup*, to cry] to denote 'stridulous breathing' by Francis Home (1719–1813) of Edinburgh in 1765 in his *An Inquiry into the Nature, Cause and Cure of Croup.* Pierre Bretonneau (1771–1862) of Tours, France, introduced the term 'diphtheria' for the disease in 1826 and performed tracheostomy for croup.

Crouzon Disease Craniofacial dysostosis and hypertelorism, due to autosomal dominant inheritance. Described by French neurologist, Octave Crouzon (1874–1938) in 1912.

Crow Sign Compression of the internal jugular vein on the normal side, in cases of lateral sinus thrombosis, causes engorgement of retinal vessels. Described by American otorhinologist, Samuel Jones Crowe (1883–1955), of Johns Hopkins Medical School.

Crozier, John Beattie (1849–1921) Physician from Toronto who emigrated to England. He published several works on philosophy and sociology including, *Civilisation and Progress* (1885), *The Wheel of Wealth* (1906) and *Sociology Applied to Practical Politics* in 1911.

Cruchet, Jean René (1875–1959) French surgeon from Bordeaux. He described epidemic encephalitis lethargica in 1917. The disease was described 13 days later by Constantin von Economo (1876–1931) and is known as von Economo disease.

Cruikshank, William (1745–1800) Surgeon and anatomist from Edinburgh. He came to London on the initiative of David Pitcairn (1749–1809) in 1771 and became librarian to John Hunter (1728–1793). He published *Anatomy of the Absorbant Vessels of the Human Body.* He demonstrated the passage of the impregnated ovum through the fallopian tube in 1778.

Cruise Operation An operation for chronic glaucoma by making a corneoscleral wedge-shaped opening without iridectomy. Originated by London ophthalmologist, Sir Richard Robert Cruise (1876–1946).

Crush Syndrome Acute tubular necrosis associated with myoglobinuria as a result of crush injury to soft tissues. Described by Seigo Minami of Tokyo in 1923. Its occurrence in victims of air raids during World War ll was described by Eric George Lapthorne Bywaters (b 1910) of England in 1941. The relationship of crush injury to shock was experimentally investigated by Baltimore surgeon, George Walton Duncan (b 1914) in 1942.

Cruveilhier Disease Amyotrophic lateral sclerosis, a form of progressive muscular atrophy, described by Jean Cruveilhier (1791–1873) in 1853. *See amyotrophic lateral sclerosis.*

Cruveilhier, Jean (1791–1873) Son of an army surgeon from Limoges, and a pupil of Guillaume Dupuytren (1777–1835). He became professor of pathology at Montpellier in 1824, and was appointed professor of pathological anatomy at Paris in 1836. He gave the first description of disseminated sclerosis or multiple sclerosis in 1840, and also described a form of amyotrophic lateral sclerosis (Cruveilhier disease) in 1853. *See amyotrophic lateral sclerosis.*

Cruveilhier–Baumgarten Disease Jean Cruveilhier (1791–1873) of Paris described the flow of blood from a dilated portal space at the origin of the left branch of the portal vein within the liver to the anterior abdominal wall in cases of cirrhosis, in 1835. A full description was given by American physician, Paul C. Baumgarten (1873–1945) in 1891, and it was named Cruveilhier–Baumgarten disease. Baumgarten was a founder member of the Association of Physicians and he was physician at Harvard (1897–1898) and Johns Hopkins (1903–1907) hospitals.

Cruz, Osvaldo Gonçalves (1872–1917) Bacteriologist in Rio de Janeiro after whom the causative organism of South

American trypanosomiasis, *Trypanasoma cruzi*, is named. Carlos Justiniano Ribeiro Chagas (1879–1934), who worked at the Osvaldo Cruz Institute, discovered the pathogenic protozoan in 1909 and the disease was named Chagas disease.

Cryolite [Greek: *kryos*, frost + *lithos*, stone] Sodium aluminum fluoride, a rare mineral found mostly in Greenland. *See fluorosis*.

Cryophorus [Greek: *kryos*, frost] An instrument to measure the relationship between evaporation at low temperatures and the production of cold. Invented by an English physician and chemist, William Hyde Wollaston (1766–1828) in 1812.

Cryoprecipitate [Greek: *kryos*, frost] Observed as a gelatinous material in frozen plasma which remained undissolved when the plasma was thawed. It was later found to be a globulin with significant antihemophilic properties. Judith Pool (1919–1975), a graduate of Chicago University, and colleagues demonstrated that a proportion of the substance contained factor VIII, and they named it 'cryoprecipitate' in 1959.

Cryoscopy [Greek: *kryos*, frost + *skopein*, to view] The use of the freezing point of urine as a diagnostic test was established by Baron Alexander von Sandor Koryanyi (b 1886) of Budapest in 1895. *See osmolarity*.

Cryptococcus neoformans A fungus that was described in fruit juice in Italy by F. Sanfelice in 1895. A subacute form of infection of the nervous system caused by the organism was described in 1895 by Abraham Buschke (1868–1943), a dermatologist in Berlin.

Cryptorchidism [Greek: *kryptos*, hidden + *orchis*, testis] Undescended testis, treated with nearly 40 different surgical operations until the turn of the 19th century. B. Shapiro of Germany started treating it with an anterior pituitary-like substance isolated from the urine of pregnant women, in 1930. *See orchiopexy*.

Crystallization [Greek: *krystallos*, ice] The geometrical law of crystallization was discovered by French mineralogist, René Just Hauy (1743–1822) in 1781.

Crystallography [Greek: *krystallos*, ice + *graphein*, to write] *See X-ray crystallography*.

Crystalloid [Greek: *krystallos*, ice + *eidos*, resemblance] An early account of crystals was given by Robert Hooke (1635–1703) in his *Micrographia* published in 1665. Further work was carried out by Erasmus Bartholin (1625–1698) of

Copenhagen. In his *Experimenta Crystalli Islandici dissiaclastici* he described the properties of double refraction and rhomboidal cleavage of Iceland spar or calcite. Geometrical forms were observed by the anatomist Niels Steno (1638–1686) in 1665. The fact that different crystals were present in different salts was demonstrated by Anton van Leeuwenhoek (1632–1723) in 1695. *See colloid chemistry*.

Ctesias Historian and physician from Cnidos. He was physician to Artaxerxes II for 17 years during the war with his brother Cyrus the Younger around AD 404. He wrote a history of the Persians and Assyrians.

Ctesibus A scholar who studied physics at the Alexandrian school in 300 BC. He laid the foundation for hydromechanics with his inventions of a hydraulic pneumatic machine, a siphon and a hand-operated fire engine. He was also the inventor of the clepsydra or water clock.

Cullen Sign A discoloration of the skin around the umbilicus in cases of ruptured ectopic pregnancy. Described by Canadian-born American gynecologist, Thomas Stephen Cullen (1868–1953), in 1916. He was professor of clinical gynecology at Johns Hopkins Hospital in 1939.

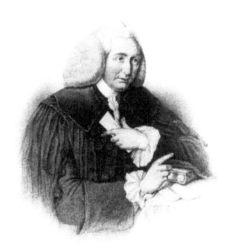

William Cullen (1710–1790). Courtesy of the National Library of Medicine

Cullen, William (1710–1790) Scottish physician, who was first a barber and then became an apothecary, before he graduated in medicine in 1740. He wrote *Synopsis Nosolo-giae Practicae* in 1769 which divided disease into fevers, neuroses, cachexias and local disorders. In 1744 he was instrumental in forming the first medical school in Glasgow, to which he was appointed professor of medicine in 1751. He later moved to Edinburgh as professor of medicine in 1763, and was the first to give clinical infirmary lectures in the vernacular instead of Latin. His other publications include *Institutions of Medicine* (1772), *First Lines of the Practice of Physic* (1778–1779) and *Treatise of Materia Medica* (1789).

Culpepper, Nicholas (1616–1653) Son of a Sussex clergyman who was disinherited by his family for becoming a physician instead of a clergyman. He was also a herbalist and astrologer in London. In 1649 he published a book on herbal remedies, which was denounced by the Royal College of Physicians. However, his book became one of the most popular works on herbal medicine and ran to several editions for the next three centuries. It was the first on medicine to be published in the American colonies, as *The English Physician.*

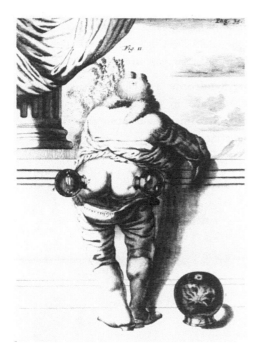

From F. Dekkers, dry-cupping bells on buttocks. Courtesy of the National Library of Medicine

Cuming, William (1714–1788) Physician from Edinburgh who settled in Dorchester and contributed to Hutchin's History of Dorset.

Cuneiform Inscriptions [Latin: *cuneus*, wedge] Writings resembling arrowheads, on clay tablets developed by the Sumerians around 3000 BC. Thousands of clay tablets related to Assyrian culture were found in the remains of the royal library of the King of Assyria, Ashurbanipul (668–626 BC) at Nineveh in the late 19th century. The texts were studied by Campbell Thompson in 1906 and elucidated many historical, medical, astronomical, social, literary and religious aspects of ancient Assyria. *See Sumerian medicine.*

Cunningham, William Physician from London who lived

in Norwich around 1559. He returned to London and became a lecturer at Surgeon's Hall in 1563. He also practiced the art of copper engraving and published *A Cosmo-graphical glass containing the Principles of Cosmography, Geography, Hydrography or Navigation* in 1559. He wrote a treatise on Hippocratic works.

Cupping A mode of treatment for diseases by drawing blood, practiced since the time of Hippocrates (460–377 BC). Glass, horn and copper instruments were used by ancient physicians. Wet cupping required incisions, and early descriptions suggest that it may have been similar to incisions currently practiced for hemotoma or pus formation. Dry cupping involved applying a heated cupping glass to the skin to draw blood to the surface by inducing hyperemia. *See blood letting.*

Cuprum Vitriolatum Copper sulfate, used as an astringent in the treatment of ulcer, tumor and an inflamed urethra.

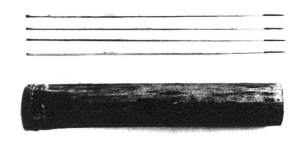

Curare-tipped darts and blow-pipe

Curare A nonspecific term for a group of South American arrow poisons called *woorara* and obtained from the roots of the vine, *Strychnos toxifera.* The first mention was made by an Italian scholar and historian, Peter Martyr Angherius (1455–1526) in 1516. The effects of the poison known as *woorali* were described by Sir Walter Raleigh (1552–1618) on his voyage to British Guiana in 1595. Charles Marie de la Condamine (1701–1704), a French scientist and explorer, brought it from the Amazon to Europe around 1743. Alexander von Humboldt (1769–1859) was one of the first to describe the poison in detail in 1799. In 1811 Sir Benjamin Brodie (1783–1862), in his experiments on animals, used it to paralyze and kept them alive by maintaining their respiration with bellows. *Woorali* was described as a poison 'that destroys life so gently, that the victim appears to be in no pain whatever' by Charles Waterton (1782–1865) in *Wanderings in South America,* published in 1825. Its paralyzing effect on the myoneural junction in frogs was demonstrated by Claude Bernard (1813–1878) in 1840. It was first used in medical practice to relax the muscles in rabies in 1838, in tetanus in 1858, and in epilepsy in 1860. It was used during surgery by German physician, Laewen of Zwickau, to produce muscle relaxation in 1912. However, the significance of Laewen's discovery went unnoticed for two decades. In 1935, Harold King, a Welsh chemist obtained a pure form, D-tubocurarine, and Archibald R. McIntyre and A.E. Bennett obtained the same substance from the bark of *Chondodendron tomentosum* from Ecuador in 1939. A standardized form, called Intocostrin, was produced in the same year. Frederick Prescott demonstrated its clinical use through self-experimentation. Scott M. Smith, a surgeon from Utah, also conducted experiments on himself in 1943, and the drug, as tubocurarine chloride, subsequently became established as a muscle relaxant in anesthesia. *See arrow poisons.*

Curie, Marie (1867–1934) The discoverer of radium. She was the daughter of a Polish professor, Sklodowska, from Warsaw. She came to Paris in 1891 and started working at the Paris faculty with Pierre Curie (1859–1906), whom she married in 1895. The couple met while working with Henri Becquerel (1852–1908), who discovered polonium and radium from pitchblend in 1893. The team discovered radioactivity in 1903, for which they were awarded the Nobel Prize in 1911. Marie succeeded her husband as professor at the Paris Sorbonne in 1906.

Curie, Pierre (1859–1906) He married Marie Sklodowska (1867–1934) in 1895, and the couple worked with Henri Becquerel (1852–1908) to discover radioactivity in 1903. He also identified α, β and γ rays and was later appointed professor at the Paris Sorbonne in 1904. He suffered radioactive injuries from his work and three years after his historic discovery, he was run over by a brewer's cart and died.

Curling Ulcer *See Curling, Thomas Blizard.*

Curling, Thomas Blizard (1811–1888) London surgeon from Tavistock Place, and a nephew of London physician Sir William Blizard (1743–1835). He joined the London Hospital as an assistant surgeon in 1834 at the age of 23 years, and was made full surgeon in 1849, a post which he held for the next 20 years. He was the first to give an accurate clinical description of cretinism in 1850. He discovered acute duodenal ulceration associated with severe burns (Curling ulcer) in 1842 and published *Diseases of the Testis* and *Diseases of Rectum*.

Currie, James (1756–1805) Physician from Dumfries in Scotland, mainly known for his methods of inducing hypothermia for treating disease. He gave a presentation on

the methods of lowering the body temperature at a Royal College of Physicians' meeting in London in 1797. This was based on his experience of over 20 years. He was also one of the first to employ the thermometer in the management of febrile diseases. His work *Medical Reports on the Effects of Water, Cold and Warm as a Remedy in Febrile Diseases* was published in 1797. He also published an edition of Burns' works with a biography of the poet.

Curshmann–Batten–Steinert Syndrome Myotonia dystrophica, consisting of frontal baldness, testicular atrophy, dystrophy of sternomastoid muscles and myotonia of lingual and thenar muscles. Described by F.E. Batten (1865–1918), a neurologist at Queens Square, London in 1909. German physician, Hans Steinert, also described it in the same year. Hans Curshmann (1846–1910), professor of medicine in Leipzig, gave an account in 1912.

Cushing Syndrome The clinical manifestations of basophilic adenoma in the anterior pituitary gland were described by American neurosurgeon, Harvey Williams Cushing (1869–1939) in 1932.

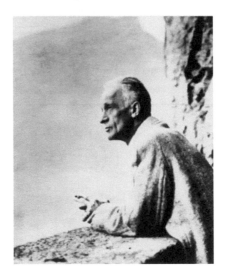

Harvey Williams Cushing (1869–1939). Courtesy of the National Library of Medicine

Cushing, Harvey Williams (1869–1939) Eminent American neurosurgeon, born in Cleveland, Ohio and graduated from Harvard Medical School and Yale College. He completed his internship at Massachusetts General Hospital and worked with William Halstead (1852–1922) at Johns Hopkins, and was appointed professor of neurosurgery at Yale in 1932. His main interest was the pituitary gland and its related disorders. He commenced his experiments on the gland around 1905 and performed the first successful removal of a pituitary gland in an acromegalic patient in

1909. He also wrote a biography of Sir William Osler (1849–1919) in 1914. *See acromegaly, Cushing syndrome.*

Cushing, Hayward Warren (1854–1934) Boston surgeon who introduced a mattress type of continuous invaginating intestinal suture (Cushing suture).

Cushny, Arthur Robertson (1866–1926) British pharmacologist who qualified from Aberdeen in 1889. He served for a brief period as professor of pharmacology at the University of Michigan before returning to London in 1904. He held a professorship first at University College London and later at Edinburgh. His contributions include *The Secretion of Urine* (1917) and *Of Pharmacology and Therapeutics* (1899).

Cuspinian, John (1473–1529) German physician whose real name was Speishammer. He was a favorite of the German Emperor Maximilian I (1459–1519) who made him head of the senate. He published several medical treatises.

Cuvier, Georges Leopold (1769–1832) Born in Paris and considered the founder of vertebrate paleontology. He was the son of a Swiss officer in the French army in Würtemberg. He studied in Stuttgart and became an assistant at the Natural History Museum of Paris in 1795. He published several important works on comparative anatomy and fossil bones and described over 5000 species of fish. After working initially with Jean Baptiste Lamarck (1744–1829) he later became an opponent of Lamarck's theories. The four major divisions of the animal kingdom – Vertebrata, Mollusca, Articulata and Radiata – were proposed by him in 1817. He held several prestigious positions including the post of Minister of the Interior, Director of Educational Reforms and Chancellor of the University of Paris. His publications include *Leçons de Anatomie Comparée* (1801–1805), *L'Anatomie des Mollusques* (1816), *Les Ossements fossiles des quadrupedes* (1812), *Historie Naturale des Poissons* (1828–1849) and *Le Regne Animal distribue d'aprés son Organisatione* (1817).

Cyanotic Heart Disease [Greek: *kyanos*, dark blue] *See Fallot tetralogy, pediatric cardiology.*

Cybernetics [Greek: *kybernetes*, director or helmsman] Control of functions and communications through feedback or self-regulating mechanisms in animals and machines. Term coined by American mathematician, Norbert Wiener (1894–1964) in 1948. Sir Matthew Hale (1606– 1676), Lord Chief Justice of London, suggested this by comparing animals and artificial engines.

Cyclamate Introduced as an artificial sweetener in 1950 and banned as a food additive in the USA in 1969 because of an association with bladder tumors in animals.

Cyclic Adenosine Monophosphate *See AMP.*

Cyclic Albuminuria *See albuminuria, benign albuminuria.*

Cyclophosphamide Introduced into therapeutics by Herbert Arnold and co-workers in 1958. It was used in the treatment of Burkitt lymphoma by Denis Parsons Burkitt (1911–1993) of Enniskillen, Northern Ireland in 1960. *See cancer therapy.*

Cyclopropane [Greek: *kyklos*, circle or ring] Trimethylene, prepared by August von Freund (1835–1892) in 1882. It was introduced as a local anesthetic by Velyien Ewart Henderson (1877–1945) and George Herbert William Lucas (b 1894) of Toronto in 1929. The first clinical use in general anesthesia was achieved by Alan Joan Styles in 1934.

Cycloserine Introduced as first-line treatment in tuberculosis by P.B. Storey in 1958.

Cyclosporin [Greek: *kyklos*, circle or ring + *spora*, seed] A group of workers from Basel, Switzerland found a fungus in two samples of soil which they took from Wisconsin and Norway in 1969. In their search for a new antibiotic they isolated cyclosporin from it. Jean Borel later noted the immunosuppressive property and tried it on animals. As a result, it was introduced to overcome the rejection reaction in organ transplantation in 1978.

Cyclothymia Alternating moods of depression and joy. Termed 'cyclothymia' in psychiatry by Karl Kahlbaum (1828–1899), a German psychiatrist, around 1860.

Cyclotron A chamber for bombardment of nuclei with deuterons or neutrons to produce artificial radioactivity. Developed by Ernest Orlando Lawrence (1901–1958) in California in 1931. He received the Nobel Prize in 1940.

Cyon, Elie de (1842–1912) Russian physiologist who demonstrated the cardioinhibitor and cardioaccelerator effects of the two autonomic outflows to the heart in 1866.

Cyrtometer Instrument made of jointed whale bone, for tracing the outline of the chest wall on paper during respiration. Devised by Eugène Joseph Woillez (1811–1882) of Paris, around 1860.

Cystecercosis *See Taenia worms.*

Cystic Fibrosis Cystic fibrosis of the pancreas was described by Guido Fanconi (1892–1979), Swiss professor of pediatrics at the University of Zurich. The disease also bears the name (Andersen syndrome) of an American pediatrician, Dorothy H. Andersen (1901–1963), who gave another description. The gene marker for cystic fibrosis was discovered on chromosome 7 in 1985.

Cysticercosis [Greek: *kystis*, bladder + *kerkos*, tail + *eidos*, form] Numerous vesicles were found in the dura mater of an epileptic priest by Rumler in 1588. Its presence in the vitreous humor was demonstrated on ophthalmoscopy by Albrecht von Graefe (1828–1870) in 1860. Cysticercosis as a cause of epilepsy was identified by a group of British army doctors led by W.P. MacArthur in 1930.

Cystine [Greek: *kystis*, bladder] Amino acid isolated from urinary calculi by an English physician and chemist, William Hyde Wollaston (1766–1828) in 1810. It was obtained from a protein hydrolysate of hair by Carl Thore Morner in 1899.

Cystinosis Dwarfing and rickets, described by Swiss physiologist, Emil Aberhalden (1877–1950) in 1903. The presence of amino acids in the urine and cystine crystals in the bone marrow of patients with cystinosis was demonstrated by Dutch pathologist, G.O.E. Lignac (1891–1954) in 1924. *See Aberhalden–Fanconi syndrome.*

Cystinuria [Greek: *kystis*, bladder + *oureon*, urine] Bladder stones in patients with cystinuria were noted by William Hyde Wollaston (1766–1828) in 1810. A cystine stone from the bladder of a boy of six years was removed by Julius Muller in 1852. *See aminoaciduria.*

Cystocele [Greek: *kystis*, bladder + *kele*, tumor + *koilia*, hollow] Stoltz operation for cystocele, by denuding a patch on the anterior abdominal wall and running a purse string suture around the edge was designed by French gynecologist, Joseph A. Stoltz (1803–1896).

Cystogram [Greek: *kystis*, bladder + *graphein*, to write] Radiological visualization of the bladder, or cystogram, was achieved by Friedrich Voelcker (1872–1955) and Alexander von Lichtenberg (1880–1949). An apparatus consisting of a catheter, manometer and a moving strip of bromide paper, to measure and record the behavior of the bladder and its sphincters was designed by Derek Ernest Denny-Brown (1901–1980) and E.G. Robertson in 1933. They used this to study the functioning of the bladder and sphincters following complete transection of the spinal cord. Stewart later developed the method into a cystometer in 1942.

Cystosarcoma Phylloides *See Brodie tumor.*

Cystoscopy [Greek: *kystis*, bladder + *skopein*, to look] An attempt to look into the human urethra and bladder was made by Phillip Bozzoni (1773–1809) of Frankfurt in 1805. His method was improved by Gascon P.S. Segalas (1792–1875) in 1826. Further work was pioneered by Jean Antonin

Desormeaux (d 1894) of Paris in 1865. The first electrically-lit cystoscope was devised by Max Nitze (1848–1907) of Berlin in 1877, and an improved form was introduced by David Newman of Glasgow Royal Infirmary in 1883. Joseph Leiter, a Viennese instrument maker, joined with Nitze and perfected a practical cystoscope that was marketed in 1880. The practical visualization of the interior of the bladder was made possible by Hartwig of Berlin, who placed an Edison light into a cystoscope in 1887. The first American-made cystoscope was constructed by Reinhold Wappler and William K. Otis of New York in 1900. The Brown–Buerger cystoscope, which helped to irrigate as well as observe the bladder during the procedure, was devised by Leo Buerger (1879–1943) in 1909. Application of high frequency current through a Nitze cystoscope for destruction of bladder tumors was described by New York surgeon, Edwin Beer (1876–1938) in 1910.

Cystotomy [Greek: *kystis*, bladder + *tome*, to cut] The first suprapubic cystotomy was performed by French surgeon, Pierre Franco (1500–1561) in 1556.

Cytoarchitronics Study of cell structure and layers of specific areas of the brain pioneered by Alfred Campbell (in 1905) and Lewis Bevan (in 1909).

Cytochrome [Greek: *kytos*, hollow + *chroma*, color] A hydrogen acceptor in cellular respiration, discovered by C.A. MacMunn, who called it 'histohematin' in 1886. His discovery was forgotten for the next four decades, until it was rediscovered and named by a British biochemist of Polish origin, David Keilin (1887–1963) in 1925.

Cytochrome Oxidase Identified by German professor of biochemistry in Freiburg, Otto Heinrich Warburg (1883–1970), who called it *atmungsferment* (respiratory enzyme), in 1934. *See cytochrome.*

Cytochrome Reductase Enzyme isolated from yeast by E. Haas, B.L. Horecker and T.R. Hogness, in 1940.

Cytogenetics [Greek: *kytos*, hollow + *genos*, offspring] Branch of genetics devoted to study of cellular constituents of heredity, i.e. chromosomes. *See genetic engineering.*

Cytology [Greek: *kytos*, hollow + *logos*, discourse] Fragments of malignant tissue in the sputum were recognized by Walter Hayle Walshe (1812–1892) of London in 1843. Identification of malignant cells in body fluids was made by F. Donaldson, who described his findings in *The Practical Application of Microscope to Cancer* published in 1853. Malignant cells were identified in sputum by Lionel S. Beale (1828–1906) of King's College in 1860, and in gastric washings by O. Rosenbach (1851–1907) of Germany in 1882. The use of cytology in a clinical setting was introduced by George Nicholas Papanicolaou (1883–1962), who investigated the normal cyclical changes of the vaginal epithelium with Charles Rupert Stockard (1879–1939) of New York and described the role of the vaginal smear in the diagnosis of cancer in 1928.

Cytomegalovirus (CMV) Noted in the early 1900s as an important cause of brain damage in newborn infants and a common cause of microcephaly. It was isolated in 1956 independently by G. Margaret Smith and co-workers, W.P. Rowe, J.W. Hartley, S. Waterman, T.H. Weller and J.C. Macauley.

Cytoplasm [Greek: *kytos*, cell or hollow + *plasma*, something molded] The part of the cell within the cell membrane, but outside the nucleus. Term coined by Edouard Adolf Strasburger (1844–1912) in 1882. *See cell, protoplasm.*

Czermak, Johann Nepomuk (1828–1873) Professor of comparative anatomy and a physiologist at Jena who devoted his time to the study of the minute anatomy of teeth. He improved the laryngoscope invented by Manuel Patricio Rodriguez (1805–1906) and popularized its use.

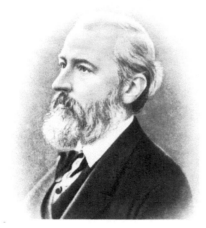

Johann Nepomuk Czermak (1828–1873). Courtesy of the National Library of Medicine

Czerny, Adalbert (1863–1941) Pediatrician in Berlin who described deficiency anemia (Czerny anemia) seen in infants with a deficient diet.

Czerny, Vincenz (1842–1916) Assistant to Theodor Billroth (1829–1894) who became the professor of surgery at Heidelberg. He successfully resected the esophagus in a human in 1877, and removed a cancer of the large bowel. He introduced the vaginal operation for carcinoma of the uterus in 1878.

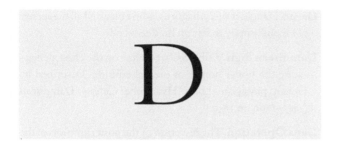

D'Acosta, Jose (1539–1600) *See altitude sickness.*

D'Arsonval, Jacques Arsene (1851–1940) The inventor of the reflecting galvanometer (Arsonval galvanometer). He was born to a French noble family at Borie and chose medicine as his career. He introduced high frequency electrotherapy in 1892. He also used electrotherapy for heating tissues, later developed into diathermy in the 1920s.

D'Herelle, Felix (1873–1949) Canadian bacteriologist from Montreal who was a professor at Yale from 1926 to 1933. In 1915 he discovered the bacteriophage. *See Twort–Herelle Phenomenon.*

Da Costa Syndrome (Syn. effort syndrome, neurocirculatory asthenia, cardiovascular neurosis, soldier's heart) Irritable heart amongst soldiers, noted by Arthur Bowen Richards Myers (1838–1921) in 1869. The same condition amongst soldiers during the American Civil War was described by Jacob Mendes Da Costa (1833–1900) of Jefferson Medical College, Philadelphia, in 1871. Sir Thomas Lewis (1881–1945) described it as 'effort syndrome' in 1917. Paul Wood (1907–1962), an eminent English cardiologist, attributed the somatic symptoms to psychoneurosis arising out of fear, in 1941.

Da Costa, Jacob Mendes (1833–1900) Born in the West Indies to parents of Portuguese origin. In 1848 he graduated from Jefferson College, Philadelphia, where he was later professor of medicine. He worked on functional diseases of the heart and described effort syndrome in soldiers, in 1871. He also wrote a standard treatise on diagnosis of disease in 1864. *See Da Costa syndrome.*

Da Vinci, Leonardo *See Leonardo Da Vinci.*

Dacron Used in modern arterial surgery, including the repair of aneurysms. Introduced by Emerick D. Szilagyi (b 1910) and co-workers in 1958.

Dagley, Stanley (b 1916) English microbiologist from Burton-on-Trent who worked with Cyril Norman Hinshelwood (1897–1967) at Oxford. He demonstrated that the bacterium *Aerobacter aerogenes* required carbon dioxide for its metabolism. He later became professor of biochemistry at the University of Minnesota and did research on citrate lyase, which converts citrate into oxaloacetate and acetic acid.

Dakin Solution Antiseptic containing sodium hypochlorite. Widely used for treating wounds in the two World Wars and developed by London chemist, Henry Drysdale Dakin (1880–1952).

Dakin, Henry Drysdale (1880–1952) English chemist, born in London. He trained in Marburg under Albrecht Kossel (1853–1927), professor of physiology at Hamburg, with whom he isolated the enzyme arginase. He independently synthesized epinephrine in 1906 and isolated a pyrrole, an intermediate in heme synthesis, in 1931. He was a pioneer in the study of protein structure and worked at the Rockefeller Center in the USA. *See Dakin solution.*

Dale, David (1739–1806) Scottish industrialist and philanthropist from Ayrshire who provided schooling and shelter for hundreds of poor children from Glasgow. He was also a director of the Glasgow Royal Infirmary, founded in 1794.

Dale, Samuel (1659–1739) Apothecary from Braintree, Essex who was made licentiate of the Royal College of Physicians in 1730. He wrote *Pharmocologia seu Manudictio Matriam Medicam* (1693) and several other works.

Dale, Sir Henry Hallett (1875–1968) Eminent British physiologist and experimental pharmacologist who demonstrated in 1909 that the active principle of the pituitary produced contraction of the smooth muscles of the arteries, uterus and spleen. He joined the Wellcome Research Laboratories in 1914 and was appointed director of the Department of Biochemistry and Pharmacology at the National Institute of Medical Research in 1924. During the period 1914 to 1929 he isolated the active principle of ergot, elucidated the action of histamine and adrenaline, and carried out important studies on the release of acetyl choline at voluntary motor nerve endings. The Nobel Prize for work on chemical transmission of nerves was shared by Dale and Otto Loewi (1873–1961), a German pharmacologist, in 1936. Dale was also Director of the Wellcome Trust, the President of the Royal Society from 1940 to 1945 and the President of the Penicillin Committee in 1941.

Dalechamp, James (1513–1588) Born in Caen, he practiced as a physician at Lyons from 1552 to 1558. He wrote *De Morbis Acutis* (1556), *Chirugie Francois* in 1559 and other works.

Dalen, Johan Albin (1866–1940) Swedish ophthalmologist who described small white spots on the retina (Dalen spots) and nodules in the pigmented epithelium of the choroid and iris (Dalen nodules) in sympathetic ophthalmitis.

Dalldorf Test Test for capillary fragility in which a suction cup is applied to the arm and the number of petechiae produced are counted over a fixed period of time. Introduced by New York pathologist, Gilbert Julius Dalldorf (b 1900). He also isolated the coxsackie virus in 1948.

Dalrymple Sign Abnormal widening of the palpebral fissure seen in exophthalmic goiter. Described by English oculist, John Dalrymple (1804–1852) in 1834.

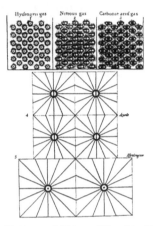

Picture of atoms. F.J. Moore, *A History of Chemistry* (1918). McGraw Hill, New York

Dalton, John (1766–1844) Eminent English chemist, the son of a hand-loom weaver in Eaglesfield, Cumbria. He investigated his own color-blindness and weather. In 1787, during a study of climate in the Lake District, he became interested in gases which led him to postulate some important laws. His law of partial pressures is now universally known as Dalton Law. He developed his theory of atoms in 1801 and determined the atomic weight of various elements. His first observations on the subject, *Inquiry into the Relative Weight of the Ultimate Particles* was submitted to the Philosophical Society in 1803. He published his *New System of Chemical Philosophy* in 1808 and is considered the father of atomic theory.

Daltonism (Syn. Color-blindness) *See Dalton, John, color vision.*

Dam, Carl Peter Henrik (1895–1976) Danish biochemist from Copenhagen who moved to America in 1940. He became a member of the Rockefeller Institute for Medical Research in 1945. He discovered 'antihemorrhagic factor' in 1929 and named it vitamin K in 1934. He was awarded the Nobel Prize for Medicine or Physiology in 1943 with Edward Adelbert Doisy (1893–1986), a biochemist from Illinois, for his work on the structure of vitamin K.

Damo Daughter of Pythagorus, who entrusted all the secrets of his philosophy to her on his death bed.

Damoiseau Sign Visible S-shaped line on the chest, demarcating the upper border of pleural effusion. Described by French physician, Louis Hyacinthe Celeste Damoiseau (1815–1890) in 1850.

Dana Operation The resection of the posterior roots of the spinal nerves as treatment for intractable pain, athetosis, or spastic paralysis. Designed by New York neurologist, Charles Loomes Dana (1852–1935).

Dana Syndrome (Syn. Putnam disease, subacute combined degeneration of the cord) A form of degenerative change of the spinal cord associated with pernicious anemia. First described in 1891 independently by Charles Loomes Dana (1852–1935) of New York, and James Jackson Putnam (1846–1918) of Boston. It was later reviewed and described by Ludwig Lichtheim (1845–1928) of Germany in 1897.

Dana, Charles Loomes (1852–1935) New York neurologist who described subacute combined degeneration of the cord (Dana syndrome) in 1891. He also published a catalogue of poems written by doctors, with biological notes, *Poetry and the Doctors,* in 1916.

Dance Sign Empty right iliac fossa found in children with intussusception. Described by French physician, Jean Baptise Hippolyte Dance (1797–1832).

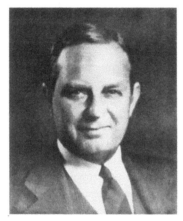

Walter Edward Dandy (1886–1946). Courtesy of the National Library of Medicine

Dandy, Walter Edward (1886–1946) American neurosurgeon from Johns Hopkins Hospital who in 1918 devised the method of introducing air into the cerebral ventricles for visualizing them on X-rays. He also performed partial resection of the sensory root of the trigeminal ganglion as treatment of trigeminal neuralgia in 1934. *See Dandy–Walker syndrome.*

Dandy–Walker Syndrome Failure or obstruction of the foramen of Luschka and Magendie giving rise to hydrocephalus. Described independently by two American neurosurgeons, Walter Edward Dandy (1886–1946) in 1921, and Arthur Earl Walker (b 1907) of Johns Hopkins Hospital in 1944.

Dangerous Drugs Act Passed in England in 1951 and amended in 1953, to control the import, production and use of narcotic substances. Another act was introduced in 1967 to control drug addiction that stipulated the compulsory registration of drug addicts by medical practitioners.

Danielli, James Frederick (1911–1984) British cell biologist, born at Wembley and educated at University College London. He is known for his work on the role of vitamin C in wound healing, aging and the permeability of biological membranes.

Danielssen Disease A form of anesthetic polyneuritis in leprosy. Described by Norwegian physician, Daniel Cornelius Danielssen (1815–1894).

Danlos, Henri Alexandre (1844–1912) The first to apply radium treatment for lupus of the skin in 1901. He described Ehlers–Danlos syndrome in 1908. *See Ehlers–Danlos syndrome.*

Danysz Bacillus A group of paratyphoid bacilli used for poisoning rats. Discovered by a Polish bacteriologist, Jean Danysz (1861–1928). He joined the Pasteur Institute in Paris in 1893 and worked on diseases that controlled animal pests.

Dappers, Oliver (d 1690) Physician from Amsterdam who published descriptions of Africa and Asia in 1668.

Dapsone Introduced as a treatment for leprosy by Gladwin Albert Hurst Buttle (1899–1983) and co-workers in 1938.

Daran, James (1701–1784) Physician from Gascony who wrote *Traite sur le Gonorrhoea Virulenta* in 1756.

Darier Disease (Syn. pseudoxanthoma elasticum) Hereditary form of skin disease with lax or stretched skin associated with cardiovascular and gastrointestinal abnormalities. Described by French dermatologist, Jean Ferdinand Darier (1856–1938) in 1896.

Darkshevich Fibers Fibers connecting the ophthalmic tract to the habenular nucleus, named after the Moscow neurologist, Liverij Osipovich Darkshevich (1858–1925).

Darling, Samuel Taylor (1872–1925) American pathologist who described histoplasmosis (Darling disease) while he was in Ancon in the Panama Canal zone in 1906. *See Histoplasma capsulatum.*

Darlington, Cyril Dean (1903–1981) English geneticist, born in Chorley, Lancashire and educated in Wye. He founded the Cytology Department at the John Innes Horticultural Institution in London in 1937 and became director of the Institute in 1939. He was appointed Sheridan professor of botany at Oxford in 1953 and proposed 60 genetic terms. He studied the role of chromosomes in evolution and selection and published several books including, *Elements of Genetics* with K. Mather, *Recent Advances in Cytology* (1932) and *Evolution of Genetic Systems* (1939).

Darnall Filter Made of Canton flannel for purifying drinking water, now obsolete. Devised by American army surgeon, Carl Rogers Darnall (1867–1941).

Darrow Solution A physiological electrolyte solution containing potassium. Formulated by American professor of pediatrics, Daniel Cady Darrow (1895–1965), at Duke University, North Carolina.

Darwin Tubercle *See Woolner, Thomas.*

Darwin, Charles Robert (1809–1882) The architect of evolutionary theory, born in Shrewsbury. His father, Robert Darwin, was a physician and his mother was the daughter of Josiah Wedgwood. He entered Edinburgh University in 1825 to study medicine but lost interest and returned home after two years. He joined Cambridge University in 1828 and obtained his BA degree in 1831. Soon after his graduation, at the age of 22 years, he took a voyage as a naturalist in *HMS Beagle* which lasted for four years. On his return he worked on his theory of evolution for 20 years and published his monumental work on the subject, *On the Origin of Species by Means of Natural Selection* in 1859. His other works include: *The Fertilisation of Orchids* (1862), *The Variation of Plants and Animals under Domestication* (1867), *The Descent of Man and Selection in Relation to Sex* (1871), *Expression of the Emotions in Man and Animals* (1873), *Insectivorous Plants* (1875), *Climbing Plants* (1875), *The Effects of Cross and Self Fertilisation in the Vegetable Kingdom* (1876), *The Power of Movements in Plants* (1880) and *The formation of Vegetable Mould through action of Worms* (1881). *See evolution.*

Darwin, Erasmus (1731–1802) Physician and poet, born in Elton, near Newark in Nottinghamshire. He took his degree at St John's College Cambridge in 1755 and later moved to Edinburgh. He published *The Botanic Garden* (1789), *Zoonomia or the Laws of Organic Life* (1794–1796), *Phytologia* (1799) and a tract on female education. His son, Charles Darwin, who studied medicine at Edinburgh died in 1778, leaving *An Essay on the Retrograde Motion of the Absorbent Vessels*, which was later published by his father. Charles

Darwin (1809–1882) author of the theory on evolution, was his grandson by his first marriage.

Darwin, George Howard (1845–1912) The grandson of Charles Darwin (1809–1882), born at Down, in Kent. He was formally educated in law in 1874, but took up astronomy and mathematics. His important work, *The Tides,* on their effects on the solar system, was published in 1898. He also wrote a treatise on a statistical inquiry into the effects of marriages between first cousins.

Darwin, Sir Francis (b 1848) Third son of Charles Darwin (1809–1882), born at Down, Kent. He graduated as a physician from Cambridge and helped his father in his botanical studies. He published *Foundations of the Origin of Species* in 1909 and also wrote a biography of his father.

Darwinism The theory of evolution according to which higher organisms developed from lower organisms through a process of natural selection was proposed by Charles Darwin (1809–1882) in 1859. *See Darwin, Charles, evolution.*

Dastre, Jules Albert François (1844–1917) Physiologist in Paris who demonstrated that the constriction of the blood vessels in the skin is associated with dilitation of the splanchnic blood vessels.

Dattner, Bernhard (1887–1952) Associate professor of neurology at the New York University Medical College, who designed a needle (Dattner needle) for aspirating cerebrospinal fluid. It consisted of a fine inner needle within an outer moderate-bore needle for perforating the spinal dura mater. Dattner published *The Management of Neurosyphilis* in 1944.

Dausset, Jean Baptiste Gabriel (b 1916) French immunologist and discoverer of the human leukocyte antigen (HLA) group. He was born in Toulouse and studied medicine at the University of Paris. His discovery led to recognition of the major histocompatibility complex (MHC) by George Davis Snell (b 1903). His work on skin grafting in 1967 led to the procedure of tissue typing which greatly reduced the number of rejection reactions. With Snell and Baruj Benacerraf (b 1920), a Venezuelan-born American immunologist, Dausset received the Nobel Prize for Medicine or Physiology in 1980.

Davaine, Casimir Joseph (1812–1882) French physician and microbiologist, born in St Amand-les-Eaux and studied medicine in Paris. He was an originator of the germ theory of disease before Pasteur and identified the anthrax bacillus in the blood of animals.

Davainea A genus of tapeworm found in Asiatic Russia.

Named after a French physician and microbiologist, Casimir Joseph Davaine (1812–1882).

Davenport, Charles Benedict (1866–1944) Foremost geneticist in America, based on Mendelism. He was born in Stamford, Connecticut. He graduated from Harvard University with a doctorate in philosophy in 1892 and became director of the Station for Experimental Evolution at the Carnegie Institute in Washington in 1904. He published a work on the heredity nature of epilepsy in 1911.

David Disease Pott disease of the spine, independently described by French surgeon, Jean Pierre David (1738–1774).

David, Jean Pierre (1737–1784) French professor of anatomy and surgery at Rouen. He advocated allowing sufficient time and rest for joint diseases to heal.

Davidoff, Leo Max (1898–1975) New York neurologist who developed an improved method of encephalography with Cornelius D. Dyke in 1925. They published an article 'Chronic subdural hematoma' in the *Bulletin of the Neuro-logical Institute of New York* in 1938.

Davidoff, M. Professor of forensic medicine in St Petersburg. He described the Paneth cells in the mucosa of the small intestine in 1887 that were described independently in the same year by Joseph Paneth (1857–1890), professor of physiology in Breslau.

Davie Disease *See endomyocardial fibrosis.*

Daviel Operation A modern treatment for cataract by extraction of the lens. First described by French oculist, Jacques Daviel (1696–1762).

Davies, Herbert (b 1818) Physician and cardiologist at the London Hospital who studied under René Laënnec (1781–1826) at Paris. He advocated the use of the stethoscope in England and published *Course of Lectures on Diseases of the Heart and Lungs and On the Treatment of Acute Rheumatism by Free Blistering.* He founded the Royal Chest Hospital, City Road, London.

Davies-Colley, John Neville (1842–1900) London surgeon who described the Davies-Colley operation, in which a bone wedge is removed to correct talipes.

Davis, John Staige (1872–1946) Surgeon at Baltimore who described a method (Davis graft) of splinting skin grafts in 1909. He was the first American surgeon to devote his practice to plastic surgery and he published *Plastic Surgery: Its Principles and Practice* in 1919.

Davisson, Clinton Joseph (1881–1958) Physicist from Illinois. He discovered the diffraction of electrons by crystals, which supported the wave theory of electrons.

Davson, Hugh (b 1909) English pioneer in cell physiology, born and educated in London. He published *Physiology of the Eye* (1949) and *Of General Physiology* (1951), and edited a new version of Ernest Starling's (1866–1927) *Principles of Human Physiology.*

Davy Lever A wooden sound used in the 19th century for insertion into the rectum to stop bleeding in the iliac artery. Named after London surgeon, Richard Davy (1838–1920).

Davy Test Test for detection of phenol using molybdic and sulfuric acid, devised by an Irish physician, Edmund William Davy (1826–1899).

Davy, Edward (1806–1885) Physician from Devon. He did early experiments on telegraphy and demonstrated it over a distance of one mile at Regents Park in London. He emigrated to Australia in 1838 and practiced as a physician in Victoria. His other contributions include Davy blow pipe for chemical analysis, Davy mercurial trough for gas chemistry and Davy diamond cement for repair of broken china.

Davy, Sir Humphry (1778–1829) Considered as one of the greatest English chemists. He was apprenticed to a surgeon, J.B. Borlace, in Cornwall. At the age of 17 years he began his experiments on the inhalational effects of nitrous oxide. In 1798 he joined the Medical Pneumatic Institution founded by Beddoes, to study the inhalation of gases in the treatment of disease. His *Researches, Chemical and Philosophical; Chiefly Concerning Nitrous Oxide* was published in 1799. Following this, he took charge of the laboratory at the Royal Institution at the invitation of Count Rumford, in 1801. He discovered the elements, sodium, potassium, magnesium, strontium and barium.

Dawkin, Sir William Boyd (1837–1929) Anthropologist and paleontologist from Welshpool, Montgomeryshire, who was professor of paleontology at the Victoria University Manchester for a long period. He published *Early Man in Britain and his place in the Tertiary Period* (1880) and several other works on the geology of the Isle of Man.

Daws, Rutter William (1799–1868) London astronomer who discovered many comets and the phenomenon of double stars. He also described the canals on Mars. As a child, Daws lived for a short while in Sierra Leone, where his father was governor in 1807. On his return to England he studied medicine and practiced for some time before he took up astronomy.

Dawson, Sir John William (1820–1899) Canadian geologist from Nova Scotia who graduated from Edinburgh University in 1842. He founded the Royal Society of Canada and was its first president. Dawson published *The Dawn of Life* (1875), *The Origin of the World* (1877), *The Meeting Place of Geology and History* (1894) and several other works.

Dawson, Thomas (d 1782) London physician who graduated from Glasgow in 1753. He was elected physician at the Middlesex Hospital in 1759 and later at the London Hospital in 1764. He published *Cases of Acute Rheumatism and the Gout* (1776) and *An Account of a Safe and Efficacious Medicine in Sore Eyes and Eyelids* in 1782.

Day Test Test for detecting traces of blood using guaiacum tincture. Devised by an American physician, Richard Hance Day (1813–1892).

DC Cardioverter *See cardioversion.*

DDT Dichlorodiphenyltrichloroethane, first prepared by Othman Zeider in 1874. The lethal effect of DDT on insects was demonstrated by Swiss chemist, Hermann Paul Muller (1899–1965) at the experimental laboratory of Johann Rudolf Geigy, in 1899. It was marketed as a pesticide in 1942 and Muller was awarded the Nobel Prize in Physiology or Medicine for his work in 1948. It was extensively used as a pesticide in tropical countries, but had to be replaced by other compounds around 1960, owing to its toxic effects as well as resistance to it that was developed by insects.

De Beer, Sir Gavin Rylands (1899–1972) London zoologist who graduated from Oxford and taught there from 1923 to 1928. He published *Introduction to Experimental Embryology* (1926) and *Development of the Vertebrate Skull* in 1935.

DeLee, Joseph Bolivar (1869–1942) Born in New York and graduated in 1891 from North Western University, Chicago, where he was professor of obstetrics for 40 years. He designed several obstetric instruments and was a leading figure in his field. He published *Principles and Practice of Obstetrics* in 1913.

De Morgan Spots *See Campbell De Morgan spots.*

De Morgan, Campbell Greig (1811–1876) *See Campbell De Morgan spots.*

De Musset Sign Head nodding owing to arterial pulsation in aortic insufficiency. Named after the French poet Alfred De Musset (1810–1857) who, with his brother, is supposed to have observed the sign in their mother.

de Quervain Disease A painful contraction of the thumb muscles: abductor pollicis longus and extensor pollicis brevis. Described by Swiss professor of surgery, Fritz de Quervain (1868–1940) of Bern in 1895.

de Quervain Thyroiditis An acute form of thyroiditis, described by Swiss professor of surgery, Fritz de Quervain (1868–1940) of Bern in 1904.

Deadly Nightshade *Atropa belladonna*, the plant that is the source of the alkaloid, atropine. One of the first English monographs on it, *Observations on the Use of Belladonna in Painful Disorders of the Head and Face*, was published in 1818 by John Bailey, who studied its therapeutic uses. The substance was used in ophthalmic surgery by J.A.H. Reimarus (1729–1814) of Hamburg. Extract of Bulgarian belladonna was introduced as a treatment for post-encephalitic parkinsonism in England by F.J. Newahl and C.C. Fenwick in 1937. The therapeutic action of English belladonna was proved to be identical to that of Bulgarian belladonna by D. Hill in 1938. *See Atropa belladonna*.

Deaf Mutes Scottish educator, George Dalgarmo (1626–1687) invented an alphabet for deaf mutes in 1680. One of the earliest attempts at their systematic education was made by Johan Conrad Amman (1669–1730) of Amsterdam in 1692. He published his *Surdus Loquens* in 1692. An alphabet to communicate with them was used by Abbe L'Eppe in 1771. In 1821, Johannes Purkinje (1787–1869) observed that they can hear through the bones of the skull. This observation was put into clinical use for the diagnosis of aural diseases by Berlin otologist, Johan Constantin August Lucae (1835–1911) in 1870. Further new tests for audition in deaf mutism and unilateral deafness were devised by Friedrich von Bezold (1836–1868) of Munich in 1896. *See audiology, hearing*.

Death Certificate The statutory duty of the doctor in England, to issue a certificate on a patient on whom he attended during his or her last illness, was first specified in the Births and Deaths Registration Act of 1874.

Death Rate The first recorded study in England of the death rate in both sexes was done by John Graunt (1620–1674) of London. He published the first book on vital statistics, *Natural and Political Observations Upon the Bills of Mortality* in 1662. *See vital statistics*.

Deaver, John Blair (1855–1931) American surgeon from Lancaster, Pennsylvania who described the fat-free portions of the gut and their relation to the vascular arcade in 1902. He also devised the Deaver incision for appendectomy through the sheath of the right rectus muscle.

Debout Pill Remedy for migraine, made of colchicum, quinine sulfate and digitalis. Prepared by French physician,

Emile Debout (1811–1865) around 1850.

Debove, Georges Maurice (1845–1920) Histopathologist from Paris who described the layer of cells beneath the cilia of the trachea and bronchi in 1874.

Debré Syndrome *See cat scratch fever*.

Decatorthoma An ancient term for a medicine made of ten ingredients.

Decerebrate Rigidity Early investigators, including Robert Whytt (1714–1766), Luigi Rolando (1773–1831) and Pierre Flourens (1794–1867), who observed the effect of removing the forebrain in experimental animals. Cerebellar seizures in humans resembling the effects of decerebration were observed by John Hughlings Jackson (1834–1911) in 1870. The condition of muscular rigidity of the body produced by transection of the spinal cord through the upper part of the midbrain was studied by Charles Sherrington (1857–1952) of Oxford University in 1897. He used the transected cat, which he referred to as a 'spinal animal'. He demonstrated that life could be maintained in a healthy state in such an animal, despite decerebrate rigidity.

Decidua A membranous structure produced by the uterus and discarded after parturition. First described by Fabricius ab Aquapendente (1537–1619) of Padua in his work on embryology, *De Formato Foetu*, published in 1600.

Decompression Sickness *See caisson disease*.

Decortication [Latin: *decorticare*, to peel] *See Delorme operation*.

Deen Test A test for detection of blood in gastric juice with the help of guaiac and other agents. Devised by a Dutch physiologist, Izaak Abrahamzoon van Deen (1804–1869) in 1840.

Deep Vein Thrombosis The purified fraction of the venom of the Malayan pit viper was used as a therapeutic agent for anticoagulation under the name ancrod. It was first tried as treatment for deep vein thrombosis by W.R. Bell and colleagues in 1968. Heparin was discovered by William Henry Howell (1860–1945) of Johns Hopkins University in 1918 and it was obtained in a purified form by Charles Herbert Best (1899–1978) of Toronto in 1938. It was used in treatment of venous thrombosis by Donald Walter Gordon Murray (1894–1976) and co-workers in 1937.

Defibrillation *See cardioversion, defibrillator*.

Defibrillator Pioneer work on the apparatus was done by Jean Louis Prevost (1790–1850) and F. Batelli, who induced ventricular fibrillation in the dog's heart by applying a small current and terminated the arrhythmia by giving a larger dose of current. One of the first practical electrical defibrillators to treat the irregularity of the heart was constructed by American professor of electrical engineering, William Bennett Kouwenhoven (1886–1975) of Johns Hopkins University, in 1936. The first countershock to a fibrillating human heart leading to recovery was administered by Claude Schaeffer Beck (1894–1971) and colleagues in 1945. A further advance was made by C.E. Herrod and co-workers, who presented a combined pacemaker and defibrillator in 1952. W.G. Bigelow and J.A. Hopps applied a similar device to clinical use in 1953. Following this success, Paul Maurice Zoll (b 1911) and co-workers terminated ventricular fibrillation in four patients by applying alternating countershock current in 1956. The advantage of direct current (DC) was observed over alternating current (AC) and a DC capacitor discharge capable of depolarizing the myocardium transthoracically was developed by Bernard Lowen and R. Amarasingham in 1962. The implantable defibrillator was approved by the American Food and Drug Administration in 1985.

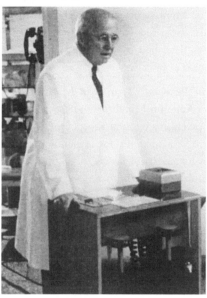

William B. Kouwenhoven (1886–1975)

Deficiency Diseases *See vitamins, accessory food factors.*

Deglutition [Latin: *de*, down + *glutire*, to swallow] The earliest description of the mechanism of deglutition was given by François Magendie (1783–1855) of Bordeaux in 1813. He included the three stages of passage of food: through the mouth, pharynx and esophagus. The swallowing reflex involved in the act of deglutition was described by Karl Hugo Kronecker (1839–1914) of Bern in 1880. The act of deglutition was studied in animals through the use of contrast medium and X-rays by American physiologist,

Walter Bradford Cannon (1871–1945), in 1902.

Deiters, Otto Friedrich Carl (1834–1863) German physician and pupil of Rudolph Virchow (1821–1902). He described the lateral nucleus of the eighth nerve and discovered astrocytes in 1863.

Dejerine Disease A form of hypertrophic interstitial neuritis in infants. Described by Swiss-born French neurologist, Joseph Jules Dejerine (1849–1917) and Jules Sottas (1866–1943) in Paris in 1893.

Dejerine-Klumpke, Augusta (1859–1927) Born in San Francisco, she was educated in Switzerland and completed her medical studies in Paris where she became the first woman intern in the French hospital system. She married another neurologist, Joseph Dejerine (1849–1917), and they worked together to make several important contributions in neurology.

Dejerine-Klumpke Syndrome (Syn. lower brachial palsy) Enophthalmos, ptosis and paralysis of the area of the ulnar nerve, following injury to the eighth cervical nerve and first thoracic root. Described by Augusta Dejerine-Klumpke (1859–1927) of Paris in 1885.

Dejerine–Roussey Syndrome Thalamic syndrome consisting of paroxysms of contralateral pain, ataxia and choreo- athetoid movements due to thrombosis or lesions of the thalamogeniculate artery. Described by Joseph Jules Dejerine (1849–1917), and Gustav Roussey (1874–1948) of Paris in 1906.

Dejerine–Sottas Syndrome A slowly progressive form of hereditary neuritis associated with kyphoscolisis, arthritis and ocular changes. Described by French neurologists, Joseph Jules Dejerine (1849–1917) and Jules Sottas (1866–1943) of Paris in 1890.

Delafield Stain A strong solution of hematoxylin, first prepared by Francis Delafield (1841–1915), a pathologist in New York.

Delayed Hypersensitivy Reaction The cellular transfer of delayed cutaneous hypersensitivity and the role of mononuclear cells in the process was demonstrated by Karl Landsteiner (1868–1943) in 1942. The role of lymphokines in delayed hypersensitivity was discovered by John David (b 1930) in 1966.

Delbet Sign An indication of adequate circulation in cases of arterial aneurysm of the limbs. Described by French surgeon, Paul Delbet (1866–1924). He considered circulation through the collateral vessels to be adequate, if nutrition to the distal limb was maintained.

Delbet, Pierre Louis Ernest (1861–1925) A surgeon in Paris who described an operation for fractured neck of the femur in which a bone graft was applied to the femoral neck.

Delbruck, Max (1906–1981) German biophysicist and pioneer in genetics of the phage. He was born in Berlin and emigrated to America in 1937. In 1946 he discovered that viruses can exchange genetic material to create new types of viruses. He formed the Phage Group for the use of the phage as an experimental tool and was awarded the Nobel Prize for Physiology or Medicine in 1969.

Delepine, Sheridan (1855–1921) Physician of Swiss origin who emigrated to Britain in 1877 and qualified in medicine from Edinburgh in 1882. He was the first curator and demonstrator at the pathology museum at St George's Hospital and the first holder of chair of pathology and bacteriology at the University of Manchester. *See microtome.*

Deletion [Latin: *delere*, to efface] A process by which the loss of a segment of a chromosome occurs. Described by an American geneticist, Theophilus Shickle Painter (1889–1969) and Joseph Hermann Muller (1890–1967) in 1929. It was recognized later as an important cause of several congenital diseases.

Delinquent *See child psychiatry.*

Delirium Tremens [Latin: *de,* away from + *lira,* furrow or track] Associated with alcoholism, and described by Thomas Sutton (1767–1835) of London in 1813. A classical description was given by John Ware (1795–1864), professor of medicine at Harvard University in 1831.

Delore Method A method of forcible manual correction of genu valgum, proposed by a French physician, Xavier Delore (1828–1916) in 1860.

Delorme Operation Decortication of the lung in empyema (pleurectomy) to allow the lung to expand fully. Advocated by French surgeon, Edmund Delorme (1847–1929) in Paris. The same operation was designed independently by American surgeon, George Ryerson Fowler (1848–1906).

Delos Greek island, supposed to have risen from the sea by the powers of Neptune, according to Greek mythology. It was the birthplace of the Greek god of health Apollo.

Delpech, Jacques Matthieu (1777–1832) A surgeon from Toulouse, he was professor of surgery in Montpellier and a pioneer of orthopedic surgery in Paris. He devised a new method of treatment of clubfoot by subcutaneous section

of the tendo achilles. He also pointed out the tubercular nature of spinal caries. He was killed by one of his patients who believed that the varicocele operation Delpech performed on him made him unsuitable for marriage.

Deltoides [Greek: *delta*] The muscle of the upper arm and scapula derives its name from its triangular shape.

Demarquay Sign The fixation of the lower end of the larynx during phonation and deglutition as a sign of syphilis of the trachea. Described by French surgeon, Jean Nicholas Demarquay (1811–1875).

Dementia [Latin: *de,* down + *mens,* mind] Phillipe Pinel (1745–1825) was one of the first to recognize intellectual deterioration as a separate entity – dementia. Jean Etienne Dominique Esquirol (1772–1840) of Toulouse, one of the first lecturers in psychiatry, studied the different stages in senile individuals in 1838. Alois Alzheimer (1864–1915) studied brains of demented and senile patients and correlated histological findings with the signs and symptoms of dementia in his research on neuropathology at Kraepelin's Clinic in Munich in 1907. Another form of presenile dementia associated with circumscribed atrophy of the brain was described by Czech psychiatrist, Arnold Pick (1851–1924) in 1892. *See subcortical dementia.*

Dementia Praecox Term used by Austrian psychiatrist, Benedict Augustin Morel (1809–1873) in 1856. It was later used in psychiatry by Emil Kraepelin (1856–1926) in 1901. The term 'schizophrenia' for dementia praecox was introduced by Eugene Bleuler (1857–1939), professor of psychiatry at Burgholzli Hospital in 1911.

Democedes (*c* 540 BC) Greek physician and native of Cnidos. He settled in the Greek colony of Croton where he wrote the first Greek treatise on medicine. Herodotus (484–407 BC), in his book of history, devoted several pages to him. This was probably the first biography of a physician. He attended Prince Polycrates of Samos and was later appointed as physician to Darius.

Democritus (470–360 BC) Greek philosopher from Abdera, a contemporary of Socrates (470–399 BC). He was the first to state, in his cosmic theory, that everything in nature, including the body and soul, consisted of atoms, the movements of which controlled all activities. He wrote treatises on medicine and anatomy, and is supposed to have lived to the age of 109 years.

Demography [Greek: *demos,* people + *graphein,* to write] The study of mankind, especially in relation to statistical data. Taking of censuses was a regular feature of the Roman empire. In 1085 William II, in his survey of most of England, mainly to record land ownership for taxation, incidentally made one of the earliest records of the English population. The Doomsday Book, which was completed at the end of his survey in 1086, reveals that there were about 2 million people in England. Sir Matthew Hale (1609–1676), an English judge from Alderly in Gloucestershire, was one of the first to propose a mechanism governing the growth of population in his treatise on the primitive organization of mankind. The first census in Ireland was taken by Sir William Petty (1623–1687), from Hampshire, who published a book on statistics, *Essays on Political Arithmetic*, in 1687. The population of England and Wales in 1700 was under 6 million and the entire population of Great Britain in 1801 was just under 11 million. The world population in 1863 was at that time estimated at 1.25 billion. English clergyman, Thomas Robert Malthus (1766–1834), in his *An Essay on the Principle of Population or A View of its Past and Present Effects* published in 1803, pointed out that the only limits to expansion of population were space and food.

Demonology It is rooted in fear of the unknown. Sorcerers used this fear to exert their influence and control people. The Assyrians, Babylonians, ancient Hindus and Egyptians all passed through a primitive stage of demonology. The power of sorcerers and witch doctors was often put to trial, when they were called upon to cure diseases that were thought to have been sent by evil spirits or sacred sources. In their efforts to cure the sick, the wiser ones, who probably observed the therapeutic effects of herbs and learned from the behavior of animals which often resorted to nature for healing, applied their observations to healing, thus paving the way for scientific medicine. The Babylonians had several demons: Dodid was their demon of abortion and Labartu was a female demon that tore children prematurely from the mother's womb. The ancient Egyptians recognized 36 separate devils and divinities, each working on different part of the body for good or evil. The Maoris believed that certain devils entered certain organs. In Australia and Tasmania, devils were believed to have the power of entering bodies and eating the liver. Tasmanians laid their sick around the corpse so that the devil would come in the night and take out the cause of the disease. Finnish mythology involved considerable disease–demon theory. They believed all diseases to be daughters of Louhiater, the demon of diseases. Their goddess, Suoneta, was a healer and renewer of flesh. In the East, Cambodians exorcised the demon of smallpox with the urine of a white horse.

Demours, Pierre (1702–1795) Ophthalmologist from Marseilles who practiced in Paris. He described the lamina basalis of the posterior cornea in 1767. This had previously been described by Jean Descemet (1732–1810).

Dendrochronology [Greek: *dendron*, tree + *chronos*, time + *logos*, discourse] A method of dating ancient pieces of wood by studying and counting the annual rings in it. Introduced by an American astronomer, Andrew Ellicott Douglass (1867–1962) of Winsor, Vermont in 1915.

Dengue Fever [Spanish: *dengue*, dandy] Derives its name from the mincing walk noted amongst those affected. It is also known as break-bone fever, *bou-bou* (terror in Arabic) and articular fever. It is mostly a disease of tropical climates and was described in Batavia in Java by the town medical officer, David Bylon, in 1779. It was described in more detail by Benjamin Rush (1745–1813) of Pennsylvania in 1780. Epidemics occurred in the West Indies and southern states of North America in 1827. One of the major epidemics started in Zanzibar in 1870 and reached most parts of Asia by 1873. The mosquito *Aedes aegypti* was shown to be a vector in its transmission by Thomas Lane Bancroft (1860–1933) in 1906. The causative agent, a filterable virus, was discovered by Percy Moreau Ashburn (1872–1940) and Charles Franklin Craig (1872–1950) in 1907. The first vaccine for prophylaxis against dengue fever was prepared by Albert Bruce Sabin, the American microbiologist of polio vaccine fame, in 1945.

Denis, Prosper Sylvian (1799–1863) *See fibrinolysis.*

Denker, Alfred (1863–1941) German otorhinologist who devised a radical operation (Denker operation) for suppuration of maxillary air sinuses.

Denman Evolution Spontaneous version of transverse presentation in obstetrics, occurring through rotation of the head and shoulder. First described by an English obstetrician, Thomas Denman (1733–1815).

Dennett, William Sawyer (1849–1924) American ophthalmologist who invented an electric light ophthalmoscope in 1885.

Dennie–Marfan Syndrome Mental retardation and spastic tetraplegia in children with congenital syphilis. Described by Bernard Jean Antonin Marfan (1858–1942), a pediatrician in Paris. Another account was given by American dermatologist, C. Dennie (1883–1971) in 1929.

Denny-Brown, Derek Ernest (1901–1980) New Zealand-born neurologist who worked with Charles Scott Sherrington (1857–1952) at Oxford. He demonstrated the reaction of a single motor neuron following its activation by a stimulus in 1929. After serving for a short period as neurologist at St Bartholomew's Hospital, he spent the rest of his career at Harvard. The first apparatus, consisting of a catheter, manometer and a moving strip of bromide paper, to measure and record the behavior of the bladder and its sphincters (cystogram) was designed by him in 1933.

Denonvilliers, Charles Pierre (1808–1872) Professor of surgery and anatomy in Paris. He described prostatoperitoneal aponeurosis in 1845.

Denovilliers Operation Plastic correction of a defective ala nasi done by transferring a triangular flap from the side of the nose. Described by Charles Pierre Denovilliers (1808–1872), professor of surgery in Paris.

Dental Caries Ancient Babylonians believed that bad teeth were caused by divine displeasure and they prescribed incantations and prayers as treatment. Aristotle (384–322 BC) advised extraction of a loose tooth by hand instead of pliers, to avoid damage to the gums. Partial denture work found in Etruscan tombs dating back to 700 BC bear witness to the antiquity of the disease and human efforts to overcome the deformity caused by it. Aulus Cornelius Celsus (25 BC–AD 50) advocated copious washing of the mouth on rising to prevent tooth decay. Rhazes (AD 850–923), an Islamic physician, was one of the first to recommend the filling of dental cavities. John of Gaddesden (1280–1361) proposed that decay of teeth was due to either humors or worms. It was a disease of all classes, Elizabeth I suffered badly from tooth decay and refused tooth extraction until the ease of the procedure was demonstrated by her dentist on the Bishop of London. John Hunter (1728–1793) was the first to recommend the complete removal of pulp before filling. The first practical dental cement, an oxyphosphate of zinc, was introduced in 1869 and the first foot-operated dentist's drill was used in 1871.

Dental Drill Invented by John Green Wood, George Washington's dentist, in 1790. The first foot-operated dentist's drill was used in 1871.

Dentistry [Latin: *dens*, tooth] Ancient Etruscans in Tuscany made remarkable dental bridges before the Christian era, which are still preserved. The record of the earliest dentist is found in a wood panel from Saqqara, Egypt, dating from 3000 BC. The title on this panel is Chief of the Toothers and of the Physicians. Galen (129–200), gave an account of diseases of the teeth in his fifth book. Albucasis (936–1013) gave probably the first illustration of dental instruments in his legendary treatise *Altasrif.* The eminent French surgeon, Ambroise Paré (1510–1590) also practiced dentistry. The first English book entirely devoted to it, *The Operator for the*

Teeth, was written by Charles Allen of York in 1685. Thomas Berdmore, a dentist to George III, wrote an important book on the teeth and gums in 1768. Another treatise was that of John Hunter (1728–1793), the *Natural History of the Human Teeth,* published in 1771. He was also the first to study teeth scientifically and to recommend the complete removal of pulp before filling. Two other important early treatises were written by Pierre Fauchard (1678–1761) of France (*Le Chirurgien Dentiste,* 1728) and the German surgeon, Phillip Pfaff (*Abhandlung von den Zahnen,* 1756). Fauchard also described pyorrhea alviolaris in 1746. This later came to be known as Riggs disease, since the treatment by scraping the teeth to the roots was proposed by American surgeon, John Mankey Riggs (1810–1885) in 1876. The first dental school in the world, Baltimore College of Dental Surgery, was established in America in 1839. Horace Wells (1815–1848) was the first to use nitrous oxide in dentistry in 1844. The Orthodontical Society of London was founded in 1856 and the Dental Hospital of London was established at Soho in 1859. The London School of Dental Surgery was founded a year later at the same site in Soho Square. The Edinburgh Dental Hospital and School was founded by John Smith (1825–1910), who inherited his father's practice as a dentist in 1851. Smith also published *A Handbook of Dental Anatomy and Surgery* in 1864 and founded the Edinburgh Dental Dispensary in 1860. The first dental X-rays were taken by William James Morton (1846–1920) in 1896. See *artificial teeth, dental caries, tooth transplantation, dental drill.*

Denuce, Jean Louis Paul (1824–1889) Professor of clinical surgery at the University of Bordeaux. He described the quadrate ligament of the superior ulnar articulation in 1854.

Denys, Jean Baptist (1640–1704) Professor of surgery in Paris who investigated the effect of blood transfusion in animals. Following his experiments on animals, he transfused 12 ounces of blood from a lamb to a dying man in 1667. See *blood transfusion.*

Deoxyribonuclease Enzyme crystallized from beef pancreas by M. Kunitz in 1950. The amino acid composition of bovine pancreatic ribonuclease was determined by the Americans, Stanford Moore (1913–1982), William Howard Stein (1911–1980) of New York, and Christian Boehmer Anfinson (b 1916) of Pennsylvania, for which they were jointly awarded the Nobel Prize for Chemistry in 1972.

Deoxyribonucleic Acid (DNA) Johann Friedrich Miescher (1844–1895) identified 'nuclein' in the cell in 1871. This was later found to be the nucleoprotein responsible for genetic transmission. The chemical distinction of these proteins in

DNA was made by Phoebus Aaron Theodore Levene (1869–1940) in 1903. DNA in a pure state was obtained by Andrei Nikolaevitch Belozersky in 1936, who also showed the presence of RNA and DNA in bacteria in 1939. The adenine and thymine bases in DNA were described by a Czech-born biochemist, Erwin Chargaff (b 1905) while he was professor of biochemistry at Columbia University, New York in the 1950s. Genetic transmission was established by Theodore Oswald Avery (1877–1955) in 1944. The occurrence of four different bases forming a code for directing the synthesis of proteins was elucidated by an American physicist of Russian origin, George Gamow (1904–1968) in 1950. X-ray diffraction photography of DNA molecules was performed by Rosalind Franklin (1920–1958) of King's College, London around 1952. Her work led to the historic discovery of the molecular structure of DNA by James Dewey Watson (b 1928), a biologist from Chicago, and Francis Harry Compton Crick (b 1918), from Northhampton, at the Cavendish Laboratory in Cambridge, England in 1953. The double helical structure of DNA was revealed by a New Zealand-born British biochemist, Maurice Hugh Frederick Wilkins (b 1916) and colleagues in the same year. Artificial synthesis of nucleic acids using enzymes was achieved by Arthur Kornberg (b 1918) from Brooklyn and co-workers in 1956. A Japanese biochemist, Reiji Okazaki (1930–1975), discovered DNA–RNA fragments in 1957, which solved the problem of how DNA was synthesized simultaneously in opposite directions, but with corresponding opposite polarity. The reverse transcriptase enzyme capable of transcribing DNA from RNA was discovered by American microbiologist, David Baltimore (b 1938) of New York in 1970 and his finding formed the basis for manipulation of the genetic code. A new method for finding the sequence of bases in nucleic acids was devised by American molecular biologist, Walter Gilbert (b 1932) of Boston, Massachusetts around 1970. The full sequence of bases in the DNA of a virus (Phi X 174) was worked out by Frederick Sanger (b 1918), an English biochemist from Rendcombe, in 1977. The first genetic map was produced by an American biologist and physician of Russian–Jewish origin, Daniel Nathans (b 1928) from Delaware, who used his method to locate a specific gene in DNA. He shared the Nobel Prize with Hamilton Orthaniel Smith (b 1931) of New York and Swiss microbiologist, Werner Arber (b 1929) in 1978. *See genetic engineering.*

Depilatories [Latin: *de*, away + *pilus*, hair] Substances used from ancient times to remove unwanted hair on the body. Athenaeus of Naucratis in Egypt in the 3rd century described this as common practice amongst Tuscans. Many ancient Roman satirists commented on the application of depilatories to the private parts of the body. Arsenic and quicklime were commonly used during Roman times.

Depression [Latin: *deprimere*, to press down] Lithium was recommended as treatment for gout by Alfred Baring Garrod (1819–1907) in 1859 and 'Lithia tablets' became an over-the-counter treatment around 1867. As periodic depression was suspected to be due to uric acid diathesis, Alexander Haig in London tried lithium for depression in 1892. When the drug Iproniazid was used for the treatment of tuberculosis in 1910 it was noted to produce an elevation of mood. This observation led to the search for similar compounds to treat depression. These were called 'psychic energizers' prior to the use of the term antidepressants. Ipro-niazid was noted to have monoamine oxidase-inhibiting properties and further research led to the discovery of other tricyclic and monoamine drugs as mainline treatment for depression. *See melancholy, lithium.*

Derbyshire Neck (Syn. thyroid goiter) Prevalent in Derbyshire during the 19th century.

Dercum Syndrome (Syn. adiposa dolorosa) A subcutaneous connective tissue disorder resulting from deposition of fat, giving rise to painful symptoms in postmenopausal women. Described by Philadelphia physician and neurologist, Francis Xavier Dercum (1856–1931) in 1889.

Dermatitis Herpetiformis Louis Adolphus Duhring (1845–1913), an American dermatologist, introduced the term in 1884 to describe a group of skin eruptions. It was later named Duhring disease after him.

Dermatology [Greek: *derma*, skin + *logos*, discourse] The first systematic treatise on skin diseases was written by Hieronymus Mercurialis (1530–1606) in 1572. The first dermatological text in England, *De Morbis Cutaneis, A Treatise on Diseases of the Skin,* was written by Daniel Turner (1666–1741) of London in 1714. Another famous early monograph was written by Robert Willan (1757–1812) from a Quaker family in Yorkshire, in 1796. His *On Cutaneous Diseases* was unfinished at the time of his death and was completed by Thomas Bateman (1778–1821). The founder of modern French dermatology was Jean-Louis Alibert (1766–1837) who described mycosis fungoides in 1806, keloid in 1810, and Aleppo boil in 1829. In Vienna, Ferdinand von Hebra (1816–1880) founded the histological approach to dermatology with his classification of skin diseases in 1845. One of his pupils, Moritz Kaposi (1837–1902), a Hungarian, completed Hebra's textbook and described several other skin conditions. He gave original descriptions of pigmented sarcoma of the skin (1872), later known as Kaposi sarcoma; diabetic dermatitis (1872); xeroderma pigmentosum (1882); and lymphoderma perniciosa (1885). Sir James Erasmus Wilson (1809–1884), a leading London dermatologist, established dermatology as a specialty in England. He was the first to describe dermatitis exfoliativa in 1890 and he also gave a classification of cutaneous disorders. He wrote *Treatise on Diseases of the Skin* in 1842, a dissector's manual in 1838 and a dermatological atlas in 1847. He delivered a series of lectures at the Royal College of Surgeons from 1871 to 1878 and donated £5000 to the Royal College of Surgeons to create the first chair of dermatology in England. He later offered to leave his fortune to his assistant Malcolm Morris, if he agreed to publish a new edition of *Treatise of Diseases of the Skin* and sustain his opposition to the suggestion that there was a parasitic cause in ringworm disease. Morris declined to take up his offer and Wilson left his fortune to another cause.

Dermatomyositis [Greek: *derma*, skin + *myos*, muscle + *itis*, inflammation] *See connective tissue disease.*

Desault, Peter (1675–1737) French physician, who published a treatise on venereal disease and another work on stones in the bladder and kidneys.

Desault, Pierre Joseph (1744–1795) French surgeon at the Hôtel Dieu, one of the first professors at the École Practique de Chirurgie in Paris. His *Oeuvres Chirurgicales* was published in three volumes in 1803 and remained as a standard work on surgery for 50 years. He was imprisoned during the revolution and later released. He died while he was the attending physician to the Dauphin.

Descartes, René (1596–1650) Philosopher, mathematician and scientist from Touraine, France. He wrote *De Homine* in 1622. His more famous work, *Discourse de la Methode,* in which he introduced the science of reasoning, was published in 1637. He explained the mechanism of the eye in his *Dioptrica* (1637), in which he compared the eye to a camera obscura. He was probably the first to suggest that reflex reactions occurred without any conscious awareness, following his observation of the reaction of batting of the eyelids in response to a threatened blow.

Descemet Membrane The posterior membrane of the cornea, described in 1758 by Jean Descemet (1732–1810), professor of anatomy in Paris.

Desensitization The first attempt to protect from hay fever by injecting an extract of pollen was made by Leonard Noon (1878–1913) in 1911.

Desmarres, Louis Auguste (1810–1882) Ophthalmologist in Paris who designed an operation (Desmarres operation) for pterigium in 1850. The curved lid retractor for examining the eyes is named after him.

Desportes, John Baptiste (1704–1748) Born in Bretagne, France, he was physician to the king. He published *Histoires des Maladies de Saint Domingue* in 1770.

Dessinius, Bernard (1510–1574) Physician in Amsterdam who wrote *De Compositoniae Medicamentorum* in 1555.

Detergents [Latin: *detergere*, to cleanse] According to early Greek physicians, medicines that cleanse viscid humors that adhere to or clog blood vessels.

Deuterium [Greek: *deuteros*, second] Hydrogen-2. Discovered by Harold Clayton Urey (b 1893) of Indiana in 1934. Deuterium oxide, or heavy water, was obtained in the same year by American physical chemist Gilbert Newton Lewis (1875–1946) of Weymouth, Massachusetts.

Deutschlaender Disease March fracture, involving the metatarsal bone (usually the 2nd), named after Hamburg surgeon, Karl Ernest Wilhelm Deutschlaender (1872–1942).

Devaux, John (1649–1729) French surgeon in Paris who published several treatises on surgery. One of his works was on preserving health by instinct.

Deventer, Hendrick van (1651–1724) Dutch obstetrician who introduced pelvimetry. He defined the oblique diameter of the pelvis and described the anteroposterior shortening of the pelvis.

Devergie Disease Pityriasis rubra, described by French physician, Marie Guillaume Devergie (1798–1879).

Deviation of the Eyes Deviation to the side of the lesion of the cerebral hemisphere was described by Swiss physician, Jean Louis Prevost (1833–1927) in 1868.

Devic Optic Neuritis Neuritis of the optic nerve accompanied by acute loss of vision, central scotoma and convulsions. Described by French physician, M.E. Devic (1858–1930) in 1894.

Devonian Period The strata belonging to the Paleozoic era, over 400 million years old, were first found in Devonshire. The term Devonian was coined by Adam Sedgwick (1785–1883), a geologist and a contemporary of Charles Darwin (1809–1882).

Devonshire Colic Lead-colic (Syn. colica pictonum or Poitou colic) Devonshire physician, Sir George Baker (1722–1809), was the first to point out that lead poisoning due to the cider presses used in Devon was the cause of lead-colic in *An Essay Concerning the Causes of the Endemic Colic in Devonshire* in 1767. *The Endemic Colic of Devonshire and Plymouth,* supporting Baker's theory, was published by Alcock in 1769. James Hardy, a physician in Barnstaple, later wrote a treatise on the colic of Somerset and Poitou in which he attributed the disease to absorption of lead used for coating drinking vessels. Conclusive evidence that colica pictonum was caused by poisoning from lead pipes (which were treated with carbonic acid) used for conveying drinking water, was provided by Hisern (1840) and Cuynat in 1843. *See colica pictonum.*

Dewar, Sir James (1843–1923) Scottish chemist from Kincardine. He was educated at Edinburgh University and later studied in Europe under the famous chemist Friedrich August Kekulé (1829–1896) in 1868. Dewar developed the theory of the pyridine ring and also prepared large quantities of liquid oxygen with his invention of the Dewar flask, in which liquefied gases could be conserved for a considerable period without evaporating. He perfected the calorimeter, invented a method of liquefying hydrogen in 1898, and made several other chemical discoveries.

Dextran First introduced as a substitute for plasma by Anders Johan Troed Gronwall and Bjorn Ingleman in 1944.

Dextrose [Latin: *dexter,* right-hand] Grape sugar. *See glucose.*

Dharmavantri An ancient Hindu god and physician, held to be equivalent to Aesculapius.

Di Gugliemo Disease A form of anemia secondary to erythroleukemia, described by Italian hematologist, G. Di Gugliemo (1886–1962).

Diabetes Insipidus [Greek: *diabainein,* to pass through + *insipidus,* tasteless] The first description was given by Peter Johann Frank (1745–1821) of Bavaria who also differentiated it from diabetes in 1794. British neurologist, Byrom Bramwell (1847–1931) from North Shields, described polydipsia associated with intracranial tumors in 1888. The relationship of lesions in the posterior lobe of the pituitary to diabetes insipidus was pointed out by a German physician, Alfred Erich Frank (1887–1957) in 1912. The role of the hypothalamus was demonstrated by Sir John Henry Biggart (1905–1979), who produced the condition in dogs by experimentally inducing lesions in the hypothalamus, in 1939. A description of familial nephrogenic diabetes insip-idus was given by Samuel Jones Gee (1839–1911) in *Contri-bution to the History of Polydipsia* in 1877.

Diabetes [Greek: *dia,* through + *bainein,* to go] The urine of diabetics was noted to attract insects, because of its sugar content, by ancient Brahmins and they named it honey urine. Around AD 100 Aretaeus gave the name 'diabetes' to the wasting disease. In *On the Causes and Symptoms of Chronic Diseases,* he gave a vivid description of the thirst, polyuria and dehydration that occurred. The symptoms of thirst and production of sweet urine were also observed by a Chinese physician, Chen Chuan in AD 643. The sweetness of urine was also observed by Thomas Willis (1621–1675) in 1674. In 1683, Johann Conrad Brunner (1653–1727) demonstrated the occurrence of polyuria and thirst in dogs following the excision of their pancreas. The sweetness of urine was shown to be due to a sugar by Matthew Dobson (1730–1784) of Yorkshire who was a physician at Liverpool Infirmary in 1775, and the sugar in the urine was shown to be glucose by Eugene Chevreul (1786–1889) of Paris in 1815. The relationship between fibrosis of the pancreas and diabetes mellitus was pointed out by John Bright in the mid-19th century. The first systematic experiments which showed that pancreatectomy led to diabetes mellitus were conducted by Joseph von Mering (1849–1908) and Oskar Minkowski (1858–1931) in 1889. Eugene Lindsay Opie (1873–1971) suggested that the antidiabetic substance was present in the islets of Langerhans in 1903. Two years later, John Rennie and Thomas Fraser of Aberdeen obtained this active substance from fish. In 1908 a research chemist in Berlin, Ludwig Zuelzer (1870–1949), treated some comatosed diabetic patients effectively with an extract of pancreas and the long search for an antidiabetic substance ended with the discovery of insulin by Sir Frederick Grant Banting (1841–1941) and Charles Herbert Best (1899–1978) in 1922. *See insulin, glycosuria.*

Diabetic Acidosis Coma in diabetes was described by William Prout (1785–1850). Acetonemia as a cause of diabetic coma was recognized by Adolf Kussmaul (1822–1902) in 1874. He also described air hunger in acidosis, which was later named Kussmaul respiration. Beta-oxybutyric acid in urine was discovered by Ernest Stedelman in 1883 and the presence of this substance in diabetic ketoacidosis was demonstrated by Adolf Magnus-Levy (1865–1955) in 1899.

Diabetic Coma *See diabetic acidosis.*

Diabetic Nephropathy Micronodular lesions in the glomeruli of the kidney, occurring in diabetic nephropathy. Described by Paul Kimmelsteil (1900–1970) and Clifford Wilson (b 1906) of America in 1936.

Diabetic Piqûre Hyperglycemia and glycosuria caused by brain trauma such as puncture of the fourth ventricle or pressure of tumors on the fourth ventricle.

Diabetic Retinopathy The first study of retinitis in cases of glycosuria was done by Henry Dewey Noyes (1832–1900) of America in 1869.

Diachrista Medicines described by Paul of Aegina (625–690) to be applied to fauces, tongue, uvula and the palate in order to clear phlegm.

Diagnosis [Greek: *dia*, through + *gnosis*, knowledge] Judgment of disease from its symptoms and signs.

Diagnostic Cytology *See cytology.*

Diagnostic Enzymology Initiated by Julius Wohlgemuth (1874–1948) who detected an increase of amylase in urine of patients with pancreatitis in 1908. The first enzyme to be used diagnostically was serum phosphatase, which was found to be elevated in bone disease by Herbert Davenport Kay (b 1893) in 1929. The elevation of serum glutamic oxaloacetic transaminase (SGOT) in myocardial infarction was demonstrated by John Samuel LaDue (1911–1980) and Felix Wroblewski (b 1921) in 1954. Elevated lactic dehydrogenase (LDH) in myocardial infarction was observed by Wroblewski in 1956. J.C. Dreyfus showed a rise of creatinine kinase (CPK) in myocardial infarction in 1960. E.S. Vessel and A.G. Bearn used electrophoresis to characterize the serum fractions of LDH in myocardial infarction in 1957. The term 'isoenzymes' to denote molecules with different physical properties but similar enzymatic properties was proposed by C.L. Markert in 1963.

Dialysis [Greek: *dia*, through + *lyein*, to loose] The first experiments on dialysis with different substances were in 1861 by Thomas Graham, a chemist in Glasgow. A dialyser that he constructed was simple and made of parchment tied to the end of a large-mouthed funnel. *See artificial kidney, peritoneal dialysis.*

Diapedesis [Greek: *diapedesis*, leap through] The mechanism of the passage of white blood cells through the walls of the capillaries was observed by William Addison (1802–1881) of Malvern, England in 1843. It was later described by a British physiologist, Augustus Volney Waller (1816–1870) in 1846. A more through study and the part played by blood cells in inflammation was carried out in 1867 by Julius Friedrich Cohnheim (1839–1884), professor of pathology at Breslau.

Diaphoresis [Greek: *dia*, through + *phoresis*, being carried] Perspiration. The role of perspiration in regulating body temperature was demonstrated by Sir Charles Blagdon (1748–1820) in 1775.

Diaphragm [Greek: *dias*, across + *phragma*, wall] Ancient physicians used the term in general to mean any partition, such as the mediastinum, palate or nasal septum. Galen (129–200) used it specifically for the diaphragm. The centrum tendinosum of the diaphragm was described by Jean Baptiste van Helmont (1577–1644), a surgeon at Louvain, in 1644.

Diaphragmatic Hernia *See hiatus hernia.*

Diarrhea [Greek: *dia*, through + *rhoea*, flow] First defined as a condition of abnormal frequency and liquidity of fecal discharges by Hippocrates. *See food poisoning, salmonellosis.*

Diastase *See amylase.*

Diastolic Blood Pressure [Greek: *dia*; through + *stolve*, to send] First measured by Strasburger using Riva-Rocci's apparatus in 1904. Sudden diminution of pulse pressure while the cuff was deflated was taken as equivalent to diastolic pressure. Russian physician, Nikolai Sergievich Korotkov (1874–1920), observed the five phases of sound heard over the artery while deflating the cuff and he took the pressure during the fourth phase, when the sound became muffled, as the value equivalent to diastolic pressure.

Diathermy [Greek: *dia*, through + *therme*, heat] In 1891 Nikola Tesla (1856–1943), an American electrical engineer, observed that heat was produced in live tissue when current was passed through it, but no clinical significance was attached to it at the time. In 1898 Jacques Arsene d'Arsonval (1851–1940) demonstrated that the contraction of muscles brought about by their intrinsic electrical activity could be reversed by applying an external current, suggesting a clinical use for electricity. Temperature rise in tissues during the application of current was documented by Karl Franz Nagelschmidt (1875–1952), who gave the present name 'diathermy' to the procedure in 1908. Diathermy for therapeutic purposes was introduced into England by Lewis Jones in the 1930s. Shortwave diathermy was introduced by Erloin Schlieshake in 1931.

Diathesis [Greek: *dia*, through + *titheni*, to place] The term denotes natural or congenital pre-disposition to a specific disease.

DIC *See disseminated intravascular coagulation.*

Dick Test Skin test to detect susceptibility to scarlet fever. Devised by George Frederick Dick and his wife Gladys Rowena Dick (1881–1963) of Johns Hopkins School of Medicine in 1924. The couple also showed hemolytic streptococci as the cause of scarlet fever in 1923.

Dick, Sir William Bart (1703–1785) A physician from

Edinburgh who cultured rhubarb, for which he received a medal from the London Society of Arts.

Dickens, Charles (1812–1870) Author immortalized through his literary works. He had a complicated medical history. In his late teens he suffered from trigeminal neuralgia and colicky abdominal pains attributed to renal stones. In 1867 he was wrongly diagnosed as having gout and in 1840 he developed an anal fissure which was operated upon without anesthesia. He was also diagnosed as having a disturbance of heart rhythm by Sir Thomas Watson from Middlesex Hospital in 1866. In 1869 he began to have transient ischemic attacks. The cause of his death was diagnosed as brain hemorrhage.

Dickenson, Edmund (1624–1701) A physician from Berkshire who wrote on philosophy and nature.

Dickey, John Stuart Anatomist from Belfast who moved to Ontario as a professor at the Western Medical College in 1912. He described the fibers of the scalenus anterior which passed through the cervical pleura, in 1911.

Dickson, Thomas (d 1784) A physician from Dumfries who graduated from Leiden (1746) and was a physician to the London Hospital (1759) where he served for 25 years.

Dicoumarol or warfarin The story of warfarin began with a cattle disease around 1920 in the midwestern United States and Canada. This disease killed hundreds of thousands of cattle and all the affected animals were noted to bleed excessively during their illness. A veterinary pathologist, Frank Schofield of Ontario, observed that all the diseased cattle had eaten moldy or spoilt sweet clover. He also recorded the symptoms of other animals which bled to death after having eaten the same plant. His observation remained unheeded until 1940 when the toxic substance, dicoumarol, was isolated from sweet clover by a biochemist Karl Paul Link of Wisconsin. This substance was later called warfarin and was used clinically for anticoagulation.

Dicrotic Pulse [Greek: *dis*, double + *crotos*, stroke] Paul of Aegina (625–690) compared the double pulse to a goat leap or dorcadissans. The term 'dorcadissans' is derived from the dorcas gazelle, which jumps in the air and takes another swifter spring before it reaches the ground. After diastole, if the pulse recurred before systole, he called it 'dicrotos' to denote that it beat twice.

Dictionary of Medicine The first printed dictionary on drugs, *Synonyma medicinae,* written by Simon de Cordo (1270–1330), was published in 1473. A dictionary of medicine compiled from Greek and Arab sources by Giacomo

Jacob de Dondi (1298–1359), *Aggregator de Medicinis Simplicibus,* appeared around the same time. Matthaus Sylvaticus (d 1342) of Mantua produced a dictionary of Greek and Arab medical terms around 1320. A Greek dictionary of ancient medical texts, including that of Hippocrates was published by Anuce Foes (1528–1595) in 1588. The first dictionary of medicine in Britain was published by Stephen Blanchard (1625–1703) in 1684. The largest early medical dictionary in three volumes was published by Robert James (1705–1776) in 1745. Panckoucke's *Dictionaries des Science Medicales* in 60 volumes was published from 1812 to 1822 in France. *A Dictionary of Practical Medicine,* compiled from 1834 to 1858, was produced by James Copeland of Orkney. Samuel Cooper (1780–1848), professor of surgery at University College London, published *A Dictionary of Surgery* in 1809 which went through seven editions during his lifetime and was translated later into German, French and Italian. One of the most quoted dictionaries of the late 19th century was that of Richard Quain (1860–1898) published in 1882. Contributors to this dictionary included Sir Thomas Clifford Allbutt, William Broadbent, Charles Brown-Sequard, Lauder Brunton, William Ewart, William Cayley, Thomas B. Curling, Langdon Down, William R. Gowers, Jonathan Hutchison, Florence Nightingale, Manson Patrick, James Paget and other important personalities in medicine. *The American Illustrated Medical Dictionary* was published by W.A. Newman Dorland in 1900 and had run to 16 editions by 1932. The first edition of the *Illustrated Dictionary of Eponymic Syndromes* was published by Stanley Jablonsky of the National Library of Medicine in 1969. A *Dictionary of Medical Eponyms* was published by B.G. Firkin and J.A. Whitworth in 1987.

Diday, Charles Paul Joseph (1812–1894) He dedicated his life to the study of syphilis and made significant contributions with Jean Alfred Fournier (1832–1914) at the famous venereal clinic in St Louis.

Dieffenbach, Johan Friedrich (1792–1847) Professor of surgery in Berlin who succeeded A.K. von Grafe (1787–1840). He devised a new method of treatment for strabismus by severing the tendons of the eye muscles. He also pioneered surgical treatment for vesicovaginal fistula.

Diemerbrock, Isbrand van (1609–1674) Dutch physician who wrote an important treatise on plague in 1646.

Dietetics Almost all the ancient physicians including Hippocrates (460–377 BC), Galen (129–200), Celsus (25 BC–AD 50), Paul of Aegina (625–690), Acturius, Averrhoes and Oribasius wrote extensively on dietetics. Galen's work ranks as the best and most complete treatise on the subject.

Roman philosopher, Cicero (106–143 BC), forbade two full meals per day and Hippocrates denounced the eating of a full dinner. Haly Abbas (930–994) specified a certain number of meals, Galen concentrated on selection of the type of food and Athenaeus of Naucratis in Egypt around 300 BC equated a good physician with a good cook. One of the early popular works in Europe was written by Isaac Judaeus (855–955) and published as *De Dieta* in 1487. The English physician Fredrick William Pavy (1829–1911), whose main interest was carbohydrate metabolism, published an important book *Treatise on Food and Dietetics* in 1874. An outstanding book in the early 20th century, *Science of Nutrition*, was published by German physiologist, Graham Lusk (1866–1932) in 1909.

Dietl, Joseph (1804–1878) A physician in Cracow who described the acute symptoms (Dietl crisis) due to partial obstruction caused by kinking of the ureter in a floating kidney.

Dieudonne Medium Agar containing defibrinated ox blood treated with caustic soda, for growing *Vibrio cholerae*. Devised by Munich bacteriologist, Adolf Dieudonné (1864–1945).

Dieulafoy Disease Gastric ulceration occurring as a complication of pneumonia. Described by G. Dieulafoy (1839–1911), a French professor of medicine at the Hôtel Dieu.

Diffraction *See electron diffraction, X-ray diffraction.*

Diffuse Interstitial Pulmonary Fibrosis A syndrome leading to dyspnea and clubbing, first reported by a Louis Hamman (1877–1946) and Arnold Rice Rich (1893–1968) of Johns Hopkins Hospital in 1944. A description in England was given by A.G. Heppleston in 1951. A review of all previous publications with additional cases was published by E.H. Rubin and R. Lubliner in 1957.

Diffusion The Scottish chemist and founder of colloid chemistry, Thomas Graham (1805–1869), started his studies on the subject around 1831. He postulated in 1846 that diffusion of gases and liquids occurred in the body through minute pores. The process of diffusion of fluids across a membrane was shown to be due to osmosis by Graham at the Bakerian Lecture he gave in 1854. *See osmosis.*

DiGeorge Syndrome Characterized by congenital absence of the thymus and parathyroid glands, leading to recurrent infection. Described by an American pediatrician, Angelo M. DiGeorge (b 1921) and co-workers in 1967.

Digestion [Latin: *digestio*, digestion] Erasistratus (340–257 BC), the founder of the Alexandrain school of anatomy, was the first to refute Aristotle's view that digestion is a process similar to cooking and proposed that food, once in the stomach was torn to pieces and pulped by peristaltic motions of the stomach wall. Gastric digestion was studied in 1752 in birds by the French naturalist, Antoine René de Reaumur (1683–1757), who was also the first to obtain gastric juice in a pure state. One of the earliest studies on the physiology was performed by Abbe Lazaro Spallanzani (1729–1799), an Italian physician, in 1780. He showed that digestion differed from putrefaction and the fermentation process of wine and demonstrated that hydrochloric acid was produced by the stomach. The presence of free hydrochloric acid in the stomach was shown by an English physician, William Prout (1785–1850) in 1823. William Beaumont (1785–1853), an American army surgeon, carried out scientific human studies on the role of gastric secretion in 1822. He did a series of analyses on gastric juice obtained from one of his patients who had a traumatic gastric fistula caused by a gunshot wound. His *Physiology of Digestion*, published in 1845, is regarded as one of the first on physiology in America. Digestive enzymes were further studied by Theodor Schwann (1810–1882) and Willy Kuhn (1837–1900). A stomach tube for withdrawing gastric secretions was designed by M. Rehfuss (b 1887) in 1914. It contained a metal capsule that sometimes damaged the gastric mucosa, and in 1921 John Alfred Ryle (1889–1950) improved this by covering the entire tip with rubber and providing perforations above the bulb. Further studies using a breakfast test meal were performed by Ryle in the same year. The appearance of amino acids in the blood after a protein meal was shown in 1906 by Otto Knut Olof Folin (1867–1934), a Swedish-born professor of biochemistry at Harvard University.

Digitalis [Latin: *digitabulum*, thimble] The foxglove, *Digitalis purpurea*, has been known for centuries as a folk remedy in Britain. The Germans call it 'fingerhut' and the Bavarian physician and botanist Leonhart Fuchs (1501–1566) Latinized the German name and called it digitalis in his *Plantarum Omnium Nomenclaturae* published in 1541. He described the medicinal use of the plant in dropsy and other conditions in 1542. J. Gerard (1545–1612) in 1597 advocated the foxglove as treatment for viscous humors affecting the chest and it was introduced into the London Pharmacopoeia in 1722, mainly through the recommendation of the British herbalist, William Salmon (d 1700). William Withering (1741–1799), a physician from Shropshire, learnt of its value in dropsy from one of his patients and started using it. By 1779 he had established a place for it in treatment of dropsy and *An Account of the Foxglove* was published in 1785. Animal experiments were performed by C.C. Schiemann in 1786. The drug was also used as an antipyretic for a short period following the recommendation of Traube and Hankel around 1869. Sir James Mackenzie (1853–1925) introduced it as treatment for atrial fibrillation around 1900.

Digitoxin Isolated from digitalis by Johann Ernest Oswald Schmieddeberg (1838–1921) in 1875. *See digitalis.*

Digoxin Isolated from the *Digitalis lanata* by Sydney Smith in 1930. *See digitalis.*

Dihydrotachysterol (AT10) Obtained by ultraviolet irradiation of ergosterol and introduced as treatment for rickets by Friedrich Holtz in 1933. It was recommended as a treatment for hypopathyroidism by Fuller Albright in 1941.

Dimercaprol (2-3-Dimercaptopropanol) British Anti Lewisite (BAL) was discovered as an antidote to the war gas lewisite during World War ll by Sir Rudolph Albert Peters and co-workers. It was later found to be effective as a chelating agent in treatment of poisoning by heavy metals. Its most frequent use in the late 19th century was for treating the toxic side-effects of arsenotherapy. *See lewisite.*

Dimitry, Theodore John (1879–1945) An ophthalmologist in New Orleans who described a method of evisceration of the eyeball followed by insertion of an artificial ball before the sclera and conjunctiva were stitched over it.

Dimmer, Friedrich (1855–1926) Viennese ophthalmologist who described a special operation for treating ectropion. He also described a form of unilateral keratitis (Dimmer keratitis) in farm workers.

Dimsdale, Thomas (1712–1800) English physician from Essex who wrote a treatise on smallpox inoculation, *Thought and General and Partial Inoculation* in 1776. He traveled to Russia to inoculate Catherine the Great in 1768 and on his return became Member of Parliament for Hertford and gave up his medical practice.

Dinitrophenol Shown to have a marked influence on metabolism by P. Cazeneuve and R. Lepine in 1885. It was introduced as a treatment for obesity by Mehrtens and Tainter in 1933. It became popular and was sold under various trade names such as Aldinol, Dinitrolac, Nitromet, Slendite and Slim. Nearly 100,000 people used it in America for a few years before its toxic side-effects were revealed.

Dinosaur The first fossil of a dinosaur was discovered by a surgeon and paleontologist from Sussex, Gideon Algernon Mantell (1790–1852), in 1822. He named it the *Iguanadon,* owing to the resemblance of its fossil teeth to the iguana. The term 'dinosaur' was coined by Richard Owen (1804–1892) in 1842 to denote extinct reptiles that lived 175 million years ago. One of the first fossil dinosaur eggs was discovered in Mongolia by Roy Chapman Andrews (1884–1960), Director of the American Museum of National History in New York.

Diocles of Carystius Greek physician around 400 BC who practiced just after Hippocrates. He wrote 16 books on medicine and anatomy and was ranked next to Hippocrates by Pliny (AD 28–79).

Diones, Peter (d 1718) A surgeon in Paris who wrote several works on anatomy and surgery.

Dioporon A medicinal preparation recommended by the African physician, Aurelianus Caelius, in the 4th century.

Dioptrics [Greek: *dia*, through + *opsis*, sight] The study of refracted and transmitted light in relation to the lens and the eye. Johannes Kepler (1571–1630) published his *Dioptrice* in 1611 and the law of refraction was discovered by Snellius or Williebrord Snell (1591–1626), a professor of mathematics at Leiden in 1624. René Descartes (1596–1650) was one of the first to explain the mechanism of the eye in his *Dioptrica* in which he compared the eye to a camera obscura in 1637.

Dioscorides, Pedanius Greek physician from Anarzaba, Turkey who lived around AD 100, during the reign of Nero. He was originally a soldier who later studied medicinal herbs and described over 600 plants in his five books on materia medica. He divided fungi into edible and poisonous groups and specified the use of plants for specific diseases. He was the first to use the term *materia medica.* A translation of his manuscripts was produced by a Jewish court physician at Cordova, Hasdai Ben Sharput, around AD 950. Another Greek text was published by Aldo Manuzio (1449–1515) in 1499.

Diphenylhydrantoin Epinutin or hydrantoin was introduced as treatment for epilepsy by American neurologists, Hiram Houston Merrit (1902–1939) of New York and Tracy Jackson Putnam (b 1894) of Boston in 1938. *See antiepileptics.*

Diphtheria [Greek: *diphthera*, leather] A specific description was given by Areatus in the first century. The first tracheotomy in diphtheria was performed by a Scottish physician George Martine (1702–1743) in 1730. A modern description was given by a Quaker physician, John Fothergill (1712–1780) of Yorkshire in his *Account of the Putrid Sore Throat* published in 1748. It is also mentioned by French physician, Marteau de Grandvilliers in his *Gangrenous Affections of the Throat* published in 1757. It was known as croup until Pierre Fidèle Bretonneau (1778–1862) of Tours, France renamed it in 1820. Diphtheria was shown to be due to the toxin and not the bacterium by a French bacteriologist, Pierre Roux (1853–1933) of Charente and Alexander Emile Jean Yersin (1863–1943) in 1889. *See Corynebacterium diphtheriae.*

Diphtheria Antitoxin Produced from the blood of infected horses by Emil Adolf von Behring (1854–1917) in 1891.

Diplegia [Greek: *di*, twice + *plege*, stroke] *See spastic diplegia.*

Diplococcus [Greek: *diploos*, double + *kokkos*, berry] The occurrence of cocci in lobar pneumonia was noted by Carl Joseph Eberth (1835–1925) in 1880, and their presence in pairs was noted by C. Talmon in 1882. The bacterium was isolated by a German physician, Albert Fraenkel (1848–1916) of Berlin in 1886 and was named *Diplococcus pneumoniae*, before its name was changed to *Streptococcus pneumoniae*, commonly called pneumococcus. Another diplococcus with Gram-negative properties was isolated from six patients with acute cerebrospinal meningitis by Anton Weichselbaum (1845–1920) of Vienna in 1887. He named it *Diplococcus intracellularis meningitides*. Weichselbaum and von Lingles-hiem of Germany independently established this organism as a cause of meningitis in 1905.

Diploid The zygotic number (2n) of chromosomes as opposed to the haploid (n) or gametic number of chromosomes. Described by Eduard Adolf Strasburger (1844–1912) in 1905.

Diploma [Greek: *diploos*, double + *lomos*, letter] Originally a charter from the prince. It was so named because it was presented folded or doubled.

Dippel, John Conrad (1672–1734) Born in Frankenstein, Germany and took his medical degree at Leiden in 1771. He claimed to have discovered the philosopher's stone, but despite this he made a major contribution to medicine with his discovery of Prussian blue.

Dipsomania [Greek: *dipso*, thirst + *mania*, madness] A craving for alcohol. *See addiction, alcohol.*

Disabled Persons (Employment) Act Intended to help overcome physical handicap in employment and other related matters, passed in Britain in 1944.

Disc Prolapse [Greek: *diskos*, disc] *See intervertebral disc prolapse.*

Disease [French: *des*, from + *aise*, ease] The skeletons of extinct animals have shown evidence of disease. Paleopathology [Greek: *palaeo*, old + *pathos*, suffering + *logos*, discourse], the study of ancient diseases through examination of mummies, fossils, osseous remains and ancient writings, contributed to the knowledge of the antiquity of disease. Coronary atherosclerosis, schistosomiasis, bone tumors, tuberculous abscesses and several other conditions have been recognized as several thousand years old. Tuberculosis of the spine, arteriosclerosis and gall stones in Egyptian mummies from 3000 BC have been shown by Sir Mark Armand Ruffer (1859–1917), a pioneer in the field. The study of papyri and clay tablets has also given insight into the nature of diseases that prevailed during ancient times.

Disinfection *See antiseptics.*

Dislocation of the Hip Joint [Latin: *dis*, apart + *locare*, to place] Henry Jacob Bigelow (1818–1890) of Massachusetts General Hospital gave the first anatomical description of the hip joint in relation to its dislocation in 1869. He also proposed the flexion method for the reduction of dislocation. *See congenital dislocation of hip joint.*

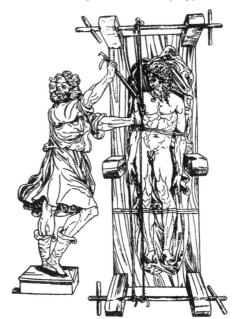

Treatment to reduce dislocation of shoulder joints. From Vidus Vidius, *Chirurgia e Graeco in Latinum Conversa* (1544)

Dislocation of the Shoulder Joint It was dealt with in detail by Hippocrates around 400 BC who stated 'I know of only one kind of dislocation, the one in which the humerus bone is to be found in the axilla region. I have never seen the shoulder dislocating outward and I disagree with those that mistakenly consider the humerus head dislocating forward, only because the patient, due to muscle weakness, has practically no deltoid fibers to cover the head substantially'. A method of reducing the shoulder joint which has been dislocated for several months was described in 1762 by Charles White (1728–1813), a Manchester surgeon and a founder of the Manchester Infirmary and Manchester Lying-in Hospital. A method of reduction of subluxation of the shoulder joint was described in 1870 by Emil Theodor Kocher (1841–1917), Swiss professor of surgery at Bern. Surgical treatment was first performed by Arthur Sidney Blundell Bankart (1879–1951), a surgeon from Exeter, in 1923. Another operation was devised in 1943 by an American orthopedic surgeon, Paul. B. Magnuson (1884–1968) of North Western Medical College.

Disodium Cromoglycate The plant *Ammi visnaga* has been used for centuries in treatment of asthma and the crude extract obtained later from its seeds was known as khellin. Sodium cromoglycate, the active ingredient of khellin, was obtained in 1967. Its trade name is Intal. It is now widely used for asthma. Khellin was introduced as a vasodilator for treatment in angina by G.V. Anrep in 1949, but it was found ineffective.

Dispensary [Latin: *dis*, apart + *pensare*, to weigh] The concept of providing medicine and care for the needy on an outpatient basis in England was proposed by a physician, John Coakley Lettsom (1744–1815). The first dispensary in England, the Royal General Dispensary, for giving medical advice and supplying medicine to the poor, was established at Aldersgate, London in 1770. About 40 dispensaries were set up in England by 1800.

Dispersion of Light [Latin: *dis*, apart + *spargene*, to scatter] Dispersion of light by a prism was demonstrated by Isaac Newton (1642–1723). He made a small hole in his darkened room to let in a ray of light and placed a prism in its path. He was surprised by the production of intense colors. James Clerk Maxwell (1831–1879) was the first to suggest a theoretical explanation in 1869. The same explanation was given independently by a German physicist, Sellmeyer in 1872. Kundt law was proposed in 1871. Further laws were proposed by Lorenz (1829–1891) of Copenhagen and H.A. Lorentz (1853–1928) of Leiden. *See absorption spectra.*

Displacement A defense mechanism in which a patient displaces his love or hate for an inappropriate person or object towards an acceptable one. First described by Sigmund Freud in 1900.

Dissecting Aneurysm A description of the dissecting aneurysm of the aorta was given by Frank Nicholls (1699–1778), physician to George II, who described its pathogenesis. The morbid anatomy was given by J. Shekelton of Dublin in 1822. P.M. Latham (1789–1875), a physician at Bartholomew's Hospital presented a case diagnosed by J. Swain, before death, in 1855. Thomas Bevill Peacock (1812–1882) of St Thomas' Hospital presented two papers and discussed its pathogenesis in 1843 and 1863.

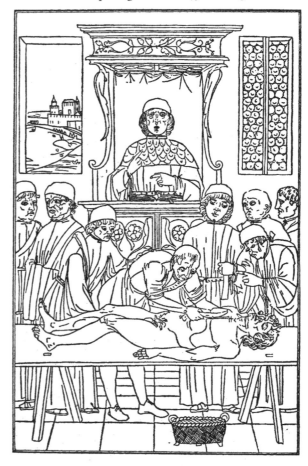

Dissection. First known picture of anatomical dissection of a human. William Sterling, *Some Apostles of Physiology*. (1902), Waterlow & Sons, London

Dissection [Latin: *dissecare*, to cut open] Anatomical knowledge of animals was obtained during ancient times through observations on sacrificed animals. The Chinese physician Pien Ch'iao is supposed to have performed the earliest human dissections a few centuries before the establishment of the Ptolemaic school of anatomy at Alexandria. Herophilus and Erasistratus recorded human dissections around 250 BC. Human dissections were banned in the Roman Empire around 150 BC and from this period up to the time of Andreas Vesalius (1515–1564) knowledge of anatomy remained patchy and inaccurate. Animal dissections were promoted during the time of Galen (129–200), as ecclesiastic and secular authorities did not approve the dissection of human corpses. The same situation continued in Islamic medicine from AD 750 –1200. Many of the observations of Galen on animals were applied to humans and went unchallenged for over 1000 years. The study and development of comparative anatomy through animal dissections contributed significantly to our present knowledge of physiology, embryology and evolution. Vesalius collected human bones from burial grounds and studied them in detail. When he started attending the University of Paris to study medicine he was dissatisfied with the lack of dissection of human bodies. He then studied anatomy on his own by dissecting cadavers which he recovered from executions and burial grounds and began to observe that many of Galen's statements were incorrect. Davis Edwardes (1502–1542) was the first to perform a recorded human dissection in England in 1531, and he published the first anatomy book in English. Dissections were commenced on a regular basis in England in the early 17th century. One of the privileges of the Royal Society was the right to claim the bodies of executed persons and a committee was formed in 1664 to undertake dissections on every execution day.

Disseminated Intravascular Coagulation (DIC) In 1834 H.M.D. de Blainville of Paris demonstrated massive intravascular clotting in experimental animals following an intravenous injection of brain tissue. This condition of defibrination was previously observed in 1772 by William Hewson (1739–1774) in obstetric patients who, after parturition, had temporary afibrinogenemia. English physiologist, Leonard Charles Woolbridge (1857–1889), in 1886 showed that by injecting tissue thromboplastin intravenously into animals their blood became incoagulable. The consumption of clotting factors – factor V (E.W. Page, 1951) and factor VIII (G.D. Penick, 1958) – with a concomitant reduction in platelets (R.C. Hartmann, 1951) and fibrinogen levels (C.A. Mills, 1921) in DIC was demonstrated by several workers. A reduction in fibrinogen levels remained the striking feature which occurred in patients with shock, septicemia and other states. An increase in fibrinogen degradation products in the blood was first observed by H. Stormorken in 1957. J.W. Cromwell and W.L. Read in 1955 were the first to demonstrate that heparinization could prevent minute clots.

Disseminated Lupus Erythematosus (DLE) *See systemic lupus erythematosius.*

Disseminated Sclerosis *See multiple sclerosis.*

Dissociation [Latin: *dis*, apart + *sociare*, to unite] A theory related to electrolytes in solution was proposed by the Dutch chemist J.H. Van't Hoff (1852–1911) in 1877 and was perfected by his pupil S.A. Arrhenius (1859–1927) in 1883. The theory of complete dissociation was proposed 20 years later by the American physical chemist A.A. Noyes. Other important workers in the early 20th century include Gilbert Newton Lewis (1875–1946) of Weymouth, Massachusetts and Danish physical chemist, Niels Janniksen Bjerrum (1879–1958).

Distillation The distillation of wines and spirits was introduced into Europe by the Arabs around AD 1150. Distillation in England began in the 15th century and an Act of Parliament to prevent unlicensed persons practicing it in England was passed in 1846. *See alcohol, wine.*

Distoma (Syn. fluke, fasciola) Derived from the Greek for 'double mouth'. The term 'fluke' for the parasite was used by Anders Adolf Retzius (1796–1860) and Fasciola was given to the genus by Carl Linnaeus (1707–1778). Several different flukes belonging to the genus have been described.

Disulfiram In 1949, when the compound tetraethylthiuram disulfide was tried as worm treatment, those who took the compound became very ill after consuming alcohol. This observation led to the development of disulfiram for treatment of chronic alcoholism. It was produced on a commercial scale by Rothstein and Binovic in 1954.

Dittel, Leopold Ritter (1815–1898) Professor of surgery in Vienna who, in 1857, described the superficial fascia of the neck, through which the external jugular vein penetrated behind the sternomastoid muscle. He also specialized in urology and described the enucleation of the enlarged lateral lobes of the prostate through an external incision in 1860.

Diuretics [Greek: *dia*, through + *ouron*, urine] A vinous preparation used as a diuretic in the treatment of dropsy was mentioned by Pliny in the 1st century. The seed of the ash tree (*Fraxinus*) taken with wine was used as a diuretic for dropsy in the 15th and 16th centuries. *Digitalis* leaves, dilute alcohol, caffeine and calomel were some of the diuretics used in the 18th and 19th centuries. The earliest synthetic diuretics were organic mercurials (mercupurin, mercuhydrin) which were introduced around 1920 and remained in use for nearly two decades. Acetozolamide became popular following publication of T.H. Maren's paper on it in 1952. Chlorothiazide was introduced by K.H. Beyer and colleagues in 1958. Spiranolactone, with antagonistic properties to aldosterone, was described by C.M. Kagawa and co-workers in 1959. Loop diuretics (furosemide, ethacrynic acid) were introduced in the early 1960s. Bumetanide was introduced independently by K. Duchin and D.L. Davis in 1974.

Diurnal Blood Pressure William H. Howell (1860–1945) first observed, in 1897, that blood pressure fell significantly during sleep.

Divers' Disease *See caisson disease.*

Diverticulosis [Latin: *dis*, apart + *vertere*, to turn] Recognition of colonic diverticular disease became common only after the introduction of the barium enema as a diagnostic test in radiology in 1914. A classic paper, *Sacculi of the Large Intestine with special reference to the Blood Vessels of the Bowel Wall*, was written by H. Drummond (1916), who discussed the mechanism of diverticulum formation.

Dix, Dorothea Lynde (1802–1887) A tireless worker who dedicated her life to the improvement of the care of the insane, both in America and in Britain. She was born in Hampden, Maine and grew up in Boston. Her lobbying led to the building of asylums for the insane who, up to that time, were inappropriately placed in almshouses or jails. Of the many institutions she founded, only Dixmont Hospital, Pennsylvania bears her name.

Dixon, Walter Ernest (1871–1931) Regius professor of physick at Cambridge who demonstrated that the alkaloid muscarine had a characteristic pattern of action that was antagonized by atropine.

DNA Fingerprinting *See genetic fingerprinting.*

DNA Polymerase Discovered by American biochemist, Arthur Kornberg (b 1918) of Brooklyn, New York. He also synthesized biologically active DNA in 1956 for which he received the Nobel Prize in 1959.

DNA *See deoxyribonucleic acid.*

Dobell Solution Antiseptic consisting of borax, sodium bicarbonate and phenol. Introduced by a London physician, Horace Benge Dobell (1828–1917).

Dobell, Clifford (1886–1949) Protozoologist who published: *Amoeba Living in Man* (1919) and *Intestinal Protozoa of Man* (1921). *See protozoa.*

Dobereiner Lamp A lamp that illuminated by the burning of hydrogen produced by the action of sulfuric acid on zinc in the presence of a platinum sponge. Invented by a German professor at Jena, Johann Wolfgang Dobereiner (1780–1849) in 1810.

Dobereiner, Johann Wolfgang (1780–1849) German professor of chemistry in Jena from 1810 to 1849. He developed the relationship of atomic weights between the elements calcium, barium and strontium. This later formed the basis for Dimitri Ivanovich Mendeleff's periodic table. *See Dobereiner lamp.*

Dobie, William Murray (1828–1915) Born in Liverpool, he was a physician at the Chester Royal Infirmary. He gave several original descriptions of the histological appearance of muscle fibers.

Dobson, Matthew (1713–1784) *See glycosuria.*

Dobzhansky, Theodosius (1900–1975) A geneticist from the Ukraine who joined Thomas Hunt Morgan (1866–1945) in America to do research on *Drosophila*, the fruit fly. He provided the experimental link between Charles Darwin's evolutionary theory and Gregor Mendel's laws of genetics. His *Genetics and the Origin of Species* was published in 1930.

Dochez, Alphonse Raymond (1882–1964) New York bacteriologist who differentiated the four different types of pneumococci on the basis of precipitin tests. He also prepared an antitoxin against scarlet fever by immunizing horses against it.

Doctor The title was first conferred by the church. It was given to Atanasius, Augustine, Ambrose and several others. The first degree of doctor given to a medical person was conferred in Salerno in the 11th century. It was conferred in England in 1207. Thomas Aquinas (1225–1274) and Roger Bacon (1214–1294) received their titles later. The first regular medical degree of Bachelor of Medicine in America was given to ten men who graduated from the College of Philadelphia in 1768. King's College, New York awarded medical degrees to two men in 1769.

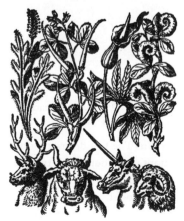

Doctrine of Signatures as depicted by Giambattista della Porta in the 16th century

Doctrine of Signatures Based on the belief that every

natural substance which possessed any medicinal value indicates, by an obvious and well marked character, the disease for which it is the remedy, or the object for which it should be employed. The lungwort was employed for complaints of the chest, since its leaves resembled the surface of the lungs. Similarly, dry yellow turmeric was used as a treatment for jaundice because of its color. Eyebright or *Euphrasia*, became popular as an eye application as its flowers resembled the pupils of the eye.

Dodart, Denys (1634–1701) A physician to the king in Paris. He published *Medicina Statica Gallica*.

Dodds, Sir Edward Charles (1899–1973) Born in Liverpool and moved to Maida Vale in London in 1911. He entered Middlesex Hospital Medical School in 1926 and later became one of the youngest professors in London at the age of 25 years. He held the chair of biochemistry at the Middlesex Hospital for nearly 40 years and discovered a highly active synthetic estrogenic compound in 1938 which he named 'stilbestrol'. *See estrogen*.

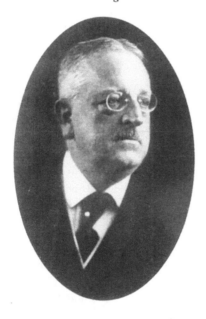

Albert Döderlein (1860–1941). Reproduced by permission of Georg Thieme, Leipzig and Prof. G. Döderlein, Jena

Döderlein Bacillus The first description of this bacillus in vaginal secretions in relation to puerperal fever was given by Albert Siegmund Gustav Döderlein (1860–1941), a German gynecologist, in 1892. The bacillus was later isolated from the feces of breastfed infants by Ernst Moro in 1900.

Dodson, Henry (d 1753) One of the first surgeons at the London Hospital.

Dog First domesticated in Mesopotamia around 10,000 BC. Excavations of predynastic graves of around 4000 BC in Egypt have shown the practice of burial of dogs with humans. The ancient Egyptian god Anubis had a dog's head and the Hindu god Dharma assumed a dog's form to guide the Padava brothers to paradise in the Sanskrit epic, *Maha-Bharata*. The god Odin of the Scandinavians rode through the air as a 'wild huntsman' followed by dogs. Cuchulin [Gaelic: *cu*, dog], the Gaelic hero, killed the dog of Hades and took its place until another dog was found and trained. In Scotland and Ireland the ancient sculptured 'dog stones' were venerated.

Dogiel, Alexander Stanislavovic (1852–1922) A neurologist and professor of histology at St Petersburg. He described nerve endings of the bulb type in 1903.

Dogliotti, Achile Mario (1897–1966) Physician from Milan. He introduced epidural anesthesia successfully into obstetric practice in 1933. He also performed the first surgical section of the pain–temperature pathway, leminiscus lateralis, for control of pain in 1938.

Dogma *See dogmatism*.

Dogmatism The dogmatist sect was founded by Thessaulus and Draco, the sons of Hippocrates, on the Greek island of Cos. Their concept, that investigations should cease as Hippocrates had already stated all the essentials, was propagated by the sect which thrived during the Alexandrian period.

Doisy, Edward Adelbert (1893–1986) A biochemist from Illinois who used fluid from the ovarian follicles of a hog's ovaries in 1924 to demonstrate the induction of pubertas praecox in immature albino rats. The first steroid hormone, estrone, was extracted in a pure state from the urine obtained during pregnancy, independently by Doisy and Adolf Friedrich Johan Butenandt (b 1903) in 1929. This was first named 'Theelin' by Doisy, who also obtained estradiol from ovarian tissue in 1935. He also contributed to diagnostic chemistry by devising a method for estimation of inorganic phosphates in the blood, while working with Boston biochemist, Richard D. Bell in 1920. His publications include *Sex Hormones* (1936) and *Sex and the Internal Secretions* (1939).

Dolbeau, Henri Ferdinand (1830–1877) Surgeon in Paris who described an operation (Dolbeau operation) for lithotomy in which the stone is crushed in the bladder through a median incision in the urethra.

Dolichostenomelia [Greek: *dolichos*, long + *stenos*, narrow] The long, slender limb features of Marfan syndrome were described as 'dolichostenomelia' by Bernard Jean Antonin Marfan (1858–1942) in 1896. *See Marfan syndrome.*

Dolitrone Introduced as an intravenous anesthetic by C.R. Thomson, J.K. Smith and H.W. Werner in 1954 and clinical trials were conducted by James Lundy in 1954. Further trials in 1956 failed to confirm it as an effective anesthetic agent.

Dolley, Read Sarah Adamson (1829–1909) One of the first few women to graduate in medicine in America. She obtained her MD from Central Medical College, New York in 1851 and served as an intern for a year at the Blockley Almshouse Hospital in Philadelphia.

Dollinger, Johann Ignas Josef (1770–1841) Born in Bavaria, he was professor of physiology in Munich in 1824. He described the thickening of the Descemet membrane in 1817.

Domagk, Gerhard (1895– 1964) German biochemist, born in Lagow, Poland and graduated in medicine from Kiel in 1921. He discovered the antibiotic, Protonsil, containing sulfanilide in 1935. He refused the Nobel Prize on the instructions of the German Nazi government in 1939. He also introduced thiosemicarbazone for tuberculosis in 1946. *See antibiotics, sulfonamides.*

Dominance The relationship of two allelomorphs in which single gene heterozygotes resemble one of the two homozygous parents (said to carry the dominant allelomorph) rather than the other (said to carry the recessive allelomorph), on an arbitrary scale distinguishing between the two phenotypes. Described by Gregor Mendel (1822–1884) in 1865.

Dominique, Jean Etienne The first lecturer in psychiatry in Paris who studied states of dementia in senile individuals in 1838.

Donald, Archibald (1860–1937) *See Manchester operation.*

Donaldson, Robert (1877–1933) Pathologist in London who devised an iodide stain (Donaldson stain) for identifying amebic cysts in stools.

Donath–Landsteiner Test A test in which serum produces hemolysis after incubation with red cells at 4°C and rewarming at 37°C. Named after German physician, Julius Donath (1870–1950) and Karl Landsteiner. *See paroxysmal hemoglobinuria.*

Donde, James or Dondus (d 1350) Physician in Padua who was known as The Aggregator because of his skill in preparing various medicines. He wrote *Promptuarium Medicinae* in 1481. He was also a skilled mechanic and constructed a clock which, as well as time, denoted various festivals and the course of the moon and sun.

Donders, Franciscus Cornelis (1818–1889) Dutch ophthalmologist and physiologist at Utrecht. He introduced prismatic and cylindrical lenses in spectacles. His *The Anomalies of Refraction and Accommodation* (1864) formed the basis for fitting eyeglasses for myopia, strabismus, hypermetropia and other conditions.

Dondi, Jacope de (1290–1359) Physician and horologist in Padua. He graduated in medicine in Padua and became a teacher there. He constructed the astronomical clock for the Prince of Padua in 1344 and in 1348 began construction of a more elaborate clock, which took 18 years to complete. His son, Giovanni de Dondi (1318–1389), was also a physician in Padua.

Donnan Equilibrium The theory relating to the distribution of different ions in solutions across a membrane. Proposed by Frederick George Donnan (1870–1956), an Irish chemist in 1911.

Donnan, Frederick George (1870–1956) Irish chemist, born in Colombo, Sri Lanka who studied science at Queen's College, Belfast. He worked under Friedrich Wilhelm Ostwald (1853–1932) in Leipzig, J.H. van't Hoff (1852–1911) in Berlin and William Ramsay (1852–1916) in London, before he was made the first Brunner professor of physical chemistry at Liverpool in 1904. He obtained an international reputation as a colloid chemist and proposed the theory of equilibrium across membranes (Donnan equilibrium) in 1911.

Donne, Alfred (1801–1878) Anatomist in Montpellier who pioneered the microscopic study of body fluids and secretions in 1837. In 1836 he described *Trichomonas vaginalis.* He observed platelets in the blood in 1842 but mistook them for fat globules.

Donnolo or Sabbatai ben Abraham (AD 913–970) Jewish physician from Otranto who practiced in the south of Italy. He wrote a work on materia medica and another on astrology in 946, in which he described the doctrine of macrocosm and microcosm. His materia medica or *Antidotarium* is the oldest known medical work in Hebrew and contains descriptions of over 120 remedies.

Donohue Syndrome A familial condition consisting of mental retardation, sexual precocity, hypertelorism and other features. Described by Canadian pathologist, W.L. Donohue (b 1906) in 1948.

Donovan Solution Containing iodides of arsenic and

mercury for application to cutaneous and venereal sores. Prepared and marketed by Irish pharmacist, Edward Donovan (1789–1837).

Donovan, Charles (1863–1951) Scottish physician and microbiologist who demonstrated the characteristic staining bodies in the spleen of patients with kala azar at autopsy in 1903. He was also the first to identify these in the splenic blood of live patients. The bodies were later recognized as protozoal parasites which were the same as those found in oriental sore. They were named Leishman–Donovan bodies.

Doppler Phenomenon The pitch of a whistle from a rapidly moving body like a locomotive was observed to be higher when the body was approaching the listener by an Austrian mathematician, Christian Doppler (1803–1853), from Salzburg. He proposed his 'Doppler principle' in a paper while he was professor of mathematics at the State Technical Academy in Prague in 1842. It was later used in radiology and other branches of science. Ultrasonic Doppler was used to study cardiac functions by S. Satomura in 1957.

Dorsey, John Syng (1783–1818) A nephew of the eminent American surgeon, Philip Syng Physick (1768–1837). He graduated from Pennsylvania in 1802 and studied surgery under Alexis Boyer (1757–1833) at Paris and John Hunter (1728–1793) in London. He published the first surgical work in America *The Elements of Surgery* in 1813.

Dosimetry [Greek: *doose*, dose + *metrein*, to measure] A system of therapeutics dealing with accurate administration of alkaloids in the form of granules of definite strength, developed in the early 19th century.

Dott, Norman McOmish (1897–1973) Scottish neurosurgeon in Edinburgh who performed the first planned operation for an intracranial aneurysm in 1932. He devised an adjustable mouth gag (Dott gag) with a tongue piece for use in intratracheal anesthesia.

Douche [French: *doucher*, to pour] A method of application of water through a jet as a form of treatment has been practiced from ancient times. Aetius of Amida recommended it for ardent fever and ophthalmic infections around AD 600. Vaginal douches with vinegar, disinfectants and water have been used as methods of contraception.

Douglas Bag Bag for collecting expired air for respiratory function studies. Devised by an English respiratory physiologist, Claude Gordon Douglas (1882–1963) in 1911.

Douglas, James (1675–1742) Physician from Scotland who later settled in London to practice midwifery. He published *A Description of the Peritoneum* (1730), *A Description of the Muscles* (1707), *A History of Lateral Operation for the Stone* (1733) and several other treatises. The rectouterine peritoneal pouch, the pouch of Douglas, is described in the work published in 1730.

Douglas, Stewart Rankin (1871–1936) London pathologist who prepared a slow-growing culture medium for the diphtheria bacillus. In 1903 he also demonstrated, with Almroth Edward Wright (1861–1947), a thermolabile substance in serum (opsonin) which acted on bacteria during phagocytosis.

Doulton, Sir Henry (1820–1897) Founder of an English pottery factory at Lambeth. He was born at Vauxhall. He is less known for his most important invention of impervious drainage pipes which replaced the unhygienic brick gulleys and brought about a revolution in sanitation.

Dover Powder A preparation of opium and ipecacuanha prepared by the doctor and buccaneer Thomas Dover (1662–1742) from Barton-on-Heath. He cleverly used ipecacuanha in proportions adequate to induce vomiting to prevent the abuse of the remedy by those who became addicted. His remedy was popular in England up to the end of the 19th century, when it was gradually replaced by aspirin. It continued to be used in Europe for a longer period. *See Dover, Thomas.*

Dover, Thomas (1662–1742) English physician and seafarer from Barton-on-Heath. During one of his own private charter voyages in 1701 he rescued Alexander Selkirk. Selkirk's experience inspired Defoe to write *Robinson Crusoe*. In 1701 Dover introduced his 'Dover powder', a preparation of opium and other ingredients such as ipecacuanha and saltpeter. Dover wrote *The Ancient Physician's Legacy to his Country* in 1733. *See Dover powder.*

Dowden Operation An operative method for femoral hernia. Devised by Edinburgh surgeon, John Wheeler Dowden (1866–1936) in 1918.

Dowman, Hugh (1740–1819) A physician and poet from Devonshire whose publications were mainly poetry.

Downes, Sir Arthur Henry (1851–1938) *See actinotherapy.*

Downes, John (1627–1694) English physician who obtained his MD from Leiden with his inaugural thesis, *Disputatio Medica Inauguralis de Affectione Hypochondrica* in 1660. He obtained an MD from Oxford and was physician to Christ's Hospital.

Down, John Langdon Haydon (1828–1896) Born in Cornwall in England, he studied pharmacy, first with his father and later at the pharmaceutical society of London. He assisted Michael Faraday in his experiments on gases. After a long illness, he returned to London as a student at the London Hospital and obtained his degree in 1858. He then became medical superintendent to the Earlswood Asylum for Idiots, and in 1859, assistant physician to the London Hospital. He published a blueprint for treatment and education of the mentally retarded and *Observations of ethnic classification of idiots* in 1866, in which he used the term 'idiocy' to denote a malady which is essentially different from insanity in both nature and treatment. He described mongolism in 1887 and this later became known as Down syndrome. *See Down syndrome.*

Down Syndrome John Langdon Haydon Down (1828–1896) of Teddington, England in 1866 proposed an ethnic classification for idiots according to their facial and body features. One of the groups, which he called Mongolian, later gave rise to the term Mongol for this group. The association between cardiac abnormalities and Down syndrome was noted by Edward Archibald Garrod (1857–1936) in 1894. Increased maternal age as a cause of mongolism or Down syndrome was shown by Lionel Sharples Penrose (1898–1972), a British geneticist, in 1938. It was the first human chromosomal abnormality (trisomy 21) to be detected – in 1959, by the French geneticist, Jerome Lejeune. The first prenatal diagnosis through amniocentesis was made in 1968.

Downy Cells Atypical lymphocytes seen in infectious mononucleosis. Described by American hematologist, Hal Downy (1877–1959) of Minneapolis in 1936.

Doyen, Eugene Louis (1859–1916) French surgeon, born at Rheims and educated in Paris. He was one of the first to use cinematography in surgical teaching in 1898. He also designed several surgical instruments that were named after him.

Doyere, Louis (1811–1863) Professor of physiology and applied zoology in France. He was the first to observe the termination of motor nerves in the muscles of insects in 1837.

Doyle, Sir Arthur Conan (1859–1930) A student of Joseph Bell (1837–1911), a surgeon in Edinburgh. Doyle, after qualifying in medicine, practiced at Southsea. He tried unsuccessfully to enter Parliament. He was later inspired by the investigative and inquiring approach of Bell to medical cases and started writing the adventures of Sherlock Holmes, which were serialized in the *Strand Magazine* from 1891 to 1893. His first work *A Study in Scarlet* was published in 1887.

Doyne, Robert Walter (1857–1916) British ophthalmologist, born in Wexford and studied medicine at Bristol Medical School and St George's Hospital. He was the first reader in ophthalmology at the University of Oxford and consultant ophthalmic surgeon to the Radcliffe Infirmary.

Draco Son of Hippocrates. He founded the dogmatist school with his brother Thessaulius. He was royal physician to Queen Roxana, the wife of Alexander the Great.

Dracunculus medinensis [Latin: *dracunculus*, little dragon] (Syn. guinea worm) Based on the narration given by Agatharchides of Knidos, a tutor of Ptolemy (150 BC), Plutarch stated that 'the people by the Red Sea suffered from a severe disease in which small snakes came out of the skin and gnawed the legs and arms and when touched drew back again into the skin and caused patients insufferable pain'. Galen (129–200) stated that he has never seen the worm but knew others who had. He mistakenly believed that the cause was a disease of the veins similar to varices. Avicenna (980–1037) and Paul of Aegina (AD 625–690) recommended attaching a lead weight to the worm so that it could gradually be drawn from the skin without being broken or having pieces of it left behind. It was first scientifically described by Hieronymus George Welsh Velscius in 1674. The mode of transmission was established by Colin Chisholm (1755–1825) in 1794. A detailed description was given by Henry Charlton Bastian (1837–1915) in 1863 and the full life cycle was elucidated by Aleksiei Pavlovich Fedchenko (1844–1873) in 1869.

Dragendorf, Georg Johann Noel (1836–1898) German professor of pharmacy at Dorpat who specialized in toxicology and published his work on the subject in 1868.

Drager, Glen A. (1917–1967) Neurologist at the National Institute of Neurological Diseases and Blindness, Bethesda, Maryland. He described Shy–Drager syndrome, a form of orthostatic hypotension, with G. Milton Shy (1919–1967) in 1960.

Dragstedt Operation Complete vagotomy and gastrojejunostomy as treatment for duodenal ulcer. Devised by American surgeon, Lester Reynold Dragstedt (1893–1975) from Montana.

Drake, Daniel (1785–1852) Professor of medicine at the Jefferson Medical College, he was a great reformer of medical education in America. He wrote *The Diseases of the Interior Valley Fever of North America* and *Practical Essays on Medical Education and Medical Profession in the United States* in 1832. He was instrumental in founding the Medical College of Ohio in 1821.

Drake, James (1667–1707) A physician and political writer, born in Cambridge. He obtained his medical degree there in 1696. He was a strong critic of the government and questioned its conduct in his newspaper *Mercurius Politicus,* for which he was prosecuted. He was a prolific writer and published *A New System of Anatomy* in 1707 and other works on politics and drama.

Dran, Henry Francis (d 1770) Surgeon from Paris who wrote *Observations on Surgery, On Gun Shot Wounds* and other important surgical works.

Draper, Henry (1837–1882) A medical graduate from New York University who became professor of physiology at the same institution. He later devoted his time to astronomy and discovered the presence of oxygen in the sun. He also published *A Textbook of Chemistry* and *On the Construction of a silvered-glass Telescope.*

Draper, John Williams (1811–1882) A physiologist and chemist from St Helens near Liverpool. He emigrated to America in 1839 and became professor of chemistry at New York University in 1850. He published *On the Forces that Produce Organisation of Plants* (1844) and *Physiology* in 1856.

Drasch, Otto (1849–1911) Professor of histology at Graz, Austria. He described the cuneiform cells in the mucous membrane of the trachea in 1886.

Dreams The Greek philosopher, Plato was probably the first to initiate the dream theory, in which he suggested the appearance of unexpressed desires in sleep. The earliest English book, *The moste pleasante arte of the interpretacion of dreames* was published by Thomas Hill of London in 1576. He recognized that they were determined by fears and wishes. J. Moreau de Tours (1804–1884) was the first to point out that the dreams offered a clue to understanding of disturbed mental functions. He also explained subjective psychological phenomena involved in them. Wilhelm Griesinger (1817–1878) also has pointed out the relationship of mental symptoms to dreams. Sigmund Freud used dreams for psychoanalysis and published *The Interpretation of Dreams* in 1900.

Drechsel Test A test for bile using phosphoric acid and cane sugar as reagents. Devised by Swiss chemist, Edmund Drechsel (1843–1897).

Dressler Syndrome (Syn. cardiotomy syndrome, post-pericardiotomy syndrome) Pericarditis, pleurisy and fever following pericardiotomy, myocardial infarction or trauma to the heart. Described by a Polish-born American cardiologist, William Dressler (1890–1969) in 1955. He was

educated in Vienna and practiced there until 1938. He emigrated to America and became the chief of the cardiac clinic at Maimonides Hospital, Brooklyn, New York.

Dreyer Test A modified form of the Widal test for diagnosis of typhoid and paratyphoid, now obsolete. Introduced by English pathologist in Oxford, Georges Dreyer (1873–1934).

Driesch, Hans Adolf Edouard (1867–1941) German physiologist and philosopher, son of a wealthy merchant in Kreuznach. He studied zoology at Freiburg and Jena and demonstrated the first cell division in a fertilized ovum of the sea-urchin in 1891.

Drift Age Another term for the early or lower Paleolithic period. It derives its name from the fact that stone implements belonging to it were found in the gravels of river-drift type.

Drinker, Phillip (1894–1972) American public health engineer who invented the iron lung in 1929 for treatment of respiratory failure in poliomyelitis.

Dropsy Paul of Aegina (625–690) described dropsy thus: 'when the liver is greatly congealed, sometimes primarily, as when it has been inflamed, indurated or otherwise affected, or when from the sympathy of the other parts, the process of sanguification ceases and the affection is called dropsy'. He was probably referring to edema or dropsy due to hepatic causes. Hippocrates (460–377 BC) described the causes and treatment due to disease of the spleen and liver and approved paracentesis thoracis and paracentesis abdominis as treatments. Ox dung, a popular remedy since ancient times, was mentioned as treatment for dropsy by Paul of Aegina and Galen (129–200). A vinous preparation as a diuretic in the treatment was mentioned by Pliny (AD 28–79). Alexander of Tralles, in AD 600, pointed out other forms of dropsy arising from the heart and kidneys. Gulielmus de Salicito (1201–1277), an Italian surgeon, noticed the association of dropsy or swelling of the body with hardened kidneys in 1275. The correlation between dropsy and albuminuria was observed by William Charles in 1811 and John Blackall (1771–1860) in 1813. Richard Bright (1789–1858) in 1827 identified the characteristic inflammation of the kidneys in cases of albuminuria and dropsy. He was also the first to differentiate between cardiac dropsy and renal dropsy.

Drowning One of the first scientific treatises on drowning, *Proposal for the Recovery of People Apparently Drowned,* was presented to the Royal Society of London by John Hunter (1728–1793) in 1776. He stressed the fact that death occurred as a result of the inability of the lungs to ventilate.

Druce, George Claridge (1850–1932) English pharmacist and botanist from Potter's Bar. He published treatises on the flora of Oxfordshire (1886), Buckinghamshire (1930) and Berkshire (1890).

Drug Interaction *See chemotherapy.*

Drug Levels *See chemotherapy.*

Drug Resistance *See bacterial resistance.*

Druid Priests amongst ancient Germans, Gauls and Britons who possessed a high degree of scientific knowledge. They are supposed to have invented water clocks. The origin of the word was pointed out by Pliny (AD 28–79) as the Greek term *drus,* which means oak. According to him, they venerated mistletoe, especially when it was found rooting in the oak tree. Cicero mentioned that they embraced the philosophy of Pythagoras (530–586 BC), including that of transmigration of souls. Druids in England opposed Caesar's invasion of Britain in 55 BC and were later persecuted by the Roman governor, Paulinius.

Drummond, Henry (1851–1897) Born in Stirling, he was a scientific explorer and teacher of spiritual philosophy. He published his literary and scientific work *Tropical Africa* in 1890. His Lowell Lectures at Boston in 1893 were published as *The Ascent of Man.*

Drummond, Sir David (1852–1932) English surgeon at Durham who devised an operation for ascites in which the surface of the parietal peritoneum was roughened to facilitate adhesions.

Drummond, Sir Jack Cecil (1891–1952) Pioneer in the field of nutritional research in England. He suggested the term 'vitamin' in 1920. He published a history of the English diet in 1939.

Drunken Driving An offense in England by the Road Traffic Act of 1972. The legal limit of alcohol was set at 80mg/100 ml. The earliest form of the breathalyzer was devised by Lallamand, Perrin and Duroy of Paris in 1860.

Drunkenness Inebriety. The earliest charge of drunkenness, around 1300 BC, is found in an Egyptian papyrus. Another early account was given by Pliny the Elder around AD 50. A classical work on the subject, *The Deipnosophists* was written by Athenaeus of Greece in AD 200. The Stoic philosopher Lucius Annaeus Seneca, around AD 50, gave a remarkable description of the effects of chronic alcoholism. *See alcohol, addiction, temperance.*

Dryopteris Felix mas The male fern, known as an abortifacient and wormicide. The powder of the root of the female fern was taken with honey by the ancients as treatment for long worms, and the root was taken to cure rupture (hernia) and ulcers. It was recommended as treatment for rickets in the 17th century. In 1775 Louis XVI paid 18,000 francs to the widow of the Swiss surgeon, Nuffer, to obtain a secret remedy against the tapeworm, and its principle content was Felix mas. Frederick the Great similarly obtained another remedy, after granting an annuity and the title of Councilor to a Swiss apothecary called Matthieu. His remedy later proved to be the same. The root of the male fern has remained as a folk medicine for inducing abortion. One of the earliest botanical works on ferns was done by Wilhelm Hofmeister (1824–1877), professor of botany in Berlin, in 1850.

Drysdale Corpuscles Transparent microscopic cells seen in the fluid of ovarian cysts. First described by American gynecologist, Thomas Murray Drysdale (1831–1904).

Duane Test The use of a candle flame and a prism to measure the degree of ocular heterophoria. Devised by Alexander Duane (1858–1926), an oculist in New York.

Dubin–Johnson Syndrome A form of chronic intermittent jaundice with pigmented liver. Described in a series of 12 patients by an American professor of pathology in Pennsylvania, I.N. Dubin and a Washington pathologist, S.B. Johnson, in 1954.

Dubini, Angelo (1813–1902) *See Ancylostoma duodenale.*

Dubois Disease The absence of a thymus, or sometimes multiple abscesses in it, in cases of congenital syphilis. Described by Paul Dubois (1795–1871) of Paris in 1850.

DuBois, Eugene Floyd (1882–1959) New York physiologist who studied basal metabolism and devised a table for calories per square meter of body surface for different ages. His *Basal Metabolism in Health and Disease* was published in 1924.

Dubois, Eugene Marie François Thomas (1858–1940) Dutch physician and paleontologist from Eijsden. He graduated from Leiden and was stationed in Java as a surgeon to the Dutch East Indian Army. During his stay in 1893 he discovered the teeth, calvarium and femur of a primitive man and this was acclaimed as the missing link in evolution. The primitive man to whom the skeleton belonged was later named *Pithecanthropus erectus.*

Dubois, Jacques (1478–1555) Professor of anatomy and surgery in Paris who was an ardent follower of Galen's system of medicine.

Dubois, Paul Charles (1848–1918) Professor of neuropathology in Bern who strongly advocated psychotherapy on the basis of rational acceptance of moral standards and principles. His method was a revival of Phillipe Pinel's (1745–1825) moral treatment.

Dubois-Reymond, Emil Heinrich (1818–1896) German professor of physiology in Berlin, who worked under Johannes Muller (1801–1858) and graduated in medicine in 1843. He demonstrated the existence of resting current in nerves in 1845. He also suggested the role of chemicals in the transmission of nerve impulses in 1877.

Dubos, René Jules (1901–1982) French bacteriologist who emigrated to America and joined Rockefeller University in 1927. He isolated one of the first antibacterial substances from *Bacillus brevis* in 1939 and named it tyrothricin. It became the first commercially produced antibiotic but was not found to be very effective. However, his work provided the impetus for the search for other antibiotics.

Dubost, Charles (b 1914) *See abdominal aneurysm.*

Duchenne Disease *See tabes dorsalis.*

Duchenne Muscular Dystrophy (Syn. pseudohypertrophic muscular dystrophy) An X-linked recessive form of progressive muscular dystrophy occurring in early childhood, mostly in boys. Described by Guillaume Benjamin Amand Duchenne (1806–1875) of Paris in 1868. The gene marker was discovered by Kay Davies and Robert Williamson in 1983 and the protein dystrophin, which was completely absent in it, was discovered by Louis M. Kunkel and Eric P. Hoffmann and co-workers in 1986. Their findings made it possible for it to be diagnosed during the early stages.

Duchenne, Guillaume Benjamin Amand (1806–1875) A neurologist from Boulogne who studied under, René Laënnec (1781–1826), Guillaume Dupuytren (1777–1835) and François Magendie (1783–1855) in Paris. He was one of the earliest workers on the electrophysiology of muscles and published *De Electerisation Locale* in 1825. Some of his other contributions include the differentiation between various forms of lead palsy and original descriptions of progressive spinal muscular atrophy, spinal pathology of anterior poliomyelitis, tabes dorsalis and pseudohypertrophic muscular dystrophy.

Duckworth Phenomenon The occurrence of respiratory arrest before cardiac arrest in certain cases of brain infection. First described by London physician, Sir Dyce Duckworth (1840–1928).

Ducrey Disease (Syn. chancroid, soft chancre) A sexually transmitted infection characterized by ulceration of the male and female external genitalia. Described by Italian professor of dermatology, Augusto Ducrey (1860–1940) in 1889. The organism responsible was later named *Haemophilus ducreyi* in his honor. A special culture medium for it was prepared by Boston physician, Lincoln Davis (b 1872), in 1903.

Ductless Glands The ductless nature of the thymus and thyroid glands was first recognized by Albrecht von Haller (1708–1777) in 1766. The concept of internal secretion – that every organ, tissue and cell secretes substances into blood that influence other parts of the body – was proposed by Theophile de Bordeu (1722–1776) of Paris in 1775. The term 'internal secretion' was first used by Claude Bernard (1813–1878) in 1855. Evidence of a humoral substance that produced an effect on a site or organ remote from its origin was presented by Arnold Adolph Berthold (1803–1861) in 1849. He transplanted a testis to a rooster that had previously had its testis removed and demonstrated the normal resumption of male sexual characteristics. In 1884 Charles Louis Xavier Arnozan (1859–1928) and Louis Vallard (1850–1935) tied the pancreatic duct and produced atrophy of the pancreas without the development of diabetes. The first direct scientific demonstration of internal secretion was provided by William Bayliss (1860–1924) and Ernest Starling (1866–1927). In 1902 they obtained a substance from the intestinal mucous membrane that had a remote action on the pancreas and named it 'secretin'. Starling coined the term 'hormone' to denote similar substances secreted by ductless glands in his Croonian Lecture to the Royal College of Physicians in 1905.

Ductus Arteriosus First described by Galen (129–200) who also suggested its spontaneous postnatal closure. His description was improved by Gabriele Falloppio (1523–1562) in 1561 and it was given its present name by Julius Caesar Arantius (1530–1589) around 1550. It was also described by the French anatomist, Botallus (1519–1587) in 1565. A detailed account was given by Giovanni Battista Carcano Leone (1536–1606) in 1574 and the mechanism of functional closure of the ductus arteriosus was proposed by Rudolph Virchow (1821–1902) in 1852. *See patent ductus arteriosus.*

Dudgeon, Leonard Stanley (1876–1938) *See cervical smear.*

Dudley, Benjamin Winslow (1785–1870) American surgeon from Kentucky who used trepanning for epilepsy in 1833.

Dudley Operation A method of treating a retroverted

uterus by suturing it to the round ligament through an abdominal opening. Devised by Emilius Clark Dudley (1850–1928), an obstetrician in Chicago, in 1894.

Dugas Test A test for dislocated shoulder in which, with the hand on the affected side placed on the opposite shoulder, the elbow cannot touch the chest. Devised by Louis Alexander Dugas (1806–1884), an American professor of surgery at the Medical College of Georgia.

Duhring Disease *See Duhring, Louis Adolphus.*

Duhring, Louis Adolphus (1849–1929) American dermatologist who wrote the first textbook of dermatology in his country. He also introduced the term dermatitis herpetiformis to describe a group of skin eruptions (Duhring disease) in 1884.

Dührssen, Alfred (1862–1933) German gynecologist, born in Heide and studied medicine in Königsberg. He introduced a vaginal operation for myomectomy and other gynecological conditions.

Duke, Clement (1845–1925) London physician who studied medicine at St Thomas' Hospital and was medical officer to Rugby School from 1871 to 1908. He differentiated between rubella and roseola infantum on the basis of etiology.

Duke, William Waddell (1883–1945) A pathologist from Kansas City who introduced a method of estimating bleeding time by making a needle puncture on the lobe of the ear and removing the blood every 30 seconds with blotting paper until it stopped. He estimated the normal bleeding time to be two to five minutes.

Duke-Elder, William Stewart (1898–1978) English ophthalmic surgeon at St George's Hospital, London in the 1920s. He became ophthalmic surgeon to the Queen. He was one of the founders of the Institute of Ophthalmology at London University in 1948 and was also its first director. He published *System of Ophthalmology* in 19 volumes from 1958 to 1976.

Dukes Classification Classification for rectal carcinoma proposed by a pathologist at St Mark's Hospital, London, Cuthbert Dukes (b 1890) in 1932.

Dulong and Petit Law The product of specific heat and atomic weight is constant for all elements. Proposed in 1818 by a French physician Alexis Therese Petit (1791–1820) and a chemist, Pierre Louis Dulong (1785–1838) of Paris.

Dumb Chironomia [Greek: *chir*, hand + *nomos*, custom] Giovanni Bonifacio wrote on a sign language for the deaf and dumb in 1616. John Bulwer was the first English person

to write a treatise on chironomia in 1644. John Wallis (1616–1703), one of the founders of the Royal Society, was a pioneer in teaching deaf-mutes through gestures and writing. Juan Pablo Bonet (1579–1633) devised and taught a new system of communication for the deaf and dumb in 1620. The first British school for the deaf and dumb was established in Edinburgh by Thomas Braidwood (1715–1806). One of the first asylums in London was established by John Townsend (1757–1826), a clergyman, at Kingston in Surrey.

Dumontpallier Test A test for detection of bile pigments using iodine as a reagent. Devised by French physician, Alphonso Dumontpallier (1826–1898).

Dumping Syndrome A symptom complex occurring after gastroenterostomy. First described by Sir Arthur Fredrick Hertz (Hurst) of Guy's Hospital in 1922.

Dunant, Jean Henry (1828–1910) *See Red Cross Society.*

Dunbar, William Phillips (1863–1922) American physician in Hamburg who studied the role of pollen in hay fever and introduced a serum against pollen in 1905.

Duncan, Andrew, Junior (1773–1832) Born in Edinburgh, he was a physician to the Royal Dispensary, founded by his father. He edited the *Medical and Surgical Journal* and also published *Edinburgh New Dispensatory* in 1803.

Duncan, Andrew (1744–1828) A physician from St Andrews, Scotland who traveled to India as a surgeon in 1768. He returned as a lecturer in Edinburgh and founded the Royal Dispensary at Richmond Street in 1776. He was President of the Royal College of Physicians and first physician to the King in Scotland in 1821. He wrote *Annals of Medical Science* and other works and was instrumental in establishing the lunatic asylum at Morningside in 1792.

Duncan, Daniel (1649–1735) A physician from Languedoc in France who wrote *La Chyme Naturalle* and other works on chemistry and anatomy. He settled in London towards the last stages of his career.

Duncan, James Matthews (1826–1890) Born in Edinburgh, he was an obstetrician and an assistant to Sir James Simpson. He moved to London in 1877 and became a leading obstetrician there. He described the peritoneal folds of the uterus (Duncan folds) in 1854.

Duncan, T. James (1884–1958) The first person to be appointed as a reader in medical mycology at London University.

Dundas, David English physician in the late 17th century who did pioneer work on rheumatic diseases of the heart and published *An account of Peculiar Diseases of the Heart,* in 1808. The 'peculiar disease' described by him was later recognized to be rheumatic heart disease.

Dung Excreta of various animals were used as medicines in ancient times. Some of these remedies include dog dung in milk for gout, and crocodile dung and rabbit dung for cure of consumption. In ancient Egypt, around 1800 BC, pessaries made of the dung of crocodiles and other animals were used to prevent pregnancy. Quintus Serenus Salmonicus used mouse dung as a poultice in AD 200, and the dung of screech owls was used for melancholy. In 300 BC Serapion of Alexandria, an opponent of Hippocratic medicine, amongst his unusual remedies also promoted the use of crocodile dung. As a result, this became the most costly excreta to obtain.

Dunham Solution Contained peptone and sodium chloride, for use in the indole test. Prepared by Edward Kellogg Dunham (1860–1922), a pathologist in New York.

Dunhill, Sir Thomas Peel (1876–1957) London surgeon and pioneer in thyroid surgery. He described the operative removal of intrathoracic tumors through a sternal approach in 1922. The Dunhill forceps used in thyroid surgery are named after him.

Dunn, Naughton (1884–1939) He trained under Robert Jones (1858–1933) at Liverpool, before becoming an orthopedic surgeon at the Royal Orthopedic Hospital at Birmingham. He described an operation for paralytic foot in which the peroneal and tibialis posterior tendons were transferred to the achilles tendon, in 1919.

Duodenal Ulcer The first description was given by George Erhard Hamberger (1697–1755) in 1746 and an account of a perforating ulcer was given by Jacopo Penada (1748–1828) in 1793. A comprehensive study was undertaken by Julius Krauss of Berlin in 1865. A modern approach to the pathogenesis and causation was made by Berkeley George Andrew Moynihan (1865–1936) of Leeds in 1910. Duodenal ulcers in infants within the first few months of life were reported by A.M. Thomas in 1924 and by J.A.L. Louden in 1925. Postmortem findings in these infants were later published in *The Lancet*. Pyloric resection was performed by Brooklyn surgeon, William Leon (b 1888) in 1938, and gastrojejunostomy became one of the commonest forms of treatment in the early 1900s. Section of supradiaphragmaic vagus nerves as treatment was performed by a Chicago surgeon, Lester Reynold Dragstedt (1893–1975) and Frederick Mitchum Owens (b 1913) in 1943. *Campylobacter pylori* was shown to be the cause of gastritis and probably duodenal ulcers by an Australian, Barry J. Marshall,

in 1984. This bacterium was renamed *Helicobacter pylori*.

Duodenostomy [Latin: *duodenarius*, twelve; Greek: *stoma*, mouth + *tome*, to cut] First performed by Carl Johan August Langenbuch (1864–1901) in 1879.

Duodenum [Latin: *duodenarius*, twelve] The first part of the intestine immediately following the stomach was described as being 12 fingers in length and breadth by the Alexandrian anatomist, Herophilus, in 344 BC. Geradus of Cremona (1147–1187), who translated Avicenna's work, was the first to give the name duodenum to it. The Greeks referred to it as *ekphysis* (growing out) in the belief that it was a diverticulum from the stomach.

Duplay Bursitis Involving the subacromial or subdeltoid bursa. Described by French surgeon, Simon Duplay (1836–1924) in 1872.

Dupré Disease A form of psychoneurosis in which the patient makes a conscious effort to control his symptoms. Described by French physician, Ernest Dupré (1862–1921).

Dupuytren Contracture The first description of the condition was given in 1818 by Felix Platter (1536–1614), a physician in Basel. A more detailed account, describing the fibrous thickening of the palmar fascia leading to contractures of the hand, was given by Guillaume Dupuytren (1777–1835) of Paris in 1831. He also devised an operation for it in 1832. It was described earlier by Sir Astley Paston Cooper (1768–1841).

Dupuytren Fracture An original description of the fracture of the lower end of the fibula was given by Guillaume Dupuytren (1777–1835) of Paris in 1819.

Dupuytren, Guillaume (1777–1835) French surgeon who became chief surgeon at the Hôtel Dieu in 1815. He was the first to excise the lower jaw in 1812, and the first to treat wry neck by subcutaneous section of the sternomastoid, in 1822. He gave original descriptions of fracture of the lower end of the fibula in 1819, congenital dislocation of the hip in 1826, and contraction due to palmar aponeurosis in 1831.

Dura Mater [Latin: *durus*, hard + *mater*, mother] The terms dura mater and pia mater, referring to the outer layers of the brain, were coined by Bishop Stephen of Antioch in his translation of the medical works of Haly Abbas (930–994). An Italian professor of anatomy in Rome, Antonio Pacchioni (1665–1726) described the arachnoid granulations of the dura mater in 1692 and proposed that it exerted a contractile force on the brain. The term 'pachymeninges' [Greek: *pachys*, thick + *meninx*, membrane] also refers to the dura mater.

Durand, Paul (1895–1961) French physician in Tunis who isolated a virus called D virus during his research on yellow fever in 1940.

Dürer, Albrecht (1471–1528) One of the earliest illustrative anatomists in Europe. His *Vier Bucher von menschlicher proportion* were published in Nuremberg in 1528. His other treatise, *De Symmetria partium in rectis formis humanorum corporum,* was published posthumously in 1532.

Duret, Henry (1849–1921) French neurosurgeon in Paris who described the arteries supplying the nuclei of the cranial nerves and the subarachnoid canals.

Duret, Lewis (1527–1586) Physician in the 16th century who was royal physician to Henry III.

Durham, Edward Herbert (1866–1945) *See agglutination.*

Durham Tube A jointed tracheotomy tube devised by English surgeon, Arthur Edward Durham (1834–1895).

Duroziez Disease Congenital mitral stenosis. Described by French physician, Louis Paul Duroziez (1826–1897), in 1877. As a student, he won the Corvisart Prize for his work on digitalis. He graduated in medicine from Paris in 1853 and was appointed chief of clinic with Jean Martin Charcot (1825–1893) in 1856.

Duroziez Sign Two separate murmurs heard over the femoral or brachial artery during the diastolic and systolic phases of the heart in aortic insufficiency. Described by French physician, Louis Paul Duroziez (1826–1897), in 1861. The mechanism of production of these murmurs was explained by Herman Ludwig Blumgart (b 1895) in 1933.

Duroziez, Paul Louis (1826–1897) French physician born in Paris and graduated from there in medicine in 1853. He became chief of the clinic at the Charité in 1856 and joined the army as a surgeon during the Franco-Prussian War in 1870. His *Traite des Maladies du Coeur* was published in 1891. *See Duroziez sign.*

Dutta Gemunu or Dutha Gamani A king of Ceylon who died in 161 BC. He is credited with having built 18 hospitals to which he formally appointed physicians.

Dutton Disease The first case of human trypanosomiasis was described by pathologist, Joseph Everett Dutton (1876–1905) of Liverpool, in 1902. He named the parasite *Trypanosoma gambiense* and the disease was later named after him.

Dutton Fever *Borrelia duttoni,* a spirochete from a tick causing African relapsing fever (Dutton fever), was identified by Joseph Everett Dutton (1876–1905) of the Liverpool

School of Tropical Medicine and John Lancelot Todd (1876–1949) in 1905. *See relapsing fever.*

Duval, Matthias Marie (1844–1907) Professor of anatomy and professor at the National School of Fine Arts in Paris. He published a work on artistic anatomy and other works. He described the gyrus dentatus and its communication with the rhinencephalon in 1881.

Duverney, Guichard Joseph (1648–1730) Professor of anatomy in Paris. He did research on the inner structure of the ear and wrote the first treatise in otology in 1683. He gave one of the first descriptions of subarachnoid hemorrhage confined to the spina theca, following autopsy of a magistrate in 1682. This patient, who died suddenly, was found to have a large clot in the theca.

Dwarf The ancient Greek poet, Philetas from the island of Cos, was a dwarf and he is supposed to have carried weights in his pockets to prevent him from being blown away. There are records of several dwarfs of less than 60 cm high in ancient Greek and Roman times. Skeletons of the Neolithic period belonging to adult pygmies, who were less than 160 cm tall, were found at a burial place at Schauffhausen in Switzerland in 1892. Jeffrey Hudson, a famous English dwarf who lived in the 17th century, is said to have measured only 45 cm. Philibert Commerson (1727–1773), a French physician who practiced in Montpellier, described finding a nation of dwarfs of around 90 cm in the interior of Madagascar. Charles Stratton (1838–1833) from Bridgeport, Connecticut, known as General Tom Thumb, was only 77.5 cm at the age of 25 years. In 1910 Bernhard Aschner (1883–1960) demonstrated that the anterior pituitary produced a substance that influenced growth. Herbert Mclean Evans (1882–1971) and Joseph Abraham Long (b 1879) discovered growth hormone in 1921 and demonstrated the gigantic overgrowth of rats treated with it. A marked stimulation of growth in a 17-year-old pituitary dwarf who was treated with the growth hormone for 10 months was shown by M.S. Raben in 1958.

Dwyer Fusion Anterior spinal fusion with staples, screws and wire. Devised by an Australian orthopedic surgeon Allen Frederick Dwyer (1920–1975) at Mater Hospital, Sydney.

Dye Dilution Curve In 1894, George Neil Stewart (1860–1930) discovered that it was possible to measure cardiac output in animals by injecting dye into a vein and analyzing the amount that appeared in arterial blood. This method was later used in the study of cardiac output in humans by an American physiologist, William Ferguson Hamilton (b 1893) and co-workers in 1932. The dye dilution curves obtained by this method were later used in diagnosis of congenital heart disease. *See cardiac output.*

Dyeing of Hair Discussed in detail by Paul of Aegina (625–690). He described the various methods as well as the choice of colors such as gold, yellow and black. Galen (129–200) remarked that such treatment does not belong to physicians, but under certain circumstances he was obliged to give this treatment to royal ladies. Silver salts were used as hair dyes by Jerome Cardan (1501–1576) of Pavia and Ambroise Paré (1510–1590) of France.

Dye Those made from purple murex were used by the Phoenicians as early as 1000 BC. Most of the other dyes used in ancient times came from sea molluscs, plants or insects. The Incas were skilled in dyeing long before the Spaniards reached Mexico and they used the scarlet coch-ineal dye. Manganese, antimomy and lead chromate were used for textiles and in printing before the discovery of aniline dyes by an English dye chemist, John Mercer (1791–1866), in 1813. Coal tar was an unwanted waste product of the gas industry until August Wilhelm Hofmann (1818–1892) in 1843 extracted aniline from it and established the dye industry. The first aniline dye, mauve, was prepared by William Henry Perkin (1838–1907), a co-worker of Hofmann in 1856. Robert Koch (1843–1910) used aniline dyes for staining specimens for microscopic studies in 1877. The inhibitory action of dyes on bacteria was demonstrated by A. Rozahegyi in 1887. Cancer of the bladder due to aniline was demonstrated by several workers including S.G. Luenberger of Basel (1912), F. Curshmann of Germany (1920) and R. Oppenheimer (1926). Acriflavin dye was synthesized by Benda in 1912 and it was introduced as an antiseptic in 1913 by Carl Hamilton Browning (1881–1972), a pupil of Paul Ehrlich (1854–1915). It was given intravenously for treatment of encephalitis lethargica by H.H. Young. The red azo dye was the first antibacterial substance noted to provide specific protection against streptoccocal infection by Gerhard Domagk (1895–1964) in 1935. The main active antibacterial component in red diazo dye was later shown to be sulfanilamide.

Dynamics The study of moving bodies. Established on a scientific basis by Galileo (1564–1642). It was also studied by Archimedes (287–212 BC) and Leonardo Da Vinci (1452–1519). Galileo conducted experiments on the movement of falling bodies, pendulums and projectiles and introduced the concept of uniform acceleration, distinguishing it from uniform velocity.

Dynamite Alfred Nobel (1833–1896) of Stockholm, the originator of the Nobel Prize, invented land mines for the Russian army, using gunpowder, and subsequently established over ten factories that manufactured nitroglycerin (for dynamite production) across Europe in 1872. In 1873 the British government granted permission for Nobel to build a factory to make it at Ardeer in Ayrshire. Maximum precautions were taken to avoid explosions and it became the only dynamite factory in the world with no record of major accidents. *See Nobel, Alfred.*

Dyschondroplasia *See Ollier disease.*

Dyscrasia [Greek: *dys*, ill or bad + *krasis*, mixture] An old term to denote abnormal composition of blood and humors.

Dysentery [Greek: *dys*, ill or bad + *enteron*, intestine] Paul of Aegina (625–690) described dysentery as 'an ulceration of the intestines, sometimes arising from the translation of tenesmus and attended with various evacuations, at first bilious and of various colors, then accordingly bloody and at last ichorous, like that which runs from dead bodies'. He recommended ashes of snail and dried dung of dogs who had eaten bones to be drunk in milk that had curdled by having pebbles put into it. Hippocrates (460–377 BC) earlier recommended purging, emetics and clysters as treatment. Herodotus (484–407 BC) described the epidemic dysentery that broke out in the Persian army while they marched through Thessaly. It is also mentioned in the *Ayur-Veda* as *Atisar*. Galen's (AD 129–200) theory that it originated from the pungent juices of bile was upheld until the 17th century and was partly responsible for the lack of further work. A more accurate and complete description was given by Calius Aurelius in the 4th century. The pathological changes related to dysentery were described by Giovanni Battista Morgagni (1682–1771) in 1747. The first report of tropical dysentery in the East Indies was given by Jacob de Bontius (1592–1631), and Willem Piso (1611–1678) obser-ved it in the West Indies in 1648. *See salmonellosis, food poisoning, amebic dysentery.*

Dyslexia [Greek: *dys*, ill or bad + *lexis*, diction] The term was suggested by Rudolf Berlin (1833–1897) in 1887. A description of a case of developmental dyslexia was given in an article in the *British Medical Journal*, 'A case of congenital word blindness' by a general practitioner, Pringle-Morgan, in 1896. It was initially thought to be due to a defect in visual processing. James Hinshelwood (1859–1919), an ophthalmologist, also subscribed to this opinion in his *Congenital Word Blindness* published in 1917. The current view is that it is a verbal deficit with speech processing difficulties.

Dystrophia Adiposa Genitalis *See Fröhlich syndrome.*

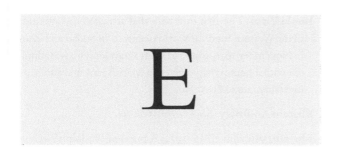

Eagleton, Wells Phillips (1865–1946) American neurologist who described cavernous sinus thrombophelibitis in relation to septicemia in 1926.

Eales Disease Characterized by sudden impairment of vision due to recurrent retinal and vitreous hemorrhage of unknown etiology. Described by an English physician, Henry Eales (1852–1913), the son of a vicar in Devon. He studied medicine at University College London and graduated in 1873. He was ophthalmic surgeon at the Midland Eye Hospital from 1878 for 35 years.

Ear One of the early important monographs on the ear, *De Aure Humana,* which included the anatomy and physiology, was published by an Italian physician and pupil of Marcello Malpighi (1628–1694), Antonio Valsalva (1666–1723) in 1704. *See hearing, audiology.*

Ear Surgery Several plastic operations were described for ear deformities in the early 1900s. An operation for prominent ears was devised by a New York surgeon, William Henry Luckett (b 1872) in 1910. The reconstruction of external ear in cases of deformity was described by a New Zealand-born British plastic surgeon, Sir Harold Delf Gillies (1882–1960) in 1937. A total reconstruction was described by a Kansas surgeon, Earl Calvin Padgett (1893–1946) in 1938. George Warren Pierce (b 1889) of San Francisco described another method in 1930.

Early American Hospitals The first hospital in the American continent, the Hospital of Immaculate Conception was built by the conqueror Cortez (1485–1554) in Mexico in 1524. The English Naval commander Sir Francis Drake (1545–1596) was a patient there for a few months following a shipwreck. The Bishop of Michoacan built the next hospital, in Santa Fe, in 1531. Seven Augustine nuns from France started a small Charity Hospital in New Orleans in 1727 and it was given a new lease in 1803. The Philadelphia General Hospital, known as the Blockly Hospital for several generations, was founded in 1731. St Phillip's Hospital in Charlestown, Carolina, was established in 1736. The Pennsylvania Hospital followed in 1756, established by a

physician, Thomas Bond (1712–1784) from Maryland, with the help of Benjamin Franklin (1706–1790). The New York Hospital received its Royal Charter in 1771 but, after a series of setbacks, was able to open only in 1791. The Boston Dispensary, offering ambulatory treatment for the poor, started in 1796. The Mulanthy Hospital, the first Catholic hospital in the United States, was established in St Louis in 1828. St Vincent's Hospital in New York was built in 1850. *See Massachusetts General Hospital.*

Early Canadian Hospitals The first hospital in Canada, in Halifax, Nova Scotia, was founded in 1750 and was granted to the city as an almshouse in 1766. Another small hospital in a four-room house, called the House of Recovery, was started by the Benevolent Society of Montreal in the early 19th century and became incorporated into the McGill Medical School in 1823. The Toronto General Hospital was built from funds obtained by melting down the medals of war heroes, following disputes about who should be awarded them. Although the hospital was established in 1820 it started functioning only in 1829.

Early Hospitals in Britain These were started mainly through charities set up by the rich for the poor. The London Hospitals were established in the following chronological order: St Bartholomew's Hospital (1123), St Thomas' Hospital (1173), Westminster Hospital (1719), Guy's Hospital (1721), St George's Hospital (1733), London Hospital (1740) and Middlesex Hospital (1745). Winchester Hospital was the first in the style of the London hospitals to be established outside London in 1723. The Royal Infirmary in Edinburgh was established in 1729. The first specialist hospital, the Eye Hospital at Moorfields, was started as a dispensary by a surgeon, John Cunningham Saunders (1773–1810) in 1805. By 1860 66 specialist hospitals were established in London. *See early American hospitals, infirmaries.*

Early Man *See Cro-Magnon, Neanderthal man, Piltdown man, anthropology.*

Earth Archelaus, a Greek philosopher who lived before the time of Socrates (470–400 BC), was the first to propose that the Earth was not flat. Anaximander (611–547 BC) of Miletus was the first among the Greeks to draw a map of the Earth giving details of its surface and to speculate on the sizes and distances of the heavenly bodies. Hipparchus, an astronomer of Bithynia who lived around 150 BC, stated that the Earth was flat at the poles. In 1779 the French naturalist, Comte Buffon (1707–1788), proposed that the Earth was originally hot before cooling, and set the age as 75,000 years. Work by several geologists over the next two centuries set the age as 4.6 billion years. *See geogeny.*

East India Company Chartered by Queen Elizabeth I in 1600 and started trading in 1612. It played a prominent part in promoting medicine during colonial times and two of its early surgeons were Gabriel Boughton, who went to Agra in 1645, and William Hamilton, who served in Delhi from 1714 to 1717. Later other surgeons, including James Lind (1716–1794), Patrick Russell (1727–1805) and Joseph Fayrer (1824–1907) served in India. Fayrer wrote the first book on poisonous snakes in India, *Thanatophidia in India,* in 1884.

Easton, John Alexander (1807–1865) He graduated from Glasgow University in 1836 and was professor of materia medica in the same institution in 1855. He held his post until his death. He is mostly known for his popular remedy known as Easton's syrup, which contained phosphate of iron, quinine, strychnine and glycerin.

Eating Disorders *See anorexia nervosa, bulimia.*

Eaton Agent The causative agent of atypical pneumonia was identified as a filterable agent transmissible to rats by American bacteriologist, Monroe Davis Eaton (b 1904) in 1944. He was born in Stockton, California and graduated in 1930 from Harvard where he was associate professor of immunology in 1947. *See atypical pneumonia.*

Eaton–Lambert Syndrome A myasthenic reaction associated with small cell carcinoma of the bronchus. First described by American neurologists at the Mayo Clinic, E.H. Lambert (b 1915) and L.M. Eaton (1905–1958) in 1956.

Ebers Papyrus Bought by an Egyptologist and novelist George Moritz Ebers (1837–1898) of Berlin in 1873 from an Arab in Luxor who claimed that he found it buried with a mummy at Thebes. Although the papyrus was written around 1500 BC, its text refers to earlier Egyptian medicine practiced since 3300 BC. It was the first of the papyri to be published. It contains descriptions of ancient medical practices, accounts of herbal medicines, demonology and mineral medicines. A German translation of the papyrus was produced by Joachim in 1890, and an incomplete translation of it was made by Cyril P. Bryan in 1930. An excellent translation of its entire contents was done by B. Ebbell in 1937.

Eberth, Carl Joseph (1825–1926) Born in Würzberg, he was a pupil of Rudolph Virchow (1821–1902). He was a bacteriologist and professor of pathology at Halle and discovered *Salmonella* as the causative organism of typhoid in 1880. He also described the broken-line appearance of cardiac muscles under the microscope, in 1866.

Ebner, Victor (1842–1925) Professor of histology and an embryologist at Innsbruck who described the serous glands in relation to the taste papillae of the tongue, in 1873.

Ebola Virus The first outbreak that attracted the attention of the Western medical world occurred in Sudan and Zaire in November 1976. It spread from a traveler who was admitted with a hemorrhagic fever to Maridi Hospital and had a mortality rate of 80–90%.

Ebstein Anomaly *See Ebstein, Wilhelm.*

Ebstein, Wilhelm (1836–1912) A pupil of Rudolph Virchow (1821–1902) and Moritz Heinrich Romberg (1795–1873), who later became professor of medicine at Göttingen. He described the congenital displacement of the tricuspid valve into the right ventricle (Ebstein anomaly) in 1866, and the hyaline degeneration of the epithelial cells in the renal tubules seen in diabetes mellitus in 1880. The first description of Ebstein anomaly in America was given by William George MacCallum (1874–1944), professor of pathology at Johns Hopkins Hospital, in 1900.

Ebstein Fever (Syn. Pel–Ebstein fever) Chronic relapsing pyrexia of Hodgkin disease. Described by a Göttingen physician, Wilhelm Ebstein (1836–1912) and a Dutch physician at Amsterdam, Pieter Klazes Pel (1852–1919) in 1887.

Ecbolics [Greek: *ekbolikos,* casting out] An ancient term for methods or substances for inducing abortion. Ergot was mentioned as an oxytocic in Adam Lonicer's *Kreuterbuch* in 1582. Desgranges, a surgeon in Lyons, mentioned the use of spurred rye in prolonged labor in 1777. John Stearns (1770–1848) of Saratoga County, New York, advocated the use of contaminated rye around 1800. *See oxytocin, prostaglandin, ergot.*

Eccles, Sir John Carew (b 1903) Australian neurophysiologist and Nobel Prize winner in medicine, born in Melbourne in 1903 and studied medicine there. He undertook postgraduate studies on a Rhodes scholarship at Oxford in 1925 and worked in Sir Charles Scott Sherrington's (1857–1952) department of physiology. He proposed that synaptic transmission in the nervous system was more an electrical than a chemical phenomenon, and demonstrated the depolarization of postsynaptic muscle in response to a neural stimulus, which he named excitatory postsynaptic potential (EPSP). He also identified inhibitory neurons and demonstrated control of the nervous system by inhibitory synapses. On his return, he was appointed professor of physiology at the Australian National University, Canberra in 1952. After his compulsory retirement in 1968 he joined the State University of New York at Buffalo and served there until 1975. He shared the Nobel Prize for his work on nervous impulses with Sir Alan Lloyd Hodgkin (b 1914) and Sir Andrew Fielding Huxley (b 1917) in 1963.

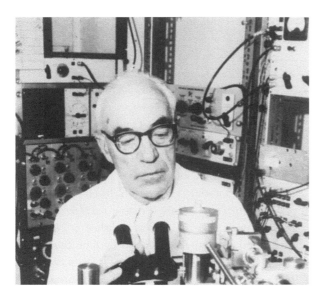

Sir John Carew Eccles. Courtesy of the National Library of Medicine

ECG *See electrocardiography.*

Echinococcus [Greek: *echinos*, sea urchin + *kokkos*, berry] The Taenia group of worms were known from ancient times and Hippocrates called them broad lumbrici. Galen (129–200) and Paul of Aegina (625–690) recommended absinthium or wormwood as treatment. The term was first used for the vesicular hydatid by Karl Asmund Rudolphi (1771–1832) in 1808. The endemic nature in Iceland was pointed out by Schleisner in 1849, and Carl Theodor Ernest von Siebold (1804–1885) demonstrated that dogs could be experimentally infected with it in 1854. The first complete life history and morphology was given by Karl Georg Friedrich Rudolph Leuckart (1823–1898) in 1860. A skin test for hydatid disease was described by an Italian physician, Tommaso Casoni (1850–1925) in 1912. A diagnostic serum test was devised by a Paris physician, Michel Weinberg (1868–1940) in 1909.

ECHO Virus (Enteric Cytopathogenic Human Orphan virus) During the 1940s several viruses were isolated from healthy subjects in the course of research. These were found not to be pathogenic to any laboratory animals and were named 'orphan' viruses. Later work revealed that they may cause aseptic meningitis and respiratory diseases in humans. The Committee of the National Foundation of Infantile Paralysis in the USA named them ECHO viruses in 1955.

Echocardiography [Greek: *echo*, returned sound + *kardia*, heart + *graphein*, to write] Ultrasound was used to record the continuous movement of the heart walls by Inge Edler and Carl Helmuth Hertz in 1954. Their device was first called the ultrasonic spectroscope, which was used to demonstrate the aortic and mitral valve movements in 1961. Their method, known as ultrasonic cardiography, was further developed by an American radiologist, Claude Joyner and a German team from Effert's laboratory in Germany. The first American textbook on echocardiography was written by Harvey Feigenbaum of Indiana. *See Doppler phenomenon.*

Echolalia [Greek: *echo*, sound + *lalein*, to babble like a child] Involuntary purposeless repetition of a word or sentence. One of the first descriptions was given by an Aberdeen clergyman, George Garden (1649–1733) in a letter *concerning a man of strange imitating nature* in 1677. It was named echo phenomenon by Moritz Heinrich Romberg (1795–1873) of Berlin in *Manual of Nervous Diseases of Man* (translated into English for the Sydenham Society by Edward H. Sieveking), published in 1853. A Berlin psychiatrist, Hugo Karl Liepmann (1863–1925) also gave a description around 1907.

Eck Fistula Ligation of the portal vein and the hepatic artery followed by the establishment of a permanent communication between the portal vein and inferior vena cava was performed by Russian physiologist, Nikolai Vladimirovich Eck (1847–1908) in 1877. It was named after him and provided a way of studying the metabolism of the body in relation to the liver.

Ecker, Alexander (1816–1887) Anatomist in Basel and Freiburg who gave an original description of several convolutions of the occipital lobe. He wrote a treatise on the movements of the brain and spinal cord in 1843 and published a monograph on the structure of the suprarenal glands in 1846.

Eclampsia [Greek: *eklampein*, to shine forth] Epigastric pain preceding eclampsia was described by a Paris physician, François Chaussier (1746–1828) in 1824. Three patients with eclampsia – one treated with leeches (who died), the other extensively bled and the third on whom no intervention was carried out – were described by Robert Harper in *The Lancet* in 1861. The presence of albumin in the urine of mothers with puerperal convulsions or eclampsia was described by John Charles Lever (1811–1858), a lecturer in midwifery at Guy's Hospital in his paper *Albumin in the Urine of Eclamptic Women*, published in 1843. A conservative method of treating it, through control of fits, sedation and quiet surroundings, was advocated by Russian obstetrician, Vasili Vasilievich Strognov (1857–1938) in 1899. An English obstetrician, Thomas Denman (1733–1815) of Bakewell, also suggested conservative management in 1793. The occurrence of shock following delivery in eclampsia was pointed out by a New York obstetrician, Harold Capron Bailey (1879–1929) in 1911.

L'Ecluse, Charles de or Clusius (1526–1609) Physician and botanist from Flanders, who became professor at the University of Leiden. His botanical works were published in Antwerp in 1601.

Ecology [Greek: *oikos*, household + *logos*, discourse] The science dealing with the study of living animals and plants in relation to their environment. One of the first recognizable works on ecology, *The Natural History and Antiquities of Selborne* by Gilbert White (1720–1793) in 1789 became the fourth best selling book in English and ran to 200 editions. F.J.A.N. Unger in 1836 demonstrated the dependence of plants on the chemical composition of the soil. The term was introduced by Heinrich Phillip August Haeckel (1834–1919) of Jena in 1866. *Ecology of the Plant,* was published in 1895 by Dane Warming (1841–1924). Animal ecology was studied by Charles Darwin (1809–1882) and Charles Sutherland Elton (1900–1991) of Liverpool, who published *Animal Ecology* (1927), *Animal Ecology and Evolution* (1930) and *The Pattern of Animal Communities* (1966).

Economo Disease *See encephalitis lethargica.*

Ecphyma [Greek: *ektos*, outside + *phyma*, swelling] Term coined by English physician, James Mason Good (1764–1827) of Epping in Essex to denote warts and corns.

ECT *See electroconvulsive therapy.*

Ectoderm [Greek: *ektos*, outside + *derma*, skin] The concept of embryonic development of organs from different germ layers was proposed in 1828 by Carl Ernst von Baer (1792–1876), a professor at St Petersburg. The germ layers were classified into ectoderm, endoderm and mesoderm by Robert Remak (1815–1865) in 1845.

Ectopia Vesicae [Greek: *ektos*, without; Latin: *vesica*, bladder] Attempts to close the opening of ectopic vesicae with skin flaps were made in 1844. Philibert Joseph Roux (1780–1854), a surgeon at the Charité Hospital in Paris, was a pioneer of plastic surgery in France and made an unsuccessful attempt in 1853. Daniel Ayres (b 1822) of Brooklyn, New York used a skin flap from the abdomen in 1858 which was partly successful. Joseph Pancoast (1805–1882) of Philadelphia had better results in the same year and Timothy Holmes introduced a successful method in 1863.

Ectopic Heart Beat *See extrasystole.*

Ectopic Pregnancy [Greek: *ektos*, outside + *topos*, place]

The first operation for extrauterine or ectopic pregnancy was reported in France in 1591. It was performed in America by a New York a surgeon, John Bard (1716–1799), in 1760. William Baynham, a country physician from Virginia, performed the second operation in 1790. A case of extrauterine pregnancy was presented by Thomas Blizard (1743–1835), a surgeon at the London Hospital, in *Transactions of the Royal Society of Edinburgh* in 1800. In 1816 John King from Edisto Island, South Carolina performed an extensive operation for abdominal pregnancy and saved both mother and child. He wrote the first book, *An Analysis of the Subject of Extra-uterine Foetation, and of the Retroversion of the Gravid Uterus,* and it was published in Norwich in 1818. Another treatise was written by John Stubbs Parry (1843–1876) of Philadelphia in 1876. Robert Lawson Tait (1845–1899) from Edinburgh performed the first successful operation of ruptured tubal pregnancy in 1883. The Cullen sign, discoloration of the skin around the umbilicus in cases of ruptured ectopic pregnancy, was described by Thomas Stephen Cullen (1868–1953) of America in 1916.

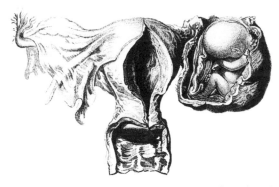

Ectopic Pregnancy. Francis H. Ramsbotham, *The Principles and Practice of Obstetric Medicine and Surgery* (1856). Churchill, London

Ectopic Secretion [Greek: *ektos*, outside + *topos*, place] Secretion of hormones by tumors of tissues other than those responsible for their normal secretion. Named by G.W. Liddle and co-workers around 1960. Ectopic adrenocorticotropic hormone production in a case of bronchial carcinoma was described by W.H. Brown in 1928.

Ectozoa [Greek: *ektos*, outside + *zoon*, animal] Term employed by early naturalists to denote external parasites.

Ectropion [Greek: *ektos*, outside + *trope*, turning] Eversion of the eyelids. Paul of Aegina (625–690) described scarring and fungus as two different causes. When it was caused by fungus he recommended local application of burnt lead washed with sulfur and he advised surgical treatment for ectropion caused by a scar. Alsaharavius (AD 980) gave a detail account but his treatment was essentially the same as that of Paul of Aegina.

Eczema [Greek: *ekzein*, to boil out] A classification of different kinds of eczema was given by an English physician, Robert Willan (1757–1812) in 1796. A classical account of eczema was given by Ferdinand von Hebra (1816–1860) of Vienna in 1860. Seborrheic eczema was described by Paul Gerson Unna (1850–1929) of Hamburg in 1887.

Eddowes Disease *See osteogenesis imperfecta.*

Edebohls, George Michael (1853–1908) New York surgeon who introduced decortication for treatment of chronic nephritis in 1901. He performed nephropexy in a movable kidney affected with chronic nephritis, in 1899.

Edelman, Adolf (1885–1939) Physician in Vienna who was one of the first to describe anemia in chronic infections. He devised a test for urobilin in urine in 1915.

Edema [Greek: *oidema*, swelling] *See dropsy.*

Eden, Sir Fredrick Morton (d 1809) A writer on statistics and politics who wrote *The State of the Poor; or the History of Laboring Classes of England, from the Conquest to the Present Time.*

Edessa A town in Mesopotamia, famous for its schools of theology in the 5th century. Nestorians gained control of the medical school and made it into a famous institution around 450. The town also had two large hospitals where the Nestorians practiced. It was captured by the Saracens in 1184.

Edinburgh Harveian Society One of the earliest medical social clubs in Scotland, founded by Andrew Duncan (1744–1828) in 1782.

Edinburgh Medical Journal *See Annals of Medicine.*

Edinburgh Medical School An army surgeon, John Monro (d 1737), was the first to suggest a medical school in Edinburgh on the lines of the medical school at Leiden. His son Alexander Monro, Primus (1697–1767) commenced formal anatomy lectures at Edinburgh. The original faculty of medicine was started in 1726 by four physicians, Andrew St Clair, John Rutherford (1695–1779), Andrew Plummer (d 1756) and John Innes (d 1733). Joseph Gibson (d 1739) was the first professor of midwifery in the same year. The buildings adjacent to the Royal Infirmary were designed by Rowland Anderson in Renaissance style in 1876. The McEwan Hall for the graduates was added to the medical school in 1888.

Edinburgh Royal Infirmary Started through voluntary contributions with six beds in a small rented house at Robertson's Close in 1729. A total of 35 patients were treated in its first year and in 1738 it joined with another hospital formed two years earlier. A Royal Charter was granted by King George II in 1736. The new hospital with 228 beds opened in 1741 and in 1829 the buildings of the old High School were incorporated. The George Watson's Hospital was selected as a new site in 1870 and the present Royal Infirmary opened in 1879.

Edinburgh University Commenced as a college by the Town Council of Edinburgh in 1581 at a site of ancient religious houses donated by Mary Queen of Scots, and with the funds provided by Robert Reid, Bishop of Orkney. It received its charter from King James VI in 1582, and 80 students were enrolled in 1583. Its first principal was appointed in 1585. Alexander Monro (1697–1767) was professor of anatomy at Edinburgh in 1721, and the Monros continued to contribute to its development through three generations. Professor of physick, John Rutherford (1695–1779), was the first to obtain permission to conduct lectures at the Infirmary in 1748. The foundation for the new buildings was laid by Francis, the Grand Master of the Masons of Scotland in 1789. Some famous medical figures from Edinburgh include: Sir Charles Bell (1774–1842), William Cullen (1710–1790), Robert Knox (1791–1862), James Y. Simpson (1811–1870), Sir Arthur Conan Doyle (1859–1930) and Benjamin Bell (1749–1806).

Edinger, Ludwig (1855–1918) German anatomist and professor at Frankfurt-am-Main. Regarded as the founder of comparative neuroanatomy. He described the nucleus of the third cranial nerve (Edinger–Westphal nucleus) in 1885.

Edinger–Westphal Nucleus *See Edinger, Ludwig, Westphal, Karl Friedrich Otto.*

Edison, Thomas Alva (1847–1931) The ingenious inventor, was born in Milan, Ohio. His family moved to Michigan in 1854, and his interest in science started with his studies on train telegraphy in 1862. His inventions include: a talking machine in 1876; a mimeograph; electrical lamps; the electrical system for New York's underground central station system; and over 1000 patents. He started experiments on X-rays soon after their discovery by Wilhelm Conrad Röntgen (1845–1923) in 1895 and chose calcium tungstate as the most suitable substance that would become luminous on exposure to X-rays, and constructed the first fluoroscope which was exhibited at the New York city electrical exhibition in 1896. His electric light played a major role in the development of the early cystoscope.

Edkins, John Sydney (1863–1940) London physiologist who proposed a hormonal theory for gastric secretion in 1905.

EDTA Ethylenediaminetetraacetic acid. A powerful chelating agent discovered by G. Schwarzenbach and H. Acker-man in 1948. The first recorded successful treatment of lead encephalopathy with EDTA was given by Sidbury to an 18-month-old baby in 1955.

Edwards Syndrome *See trisomy 18 syndrome.*

Edwards, Robert Geoffrey (b 1925) A pioneer of *in vitro* fertilization with obstetrician Patrick Christopher Steptoe (1913–1988). He was educated at the universities of Wales and Edinburgh and became reader in physiology at the University of Cambridge (1969), before he was appointed professor of reproduction there in 1985. He started his research on *in vitro* fertilization with Steptoe in 1968 and achieved the first birth of a baby ('test tube baby') in 1978.

Edwards, William Frèdèric (1777–1849) French physician who wrote an early and important work on the effect of light on the body, in 1824.

Edwin Smith Papyrus An important surgical treatise written around 1600 BC. Purchased by Edwin Smith (1822–1906) at Thebes, near Luxor in 1862, and presented to the New York Historical Society by his daughter. It was translated in 1930 and contains details of Egyptian surgical medicine from 2500 BC. It describes 48 diseases, plasters, splints for broken bones, suturing, cauterization and other methods of advanced surgical and medical practice. *See Egyptian medicine.*

EEG *See electroencephalogram.*

Effort Syndrome (Syn. cardiovascular neurosis, neurocirculatory asthenia, Da Costa syndrome) Sir Thomas Lewis (1881–1945) named it and it was noted amongst soldiers by Jacob M. Da Costa (1833–1900) of Philadelphia during the American Civil War in 1871. English cardiologist, Paul Hamilton Wood (1907–1962) in 1941 attributed the somatic symptoms to psychoneurosis arising out of fear.

Egg *See ovum.*

Ego Three psychological levels of functioning, impulses or id, ego and conscience, were described by German psychiatrist, Johan Christian Heinroth (1773–1843). He considered self-awareness as the main characteristic of the ego. The relationship and conflict between the id and ego were studied by Sigmund Freud (1856–1939), and he published *The Ego and the Id* in 1923. Anna Freud (1895–1892), a psychiatrist and the youngest daughter of Freud, advanced her father's work on the ego and wrote *The Ego and Mechanisms of Defence* in 1936, in which she gave a systematic and clear description of defense mechanisms involved in the ego.

Egyptian Chlorosis *See Anchylostoma duodenale.*

Egyptian Hieroglyphics A form of picture-writing used by the earliest dynasties in Egypt. The first form is at King Narmer's Palace. Study and deciphering was started by the French founder of Egyptology, Jean François Champollion (1790–1832). Much of Egyptian history and culture was made known through his work, and he published *Precis du Systeme Hieroglyphigue* in 1824. An attempt to decipher them in England was made by the British physician, James Young (1773–1829), whose celebrated *Egypt* appeared in the *Encyclopaedia Britannica* in 1819. *See Rosetta stone.*

Egyptian Medicine Known to have been practiced since 3500 BC. Much of the present knowledge was obtained from papyri such at the Ebers, Smith, Kahun and Hearst papyri. The Smith papyrus contains surgery and 48 descriptions of diseases. The Ebers papyrus contains 178 columns, which give mainly medical prescriptions and charms. The first of the Egyptian physicians was Imhotep who practiced medicine during the third dynasty around 3300 BC and was deified. His medicine was taken over by priests and remained the best in the ancient world until its decline around 1200 BC. Egyptian doctors were highly specialized and their tombs, from about 2500 BC, contain inscriptions such as 'eye specialist to the palace' and 'keeper of king's rectum'. The Al-Mansur Hospital, one of the earliest hospitals during the Middle Ages, was established in Cairo in 1276. It was a marvel of medicine of that period, containing wards for special diseases, clinics, lecture rooms, a library and many other parallels of a modern hospital. *See Ebers papyrus, Smith papyrus, Kahun papyrus, Hearst papyrus.*

Egyptian Mummies *See mummy.*

Ehlers–Danlos Syndrome A hereditary connective tissue disorder in a 23–year-old man, who was able to pull his skin from the pectoral area to the mouth, was described by Job Janszoon van Meekeren (1611–1666) in 1682. A modern description was given by a Danish dermatologist in Berlin, Edvard Ehlers (1863–1937) in 1901 and a French physician, Henri Alexandre Danlos (1844–1912) in 1908.

Ehrenberg, Christian Gottfried (1795–1876) German naturalist of Prussian origin, and a professor in Berlin. He was a pioneer in the microscopic study of organisms and discovered that phosphorescence in the sea was caused by living organisms. He visited Ghizzan in Egypt and other parts of Middle East and brought several specimens of plants to Europe in 1820.

Ehrenritter, Johannes (d 1790) Anatomist in Vienna who described the ganglion of the glossopharyngeal nerve in 1790. He died before his work was published.

Ehrlich, Paul (1854–1915) German bacteriologist of Jewish origin from Strzelin. He was a pioneer in hematology and chemotherapy, and made a significant contribution with his methods of staining. He used aniline dyes to stain white blood cells in 1877, and introduced the differential blood cell count in 1879. He identified reticulocytes in 1881, and gave a description of aplastic anemia in 1888. He differentiated between lymphocytic and myelogenous leukemia in 1891, and identified and named mast cells in 1863. The quantitative method of estimation of toxins in immunology and the concept of the therapeutic index were introduced by Ehrlich in 1897. His side-chain theory revolutionized thinking in chemotherapy and in 1911, in pursuit of safer therapeutic arsenic compounds, he produced neosalvarsan or neoarsphenamine, which was effective in treatment of relapsing fever, syphilis and trypanosomiasis. He shared the Nobel Prize for Physiology or Medicine with Elie Metchnikoff (1845–1916) in 1908. *See side-chain theory, chemotherapy.*

Ehrlich Test For bile pigments in the urine. Devised by Paul Ehrlich (1854–1915) in 1883.

Eichorst, Hermann (1849–1921) Physician in Zurich who gave a comprehensive account of pernicious anemia in 1878. He also described a type (Eichorst type) of progressive muscular atrophy affecting the femoral and tibial muscles.

Eichsted, Carl Ferdinand (1816–1892) *See pityriasis versicolar.*

Eijkman Institute The search for vitamins was started at the Research Laboratory for Bacteriology and Pathological Anatomy in Batavia (Jakarta). The laboratory was later named after Christian Eijkman (1858–1930), the discoverer of the cause of beriberi.

Eijkman, Christian (1858–1930) Dutch Physician from Nijkerk. While serving in the Dutch East Indies (Indonesia) he established the cause of beriberi and proposed the concept of essential food factors, later known as vitamins. His experiments on prisoners in Java showed that beriberi could be cured by taking unpolished rice. He shared the Nobel Prize with Sir Frederick Gowland Hopkins (1861–1947) in 1929. *See beriberi.*

Eileithyia Greek goddess of childbirth, whose symbols were the moon for procreation, and a cow representing fertility.

Einhorn, Albert (1856–1917) German chemist from Munich, who discovered the local anesthetic, novocaine, in 1899.

Einhorn, Max (b 1862) *See endoscopy.*

Einstein, Albert (1875–1955) Born to Jewish parents in Ulm in Bavaria. He studied mathematics at the Technical High School in Zurich from 1896 to 1900, and his initial intention was to become a secondary school teacher. He became naturalized in Switzerland in 1901 and started working as an engineer at the Swiss Patent Office in 1902. He published his first work on relativity, which stated that time and space are not absolute but merely relative to the observer, while he was attached to a Swiss university in 1905. He later became professor of physics at Berlin and proposed the special theory of relativity, the theory of Brownian movement and the quantum law of the emission and absorption of light. One of his predictions regarding deflection of light by cosmic masses was tested during the solar eclipse in May 1919, and was proved correct. He became director of the Kaiser Wilhelm Physical Institute in Berlin in 1933 but left for America a year later, during the time of Hitler's rise to power. He was appointed professor in 1940 at Princeton University at New Jersey, where he continued to work on his unified field theory until his death. *See relativity.*

Einthoven, Willem (1860–1927) Dutch physiologist and professor of physics in Leiden, who simplified measuring time-related electrical changes in tissues with his invention of the string galvanometer in 1903. It was later developed into the electrocardiograph. He also presented the first field hypothesis of clinical significance in papers in 1912 and 1913, later becoming known as the Einthoven triangle hypothesis. He was awarded the Nobel Prize for Physiology or Medicine in 1924.

Eisenmenger Syndrome A congenital anomaly of the heart associated with an over-riding aorta, patent interventricular septum and right ventricular hypertrophy. Described by German physician, Victor Eisenmenger (1864–1932), in 1897.

Elasticity [Greek: *elaunein*, to draw out] The properties of elastic bodies in relation to their motion were studied by Sir William Petty (1623–1687) around 1674. Further work was done by Robert Hooke (1635–1703) who erroneously attributed elasticity of objects to air within them. Isaac Newton's (1642–1727) work on elasticity and cohesion was published in *Optiks* in 1703.

Elbow The anatomy was described by German surgeon, Hans Carl Leopold Barkow (1798–1873), in 1841. Scottish anatomist, Alexander Monro (1697–1767) described the olecranon bursa in 1726. Radiohumeral bursitis or tennis elbow was described by Boston surgeon, Robert Bayley Osgood (1873–1956) in 1922.

Elbow Joint Transplantation The first excision of the elbow joint was performed by a French surgeon, P.F. Moreau in Bar-de-Luc, near Nancy in 1803. Elbow joint transplantation in cases of ankylosis was pioneered by Peter Ivanovitch Buchmann (1872–1948) of St Petersburg in 1908.

Elderly Care *See geriatrics.*

Electric Shock Treatment *See electrotherapy, electroconvulsive therapy.*

Electrical Anesthesia In 1890 Jacques Arsene d' Arsonval (1851–1940) showed that it was possible to use electricity to induce anesthesia. Stephan Armand Nicolas Leduc (1853–1939) in 1902 applied current between the loin and the head to produce spinal anesthesia. In this procedure, electrodes delivering a current of 135 milliamperes at 700 cycles per second were applied to the head to produce general anesthesia, but the procedure was complicated by tachycardia and hypertension, thus limiting its use.

Electrical Resistance First measured in absolute terms by Gustav R. Kirchhoff (1824–1887) in 1849. James Joule (1818–1889) devised a simple method of measuring the absolute value in 1870. Lord Kelvin (1824–1907) designed a method for measuring its value with the help of a rotating coil around 1873. *See Ohm, George Simon.*

Electricity [Greek: *elektron*, amber] The electrostatic property of amber when rubbed was observed by the Greek philosopher, Thales, around 600 BC. English physician, William Gilbert (1544–1603) of Colchester, noticed around 1600 that other substances produced the same effect. He later published *De Magnete, Magneticisque Corporibus, te de Magno Magnette Tellure, Physiologia Nova,* which established him as the initiator of the study of electricity. He was also the first to use the term. Around 1630, an Italian Jesuit, Cabaeus, made another important observation that particles that were attracted to each other often repelled each other after contact. Otto von Guericke (1602–1686) produced the first frictional machine for continuous production of electricity in 1647. Robert Boyle (1626–1691) used glass to produce a similar effect in 1676. An Englishman, S. Gray, discovered the electrical conductivity of metals in 1729. In 1791 Luigi Galvani (1737–1827) started investigating the phenomenon of twitching in frog muscle when brought into contact with two metals. The positive and negative components of electricity were first noted by a French chemist, Charles François de Cisternay du Fay (1698–1739). Andre Marie Ampere (1775–1836) suggested units for measuring electricity while he was professor at the École Polytechnique of Paris in 1775. The effect of electric current on a needle was observed by Hans Christian Oersted (1777–1851), which opened the doors for the study of electromagnetism in 1819. Michael Faraday (1791–1867) discovered the phenomenon of electromagnetic rotation in 1822, and presented *Experimental Researches on Electricity* to the Royal Society in 1831. The first practical electromagnet was constructed by an English scientist, William Sturgeon (1783–1850) of Whittington, Lancashire in 1825. The large-scale distribution of high-voltage electricity with the use of dynamos and alternators was pioneered by a Liverpool engineer of Italian origin, Sebastian Ziano de Ferranti (1864–1930).

Electrocardiogram (ECG) *See electrocardiography.*

Electrocardiography The fact that the contraction of heart muscle was accompanied by electrical activity originating in the heart muscle was demonstrated by a Swiss physiologist, Rudolph Albert von Kölliker (1817–1905), and a German anatomist, Johannes Müller (1808–1858) in 1858. They used a crude but ingenious apparatus made of the skeletal muscle of a frog and connected it to the frog's heart. They demonstrated that with each systole two contractions of the skeletal muscle were produced. In 1872 Felix Jacob Marchand (1846–1928), a pathologist at Leipzig, used a crude differential rheotome connected to a galvanometer and measured the electrical variation of the frog heart at intervals. In the same year, Theodor Wilhelm Engelmann (1843–1909), a German physiologist, made a detailed study of a frog's heart muscle using a rheotome. In 1879 John Scott Burdon-Sanderson (1828–1905), professor of medicine at Oxford, devised an improved rheotome, using a capillary electrometer designed by a German physicist, Gabriel Jonas Lippmann (1845–1921) in 1875. Sanderson used this to make a detailed study of electrical changes in the ventricles of the frog and the tortoise. The first electrocardiogram of a man, by means of a capillary electrometer, was produced by Augustus Desire Waller (1856–1922), a physiologist at St Mary's Hospital, London, in 1887. William M. Bayliss (1860–1924) and Ernest Henry Starling (1886–1927) in 1892 did further experiments and postulated that the excitation of the heart originated in the atrium and spread to the ventricle through a network. Willem Einthoven (1860–1927), a Dutch physiologist, simplified the method of measuring the time-related electrical changes of the tissues with his invention of the string galvanometer in 1903. He presented the first field hypothesis of clinical significance in two papers in 1912 and 1913, known as the Einthoven triangle hypothesis. Einthoven's string galvanometer was improved by Sir Thomas Lewis (1881–1945), who added an extra string, making it possible to record different leads. The cell membrane theory to explain the electrical properties of the muscle was put forward by a German professor of physiology at Halle, Julius Bernstein (1839–1917), in 1912. Further studies were done independently by W.H. Craib and Frank Norman Wilson (1890–1952) around 1927, and Wilson and co-workers published an important work on the genesis of the electrocardiogram in 1933. The first recording of a fetal electrocardiogram was produced by M. Cremer of Germany in 1906. Chest leads in ECG were introduced by Charles Christian Wolferth (1887–1965) and Francis Clark Wood (b 1901) in 1932, and the unipolar leads were devised by F.N. Wilson in 1934.

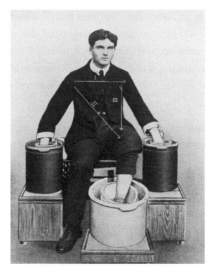

Electrical connections used in experimental electrocardiography. Sir Thomas Lewis, *Clinical Electrocardiography* (1918). Shaw and Sons, London

Electroconvulsive Therapy (ECT) The first use for mental illness was by a French physician, J.B. Le Roy in 1755. The negative correlation noted between schizophrenia and epilepsy, and the observation that schizophrenic patients improved after a fit, led Ladislaus Joseph Meduna (1896–1965) to use a convulsant drug, cardiozol, to treat mental patients in 1934. Insulin was used to impart hypoglycemic shock to psychiatric patients in the 1930s. Electrically induced convulsions were given to mental patients by Lucio Bini (1908–1964) and Ugo Cereletti (1877–1963) of Italy in 1937. Their method was introduced into England by Shepley and McGregor at Warlingham Park Hospital in 1939.

Electrode [Greek: *elektron*, amber + *hodos*, way] Term introduced by Michael Faraday (1791–1867) to denote a surface from which the electric current entered or left a body.

Electroencephalography (EEG) The evidence for electrical activity in the brain of living animals was provided by Richard Caton (1842–1926), an English neurologist from Liverpool, in 1875. Localization of electrical activity in relation to the functions of the cerebral cortex was studied by Francis Gotch (1853–1913) and Victor Alexander Haden Horsley (1857–1916) in 1892. A string galvanometer to record the electrical activity of the brain was introduced by Russian physiologist, Pravdich Neminsky (1879–1952) in 1913. He used it to record two waves of different frequencies in the brain, and named them electrocerebrograms. Hans Berger (1873–1941), a German psychiatrist, introduced the term elektrenkephalogramm in 1929. Its use in diagnosis of epilepsy was demonstrated by F.A. Gibbs and W.G. Lennox in 1935. It was used to localize intracranial tumors by William Grey Walter (1911–1977) of Britain in 1936. An early work on the subject, *Atlas of Electroencephalography*, was published by Gibbs in 1941.

Electrolysis [Greek: *elektron*, amber + *lysis*, loosening] The decomposition of water by electric current was demonstrated by van Troostwijk (1752–1837) and Deimann (1743–1808) in 1789. The earliest theory related to electrolysis was proposed by Theodor von Grotthus (1785–1822) in 1805. Johann Wilhelm Hittorf (1824–1914), a professor at the academy of Münster in Westphalia studied the rate of movement of anions and cations during electrolysis. His method was used by Friedrich Wilhelm Kohlrausch (1840–1910), a professor at the University of Würzberg, to calculate ionic velocities. Understanding was advanced by the Dutch chemist, Jacobus Henricus Van't Hoff (1852–1911) and Swedish physicist Svante August Arrhenius (1859–1927) in 1887. The laws that state that the amount of substance decomposed by electric current is proportional to the time of passage and the strength of the current was proposed by Michael Faraday (1791–1867) in 1833.

Electromagnetic Theory The effect of electric current on a needle was observed by Christian Hans Oersted (1777–1851) in 1819. Michael Faraday (1791–1867) discovered electromagnetic rotation in 1822 and presented his initial findings in *Experimental Researches on Electricity* to the Royal Society in 1831. His work led to the development of the dynamo as an alternative to the battery. Further work was published by James Clerk Maxwell (1831–1879) in the *Philosophical Transactions of the Royal Society* in 1865.

Electrometer [Greek: *elektron*, amber + *metron*, measure] Invented by a French abbot, Jean Antoine Nollet (1700–1770), professor of physics in Paris in 1747.

Electromyography (EMG) [Greek: *myos*, muscle +

graphein, to write] The method of obtaining myograms or electrical recordings of muscle was introduced by Hermann Helmholtz (1821–1894) in 1851 and improved by Jules Etienne Marey (1830–1904) of Paris around 1870. Emil du Bois Reymond (1818–1896) of Berlin was a pioneer who defined 'electrotonus' and graphically recorded tetanus in 1843. The recording of voluntary contractions of muscle on a time-related basis was improved with the invention of Julius Bernstein's (1839–1917) differential rheotome in 1890. Recording of the activity of single motor units was made possible by the introduction of concentric needle electrodes by Detlev Wulf Bronk (1887–1975) of the Rockefeller Institute in 1929.

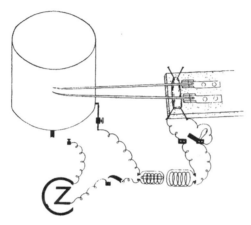

Marey's myographic forceps for electromyographic studies. Sir Edward Sharpey-Schafer, *Experimental Physiology* (1918). Longman, Green & Co., London

Electron Microscope The fundamental theory that led to the invention of the electron microscope by Ernst August Friedrich Ruska (1906–1988) and L. Marton in 1934 was originally proposed by Ernst Abbe (1840–1905) in 1873. Abbe realized that optical microscopy was limited by the fact that two separate objects cannot be distinguished if the distance between them is less than half the wavelength of the light used for illumination, Abbe law. This was overcome with the discovery of rays which had a shorter wavelength. Ruska showed that a magnetic coil can focus a beam of electrons and created the first crude electron microscope of 400x magnification in 1932. A year later he improved its power to 12,000x. The electron microscope became commercially available in England in 1935. Further development was done by a Canadian physicist, James Hillier (b 1915) in 1937. Vladimir Kosma Zworykin (1889–1982) of Russian improved it to provide 50 times the magnification of a light microscope in 1939. The first electron microscopic study of the cell, showing the endoplasmic reticulum and

mitochondria, was done in 1945 by an American cytologist, Albert Claude (b 1898) of Belgian origin. The scanning electron microscope, capable of producing three-dimensional images at a magnification of over 100,000, was developed around 1948 by an electronic engineer, Sir Charles Oatley (b 1904) of Frome in Somerset, and came into practical use in 1969. The tunneling electron microscope, based on the quantum mechanical effect or tunneling of electrons, was developed by a Swiss physicist, Heinrich Rohrer (b 1933) and Gerd Karl Binnig (b 1947) of Germany in 1980.

Electron The term was used by an Irish physicist, George Johnston Stoney (1826–1911) in 1874 to denote particles of electricity in electrolysis. Sir John Joseph Thomson (1856–1940) in 1881 determined the ratio of the charge on a cathode particle to its mass. He first called these 'corpuscles'. Measurement of the electronic charge was made by an Irish physicist, Sir John Sealy Edward Townsend (1868–1957) from Galway in 1897.

Electrophoresis A process of analysis based on the mobility of different substances in an electric field. Described by Arne Wilhelm Tiselius (1902–1971) of Stockholm in 1930. It was simplified in 1944 by Richard Laurence Millington Synge (1914), A.H. Gordon and John Porter Archer who used water on cellulose (filter paper) as a medium. Charles Dent, professor of metabolism at the University of London, used the technique to identify 60 different amino acids in 1948. Gel electrophoresis was used to assay the variation in protein sequences by New York geneticist, Richard Charles Lewontin (b 1929), in 1966. Pulse field gel electrophoresis for separation of large DNA molecules was developed by another New York geneticist, Charles Robert Cantor (b 1942) at the University of California, Berkeley. His method became an essential tool in the study of DNA in chromosomes.

Electrophysiological Studies of the Heart *See electrocardiography.*

Electrophysiology Irritability as the hallmark of living tissue was demonstrated by Francis Glisson (1597–1677), professor of physick at Cambridge in 1677. The distinction between irritability and sensitivity of living tissue was made by Albrecht von Haller (1708–1777) in 1756. Luigi Galvani (1737–1798) in 1790 showed that electrical stimulation applied to the exposed spinal cord of the frog produced contraction of the skeletal muscle and this laid the foundation for electrophysiology. In 1838 Carlo Matteucci (1811–1868), an Italian physiologist, showed that current could be made to flow from the cut end of an isolated muscle to its uncut surface if these points were connected by a galvanometer. Emil Heinrich du Bois Reymond (1818–1896), an Italian electrophysiologist, demonstrated around 1840 that the electrical state of the nerve changed when a current was passed through it. The all-or-none phenomenon, which states that once the threshold of a stimulus was reached, the response was independent of the size of the stimulus, was proposed by the American physiologist Henry Pickering Bowditch (1840–1911) in 1871. Other pioneering work was done by Wilhelm Biedermann (1852–1929), and his extensive treatise, *Elektrophysiologie,* was published in 1895. *See all-or-none phenomenon.*

Electrotherapy The earliest form of electrotherapy for neuralgia and headache involved the torpedo fish, which has electrical properties, and was done by Dioscorides in the 1st century. The Roman physician to Claudius, Scribonius Largus (AD 45), also used electricity from the ray fish to treat headache. The first application of galvanic current in therapeutics was by Carl Johann Christian Grapengiesser (1764–1846) of Berlin in 1801. Further work was done by Joseph Constantine Carpue (1764–1846) in 1803. Static electricity was employed in treatment of nervous diseases in England by Thomas Addison (1793 1860) in 1837. A. Becquerel introduced the use of current for neuralgia in 1860. Samuel Gustav Crussel (1810–1858) in 1841 and Guillaume Benjamin Amand Duchenne of Bologne (1806–1875) in 1855 popularized its use in treatment. One of the earliest modern works, *A New Induction Current in Medical Electricity,* was published by William James Morton of New York in 1881. High frequency current was introduced by Arsene D'Arsonval (1851–1940) in 1887. *See electroconvulsive therapy (ECT), cardioversion.*

Elementary Education The Act of Elementary Education, passed in 1870, marked the starting point of the modern system of state education in England. It stated that the cost of education should be borne by the local rates except in areas where adequate schools existed through voluntary contributions.

Elements The concept of an element was proposed by Anaxagoras who lived around 500–427 BC, and the term was coined by Plato (428–348 BC). Empedocles proposed the theory of four elements – fire, air, earth and water – around 450 BC, at least half a century before Aristotle. Seven metallic elements were known to the ancients before the Christian era – gold, silver, copper, lead, tin, iron and mercury. The word was used in its modern scientific sense by Robert Boyle (1627–1691) in 1662. In 1789 Antoine Lavoisier (1743–1794) defined an element as 'a substance that cannot be split up into a simpler form by any means'. As science progressed, many substances that were thought to be elements were split up to reveal their compound nature. Sir Humphry Davy (1778–1829) decomposed caustic potash by electrolysis, and in 1783 Henry Cavendish (1731–1794) demonstrated that water is a compound and not an element, as was previously thought.

Elephant Discovery of fossilized bones of elephants was reported in Sussex, England in 1739. In 1820 exploration of caves at Kirkdale in Yorkshire by the geologist, William Buckland (1784–1856), revealed fossil remains of elephants that had lived before the catastrophic change in climate occurred. An anatomical treatise on it, *An Anatomical Account of the Elephant Accidentally Burnt* was published by A. Molyneux in 1696. Patrick Blair (1666–1728), a British physician, dissected one and published his work in 1710. *Some Anatomical Observations made upon the Elephant* was published by English physician, William Stukeley (1687–1765) from Lincolnshire in 1723. Work comparing fossil and modern elephants was done by the anatomist George Cuvier (1769–1832) in 1800.

Elephant Man Joseph Merick (1860–1890) was grossly deformed by neurofibromatosis and was exhibited to the public for a fee. He was rescued by the London surgeon Frederick Treves (1853–1923), and given a permanent place at the London Hospital. Treves wrote a biography of him, *Elephant Man* in 1923.

Elephantiasis [Greek: *elephas,* elephant] First mentioned by the Roman poet Carus Lucretius who said '*est eliphas morbus*' around 100 BC. Earlier references confused elephantiasis and leprosy, and Pliny stated that elephantiasis was not known in Italy until the days of Pompeii when it was imported from Egypt. Aulus Cornelius Celsus (25 BC–AD 50) considered it to be chronic and recommended remedies such as exercise, baths and rubbing of the body with pounded plantain. Aretaeus (*c* AD 100) gave a detailed description, and pointed out the resemblance of the eyebrows to the mane of a lion, hence the name, morbus leonicus. Aretaeus, Paul of Aegina (AD 625–690) and other ancient authors recommended the flesh of vipers in broth to be taken internally and applied externally. Galen (AD 129–200), in his *De Causis Morborum,* gave a vivid description of the facial features. According to him it was prevalent in Alexandria, owing to the high local temperature and food of the inhabitants. Acturius of Byzantine, around AD 1300, considered it to be a cancer of the whole body, and stated that lepra, elephantiasis, psora and impetigo were different grades of malignancy of the same disease. Avicenna (980–1037),

Serapion Junior or ibn Serabi (c 1070) and Avenzoar (1113–1162) described it as 'lepra'. Albucasis (AD 980) described four varieties, leonina, elephantia, serpatina and vulpia. Filariasis was known to the ancients, and Islamic physicians gave a good description as *da-al fil*, which meant elephantine disease. The Latin translation of the Arab work named it 'elephantiasis'. The term during modern times has been confined to infection by the filarial worm, *Filaria sanguinis-hominis* or *Wuchereria bancrofti*. See *filariasis, scrotal elephantiasis, leprosy*.

Eleventh Cranial Nerve *See spinal accessory nerve.*

d'Elhueyar y de Suvisa, Fausto (1755–1833) Spanish chemist who studied medicine at Paris before studying metallurgy. He isolated tungsten (named, wolfram) from wolframite with his brother Juan Jose, in 1790.

Elixir The term *al-iksir* was used by Arab alchemists to denote a medium through which transmutation was effected, and later believed to be connected to the attainment of eternal youth.

Ellenbog, Ulrich (1440–1499) Austrian physician who wrote the first book on toxicology and industrial hygiene in 1473.

Eller, John Theodore de Brockhusen (1689–1759) German physician from Anhalt, who studied under Hermann Boerhaave (1668–1738) in Leiden. He later became royal physician to the Prince of Anhalt and Frederick I, King of Prussia.

Ellermann, Wilhelm (1871–1924) Danish pathologist in Copenhagen who demonstrated that leukemia could be produced by a filterable agent in 1908. He also designed a skin test with tuberculin of various dilutions to gauge the severity of the disease.

Elliot Smith, Grafton (1871–1937) Australian anthropologist and neurologist who was a professor of anatomy in Cairo (1900), Manchester (1909) and University College (1919). He wrote *Human History* in 1930

Elliot, George Thompson (1851–1931) American dermatologist in New York who described the Elliot sign of induration at the periphery of certain syphilitic skin lesions.

Elliot, John (d 1787) Scottish physician from Peebles who joined a private warship as a physician and made his fortune.

Elliotson, John (1791–1868) Professor of surgery at the University of London who revived mesmerism and used it as a form of anesthesia during surgery. Owing to opposition from his peers, he resigned but continued to promote the practice of mesmerism. He was also one of the first physicians to use the stethoscope in clinical medicine.

Ellis, George Viner (1812–1900) Physician at University College London. He published *Demonstrations of Anatomy* in 1840.

Ellis, Henry Havelock (1859–1939) Psychologist from Croydon who studied medicine at St Thomas' Hospital, London. After a period in New South Wales, he graduated in medicine at the age of 30 years. However, he soon gave up his practice and turned to research and writing. He published *A Study of British Genius* in 1904, and *The Criminal* in 1910. He was a pioneer in the study of sexual psychology and published six volumes of *Studies in Psychology of Sex* (1899–1910), *Impressions and Comments* in three series (1914 to 1924), *Affirmations* (1898) and other works.

Ellis, Sir Arthur William Mickle (1883–1966) Canadian-born London physician who gave a classification of Bright disease based on clinical and histological features in 1942. He was the first professor of medicine at the London Hospital.

Ellis–van Creveld Syndrome A congenital condition associated with dyschondroplasia, polydactyly, ectodermal dysplasia and cardiac malformations. Described by British physician, Richard White Bernard Ellis (1902–1966) at Guy's Hospital and Dutch pediatrician, S. van Creveld (b 1894) in 1940.

Elman Test Used for quantitative analysis of serum amylase. Devised by American surgeon, Robert Elman (b 1897) in 1927. See *amylase*.

Eloy, Nicholas Francis Joseph (1714–1788) Born in Mons, a physician to Prince Charles of Lorraine. He wrote several medical treatises.

Elsberg, Charles Albert (1871–1948) American pioneer in neurosurgery in New York. He published several papers on olfactory sensation and vision in 1938. His first book on neurosurgery was published in 1916.

Elsholtz, Johann Sigmund (1623–1688) German physician who wrote an early treatise on blood transfusion in 1665. See *phosphorus*.

Elvejhem, Conrad (1901–1962) American biochemist, born and educated in Wisconsin. He demonstrated the effect of nicotinic acid in preventing pellagra in 1938. He also showed that elements such as copper, cobalt and zinc were essential to nutrition. See *nicotinic acid*.

Ely Sign A sign for detecting hip lesion or psoas muscle irritation by flexing the hip. Described by American orthopedic surgeon, Leonard Wheeler Ely (1868–1944) from San Francisco.

Elyot, Sir Thomas (1490–1546) A medical graduate from Oxford who, for a time, was an ambassador to the Court of Charles V. He wrote *The Boke named the Governour* in 1531, which was the first treatise on ethics in English, and *Castel of Helth* in 1539, which contained prescriptions for various ailments, some of which he himself suffered.

Embalmer In ancient Egypt they were probably members of the medical profession as well as priests. According to Pliny (AD 29–79) they examined bodies during the process of embalming and made a study of the diseases from which the person had died. They also had a high degree of knowledge of anatomy and individually embalmed separate organs, such as the intestines, and described them. *See embalming.*

Embalming In Egypt, this originated from the belief that the soul could return to its body, if the body was well preserved. In Israel too physicians embalmed bodies around 1600 BC. A pioneer of modern embalming was Frederik Ruysch (1638–1731), professor of anatomy in Amsterdam from 1666 to 1731. The famous English surgeon, John Hunter (1728–1793), practiced Ruysch's art of embalming by injecting camphorated spirits of wine into arteries and veins. A book on the subject, *The Art of Embalming,* was published by Thomas Greenhill, a surgeon who practiced in Bloomsbury, London in 1730. *See embalmer.*

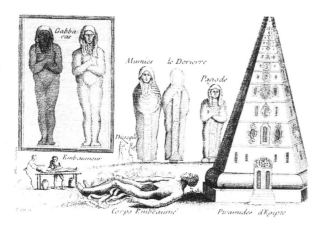

Egyptian embalming practices. Courtesy of the National Library of Medicine

Embolectomy [Greek: *embolos*, plug + *ektome*, excision] The first attempt at pulmonary embolectomy was made by Friedrich Trendelenburg (1844–1924) in 1908. The procedure he described (Tredelenburg operation) was successfully carried out 16 years later by Martin Kirschner

(1879–1942) in 1924. A successful embolectomy of the femoral artery was performed by Einar Samuel Henrick Key (1872–1954) of Germany in 1912, and aortic embolectomy was performed a year later by Fritz Baur. Arterial embolectomy through a balloon catheter was devised by Thomas Fogarty and colleagues in 1963.

Embolic Nephritis Hematuria with focal glomerular lesions in the kidney due to minute bacterial emboli from endocardial vegetations in bacterial endocarditis. Observed by Max Hermann Friedrich Loehlein (1877–1921) of Leipzig in 1907. It was described earlier as hemorrhagic nephritis by Harbitz of Germany in 1899. Emanuel Libman (1872–1946) referred to the lesions as 'embolic glomerular lesions of subacute bacterial endocarditis' in 1923.

Embolism [Greek: *embolos*, plug] The term to denote detached blood clots which blocked blood vessels was first used by Rudolph Virchow (1821–1902) in 1848. Charles Delucina Meigs (1792–1869), professor of midwifery at Jefferson Medical College, was the first to recognize it as a cause of maternal death, in 1849. Cardiac source of emboli was noted by William Senhouse Kirkes (1823–1864), a physician at St Bartholomew's Hospital in *On some of the Principal Effects from the Fibrinous Deposits from the Interior of the Heart* in 1852. Diagnosis of mesenteric embolism in a living subject was made by Adolf Kussmaul (1822–1909) in 1864. Fat embolism due to fractured bones or as a result of orthopedic operations was observed by H. L. Davis and C. G. Goodchild in 1936. *See embolectomy.*

Embryology [Greek: *em*, within + *bryein*, to swell + *logos*, discourse] A study of embryos was performed by Aristotle and he described them in *De Generatione Animalium* around 350 BC. The term was first admitted into the French language by the Academie in 1762, and came into English use in the 19th century. Several structures, such as the ductus arteriosus and heart valves, were described during embryonic development by Giulio Cesare Aranzio (1530–1589) in 1564. Fabricius ab Aquapendente (1533–1619), a pupil of Gabriele Falloppio (1523–1562), made his largest contribution to embryology with his work on its development in lower animals. He was also probably the first to describe the uterine decidua. His work on embryology *De Formato Foetu* was published in 1600. Caspar Friedrich Wolff (1733–1794) of Berlin, at the age of 26 years, published *Theorica Generiationis* in 1759, which ended the preformation theory and opened the doors to modern embryology. Wolff's work was opposed by many learned men, including Albrecht Haller (1708–1777) who supported the preformation theory. The human ovum was described in 1827 by Karl Ernst von Baer (1792–1876) of Estonia, who also discovered the notochord and established the theory of germ cell layers. The segmentation of the frog's ovum was described by Jean Louis Prevost (1790–1850) in 1827. A book on comparative embryology was written by Rudolph Albert von Kolliker (1871–1905), and a classic work was produced by Wilhelm His (1831–1904) in 1874. Ernst Heinrich Phillip August Haeckel (1834–1919) of Jena, an embryologist and founder of modern morphology, published *Anthropogenie*, another classic treatise, in 1875. The union of the spermatozoon and the ovum was described by August Oscar Hertwig (1849–1922) in 1876, and the youngest human embryo of 13 days was described by Hungarian gynecologist, Peters Hubert in 1899. The first work on experimental embryology in English was published by Thomas Hunt Morgan (1866–1945) in 1897.

Emergency Medical Services *See Accident and Emergency services.*

Emerson, Gladys Anderson (b 1903) American biochemist from Caldwell, Kansas, whose main research was on nutrition. She isolated vitamin E in a pure form and studied diseases caused by vitamin B complex deficiency. She was professor of nutrition at the University of California in Los Angeles in 1956.

Emery Test A modified Wasserman test for syphilis. Devised by English physician, D. Walter Emery (1870–1923), in 1910.

Emesis [Greek: *emein*, to vomit] Vomiting was used in the past for getting rid of excess humors of the body. A painting from 500 BC, showing this treatment in a young man, can be seen at the Martin von Wagner Museum at Würzburg University. *See hematemesis, hyperemesis.*

Emetine Joseph Pelletier (1788–1842) French chemist in Paris, while working with François Magendie (1783–1855) and Joseph Bienaime Caventou (1795–1877), isolated the alkaloid emetine from ipecacuanha imported from South America, in 1817. Sir Leonard Rogers (1868–1962), a London pathologist, was the first to prescribe it as treatment in amebiasis. The curative effect against schistosomiasis was demonstrated in 1913.

EMG *See electromyogram.*

Emin Pasha (1840–1892) German physician of Jewish origin who practiced at Scutari. He was known in his country as Eduard Schnitzer before he converted to the Muslim religion. He was chief medical officer to the equatorial province and later became its governor. He wrote several valuable treatises on geography and traveled extensively

in the Middle East and Africa until he was killed by Arabs in Manyema.

Emmons Method Used for determining cell diameter and devised in 1927 by Canadian physician, Frank Williams Emmons (b 1896).

Emmons, Wilson Chester (1900–1985) The first trained mycologist to be employed by the United States Department of Health. He proposed a generic classification of dermatophytes in 1934.

Emotions Charles Darwin (1809–1882) in his *Expressions of the Emotions in Man and Animals* published in 1872 arrived at the conclusion that 'the expressive actions exhibited by man and the lower animals are innate or inherited'. William James (1842–1910), an American psychologist of Harvard University, in 1884 proposed the theory of emotion, in which he explained emotional experience in terms of bodily accompaniments.

Empedocles of Agrigentum A pupil of Pythagoras (530–586 BC), he was a physician, philosopher and poet. He and Alcmaeon enunciated the doctrine of the four elements: earth, water, fire and air. He also proposed the theory of respiration, sight and hearing in relation to the function of the brain. The concept that life was a gradual process and that plants evolved before animals, and imperfect forms were gradually replaced by perfect forms, was proposed by him. This earned him the title of the first evolutionist. He was also the first to demonstrate that air has weight.

Empirics The School of Empirics was founded in Greece during the immediate post-Hippocratic times by the Greek philosopher, Pyrrho (d 288 BC) of Elis. It was born out of Skepticism and was based on the principle that there is no certainty of anything, no true knowledge of phenomena, and that experience alone can be the guide.

Emphysema [Greek: *em*, into + *physa*, bellows] Term used by many ancient physicians including Galen (129–200) to denote a collection of flatulent spirits (air or gas) in any organ, such as the skin, muscle or intestine. The earliest pathological account of emphysema of the lung was given by Sir John Floyer (1649–1734) in 1698. Since Floyer himself suffered from it he was able to give a classic description. John Millar (1733–1805) described it in 1769. A post-mortem account of the emphysematous appearance of the lung in asthma was given by Sir William Watson (1715–1787) in 1746. A clinical description in chronic obstructive pulmonary disease was given by Matthew Baillie (1760–1823) in 1797. He had published *Morbid Anatomy* in 1793, which contained illustrations of emphysema of the lungs at the postmortem of Samuel Johnson (1709–1784). The role of straining or coughing as a cause was proposed by Sir William Jenner (1815–1898) in 1845. Pearson Irvine in 1877 contended that it was mainly due to bronchial pressure. Inspiratory distension due to bronchitis as a predisposing cause was suggested by McVail of Glasgow in 1884.

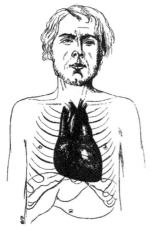

Position of heart and blood vessels in emphysema. J. Russel Reynolds, *A System of Medicine* (1877). MacMillan, London

Empyema [Greek: *em*, in + *pyos*, pus] Hippocrates, in his book of prognostics, gave a striking picture of empyema and recommended an incision be made into the chest wall to drain the fluid. This was probably the first description of paracentesis thoracis. Although Aretaeus, around AD 150, gave a good description of empyema thoracis, he recommended conservative management and mentioned that pus may be evacuated by communicating with the windpipe. Like many other ancient physicians of his time he also advocated diet and a sea voyage as treatment. The value of milk in empyema and phthisis was stressed since ancient times, and Galen (129–200) wrote 'ancients let consumptive patients suck a woman'. Cautery or burning of the chest wall was recommended as treatment by Galen and Paul of Aegina (AD 625–690). Avezoar (1113–1162) practiced cautery and paracentesis of the chest. Paul of Aegina stated that it is formed in the cavities of the chest or pleura, and described its symptoms as 'weight in the chest, an intense dry cough with pain and sometimes with fluid, and attacks of fever'. Thoracotomy, initially recommended by Hippocrates, was revived by Ernest George Ferdinand von Kuster (1839–1930) in 1889. Continuous aspiration was introduced by an English surgeon, Frederick Charles Cresswell Hewitt in 1876. Extensive rib resection was performed by Max Schede in 1890, and decortication of the lung was performed by Edmond Delorme (1847–1929) in 1894.

Emulsification The principle was unknowingly used by the ancients when they used fine earth for washing. The most common use of it in modern times is in soap. The behavior of emulsions in relation to solubility and surface tension was studied independently by: American colloid chemist, Wilder D. Bancroft, J.H. Hildebrand of California and W.D. Harkins of Chicago. The solubility theory was proposed by Bancroft in 1913, and the molecular-wedge hypothesis was put forward by Harkins and Hildebrand in 1923. A novel way of forming emulsions using ultrasonic waves was invented in 1923 by a French physicist, Langevin.

Emulsin Albuminoid material which catalyzed hydrolysis of the glucoside, amygdalin. Isolated from bitter almonds by Jean Pierre Robiquet (1780–1840) in 1813. Justus von Liebig (1803–1873) and Friedrich Wohler (1800–1882) studied it and named it emulsin in 1837.

Emulsion *See emulsification.*

Enalapril *See angiotensin converting enzyme inhibitors.*

Encephalitis Lethargica [Greek: *enkephalos*, brain + *itis*, inflammation] Although it was probably noted in the 16th century, it received attention only in 1917 when cases began to appear in Austria and France. In the 1920s an epidemic occurred on a worldwide basis. The first cases in Austria were described by Austrian neurologist, K. von Economo (1876–1931) in 1917, and it was named after him. It had a mortality of about 50%, but a number of patients with non-fatal disease later developed parkinsonism. The epidemic waned around 1928 and disappeared by 1930. The dramatic beneficial effect of the drug L-Dopa on patients with post-encephalitic parkinsonism was shown by British neurologist, Oliver Sacks (b 1933) in the 1960s.

Encephalography [Greek: *enkephalos*, brain + *graphein*, to write] A method of radiologically visualizing the spinal cord and ventricles by introducing air through a lumbar puncture. Devised by Walter Edward Dandy (1886–1946) of Missouri who was professor of neurosurgery at Johns Hopkins, and Erik Lysholm (1891–1947) in 1918. *See air ventriculography.*

Encyclopedia The first encyclopedia of medicine and natural science was compiled by Pliny the Elder in the 1st century. It contained over 20,000 entries compiled from over 2000 books and has continued to be quoted. Bishop Isidore of Seville (AD 560–636) produced an encyclopedia of all sciences which was widely used for centuries. Other similar books were produced by Alcuin (735–804) and Rabanus Maurus (776–876) of Germany. French Dominican monk, Vincent de Beauvais (1190–1264) under the patronage of Louis IX, gathered knowledge of the

Middle Ages in his *Speculum Majus.* Another voluminous encyclopedic work consisting of 12 folio volumes covering animal, vegetable and mineral subjects was produced by Ulyssi Aldrovando (1522–1605) of Bologna in 1598. *Lexicon Technicum,* which contained details of over 8000 scientific terms, was published by English mathematician and divine, John Harris (d 1719) in 1704. *Encyclopaedia Britannica* was published in three volumes in 1771. Other encyclopedias of medicine published in the 19th century include: *Cyclopaedia of Practical Medicine* by Sir John Forbes (1787–1861); another by R.B. Todd, from 1835 to 1859; *Dictionaries des Science Medicales* in 60 volumes by Charles L.F. Panckoucke, *A Dictionary of Practical Medicine* by James Copeland of Orkney. One of the most quoted dictionaries of the late 19th century was that of Richard Quain (1816–1898) which appeared in 1882.

End Artery Term introduced by Julius Friedrich Cohnheim (1839–1884) in 1860 to denote an artery which was essential for a circumscribed area. If the artery were occluded the area would die.

Endarterectomy [Greek: *endo,* within; Latin: *arteria,* artery; Greek: *ektome,* excision] *See carotid endarterectomy.*

Endarteritis Obliterans [Greek: *endo,* within + *itis,* inflammation; Latin: *arteria,* artery + *oblitaratus,* erased] *See Buerger disease.*

Endemic Typhus [Greek: *en,* in + *demos,* people] *See murine typhus.*

Enders, John Franklin (1897–1985) American bacteriologist from Hartford, Connecticut, who studied bacteriology. He cultivated the polio virus in human tissue at his laboratory for poliomyelitis research which he founded in 1946. His work led to the development of the polio vaccine by Jonas Salk, and he was awarded the Nobel Prize for Physiology or Medicine in 1954. He also developed a vaccine for measles in 1962.

Endocarditis [Greek: *endo,* within + *kardia,* heart + *itis,* inflammation] Early pathological observations on rheumatic carditis were made by Raymond de Vieussens (1641–1715), Lazarus Riverius (1589–1655) and Giovanni Battista Morgagni (1682–1771) in 1761. John Hunter (1728–1793) gave a classic description of the specimens of mitral and aortic disease in his museum. The term 'rheumatic' was applied to the heart disease by David Pitcairn (1749–1809) in 1788. English physician, David Dundas, did pioneer work on rheumatic diseases of the heart and published *An account of Peculiar Diseases of the Heart* in 1808. The 'peculiar disease' he described was later recognized as rheumatic heart disease.

The term 'endocarditis' was used by Jean B. Bouillaud (1796–1881) in 1835. Jean Nicolas Corvisart (1755–1821) used the term 'vegetations' to refer to nodular valvular lesions which are now recognized to be of bacterial origin. Peripheral emboli caused by valvular vegetations were recognized by William Senhouse Kirkes (1823–1864) of England in 1842. Emanuel Frederick Hagbarth Winge (1827–1894) of Norway demonstrated the bacterial origin of ulcerative endocarditis in 1869. Hematuria with specific focal glomerular lesions in the kidney due to minute bacterial emboli from endocardial vegetations in bacterial endocarditis was observed by Max Hermann Friedrich Löhlein (1877–1921) in 1910. It was also observed and described as hemorrhagic nephritis by Harbitz of Germany in 1899. New York physician, Emanuel Libman (1872–1946), later referred to the lesions as 'embolic glomerular lesions of subacute bacterial endocarditis' in 1923. *See subacute bacterial endocarditis.*

Endocardium [Greek: *endo,* within + *kardia,* heart] The inner lining of the heart, named by Jean Bouillaud (1796–1881) in 1835. *See endocarditis.*

Endocrinology [Greek: *endo,* within + *krineien,* to separate + *logos,* discourse] A pioneer was Swiss anatomist, Johann Conrad Brunner (1653–1727). He produced the symptoms of thirst and polyuria indicative of diabetes in dogs by surgical excision of their pancreas and published *Glandula Pituitaria* in 1688. His *Glandula Duodeni seu pancreas Secundum detectum* was published in 1715. The concept of internal or endocrine secretion, in which an organ or tissue discharges its secretion directly into the bloodstream to influence other parts of the body, was proposed by Théophile de Bordeu (1722–1776) of Paris in 1775. Scientific evidence of a humoral substance that produced an effect on a site or organ remote from its origin was presented by Arnold Adolph Berthhold (1803–1861) of Göttingen in 1849. He transplanted the testis to a rooster which previously had its testis removed and showed normal resumption of male sexual characteristics. George Oliver (1841–1915) and Edward Sharpey-Schafer (1850–1935) in England in 1895 demonstrated that extracts of the suprarenal gland, when injected intravenously, produced a contraction of the arteries and acceleration of the heart rate, thereby increasing blood pressure. The active substance in their extract was named 'adrenaline' in England. John Jacob Abel (1857–1938) of Johns Hopkins Medical School independently isolated the same active substance in 1899 and called it 'epinephrine'. William M. Bayliss (1860–1924) and Ernest Henry Starling (1866–1927) in 1902 obtained a substance from the intestinal mucous membrane which had a remote action on the pancreas. They named it 'secretin', and coined the term 'hormone' to denote similar substances. Fuller Albright (1900– 1969), known as the father of endocrinology in America, did most of his work on the subject at the Massachusetts General Hospital in the early 1900s. His main interests were bone diseases and the parathyroid gland and he described vitamin D-resistant rickets, osteomalacia of steatorrhea, idiopathic hypoparathyroidism, bone changes in kidney disease and other important endocrinological entities. Endocrinology in America received a definite footing with the formation of the Association for the Study of Internal Secretions in 1917, and its official publication *Endocrinology* appeared in the same year. *Journal of Clinical Endocrinology* was founded in America in 1941, and was renamed *The Journal of Clinical Endocrinology and Metabolism* in 1952. In England the *Journal of Endocrinology* was founded in 1938 and the Society for Endocrinology was formed in 1946. *See ductless glands, internal secretions, hormones.*

Endoderm [Greek: *endo*, within + *derma*, skin] The concept of the embryonic development of organs from different germ layers was proposed in 1828 by Carl Ernst von Baer (1792–1876), a professor at St Petersburg. The germ layers were classified into ectoderm, endoderm and mesoderm by Robert Remak (1815–1865) in 1845.

Endometriosis [Greek: *en*, within + *metra*, womb + *osis*, condition] Ovarian endometriosis was described by W.W. Russel in 1898 and D.B. Casler at Johns Hopkins in 1919. A detailed account of pelvic endometriosis was given in 1921 by New York gynecologist, John Albertson Sampson (1873–1946).

Endometrium The normal cyclical changes in the endometrium, previously thought to be due to inflammation, were described by two Viennese gynecologists, Ludwig Adler (1876–1958) and Fritz Hitschmann (1870–1926) in 1907.

Endomixis [Greek: *endo*, within + *mixis*, mixing] A process of replacement of a macronucleus by a micronucleus in infusoria was described by Woodruff in 1917.

Endomyocardial Fibrosis [Greek: *endo*, within + *mys*, muscle + *kardia*, heart; Latin: *fibra*, band] A fatal form of fibrosis of the endocardium leading to intractable heart failure (Davies disease) was described in children and young adults in Uganda by J.N.P. Davies, in 1948.

Endonucleases Bacterial enzymes capable of splitting DNA strands. Isolated and demonstrated by New York biochemist, Hamilton Othaniel Smith (b 1931).

Endoscopy [Greek: *endo*, within + *skopein*, to look] The first esophagoscopy was attempted by Adolf Kussmaul (1822–1902) in 1868. He used a modified Desomeaux urethroscope to diagnose a case of carcinoma of the esophagus. An early esophagoscope was invented by the English otorhinologist, Sir Morell Mackenzie (1837–1892) in 1880. New York physician, Max Einhorn (b 1862) in 1902 perfected an esophagoscope equipped with incandescent lighting. The first fiber optic instrument for transmission of light and images was devised and patented by John Logie Baird in 1928. A flexible fiber optic esophagoscope was described by P.A. LoPresti and A.M. Hilmi in 1964. The first flexible fiber optic endoscopy was performed on a patient in Michigan University by Hirschowitz in February 1957. *See fiber optic endoscopy.*

Endosmosis [Greek: *endo*, within + *osmos*, impulse] A process of attraction of a lighter medium to a denser medium through a membrane was described by René Jochium Henry Dutrochet (1776–1847) in 1826. If the movement took place from outside to inside he called it endosmosis and the reverse was named exosmosis.

Endospores [Greek: *endo*, within + *sporos*, seed] The formation of intracellular spores was observed by Ferdinand Julius Cohn (1828–1898) in 1875, and the process was studied in greater detail by Robert Koch (1843–1910) in 1876.

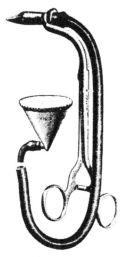

Funnel with tube for endotracheal anaesthesia. P J Flagg, *The Art of Anaesthesia* (1916). Lippincot, Philadelphia

Endotracheal Anesthesia [Greek: *endo*, within; Latin: *trachia*, windpipe] Andreas Vesalius (1514–1564) was the first to pass a tube into the trachea of an animal in 1542, and Robert Hook (1635–1703) gave a demonstration of the procedure before the Royal Society in 1587. London physician,

Charles Kite (1768–1811) of Gravesend described nasal and oral intubation for resuscitating those who were drowned in 1788. The endotracheal tube was introduced through a tracheostomy wound for inducing anesthesia in animals by John Snow (1813–1858) in 1858. German surgeon, Friedrich Trendelenburg (1844–1924) produced continuous anesthesia by tracheotomy and introducing a cannula with an inflatable cushion in 1873. Intubation of upper laryngeal orifice and trachea through the mouth was performed by a Glasgow surgeon, William Macewen (1848–1924), in 1878. Franz Kuhn (1866–1929) improved the technique using a flexible metal tube introduced with the use of a curved guide through the mouth in 1901. The use of ether for endotracheal insufflation was pioneered by Cassel of Germany in 1900 and Charles Albert Elsberg (b 1871) of New York in 1909. This method was further improved in the same year by Samuel James Meltzer (1851–1920) and John Auer (1875–1948) at the Rockefeller Institute, New York. Sir Robert Kelly (1879–1944), a Liverpool surgeon, following his visit to America in 1910, introduced the method into England. He also developed an apparatus to pass a mixture of warm moist air and ether down to the bifurcation of the trachea. His apparatus was modified by Francis Shipway (1875–1968) of Guy's Hospital in 1916. The use of endotracheal anesthesia was perfected by Sir Ivan Whiteside Magill (1888–1986) and he used it extensively in the treatment of facial injuries during World War 1. *See anesthesia.*

Endotracheal Intubation [Greek: *endo*, within; Late Latin: *trachia*, windpipe; Latin: *tuba*, a pipe] The first practical laryngoscope which enabled endotracheal intubation was designed by American laryngologist, Chevalier-Jackson (1865–1958) of Pittsburgh, and improved by Sir Ivan Whiteside Magill (1888–1986). Another laryngoscope was devised by Robert Reynolds Macintosh (b 1897), the first Nuffield professor of anesthetics at Oxford. His assistant, Freda Pratt Bannister helped to develop the direct laryngoscope and improved tracheal intubation in 1944. *See endotracheal anesthesia.*

Enema [Greek: *eniémi*, I throw in] The clyster was used in ancient times by the Greeks to administer astringents, emollients, nutrients, antihelmintics and antispasmodics. One of the earlier forms of enema was devised by the Mongols, who used a cow horn with a bladder fixed to its broad end to pump the medicinal substances.

Energy [Greek: *energein*, to be active] The term 'energy' to denote the present equivalent of kinetic energy was proposed in 1802 by English Quaker physician, Thomas Young (1773–1829). Pioneer work was done by the German physicist, Herman von Helmholtz (1821–1894) around 1850. The term was applied to cover a larger area in physics by Macquorn Rankine (1820–1872) in 1854. The word was used in the present scientific context later in the same year by Lord Kelvin (1824–1907).

Engelmann, Theodor Wilhelm (1843–1909) Professor of biology in Berlin who described the transparent homogeneous layer found on either side of the Krause membrane in 1893.

Englisch, Josef (1835–1915) A physician in Vienna who described the petro-occipital venous sinus in 1863.

English, Thomas Dunn (1819–1902) American physician and playwright. He wrote over 50 plays, but he is known more for his poem, *Ben Bolt.*

Engraving Prints from engraved copper plates were made in Germany in 1450. Thomas Geminus, a London engraver and physician in the 16th century published one of the earliest English illustrated anatomical textbooks, *Compendiosa totius anatomie delinreato* in 1545. Other anatomists, such as Carlo Ruini (1530–1598), Bartholomew Eustachio (1524–1574) and Godfrey Bidloo (1649–1598), engraved their own plates. The method of engraving on glass started in the 18th century and was perfected by Bourdier of Paris in 1799.

Enkephalin Naturally occurring opiate-like analgesic substances in the body. Discovered and named by German biochemist, Hans Walther Kosterlitz (b 1903) from Heidelberg, who was professor of pharmacology at the University of Aberdeen in the late 1960s. Further advance was made by an American psychiatrist and pharmacologist, Solomon Halbert Snyder (b 1938) who demonstrated the presence of opiate receptors in nervous tissue in 1973.

Ent, Sir George (1604–1689) A physician from Sandwich, England, educated at Sidney College Cambridge and took his doctor's degree at Padua. He wrote *Apologia pro Circulatione Sanguinis* and other medical works, and was knighted by Charles II.

Enteric Cytopathogenic Human Orphan Viruses *See ECHO virus.*

Enteric Fever [Greek: *enteron*, gut] A term for typhoid, coined by Charles Ritchie (1799–1878) of England in 1846. A description of the epidemic illness was given by Thomas Willis (1671–1775) in 1659. The name 'typhoid' was used by Pierre Charles Alexander Louis (1787–1872) of Paris. He also described the occurrence of rose spots in the illness in 1829. The contagious nature was pointed out by an American physician, Nathan Smith (1762–1829) in

A Practical Essay on Typhus Fever, published in 1842. A clear differentiation between typhus and typhoid fever was made by Alexander Patrick Stewart (1813–1883) in 1840, and the causative organism, *Salmonella typhi,* was discovered by Carl Joseph Eberth (1835–1926) in 1880.

Enterocele [Greek: *enteron,* gut + *koilos,* hollow] Protrusion of the bowel occasioned by a rupture of the peritoneum, or relaxation of the muscle. Described by Paul of Aegina (625–690). When the intestines remained in the groin, he called it bubonocele, and when they descended into the scrotum he named it enterocele.

Enterotomy [Greek: *enteron,* gut + *tome,* cutting] A procedure for opening an obstructed bowel above the site of obstruction and allowing its contents to escape. First suggested by Mannoury in 1819. The procedure was first performed by Auguste Nelaton (1807–1873) of Paris in 1840.

Entomology [Greek: *entomon,* insect + *logos,* discourse] The study of insects. Established as a science by Jan Swammerdam (1637–1680), a Dutch naturalist and graduate in medicine from Leiden who was one of the first microscopists, and proposed a system of classification of insects. His *Historia insectorum generalis* was published in 1669. Another founding work, *Memoires pour servir a l historie des insectes,* was published by Antoine F. Rene de Reaumer (1683–1757) of La Rochelle in 1734, and a classification of insects was proposed by Carl Linnaeus (1707–1778) in 1739. An early English treatise, *The English Moths and Butterflies,* was written by Benjamin Wilkes in 1748. The Entomological Society was established in London in 1833.

Entropy [Greek: *en,* in + *tropein,* to turn] Term used to denote the degradation of energy in a closed system by Rudolf Clausius (1822–1888), professor of physics at Bonn and a contemporary of James Joule (1818–1889) in 1865.

Environmental Laws [French: *environ,* about] Several acts of Parliament were passed in Britain in the 19th century to preserve the environment. River Pollution Prevention Acts, to maintain the purity of lakes, canals, streams, waterways and rivers, were passed in 1876 and 1893. The Canal Boat Acts of 1877 and 1884 required that any boat used on water as a dwelling must be registered. The Alkali Acts to control emission of gases into the atmosphere were enacted in 1863 and 1874.

Enzyme [Greek: *en,* in + *zyme,* leaven] Term used in 1878 by Willy Kuhne (1821–1901) to denote a class of organic substances that activated a chemical change. The first enzyme, diastase or amylase, was isolated by Anselme Payen (1795–1871) in 1833. In 1897 Eduard Buchner (d 1917), professor of chemistry in Berlin, extracted zymase from yeast, and demonstrated that fermentation of sugar could be effected with it in the absence of living yeast cells. A crystalline form of the enzyme urease was prepared by James Batcheller Sumner (1887–1955) of Cornell University in 1926. The crystalline form of pepsin was prepared by John Howard Northrop (1891–1987), Wendell Meredith Stanley (1904–1971) and co-workers at the Rockefeller Institute in 1930. They received the Nobel Prize for their work on enzymes in 1946. The concept that specific genes control production of specific enzymes was developed by American biogeneticist, George Wells Beadle (1903–1989) around 1940. Existence of a complex between enzyme and substrate was shown in 1942 by American biophysicist Britton Chance (b 1913) of Pennsylvania, educated at the University of Cambridge in England.

Enzymology *See diagnostic enzymology, enzyme.*

Eocene Period [Greek: *eos,* dawn + *cene,* recent] A geological age in Earth history, identified and named by the British geologist, Charles Lyell (1797–1875), in 1833.

Eosinophilia [Greek: *eos,* dawn + *philein,* to love] *See tropical pulmonary eosinophilia.*

Eosinophilic Granuloma [Greek: *eos,* dawn + *philein,* to love; Latin: *granum,* grain] *See Wegener granulomatosis.*

Ephedrine A herbal drug called *Ma Hung,* obtained from *Ephedra.* First used by the Red Emperor of China for various ailments, such as breathing difficulties and fevers. For over 2000 years the ancient Chinese also used it for anaphylaxis. It was found to contain the alkaloid ephedrine. It was isolated from *Ephedra vulgaris* by Nagajosi Nagai (1844–1929) in 1887.

Ephesus A city in modern Turkey, founded by the Ionians in 1043 BC. It contained the famous temple of Diana and was the birthplace of Soranus, a surgeon in AD 200.

Epicharmus Poet, philosopher and disciple of Pythagoras (530–586 BC).

Epictatus Stoic philosopher who lived around the time of Emperor Nero (d AD 68) in Rome. He suggested the immortality of the soul, and was against suicide.

Epicurean Philosophy based on the teachings of Epicurus (341–271 BC) of Gargettus, near Athens. He stated that the greatest good, consisting of peace of mind came from virtue, and this prevented disquiet or unhappiness. The term was later adopted to represent deriving happiness from sensual pleasures.

Epicurus (341–271 BC) Greek philosopher from Gargettus, near Athens and the founder of the Epicurean School. *See Epicurean.*

Epidaurus Greek city-state in the Peloponnese, which was a center of the cult of Aesculapius in 600 BC. It had many sanitariums, one of which still remains, and had over 180 rooms, dormitories and a bathing complex.

Epidemic Louse-Borne Typhus *See typhus, factory fever.*

Epidemics [Greek: *epi*, upon + *demos*, people] Have been recorded since ancient times. The Greeks considered Apollo, the god of health, to be a bringer of pestilence. One of the earliest plagues struck around 1000 BC in Israel, killing over 50,000 people. Another started in Ethiopia and reached Athens around 430 BC, during the time of the Greek statesman, Pericles (d 429 BC). Hippocrates (460–377 BC) made no specific reference to this, although he wrote a treatise on epidemics. A description by the Greek historian Thucyclides (469–391 BC) of Athens, suggests that it may have been scarlet fever. A severe epidemic of malaria struck Rome in 100 BC, and another occurred in AD 79. Thereafter, several epidemics of malaria plagued Rome. The epidemic that occurred in AD 165 was described by Galen (AD 129–200), although he fled from Rome during it. From his description, many historians believe that this was the first outbreak of smallpox in Rome. An outbreak of bubonic plague, which started in Egypt, reached Rome around AD 540, killing over 10,000 people per day at its peak, and lasted for nearly 50 years. *See epidemiology, malaria, Asiatic cholera, bubonic plague.*

Epidemiology [Greek: *epi*, upon + *demos*, people + *logos*, treatise] The first scientific explanation and description of how a disease spreads from person to person, and from place to place, was given by a Danish physician, Peter Ludwig Panum (1820–1885). His report, submitted to the Danish government in 1847 on the epidemic of measles in the Faeroe Islands, is considered a classic. The first scientific work in England was done by John Snow (1813–1858), an anesthetist and epidemiologist. He started his medical studies in Newcastle Infirmary, where he developed his interest in the epidemiology of cholera. He moved to London in 1836 and graduated in medicine in 1844. During the cholera outbreaks of 1848 and 1854 in London, he carried out epidemiological investigations and traced the source of one of the outbreaks to a sewage-contaminated well in Soho. His pioneering work led to identification of other sources of cholera and helped to abort several epidemics. A historic view, *Epidemics and crowd diseases; an introduction to the history of epidemiology,* was published in 1935 by Major

Greenwood (1880–1949), professor of medical statistics and epidemi-ology at the London School of Hygiene and Tropical Medicine.

Epidermolysis Bullosa Autosomal recessive disease in which bullous lesions of the skin occur from minor trauma. Described in 1882 by German professor of medicine, Johannes Karl August Eugen Alfred Goldscheider (1858–1935) in Berlin.

Epididymis [Greek: *epi*, upon + *didymos*, double or twofold] The paired structure related to the testis was given its current name by Herophilus around 300 BC.

Epidural Anesthesia [Greek: *epi*, upon; Latin: *dura*, hard] J. Leonard Corning (185–1923) of America discovered that the introduction of a local anesthetic into the epidural space caused anesthesia of the spinal nerves in 1885. Papers on anesthesia produced by injection through the sacral hiatus were published by Fernard Cathelin (b 1873) of Paris in 1901 and A. Lawen in 1910. The first operative delivery in obstetrics under a spinal block was performed by Kreis in 1901. In 1909 W. von Stoeckel introduced the method of injecting cocaine into the extradural space via the sacral canal, and H. Schimpert of Germany used a segmental nerve block at the costal margin to reduce uterine pain in 1911. Fidel Pages Miraw (d 1924) from Lima was the first anesthetist to use the lumbar route, in 1921, and his method was revived by Achille Mario Dogliotti (1897–1966) of Milan in 1933. An accurate description of the nerve supply related to uterine pain was given by J.G.P. Cleland, who employed a series of paravertebral and low caudal blocks in obstetrics in 1933. It was successfully introduced into obstetric practice in the same year by Dogliotti. Peritoneal infiltration of the branches of the pudendal nerve, the perineal branches of the small sciatic nerve and the labial branch of the ilioinguinal nerve with novocaine for pelvic delivery, was described by C.P. Sheldon in the *New England Journal of Medicine* in March 1941, and the technique was used in England in 1945.

Epigenesis [Greek: *epi*, upon + *genesis*, descent] The theory that new structures arise in the course of development, as opposed to preformation theory, was put forward by Casper Friedrich Wolff (1733–1794) in 1759. *See preformation theory.*

Epiglottis [Greek: *epi*, upon + *glossa*, tongue] Its role in swallowing was first studied by the French physician François Magendie (1783–1855) from Bordeaux.

Epilation [Greek: *epi*, upon + *pilus*, hair] A method of treatment for ringworm infection, introduced during the late 18th century. Various methods were used to peel off the affected skin, which resulted in significant trauma. Leopold Freund (1868–1944) first observed the effect of X-rays on the skin in the condition in 1896, and R.J.A. Sabouraud (1864–1938) introduced epilation using X-rays in 1903. An X-ray apparatus for epilation was designed by A.L. Dean, who unfortunately died from X-ray injuries in 1904. The use of X-rays for epilation was continued up to the early 1920s.

Epilepsy [Greek: *epi*, upon + *lepsis*, seizing] (Syn. sacred disease, falling sickness) Hippocrates (460–377 BC) disputed the common belief that epilepsy or *morbus sacer* was due to demonic influence. He also pointed out that inferior animals such as goats suffered from it, and were found to have water in the brain. He believed that the attacks occurring before puberty were easier to cure than those occurring after puberty which were intractable. It was also paradoxically called the 'sacred disease' during these times and various amulets were used in treatment. The Roman poet, Carus Lucretius, gave an accurate description of the symptoms and signs around 50 BC. Aulus Cornelius Celsus (25 BC–AD 50) recommended bleeding and use of hellebore as treatment. Later in the same century Aretaeus dealt with acute and chronic epilepsy and mentioned the use of copper as a treatment. Agate was used by ancient physicians as a diagnostic test, as its smell was supposed to bring on an attack. The influence of the full moon on attacks was credited by several physicians, including Galen (AD 129–200) and Antyllus (*c* AD 250). Aurelianus Caelius, in the 4th century, gave a complete account in which he advocated a light diet, abstinence from wine, gentle exercise and a change of environment or sea voyage. He also denounced the practice of applying fire or other hot things to the head as treatment. The first monograph on it in English, *Cases of Epilepsy, Hysteric Fits, and St Vitus Dance, with the Process of Cure* (1746) was published by John Andree, a physician at the London Infirmary which later became the London Hospital. *See antiepileptics, sacred disease, grand mal, falling sickness, aura.*

Epiloia In 1880, Desire Magloire Bourneville (1840–1909), a physician in Paris, was the first to describe adenoma sebaceum associated with mental deficiency and epilepsy, also known as epiloia. *See adenoma sebaceum.*

Epinephrine [Greek: *epi*, upon + *nephros*, kidney] Chemical extraction of the active principle of the suprarenal gland was performed by John Jacob Abel (1857–1938) of Johns Hopkins Medical School in 1898. He named it 'epinephrine', known as adrenaline in England. Intracardiac injection as treatment for cardiac standstill was introduced in the early 1920s. *See Henry Dale, Ulf von Euler.*

Epinutin Diphenylhydantoin, introduced as treatment for epilepsy by Hiram Houston Merrit (1902–1979) and Tracy J. Putnam (B 1894) in 1938. *See antiepileptics.*

Epinyctides Described as a bad species of pustule by Paul of Aegina (625–690).

Epiploic [Greek: *epiloon*, net] The greater omentum was named epiploon by Galen (AD 129–200) because of its appearance of fat held in the form of a network on the blood vessels.

Episiotomy [Greek: *epi*, upon + *tome*, cutting] The first incision of a rigid perineum which was likely to tear during delivery of the child was performed by an obstetrician in Dublin, Sir Fielding Ould (1710–1789). The first in America was performed by Valentine Taliaferro in 1851.

Epispadias [Greek: *epi*, upon + *spadon*, rent] A congenital condition considered at one time to be incurable. First successfully treated using reversed flap surgery by Auguste Nelaton (1807–1873) of Paris in 1852. Another method of operative treatment was described in 1869 by Karl Thiersch (1822–1895), professor of surgery at Erlangen.

Epistaxis Profuse bleeding from the nose was thought by Hippocrates (460–377 BC) to be due to a disposition to convulsions, and he prescribed venesection as treatment. Galen (129–200) proposed that convulsions occurred as a result of undue application of cold to stop the bleeding. He also considered bleeding from the nose during fevers to be an unfavorable symptom. Aetius of Amida, around AD 600, recommended the encouragement of bleeding by irritating the nostrils with a stalk of grass. As recently as 1825 a chemist at Leamington was selling 'moss from a dead man's skull'. This, in a dried powdered form, was in use for centuries as snuff for treating epistaxis.

Epithelioma [Greek: *epi*, upon + *thele*, papilla] Term coined by Adolph Hanover (1814–1894) to denote the skin lesions which he observed in 1852.

Epithelium [Greek: *epi*, upon + *thele*, papilla] Term first used to refer to the skin on the papilla of the lips by Frederic Ruysch (1638–1731) in 1670. It was introduced into histology by Jacob Henle (1809–1885) in 1844.

Epizootic Lymphangitis [Greek: *epi*, upon + *zoon*, animal + *itis*, inflammation; Latin: *lympha*, water] A condition of horses caused by *Histoplasma farciminosus*, which reached England through army horses from South Africa during the Boer War. The first case was noted in Aldershot in 1902 and it led to other outbreaks.

Eppinger, Hans (1879–1946) Viennese physician who described the electrocardiographic changes of bundle branch block in 1910.

Epsom Salts The medicinal values of Epsom spring water was discovered during the time of Queen Elizabeth I in the 16th century, and the Epsom spa became famous in 1640. London physician, Nehemiah Grew (1641–1712), wrote a treatise on Epsom salts in 1675, and a factory to extract them was established in 1700. Their use as medicine was very popular during the 19th century.

Epstein, Alois (1849–1919) Pediatric professor from Prague who was director of the Children's Clinic in his city.

Epstein, Sir Michael Anthony (b 1921) English microbiologist, born in London and educated at Trinity College, Cambridge. He joined the Middlesex Medical School as a reader at the end of World War ll, and became professor of experimental pathology at the University of Bristol in 1968. He discovered a new virus, responsible for infectious mononucleosis as well as some forms of cancer, in 1964. This was the first virus found to be associated with cancer.

Epstein–Barr Virus The causative organism of infectious mononucleosis. Discovered by London microbiologist, Sir Michael Anthony Epstein (b 1921) and Yvonne M. Barr (b 1932) in 1964. Barr obtained her PhD from the University of London in 1966.

Equine Encephalomyelitis Observed as a summer illness affecting horses and mules in western and eastern parts of America, Venezuela and the Caribbean. K.F. Meyer and co-workers pointed out the possibility of it being transmitted to humans in 1931, and a large epidemic occurred amongst humans in north-central America and adjacent parts of Canada in 1941. Several strains of the causative virus were isolated from 1931 to 1938.

Erasistratus (340–257 BC) One of the first anatomists at the Alexandrian School, born at Iulis on the island of Ceos. His father was a physician to Seleucus I Nicator, the King of Syria. He was a pupil of Metrodorus, and son-in-law of Aristotle (384–322 BC) in Athens. He later studied medicine at Cos under a physician of the dogmatic sect, Prax-agorus, and joined the Alexandrian School where he started dissecting human bodies and accurately described complicated structures such as the convolutions and the ventricles of the brain. He was an able physician who described morbid hunger and named it 'bulimia'.

Eratosthenes (274–194 BC) A librarian at the University of Alexandria who made significant contributions to mathematics. He invented an instrument for duplicating the cube, measured the circumference of the Earth and calculated its distance from the sun and the moon using simple calculations. He estimated the distance from the Atlantic to the eastern ocean as 7800 miles, and the distance of Cinnamon Land, or Tabrobane (Sri Lanka), from Thule as 3800 miles. He was blinded by an eye disease and committed suicide.

Erb Palsy Brachial palsy. Described by the English obstetrician, William Smellie (1697–1763) and by Guillaume Duchenne (1806–1875) in 1855. Another account was given in 1874 by Wilhelm Erb (1840–1921) after whom it is named.

Erb, Wilhelm Heinrich (1840–1921) German neurologist from Bavaria, and professor at Heidelberg, who described brachial palsy in 1874 and syphilitic spinal paralysis in 1875. He discovered the absence of knee jerk in spinal syphilis. He developed electrotherapy as treatment for nervous diseases in 1882.

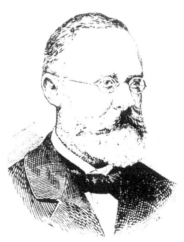

Wilhelm Heinrich Erb (1840–1921). Courtesy of the National Library of Medicine

Ercker, Lazarus (1530–1593) Bohemian metallurgist who wrote the first treatise on mining and metallurgical chemistry, *Bescherubung allerfurnemisten minerlischen Ertzt und Berkwerksarten,* in 1574. He was superintendent of the mines of the Holy Roman Empire and Bohemia, under Rudolf II.

Erdheim, Jakob (1874–1937) Physician from Vienna who described parathyroid adenoma in relation to osteomalacia in 1903.

Ergometrine Active extract of ergot, isolated by a London chemist, Harold Ward Dudley (1887–1935) and an English surgeon, John Chasser Moir (1900–1977), in 1935. Moir used it intravenously, before the delivery of the placenta in mothers, in 1943.

Ergosterol A phytosterol present in ergot, yeast and other fungi. Its antirachitic properties after irradiation with ultraviolet were demonstrated by Otto Rosenheim (1871–1955) and Thomas Arthur Webster in 1926. Robert Benedict Bourdillon (1889–1971) also showed its conversion to calciferol or vitamin D_2 after irradiation in 1929.

Ergotinine Discovered in 1888 by French physician, Charles Tanret (1847–1917), who isolated it from ergot of rye, *Claviceps purpurea.*

Ergot [Old French: *argot*, cock spur] The ancient Chinese knew of the abortifacient effect of the rye fungus, *Claviceps purpurea.* The first person to record its specific use in midwifery was Adam Lonicer of Frankfurt-am-Main in his *Krauterbuch,* published in 1582. It was used in obstetrics around 1770 in France, and was introduced into England for that purpose in 1807. John Stearns (1770–1848), the first President of the New York Academy of Medicine, introduced it into obstetrics in America in 1807. *See ergotamine, ergotism.*

Ergotamine [Old French: *argot*, cock spur; Greek: *ammoniakon,* resinous gum] First isolated from the fungus *Claviceps purpurea* by Karl Spiro (1867–1932) and Arthur Stoll (1887–1971) in 1921. Its action on the uterus was studied by Sir John Henry Gaddum (1900–1965) in 1926. Ergotamine tartrate was observed to relieve migraine by Tzanck in 1928. Its therapeutic use in migraine was shown by W.G. Lennox of America in 1934.

Ergotism [Old French: *argot*, cock spur] It was known as an obstetric remedy to the Chinese around 1000 BC. The use of barley in many ancient remedies suggests that the ergot fungus was unknowingly used by the ancients in childbirth and other conditions. The poisonous properties of molds growing on grain were described by Galen (129–200) who was probably the first physician to recognize the fungus. A reference to it in midwifery was made by Adam Lonicer or Lornicerus, a German botanist, in 1582. Casper Bauhin (1560–1624) described and illustrated the fungus. Epidemics of ergot poisoning due to infected rye or barley have been recorded since the Middle Ages. The first recorded outbreak occurred in France, at Limoges in AD 591. The symptoms of intense irritation and burning which led to dancing were interpreted as demonic possession. In 1085 Pope Urban II designated St Anthony as the saint against the disease and it came to be known as *ignus sacer* (holy fire) or St Anthony's fire. The first suggestion that it was due to contamination of rye by biological agents was made by the Parisian herbal physician Denis Dodart in 1676. In his letter to the Royal Academy of Sciences Paris, he pointed out that

degenerating rye contained an external agent. One of the last outbreaks in England occurred in Manchester in 1927. The fungus was named *Claviceps purpurea.*

Erichsen, Sir John Eric (1818–1896) Surgeon at University College, London, who described post-traumatic neurosis and whiplash injury following railway accidents, in 1866. He published *The Science and Art of Surgery* in 1853.

Erlanger, Joseph (1874–1965) American physiologist from San Francisco who was educated at Johns Hopkins Medical School. He became professor of physiology at Wisconsin in 1906, before he was appointed to the chair at Washington University, St Louis in 1910. He studied nerve conduction with Herbert Spencer Gasser (1888–1963) of the Rockefeller Institute, and proved that the velocity of the impulse was proportional to the diameter of the nerve fiber, for which he shared the Nobel Prize with Gasser in 1944. During his work on the heart, Erlanger tied the bundle of His and demonstrated various degrees of heart block.

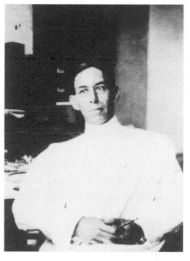

Joseph Erlanger (1874-1965). Courtesy of the National Library of Medicine

Ernest, Paul (1859–1937) *See Babes–Ernest granules.*

Erotomania [Greek: *eros,* love + *mania,* madness] *See nymphomania.*

Ersepeloid A description was given by the surgeon, Anton Julius Friedrich Rosenbach (1842–1923) at Göttingen.

Erysipelas [Greek: *erythros,* red + *pella,* skin] Hippocrates pointed out the danger of it being translated to internal parts, by which he probably meant septicemia. Galen (129–200) gave an extensive account of its symptoms and signs. He advocated various cataplasms as treatment. Serapion described it accurately as *al massire.* It was confused with ergotism in the 17th century and was also known as St Anthony's fire in England. The bacterial cause was discovered by Friedrich Fehleisen (1854–1924) in 1886.

Erythroblastosis Fetalis [Greek: *erythros*, red + *blastos*, bud] Hemolytic disease of the newborn. It was described by the Scottish pioneer of antenatal care, John William Ballantyne (1861–1923), in *Deformities of the Foetus*, published in 1895. It was first shown to be due to isoimmunization of the mother by a corpuscular factor (rhesus factor) in the fetus by Karl Landsteiner (1868–1943) and Alexander Solomon Wiener (b 1907) in 1940. The mechanism of production of hemolysis due to rhesus (Rh) incompatibility was further studied and explained by Philip Levine (1900–1987) and colleagues in 1941. Exchange transfusion as treatment was introduced by Louis Klein Diamond (b 1902) in 1948. Intrauterine transfusion of the fetus was pioneered by Albert William Liley of England in 1963.

Erythrocytosis [Greek: *erythros*, red + *kytos*, cell or hollow] Caused by renal disease, and described by German physician, Felix Gaisbock in 1922. The first clear evidence of the causal relationship between renal disease and erythrocytosis was provided by K.D. Fairley in 1945. He described two cases caused by renal carcinoma and demonstrated its remission by the removal of these tumors. Erythrocytosis due to massive renal cysts was shown by G.W. Cooper and W.B. Tuttle in 1957. Polycystic kidney causing it was described by C.W. Gurney in 1960.

Erythromelalgia Red neuralgia, a condition associated with painful feet. Mentioned by Robert Graves (1796–1853) in 1848. It was described in detail and named by American neurologist, Silas Weir Mitchell (1829–1914) of Philadelphia in 1872.

Erythromycin [Greek: *erythros*, red + *mykes*, fungus] Antibiotic first obtained from *Streptomyces erythreus* by James Myrlin McGuire and colleagues in 1952.

Erythropoiesis [Greek: *erythros*, red + *poiesis*, making] First shown to take place in the bone marrow, independently by Ernest Neumann (1834–1918) and Giulio Bizzozero (1846–1901), in 1868. *See erythoropoietin.*

Erythropoietin An increase in peripheral red blood cells in normal rabbits injected with plasma from rabbits made anemic through bleeding was shown by P. Carnot, professor of medicine in Paris, and G. Deflandre in 1906. They named the substance hemopoietin. As this humoral agent regulated erythropoiesis it was renamed erythropoietin by Finnish workers E. Bonsdorff and E. Jalavista in 1948. Kurt Reisman demonstrated it through his experiments in 1950, and his findings were confirmed by Erslev (1953) and Borsook

(1954). The first suggestion that it came from the kidneys was made by L.O. Jacobson in 1957. Naets showed its complete cessation in nephrectomized dogs in 1958. The first attempt to prepare it from renal tissue *in vitro* was made by D.G. Pennington in England in 1961. He also explained its role in the pathogenesis of anemia due to chronic renal failure earlier in the same year. It was prepared by a Polish worker, Z. Kuratowska, in 1964. *See erythrocytosis.*

Escherichia coli A bacterium named after the German bacteriologist, Theodore Escherich (1857–1911), who gave the first account of the bacillus infection in children in 1885.

Esmarch Bandage Made of rubber and used for application to limbs, especially to reduce blood loss. Designed by a military surgeon, Johann Friedrich August von Esmarch (1823–1908). He was born at Tonning in Schleswig-Holstein and graduated in medicine from Göttingen in 1848. He published *First Aid to the Injured* (1875) and *Bullet Wounds*. Through his second marriage to Princess Henriette von Schleswig-Holstein, he became the uncle of Emperor William II.

Esophageal Atresia Associated with tracheoesophageal fistula in a two-year-old baby was described by a physician-general to the army, Thomas Gibson (1647–1722), of Brampton, Westmoreland, in *Anatomy of Human Bodies Epitomized* published in 1697. Another English physician, William Durston, has also been credited with the first description of the condition in 1670. The esophageal lesion mentioned by Durston had only a vague resemblance to that described by Gibson. The next case was reported by a physician named Martin in 1821. A series of 43 cases was presented by Morrel MacKenzie (1837–1892) in 1884. Tracheoesophageal fistula without esophageal atresia was recognized by D.S. Lamb of Philadelphia in 1873. Gastrostomy as treatment was introduced into England by Steele in 1888. Sir Arthur Keith (1866–1955) traced 14 specimens in the London museums and gave an accurate description in 1910. A landmark in pediatric surgery was established when N Logan Levin (b 1902) and William E. Ladd (1880–1967) performed a multiple stage procedure to save two infants in 1939. The first successful anastomosis was performed by Cameron Haight (1901–1970) and Harry A. Towsley in 1941. P.M. Engel and co-workers in 1970 reported the first case of a woman with tracheoesophageal fistula who survived to adulthood and gave birth to a daughter with an identical lesion.

Esophageal Carcinoma Vincenz Czerny (1842–1916), an assistant to Theodore Billroth (1829–1894), performed the first resection of the cervical part of esophagus for carcinoma in 1877. Friedrich Voelcker (1872–1955) resected eso-phageal carcinoma through the abdominal route in 1908, and his technique was employed by Kummel (1910) and Bircher in 1918. Successful resection of thoracic esophagus for carcinoma was performed by a New York surgeon Franz Torek (1861–1938) in 1913. Following this, he constructed an artificial tube to connect the esophagus to the stomach, and his patient survived for 13 years without any recurrence of malignancy. No further surgical success was recorded until Grey Turner reported a case in 1933. Around this time, T. Ohsawa of Japan performed over 101 operations, although only 8 patients survived. The first successful esophageal resection and immediate anastomosis in England was performed by Russell Claude Brock (1903–1980) in 1942. The first successful resection and esophagogastrostomy for carcinoma of the lower end of the esophagus in England was performed by Vernon Thompson in 1945. A method of resecting carcinoma of the middle third of the esophagus was described by Ivor Lewis in 1946. *See esophagectomy.*

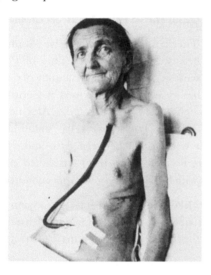

Esophageal carcinoma in Torek's first patient to be treated by resection of the middle third of the esophagus (1913)

Esophageal Manometry Performed in humans to study esophageal motility by Karl Hugo Krönecker (1839–1914) and Samuel James Meltzer (1851–1920) in 1884. Their work was revived by P. Kramer and F.J. Ingelfinger of Boston in 1949. A miniature recording device was designed by O.H. Gauer in 1950.

Esophageal Resection *See esophagectomy, esophageal carcinoma.*

Esophageal Rupture Emesis leading to a fatal rupture of the esophagus was described by Herman Boerhaave (1668–1738) in 1724. Hematemesis due to post-emetic

mucosal laceration of the lower end of the esophagus and gastric cardia was recognized by Boston pathologist, Kenneth G. Mallory (b 1900) and American physician, Konrad Weiss (1898–1942) in 1929. *See Boerhaave syndrome.*

Esophageal Sarcoma [Greek: *oisein*, to carry + *phagema*, food + *sarkos*, fleshy] Rare tumor investigated by Dvorak, who produced a series of 15 cases in 1931. Most were leiomyosarcomas or fibrosarcomas. D.E. Clarke recorded a successful resection of esophageal sarcoma in 1947.

Esophageal Stricture The first expanding dilator for treating esophageal stricture was developed by English physician, Josiah Cox Russel, in 1898. Another dilator made of metal was devised by American professor of medicine at the Mayo Foundation, Henry Stanley Plummer (1874–1937), in 1920. Gastrotomy in a case was performed in America by Frank Fontaine Maury (1840–1879) in 1870. New York surgeon, Robert Abbey (1851–1928), devised a method around 1890 of dilating it retrogradely, by opening the stomach to receive a 'string saw' through the buccal cavity to cut the remaining tissue contributing to the stricture.

Esophageal Varices Since Galen noted an instance of bleeding from the esophagus no specific mention of the condition was made until Antoine Portal (1742–1832) noticed the condition in 1803. Peter Frank (1745–1821) observed the relation of gastric hemorrhage secondary to portal hypertension in 1820. The first scientific account of hemorrhage from dilated esophageal veins was given by Karl Rokintansky (1804–1878) of Vienna in 1840.

Esophagectomy [Greek: *oisein*, to carry + *phagema*, food + *tomos*, to cut] Experimental resection of the esophagus in animals was done by Theodore Billroth (1829–1894) in 1871, and his assistant Vincenz Czerny (1842–1916) performed the first resection of the cervical part of esophagus for carcinoma in 1877. German surgeon, Friedrich Voelcker (1872–1955) resected esophageal carcinoma through an abdominal route in 1908. *See esophageal carcinoma.*

Esophagitis [Greek: *oisein*, to carry + *phagema*, food + *itis*, inflammation] *See reflux esophagitis.*

Esophagoscopy [Greek: *oisein*, to carry + *phagema*, food + *skopein*, to view] First use of an esophagoscope was reported in 1837 at the Edinburgh Royal Infirmary, to extract a padlock that had been swallowed. The instrument was specially devised by an instrument maker by the name of Macleod. An attempt to view the esophagus was made by two otorhinologists, F. Semeleder (1832–1901) and Karl Stoerk (1832–1899) of Vienna in 1866. Semeleder designed spoon-shaped forceps with a laryngeal mirror attached at one end, and offered himself as a subject for Stoerk to visualize his esophagus, but their efforts failed. An esophagoscope made of two telescopic metal tubes devised by Walderburg, was demonstrated by Stoerk at the Society of Physicians in Vienna in 1871. A speculum type was designed by the English otorhinologist, Sir Morell Mackenzie (1837–1892) in 1880, and the use of electric light to examine the esophagus was introduced by J. von Mikulicz-Radecki (1850–1905) in 1881. An attempt to introduce it into routine use was made by Adolf Kussmaul (1822–1902), who modified the Desomeaux urethroscope to diagnose a case of esophageal carcinoma in 1868. Max Einhorn (b-1862) perfected it with incandescent lighting in 1902. William Hill made a valuable contribution by adding a dilating speculum in 1918. A flexible fiber optic esophagoscope was described by P.A. LoPresti and A.M. Hilmi in 1964. *See fiber optic endoscopy.*

Esophagotomy [Greek: *oisein*, to carry + *phagema*, food + *tomos*, to cut] The first recorded procedure was performed by James Syme (1799–1870) to remove a mutton bone from the esophagus in 1861.

Esophagus [Greek: *oisein*, to carry + *phagema*, food] *See esophageal atresia, esophagitis, esophagoscopy, esophageal rupture, esophageal manometry, esophageal carcinoma.*

Esquirol, Jean Etienne Dominique (1772–1840) Born in Toulouse, a French physician and pioneer in mental disease. He was one of the first lecturers in psychiatry at the Salpêtrière in 1811. He was also one of the first to note adult psychiatric illnesses in children and to investigate dementia in senile states.

Essential Amino Acids Of the first 20 amino acids discovered, ten were found to be essential in rats by American biochemist, William Cumming Rose (1887–1984), in 1937. He later established that only eight were essential in humans. *See amino acids.*

Essential Fatty Acids The 'fat deficiency disease' in rats due to lack of certain unsaturated fatty acids was described by George Oswald Burr (b 1896) and Mildred M. Burr of America in 1929. These were identified as linoleic, linolenic and arachidonic acids, and were collectively named 'vitamin F'. Their role in human nutrition was shown by Ida Smedly-Maclean and colleagues in London in 1943. The different pathways of unsaturated and saturated fatty acids were demonstrated using deuterium, by a German-born American biochemist, Rudolf Schoenheimer (1898–1941) of Columbia University, in 1937.

Essential Hypertension The introduction of the sphygmomanometer into clinical medicine by Samuel Siegfried von Basch (1837–1905) in 1893 led to the recognition of 'essential hypertension'. He made over 100,000 blood pressure estimations and gave the name 'latent arteriosclerosis' to what is now known as essential hypertension. Continued hypertension as a cause of atherosclerosis was described by Henri Huchard (1844–1910) of Paris in 1887. The subject was extensively studied by Thomas Clifford Allbutt (1836–1925) in England around 1900, and Huchard in 1899. Theodore Caldwell Janeway (1872–1917) did work on it in America in 1904. The malignant phase was described by T. Fahr of Berlin in 1925. Racial predisposition was studied by Harris of America who found that it was rare in Chinese and Orientals, in 1927. He also found that it was rarely found in Africans, whereas it was very common in blacks living in cities of America. Nye in 1937 noted that hypertension was completely absent in Australian Aborigines. Sir George White Pickering (1904–1980), Regius professor of medicine at Oxford in 1956, pointed out the protein nature of renin and its role in hypertension. His important work, *The Nature of Hypertension*, was published in 1960.

Essential Unsaturated Fatty Acids *See essential fatty acids.*

Esthetics [Greek: *aisthenasthai*, to perceive] Study of perception of beauty, known since the time of Plato. In the modern sense, it denotes the critical study of perception or taste for beauty and art, and was used by German professor of philosophy at Frankfurt-an-Oder, Alexander Gottlieb Baumgarten (1714–1762). His unfinished treatise *Aesthetica* was written between 1750 and 1758. Gustav Theodore Fechner (1801–1887) established experimental esthetics with his *Vorschule der Aesthetik* published in 1876.

Estlander, Jakob August (1831–1881) A surgeon in Helsinki who described an operation for double harelip. He also resected the ribs lying over empyema (Estlander operation).

Estrogen [Greek: *oistros*, gadfly + *genos*, descent] In 1911 Eugen Steinach (1861–1944) successfully transplanted ovaries. Crude extracts of ovary and placenta were used to promote uterine growth by Adler in 1912. A method of extraction, quantitative assay and purification of female hormone preparations was announced by American physicians, Edgar van Nuys Allen (1900–1961) and Edward Adelbert Doisy (1893–1986) in 1923. Estrogen in pregnant urine was observed by Bernhardt Zondek (1891–1967) in 1927. Estrone, the first steroid hormone in a pure state, was extracted from urine in pregnancy independently by Doisy and Adolf Friedrich Johan Butenandt in 1929. In 1930 Selmar Asch-heim (1878–1965) and Zondek found pregnant mare's urine to be a better source and this led to commercial preparation of the hormone. Estriol was obtained from urine by Guy Frederick Marrian (1904–1981) of University College in 1930, and Doisy obtained estradiol from ovarian tissue in 1935. Progesterone was obtained from the corpus luteum of sow's ovaries by Butenandt in 1934. 50,000 sows were used to obtain 20 mg of pure progesterone and this motivated the search for synthetic estrogens. Sir Edward Charles Dodds (1899–1973) produced the synthetic estrogen, stilboestrol, in 1938. *See synthetic estrogen.*

Ethambutol A synthetic compound with antituberculous activity in mice. Discovered by J.P. Thomas and co-workers in America in 1961.

Ether 'Sweet oil of vitriol' (Syn. sulfuric ether). First prepared by treating oil of vitriol (sulfuric acid) with distilled sprits (alcohol) by Valerius Cordus (1515–1544) of Leipzig in 1540. In 1729 a German chemist distilled ether while he was working in London. Ernst Stahl (1660–1734) of Berlin also prepared it in 1731, and it came to be commonly known as sulfuric ether. The first mention of its use for relief of pain was made by Paracelsus (1493–1541) of Switzerland, who recommended its internal use in preference to opium. The first recorded use of ether as an anesthetic was by a student, William E. Clark of Berkshire Medical College. He administered it to a patient whose tooth was extracted by Elijah Pope of Rochester in 1842. It was next used as an inhalational anesthetic by an American, Crawford Williamson Long (1815–1878), in 1843, but he failed to publish his findings. Charles T. Jackson, a chemist in Boston, observed its anesthetic properties and conveyed his findings to William Thomas Green Morton (1819–1868), a dentist, in 1846. Morton then proposed it for surgical operations. A tumor in the neck of a patient was removed under its influence by a Boston surgeon, John Collins Warren (1778–1856) on 17 October 1846. It was first used as surgical anesthesia using Squire's inhaler in England in 1846 by Robert Liston (1794–1847) at University College Hospital. The first documented use of ether in England, however, was by Francis Boott a Boston-born physician who, on the advice given in a letter by the son of Henry Bigelow, professor of materia medica in Boston, used it in dental surgery two days before the demonstration by Liston. Joseph Malgaigne (1806–1865) used it in France in 1847. Its use in rectal anesthesia was demonstrated by the Russian surgeon, Nikolai Pirogoff (1810–1881) in 1847. Its use was limited owing to the damage caused to local tissues. Pirogoff later produced an apparatus to warm ether and introduce it in the form of vapor into the rectum. In 1855 Dudley Buxton devised an improved apparatus with a similar function but, again, the local side-effects continued to predominate. A new

technique of mixing ether with olive oil was introduced in 1913 by James T. Gwathmey (1863–1944), and this overcame the problem. Its use for endotracheal insufflation was pioneered by Cassel of Germany in 1900, and later by Charles A. Elsberg of New York in 1909. This method was improved by Samuel James Meltzer (1851–1920) and John Auer (1875–1948) at the Rockefeller Institute, New York. Sir Robert Ernest Kelly (1879–1944), a surgeon from Liverpool, following his visit to America in 1910, introduced the method into England. L. Burkhardt was the first to use intravenous anesthetics, chloroform and ether, in 1909. Kelly later developed an apparatus and it was modified by Francis Edward Shipway (1875–1968) of Guy's Hospital in 1916. Thomas Joseph Clover (1825–1882) further modernized the technique by introducing the Clover inhaler for administering ether and chloroform in 1876. English anesthetist, Sir Dennis Brown (1892–1967) designed the ether inhaler (Dennis Brown Inhaler) in 1928. *See anesthesia.*

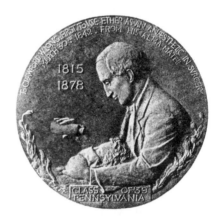

Crawford Williamson Long administering ether. Courtesy of the National Library of Medicine

Ether Theory In 1803, English physician, Thomas Young (1773–1829), proposed ether as a hypothetical invisible substance or medium in space through which light traveled in waves. In 1888 Albert A. Michelson (1852–1931) and his pupil Edward Williams Morley (1853–1923) attempted to determine the velocity of the Earth by measuring the velocity of light in relation to the ether. Their work showed that the velocity of light was the same in all directions and was independent of the motion of the Earth. In 1905 Albert Einstein (1879–1955) discarded the ether theory in his calculations and concluded that speed can be measured only in relation to another object.

Ethics of Human Experimentation The first directive on informed consent in human experimentation was issued by the Prussian Minister of the Interior in 1891. In his instructions to all prisons giving tuberculin as treatment for tuberculosis, he specified that it should not be given against the person's will. The case of Albert Neisser (1855–1916), the discoverer of the gonococcus and professor of venereology at Breslau, was one of the first to highlight the ethics related to human experimentation and informed consent. In 1898, in his search for a means of prevention of syphilis, Neisser injected the serum of syphilitic patients into patients who were admitted for other medical conditions, without informing them. Some of these patients developed syphilis and Neisser concluded that the serum was not effective. He claimed that the patients had contracted syphilis elsewhere. Neisser was investigated by the public prosecutor and was fined by the Royal Disciplinary Court. Following the publicity of this case, Albert Moll collected a list of over 600 such instances of unethical research in his *Physicians Ethics*. He also advocated the procedure of gaining informed consent for human experimentation. The Prussian Parliament debated the issue further and commissioned a report from the Scientific Medical Office of Health, which included Rudolph Virchow (1821–1902) and other eminent physicians. As a result of their work, regulations on human experiments based on ethics were issued by the government to all hospitals and clinics in 1900. The first document that outlined ethical regulations on human experimentation based on informed consent followed the Nuremberg medical trials in 1947. This Nuremberg Code laid down ten standards to which physicians were expected to conform when carrying out research on humans. The Declaration of Helsinki, which was derived from the Nuremberg Code, was passed by the World Medical Assembly in Helsinki in 1964. The Helsinki Declaration contained further guidelines on biomedical research involving human subjects.

Ethics The study of ideal conduct, classed as a branch of philosophy. The first treatise in English, *The Boke named the Gouernour*, was published in 1531 by English physician, Sir Thomas Elyot (1490–1546). One of the earliest books, *Ethics*, was written by Baruch Spinoza (1632–1677), a Dutch philosopher of Jewish descent in Amsterdam. Spinoza dealt with metaphysics, psychology and ethics. *See moral philosophy, ethics of human experimentation.*

Ethnology [Greek: *ethnos*, nation + *logos*, discourse] A branch of anthropology that deals with distinct characteristics of mankind, their modifications, and the causes of their distribution. *Researches on the Physical History of Mankind* by British physician and anthropologist, James Cowles Prichard (1786–1848) was an early treatise on the subject published in 1841. The Ethnological Society in England was established in 1843. R.G. Latham's, *Ethnology of the British*

Empire, appeared in 1851. A series of lectures was started at the Royal Institution by Thomas Huxley (1825–1895) in 1866.

Ethology The study of animal behavior. Developed by Austrian zoologist, Konrad Zacharias Lorenz (1903–1989). In *On Aggression* (1963), he argued that behavior in man is inherited and can be channeled to other productive activities. The behavior of humans was described by English ethologist, Desmond John Morris (b 1928) of Wiltshire in *The Naked Ape*, published in 1967. The first chair of ethology at Cambridge was created in 1966, to which William Homan Thorpe (1902–1986) was appointed. He wrote *Learning and Instincts in Animals* in 1956.

Ethryg or Etheridge, George (d 1588) Oxford physician who wrote *Hypomnemata, seu Observationes Medicamentorum quae hac aetate in ususunt.*

Ethylene Introduced as a general anesthetic by a Chicago surgeon Arno Benedict Luckhardt (b 1885) in 1923.

Etienne, Charles (1503–1564) Born in Paris, he was the first to detect the valves at the orifices of hepatic veins, and to describe the central canal of the spinal cord.

Etiology [Greek: *aitia*, cause + *logos*, discourse] Diseases were attributed to demons or divine forces during ancients times and Hippocrates (460–377 BC) set medicine on a scientific footing. The preformation theory and theory of spontaneous generation prevailed until the germ theory of disease began to appear in the 16th century. Girolamo Fracastro or Fracastorius (1478–1553), a physician of Verona, proposed a possible infectious etiology for diseases in *Contagium Vivum* published in 1546. Demonstration that disease is associated with living microorganisms was provided by Agostino Bassi (1773–1856) of Lodi with his work on silkworms in 1835. Puerperal fever was one of the first human diseases to be investigated for an infective cause. Oliver Wendell Holmes (1809–1894) pointed out the contagious nature of puerperal fever in *On the Contagiousness of Puerperal fever* in 1842 and Ignaz Semmelweiss (1818–1865) of Vienna demonstrated contamination as a cause of the disease in 1847. The germ theory was proved by Louis Pasteur (1822–1895). Study of occupation as a cause of disease was pioneered by Bernardino Ramazzini (1633–1714) in 1700. Chemicals as a cause of cancer and other diseases was recognized in the 18th century.

Etruscans Ancient indigenous people from Eturia in Italy, now known as Tuscany. They were a highly civilized race from whom the Romans derived most of their laws and customs. Some remarkable specimens of dental bridge work done by them before the Christian era are now preserved in the museum of Corneto.

Euclid A mathematician from Alexandria who lived around 300 BC. He wrote 13 books on mathematics containing problems with theorems and illustrations which remained as standard works on geometry for over 2000 years. He was held in high esteem by Plato and Ptolemy, who later became his pupil. An early translation of his work into Latin was by Gerard of Cremona (1147–1187), who obtained a thorough knowledge of Arabic at Toledo in central Spain. Another, *Elements,* from Arabic was by Adelard of Bath in 1142. The first printed mathematical book, a translation of Euclid's *Elements* was published by Johannes Campanus in 1482, and a Greek edition appeared in Basel in 1533.

Eudemius A Roman physician in 15 BC. He made observations on hydrophobia and pointed out its poor prognosis. He was executed by order of Tiberius.

Eudiometer An instrument to measure the purity or quantity of oxygen in air, devised by Joseph Priestley (1733–1804) in 1772.

Eudoxus (400–360 BC) A scientist and philosopher from Cnidos. He was a pupil of Plato (428–348 BC) and he learnt astronomy at Heliopolis in Egypt. He established a school and observatory at Cnidos, and proposed the theory of homoconcentric spheres, which exerted an immense influence on astronomy for the next 2000 years.

Eugenics [Greek: *eu,* well + *genos,* birth] Sir Francis Galton (1822–1911), a cousin of Charles Darwin (1809–1882), coined the term in 1883 to 'denote the study of agencies under social control that may improve or impair the racial qualities of future generations, either physically or mentally'. He tried to find an association between heredity and intelligence by measuring characteristics of parents and their offspring.

Euler, Ulf Svante von (1905–1983) Swedish pharmacologist and pioneer in neurotransmission, for which he was awarded the Nobel Prize in 1970. He observed raised levels of catecholamines in patients with pheochromocytoma in 1950. He isolated a biologically active lipid, which he named 'prostaglandin' in the belief that this lipid-soluble acid came from the prostate. The neurotransmitter of the sympathetic nervous system, noradrenaline, was isolated and studied by him in the 1940s.

Eunapius A physician and historian in the 4th century who wrote a book on ancient philosophers and a history of the Caesars.

Eunuch The practice of castration was known in China around 1100 BC. During the Roman era, according to Juvenal, women enjoyed sex with eunuchs to avoid pregnancy. Male castrati were used for their soprano voices up to the early 19th century in Europe.

Eurich, Frederick William (1867–1945) A physician at the Royal Bradford Infirmary who was the first to cultivate the anthrax bacillus from wool.

European Medicine Aesculapius, according to Greek legend, was the son of Apollo, the sun god, and Coronis, a mortal woman. Aesculapius was probably a man who lived around 1200 BC and came to be worshipped after his death. His priests practiced medicine which initially involved mysticism and magic, but later gave way to physical medicine, with baths in mineral springs, massage, blood letting and use of therapeutics such as iron, milk and honey. The first system of modern medicine was established by Hippocrates, from the Greek island of Cos, in 400 BC. Galen (129–200) greatly influenced the practice of medicine for hundreds of years. He explained bodily health on the basis of a system of four humors, did away with metallic remedies and promoted herbal cures. His system of medicine was supported by the church and remained unquestioned for 1500 years, until Paracelsus (1493–1541) rebelled against it. One of the main contributions of Paracelsus was his proposal of a specific remedy for each disease. He introduced mercury as treatment for syphilis. During the Middle Ages, from AD 900 to AD 1200, the Arabs dominated medicine. From the 15th century onwards, Europe took the lead with works of notable men such as Andreas Vesalius, Marcello Malpighi, William Harvey and Sanctorio Sanctorius.

Eurotransplant An organization for tissue typing potential donors and cadavers, to computer-match them with recipients. Established in Stockholm in 1966.

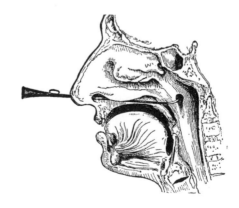

Catheter in Eustachian tube. George P. Field, *A Manual of Diseases of the Ear* (1894). Baillière, Tindall and Cox, London

Eustachian Tube A passage lined by mucosa connecting the middle ear with the nasopharynx. Described by Bartolommeo Eustachio (1524–1574), an Italian anatomist in 1562. Its role during swallowing was described in 1861 by Joseph Toynbee (1815–1866), the first aural surgeon at St Mary's Hospital, London.

Eustachio, Bartolommeo (1524–1574) Professor in Rome who completed a superb set of anatomical plates, *Tabulae Anatomica*, in 1552. His drawings remained unpublished in the Papal library until the Pope gave them to his physician, Giovanni Maria Lancisi (1654–1720). With the advice of Giovanni Battista Morgagni (1682–1771), he published them in 1714. These were the first anatomical plates to be produced on copper. He also discovered the Eustachian tube, the Eustachian valve in the fetus, the thoracic duct, the suprarenal bodies and the abducent nerve.

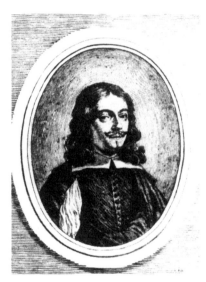

Eustachio (1534–1574). Courtesy of the National Library of Medicine

Eustachius, Ferdinand Son of the famous anatomist, Bartolommeo Eustachio (1524–1574). He maintained that medical art is of no use in prolonging life. He published *De vitae humane facultate medica prorogatione*, dedicated to Pope Sixtus V, in 1589.

Eutychius (AD 876–950) Christian physician in Cairo who wrote annals from the beginning of the world to AD 900.

Evan Syndrome Autoimmune hemolytic anemia and thrombocytopenia. Described in 1955 by American physician, Robert S. Evan of Seattle.

Evans Blue A diazo dye used to estimate blood volume and cardiac output. Developed by American physiologist, Herbert McLean Evans (1882–1971).

Evans, Dillwyn (1910–1974) British orthopedic surgeon from Cardiff. He described lateral wedge tarsectomy and medical release as treatment of clubfoot.

Evans, William Of the National Heart Hospital, London, he classified different types of stenosis and atresia of the aortic arch in 1933, and described familial cardiomegaly in 1949.

Eve, Frank Cecil (1871–1952) A physician at Hull, who described a method of artificial respiration as first aid in 1932.

Eve, Sir Frederick (1853–1916) English surgeon who described a case of intersigmoid hernia in 1880.

Evolution [Latin: *evolvere*, to unroll] The concept that plants evolved before animals, and imperfect forms were gradually replaced by perfect forms was proposed by Empedocles of Agrigentum around 450 BC. The Roman poet, Lucretius (98–55 BC) in his grand poem *De Rerum Natura*, written around 80 BC, reflected the principle of the survival of the fittest in life. Count Buffon, also known as George Louis Leclerc (1707–1788), proposed the idea of evolution by pointing out that life forms in the animal kingdom were successively derived from one another. He also suggested that the earliest life forms originated from the polar regions and the ocean. Pioneers of modern evolution theory were Herbert Spencer (1820–1903), Alfred Russell Wallace (1823–1913) and Charles Darwin (1809–1882). The phrase 'survival of the fittest' and the word 'evolution' were coined by Spencer. Both Wallace and Darwin drew their inspiration from the work of an English clergyman Thomas Robert Malthus (1766–1834) who wrote *An Essay on the Principle of Population or A View of its Past and Present Effects* in 1803. Malthus argued that the only limits to expansion of a population were space and food, implying the survival of the fittest. Although Darwin commenced his work in 1838, Wallace independently came to the same conclusion one year before Darwin published his work. Spencer proposed the concept of evolution in his article *The Development Hypothesis,* which appeared in the *Leader* in 1852. He suggested the possibility of transmutation of species. *On the Origin of Species by Natural Selection* was published by Darwin in 1859, after 20 years of work.

Ewald Test *See Ewald, Carl Anton.*

Ewald, Carl Anton (1845–1915) A gastroenterologist from Berlin who worked on secretions of the stomach, by intubation. He also designed the Ewald test meal, which was commonly used for gastric analysis during the 1940s. In this, various forms of food were given followed by analysis of the gastric aspirate at regular interval for the first two hours.

Ewart Sign Pulmonary collapse at the left base in pericardial effusion. Described in 1896 by English physician, William Ewart (1848–1929) at the Brompton Hospital for Consumption and Diseases of the Chest.

Ewing Sarcoma James Ewing (1866–1943), professor of oncology at Cornell University Medical College, New York City, described an endothelial tumor of the shaft of long bones in 1920 that now bears his name. His work against cancer was internationally recognized and he was portrayed on the cover of *Time* magazine. He published his important treatise, *Neoplastic Diseases,* in 1919.

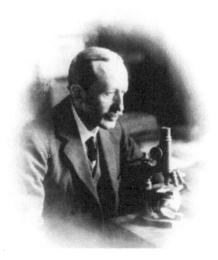

James Ewing (1866–1943). Courtesy of the National Library of Medicine

Ewins, Arthur James (1882–1957) English chemist, born in Norwood and educated at the Chelsea Polytechnic, London. He isolated the neurotransmitter acetylcholine with Henry Hallet Dale (1875–1958) in 1914. His work led to the development of the antibiotic, sulfapyridine, which was the first successful treatment for gonorrhea.

Exanthemata [Greek: *ex*, out of + *anthos*, flower] According to Galen (129–200), the term applied to all ulcerative and rough conditions of the skin. He also pointed it out as a common symptom of plague. Aetius of Amida in AD 600 gave an interesting account of fevers that were accompanied by exanthemata. Aulus Cornelius Celsus (25 BC–AD 50) described it under the generic name *pustulae.*

Exercise The effects and benefits of exercise have been studied extensively by almost all famous medical personalities from ancient times. Paul of Aegina (625–690) described it as 'violent motion, with its limit to violence, being hurried respiration'. Galen (AD 129–200) dealt extensively with it in his second book of the *Hygiena.* The beneficial effects

were pointed out by Paul of Aegina, Aetius of Amida (AD 502–575), Oribasius (AD 326–403), Haly Abbas (930–994), Avicenna (980–1037) and others. Oribasius, in his *Pergamos,* consisting of 70 books, gave several forms and discussed the merits of each. He recommended horse riding, since it strengthened the stomach muscles, above all other forms of exercise, and made the senses more acute. An English teacher at Manchester Grammar School and physician, Thomas Cogan (1545–1607) in his *Haven of Health* (1584) pointed out the advantages for the body and serious study for the mind. *See gymnasium, sports medicine.*

Exner, Siegmund (1846–1926) Professor of physiology at the University of Vienna, who described the superficial tangential layer of the molecular cerebral cortex in 1881.

Exophthalmic Goiter (Syn. Graves disease, Parry disease) Caleb Hillier Parry (1755–1822), a Bath physician, gave the first detailed account of exophthalmic goiter of the thyroid in 1786. He continued to study it and published eight more cases in 1825. Another early account was given by Guiseppe Flajani (1741–1808), an Italian physician in Rome, in 1802. Robert James Graves (1796–1853), a Dublin physician, gave an account of three more cases in 1835. Carl Adolph Basedow (1799–1854), from Merseberg near Leipzig, described four more cases in 1840. It is known as Basedow disease in Germany. The first thyroidectomy for exophthalmic goiter was performed by a German surgeon, Ludwig Reich (1849–1930), in 1880. The term was coined in 1908 by an American professor of medicine, George Dock, at Tulane, University of Louisiana, New Orleans.

Exophthalmic Ophthalmoplegia Also known as malignant exophthalmos. Described as a separate entity from Graves exophthalmos in 1938 by the British neurologist, Walter Russell Brain (1895–1966), Baron of Eynsham, and H.M. Turnbull.

Exosmosis [Greek: *ex*, without + *osmos*, impulse] A process of attraction of a lighter medium to a denser medium through a membrane. Described by Henri Joachim Dutrochet (1776–1847) in 1826. If the movement took place from outside to inside he called it endosmosis and the reverse process was named exosmosis.

Experimental Psychology The concept was introduced by German psychologist, Wilhelm Max Wundt (1832–1920) in *Beitrage der Sinneswahrneh,* published in 1862. The Society of Experimental Psychology in America was founded in 1904 by Edward Bradford Titchener (1867–1927), a naturalized American psychologist from Chichester, England. He also wrote an important work, *Experimental*

Psychology (1901–1905), in four volumes. The first chair of experimental psychology at Cambridge in England was occupied by Frederick Charles Bartlett (1889–1969) in 1931. Its origin and progress was traced by Edwin (1886–1968) of Harvard in *History of Experimental Psychology*, published in 1929. *See psychology.*

Expiration [Latin: *ex*, out + *spirare*, to breathe] *See respiration, lung function.*

Explosives Act of 1875 Passed in England to prevent accidental explosions in harbors and factories and during the transport of dynamite.

Exsanguine [Latin: *ex*, without + *sanguis*, blood] An old term for anemic.

Extracorporeal Circulation [Latin: *extra*, outside + *corpus*, body] *See heart-lung machine.*

Extracorporeal Cooling [Latin: *extra*, outside + *corpus*, body] A method of allowing the blood from a cannulated artery to pass through tubing immersed in a cooling medium and to be returned to a vein. Described by J. Boerema and colleagues in 1951. In 1954 Donald Nixon Ross (b 1922) suggested withdrawal of blood from a vein instead of an artery, and Russell Claude Brock (1903–1930) devised a method to cool the blood through the venous system without cannulating the artery in 1956.

Extradural Block [Greek: *ex*, out + *dura*, hard] A block of nerve roots between the dura and the vertebral canal as a form of regional anesthesia. Introduced by James Leonard Corning (1855–1923) of New York, and first tried in dogs by Fernard Cathelin (b 1873) in 1901. It was applied to clinical surgery by Fidel Miraë Pages (d 1924) in 1921 and Achile Mario Dogliotti in 1931, and popularized in England by C. J. Massey Dawkins in 1945.

Extrasystole [Greek: *ex*, out + *systole*, a drawing together] Word coined in 1894 by Theodore Wilhelm Engleman (1843–1909) during his observation of extra heart beats in animals. Arthur Robertson Cushny (1866–1926) and Karel Friedrich Wenkebach (1864–1940) independently related extrasystoles to an irregular pulse, in 1899 and 1900, respectively. One of the first recordings on an electrocardiogram was made by William Einthoven (1860–1927) in 1906.

Extrauterine Pregnancy *See ectopic pregnancy.*

Eye Egyptian papyri show that oculists were assigned separately to look after the left and right eyes of the king. Aristotle, in *Historia Animalium,* described the visible outer parts of the eye, and Herophilus wrote a treatise on the eye, *Periophthalmon* in 300 BC. In the 1st century, Rufus of Ephesus, in *On Naming the Parts of the Body,* described the structure of the eye. Galen (129–200) described the structure in more detail in *On the Utility of the parts of the Human Body.* He described seven layers, which are now interpreted as the conjunctiva, cornea, sclera, anterior uvea, anterior sheet of capsule, choroid membrane and retina. The earliest detailed diagram was done by an Arab, Hunanin ibn Ishak (AD 809–877), in *Book of the Ten Treatises of the Eye.* This rare manuscript was transcribed in Syria in AD 1197 from an earlier manuscript found in the private library of Taimur Pasha in Cairo. The earliest accounts on the anatomy in Europe are found in the works of Benevenutus Grassus (AD 1100) and Roger Bacon (1214–1294). Felix Platter (1536–1614), a physician in Basel, gave the most accurate description of the anatomy in his treatise published in 1583. *See ophthalmology.*

Eye Examination *See ophthalmoscope, amblyoscope, slit lamp, gonioscopy, skiascopy.*

F

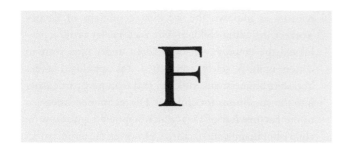

Faber, Knud Heldge (1862–1956) Danish physician who described small, pale (microcytic hypochromic) red blood cells, acholorhydria and glossitis associated with chronic iron deficiency anemia (Faber syndrome) in 1909.

Fabiola Roman woman who converted to Christianity. She devoted her life to working for the poor and sick, and built the first Christian hospital in Rome in AD 390. She is supposed to be the first recorded woman surgeon.

Fabism [Latin: *fabella*, small bean] A form of acute hemolytic anemia in the Italian district of Calabria, the Balkans and North Africa, from eating beans, *Vicia faba,* or inhalation of pollen. Observed and studied in detail by L. Preti of Germany in 1927. It was also investigated by T. McCrae and J.C. Uller in 1933. A hereditary factor in the susceptibility was demonstrated by J.E. Hutton of America in 1937. The mechanism of hemolysis was later proved to be due to glucose-6-phosphate dehydrogenase deficiency. *See lathyrism.*

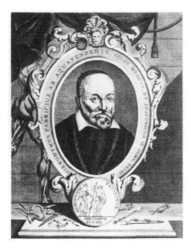

Fabricius ab Aquapendente (1537–1619). William Stirling, *Some Apostles of Physiology* (1902). Waterlow & Sons, London

Fabricius ab Aquapendente or Girolamo, Fabrizio (1537–1619) A medical graduate from Padua, pupil of Gabriele Falloppio (1523–1562) and teacher of William Harvey (1578–1657). He succeeded Falloppio as professor of anatomy in Padua in 1565, and continued to teach there

until his death. His largest contribution to science was on the development of the embryo in lower animals. The site of egg production in the hen was identified and named 'ovarium' by him in 1600. He also described uterine decidua, and his work on embryology, *De Formato Foetu,* was published in 1600. He gave accurate illustrations of the eye, and described the accommodation reflex. A collection of his surgical works, *Oeuvres Chirurgigales* was published in 1666.

Fabricius, Johann Christian (1745–1808) French entomologist and a student of Carl Linnaeus (1707–1778) who established a system of entomology using mouthparts of insects as the basis.

Fabricius Ship The fanciful resemblance of the shape of the occipital, sphenoidal and frontal bones to a ship. Named after the anatomist Fabricius ab Aquapendente (1537–1619) of Padua.

Fabry Disease X-linked condition, leading to absence of α-galactosyl hydrolase. This results in renal failure, corneal opacities and multiple skin lesions. Described by German dermatologist, J. Fabry (1860–1930) in 1898. An account in England was given by W. Anderson in the same year.

Fabry, Wilhelm or Hildanus, Fabricius (1560–1634) German surgeon, and father of surgery in Germany. He recommended amputation above the diseased part of a limb, and was the first to amputate a thigh. *Century of Surgical Cases* contained a collection of his surgical records from 1606. His other works include a monograph on gangrene (1593) and a treatise on lithotomy (1626).

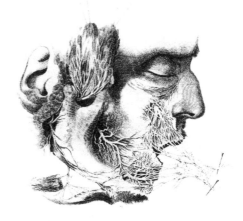

Part of facial nerve or seventh cranial nerve and fifth nerve. Sir Charles Bell, *The Nervous System of the Human Body* (1844). Henry Renshaw, London

Facial Nerve [Latin: *facies*, face] The canal of the facial nerve was described by Gabriele Falloppio (1523–1562). Facial palsy arising from nuclear and infranuclear lesions of the facial nerve (Bell palsy) was described by Sir Charles Bell (1774–1842) in 1821.

Facial Surgery *See rhinoplasty, cleft palate.*

Facial Treatment Cosmetic treatment of the face was practiced by ancient physicians, including Galen (129–200), Aulus Cornelius Celsus (25 BC–AD 50), Paul of Aegina (625–690), Aetius (502–575), Oribasius (326–403) and Haly Abbas (930–994). Paul of Aegina recommended a decoction of the ichthyocollo plant for wrinkles, and application of bruised beans for darkness of the face. Aetius gave a long list of applications for facial complaints, and Haly Abbas recommended bitter almonds and wild cucumber applications.

Facies Hippocratica A peculiar expression of the face mentioned by Hippocrates (460–377 BC) in patients with cholera, wasting diseases and starvation, before impending death. It is described by him as 'a sharp nose, hollow eyes, collapsed temples; the ears cold, contracted and their lobes turned out; the skin about the forehead being rough, distended and parched; the color of the whole face being green, black, livid, or lead colored'.

Factor V Until 1903 the classic theory of blood clotting postulated only four factors: thrombokinase, prothrombin, fibrinogen and calcium. A fifth factor was discovered by Paul Arnor Owren (b 1905) of Scandinavia in 1944, who named it factor V in 1947. A congenital form of factor V deficiency was described by him in the same year.

Factor VIII Antihemophilic globulin (AHG), effective in promoting coagulation in hemophiliacs, isolated from the plasma of normal humans by Francis Henry Laskey Taylor (1900–1959) and Jackson Arthur Patek (b 1904) in 1937. Until 1954 the main treatment for hemophiliacs was still transfusion of whole blood or fresh frozen plasma. In 1953 Robert Gwyn Macfarlane (1907–1987) of Oxford obtained factor VIII fraction from bovine blood. The first successful trial of bovine AHG was given to three hemophilic volunteers by Rosemary Peyton Biggs and Macfarlane in 1954. It was later isolated in a more pure form from human plasma and became the mainstay in the treatment of hemophilia.

Factor X The first factor common to both intrinsic and extrinsic pathways in clotting. Discovered by T.P. Telfer, K.W. Densen and D.R. Wright in 1956.

Factory Acts During the 19th century important men, such as Jeremy Bentham (1748–1832), Michael Sadler (1861–1943), Lord Shaftesbury or Anthony Ashley Cooper (1801–1885) and Robert Owen (1771–1858), brought in

reforms to improve the working conditions of factory workers, including children. The Factory Act of 1819, prohibited the employment of children under nine years in cotton mills. A select committee was appointed under Yorkshire businessman, Sadler, in 1831 to inquire particularly into the conditions for children. His recommendation led to the Factory Act of 1833 which imposed regulations on child labor in mills and factories. However, the pitiful working conditions for children continued in mines where they labored for long hours, some only seeing daylight on Sundays. A Royal Commission was appointed to address this situation in 1840. The Miner's Act was passed through the efforts of Lord Shaftesbury in 1842. Compensation to workers who sustained injury was effected through the Employer's Liability Act of 1880. Another Royal Commission of 1876 resulted in the Factory and Workshop Act of 1878. Further Acts were passed in 1906, 1936 and 1961. The Health and Safety at Work Act was enacted in 1974.

Factory Fever (Syn. epidemic typhus) Named because it was common in the barracks of factory workers, owing to poor hygiene and crowded living conditions in the 18th century. An epidemic at Radcliffe near Manchester in 1784 focused attention on the problem, and a Manchester practitioner, Thomas Percival (1740–1804), was appointed to inquire into the conditions of the workers. He formed a voluntary organization, the Manchester Board of Health, to supervise medical conditions of workers.

Fagge, Charles Hilton (1838–1933) Physician at Guy's Hospital in London. He described sporadic cretinism, and gave an exhaustive account of presystolic murmurs in 1871. He described ankylosing spondylitis at necropsy as 'poker back' in 1877.

Fagon, Guy Crescent (1632–1713) Physician in Paris who defended the theory of the circulation of blood. He was physician to King Louis XIV.

Fahr Disease Intracerebral calcification of the small vessels of the deep cortex and lenticular and dentate nuclei. Described by German dermatologist, Karl Theodore Fahr (1877–1945) in 1930. A similar condition was mentioned by Rudolph Virchow (1821–1902) in 1855.

Fahraeus, Robin Sanno (1888–1968) Pathologist in Hamburg who studied sedimentation properties of blood.

Fahrenheit, Gabriel Daniel (1686–1736) Experimental philosopher and son of a wealthy merchant at Danzig in Prussia. In 1717 he moved to Amsterdam, where he trained as an instrument maker. He improved the thermometer by using mercury instead of spirits of wine in 1720 and introduced a new scale for temperature, with the freezing point of water at 32 °.

Falciform Ligament [Latin: *falx*, sickle + *forma*, shape + *ligamentum*, bandage] A description was given in 1803 by William Hey (1736–1819), a contemporary of John Hunter (1728–1793), at St George's Hospital.

Falconer, Hugh (1808–1865) Scottish paleontologist from Forres who studied medicine at Aberdeen and Edinburgh, before he went to India as an assistant surgeon to the Bengal medical establishment in 1830. He was later professor of botany at the Medical College of Calcutta and wrote several works on botany.

Falconet, Camillus (1671–1762) French physician from Lyons and a bibliomaniac. He published a translation of Villemot's *Systema Planetorum*.

Falling Sickness Caelius Aurelianus in the 4th century described epilepsy thus: 'patient falls to the ground, unconscious and not susceptible to pain'. Hildegard of Bingen (1098–1179) and others also described 'falling' during an attack. *See epilepsy.*

Fallopian Tubes Described by the Italian anatomist, Gabriele Falloppio (1523–1562), in 1561. Insufflation of the Fallopian tubes was suggested in an editorial in the *Revue Medico-Chirugicale de Paris* in 1849. The method of assessing their patency, salpingography, was devised by William Cary Hollenback (b 1883) of America in 1914. Isador Clinton Rubin (1883–1958) used the tubal insufflation method for treating sterility resulting from their occlusion, in 1920.

Falloppio, Gabriele (1523–1562) Italian anatomist from Modena, a pupil of Andreas Vesalius (1514–1564), and teacher of Fabrizio ab Aquapendente (1533–1619). He discovered the Fallopian tubes of the ovaries, the semicircular canals of the ear, the chorda tympani and the trigeminal, auditory and glossopharyngeal nerves. He also coined the terms 'vagina' and 'placenta'.

Fallot Tetralogy The first description was given by Niels Stenson (1638–1686) in 1671. It was described by Eduard Sandifort (1742–1814) in 1771. An account of congenital cyanotic heart disease was given by John Richard Farre (1775–1862) of England in 1814. Thomas Peacock (1812–1882) of London also described it in his treatise on malformations of the heart in 1858. Etienne Louis Arthur Fallot (1850–1911) of France wrote a series of papers in 1888 describing four abnormalities found at autopsy in children dying of cyanotic heart disease. His description of the syndrome which bears his name consisted of outflow obstruction to the right ventricle, ventricular septal defect, right ventricular hypertrophy and dextroposition of the aorta. The Blalock–Taussig shunt, the first surgical operation for Fallot tetralogy, was performed by Alfred Blalock (1899–1964) and Helen Taussig (1898–1986) of Johns Hopkins Hospital in 1945.

Falret, Jean Pierre (1794–1870) French psychiatrist who recognized the alternating moods of excitement and depression. He named this *la folie circulaire* in 1854.

False Teeth *See artificial teeth.*

Falta, Wilhelm (1875–1950) Bohemian physician who practiced in Vienna. He wrote an early systematic treatise on endocrine disorders which was translated into English in 1915.

Falx Cerebri [Latin: *falx*, sickle; Greek: *cerebrum*, the brain] The structure in the brain derives its name from its shape, resembling a sickle or pruning knife.

Familial Benign Pemphigus A chronic bullous dermatosis affecting the neck, axilla, groin and perianal region. Described by William Howard Hailey (b 1898) and Hugh Edward Hailey (b 1909) in 1939.

Familial Hemorrhagic Telengiectasis Multiple telengiectatic lesions of the face and upper gastrointestinal tract, with a bleeding tendency. Described independently by Henri Joules Louis Marie Rendu (1844–1902) of Paris (1896), Frederick Parkes Weber (1863–1962) of Edinburgh (1904) and Sir William Osler (1849–1919) in 1907.

Familial Hypercholesterolemia *See cholesterolemia, familial.*

Familial Periodic Paralysis Intermittent paralysis and loss of deep reflexes was described by Alexander Westphal (1863–1941) in 1885. H. Oppenheim (1858–1919) described it in 1891, and Schmidt wrote a monograph in 1919.

Fanconi Syndrome Widespread deposition of cystine crystals were described during autopsy of children who died of resistant rickets, polyuria, aminoaciduria, renal glycosuria and acidosis by Swiss physiologist, Emil Aberhalden (1877–1950) in 1903. G.O.E. Lignac, a Dutch pathologist, investigated it in 1924, and the disease in live children was described by a Swiss pediatrician, Guido Fanconi (1882–1979) of Zurich in 1946.

Fanconi, Guido (1892–1979) Swiss professor of pediatrics at the University of Zurich. He described renal tubular dysfunction (Fanconi syndrome) leading to aminoaciduria and cystic fibrosis of the pancreas in 1946. *See Fanconi syndrome.*

Fantus, Bernhard (1874–1940) A physician at Cook County Hospital, Chicago. He coined the term 'blood bank' in 1937.

Farabeuf, Louis Hubert (1841–1910) Professor of anatomy at the Faculty of Medicine in Paris. He described the triangle in the upper part of the neck, bounded by the internal jugular vein, the facial vein and the hypoglossal nerve, later named after him.

Faraday, Michael (1791–1867) Born in Newington, Surrey, son of a blacksmith from Yorkshire. At the age of 12, he worked as an errand boy to a bookseller, who promoted him to bookbinder's apprentice in 1804. He started attending Sir Humphry Davy's (1778–1829) lectures, and became so interested in chemistry that he joined the Royal Institution as a laboratory assistant in 1813. He published his observations on ether in *The Quarterly Journal of Science and Arts* in 1818. He made many important discoveries in chemistry and physics. He pioneered electrolysis and introduced the terms electrode, cathode and anode. He liquefied carbon dioxide using pressure in 1823, and condensed chlorine into a liquid in the same year. He discovered electromagnetic rotation in 1822, and presented his first series of *Experimental Researches on Electricity* to the Royal Society in 1831. He succeeded Davy at the Royal Institute in 1825.

Farmer's Lung The earliest description of the symptoms caused by moldy hay is found in Bernardino Ramazzini's (1633–1714) book on occupational diseases published in 1700. It was also known to Sveinn Palsson, a country physician in Iceland, who described it as Heysott, meaning hay sickness, in 1790. Manchester physician, Charles Harrison Blackley (1820–1900), described it in detail in his book on hay asthma in 1873. In 1861 J.H. Salisbury of Ohio made the first attempt to establish a diagnosis by skin testing. J.M. Cambell, in his article 'Acute symptoms following work with hay' in the *British Medical Journal* in 1932, described five cases from Cumbria. It was registered in 1965 as a prescribed occupational disease under the National Insurance Industrial Injuries Act of 1945. The causative organism, an aerobic thermophilic actinomycete, was identified and named *Micropolyspora faeni* in 1968.

Farmer, Chester Jefferson (1886–1969) Chicago chemist who worked with Otto Knut Olof Folin (1867–1934) to develop microchemical assay methods for urea, creatinine and other substances.

Farnham, Nicholas de (d 1257) Professor of medicine in Paris and Bologna. He was educated in Oxford and completed his medical studies in Paris. He returned to England in 1229 and was appointed professor at Oxford by Henry III. He was elected Bishop of Durham in 1241 and moved to Stockton-on-Tees in 1249.

Farr Forceps Bone holding forceps devised by American surgeon, Robert Emmet Farr (1875–1932) in 1918. He also designed a mouth-gag for use in anesthesia in 1914.

Farr, William (1807–1883) Statistician and physician from Kenley, Shropshire. He was the compiler to the Registrar General's Office in London appointed by Edwin Chadwick (1800–1890) in 1839, and did the first scientific study on vital statistics.

Farre, Arthur (1811–1887) Professor of midwifery at King's College London. The line of attachment of the mesovarium to the ovary is named after him.

Farre, John Richard (1775–1862) London physician who wrote a monograph on congenital diseases of the heart in 1814.

Farrer, William James (1845–1906) Botanist from Cumbria who graduated in medicine from Cambridge. He emigrated to Australia in 1870 and contributed significantly to the development of the wheat industry there.

Fasciculus Gracilis [Latin: *fasciculus*, small bundle + *gracilis*, tender] Structure at the posterior column of the spinal cord. Described by Friedrich Goll (1829–1903), a neuroanatomist in Zurich and a contemporary of Rudolph Virchow (1821–1902), Rudolf Albert von Kölliker (1817–1905) and Claude Bernard (1813–1878) in 1868.

Fasciola hepatica [Latin: *fasciola*, a strip of cloth, or small bandage; Greek: *hepatos,* liver] D.F. Weinland observed the cercaria of the parasite in snails in 1873. The complete life cycle was elucidated by W. Thomas and K. G. F. Rudolf Leuckart (1823–1898) in 1883.

Fasciolopsis buski [Latin: *fasciola*, a strip of cloth, or small bandage] An intestinal parasite, discovered in the duodenum in 1843 by George Busk (1807–1886) of King's College Hospital, London. He described it in *Diseases of the Liver*, published in 1845. Cirrhosis of the liver due to the same parasite (Budd disease) was described by George Budd (1808–1882) in 1843.

Fat Embolism Pulmonary fat embolism was described by a German pathologist, Friedrich Albert Zenker (1825–1898) in 1862. Its role in traumatic shock was explained by a Boston physician, William Townsend Porter (b 1862) in 1917. Two fatal cases were described by New York surgeon, Arthur Wells Elting (b 1872) in 1925. Fat embolism as a result of fractured bones or orthopedic operations, was observed and studied by H.L. Davis and C.G. Goodchild in 1936.

Fatigue Syndrome [Latin: *fatigare*, to weary] *See chronic fatigue syndrome.*

Fatless Meat A low calorie, low cholesterol alternative to natural meat was prepared after 15 years of research by an Australian butcher, Dallas Chapman in 1988. It contained 96% less cholesterol than normal meat.

Fats *See fatty acids.*

Fat Soluble Vitamins *See vitamin A, vitamin D.*

Fatty Acids Michel Eugene Chevril (1786–1889) of Paris conducted a study on animal fat in 1823. He discovered that it was composed of fatty acids and glycerol.

Fatty Degeneration The true nature of this pathological process was described by Jones Quain (1785–1851) in the *Medico-Chirugical Transactions* in 1850. He identified some of the causes: impaired general and local nutrition, blood disorders and diseases of nutrient vessels. His findings were confirmed 20 years later by Carl von Voit (1831–1908) of Munich in 1871.

Fauchard Disease Alviodental periostitis, described by a French dental surgeon, Pierre Fauchard (1678–1761).

Fauchard, Pierre (1678–1761) French dental surgeon who wrote a textbook of dental surgery, *Le Chirugian Dentiste,* in 1728. *See dentistry.*

Faulds, Henry (1844–1930) Inventor of the method of identification using fingerprints, who graduated from Anderson's College, Glasgow in 1871. He served for a short period in India and returned to Britain in 1874. He published his fingerprint method of identification in *Nature* on 28 October 1880.

Fauvel Granules Peribronchitic abscesses, described by French physician, Sulpice Antoine Fauvel (1813–1884) in 1843.

Fauvel, Suplice Antoine (1813–1884) French physician born in Paris. He was Chief of Clinic at the Hôtel Dieu, and later professor of medicine at the school of medicine at Constantinople. He founded *Gazette Medicale d'Orient* in 1856. He gave a classic description of mitral stenosis in 1843.

Fauvre, Jean Louis (1863–1944) French surgeon who described a new method of hysterectomy in 1897.

Favaloro, G. Rene (b 1923) The founder of coronary artery bypass surgery, born at la Plata, Argentina. After practicing primary care in his rural community, he studied surgery at the Cleveland Clinic in 1962. He performed the first coronary artery bypass in a woman in 1967. *See coronary artery bypass graft.*

Favism [Italian: *fava,* bean] *See fabism.*

Favre, Maurice (1876–1955) Professor of pathological anatomy at Lyons, who, along with French physicians, Joseph Nicholas (1868–1960) and Joseph Durand (b 1876), gave the first important description of lymphogranuloma venereum (Favre disease) in 1913. He also classified diseases of the reticuloendothelial system.

Favus or ringworm [Latin: *favus,* honeycomb] Described by Paul of Aegina (625–690) as 'swelling of skin, having perforations through which honey-like fluid discharged'. He advocated application of dried grapes or tender fig leaves in honey as treatment. Galen (129–200) wrote two volumes on favus involving the face and scalp. *Favus scutula,* was first observed by Robert Remak (1815–1865) during his work at the Charité Hospital in Berlin. However, he did not realize its fungal nature until Johann Lucas Schonlein (1793–1864) described it in 1839. David Gruby (1810–1898) described it as *la vrai teigne* in 1841. The first work on ringworm of the hands and feet was published by Djelaleddin-Moukhtar, a physician to the Ottoman army, in 1892.

Faxon Incision Used for draining subphrenic abscess. Described by a Boston surgeon, Henry Hardwick Faxon (b 1899) in 1941.

Febricula A term for simple fever lasting for not more than a few days, with no apparent cause.

Febrifuge [Latin: *febris,* fever + *fugare,* to drive away] A synonym for antipyretic. *See antipyretic.*

Febrile Albuminuria The occurrence of albuminuria in fevers was described by Martin Solon of Paris in 1838, and it was named by Carl Gerhardt (1833–1902) of Germany in 1868. *See albuminuria, benign albuminuria.*

Febris Synocha An old term for a group of continued inflammatory fevers.

Fecal Estimation of Fats A method of estimating total fats in the feces was proposed by Philadelphia physician, Gordon Joel Saxon (b 1879) in 1914.

Feces Examination A flotation technique for examination of helminthic ova was devised by a British physician and parasitologist, Clayton Arbuthnot Lane (1868–1949) who worked in India. A test for occult blood in feces, using Barbados aloin and other reagents, was devised by Swiss physician, Otto Rossel (1875–1911).

Fechner, Gustav Theodor (1801–1887) German psychologist from Lusatia. He studied the various modalities of subjective sensation in relation to external physical stimuli. His findings, combined with the previous work of Ernst Heinrich Weber (1795–1878), led to the formulation of a psychophysical law that the intensity of a subjective sensation is proportional to the logarithm of the corresponding physical stimulus. He wrote *Element der Psycho-physick* in 1860. His work led to the development of experimental psychology.

Fecundity [Latin: *fecundus*, fertile] An important factor to the ancients. They designated several gods and goddesses as guardians of fertility. Baal or Balder, the god, was also a source of fertility, and was worshipped by the Phoenicians in the form of a conical stone.

Fede Disease Sublingual fibroma, described by Italian physician, Francesco Fede (1832–1913).

Federici Sign Intestinal sounds heard on auscultation of the abdomen in cases of intestinal perforation, with gas in the peritoneal cavity. Described by Italian physician in Palmero, Cesare Federici (1832–1892).

Feeblemindedness *See idiocy, Down syndrome.*

Feedback Mechanism The concept of a self-regulatory system for the body was proposed by Russian psychologist, Piotre Kuzmich Anokhin (1897–1974). The term 'feedback' was used by American mathematician, Norbert Wiener (1894–1964). Early experimental work on biofeedback mechanisms was done by N.E. Miller in 1968.

Feer Disease *See acrodynia.*

Fees The professional income of physicians is a topic of great antiquity and interest. Pliny, in the 1st century, stated the following incomes for Roman physicians: Albutius, Arrantius, Calpetanus and Rubrius each earned 250,000 sesteres per annum. Quintus Stertinus received 500,000 sesteres from the emperor and his private practice brought him 600,000 sesteres. He and his brother, an Imperial physician, between them left 30 million sesteres, despite lavish living. Manilus Cortunus, according to Pliny, paid a sum equivalent to $350,000 to a doctor for curing his skin disease. The English surgeon, John of Arderne (1307–1360), is said to have charged enormous fees, which sometimes consisted of ransoms meant for knights held by Turks during the Crusades. He was probably the model for Chaucer's 'Doctor of Physick' who had a love for gold. During the 17th century the average fee for an English physician was 10 shillings, worth about $500 today. Richard Mead (1673–1754) charged a guinea, and the annual salary of a professor of physick at Cambridge in 1626 was 40 pounds. A 20-mile visit to a patient carried a fee of 12 shillings, and an out-of-area visit lasting two days cost one pound and ten shillings.

An English surgeon's fee for a one-mile visit in 1700 was 12 pence, and he charged 5 pounds for an amputation. At the end of the 18th century practitioners of physick and surgery in the State of New York charged $1 for an ordinary visit and $1.25 for a single dose of medicine. Amputation of a joint cost $100 and the fee was the same for excision of the eye or for operating on an aneurysm. The fee for a normal delivery was $25. The fee for a physician's visit in France during the mid-19th century was 1 franc. The average annual earnings of a physician in Germany at the end of the 19th century was 3000 marks.

Fehleisen, Friedrich (1854–1924) German physician who identified *Streptococcus* as the cause of erysipelas in 1886.

Fehling Operation Used in the treatment of prolapse of uterus. Devised by a German gynecologist, Hermann Johannes Karl Fehling (1847–1925) in 1881.

Fehling Test A test for sugar in the urine. Devised by a German chemist, Hermann Christian von Fehling (1812–1885) in 1848.

Feldberg, Wilhelm Siegmund (b 1900) English physiologist who demonstrated the role of acetylcholine in transmission of neuron to neuron impulses of the sympathetic ganglia, with Sir John Henry Gaddum (1900–1965) in 1965.

Feldi, Fortunato (1550–1630) Italian physician who wrote an early important work on medical jurisprudence in 1602.

Feleki Instrument A device for massaging the prostate gland, devised by Hungarian urologist, Hugo von Feleki (1861–1932) from Budapest.

Felix, Arthur (1887–1956) Polish bacteriologist who, while working with Edmund Weil (1880–1922) in 1916 in eastern Galicia, devised an agglutinin reaction for diagnosis of typhus. They noted the presence of a proteus-like organism in the urine of a patient with typhus. They demonstrated that this organism agglutinated the sera of other patients with typhus and named it 'proteus X'. *See Weil–Felix reaction.*

Fell, George Edward (1850–1918) American physician in Buffalo who described an apparatus for performing artificial respiration during surgery without collapsing the lung.

Felty Syndrome Lymphadenopathy, leukopenia and hypersplenism associated with rheumatoid arthritis. Described in 1924 in five patients by American physician, Augustus Roi Felty (1895–1964) of Johns Hopkins Hospital.

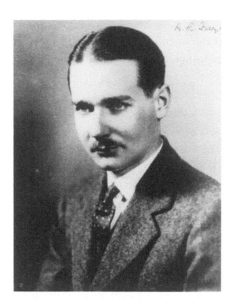

Augustus Felty (1895–1964). Courtesy of the National Library of Medicine

Female Medical College of Pennsylvania Founded exclusively for women by a group of Quakers in 1850. One of its first graduates, Anne Preston (1813–1872), was a pioneer in medical education for women. She was professor of physiology and hygiene at the college for 20 years until her death. Because of the unrecognized status of the college, its students were barred from clinical training in hospitals in Philadelphia. To overcome this, Preston founded the Woman's Hospital 1861, later renamed Woman's Medical College of Pennsylvania, in 1868. The college remains as a coeducational institute, Medical College of Pennsylvania.

Femoral Artery [Latin: *femur*, thigh; Greek: *aer*, air + *terein*, to preserve] Astley Paston Cooper (1768–1841) of Guy's Hospital was the first to perform successful ligation of the external iliac artery for a femoral aneurysm in 1808. The first successful ligation of the femoral artery in America was performed by Wright Post (1766–1822) of Long Island, New York in 1796. He used the method described by John Hunter (1728–1793). Henry U. Onderdonk of America tied the internal iliac artery in 1813. End-to-end suture of the femoral artery was performed by John Benjamin Murphy (1857–1916) of America in 1896. Successful embolectomy was carried out by Einar Samuel Henrick Key (1872–1954) of Stockholm in 1912.

Femoral Fractures An anterior suspensory splint for fracture of the femur was devised by American orthopedic surgeon, Ryno Nathan Smith (1797–1877), in 1860. Nicholson Senn (1844–1908), an orthopedic surgeon of

Swiss origin in Wisconsin, advocated reduction and permanent fixation of a fractured neck of the femur by nailing. Artificial impac-tion to promote healing in cases of fractured neck of the femur was performed by Frederick Jay Cotton (1869–1938) in 1909. Skin traction as treatment was introduced by Hamilton Russell (1860–1933), a student of Joseph Lister (1827–1912), who emigrated to Australia in 1933 and practiced as a surgeon in Melbourne.

Femoral Hernia Observed by Phillipe Verheyen (1648–1710) of Belgium, also known as Phillipus, in 1710. An operation for strangulated femoral hernia was described by Antonio de Gimbernat (1734–1816) of Spain in 1793. Another operation was designed by James Luke (1798–1881), a surgeon at the London Hospital, in 1841. Edoardo Bassini of Italy (1847–1924) described an operative procedure for uncomplicated femoral hernia in 1893, and this now bears his name. Charles Barret Lockwood (1856–1914) in London designed another in the same year. The Battle method was devised by William Henry Battle (1855–1936) of London in 1901. Others who described their own surgical methods include George Lothison (1898) and Arnold Kirkpatrick Henry (1936).

Femtochemistry The study of chemical reactions that take place on a timescale of a fraction of a second. Pioneered by American physical chemist, Richard Barry Bernstein (1923–1990) of Long Island, New York in 1955.

Fenger Operation Used for relief of ureteral stricture causing hydronephrosis. Devised by Chicago surgeon, Frederic Fenger (1840–1902) in 1894. He described vaginal hysterectomy in 1882.

Fenwick Disease Atrophy of the stomach occurring in association with pernicious anemia. Described by Samuel Fenwick (1821–1902) from Newcastle upon Tyne, who became an eminent physician at the London Hospital. He wrote *The Morbid States of the Stomach and Duodenum*, *The Student's Guide to Medical Diagnosis* and *Outlines of Medical Treatment*.

Fereol Nodes Subcutaneous nodes seen in acute rheumatism. Described by French physician, Louis Henry Felix Fereol (1825–1921).

Ferguson, Alexander Hugh (1853–1912) Chicago surgeon who specialized in treatment of hernia. He described a radical cure for femoral hernia in 1895.

Ferguson, James Haig (1862–1934) *See Haig Ferguson forceps, antenatal care.*

Ferguson, Robert (1799–1865) Graduated in medicine from Edinburgh in 1823, and later moved to London, where he founded the *London Medical Gazette* in 1827. He was first professor of midwifery at King's College London in 1831.

Fergusson, Sir William (1808–1877) Scottish surgeon and pupil of Robert Knox (1791–1862). He wrote *System of Practical Surgery* in 1857. He also devised several surgical instruments, including a vaginal speculum, a mouth gag and lion forceps. He practiced conservative surgery and avoided amputation whenever possible. He was the first in Scotland to tie the subclavian artery, while he was a surgeon at the Edinburgh Royal Infirmary, and excised the head of the femur for incurable disease of the hip in 1845. His *Progress of Anatomy and Surgery During the Present Century,* is an important book on medical history, published in 1867.

Fermentation [Latin: *fermentum*, ferment] Used to produce beer and known to the Sumerians and Babylonians. Brewing was a trade under the Pharaohs in ancient Egypt. Remains of fermented wine have been found in Danish graves from the time of Christ. Thomas Willis (1621–1675) in 1659 observe the resemblance between putrefaction and fermentation. In 1787 an Italian, Giovanni Mattia Fabroni, studied it, and noted that air was not necessary. The earliest demonstration of the role of yeast was by Charles Cagniard de Latour (1777–1859) of France in 1838. Louis Pasteur's (1822–1895) work on it commenced around 1855 and led to the discovery of yeast and bacteria, and put an end to the theory of spontaneous generation. Further work was done by the French physiologist Claude Bernard (1813–1878) in Paris in 1877. Eduard Buchner (1860–1917), professor of chemistry in Berlin, performed the first extraction of the enzyme zymase from yeast in 1897 and demonstrated its capability of breaking down sugar in the absence of yeast. *See fermentology.*

Fermentology The study of the organisms producing fermentation. The first description and drawings of yeast cells were submitted to the Royal Society of London by Dutch microscopist, Anton van Leeuwenhoek (1632–1723) in 1680. The Swedish botanist, Carl Linnaeus (1707–1778) suspected that fermentation was caused by microscopic living organisms but failed to prove it. Fermentation was explained on a chemical basis by Antoine Lavoisier (1743–1794). The equation for fermentation involving decomposition of the hexose molecule was proposed by Joseph Louis Gay-Lussac (1778–1850) in 1810. The yeast in beer was shown to belong to the vegetable kingdom by Cagnaird-Latour (1777–1859) in 1837. His theory was

proved in the same year by Schwann (1810–1882). Final proof that fermentation was due to living organisms was provided by Louis Pasteur (1822–1895) in 1857.

Fermi, Enrico (1901–1954) *See nuclear reactor.*

Fern *See male fern.*

Fernel, Jean François (1506–1558) Born in Mont Didier in France, he was an eminent physician who attended King Henry II and Catherine de Medici. In 1554 he published *Universa Medica*, which remained a standard textbook of medicine for over a century. He was also one of the first to treat gonorrhea and syphilis as two distinct diseases. He coined the Latin words which gave birth to 'physiology' and 'pathology'.

Ferrein, Antoine (1693–1769) A graduate of Montpellier and professor of surgery and anatomy at the Jardin des Plantes in Paris. He described the cortical pyramids of the kidney and bile canaliculi, which are unconnected to hepatic lobules. Both have been named after him.

Ferriar, John (1761–1815) A physician from Roxburghshire who established a practice in Manchester. He published a poem *The Bibliomaniac.*

Ferrier, Sir David (1843–1928) Neurologist from Aberdeen, Scotland. He qualified in medicine from Edinburgh with a gold medal for his doctoral thesis on comparative anatomy of the brain in 1870. He became professor of nervous pathology at King's College London in 1876. He was a pioneer in the study of the localization of cerebral function and wrote *Functions of the Brain* in 1876 and *Localization of Cerebral Disease* in 1878. He was founding editor of the journal *Brain* and received his knighthood in 1911.

Fertilization [Latin: *fertilis*, fertile] In 1779, Lazzaro Spallanzani (1729–1799) proposed that a sperm must make physical contact with the egg for fertilization to take place. It was first observed by English biologist, Martin Barry (1802–1855), in 1843. In 1875, a German biologist, Oscar Hertwig (1849–1922), while working on the eggs and spermatozoa of the sea urchin in his small laboratory in the Mediterranean, proved that the process involved the union of two nuclei.

Fetal Alcohol Syndrome Occurring as a result of maternal alcohol ingestion. Described by William Charles Sullivan (1869–1926) in 1899.

Fetal Circulation [Latin: *fetus*, offspring] Galen (129–200) initiated study of fetal circulation with his findings of the foramen ovale, its valve and the ductus arteriosus. His description of the ductus arteriosus was improved by Gabriele Falloppio (1523–1562) in 1561. Bartolommeo Eustachio (1520–1574) described the Eustachian membrane in 1563. The ductus venosus was discovered by Giulio Cesare Aranzi (1530–1589) in 1564. A detailed account of the ductus arteriosus and foramen ovale was given by Leone Giambattista Carcano (1536–1606) in 1574. Fabricius ab Aquapendente (1537–1619) constructed the first picture of fetal circulation in his *De Formato Feto* in 1600, and William Harvey (1578–1657), his pupil, completed the account in 1628. The physiology was studied in lambs by J. Cohnstein and Nathan Zuntz (1847–1920) in 1888. It was advanced in 1927 by A. Huggett who demonstrated that it was possible to deliver the fetus still attached to the mother with an intact umbilical cord. Raphael Bienvenu Sabatier (1732–1811) proposed that oxygenated blood from the placenta brought by the umbilical vein passed through the heart without mixing, to supply the head. In 1938 Joseph Barcroft, D.H. Barron and Kenneth J. Franklin of the Nuffield Institute, Oxford performed cineangiography on fetal lambs and proved this. They showed that the crista dividens diverted the larger proportion of the oxygenated blood from the inferior vena cava through the foramen ovale into the left atrium, while the smaller stream reached the right ventricle via the superior vena cava. One of the best historic accounts is given in the first chapter of *The Foetal Circulation* by Alfred E. Barclay, Kenneth J. Franklin and Majorie Prichard, published in 1944.

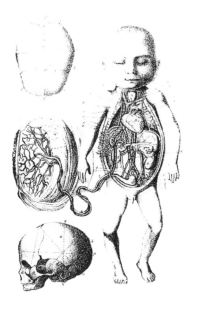

Fetal circulation. Alfred Armand L.M. Velpeau, *A Complete Treatise in Midwifery* (1852). Lindsay & Blakiston, Philadelphia

Fetal Diagnosis The blood drawn from the umbilical cord was used for diagnosis of disease in the fetus by Fernand Daffos in 1983. *See amniocentesis.*

Fetal Electrocardiogram The first recording was reported by Max Cremer (1865–1935) of Germany in 1906.

Fetal Electroencephalography The intrauterine electroencephalogram (EEG) of the fetus was recorded by D.B. Lindsley in 1942. Further fetal EEGs in 75 women at varying stages of gestation were obtained by R.L. Bernsteine and W.J. Borokowsky in 1959. A method of applying electrodes through the vagina was described by E. Huhmer and P.A. Javinen in 1963.

Fetal Heart Sounds First heard in a pregnant woman in her fifth month of pregnancy by François Mayor, a surgeon from Geneva, in 1818. By 1830 the auscultation of fetal heart sounds had become established as a part of antenatal examination. A special head stethoscope, to monitor them while both hands were free to examine the mother or deliver the child, was designed by Chicago obstetrician, David Sweeny Hills (1873–1942) in 1917. A claim to this invention was also made by Hill's colleague, Joseph Bolivar DeLee (1969–1942) of New York.

Fetal Hemoglobin Shown to be different from adult hemoglobin by Joseph Barcroft (1872–1947) in 1933. Its greater affinity for oxygen was demonstrated by N.J. Eastman and co-workers in the same year.

Fetal Surgery The first surgery on a fetus before its birth was performed in 1984 by William H. Clewall, a surgeon from Colorado Health Sciences Center in Denver.

Fetish [Portuguese: *feitico,* charm or amulet] Africans used fetishes such as claws, fangs, roots or stones, believed to be inhabited by spirits, as a remedy. Various forms were used in the past for treatment of disease. *See amulets.*

Fetishism Primitive religion that believed in fetishes. Also a form of sexual deviation in which a person obtains sexual gratification by seeing or feeling an object (fetish) such as male or female clothes, ornaments, cosmetics. German psychiatrist, Richard Kraft-Ebing (1840–1902), described several cases in *Psychopathia Sexualis,* published in 1886.

Fetography [Latin: *fetus,* offspring; Greek: *graphein,* to write] Visualization of soft tissues of the fetus using an oil-soluble contrast medium with an affinity for the vernix caesiosa was described by Utzuki and Hashidzume in 1941. During their procedure on three cases of hydramnios with fetal death, they managed to identify the fetal sex and note other abnormalities such as polydactyly, and some details of the face. The term was used to refer to the procedure by Erbsloh in 1942. It was revived by O. Aguero and I. Zighelboim in 1970.

Fetoscopy [Latin: *fetus*, offspring + *skopein*, to look] Visualization of the fetus *in utero* was achieved by introducing an instrument through the cervical canal by B. Westin in 1954. All three of his patients underwent termination of pregnancy. His device was later developed into a fiber optic telescope with a light source by Wolf of Germany and Mayer and Phelps of England in the early 1970s.

Fetus *See fetography, fetoscopy, fetal circulation, fetal heart sounds, fetal alcohol syndrome.*

Fever Considered by most ancient physicians as a 'preternatural' increase of the innate, or animal heat which was the power by which the soul performed all the functions of the body. This view was held by physicians from the time of Hippocrates (460–377 BC) to that of Galen (AD 129– 200). Erasistratus considered that fever and inflammation were identical in 300 BC. Haly Abbas (930–994), the Persian physician, described it as preternatural heat from the heart which diffused to all parts of the body through the arteries. An early monograph was published by Daniel Sennert (1572–1637), professor of medicine at Wittenberg, in 1627. John Huxam (1692–1768) of Devonshire wrote an important treatise in 1750, which was followed by another, *Observations on Fevers*, by London physician, John Clark (1744–1805), in 1780. Thomas Southwood Smith (1788– 1861), an English Unitarian minister who observed epidemics of fever at the London Fever Hospital, published *A Treatise on Fever* in 1830. *A Treatise on the Continued Fevers of Great Britain* was written by London physician, Charles Murchison (1830–1879) in 1862. *See clinical thermometry.*

Fever Therapy *See artificial fever.*

Fexism A type of cretinism found in Styria in Austria.

Fiber Optic Endoscopy [Latin: *fibra*, band; Greek: *opsis*, sight + *en*, in + *skopein*, look] The first flexible fiber optic endoscope was used on a patient in Michigan University by Basil I. Hirschowitz in 1957. The flexible fiber optic esophagoscope was designed by P.A. LoPresti and A.M. Hilmi of America in 1964. *See endoscopy, esophagoscopy.*

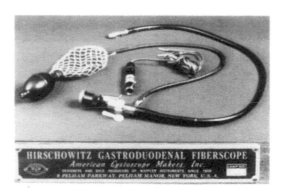

Fiber optic endoscope

Fibiger, Jonannes Andreas Grib (1867–1928) Experimental pathologist from Copenhagen, and a pioneer in the study of carcinogenesis. He demonstrated the carcinogenic effect of nematodes on the stomach of rodents in 1913, later found to be incorrect. He studied the role of coal tar in causing cancer and received the Nobel Prize for Medicine or Physiology in 1926.

Fibonacci, Leonardo (1172–1250) A distinguished mathematician from Pisa. He introduced the Indian system of decimals into Europe and discovered the Fibonacci sequence of integrals. He wrote *Liber Quadratorum* in 1225.

Fibrillation [Latin: *fibrilla*, small fibers] *See atrial fibrillation, ventricular fibrillation.*

Fibrin [Latin: *fibra*, band] Component of blood that facilitates the coagulation of blood and serous fluids was extracted by Andrew Buchanan (1798–1882) of London in 1845.

Fibrinogen [Latin: *fibra*, band + *genos*, descent] Its role in the clotting of blood was demonstrated by William Hewson (1739–1774), a British hematologist, in 1771. The splitting of fibrinogen into fibrin and other products was shown by Olof Hammarsten (1841–1932) in 1875. Large amounts in infiltrated lung tissue of patients with pneumonia was demonstrated by H. Rolleston in 1892.

Fibrinogen Degradation Product (FDP) Identified by H. Stormorken in 1957. Detection of elevated FDP levels in defibrination syndrome or other fibrinolytic states was made by H.C. Ferreira and L.G. Murat in 1963. *See disseminated intravascular coagulation (DIC), fibrinolysis.*

Fibrinolysis John Hunter (1728–1793) in his *A Treatise on the Blood, Inflammation and Gunshot Wounds*, published in 1794, mentioned that animals killed by electricity or lightning or killed after they had run hard, had blood that did not clot. Prosper Sylvian Denis (1799–1863), a biochemist at Paris, observed in 1838 that blood obtained through wet-cupping redissolved in less than 24 hours. The term was used by French physician, Albert Dastre (1844–1917), who observed the reduction in fibrin during phlebotomy in dogs in 1893. Spontaneous fibrinolytic activity in the globulin fraction of ox blood was observed by Sven Gustaf Hedin (1859–1933) in 1903. In 1906 Paul Oskar Morawitz (1879–1936) demonstrated that blood of victims of sudden death contained no fibrinogen and that this blood could destroy the fibrinogen and fibrin of normal blood. The modern scientific explanation was given by Robert Gwyn Macfarlane (1907–1987) of Oxford in 1937.

Fibroid [Latin: *fibra*, band + *oides*, form] Washington Lemuel Atlee (1808–1878), a surgeon from Pennsylvania, was a pioneer in surgical treatment of uterine fibroids in America. It was introduced into France by an eminent gynecologist in Paris, Eugene Koeberlé (1828–1915) in 1863. The method of enucleation of subperitoneal uterine fibroids through the vaginal route was introduced by Vincenz Czerny (1842–1915) of Germany in 1881. *Enucleation of Uterine Fibroids* was published by a British gynecologist, William Alexander (1844–1919) in 1898.

Fibula [Latin: *fibula*, buckle or clasp] The lesser bone of the shank was called 'sura' by Aulus Cornelius Celsus (25 BC–AD 50). Since it appeared to join the muscles of the leg like a clasp, it was named *fibula* in Latin. This is also the name of an ancient surgical instrument or a form of treatment for wounds. The instrument derives its name from its resemblance to a Roman clasp or buckle. Celsus stated that 'if there be a wound in the flesh that gapes and cannot be easily closed, it is improper to sew it, and you must apply a fibula'. According to Guido Guidi (1508–1569), these fibulas were circular or semicircular devices fitted with hooks to hold the skin in place. Gabriele Falloppio (1523–1562) believed that it simply meant the process of sewing a wound with needle and thread.

Fick, Adolf Eugen (1829–1901) German physiologist and professor in Zurich, born in Kassel, and studied medicine at Marburg. His graduation thesis was on astigmatism. He studied the physiology and physics of vision and analyzed the blind spot of the eye. He later studied quantitative hemodynamics, and became the first to calculate cardiac output by estimating the difference of oxygen content between arterial and venous blood, in 1870.

Fiedler Myocarditis Fatal myocarditis associated with infiltration of the myocardium by leukocytes, lymphocytes, or multinucleate giant cells. Described by Carl Ludwig Alfred Fiedler (1835–1921) of Germany in 1900.

Fiedler, Carl Ludwig Alfred (1835–1921) He described a fatal form of myocarditis with sudden death in 1899 that was named after him.

Fielding, George Hunsley (1801–1871) An ophthalmologist who practiced in Tunbridge Wells. The tapetum, a layer found in the retina, is named after him (Fielding membrane).

Fienus, Thomas (1566–1631) Born in Antwerp, he was professor of medicine at Louvain. He wrote *De Viribus Imaginationis* and *De Formatione & Animatione Foetus.*

Filaria [Latin: *filum*, thread] *See filariasis.*

Filariasis [Latin: *filum*, thread] The disease was known to the ancients, and Arab physicians gave a good description of it as *da-al fil*, which meant elephantine disease or elephantiasis. A modern account as hematochyluria, was given by Chapotin of Paris, who observed it in Mauritius in 1815. The laval nematode was isolated in the chylous fluid of the tunica vaginalis in a patient from Havana with hydrocele by Jean Nicolas Demarquay (1811–1875) in 1863. The same organism was later found in the urine of a number of patients with hematuria by Otto Edouard Heinrich Wücherer (1820–1873), in 1866. The nematode was also discovered in a patient with chyluria from Calcutta by Timothy Richard Lewis (1841–1886) in 1868. Lewis later found the parasite in the blood of a patient suffering from chronic diarrhea in 1870 and gave it the name *Filaria sanguinis-hominis.* The organism in its male and female forms was found in the blood of a Bengali patient with elephantiasis of the scrotum by a physician, Edward Gayer, during his work in Calcutta in 1877. The adult form of the nematode was identified in Brisbane by Joseph Bancroft (1836–1894) in 1876, and the parasite was named *Filaria bancrofti* by Thomas Spencer Cobbold (1828–1886). The worm was later named *Wuchereria bancrofti.* The periodical appearance of filaria in the blood, of diagnostic significance, was discovered by Sir Patrick Manson (1844–1922) while he was at Amoy in China in 1876.

Filatov, Nils Feodorovich (1847–1902) Pediatrician from Moscow who described the characteristic features of lymphadenopathy and fever seen in infectious mononucleosis, in 1887. He also described the early sign of Koplik spots in measles.

Filatov, Vladimir Petrovich (1875–1956) Russian surgeon who introduced the pedicle flap in plastic surgery. He also pioneered corneal transplant and tissue surgery.

Fildes, Sir Paul Gordon (1882–1971) London pathologist who established that females do not suffer from hemophilia. He also devised a blood extract culture medium (Fildes medium) for growing bacteria. *See paraaminobenzoic acid.*

Filterable Virus Minute particles in stained smears of vaccinal lesions were observed by a Scottish pathologist, John Brown Buist (1846–1915) in 1886. The first evidence for the existence of particles smaller than bacteria, capable of producing disease, was presented by Russian botanist, Dmitri Iosifovich Ivanovski (1864–1920) in 1892. During his investigation of mosaic disease of the tobacco plant, he discovered that the sap of the diseased plant was still capable of transmitting the disease despite its treatment through a bacterial filter. His findings were not taken seriously until Wilhelm Martinus Beijerinck (1851–1931) revived the interest in 1898. In *Ueber ein Contagium Vivum Fluidum*, he once again demonstrated the filterability of the agent of tobacco mosaic disease. In the same year, Friedrich August Johann Löffler (1852–1915) and Paul Frosch (1860–1928) demonstrated the filterability of the agent that produced foot-and-mouth disease. This was an important landmark in virology, as it was the first disease in animals shown to be caused by a filterable agent. In 1904 minute bodies from smears taken from fowl-pox lesions were seen by A. Borrel, who claimed these to be viruses. Similar particles were seen by Enrique Paschen (1860–1936) in 1906 and these were later confirmed to be viruses. The influenza of swine was shown to be due to a virus by American virologist, Richard Edwin Shope (1901–1966). A method of growing viruses on tissue culture was discovered by American physiologists, Thomas Huckle Weller (b.1915) and Frederick Chapman Robins (b 1916), who shared the Nobel Prize for their work in 1954. The protein and nucleic acid components of a virus were demonstrated by a German-born American biochemist, Heinz Frankel-Conrat, in 1955.

Filter [French: *filtrer*, to strain] *See bacterial filter.*

Filtration A method of water purification to remove bacteria, introduced by Robert Koch (1843–1910) in 1892. *See bacterial filter, filterable virus, ultrafiltration.*

Finch, Sir John (1626–1682) The son of a Speaker of the House in Parliament who studied arts at Oxford and Cambridge. He later obtained his medical degree from Padua and held several political positions, including that of

English Consul at Padua, Minister to the Grand Duke of Tuscany and Ambassador at Constantinople.

Findlay, William (1846–1917) Physician from Kilmarnock in Scotland who practiced in Glasgow. He published several literary works and poems including: *The Epistles of Noah* (1883), *In My City Garden* (1895), *Ayrshire Idylls of Other Days* (1896) and *Robert Burns and the Medical Profession* in 1898.

Fingerprints Johannes Evangelista Purkinje (1787–1869) classified them in 1832, and Henry Faulds (1844–1930) was the first to publish the fingerprint method of identification in *Nature* on 28 October 1880. Francis Galton (1822–1911) later published a work on the use of fingerprints in identification in 1892. A complete system of identification of humans by fingerprints was introduced by Sir Edward Richard Henry (1850–1931) in 1900.

Finkelstein, Heinrich (1865–1942) Pediatrician in Berlin who formulated a protein-rich albumin milk extract (Finkelstein feeding) for patients requiring a high protein diet.

Finlay, Carlos Juan (1833–1915) Cuban physician who proved in 1881 that *Aedes aegypti*, a species of mosquito, was the carrier of arbor virus which causes yellow fever.

Finlay, Robert Bannatyne (1842–1929) The first Viscount of Nairn, was a medical graduate from Edinburgh who gave up medicine for law soon after his graduation. He practiced law for nearly half a century before he was appointed Lord Chancellor in 1916.

Finlayson, James (1840–1906) Physician from Glasgow who wrote *Clinical Manual for the Study of Medical Cases.*

Finney, John Millar Turpin (1863–1942) American surgeon at Baltimore who described a method of pyloroplasty in 1902.

Finnish Medicine During ancient times, medicine in Finland depended on the disease demon. The Finns believed that all diseases were daughters of Louhiater, the demon of diseases. Their goddess Suoneta was the healer and renewer of flesh. The 'Tietajet', or the learned, and 'Noijat', or sorcerers, claimed to cure disease by expelling the demon with incantations and magic.

Finochietto Tourniquet Made of metal and controlled by a screw for arresting hemorrhage from the scalp. Devised by an Argentinean surgeon at Buenos Aires, Enrique Finochietto (1881–1948).

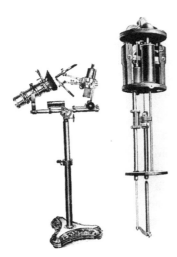

Finsen-Reyn form of lamp. P. Hall, *Ultra-Violet Rays in the Treatment and Cure of Disease* (1924). Heinemann, London

Finsen, Niels Ryberg (1861–1904) Danish physician and Nobel laureate, born in the Faeroe Islands, where his father was the governor. He graduated in medicine from Copenhagen and demonstrated the bactericidal effect of sunlight. He also developed ultraviolet treatment for lupus vulgaris in 1890. The Finsen lamp was installed at the London Hospital in 1900. He died of constrictive pericarditis at the age of 44 years.

Finsterer, Hans (1877–1955) A surgeon in Vienna who devised a Pólya type of operation or gastroenterostomy in 1918. *See Pólya gastrectomy.*

Fiorelli, Guiseppe (1823–1896) Professor of archeology in Naples. He excavated the ancient city of Pompeii. One of the oldest surviving calendars made of marble columns with the months of the year inscribed on it, compasses and other instruments used in mensuration, were found in Pompeii.

Firearms Injuries from firearms started appearing in the 15th century, and several medical men, including Ambroise Paré (1510–1590) and John Hunter (1728–1793), wrote extensively on gunshot wounds. The first known gun, a small cannon, was made in China in 1277. Gunpowder was invented in the 14th century. A medical interest in treating gunshot wounds started in the 14th century. The Colt revolver, first used during the Mexican war, was invented by Samuel Colt, an American chemist and inventor from Hartford, Connecticut in 1834. The Gatling machine gun was invented by Jordan Richard Gatling (1818–1903), a medical practitioner from North Carolina during the American Civil War in 1862. Pistols were manufactured on a larger scale in America during the mid-19th century. John Moses Browning (1855–1926), the son of a gunsmith from Ogden, Utah, invented the breech-loading single shot rifle in 1879, the Browning automatic pistol in 1911, the Browning machine gun in 1917 and the Browning automatic rifle in 1918. The submachine gun, known as the 'tommy gun' was patented by a retired army officer, John T. Thompson in 1920. *See gunshot wounds.*

First Aid The first book, *Helps for Suddain Accidents Endangering Life, by which those that live farre from Physicians or Chirurgions may happily preserve the life of a poore Friend or Neighbour till such a man may be had to perfect the cure*, was written by Stephen Bradwell of England in 1633. The modern ambulance service was initiated by the Order of St John of Jerusalem, a society that was revived in England in 1831. This order established the St John's Ambulance Association in 1877 that spread instruction in first aid and organized the transport of helpless patients. An early paper on first aid, *Observations on the preliminary care and attention necessary for accidental bodily injuries and mutilations occurring in mines and establishments where many people are employed*, was presented at St John's Gate by the Surgeon-General Thomas Laymon in 1874. The first manual of instruction was published in 1879 and 26,000 copies of it were sold at once.

Fischer, Edmond Henri (b 1920) American biochemist, born in Shanghai, China and educated in Geneva and Basel before he moved to America in 1953. In 1955, while working with Erwin Krebs (b 1918), he showed that phosphorylation and dephosphorylation processes were key factors in the activation of glycogen phosphorylase by adenylic acid. Fischer and Krebs shared the Nobel Prize for Physiology or Medicine in 1992.

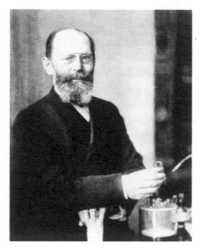

Emil Hermann Fischer (1852–1919). Courtesy of the National Library of Medicine

Fischer, Emil Hermann (1852–1919) Nobel laureate, born at Euskirchen in Prussia, and educated in Bonn and Strasburg. He discovered a new compound of hydrogen and nitrogen which he called hydraxane in 1875. He was also a teacher of Emil Aberhalden (1877–1950). He succeeded in breaking down albumin into compounds of ammonia (amino acids) in 1889. He successfully linked 18 amino acids in 1902, and synthesized the first barbiturate, veronal, with Josef von Mering (1849–1908) in the same year.

Fischer, Hans (1881–1945) Professor of organic chemistry at Munich, born in Frankfurt. His main research was on porphyrins, hemins and related compounds, and he achieved the first synthesis of hemin, for which he was awarded the Nobel Prize in 1930.

Fish Skin Disease or ichthyosis [Greek: *ichthyos*, fish] A skin condition resembling the scaly skin of the fish. Described by John Machin (d 1715). London dermatologist, Erasmus Wilson (1809–1884) described it under the name 'fish skin disease' or 'porcupine disease' in 1842.

Fishbein, Morris (1889–1976) American physician from Rush Medical College. He was a medical journalist and a reformer of the American medical system. He was editor of *The Journal of the American Medical Association* from 1925 to 1949.

Fishberg Test A concentration test for renal function. Devised by New York physician, Arthur Maurice Fishberg (b 1898) in 1930.

Fisher Murmur A systolic murmur heard in the anterior fontanel or the temporal region in cases of rickets. Described by New York physician, Louis Fisher (b 1864).

Fisher Syndrome A variant of Guillain–Barré syndrome, associated with external ophthalmoplegia, ataxia and loss of tendon reflexes. First described by Miller Fisher in the *New England Journal of Medicine* in 1956.

Fisher, Sir Ronald Aylmer (1890–1962) Professor of genetics and a statistician from East Finchley, London, who did pioneering work on blood groups as possible genetic markers. His *Statistical Methods for Research Workers* published in 1925, became the standard work on the application of statistics in research. He was professor of eugenics at University College London in 1933, and was professor of genetics at Cambridge in 1943.

Fisher, Theodore (1863–1949) London physician who described a systolic murmur heard in cases of adherent pericardium, later found to be associated with mitral stenosis.

Fission [Latin: *fissus*, cleft] German physicists, Otto Hahn (1879–1968) and Fritz Strassmann in 1938 observed that one of the products resulting from bombardment of uranium with neutrons was barium. The uranium atom during the process split into two parts of comparable mass with the release of an enormous amount of energy. This formed the basis for the development of the devastating atomic bomb used on Japan during World War ll.

Fistula [Latin: *fistula*, pipe] Described by Hippocrates (460–377 BC) in *De Fistules*. Aulus Cornelius Celsus (25 BC–AD 50) advised the inspection of fistula with a probe or sound. Paul of Aegina (625–690) stated that, if a fistula terminated in a bone it could not be cured without a surgical operation. Avicenna (980–1037), Aetius of Amida (502–575) and other ancient physicians pointed out the value of surgery. Artificial and pathological fistulae in various parts of the alimentary canal were used by several early workers to study digestion. Regnier de Graaf (1641–1673) used this experimental method in 1670. American army surgeon, William Beaumont (1785–1853) of Connecticut, performed scientific studies on the role of gastric secretions through a traumatic gastric fistula of one his patients in 1822.

Fistula in Ano *See anal fistula.*

Fistula Lachrymalis Obstruction of the ductus nasalis. Examined in detail by Percivall Pott (1714–1788). Dominique Anel (1679–1725) in 1712 devised a syringe for the injection of the lachrymal duct and he was the first to cannulate it. A screw was invented by Fabricius ab Aquapen-dente (1537–1619) to compress the lachrymal sac. Sir William Blizard (1743–1835) in 1780 proposed the injection of mercury to overcome obstruction of the lachrymal duct.

Fitz, Reginald Heber (1843–1913) A pathologist at Harvard Medical School and visiting physician to Massachusetts General Hospital. He described the diagnostic symptoms and signs due to inflammation of the vermiform appendix, and named the condition 'appendicitis'. His *Perforating Inflammation of the Vermiform Appendix: With Special Reference to Its Early Diagnosis and Treatment* was published in 1886.

Fitzgerald, George Francis (1851–1901) English physicist who proposed the contraction hypothesis related to electrostatic phenomena, in 1893.

Fitzroy, Robert (1805–1865) Commander of the *Beagle*, which carried Charles Darwin (1809–1882) on his voyage in 1831. Born at Ampton Hill, Suffolk, he became the first director of the London Meteorological Office in 1855, and invented the Fitzroy barometer. He wrote *The Weather Book* in 1863 which contained sophisticated pictures of storms similar to present satellite pictures.

Fixatives [Latin: *fixus*, fixed] Chromic acid was used for fixing tissues in 1840. Acetic acid was used to fix nuclei by Robert Remak (1815–1865) in 1854 and potassium dichromate was introduced as a cytological fixative by Heinrich Muller (1820–1864) in 1859. A new method of dehydration at low temperatures, called freeze-drying, was introduced by Richard Altman (1852–1900) in 1894.

Fixes, Anthony (1690–1765) Physician from Montpellier who published several works including *Opera medica, Leçons de Chyme, Tractatus de Febribus* and *Tractatus de physiologia*.

Fizeau, Armand Hippolyte Louis (1819–1896) French physicist, born into a wealthy family in Paris. He measured the velocity of light in the laboratory without using astronomical distances or phenomena, in 1849. He demonstrated the use of the Doppler principle in estimation of star velocity. He took the first daguerreotype photograph of the sun in 1845.

Flack, William Martin (1882–1931) Born in Kent, he was an English physiologist and director of medical research for the Royal Air Force. He discovered the sino-atrial node of the heart while working with Sir Arthur Keith (1866–1955).

Flagella [Latin: *flagellum*, whip] Structures in bacteria allowing them to move. Noted by Friedrich August Johannes Löffler (1852–1915) in 1890. The *Proteus* bacillus in its normal flagellated form was shown to grow on nutrient agar like a thin spreading film, resembling mist produced by breathing on a glass. The antigen belonging to it was named 'H' to denote the 'breath' form, by Edmund Weil (1880–1922) and Arthur Felix (1887–1956) in 1917.

Flajani Disease Exophthalmic goiter, named after Italian surgeon, Guiseppe Flajani (1741–1808), who described the condition in 1802.

Flavin Adenine Nucleotide (FAD) The presence of this co-enzyme in animal tissues was discovered by Hans Adolf Krebs (1900–1982) in 1933, and a purified form was obtained from sheep kidney by Otto Heinrich Warburg (1883–1970). The synthetic pathway was worked out by American biochemist, Arthur Kornberg (b 1918) of Brooklyn, New York.

Flavoprotein [Latin: *flavus*, yellow] The first flavoprotein, or 'yellow enzyme', was isolated by Otto Heinrich Warburg (1883–1970) and Walter Christian (1907–1955) in 1932, and crystallized by Axel Hugo Theodor Theorell (1903– 1982) in 1935. Their work formed the basis for further research on the cytochrome system of the cell.

Flea-Borne Typhus *See murine typhus.*

Flechsig, Paul Emile (1847–1929) Born in Bohemia, he was a neuropsychiatrist at Leipzig. The tractus spinocerebellaris dorsalis of the spinal cord is named after him, (Flechsig tract).

Fleischer, Bruno Richard (1848–1904) A physician at Munich who described march hemoglobinuria. *See Kayser–Fleischer ring.*

Fleming, Alexander (1823–1878) London physician who investigated the properties of the plant *Aconitum* and prepared a tincture in 1845.

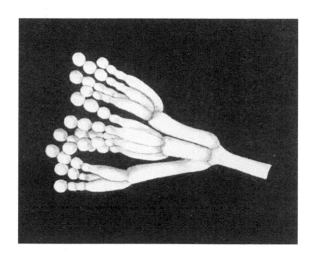

Alexander Fleming's *Penicillium notatum*. Sir Alexander Fleming, *Penicillin, its Practical Application* (1946). Butterworth, London

Fleming, Sir Alexander (1881–1955) Scottish bacteriologist from Loudoun in Ayrshire. He received his education at Kilmarnock and worked as a shipping clerk for five years until 1902. He qualified as a surgeon at St Mary's Hospital in Paddington, London and spent the rest of his career there. He discovered lysozyme in tears and mucus, and demonstrated its antibacterial properties in 1922. In 1928 he noticed by chance that *Penicillium* mold inhibited the growth of staphylococci on his culture plate. His finding was put into clinical use by Walter Florey (1895–1968), Boris Chain (1906–1979) and Edward Penley Abraham (b 1913) who demonstrated the effect of penicillin on nine patients in 1941. *See penicillin.*

Flemming, Walther (1843–1905) German histologist from Sachsenberg. He observed in 1875 a minute paired body in the ovum of the *Anodon*, lying outside the nucleus. The structure was later named the 'centrosome' by Theodor Boveri (1862–1915) in 1888. Flemming also used the term 'chromatin' and he gave a classical description of mitosis in *Zellsubstanz, Kern und Zelltheilung*, published in 1882.

Fletcher, Sir Walter Morley (1873–1933) English physiologist in Liverpool who devised a test for lactic acid in the muscle in 1907.

Flexner, Abraham (1866–1959) Brother of Simon Flexner (1863–1946), and one of the greatest reformers of medical education in America, although he was not formally educated in medicine. He undertook the task of studying the system of medical education in America in 1908, and produced a report in 1910 which led to significant reforms.

Flexner, Simon (1863–1946) American bacteriologist from Louisville, Kentucky, who became the first Director of the Rockefeller Institute in 1903. He discussed the causative organism of dysentery, *Shigella flexneri,* in 1900. He also prepared antiserum for treatment of cerebrospinal meningitis in 1908.

Flint Tools Used by prehistoric man. Georgius Agricola (1558) and Conrad Gesner (1565) described some stone axes and arrowheads but failed to give an adequate explanation for their origin. The first correct explanation was given by a physician from Tuscany, Michel Mercati (1593). English archeologist, John Frere, discovered stone flints and bones of large animals at Hoxne, Suffolk, in 1797, and proposed that these belonged to the remote past. His findings were ignored for nearly half a century until Boucher de Perthes (1788–1868) made similar findings at Abbeville, France in 1838. *See Abbeville.*

Flint, Austin (1812–1886) New York authority on clinical medicine and auscultation. He described many physical signs, including the apical mid-diastolic or presystolic functional murmur originating from the mitral valve in patients with aortic stenosis, in 1862. This murmur is now known by his name.

Flint, Austin, Junior (1836–1915) Son of an eminent cardiologist of the same name from New York. He was a founder of Bellevue Hospital Medical College, where he became professor of physiology. The vascular arches at the bases of the pyramids of the kidneys, Flint arcade, were named after him.

Flood, Valentine (1800–1847) Dublin tutor at the Windmill Street School of Anatomy in London for some time before he returned to Ireland to serve at the Richmond Hospital School. He discovered the superior glenohumeral ligament of the shoulder joint in 1829 which now bears his name.

Floppy Mitral Valve *See systolic click.*

Florence Test Test for detecting spermatic fluid using iodine. Devised by French physician, Albert Florence (1851–1927) from Lyons.

Florey, Howard Walter (1895–1968) Australian pathologist from Adelaide who became professor of pathology at Oxford in 1935. While working with Sir Ernest Boris Chain (1906–1979), he produced a pure extract of penicillin from *Penicillium notatum* in 1940. Their work led to the production of sufficient penicillin for clinical treatment of infections. Florey shared the Nobel Prize with Alexander Fleming (1881–1955) and Chain in 1945.

Florsdorf, Earl William (1904–1958) American bacteriologist in Philadelphia who devised (with Stuart Mudd) an apparatus for preserving serum, tissues and other biological materials through freezing and dehydration with a vacuum pump.

Flourens, Marie Jean Pierre (1794–1867) French physiologist in Paris, the first to conduct animal experiments on extirpation of different parts of the brain, in 1824. He identified the respiratory center in the medulla oblongata in 1837, and pioneered experiments on decerebrate rigidity. He demonstrated the anesthetic effect of chloroform on small animals in 1847.

Flower, Sir William Henry (1831–1899) Born in Stratford-upon-Avon, and graduated from London University. He was a surgeon during the Crimean War and later became the Curator of the Museum of the Royal College of Surgeons in 1861. He succeeded Richard Owen (1804–1892) as the Director of the Museum of Natural History at Kensington in 1884. He was a foremost authority on mammals and an anthropologist.

Floyer, Sir John (1649–1734) English physician, who wrote a treatise on asthma in 1698, in which he described perfumes or scents as a precipitating cause. He suffered from emphysema and gave a classic description of it. He introduced a method of documenting the pulse count, with the invention of his pulse watch in 1707. He wrote the first monograph on geriatrics, *Medicina Gerocomica,* in 1724.

Flucytosine Synthesized in 1957 and introduced as an antifungal agent by J. Berger and R. Duchinsky in 1962.

Fludd, Robert (1574–1637) Born in Kent, he graduated in medicine from Oxford and practiced in London. He was a propagator of medical mystics and a member of the Society of the Rosy Cross (a Rosicrucian) which advocated mystic healing and the pursuit of alchemy. He wrote *Philosophia Moysaica* in 1638.

Fludrocortisone Acetate A 9-halogenated synthetic steroid, prepared by J. Fried and E.F. Sabo of America in 1953.

Fluhrer, William Francis (1870–1932) New York surgeon who designed a probe (Fluhrer probe) made of aluminum for exploring gunshot injuries of the brain.

Flukes They have been known since ancient times as parasitic in humans and animals. They were described as 'broad lumbrici' by Hippocrates. Galen (129–200), and Paul of Aegina (625–690) recommended absinthium or wormwood as treatment. *See bilharziasis.*

Fluorescein Early radioisotopic agent used in diagnostic neuroradiology. Introduced by George Eugene Moore (b 1922) in 1947.

Fluorine [Latin: *fluere*, to flow] Its presence in fluorspar, giving it fluorescence, was noted by Georgius Agricola (1494–1555) in 1529. Several workers in the 19th century who tried to identify this fourth halogen were taken ill in the course of their investigations and the Belgian chemists, P. Louyet (1846) and J. Nickles (1869) died. Fluorine was isolated by Henri Ferdinand Moissan (1852–1907), a French chemist, in 1886. The chemistry of fluorine compounds was studied by London chemist, Harry Julius Emelius (b 1903), professor of inorganic chemistry at Cambridge.

Fluoroscope The X-ray fluoroscope was constructed by Thomas Alva Edison (1847–1931), and exhibited at the New York City Electrical Exhibition in 1896. Fluoroscopy was first used to study the act of deglutition in animals by Walter Bradford Cannon (1871–1945) of Harvard University in 1898. *See tungsten.*

Fluorosis Mottled teeth due to endemic fluorosis in Colorado was described by G.V. Black and F.S. McKay in 1916. An important experimental and clinical study of bones and ligaments in fluorosis was done by P.F. Moller and S.V. Gudjonsson at the Radiology Department of Copenhagen State Hospital in 1932. Fluorosis in the bones and ligaments of cryolite workers was observed by Gudjonsson in 1933. Mottling of teeth in infants born to mothers who worked in the cryolite industry in Copenhagen was observed by K. Roholm in 1937. An outbreak of fluorosis occurred in workers at the aluminum factory at Fort William in Scotland and in livestock in its vicinity in 1949. The organic combination of fluoride in bone was shown by London biochemist, Sir Rudolf Albert Peters (1889–1982) in 1969.

Fluorspar Calcium fluoride, discovered by Georgius Agricola (1494–1555). Some varieties had a delicate violet sheen, which gave rise to the origin of the word 'fluorescence'.

Blue John or Derbyshire spar, used for ornamental purposes, was first mined at Castleton in England.

Flurouracil Introduced as a tumor inhibitory compound by Charles Heidelberger (b 1920) and co-workers in 1957.

Flutter *See atrial flutter.*

Fodere, François Emmanuel (1764–1835) French surgeon in Paris who wrote several treatises on public health and medical jurisprudence. He published a work on thyroid goiter in 1792.

Foerster, Otfried (1873–1941) Neurologist in Breslau who advocated intradural division of the posterior nerve roots as treatment for pain.

Foetor Oris An old term for halitosis.

Fogarty Catheter A balloon catheter for arterial embolectomy, introduced by Thomas J. Fogarty of the Oregon Medical School, Portland and J.J. Cranley in 1963.

Foix Syndrome Ophthalmoplegia due to paralysis of the third, fourth, fifth and sixth cranial nerves, secondary to pathology in the lateral wall of the cavernous sinus. First described by French neurologist, Charles Foix (1882–1927) in 1922.

Foley, Frederic Eugene Basil (1891–1966) American urologist in Minnesota who designed a pneumatic cold punch resectoscope in 1940 for removal of the prostate through the urethra. He also designed a plastic operation for hydronephrosis caused by stricture at the ureteropelvic junction in 1937. The indwelling urethral catheter with an inflatable balloon at the tip is named after him.

Folic Acid [Latin: *folium*, leaf] Named because of its presence in green leaves. It was isolated from spinach and later from yeast and liver, and named the *L. caesi* factor, because of its influence on growth of *Lactobacillus caesi*. The hemopoietic effects of folic acid were observed by Lucy Wills (1888–1964) in 1931. The chemical structure was elucidated by Robert Crane Angier (b 1917) and colleagues in America who synthesized it in 1945. Tom Douglas Spies (1902–1960) tried folic acid on patients with nutritional macrocytic anemia and obtained a dramatic response in 1946.

Folie Circulare Jean Pierre Falret (1794–1870) a French psychiatrist at Paris, was one of the first to recognize that alternating moods of excitement occurred in patients with depression. He named it in 1854.

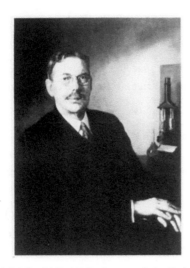

Otto Knut Olof Folin (1867–1934). Courtesy of the National Library of Medicine

Folin, Otto Knut Olof (1867–1934) Swedish-born professor of biochemistry at Harvard University who demonstrated the importance of amino acids in human digestion and metabolism in 1906. He showed that amino acids appeared in blood after a protein meal. He improved the microchemical method of estimation of blood glucose, which was devised by a Swedish biochemist, Ivor Christian Bang (1869–1918) in 1913. His colorimetric method was later developed to measure urea nitrogen and uric acid in the blood around 1919.

Folin-Wu Method *See blood glucose.*

Folius, Caesilus (1616–1650) *See Folli, Cecilio.*

Folkers, Karl August (b 1906) American biochemist from Decatur, Illinois. He was a pioneer in study of the structure and function of vitamins. Vitamin B_6 was first synthesized by Folkers and Stanton Avery Harris (b 1902) in 1939. He was also one of the first, with Mary Shaw Shorb (b 1907), to use injections of vitamin B_{12} as treatment for pernicious anemia in 1947. The structure of streptomycin was worked out by him in 1948, and he isolated mevalonic acid, a key intermediate in the synthesis of steroids in 1956.

Folklore Superstitions, handed down through generations, influenced family and community medicine during the Middle Ages and later. In Suffolk, a child with whooping cough was held face down in a hole dug in a meadow. In Norfolk, a spider tied to muslin was pinned to the mantelpiece for the same purpose. In Selbourne, children were passed through a cleft in an ash tree to cure hernia. Children with spinal deformities and skin diseases were passed though a hole in a stone in Cornwall. Similar superstitions exist across the world.

Folks, Martin (1690–1764) English philosopher from Westminster, who was vice-president of the Royal Society. He succeeded Sir Hans Sloane (1660–1753) as the President of the Royal Society.

Folli, Cecilio or Folius (1615–1660) Professor of anatomy in Venice. The auditory ossicle or processus anterior malleoli (Folli process) is named after him.

Folli, Francesco (1624–1685) Italian physician who advocated blood transfusion in 1680.

Follicle Stimulating Hormone [Latin: *folliculus*, little bag] Edgar Allen (1892–1943) of St Louis and Edward A. Doisy (1893–1986) of Illinois used ovarian follicle fluid from hog ovaries and produced pubertus praecox in immature albino rats in 1924. In 1927 Robert T. Frank and colleagues demonstrated that an identical potent hormone could be obtained from the follicle, corpus luteum, placenta and blood of pregnant women.

Follin, François Anthime Eugene (1823–1867) A surgeon from Paris who described small bodies consisting of isolated portions of Wolffian tubules in the paravarium in 1850. They were named Follin grains.

Foltz, Jean Charles Eugene (1822–1876) Professor of anatomy in Lyons in France, who described the valvular constrictions at the entry of lachrymal ducts in 1862.

Fomentation [Latin: *fomentum*, poultice] The application of flannels, cloths or sponges moistened with hot water or medicinal substances, to the surface of the body. It was a popular home remedy for many conditions at the end of the 19th century.

Fontaine Cannula Used for draining ascites, and devised by American physician, Bryce Washington Fontaine (1877–1926) of Memphis in 1925.

Fontana, Abbada Felix Ferdinand Gaspar (1730–1805) Anatomist from the University of Pisa, who founded and was first Director of the Natural History Museum in Florence. He described the Fontana canal, a circle made of spaces at the junction of the cornea, iris and sclera with the ciliary canal.

Fontanelle [French: *fontanelle*, little fountain] A point where the sagittal and frontal sutures join. Used during the Middle Ages to apply cautery to cure cerebral and ocular diseases.

Food Additives Safranine is one of the oldest known dyes used as a coloring agent for food. When industrial food production started in the mid-19th century, industrial dyes became an important source for food additives. Metal salts of copper and mercury were used for coloring, and butter yellow derived from benzene was a coloring agent used to make butter a deeper yellow. Some common additives were ripening agents, such as diaminozide, which made apples look a deeper red; taste stimulators, such as glutamates; vitamin C as an antioxidant; and emulsifiers. Diaminozide was found to be carcinogenic to animals in 1988 and was withdrawn. Glutamates were identified to cause symptoms which were later labeled as 'Chinese restaurant syndrome' in 1988. The food and drug acts passed later in both America and Britain helped to regulate their use. *See Food and Drugs Act, adulteration of food*.

Food and Drug Act (America) In 1901 ten children died after being injected with contaminated antitetanus vaccine. Following this incident the American Medical Association and other bodies agitated for control of drugs and the first Food and Drug Act was passed in 1906. The Food and Drugs Administration (FDA) became an independent regulatory agency in 1927.

Food and Drugs Act (Britain) The first proposal to prevent adulteration and to control the standard of food offered in the marketplace was passed under the Sale of Food and Drugs Act in 1875. It was amended several times over the next 50 years and a more substantial Act, which also covered food handling, was passed in 1938. The UK Food and Drugs Act 1955 is more comprehensive.

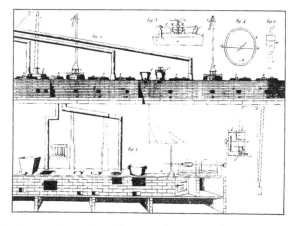

Food preservation equipment in Appert's factory, around 1830

Food Industry The use of snow and cold to preserve food was practiced in ancient Rome and by the Incas. A hindrance to mass production, supply and distribution of food in the past was lack of a practical method for storing large quantities. A mixture of snow and saltpeter as a refrigerating compound was used by an Italian, Zimara, in 1660, and the first ice was made industrially by freezing water with a

vacuum pump by Sir John Leslie (1766–1822), professor of physics at Edinburgh in 1810. His invention led to the use of steam machines and electricity for ice to be mass produced. Large cold storage rooms for preserving food started to be established around 1830. A method of preserving meat and vegetables by excluding air from containers was discovered by a French confectioner, Nicolas François Appert (1749–1841). Joseph Louis Gay-Lussac (1778–1850) examined Appert's bottles and found that they were devoid of oxygen, and concluded that oxygen caused putrefaction. Appert was one of the first to use the autoclave for sterilization in 1810, and opened the first canning factory in the world in 1812. The era of modern refrigeration began with the invention of a compression method using ammonia by a French engineer, Ferdinand Carre in 1857. Freon as a non-toxic and non-inflammable agent for domestic refrigerators was introduced by American scientist, Thomas Midgley (1889–1944) of Beaver Falls, Pennsylvania, around 1923. Plastic bottles for storage were developed by Swiss chemist, G.W.A. Kahlbaum, in 1888. The first breakfast cereal was made from shredded wheat by Henry Perky of Denver, Colorado in 1893, from an account by a person with indigestion, who took boiled wheat soaked in milk every morning to sooth his stomach. William Kellogg (1852–1943), a physician from Tyrone in Michigan, introduced the method of flaking wheat into crisp flakes in 1894. Corn flakes were marketed by mail order by Kellogg's food company in 1898. He established an industrial plant at Gloucester, Massachusetts in 1923. The production of uncooked frozen food on a commercial scale was introduced by an American leather merchant, Clarence Birdseye (1886–1956) of Brooklyn, New York in 1917. Sliced bread was introduced in 1930 and the Postum Company marketing frozen food in the same year. *See food irradiation, adulteration of food*.

Food Irradiation The use of X-rays to prevent decay of food was suggested as early as 1896, by Wilhelm Röntgen (1845–1923) and Antoine Becquerel (1852–1908). The Nuclear Materials Equipment Corporation of America started radiating bacon and potatoes with cobalt-60 to preserve them, in 1968, but the method came into use on a large scale only in the early 1980s.

Food Poisoning Ailments caused by agents transmitted by food or drink. Ancient Egyptians were forbidden to eat pork, because it caused disease. Food poisoning is mentioned in the works of Hippocrates (460–377 BC), and the Roman poets, Horace (65–8 BC) and Ovid (43 BC–AD17). Albrecht von Haller (1708–1777) studied the effects of decomposed proteins eaten by animals. The effect of putrid food on animals was also studied by Marie H.B. Gaspard (1822), François Magendie (1823) and Peter Ludwig Panum (1820–1885). A poisonous substance was noted in decaying fish by Burrows in 1814, and was found to be from alkaloids by Francesco Selmi, who named them ptomaines in 1872. Italian chemist, Nencki, isolated ptomaines in 1876. Otto Bollinger (1843–1909) stressed the importance of meat poisoning, which he called 'sepsis intestinalis' in 1877. The first investigation into the etiology of meat poisoning was made by Johne during an outbreak at Lauterbach in 1884, and a bacillus similar to anthrax was isolated as the cause. An important landmark in bacterial food poisoning was the discovery of *Bacillus enteritidis* as a cause of meat poisoning by August Gaertner (1848–1934), during an outbreak at Frankenhausen in 1888. This organism was renamed *Salmonella enteritidis*. In 1939 food poisoning became a notifiable disease in Britain under section 17 of the Food and Drugs Act. *See salmonellosis, typhoid bacillus, staphylococcal food poisoning, botulism.*

Foot-and-Mouth Disease The first disease in animals shown to be caused by a filterable agent by Friedrich Johann August Löffler (1852–1915) and Paul Frösch (1860–1928), in 1897. The ultramicroscopic nature of the virus was demonstrated by the same workers during later experiments using Berkefeld filters.

Foote, Edward Bliss (1829–1906) A medical graduate from Pennsylvania who promoted public education on contraception in the latter half of the 19th century. He published *Medical Common Sense* in 1860, and a small pamphlet on contraceptive methods, *Words in Pearl.* Following the enactment of Comstock's law, prohibiting distribution of material on contraception by mail in America, Foote was found guilty in 1876 and was heavily fined.

Foramen of Bochdalek A persisting embryonic pleuroperitoneal canal in the left posterolateral part of the diaphragm. Described in 1848 by Vincent Bochdalek (1801–1883), an anatomist of Prague.

Foramen of Magendie A foramen of the brain, described by François Magendie (1783–1855) of France in 1828.

Foramen of Monro [Latin: *foro,* to bore] The communication between the lateral ventricles and the third ventricle of the brain was discovered by Alexander Monro (1733–1817) of Edinburgh in 1783. This was later named after him.

Foramen of Winslow [Latin: *foro,* to bore] The foramen between the greater and lesser sacs of the peritoneum was described in 1732 by Jacobus Winslow (1669–1760), professor of anatomy in Paris.

Foramen Ovale [Latin: *foro,* to bore] *See atrial septal defect, congenital heart disease, fetal circulation.*

Forbes, Sir John (1787–1861) English physician who wrote *Cyclopaedia of Practical Medicine* from 1833 to 1835. He was the founder of the Sydenham Society.

Forceps [Latin: *forceps,* tongs] In 1813, a family living at Woodham Mortimer Hall, near Malden in Essex, uncovered a strange set of instruments under the floorboards in a room in their house. These were later identified by Henry Cawardine, a local surgeon at Essex, as obstetric forceps which had belonged to Peter Chamberlain (1632–1720). Chamberlain had lived at Mortimer Hall during the reign of Charles II. Obstetric forceps were probably invented by William Chamberlain, who came to England from France as a Huguenot refugee in 1569, and kept as a family secret. Hugh Chamberlain, the son of Peter, tried to sell the secret to François Mauriceau (1637–1709). Hugh later settled in Amsterdam and sold the secret to a Dutch obstetrician, Roger van Roonhuysen. It was in turn sold to a closed circle of surgeons in Amsterdam who were prepared to pay the asking price. Edmund Chapman, a surgeon from Essex, published an illustration of Chamberlain's instrument in 1735. Some years later, John Peter Rathlaw, a Dutch surgeon who studied under William Cheselden (1688–1752) in London, returned to Amsterdam and managed to gain access to the secret and published it in 1747. Since then many workers have designed forceps, and one of the earliest models was designed by M. du See of Paris, around 1740. William Smellie (1697–1763), the Scottish surgeon from Lanark, designed straight forceps in 1750, and described other longer forceps in 1754. Curved forceps was described by André Leveret (1703–1780) in 1751. Other types designed by various surgeons include those of: Jean Palfyn (1650–1730) in 1720, John Aitkin of Edinburgh in 1786, Haighton (1790), van de Laar (1777), John Leake (1729–1792) in 1774, Busch (1798), Uytterhoven (1805), Baumer (1849), Ziegler (1850), Murphy (1860), Grey Hewitt (1861), Reid (1878), Corning (1880), Poullet (1881), Etienne Tarnier (1828–1897) in 1881, McFerran (1884), Fry (1889), Sloan (1889), Cameron (1893), Fraenkel (1819) and Christian Kielland (1915).

Forceps Deceptoria An ancient surgical instrument, used for incision, which the surgeon held in his hands and was unperceived by the patient.

Forceps, Artery *See artery forceps.*

Forchheimer Sign A reddish eruption on the soft palate in cases of rubella. First described by American physician, Frederick Forchheimer (1853–1913) of Cincinnati in 1892.

Forcipressure [Latin: *forceps*, tongs + *pressare*, to press] A method of crushing blood vessels by forceps during surgery, to arrest bleeding. Devised by Sir Thomas Spencer Wells (1818–1897), an eminent gynecologist from St Albans, Hertfordshire. He also devised his own forceps which was later named Spencer Wells forceps. *See artery forceps.*

Ford, Edmund Brisco (1901–1988) English geneticist, born at Papcastle, Cumbria. He showed that the expression of a trait was under genetic control, and selection could change its inheritance to dominance or recessivity. He wrote *Mendelism and Evolution* in 1931.

Fordyce Disease Miliary bodies on the mucous membrane of the lips and the oral cavity. Described by New York dermatologist, John Addison Fordyce (1858–1925), in 1896.

Forearm Fracture The method of intermedullary fixation of this fracture was pioneered by George Schone (1875–1960), an orthopedic surgeon in Berlin in 1913. *See Colles fracture.*

Forel, Auguste (1848–1931) Professor of psychiatry in Zurich who, in 1905, published *The Sexual Problem,* which became a standard work on sexual psychology. He was also an authority on the psychology of ants. Decussation between the red nuclei of the brain is named Forel decussation.

Forensic Medicine [Latin: *forensis*, pertaining to the forum] Medical jurisprudence is a relatively new specialty, originating in 1507 when the Bishop of Bamberg introduced a penal code requiring production of medical evidence in certain cases. In 1532 Charles V introduced a code for magistrates to call for medical evidence in cases of assault, infanticide, pretended pregnancy, simulated diseases and pois-oning. The first work on forensic medicine, *Constituto Criminalis Cardina,* was published in 1553 in Germany. The first judicial postmortem was held by the French surgeon, Ambroise Paré around 1565. Another pioneer of medical jurisprudence in France was Antoine Louis (1723–1792). Alfred Swaine Taylor (1806–1880) an English forensic scientist, occupied the first chair of medical jurisprudence at Guy's Hospital in 1831 and wrote *Elements of Medical Jurisprudence* in 1836. Other English classics include: *Principles of Forensic Medicine* (1844) by William Augustus Guy (1810–1885); *Medical Jurisprudence for India* by Chever (1856); Ogston's *Lectures on Medical Jurisprudence* (1878); and Dixon Mann's *Forensic Medicine and Toxicology* (1893). Other famous British medical forensic scientists include Robert Christison (1797–1882), Harvey Littlejohn (d 1927) and Sir Alfred Sidney Smith (1883–1969). A pioneer in France was Paul Camile Hippolyte Brouardel (1837–1906), who wrote several treatises.

Forestus, Peter (1522–1597) Dutch physician who became a professor at Leiden. His work on medicine was printed in Frankfurt in 1623.

Forlanini, Carlo (1847–1918) Italian surgeon who established induction of pneumothorax as a regular treatment for pulmonary tuberculosis, in 1888. Following his work, artificial pneumothorax became part of treatment for pulmonary tuberculosis until the 1930s.

Formad Kidney An enlarged deformed kidney was observed in some cases of chronic alcoholism by American physician, Henry F. Formad (1847–1892), in 1886.

Formalin Formaldehyde was introduced as an agent for tissue fixation in histology by F. Blum in 1893.

Forman, Simon (1552–1611) A quack doctor and astrologer from Wiltshire. He studied at Magdalen College, Oxford and in 1583 set up a practice in London selling love potions and other quack remedies. He left a manuscript on Shakespeare's plays, *Booke of Plaies.*

Formic Acid [Latin: *formica*, ant] Discovered in 1774 by Karl Wilhelm Scheele (1742–1786), an eminent Swedish chemist.

Formulary [Latin: *forma*, form] A collection of recipes, formulae and prescriptions not sufficiently important to be included in the *US Pharmacopoeia* was compiled by the American Pharmaceutical Association, and recognized as the book of official standards by the Pure Food and Drugs Act in 1906. The *British National Formulary* (BNF) was developed from the National (War) formulary, and was published in 1949. It was later designed as a handbook for prescribers in the late 1970s, and the new style appeared in 1981.

Forneau 309 A trypanocidal preparation, Bayer 205, was produced by the Germans who kept the structure of the compound a secret. In 1923, Ernest Forneau, a French physician, produced a compound called Moranyl or Forneau 309, which was later found to be identical to Bayer 205.

Fornication [Latin: *fornix*, arch] During Roman times, when prostitution was acceptable amongst the upper classes, common prostitutes were looked down upon and took refuge under large arched pits or vaults called *fornices.* The term for sex outside marriage takes its origin from this.

Forssell, Carl Gosta Abrahamson (1876–1950) A radiologist in Stockholm who pioneered radium treatment for cancer of the uterus. He described a space between the mucosal folds in the pyloric antrum (Forssell sinus) seen on the radiograph.

Forssmann, John (1868–1947) Swedish pathologist who prepared a heterophile antigen for producing sheep red cell hemolysin in 1929.

Forssmann Antigen A heterophile antigen producing sheep red cell hemolysin. Prepared by Swedish pathologist, John Forssmann (1868–1947) in 1929.

Forssmann, Werner Theodor Otto (1904–1979) Born in Germany, he performed cardiac catheterization in animals while at a small Red Cross hospital, Auguste Viktoria Home, near Berlin in 1929. He later catheterized himself through a vein using a ureteral catheter, and confirmed the position of the catheter in the right auricle by X-ray, thus achieving the first catheterization of the human heart *in vivo*. He shared the Nobel Prize with André Cournand and Dickinson Richards in 1954.

Foshay, Lee (1896–1960) Bacteriologist in Cincinnati who devised a skin test for the diagnosis of tularemia, and prepared a serum for its treatment.

Fossil [Latin: *fossilis*, dug up] The petrified remains of plants or animals. Greek philosopher, Xenophanes (600 BC), was the first to observe fossil seashells in the mountains, and inferred that the Earth's surface must have fallen and risen from the sea in the past. For a long time the finding of fossils and shells on land was attributed to Noah's flood. Avicenna (980–1037) and Albertus Magnus (1193–1280) believed that they were substances of a non-organic nature. This was opposed by Leonardo Da Vinci (1452–1519) and Girolamo Fracastoro (1483–1553), who attributed them to extinct organisms. The first work on fossils in relation to geology was done in 1565 by Conrad Gesner (1516–1565), a physician from Zurich. His *Hortorum Germaniae Descripto Historia Animalium* (1551–1621) published in five volumes, earned him the name of the 'modern Pliny'. Study of fossils in paleontology was established as a branch of science by Georges Cuvier (1769–1832) of Paris, around 1800. Certain layers of the Earth were shown to have characteristic series of fossils by a civil engineer, William Smith (1769–1839), in *Stratigraphical Organized System of Fossils* published in 1817. He also published the first colored geological map of England in 1815.

Foster Kennedy Syndrome *See Kennedy, Robert Foster.*

Foster, Samuel (d 1652) English mathematician who was educated at Emmanuel College Cambridge and became professor of astronomy at Gresham College in 1636. He was one of the first members of the Royal Society.

Foster, Sir Michael (1836–1907) Considered as one of the founders of modern physiology in England. He was instrumental in establishing the *Journal of Physiology* in 1878, and took a leading role in holding the first International Physiology Congress at Basel in 1889. He produced an authoritative book of physiology, *Textbook of Physiology*, in 1877.

Fothergill Disease *See trigeminal neuralgia, Fothergill, John.*

Fothergill Operation A procedure involving anterior colporrhaphy combined with amputation of the cervix. Designed by English gynecologist, William Edward Fothergill (1865–1926) of Manchester in 1915.

Fothergill, John (1712–1780) A Quaker physician from Yorkshire who established a successful practice in London and had a magnificent botanical garden at Upton, Essex. He gave an original description of diphtheric sore throat in *Account of the Putrid Sore Throat* in 1748. He also described trigeminal neuralgia as, *Of a painful affection of the face* in 1773.

Foucault, Jean Bernard Leon (1819–1868) French physicist who initially studied medicine in Paris, but later changed to physics and other sciences. He demonstrated in 1850 that the velocity of light in different media varied inversely as their refractive indices. He also invented a gyroscope in 1852, and made several other contributions to the study of light and electricity.

Fouchet Reagent Used in testing for the presence of bilirubin in urine. Prepared by French chemist and physician, Andre Fouchet (b 1894) in 1917.

Foundling Hospitals The first person to declare child murder a crime and offer state protection and support to infants was the Emperor Constantine (AD 331). Emperor Justinian in AD 529 declared foundlings to be free and forbade them to be treated as slaves. St Goar described an establishment for orphans that existed around AD 600 in Triers in Germany. Similar establishments were founded at Anjou and Angers in France in the 7th century. The Institution of Foundlings, or the Hospital of the Holy Ghost, at Montpellier was established in 1180. The Spedale Degle Innocenti in Florence was founded in 1316 by a monk called Pollini. A proposal for a foundling hospital in England was made in 1687, but it was not established until 1739, through a charter from King George II, after a petition from Captain Thomas Coram (1668–1751).

Fourcroy, Antoine François (1755–1809) French chemist and physician who obtained his medical degree in Paris in 1780. He gave an account of lumpy tissues in a body on opening a grave at the Cemetery of Innocents in Paris in 1787. He named it 'adipocere', and presented his findings to the Academie des Sciences in Paris in 1789. He worked with another French chemist, Vanquelin (1763–1829), in isolating urea in 1808, and discovered the element iridium.

Fourier, Jean Baptiste (1768–1830) French physicist who defined thermal conductivity and invented an equation to calculate it in 1822. He introduced the Fourier series, a function in trigonometry, in *Theorie de Analitique de la Chalier,* published in 1822.

Fournier, Jean Alfred (1832–1914) Professor in the Paris faculty who made several important contributions to the study of syphilis. He worked with Paul Diday (1812–1894) at the famous St Louis venereal clinic in Paris and made a special study of congenital syphilis. Fulminating gangrene of the scrotum and perineum in diabetic patients is named after him.

Fovea [Latin: *fovea*, depression] Structure in the retina, described by an optic surgeon Francesco Buzzi (1751–1805) of Milan in 1782.

Foville Syndrome Abducens nerve and facial nerve paralysis with contralateral hemiplegia due to a pontine lesion. Described by French neurologist, Achille Louis François Foville (1799–1878) in 1858.

Foville, Achille Louis (1799–1878) A neuropsychiatrist from Pontoise, France who described Foville syndrome. The connection between the caudate nucleus and the thalamus was named Foville fasciculus. *See Foville syndrome.*

Fowler Operation Decortication of the lung in empyema (pleurectomy) to allow the lung to expand fully. Designed by New York surgeon, George Ryerson Fowler (1848–1906) in 1901.

Fowler Procedure Osteotomy of metatarsal heads. A procedure described by Edsan Brady Fowler (1865–1942), a surgeon from Evanston, Illinois.

Fowler Position A head-up position to allow drainage of fluid into the pelvis in cases of peritonitis. Described by George Ryerson Fowler (1848–1906), a surgeon from Brooklyn, New York.

Fowler Solution A genome remedy containing arsenic. Introduced by English physician, Thomas Fowler (1736–1801) of York in 1786.

Fowler, A. (1868–1940) Astronomer and spectroscopist who was an assistant to Sir Norman Lockyer (1836–1920) during his early career. He made significant contributions to the study of atomic structure and interpreted the constant proposed by Johannes Robert Rydberg (1854–1919).

Fowler, Lydia Folger (1822–1879) The second medical woman in America to receive an MD degree from Central Medical College, Rochester, New York. She became the first woman to hold a professorship in America with her appointment to the chair of midwifery at Central Medical College in 1851.

Fowler, Sir James Kingston (1852–1934) London physician who pointed out the association between throat infections and acute rheumatism in 1880. He proposed that pulmonary tuberculosis spread from the apex of the dorsal lobe along the greater fissure to the periphery (Fowler law).

Fox, George Henry (1846–1937) Dermatologist in New York who published a photographic atlas of skin diseases in 1880. A form of itchy papular eruption at the sites of apocrine glands, especially in the axilla (Fox–Fordyce disease) was described by him and John Addison Fordyce (1858–1925) in 1902.

Fox, William Tilbury (1836–1879) A leading London dermatologist who published the first book on fungi of medical importance, *Skin Diseases of Parasitic Origin* in 1863 and *A Treatise on Skin Diseases* in 1864.

Foxglove *Digitalis purpurea* has been known since the Middle Ages as foxes glew, foxes bells, bloody fingers and dead man's bells. The Germans called it fingerhut, and the current name was derived by Latinizing this word. Leonhart Fuchs (1501–1566) in 1542 described its medicinal use in dropsy and other conditions. William Withering (1741–1799), a physician from Shropshire, learnt of its value in dropsy from one of his patients and started using it. By 1779 Withering had established a place for digitalis in the treatment of dropsy and published *An Account of the Foxglove* in 1785. *See digitalis, digitoxin, digoxin.*

Fracastoro, Girolamo or Fracastorius (1478–1553) Italian physician from Verona who proposed a possible cause for infectious diseases in *De contagionibus,* published in 1546. He also introduced the term 'syphilis' in *Syphilidis sive de morbo Gallico,* published in three books in 1530. He died of apoplexy at the age of 70 years.

Fractional Test Meal Study of digestion by withdrawal of a test meal from the stomach was made possible with the invention of the stomach tube designed by Martin Emil Rehfuss (b 1887) in 1914. Before his time gastric contents had to be analyzed through artificial or traumatic fistulae. Rehfuss' tube contained a metal capsule that sometimes damaged the gastric mucosa and in 1921 John Alfred Ryle (1889–1950) improved it by covering the entire tip with rubber and providing perforations above the bulb. Further studies on gastric secretions using a breakfast test meal were done by Ryle in 1921.

Fracture [Latin: *frangere*, to break] Ancient Egyptians had various methods of treating broken bones, and the Edwin Smith papyrus describes some splints they used before 1500 BC. Hindu Brahmin surgeons also treated fractures with great skill. Paul of Aegina (625–690) defined fracture as 'a division of the bone, or a rupture, or excision of it, produced by external violence'. He called a transverse fracture through the full thickness of the bone 'cucumeratim' or 'caulatim', as he compared it to cucumber and cabbage which broke in a similar manner. A longitudinal break of the bone was called 'Scandulatim' by ancient surgeons. 'Polalentatin' is a term for a fracture into small pieces. Hippocrates (460–377 BC) dealt with them in *De Fracturis,* and Galen (AD 129–200) wrote extensively on fractures and treatment of long bones. Fabricius Hildanus (1560–1634) quoted a case history given by Sarazzin, a physician from Lyons, in which a 60-year-old gouty patient fractured his finger while putting on his gloves. This is probably the earliest description of a pathological fracture. A case of multiple pathological fractures in a nun with cancer of the breast was described by M. Louis of Paris in the 17th century. Samuel Cooper (1780–1848), in his *Dictionary of Practical Surgery,* published in 1809, devoted over 50 pages to the subject.

Fraenkel, Carl (1861–1915) German bacteriologist who described the characteristic pathology in smaller arteries and arterioles found in lesions resulting from typhus. He also demonstrated artificial immunity to diphtheria in guinea pigs by injecting them with attenuated strains of the bacillus in 1890.

Fraenkel, Henri (1864–1934) An ophthalmologist in Paris. He described the upward rolling movement of the eye during an attempt to close the eyelids in cases of lower motor neuron paralysis of the facial nerve.

Fraenkel-Conrat, Heinz (b 1910) American molecular biologist, born in Breslau, Germany, where he studied medicine before he came to Edinburgh to study biochemistry. He moved to America in 1936, and was appointed professor of virology at the University of California at Berkeley in 1958. His work on the tobacco mosaic virus proved that it could be reconstituted from protein and nucleic acid components, thus raising the possibility of a 'living chemical' in molecular biology.

Frambesia [French: *framboise,* raspberry] The disease, later known as yaws, was named 'frambesia' by François Boiffer

de Sauvages (1706–1767) in 1759. It is described by London dermatologist Erasmus Wilson (1809–1884) in 1885 as a skin eruption of reddish yellow tubercle-like lesions which gradually develop into a moist exuding fungus without constitutional symptoms, in his contribution to *Quain's Dictionary of Medicine.* It was noted to be peculiar to Africans and the people of the West Indies.

Frampton, Algernon (1766–1842) A physician from Wiltshire, elected in 1800 to the London Hospital, where he served for 40 years. He was the author of *Modern Practice of Physic,* which reached its 11th edition by 1853. He died in Hackney, where Frampton Park Road is named after him.

Francis Triad Nasal polyps, asthma and hypersensitivity to aspirin. Described by an Australian-born British physician, C.A. Francis (1898–1951). He graduated from St Bartholomew's Hospital in 1925 and was one of the first to recognize aspirin as a cause of asthma.

Francis, Edward (1872–1957) American bacteriologist who demonstrated the transmission of tularemia from man to rodents and named the disease.

Francis, Wakefield John (1789–1861) American physician, known for his Francis Triple X Pill, which consisted of mercury and aloes.

Francis, William (1878–1959) A medical graduate of Johns Hopkins, and Osler Librarian at McGill University. He played a major role in compiling *Bibilotheca Oslerina.*

Franck, George (1643–1704) German physician, born in Naumburg. He was also a poet and wrote verses in Latin, Greek, Hebrew and German. He became professor of physick in Heidelberg and wrote *Flora Francicia* and *Satyrae Medicae.*

Franck, Jacob (1856–1936) A physician in Chicago who described the prolongation of the clotting time in some cases of cirrhosis of the liver.

Francke Sign Red streaks near the border of the gums in influenza. Described by German physician, Ernst Francke (1859–1920).

Franco, Pierre (1500–1561) French surgeon who introduced the method of suprapubic cystotomy for removal of stones in 1550. He published one of the earliest monographs on hernia in 1561.

Frank Operation A method of subcutaneous symphysiotomy. Described by German gynecologist, Fritz Frank (1856–1923) in 1907.

Frank, Alfred Erich (1887–1957) *See diabetes insipidus.*

Frank, Peter Johann (1745–1821) Bavarian physician who published a work on modern public hygiene, *Complete System of Medical Polity* in German in 1777. He was the first to focus his studies on diseases of the spinal cord in 1792, and also the first to describe diabetes insipidus and differentiate it from diabetes mellitus in 1794.

Frank, Rudolf (1862–1913) A surgeon in Vienna who described a method of gastrotomy in which a part of the stomach was drawn through the chest wall and a tube inserted into it to maintain a passage.

Fränkel, Albert (1848–1916) German physician in Berlin who isolated the pneumococcus bacterium in 1886.

Fränkel, Bernhard (1837–1911) German laryngologist who devised a nasal speculum which is named after him. He also designed the Frankel test, in which the patient's head is positioned so that pus can be seen in the middle meatus in cases of suppuration of the anterior accessory sinuses.

Frankel-Hochwart, Lothar von (1862–1914) A neurologist in Vienna. He described cochlear, vestibular and trigeminal lesions (Syn. polyneuritis cerebralis menieriformis, Frankel-Hochwart disease) seen in early syphilis.

Frankelin, James An apothecary in London who was executed for murdering the poet, Sir Thomas Overbury (1581–1613). Overbury died of arsenic and mercurial poisoning given by Frankelin and his assistant, Richard Weston, in 1613.

Frankenhauser, Ferdinand (1869–1894) German professor of gynecology at Jena who described the cervical sympathetic ganglion of the uterus in 1867.

Frankland, Sir Edward (1825–1899) An eminent organic chemist from Lancashire, who developed the theory of valence in 1852. The presence of helium in the sun's atmosphere was discovered by Frankland and Sir Norman Lockyer (1836–1920) in 1868. *See valence.*

Franklin, Benjamin (1706–1790) A scientist and statesman from Boston who was intimately connected with medicine, although he was not formally trained. He invented the bifocal lens in 1785, and pioneered the treatment of nervous diseases using electricity. He also wrote on many medical subjects, such as deafness, gout and inoculation for smallpox. He was the founder and first President of the Pennsylvania Hospital in 1751. He was later commissioned to reorganize medical education in America and brought in several reforms.

Franklin, E.C. (1929–1982) *See heavy chain disease.*

Fraser, Sir Thomas Richard (1841–1919) A physician from Edinburgh who investigated the kombe poison from Africa and demonstrated its therapeutic effect on dropsy in 1885.

Fraunhofer Lines Dark lines in the solar spectrum, observed and measured with the help of a spectroscope by Munich optician, Joseph von Fraunhofer (1787–1826) in 1814. This observation later led to the identification of many elements.

Frazer, Sir James George (1854–1941) Professor of social anthropology at Cambridge in 1908. He published *Totemism* (1884), *Totemism and Exogamy* (1911) and *Magic and Religion* (1944).

Frederici Sign Heart sounds auscultated in the abdominal cavity in cases of intestinal perforation with gas in the peritoneal cavity. First described by Italian physician, Cesare Frederici (1832–1892).

Fredericq Sign A red line in the gum occurring in the presence of pulmonary tuberculosis. Described by Belgian physician, Louis Auguste Fredericq (1815–1853).

Free Electron Laser A device for producing photon emission beams by passing electrons through a magnetic field. Invented by American physicist, John Madey, around 1972. His invention provided the laser system for precise surgery. *See laser.*

Freeman, Walter (1895–1972) A neurosurgeon from Philadelphia who advocated prefrontal lobotomy in cases of specific mental diseases in 1942.

Freer Operation Surgical correction of deflected nasal septum. Described by a Chicago surgeon, Otto Tiger Freer (1857–1932) in 1903.

Freeze Drying A method of using cold to dehydrate food, practiced from ancient times. The first machine was invented by a German, Karl P.G. von Linde, in 1893. It was exhibited at the Universal Exhibition in 1900 and bought by Jacques Arsene d'Arsonval (1851–1940) who used it to prepare meat for the table. The process was adapted for preservation of biological medical products such as vaccines, tissue and serum in the 1940s.

Freezing Point Anders Celsius (1704–1744), a Swedish astronomer and physicist, defined the boiling point of water as 100 degrees and the freezing point as zero, in *Observationer om tvenne bestandiga grader par en Thermometer,* in 1742. The freezing point was also fixed at zero by René Antoine de Reaumer (1783–1757), a mathematician from La Rochelle who invented a thermometer using alcohol instead of mercury. English physician, Sir Charles Blagden (1748–1820) from Gloucestershire, discovered in 1788, that the depression of freezing point in a solution is proportional to the concentration of solutes. James Thomson (1822–1892) from Belfast, a physicist and brother of Lord Kelvin (1824–1907), discovered the effect of pressure on the freezing point of water. The effect of molecular quantities of solvent on it was described by Raoult (1830–1901) in 1883. Bernard of Paris was one of the first to use freezing point depression to calculate the concentration of solutes in urine and blood in 1902. Ernst Otto Beckmann (1853–1923), a German organic chemist in Leipzig, devised an apparatus for measuring freezing and boiling points and invented a sensitive thermometer which bears his name.

Frei Test A diagnostic intradermal skin test for lymphogranuloma inguinale, devised by a German dermatologist, Wilhelm Siegmund Frei (1885–1943), in 1925. After a period as professor of dermatology at Berlin-Spandau, he emigrated to America and became resident physician at the Montfiore Hospital, New York.

Freiberg Disease *See Kohler disease.*

Freke, John (1688–1756) London physician who described progressive myositis ossificans in 1740.

French Gonorrhea The term was first used in 1553 by Paracelsus (1493–1541) to denote syphilis. His terminology created confusion between syphilis and gonorrhea for the next three centuries. *See venereal diseases.*

French Letters *See condom.*

Frenkel, S. Heinrich (1860–1931) Medical superintendent at the Freihoff Sanatorium in Switzerland. He advocated the use of extensive physiotherapy for neurological disease with his introduction of exercises for tabetic ataxia in 1890. His *The Treatment of Tabetic Ataxia by Means of Systematic Exercise* was translated into English by L. Freyberger in 1902.

Frerichs, Friedrich Theodor von (1819–1885) Born in Aurich, he graduated from Göttingen in 1841, and held professorships at the universities of Breslau (1852), Göttingen (1848) and Kiel (1850). He discovered leucine and tyrosine in the urine of patients and described acute liver atrophy in 1855. *See carcinoma of the gallbladder.*

Fresenius, Karl Remigius (1818–1897) German pioneer in analytical chemistry, born in Frankfurt, and educated in Bonn. He later studied under Justus von Liebig (1803–1873) at Giessen and designed a systematic way of identifying compounds by precipitating various radicals. His work was published in English as *Elementary Instruction in Qualitative Analysis* in 1841.

Fresnel, Jean Augustine (1788–1827) French physicist from Broglie who developed Newton's wave theory of light. He invented the compound lighthouse lens and published a monumental work on optics, *Oeuvres Completes* in three volumes.

Freud, Anna (1895–1992) A psychiatrist and the youngest daughter of Sigmund Freud (1856–1939). She advanced her father's work on the ego and wrote *The Ego and Mechanisms of Defence* in 1936, in which she gave a systematic and clear description of defense mechanisms involved in the ego. She escaped with her father from Nazi Germany in 1938 and settled in London. Here, while working with children, she applied her father's psychoanalysis to child psychiatry. One of her last works, *Normality and Pathology in Childhood,* was published in 1968.

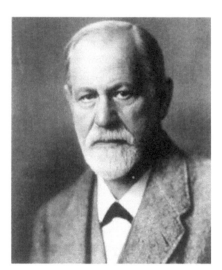

Sigmund Freud (1856–1939)

Freud, Sigmund (1856–1939) The founder of psychoanalysis, born to a Jewish family in Freiburg. His family emigrated to Vienna when he was three years old. He later graduated from the medical school in Vienna in 1881 and joined the Allgemein Krankenhaus in 1882. In 1885 he traveled to Paris where he became a pupil of Jean Martin Charcot (1825–1893). After spending nearly a year with Charcot he returned to Vienna and established his own practice where he pioneered hypnosis and electrotherapy. He met Josef Breuer (1842–1945) who, in his initial interviews with a patient Anna O (pseudonym) in 1881, used hypnosis to bring out her experiences which coincided with her symptoms. Breuer called this method the 'talking cure', and discussed it with Freud who conceived the idea of psychoanalysis from this. Freud and Breuer jointly published their findings in a preliminary communication, *On the Psychic Mechanisms of Hysterical Phenomena* in 1893. Freud regularly met with other psychiatrists such as Wilhelm Stekel (1868–1940), Carl Jung (1875–1961), Alfred Adler (1870–1937) and Eugene Bleuler (1857–1939) and their meetings led to the formation of the Psychoanalytic Society in 1907. Freud escaped from Nazi Germany in 1938, and settled in Lon-don, but died of carcinoma of the jaw within a year.

Freund Anomaly A limitation in expansion of the apex of the lung occurring because of shortening of the first rib and leading to narrowing of the thoracic inlet. Described by German gynecologist, Hermann Wolfgang Freund (1859–1925).

Freund, Jules Thomas (1891–1960) Hungarian bacteriologist who emigrated to America. He devised an adjuvant for increasing antibody production in animals.

Freund, Leopold (1868–1944) *See radiotherapy.*

Freund, Wilhelm Alexander (1833–1918) German surgeon who introduced abdominal hysterectomy as treatment for cancer of the uterus in 1913.

Frey Syndrome Auriculotemporal syndrome, in which flushing and sweating accompanied by a warm feeling over the distribution of the auriculotemporal nerve occurs during eating owing to injury to the parotid or seventh nerve palsy. Described by Polish physician, Lucie Frey (1889–1944).

Frey, Heinrich (1822–1900) Professor of histology at Zurich who described the crypts at the bottom of the gastric glands (Frey gastric follicles) in 1859.

Frey, Walter (b 1884) A physician from Kiel who demonstrated the effectiveness of quinidine in auricular fibrillation in 1918.

Freyer, Sir Peter Johnston (1851–1921) Irish surgeon who joined the Indian Medical Service in 1875. In 1897 he joined St Peter's Hospital in London as a surgeon and devised the suprapubic method of prostatectomy, described in detail in *Archives Internationales de Chirurgie* in 1914. *See prostatectomy.*

Fricke, Johann Karl Georg (1790–1841) A surgeon in Hamburg and a pioneer in plastic surgery. He described a pedicle graft operation for correcting cicatricial ectropion of the eyelid in 1829.

Friderichsen Syndrome   *See Waterhouse–Friderichsen syndrome.*

Frieben, Ernest August Franz Albert (b 1875) German physician who described the first case of cancer caused by X-rays, in 1902.

Friedländer Bacillus A bacillus isolated from a series of patients with pneumonia by Karl Friedländer (1847–1887) in 1882. The bacteria were later identified as *Klebsiella pneumoniae.*

Friedländer, Karl (1847–1887) Professor of surgery in Berlin who described the cells of the uterine decidua (Friedländer decidual cells) in 1870 and isolated a new bacillus, Friedländer bacillus, in 1882.

Friedman, Maurice Harold (1903–1991) Born in East Chicago, Indiana and graduated in medicine from the University of Chicago in 1932. He described a test for pregnancy (Friedman test) with Maxwell Edward Lapham (1899–1983) in 1931. In this test the urine of a woman was injected into a mature, female virgin rabbit. In positive cases the mature follicles of the animal's ovary ruptured within 48 hours.

Friedmann Disease A form of relapsing infantile spinal paralysis, described by German physician, Max Friedmann (1858–1925).

Friedrich Ataxia (Syn. hereditary ataxic paraplegia, hereditary ataxia) Speech impairment, lateral curvature of the spine and swaying of the body with irregular movements. Described by Nikolaus Friedrich (1825–1882), a German physician in Heidelberg in 1863. Death due to a cardiac cause in Friedrich ataxia was described by G.N. Pitt of Guy's Hospital in 1886.

Friedrich, Nikolaus (1825–1882) A German physician in Heidelberg, who described hereditary ataxia (Friedrich ataxia) in 1863. *See Friedrich ataxia.*

Friedrich, Nikolaus Anton Senior (1761–1836) German physician who described facial paralysis in 1795.

Friedrich, Paul Leopold (1864–1916) German surgeon who described the method of pneumolysis in which pleural adhesions are surgically divided.

Friend, John (1675–1728) Born in Croton, Northamptonshire and educated at Westminster School. He gave one of the earliest descriptions of hydrocephalus to the Royal Society in 1699. He was professor of chemistry at Oxford in 1704 and a year later went to Spain as an army surgeon. In 1722 he was elected as Member of Parliament for Launceston and later became physician to the Queen. Amongst his other contributions to medicine he wrote a history of physick in two volumes.

Fries, Elias Magnus (1794–1878) Swedish pioneer in mycology. His publications include *Systema Mycologium* (1821–1832), *Observationes Mycologicae* (1815–1818) and other works on lichens and fungi. He was professor of botany at Uppsala in 1835.

Fringe Medicine *See alternative medicine.*

Fritsch Catheter A double-channeled uterine catheter, designed by German gynecologist, Heinrich Fritsch (1844–1915).

Frisch, Karl von (1886–1982) A medical student in Vienna, before he studied zoology in Munich. His early work was on comparative study of vision in animals and humans, and he demonstrated that the visual acuity of fish was superior to that of humans in 1910. He also studied the behavioral pattern of bees and was awarded the Nobel Prize in Physiology or Medicine with Konrad Lorenz (1903–1989) and Nikolaas Tinbergen (1907–1988) in 1973

Fritsch, Theodor (1838–1897) A military surgeon during the Prussian–Danish war in 1867. While attending soldiers suffering from brain injury, he noted that stimulation of one side of the brain caused the opposite side to twitch. He later joined Eduard Hitzig (1838–1907), another neurologist, and did experiments on the stimulation of the brain in dogs. Their paper, published in 1870, paved the way for neurophysiology.

Fröhlich Syndrome Dystrophia adiposa genitalis. First described in a 17-year-old woman with a craniopharyngioma by the Parisian neurologist and pupil of Jean Martin Charcot (1825–1893), Joseph Babinski (1857–1932), in 1900. In the following year an Austrian physician, Alfred Fröhlich (1871–1953) of Vienna, described a similar case in a boy of 14 years as *A case of Tumor of the Hypophysis without Acromegaly.* Subsequently the same syndrome (Fröhlich syndrome) in children, characterized by adiposity, retarded growth and arrested development of the genitals associated with lesions of the hypothalamus, was described by other workers.

Fröhlich, Alfred (1871–1953) A pupil of Jean Martin Charcot (1825–1893) and an eminent neurologist. He described sexual infantilism and obesity secondary to lesions of the hypothalamus in 1900. *See Fröhlich syndrome.*

Froin Syndrome An inflammation of the meninges with obstruction of the spinal subarachnoid space associated with a coagulable state of the cerebrospinal fluid. Described by French physician, Georges Froin (1874–1932), in Paris in 1903.

Frommann, Carl Friedrich Wilhelm (1831–1892) Professor of histology at Jena who demonstrated in 1876 the striations

in the axis cylinders of the nerve cell (Frommann striae), using silver nitrate stain.

Frommel Operation Treatment for retroversion of the uterus by shortening the uterosacral ligaments. Devised by German gynecologist, Richard Frommel (1854–1912) in 1890.

Frommer Test *See acetone.*

Frontal Leukotomy *See frontal lobotomy.*

Frontal Lobe [Latin: *frons,* forehead] Galen (129–200) considered the frontal lobe to be the seat of the soul and source of animal spirits. Albertus Magnus (1193–1280) attributed memory, imagination and common sense to it. Changes in intellect and personality following cerebral injury have been observed over the past 200 years. J. W. Harlow in 1848 noted this syndrome in one of his patients whose frontal lobe was accidentally pierced with an iron bar. The inability to comprehend the nature of a grave situation in patients with frontal lobe lesions was noted by C. K. Hoffmann in 1869. Change in character in these patients were observed by Moses Allen Starr (1854–1932) of America (1884), L. Welt (1887) and M. Jastrowitz of Germany (1888). The symptomatology of frontal lobe lesions was studied in detail by P. Schuster of Germany in 1902, and its relation to intelligence was shown by Karl Spencer Lashley (1890–1958) of America in 1929. The grasp reflex in frontal lobe lesions was studied by Schuster and H. Pineas in 1926. Further investigation of the grasp reflex was done by H. Seyffarth and D. Denny-Brown (1901–1980) in 1948.

Frontal Lobe Syndrome *See frontal lobe.*

Frontal Lobectomy The first studies on the effect of unilateral lobectomy on patients were performed independently in 1932 by Canadian neurosurgeon, Wilder Graves Penfield (1891–1976) and J. Evans, and W. J. German and J. C. Fox. Further cases as treatment for tumors were described by Richard M. Brickner (1932) and S. S. Ackerly (1935).

Frontal Lobotomy Performed on four mental patients at a Swiss mental hospital by G. Burckhard in 1890. Change in behavior after it was observed and described by Leonardo Bianchi (1848–1919). The method was proposed as regular treatment for mental diseases by Egas Abreu Freire Moniz (1875–1955) in the early 1930s. He believed that morbid ideas stimulated the neurons and maintained a vicious cycle and that any alteration of the frontal lobes could interrupt this cycle. His theory was supported by experiments on the frontal lobes of monkeys by John Farquhar Fulton (1899–1960) and C. F. Jacobsen of Yale University in 1935. They noted that the monkeys became more manageable after section of their prefrontal lobes. The first frontal lobotomy on a patient was performed by Moniz, and Portuguese surgeon, Almeida Lima, in 1935. It was later advocated as treatment in cases of specific mental diseases by American neurosurgeon, Walter Freeman (1895–1972) of Philadelphia.

Froriep, August (1849–1917) A physiologist at Tübingen who described a dorsal root ganglion (Froriep ganglion) found inconsistently at a position posterior to the hypoglossal nerve.

Frozen Food The production of uncooked frozen food on a commercial scale was introduced by American leather merchant, Clarence Birdseye (1886–1956) of Brooklyn, New York. He established an industrial plant at Gloucester, Massachusetts in 1923. *See food industry.*

Frozen Sections Pieter de Riemer (1760–1831) was the first to use the technique of freezing to produce fine sections of tissue in 1818. His method was later used for producing anatomical illustrations by the Russian surgeon Nikolai Ivanovich Pirogov (1852) and Christian Braune (1831–1892) in 1872. It was further developed by Richard Altmann (1852–1900) of Leipzig in 1894. *See fixatives.*

Frozen Shoulder Syndrome A description was given by Simon Duplay (1836–1924) of Germany in 1872.

Fructosuria [Latin: *fructus,* fruit; Greek: *ouron,* urine] A colorimetric test for fructose in urine and blood, devised by American biochemist, Joseph Hyram Roe in 1934. The first series of 40 cases of this rare familial disorder was presented by M. Lasker and colleagues in 1936.

Frugard, Roger (b 1170) Physician at the Salerno School who practiced suturing of the intestines, trepanning of the sternum and recommended sea sponge for treatment of bronchocele (goiter). His *Practica Chirurgiae* (1220) remained as standard work for several centuries.

Fuchs, Ernest (1851–1930) An ophthalmologist in Vienna who described depressions on the anterior surface of the iris near the pupillary border (stomata of Fuchs) in 1885. Peripheral atrophy of the optic nerve (Fuchs nerve) is named after him.

Fuchs, Leonhart (1501–1566) A native of Bavaria and professor of medicine at the University of Ingolstadt. Apart from medicine, his other interest was botany and he published *Historia Stirpium* in 1542. This is one of the most highly illustrated botanical works of the 16th century, containing over 500 woodcuts. The genus *Fuchsia* is named after him.

Fuchs Atrophy A specific condition involving peripheral atrophy of the optic nerve. First described by a German oculist, Ernst Fuchs (1851–1930) in 1885.

Fuerbringer, Paul (1849–1930) A German physician in Berlin. He differentiated the subphrenic abscess from a supradiaphragmatic one, by inserting a needle into the abscess and noting its movements during respiration.

Fuller Operation A method of suprapubic enucleation of the prostate gland. Described by New York surgeon, Eugene Fuller (1858–1930), in 1895.

Fulton, John Farquhar (1899–1960) Professor of physiology at Yale University and a medical historian. His *Physiology of the Nervous System* published in 1938, contains the most comprehensive bibliography and author index on the subject.

Fumigation [Latin: *fumigare,* to smoke] A method of employing certain volatile medicinal agents as vapor for disinfection and treatment of diseases. Practiced since ancient times. Fumigating houses to get rid of pests were used by the Chinese in 600 BC. Acron, a physician from Sicily in AD 444, introduced fumigation to control pestilence. Avicenna (980–1037) described fumigation of the uterus as a method of abortion, and this was practiced abundantly later in the 16th century. Apparatus was described by the French surgeon, Ambroise Paré (1510–1590). Mercurial fumigation was used to treat primary and secondary syphilis in the 18th and 19th centuries.

Funduscopy [Latin: *fundus,* bottom or base; Greek: *skopein,* to view] Ernest Wilhelm von Ritter Brucke (1819–1892), a leading physiologist in Europe during the 19th century, visualized the fundus of the eye with artificial light. The ophthalmoscope, an instrument to visualize the fundus of the eye, was designed by Charles Babbage (1792–1881), the originator of the calculating machine, in 1821. In 1848 a medical student named Cushing observed that, in certain conditions, he was able to see the light reflex from the human eye and the light was not entirely absorbed by the choroid, as was previously thought. His observation was brought to the attention of Babbage, who then constructed an instrument with the same basic principle as the modern ophthalmoscope. He gave it to a veterinary surgeon who is supposed to have seen the fundus with it, but he failed to appreciate its significance. It was re-discovered by Hermann Helmholtz (1821–1914) in 1851 and he was credited for its invention. His ophthalmoscope was modified by Ruete in 1852 and since then several models have been produced. The use of the ophthalmoscope in neurology was pioneered by the eminent British neurologist, Sir William Gowers (1845–1915).

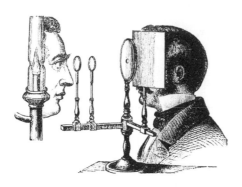

Funduscopy with the use of a light, concave mirror and two lenses. Jules Bernstein, *The Five Senses of Man* (1876). T. Fisher Unwin, London

Fungal Disease [Latin: *fungus*, mushroom] Madura foot caused by a fungus was described over 3000 years ago in the *Athara-Veda*. Diseases due to fungi were also known to the ancient Greeks and Hippocrates (460–377 BC) gave a description of thrush. Agostino Bassi (1773–1856), an Italian lawyer who later became a farmer, demonstrated the fungal cause of muscardine in silkworms in 1835. His description was probably the first on pathogenesis induced by germs, and the fungus he discovered was named *Beauveria bassiana*. Bernhard Rudolph Conrad von Langenbeck (1810–1887) observed candidosis in 1839. Frederick Theodor Berg (1806–1887) discovered the fungus in thrush in 1841. David Gruby (1810–1848) independently identified the organism of thrush around the same time. It was initially named *Oidium albicans* by C. Robin in 1853. The first fungal toxin, muscaria, was isolated by a German pharmacologist, Johann Ernst Oswald Schmiedeberg in 1869. The first case of histoplasmosis due to *Histoplasma capsulatum* was recognized at postmortem in 1905. An outbreak of pneumonia due to *Histoplasma* infection from a storm cellar occurred in Oklahoma in 1944. Up to 1945 only 17 cases were recorded worldwide, but by 1960 nearly 1000 deaths had occurred from histoplasmosis in America alone. *Achorion schönleini*, causing favus, was described by Robert Remak (1815–1865), who named it in honor of his professor, Johann Lucas Schönlein (1793–1864) in 1839. Coccidiomycosis was noted in South America and later in southern California. It was studied by E.C. Dickson in 1915 who thought that the disease was a mild form of tuberculosis, owing to the healed pulmonary lesions noted to be associated with it. The causative fungus was later named *Coccidioides imitis*. The 'San Joaquin valley fever' of California was identified to be a milder form of coccidiomycosis by Myrnie A. Gifford in 1936. Hundreds of other fungi cause diseases in plants, animals and man. *See poisonous fungi, actinomyces, candidosis.*

Fungus as Source of Medicine The use of barley in many ancient remedies suggests that the ergot fungus was unknowingly used by the ancients in childbirth and other conditions. The active substance, ergotamine, was isolated from the ergot fungus, *Claviceps purpurea,* by Karl Spiro (1867–1932) and Arthur Stroll (1887–1971) in 1921, and was introduced as treatment in migraine and obstetrics. The antibacterial action of the mold *Penicillium notatum* was first observed by Alexander Fleming (1881–1955) in 1928, and led to the discovery of penicillin. Streptomycin was isolated from *Actinomyces griseus* in 1943 and the fungus was renamed *Streptomyces*. Jean Borel, a researcher at the Sandoz Institute, later noted the immunosuppressive property of cyclosporin, and this was introduced to overcome rejection in organ transplantation in 1978. Actinomycin C was isolated from *Streptomyces chrysomallus* by Brockman in 1960, and was used to treat acute rejection reactions following organ transplants. Fungizone or amphotericin B, a potent antifungal agent, was produced from a culture of *Streptomyces nodosus* from Venezuela, by W. Gold, H.A. Stout and colleagues in 1956.

Funk, Casimir (1884–1967) Polish chemist, born in Warsaw, and educated in Berlin and Bern. From 1910 to 1913 he worked as a research assistant at the Lister Institute in London, where he began his work on beriberi. He was the first to isolate the anti-beriberi factor in 1911, and also coined the term 'vitamine'.

Furbringer, Paul (1949–1930) A physician from Berlin, who demonstrated the diagnostic value of the spinal tap. He also described the Furbringer sign, in which a needle inserted into a subphrenic abscess moved with respiration. He used this to differentiate the condition from an abscess above the diaphragm, where the needle showed no movement with respiration.

Furor Uterinus Described as 'an unseemly distemper, which is wont to seize up on maids, especially those of riper years, and sometimes widows too. They who are troubled with it, throw off the common veil of modesty and decency, and delight only in lascivious obscene discourses. They covet a man greedily, and even furiously, and omit no inviting temptations that may induce them to satisfy their desires' by Stephen Blancard (1650–1702) in his first medical dictionary in Britain, published in 1684. *See nymphomania.*

Furstner Disease Pseudospastic paralysis with tremors. Described by a German psychiatrist, Carl Furstner (1848–1906).

G

Gabriel, William Bashall (b 1893) *See rectal biopsy.*

Gad, Johannes (1842–1926) German surgeon who studied the relationship of lactic acid to muscle contraction in 1893.

Gaddesden, John (1280–1361) English physician from Hertfordshire who was educated at Merton College, Cambridge and Montpellier. He became Prebendary at St Paul's and attended Edward III. He wrote *Rosa Angelica practica medicinea capite ad pedis* (The practice of medicine from head to foot) which was used by doctors, priests and laymen. It also contains a mixture of superstition and absurdities.

Gaddum, Sir John Henry (1900–1965) British pharmacologist who did pioneering work on the role of chemical agents in the transmission of nerve impulse at synapses. He also demonstrated the competitive antagonistic effects of drugs in 1917.

Gadolin, Johann (1760–1862) Finnish chemist, born in Turku, and became professor of chemistry at Uppsala in 1797. He investigated rare earth metals and isolated yttrium from a black mineral from Ytterby, Sweden in 1794. Another rare metal, gadolinium, is named after him.

Gadolinium The rare element used in magnetic resonance scanning. Isolated in a pure state in 1886 by a chemist, Jean Charles Gallisard de Marignac (d 1894) of Stockholm, who named it after the Finnish chemist, Johann Gadolin (1760–1862).

Gaenslen, Frederick Julius (1877–1937) American surgeon in Milwaukee who described a method of subtrochanteric osteotomy for irreducible dislocation of the hip in 1935.

Gaertner, August Anton Hieronymus (1848–1934) *See Gärtner, Anton Hieronymus.*

Gaffky, George (1850–1918) German bacteriologist, born in Hannover and educated in Berlin, where he obtained his doctorate in medicine in 1873. He was Robert Koch's (1843–1910) assistant from 1880 to 1885, and was appointed to the chair of hygiene at Giessen in 1888. He obtained a pure culture of *Salmonella typhi* and demonstrated it to be the cause of typhoid in 1884. He was director of the Koch's Institute in 1912.

Gahn, Johann Gottlieb (1745–1818) Swedish chemist who discovered selenium, and isolated manganese. The phosphoric acid content of bone was demonstrated by him and Carl Wilhelm Scheele (1732–1786).

Gaillard, François Lucien (1805–1869) French surgeon at Poitiers who described a surgical method for treatment of ectropion.

Gaines, Walter Lee (b 1881) American endocrinologist who demonstrated the action of the pituitary in lactation in 1915.

Gairdner, William Tennant (1824–1907) Regius professor of medicine at Glasgow University. He wrote an important treatise on cardiac murmurs in 1861. He also differentiated between postoperative pneumonia and pulmonary collapse in 1854.

Gajdusek, Daniel Carleton (b 1923) American virologist, born in Yonkers, New York and studied medicine at Harvard. He identified a form of spongiform encephalopathy (kuru) amongst the cannibal Fore tribe in an isolated area of the Eastern Highlands of Papua New Guinea, while working with V. Zigas in 1957. He showed the transmission of a viral disease of the central nervous system of humans to another species, which earned him the Nobel Prize for Physiology or Medicine in 1976.

Galactosemia [Greek: *galaktos*, milk] The first clear account was given by Friedrich Goppert (1870–1927) of Berlin in 1917.

Galatio, Antonio (1444–1516) Greek physician who wrote several treatises, including *De situ Elementorum* and *De situ Terrarum.*

Gale, Thomas (1507–1587) English surgeon who attended King Henry's army. He wrote *An Excellent Treatise on Wounds made with Gunneshot* (1563), *Certaine Workes of Chirurgie, newlie compiled and published by Thomas Gale, Maister in Surgerie* (1586) and other treatises on practical surgery and tumors.

Galeano, Joseph (1605–1675) Italian physician and poet from Palermo who published several works on medicine and poetry.

Galeati, Domenico Gusmano (1686–1775) Italian surgeon in Bologna. The intestinal glands of the simple tubular type are named after him (Galeati glands).

Galen, Claudius (AD 129–200) The most famous of the Roman physicians, born in Pergamum in Asia Minor. He first practiced as a surgeon in his home town, Pergamum, but moved to Rome in AD 162 where he became state physician to Marcus Aurelius. For an unknown reason, at the height of his fame in Rome, he returned home in AD 166. Later, at the request of Marcus Aurelius, he returned to Rome and practiced there until his death. He founded the Galenic system of medicine which was followed for the next 1500 years until it was questioned by Andreas Vesalius (1515–1564) and Paracelsus (1493–1541). Galen described 347 herbal remedies, which earned him the title of father of pharmacology. He wrote extensively on a wide range of subjects in medicine and about 500 works are attributed to him.

Galenic Medicine   Medications containing organic ingredients, as opposed to pure chemicals.

Galileo, Galilei (1564–1642) Born to a noble family in Pisa and studied medicine before he changed to mathematics and physics. At the age of 25 years he became professor of mathematics at Pisa and moved to Padua in 1592. He constructed one of the first telescopes, based on the Dutch pattern, and used it in astronomy to discover black spots on the sun, hills and valleys on the moon and the Milky Way. He discovered the satellites of Jupiter in 1610. His scientific ideas were not in conformity with church doctrine and he spent a short period in prison and his books were publicly burnt. His principal works include: *The Operations of the compass, Nuncus Siderius, On the Tepidation of the Moon, Discourse on Solar Spots, Mathematical Discourses and Demonstrations* and *Treatise of the Mundane System*. He is considered the father of the science of moving bodies, or dynamics. He conducted experiments on the movement of falling bodies, pendulums and projectiles, and introduced the concept of uniform acceleration and distinguished it from uniform velocity.

Gall, Franz Joseph (1758–1828) Physician from Germany who described the structure of the brain on a scientific basis. He proposed that the gray matter was the active and essential instrument of the nervous system, and the white matter mainly formed the connecting links. His teachings were overshadowed by Galen's (129–200) theory of 'animal spirits', and he became disillusioned, and later practiced phrenology in Vienna. He had his own medical museum while he was physician at Würtemberg. He directed that his funeral should not be attended by clergymen and that his head should be dissected and exhibited at his museum.

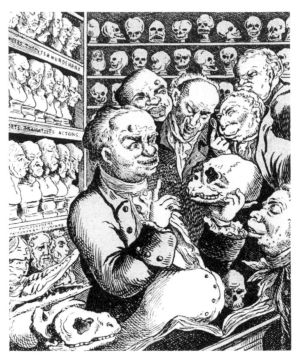

Gall and disciples. Lucien Nass, *Curiosités Médico-Artistiques* (1907). Albin Michel, Paris

Gallbladder   The spiral folds of mucous membrane in the neck of the gallbladder and the cystic duct were described by the German surgeon, Lorenz Heister (1683–1758) in 1717. Carcinoma of the gallbladder was mentioned by Maximillian Stoll (1742–1787) of Swabia in 1777, and the association between gallstones and cancer was suggested by Friedrich Theodor von Frerichs (1819–1885) of Aurich in *Clinical Treatise on Diseases of the Liver* published in 1861. The suggestion that a distended gallbladder could be relieved by a puncture was made in 1743 by Jean-Louis Petit (1674–1750), a leading surgeon in Paris. The first cholecystostomy was performed in 1867 by John Stoughton Bobbs (1809–1870) of Indianapolis. The second was performed by James Marion Sims (1813–1883) of America in 1878, but his patient died. The method described by Sims was successfully used by Lawson Tait (1845–1899) in 1879. Successful removal was performed by Carl Johan August Langenbuch (1864–1901) in 1882. The outpouching of the gallbladder near its junction with the cystic duct (Hartmann pouch) was described in 1891 by Henri Albert Charles Antoine Hartmann (1860–1952), professor of surgery in Paris. In 1928 a Chicago physiologist, Andrew Conway Ivy (b 1893), and Erie Oldberg demonstrated that when acid is injected into the duodenum a substance is released into the blood which causes the gallbladder to contract. This substance was later named 'cholecystokinin' by Ivy. *See gallstone.*

Galleazi Fracture or Dislocation Fracture of the radius accompanied by dislocation of the radio-ulnar joint. Described by an orthopedic surgeon in Milan, Ricardo Galleazi (1856–1952), in 1934.

Galleazi, Ricardo (1866–1952) Italian orthopedic surgeon and director of the famous Istituto dei Rachitici in Milan. He reviewed over 12,000 cases of congenital dislocation of the hip and devised a method of treating structural scoliosis in 1929.

Galleoti, Gino (1867–1921) Italian bacteriologist who prepared a vaccine for *Pasteurella pestis* by treating the bacteria with caustic soda.

Gallie, William Edward (1882–1959) Canadian professor of surgery at Toronto who introduced fascial sutures for surgery of inguinal hernia in 1927.

Gallium Element observed spectroscopically in 1875 by French physical chemist, Paul Emile Lecoq de Boisbaudran (1838–1912) of Cognac. He isolated it later in the same year and named it in honor of his country. A spectroscopic study of 35 other elements, *Spectres lumineux,* was published by him in 1874. Gallium was the first element to be discovered on the basis of the periodic table proposed by Dmitri Ivanovich Mendeleev (1834–1907). It is used in medicine for isotope scanning to detect infections.

Gallop Rhythm Rhythm of the failing heart on auscultation, studied and explained in 1875 by Pierre Carl Edouard Potain (1825–1901), of Paris.

Gallstone Observed in Egyptian mummies from 3000 BC. They were described by Gentile la Foligno, a professor at Padua in his *Consilia* in 1340. Removal from a living patient was performed by Hildanus Fabricius (1560–1634) in 1618. An important early study was performed by Bernard Naunyn (1839–1925) who published his findings in *Klinik der Cholelithiasis* in 1892. He advocated drainage of the bile duct in cases of cholestasis due to gallstones in 1898. Cholecystotomy was described by American surgeon, John Stoughton Bobbs (1809–1870).

Galton, Sir Francis (1822–1911) English biologist and cousin of Charles Darwin (1809–1882), born in Birmingham, and educated at King's College, London and Trinity College, Cambridge. He coined the term 'eugenics' in 1883 to 'denote the study of agencies under social control that may improve or impair the racial qualities of future generations, either physically or mentally'. In 1892 he proposed fingerprints as means of identifying criminals, and conducted the first statistical study of biological variation and inheritance in 1889. He wrote *Narrative of an Explorer in Native South Africa* and *Art of Travel* following his explorations in Africa in 1855. His other works include: *Metereographica* (1863), *Hereditary Genius* (1869), *Natural Inheritance* (1889) and *Finger Prints* (1892). He was the first to publish a newspaper weather map in *The Times* in 1875.

Galvani, Luigi (1737–1798) Italian physician, born in Bologna, and became professor of obstetrics there in 1782. He studied bioelectric effects using frogs' legs in 1786. In 1791 he investigated the twitching of frog muscle produced by being brought into contact with two metals, a phenomenon that was first noticed by his wife. His subsequent studies led him to believe that muscle or nerve generated electricity. His work led to the construction of the Voltaic pile by Alessandro Volta (1745–1827) in 1800, and laid the foundation for electrophysiology. Galvani wrote *Aloysis Galvani de Viribus Electricitatis in Motu Musculari Commentarius* in 1791.

Galvanism Another term for electricity, derived from the name of Luigi Galvani (1737–1798), an Italian physician who demonstrated the presence and conduction of electricity in animal tissue in 1791.

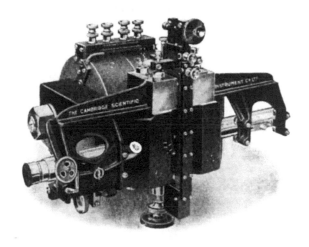

String Galvanometer. Thomas Lewis, *Clinical Electrocardiography* (1918). Shaw & Sons, London

Galvanometer The tangent galvanometer was the earliest device used for measuring electric current. Hermann Ludwig Ferdinand von Helmholtz (1821-1894) improved it by adding two coaxial cables, and the first practical moving coil galvanometer was constructed by William Sturgeon (1783-1850) of Whittington, Lancashire in 1836. This was followed by Wilhelm Weber's (1804-1891) electrodynamometer in 1840 and was further developed by Lord Kelvin (1824-1907) and James Joule (1818-1899) in 1883. An improved form, known as the d'Arsonval galvanometer, was produced by Jacques Arsene d'Arsonval (1851-1940) in 1880. Willem Einthoven (1860-1927), a Dutch physiologist and professor of physics in Leiden, was the first to apply a modified string galvanometer to measure time-related electrical changes in living tissues in 1903. His instrument was later developed into the electrocardiograph.

Gametes [Greek: *gamete*, wife + *gametes*, husband] During the times of Galen (129–200) and Aristotle (384–322 BC), fertilization of the ovum or female gamete was thought to take place by a mystic process called 'aura seminalis'. It was believed that the ovum was complete in itself and was capable of producing an embryo after a suitable stimulus was received. This view, called 'preformation', was held until the 16th century. Amphimixis [Greek: *amphi*, both + *mixis*, mingling], a process of reproduction by the fusion of two gametes during fertilization, was described by August Friedrich Leopold Weismann (1834–1914) of Jena in 1891. Haploidy, or the presence of half the original number of chromosomes in a gametic cell, was discovered by Edouard Joseph Louis Beneden (1845–1910) of Belgium in 1887. Heterozygosity, with a zygote being derived from gametes of dissimilar genes, was described and named by William Bateson (1861–1926) in 1902. Homozygosity, with a zygote developed from the union of gametes identical in the quality, quantity and arrangement of genes, was also described and named by Bateson. The diploid or zygotic number (2n) of chromosomes as opposed to the haploid (n) or gametic number was described by Eduard Adolf Strasburger (1844–1912) in 1905. The first successful *in vitro* fertilization of human gametes was done by Robert Geoffrey Edwards (b 1925) and Patrick Christopher Steptoe (1913–1988) in 1969.

Gamgee Tissue The principle of an absorbent dressing which kept the wound dry was demonstrated in 1880 by Joseph Samson Gamgee (1828–1886), a surgeon at Queen's Hospital, Birmingham. His dressing, consisting of a layer of absorbent cotton between two layers of absorbent gauze, was known as Gamgee tissue.

Gamma Helmet A device for delivering precise radiation to brain tumors using cobalt-60. Invented by Swedish physicists, Lars Leksell and Borje Larsson, in 1968.

Gamma or γ The third letter of the Greek alphabet, sometimes used to denote the third member of a group or series.

Gamma Ray Following the discovery of the radiation properties of uranium by Ernest Rutherford (1871–1937) in 1899, a new type of ray, gamma ray, more penetrating than alpha, beta or X-rays, was discovered by French physicist,

Paul Ulrich Villard (b 1860) of Lyons in 1900. The wavelength of gamma rays was measured by American physicist, Arthur Holly Compton (1892–1962) of Ohio, and C.D. Ellis, around 1915.

Gammaglobulin The three components of globulin, alpha, beta and gamma, were classified according to their mobility during electrophoresis by the Swedish biochemist, Arne Wilhelm Kaurin Tiselius (1902–1971) in 1937. He developed preparative electrophoresis in 1943 and electrokinetic filtration in 1947. He was awarded the Nobel Prize for Chemistry in 1948, and was made president of the Nobel Foundation in 1960.

Gamow, George (1904–1968) Russian-born American physicist, and professor at Leningrad who made important discoveries in molecular biology and cosmology. He moved to American and was professor of physics at George Washington University from 1932 to 1955 and at Colorado from 1956 to 1968. In 1946 he proposed the Big Bang Theory for the creation of the universe. He determined the order of the four nucleic acid bases in DNA in 1950.

Ganglion [Greek: *ganglion*, knot] The dangers of opening round tumors of the nerve tendon were pointed out by Hippocrates (460–377 BC). The term 'ganglion' was first used by Galen (129–200) to denote a pathological swelling of a nerve. Antyllus (*c* AD 250) recommended the entire excision of a ganglion tumor as treatment.

Ganglion of Ribes The uppermost sympathetic ganglion situated on the anterior communicating artery of the circle of Willis. Described in 1817 by army surgeon, François Ribes (1765–1845) of Toulouse.

Gangrene [Greek: *gangraina*, an eating sore] Ancient Greek physicians used the term for cancer. One of the first rational theories of pathogenesis, 'if morbid residue fails to be evacuated by mouth, rectum, urethra or skin pore, it will result in an eruption tumor or gangrene', was proposed by Hippocrates (460–377 BC). The Greek surgeon Archigenes, who lived around AD 100, was one of the first to start amputating limbs for indications such as gangrene and malignant tumors. Paul of Aegina (625–690) described it as 'mortifications arising from the violence of inflammation, when they are not yet formed, but forming. If such a state is not speedily cured, the affected part dies and the disease seizing upon surrounding parts, kills the person'. When the affected part became insensitive, he called it 'sphacelus'. Bleeding or venesection as treatment was recommended by Galen (129–200), Paul of Aegina and others. Alsaharavius (AD 980) recommended amputation if bleeding failed to cure the lesion. Fabricius Hildanus (1560–1624) wrote a monograph on it in 1593. A classic treatise was written by M. Victor François of Mons in 1832. François Quesnay (1694–1774), a French surgeon in Paris, suggested an arterial cause in his *Traite de la Gangrene* published in 1739. Hebred in 1817 proposed that it was caused by an obstacle to the interior of the blood vessels. Embolism as a cause was pointed out by H. Ball in *Thesis de Paris* published in 1862. *Clostridium welchii* as the cause of gas gangrene was identified by William Henry Welch (1850–1934) in 1892.

Ganja (*Cannabis sativa*) A Hindustani term for Indian hemp or cannabis. Ancient Chinese herbals referred to it as *Rh-ya*, in the 5th century. The Hindu medical works of Susruta and Charaka mentioned it as *B'hanga*, a remedy for many conditions. The Muhammadan sect of assassins during the Crusades used it, and referred to it as *hashishin*. The plant was introduced to Europe around 1563.

Ganser, Sigbert Joseph Maria (1853–1931) German psychiatrist, born in Dresden and later became professor of neurology there. He described Ganser syndrome, a form of acute hallucinatory mania in prisoners, in 1898.

Gant Clamp Angled clamp used in hemorrhoidectomy. Devised by New York surgeon, Samuel Goodwin Gant (1870–1944).

Gant, Frederick James (1825–1905) London surgeon who performed subtrochanteric osteotomy (Gant operation) for ankylosis of the hip joint.

Garcia, Manuel Patricio Rodriguez (1805–1906) Inventor of the laryngoscope. He was born to a famous family of musicians in Madrid. He was appointed professor in Paris in 1830 and wrote *Memoir on the Human Voice* in 1840. He constructed the first laryngoscope, consisting of two mirrors, in 1854. He later settled in London and died at the age of 101 years.

Garden, Alexander (1730–1791) A biologist from Edinburgh who moved to Charlestown, South Carolina and practiced as a physician. During his 20-year stay in America he discovered several botanical species before returning to Edinburgh during the last few years of his life.

Gardner Syndrome A hereditary autosomal dominant condition associated with colonic polyposis and increased risk of carcinoma. Described in 1951 by American geneticist, Eldon J. Gardner (b 1909), professor of zoology at Utah State University.

Garengeot, Rene Jacques Croissant de (1688–1759) Surgeon from Brittany who wrote *Traites des Operationes de Chirurgie, Myotomie Humain* and other works.

Gargoylism or Hurler Syndrome A hereditary disease due to a disturbance of mucopolysaccharide metabolism. Described in 1917 in two brothers by a Canadian professor of medicine, Charles Hunter (1872–1955). Further features, including corneal opacity and mental retardation, were observed in 1919 in two infants by German pediatrician, Gertrude Hurler.

Garland, George Minot (1848–1926) Physician in Boston who described a triangular area (Garland triangle) of dullness to percussion in cases of moderate-sized pleural effusion.

Garnet, Thomas (1766–1802) Physician from Cumbria who practiced in Yorkshire, Liverpool, Manchester and Glasgow. He eventually settled in Great Marlborough Street, London, and conducted lectures at his own house. He wrote *A Lecture on Health, An Analysis of the Mineral Waters of Harrogate, Outlines of Chemistry* and other treatises.

Garré, Carl (1857–1928) Swiss surgeon who described a form of chronic non-suppurative sclerosing osteomyelitis (Garré disease).

Garrison and Morton Medical Bibliography Compiled by Leslie T. Morton from Fielding Hudson Garrison's work, which provided over 4200 items of bibliography. Morton, on the editorial staff of the *British Medical Journal,* added over 1600 items and published the first edition in 1949.

Garrison, Fielding Hudson (1870–1935) A leading American medical historian. He was born in Washington and graduated in arts from Johns Hopkins University in 1890. He completed his medical studies at Georgetown University and became a lecturer on the history of medicine at the Welch Medical Library, and its librarian, in 1928. He moved to Baltimore as a lecturer on the history of medicine at Johns Hopkins University in 1930. He originated the *Bulletin of the Institute of the History of Medicine* with Henry Ernest Sigerist (1891–1957) of Yale University, in 1933. His most important book, *Introduction to the History of Medicine,* was published in 1913.

Garrod, Dorothy Anne Elizabeth (1892–1968) The first woman to be appointed to a professorial chair at Cambridge, in 1939. She was the daughter of physician Sir Archibald Garrod (1857–1936) and an expert on the Paleolithic age.

Garrod, Sir Alfred Baring (1819–1907) Consulting physician to King's College London and vice-president of the Royal

College of Physicians. He discovered excess uric acid in the blood of patients with gout. He introduced the thread test for uric acid and also coined the term 'rheumatoid arthritis'.

Garrod, Sir Archibald Edward (1857–1936) London physician, educated at Oxford and St Bartholomew's Hospital. He was a pioneer (1909) in the study of inborn errors of metabolism including alkaptonuria, cystinuria and pentosuria. He succeeded Sir William Osler (1849–1919) as regius professor of medicine at Oxford and wrote *The Inborn Factors in Disease* in 1931.

Garth, Sir Samuel (1661–1718) Physician from Yorkshire who was educated at Peterhouse, Cambridge. He was physician to King George I, and physician-general to the army. He wrote *The Dispensary,* a poem containing a lively satire on apothecaries and physicians, in 1669.

Garthshore, Maxwell (1732–1812) Physician and accoucheur from Kircudbright, Scotland, who moved to London as physician to the British Lying-in Hospital in 1763.

Gärtner, August Anton Hieronymus (1848–1934) A microbiologist who discovered a bacterium that caused meat poisoning, and named it *Bacillus enteritidis* in 1888. It was later renamed *Salmonella enteritidis.*

Gartner, Hermann Treschow (1785–1827) The elder brother of the embryologist Benjamin Gartner, born in the West Indies and graduated from Copenhagen, before he joined the Norwegian army as a surgeon. He described the ductus epo-ophori (canal of Gartner) that had been observed by Marcello Malpighi (1628–1694) in 1681.

Garve, Christian (1742–1798) German physiologist from Breslau who translated the works of Aristotle (384–322 BC) and Cicero (106–143 BC).

Gas Gangrene The gas-producing bacillus in gangrene was identified by William Henry Welch (1850–1934), a pathologist at Bellevue Hospital, New York, in 1892.

Gas Laws In 1662 Robert Boyle (1627–1691), an English chemist, stated that volume and pressure varied inversely if temperature remained constant. Joseph Louis Gay-Lussac (1778–1850), a French chemist, proposed that volume varied directly with temperature if pressure remained constant. Jacobus Henricus van't Hoff (1852–1911), a Dutch chemist, showed that solutions and gases behaved similarly, in 1877. Lorenzo Avogadro (1776–1856), an Italian physicist, proposed that equal volumes of all gases under the same temperature and pressure contained the same number of molecules, in 1811. *See Charles Law.*

Gas Term coined by Jean Baptiste van Helmont (1577–1644) to refer to carbon dioxide. A systematic study of the diffusion of gases was done by the eminent Scottish chemist, Thomas Graham (1805–1869) of Glasgow. *See gas laws.*

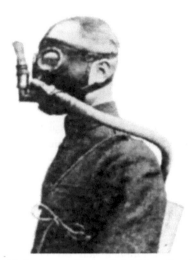

French Artillery Mask. Amos A Fries and C J West, *Chemical Warfare* (1921).McGraw-Hill, New York

Gas Warfare Suffocating gases were used to fight wars from ancient times. The Spartans burnt wood saturated with pitch and sulfur under the city walls to break the defense of the Athenians around 400 BC. The use of poison gas in warfare is also mentioned in China, dating back to 300 BC. The use of sulfur dioxide during the Crimean War was suggested by Lord Dunald in 1855, but was vetoed. The Hague Conference expounded the dangers in 1899. The Germans used phosgene, a mixture of chlorine and mustard gas in World War 1. The Allies adopted gas warfare in May 1916. Helmets lined with cotton impregnated with sodium phenolate were devised in Britain to overcome phosgene attack. Tear gas, containing chlorides and bromides of toluene, was developed by the British and French. Chloropicrin, known as the vomiting and sneezing gas, entered the gas warfare armamentarium during this period. An arsenic compound, lewisite, was discovered in 1919 by W. Lee Lewis (1879–1943) of North Western University, America. *See British anti-lewisite.*

Gasetlier, René Georges (1741–1821) French physician who had a turbulent life due to his political involvement. He wrote several minor works on medicine.

Gaskell, Walter Holbrook (1847–1914) English physiologist, born in Naples and educated at Trinity College, Cambridge. He graduated in medicine from University College, London and made physiology his career. He introduced the term 'block' in cardiology, and described the accelerator nerves of the heart in 1881. His best-known work *The Origin of the Vertebrates* was published in 1906.

Gaspard, Marie Humbert Bernard (1788–1871) *See food poisoning.*

Gassendi, Pierre (1592–1655) French philosopher and one the first members of the French Academie des Sciences, who became professor of mathematics at the College Royal in Paris in 1645. He was an early worker on the atomic theory of matter.

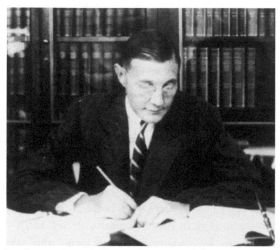

Herbert Spencer Gasser (1888–1963). Courtesy of the National Library of Medicine

Gasser, Herbert Spencer (1888–1963) American physiologist from Wisconsin who graduated in medicine from Johns Hopkins University in 1915. He became director of the Rockefeller Institute for Medical Research in 1939, and was awarded the Nobel Prize for Physiology or Medicine in 1944 for his study on the functional differentiation of nerve fibers.

Gasserian Ganglion Ganglion of the trigeminal nerve, named after Viennese anatomist, Johann Laurentius Gasser (1757–1765), by one of his students in 1765. Its involvement in herpes zoster infection of the face was described by Wilhelm Felix von Barensprung (1822–1864) in 1861. Gasserian ganglionectomy was suggested as treatment for trigeminal neuralgia by James Ewing Mears (1838–19191) in 1884, and was performed successfully by William Rose (1847–1910) in 1890. Wilfred Harris (1869–1960), a neurologist at St Mary's Hospital London, performed alcohol injection of the Gasserian ganglion through the foramen ovale for treatment of trigeminal neuralgia, around 1920. *See trigeminal neuralgia.*

Gassius, Antonius of Padua A physician in the 15th century. His treatise on health and long life, *Corona Florida,* was published in 1491.

Gastaldi, John Baptiste (1674–1747) Physician to the King of France. He wrote *Institutiones Physico-Anatomiae* and several other works.

Gastraea Theory [Greek: *gaster*, stomach or womb] Alexander Kowalewsky (1840–1901), Ernst Heinrich Phillip August Haeckel's (1834–1919) pupil, during his experimental work on amphioxus, noted that the egg cells divided and developed into a hollow space, the morula [Latin: *little mulberry*], which later invaginated to form a hollow ball or gastraea. Following this finding, many naturalists believed that the gastraea stage represented all ancestral forms of multicellular animals. This theory was developed into the celom theory [Greek: *koiloma*, cavity] by Wilhelm August Oscar Hertwig (1849–1922) and Karl Wilhelm Theodor Richard Hertwig (1850–1937), pupils of Haeckel, in 1878.

Gastrectomy [Greek: *gaster*, stomach + *ektome*, excision] Resection of the stomach for carcinoma was performed by Emile Jules Pean (1830–1898) of Paris in 1879, but was not successful. In 1881 Christian Albert Theodor Billroth (1829–1894) performed the first successful gastric resection. A complete resection of the stomach was performed by Phineas Sanborn Conner of Cincinnati in 1884, but this was unsuccessful. Carl Bernhard Schlatter (1864–1934), a German surgeon, performed the first successful total gastrectomy for carcinoma of the stomach in 1897. After this, a total of 70 cases, including one procedure of his own, were reported by W. Walters of America in 1929. A procedure of partial gastrectomy for carcinoma of the pyloric end of the stomach was devised by William James Mayo (1861–1939) in 1900. *See Billroth operation.*

Gastric Carcinoma A postmortem diagnosis in the 18th and 19th centuries, as observed by Giovanni Battista Morgagni (1682–1771) in 1761, Matthew Baillie (1761–1823) in 1793, Carl von Rokitansky (1804–1878) in 1842, Gustav Hauser in 1883 and William Henry Welch (1850–1934) in 1885. One of the best descriptions of autopsy findings was given by Hauser, and the best statistical study was done by Welch. The first successful gastroenterostomy for gastric carcinoma was performed by Anton Wolfer (1850–1917) in 1881. William Osler (1849–1919) reported 24 advanced cases of stomach cancer in 1894, out of which only one was submitted to surgery (with a fatal outcome). Until the beginning of the 20th century it was rare to see or diagnose gastric cancer before it became terminal. Osler reported his clinical experience in 150 patients in 1900. X-ray studies were employed in diagnosis around 1914. In 1909 William Carpenter McCarty (b 1880) of the Mayo Clinic, following his study on the cytology of gastric ulcers in 1907, proposed that chronic gastric ulcers were potentially precancerous.

Gastric Fistula Caused by a gunshot wound in a patient, this was used by American surgeon, William Beaumont (1785–1853), to study secretions of the stomach in 1822. The first operative treatment was performed by Albrecht Theodor Middeldorpf (1824–1868) in 1859. *See fistula.*

Gastric Freezing *See hypothermia.*

Gastric Juice Isolated from animals by René Antoine de Reaumer (1683–1757), who demonstrated its solvent effects on food in 1752. The presence of free hydrochloric acid in the stomach was shown by English physician, William Prout (1785–1850) in 1823. William Beaumont (1785–1853), an American army surgeon, carried out scientific studies on the role of human gastric secretion in 1822 and a series of analyses on gastric juice from one of his patients who had a traumatic gastric fistula caused by a gunshot wound. A stomach tube for withdrawing gastric secretions was designed by Emil Martin Rehfuss (b 1887) in 1914. It contained a metal capsule which sometimes damaged the gastric mucosa, and John Alfred Ryle (1889–1950) improved it in 1921 by covering the entire tip with rubber and providing perforations above the bulb.

Gastric Parietal Cell Antibodies Demonstrated in nearly 80% of patients with pernicious anemia by K.B. Taylor and co-workers in 1962.

Gastric Secretions *See gastric juice.*

Gastric Ulcer The first report of perforating gastric ulcer was given by English physician, Christopher Rawlinson, in 1727. A description of symptoms and morbid anatomy was given by Matthew Baillie (1761–1823) of St George's Hospital in 1793. Successful surgery was performed in Germany by Ludwig Heusner (1846–1916) in 1892 and by an English surgeon, Hastings Gilford (1861–1941), of Reading in 1893. William Carpenter McCarty (b 1880) of the Mayo Clinic did work on the cytology of gastric ulcers in 1907 and proposed that chronic gastric ulcers were potentially precancerous in 1909. Andrew George Berkeley Moynihan (1865–1936) described chronic gastric ulcer as a precancerous state in 1923. Carbinoxolone, one of the first specific drugs, was introduced by F. Avery Jones in 1965.

Gastrin [Greek: *gaster*, stomach] The chemical substance responsible for gastric secretion was identified and described by John Sydney Edkins (1863–1940) in 1906. It

was isolated by R. Gregory who also demonstrated its structure in 1966.

Gastrocnemius [Greek: *gaster*, belly + *kneme*, leg] Term used in 1600 for the calf muscle in the leg by Spigelius (1578–1625), professor of anatomy at Padua.

Gastroduodenostomy [Greek: *gaster*, stomach + *duodeni*, twelve + *tome*, cutting] Excision of the pyloric end of the stomach followed by a procedure of axial anastomosis with the duodenum, was described by Emile Jules Pean (1830–1898) of Paris in 1879. Gastroduodenostomy was performed by Mathieu Jaboulay (1860–1913) of Paris in 1892.

Gastroenterostomy For relief of pyloric stenosis. Performed by Anton Wolfer (1850–1917), a German professor of surgery in Graz, in 1881.

Gastroscopy [Greek: *gaster*, stomach + *skopein*, to view] The first attempt was made by Adolf Kussmaul (1822–1902) in 1869. A crude gastroscope, consisting of a tube which a patient could swallow, was devised by London physician, William Hill (1858–1928), in 1911. A flexible gastroscope was developed by Rudolf Schindler (1888–1968) and Wolf of America in 1932. The technique was pioneered in England by H.W. Rogers and Edwards, who published an account in 1936. In 1940 Schindler collected 22,351 cases on whom he had performed it with the original Wolf–Schindler instrument. Only one death was reported in this series. *See fiber optic endoscopy, esophagoscopy.*

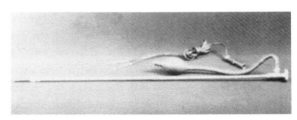

The Schindler semiflexible gastroscope (1932). *A History of Gastroenterology*, Parthenon, London

Gastrostomy [Greek: *gaster*, stomach + *tome*, cutting] First performed in a case of stricture of the esophagus by Egebert, a Norwegian surgeon, in 1837. It was revived by Charles Emmanuel Sedillot (1804–1883) of Strasbourg in 1849, and it was introduced into England by John Cooper Forster (1824–1896) of Guy's Hospital in 1858. The first in America was performed in the management of esophageal stricture by Maury Frank Fontaine (1840–1879) in 1870. A case of intestinal obstruction treated with gastrostomy was reported by Thomas Annandale (1838–1908) of Edinburgh in 1870.

Gastrotomia [Greek: *gaster*, stomach+ *tome*, cutting] An old term for laparotomy.

Gatch Method Rebreathing method of nitrous oxide–oxygen anesthesia. Described by American surgeon, Willis Dew Gatch (b 1878) in 1910.

Gates, Reginald Ruggles Canadian anthropologist who was a lecturer in biology at St Thomas' College (1912–1914) before he became professor of botany at King's College London from 1921 to 1942. In 1936 he was appointed chairman of the Bureau of Human Heredity, an international body dealing with hereditary diseases. He also took part in expeditions to the Amazon, Cuba, Mexico and the Canadian Arctic. He wrote *Human Anatomy from a Genetical Point of View* while he was a research fellow at Harvard in 1948.

Gatling, Jordan Richard (1818–1903) Medical practitioner from North Carolina who invented a gun used in the American Civil War that now bears his name. He also devised a stem plow and a machine for sowing seeds.

Gaubius, Gerome David (1705–1780) Physician from Heidelberg who succeeded Herman Boerhaave (1668–1738) at Leiden. He wrote a treatise on prescribing and a nosology.

Gaucher Disease *See Gaucher, Phillipe Charles Ernest.*

Gaucher, Phillipe Charles Ernest (1854–1918) French physician in Paris who described a familial disorder of cerebroside metabolism with large pale cells in the spleen, as Epithelioma Primitif de la Rate in 1882. He considered it to be neoplastic but Bovaird, who found similar cells in other parts of the reticuloendothelial system in 1900, regarded it as non-neoplastic. It is mostly found in Jews and manifests as pigmentation, pathological fractures, hepatosplenomegaly and thrombocytopenia. The name Gaucher disease was given to it by New York physician, Nathan Edwin Brill (1860–1925) and Frederick Samuel Mandlebaum (b 1867) in 1913.

Gauging A method of measuring the contents of any vessel in relation to its capacity for wine or other liquids, established by law by King Edward III in 1352.

Gauss Sign Unusual mobility of the uterus occurring in early pregnancy. Described by a gynecologist at Würzburg, Carl Joseph Gauss (b 1875).

Gauze A prized fabric in ancient Rome. Manufacture of gauze-like fabric commenced in Scotland in 1759. Cotton gauze was used in surgery in the 18th century.

Gavarret, Louis Dennis Jules (1809–1890) French physician who wrote one of the earliest treatises on statistics related to diseases in 1840.

Gay Glands Found in the perianal region. Described by John Gay (1812–1885), a surgeon at the Royal Northern Hospital, London.

Gay, Frederick Parker (1874–1939) American pathologist who studied the cell count in cerebrospinal fluid in poliomyelitis.

Gay-Lussac, Joseph Louis (1778–1850) Eminent French chemist, born in Saint Leonard, Haute Vienne. He became an assistant to Claude Berthollet (1749–1822) in 1800. He proposed the law of gases in 1808 that states that volume varies directly with temperature if pressure remains constant. This is known as Charles Law in England. Gay-Lussac also prepared hydroiodic acid, iodic acid and cyanogen.

Gayton, Edmund (1608–1666) London physician who wrote *Pleasant Notes upon Don Quixote* in 1654 and *The Religion of a Physician* in 1663.

Geber or Abu Musa Jabir ibn Hayyan (b 721) Arab chemist and founder of alchemy, born at Tus near Meshed and served at the Court of Harun Al-Rashid. He is credited with the discovery of nitric acid . The word 'gibberish' is derived from his name to denote unintelligible jargon used by alchemists.

Geddes, Sir Patrick (1854–1932) Born in Perth, Scotland, he was a botanist and pioneer in experimental sociology, who established the world's first sociological laboratory in Edinburgh in 1892. He was one of the first modern town planners and wrote *City Development* in 1904. His *The Evolution of Sex* was published in 1889.

Gee, Samuel Jones (1839–1911) Physician at the Hospital for Sick Children, Great Ormond Street, London. He graduated from the University of London in 1861. He described infantile celiac disease (Gee disease) in 1888, and published *Auscultation and Percussion* in 1870. He worked as a physician in St Bartholomew's Hospital in 1878 and was made a consultant physician there in 1904.

Gegenbaur, Carl (1826–1903) German comparative anatomist, born in Würzburg, where he graduated in medicine in 1851. He became a professor at Jena in 1856. He demonstrated the unicellular nature of the ovum in vertebrates in 1861 and described osteoblasts in 1885.

Geiger Counter An ionization chamber for measuring radiation or alpha particles. Constructed in 1928 by German professors, Hans Wilhelm Geiger (1882–1945) and Erwin Muller of Tübingen University.

Geiger, Phillip Laurence (1785–1836) German chemist who isolated atropine in 1833. *See conine.*

Geikie, James (1839–1915) Scottish geologist and brother of Sir Archibald Geikie (1835–1924). He was professor of geology in Edinburgh (1882–1914) and wrote: *Prehistoric Europe* (1881), *Earth Sculpture or the Origin of Land forms* (1898) and *The Great Ice Age* (1874).

Geikie, Sir Archibald (1835–1924) Eminent Scottish geologist in Edinburgh. He was the first chair of geology at Edinburgh University in 1871, a post which he held for over ten years. He published *Outlines of Geology* (1879), which passed through several editions.

Geissler Tube The first effective vacuum device through which rarefied gases could be visualized using electricity. Invented by a German physicist, Heinrich Geissler (1814–1879) of Saxony in 1855. Sir William Crookes (1832–1919) modified it and used it to produce cathode rays in 1861.

Gelineau Disease *See narcolepsy.*

Gelle Test Test to demonstrate that deafness due to a bone conduction defect is not affected by pressure over the external auditory canal. Devised by French surgeon, Marie Ernst Gelle (1834–1923).

Gellhorn, George (1870–1936) American gynecologist of St Louis who described a method of vaginal hysterectomy under local anesthesia in 1930.

Gèly, Jules Aristide (1806–1861) French surgeon who described a method of intestinal suture in 1844.

Geminus, Thomas (d 1562) Physician and engraver in London who published one of the earliest illustrated anatomical textbooks in England, *Compendiosa Totius Anatomie Delinreato,* in 1545. This contained several plates on anatomy by Vesalius.

Gemma, Reinier (1508–1555) Dutch physician and mathematician who became professor of physick at Louvain. Most of his treatises were on mathematics.

Gene [Greek: *genos,* descent] A structure to which the properties of inheritance may be attributed was described and named by Danish botanist, Wilhelm Ludwig Johannson (1857–1927), in 1909. *See chromosomes.*

Gene Markers DNA sequencing to develop gene markers for genetic diseases was developed by Ronald W. Davis and Mark H. Skolnick in 1978. The marker for Duchenne

muscular dystrophy was discovered by Kay Davies and Robert Williamson in 1983, and that for cystic fibrosis was identified on chromosome 7 in 1985.

Genealogy [Greek: *genos,* birth or descent + *logos,* discourse] The first mention of descent or pedigree is given in the Bible in Genesis. An early modern work, *Theratum Geneologicum,* was published by Henninges at Magdeburg in 1598.

General Medical Council (GMC) of the United Kingdom. The forerunner of the GMC was the General Council of Medical Education and Registration of the United Kingdom, established in 1858. Prior to the Medical Act, which led to the formation of the council, there were over 19 licensing bodies in the UK which did not reciprocate or recognize each others' qualifications. When the GMC was formed it had 24 members, with Sir Benjamin Brodie (1783–1862) as its first President. The first woman member, Christine Murrell (1874–1933), was elected in 1933.

General Nursing Council Established under the Nurses Registration Act in 1919. *See nursing.*

General Paralysis of the Insane First recognized by Thomas Willis (1621–1675) in 1672, and described by John Haslam (1764–1844), a superintendent of Bethlehem Mental Asylum from 1795 to 1816. Haslam examined the brains of the diseased insane at autopsy and recorded changes due to syphilis. Pathological lesions in the brain of psychotic patients suffering from general paralysis were shown by Louis Florentine Calmiel (1798–1895).

General Practitioner Term introduced around 1820 in England for medical practitioners who practiced all branches of medicine including surgery, midwifery, pharmacy and medicine. The first attempt to represent their interests was made by the formation of the Associated Medical and Surgical Practitioners in 1826. A common register for all doctors practicing medicine, surgery and its branches was established in 1858. The uniform role of general practitioners in providing health care to the community was established when the National Health Service Act was passed in 1948. This led to a majority of the population being registered with a general practitioner. *See Royal College of General Practitioners.*

Genetic Engineering The transfer of genetic material from one bacterial strain of *Salmonella* to another through transduction was demonstrated by American geneticists, Norton David Zinder (b 1928) and Joshua Lederberg (b 1925) in Wisconsin in 1952. Synthesis of DNA in *Escherichia coli* was studied by Matthew Stanley Meselson (b 1930) of Colorado and Franklin William Stahl (b 1929), a molecular biologist and professor at the University of Missouri, in 1958. The method of inserting new genetic information into viral DNA was developed by David Archer Jackson and Robert Symons in 1972. Fusion of a segment of human DNA, synthesized in the laboratory, into *E. coli* was performed by Herbert Wayne Boyer (b 1936) and Stanley H. Cohen of America, in 1973. A method of obtaining enzymes from genetically active bacterial gene fragments was discovered by an American molecular biologist, Hamilton Othaniel Smith (b 1931) in the 1970s. Successful introduction of a human gene into the germ line of a mouse (transgenic mice) was achieved by an American molecular biologist from New Jersey, Ralph Lawrence Brinster (b 1932) and New York geneticist, Richard de Forest Palmiter (b 1942), in the late 1970s. Transfer of genes between cells of different mammalian species was achieved by an American molecular biologist from Brooklyn, New York, Paul Berg (b 1926), in 1978. The world's first license to market living organisms modified by genetic engineering was issued by the US Agriculture Department in 1986, and the first genetically engineered vaccine for hepatitis B was approved by the US Food and Drug Administration (FDA) in the same year. Insulin was the first genetically engineered hormone to be marketed, in 1982, and was followed by genetically engineered growth hormone in 1985. *Reshaping Life: Key Issues in Genetic Engineering,* was published by Australian immunologist, Sir Gustav Joseph Victor Nossal (b 1931) in 1984.

Genetic Fingerprinting Identification of unique core sequences in DNA was discovered by English molecular biochemist, Alec Jeffreys (b 1950), in 1984. The technique involves digestion of a DNA sample from an individual with specific endonuclease enzymes and electrophoresis. The first conviction of a criminal in England, based on genetic fingerprinting, was achieved in 1987.

Genetical Society Founded by William Bateson (1861–1926) in 1919. Its first meeting was attended by 34 members and held in Cambridge in the same year.

Genetics [Greek: *genos*, origin or descent] Term coined by William Bateson (1861–1926) in 1906. The science of genetics was founded by Gregor Mendel (1822–1884), an Augustinian monk who worked on hybridization of pea plants from 1856, publishing his epoch-making work in 1865. This went unheeded until Bateson published *Mendel's Principles of Heredity* in 1902. The fact that the number of chromosomes was constant for each cell in a given body, and also probably characteristic of each species, was pointed out by a Belgian cytologist, Edouard van Beneden

(1845–1910) in 1887. Sex-linked inheritance was shown by a geneticist from Kentucky, Thomas Hunt Morgan (1866–1945), during his work on *Drosophila* in 1910. The first chair of genetics was created at Cambridge in 1912 by an anonymous donor in memory of the British Prime Minister from 1902 to 1905, Arthur James Balfour (1848–1930) and his brother Maitland Balfour (1851–1882), who was an embryologist. Reginald Crundall Punnett (1875–1967) of Tonbridge, a contemporary of Bateson, was appointed as its first professor. He published *Mendelism* in 1905. *See hybridization, chromosomes.*

Geneva Convention During the battle of Detingen in 1743, Sir John Pringle, the founder of modern military medicine in England, proposed that military hospitals both on the English and French sides should observe neutrality in order to care for the wounded. This proposal was loosely followed until the Geneva Convention, initiated by French philanthropist and humanist, Henri Dunant (1828–1910), was signed in 1864 by 26 delegates from 13 countries. A second Geneva Convention to settle issues arising from the first was held in 1868. *See Red Cross.*

Gengou, Octave (1875–1957) Belgian bacteriologist who demonstrated (with J.B.V. Bordet) the fixation of complement during an antigen–antibody reaction. They also identified the pertussis bacterium as the cause of whooping cough.

Genital Herpes *See herpes genitalis.*

Genital Warts *See condylomata accuminata.*

Genitourinary Medicine An early authority was Persian physician, Rhazes (850–932) who considered that hematuria was a symptom of bladder disease, and wrote at length on urethral stricture. He devised catheters with lateral holes for draining pus and used a catheter of lead instead of bronze whenever flexibility was needed. The founder of modern genitourinary surgery was a professor in Paris, Felix Guyon (1831–1920), who published his lectures in 1881 and a treatise on surgical diseases of the bladder and prostate in 1888. His contribution was followed by a classic work by Joaquin Dominguez Albarran (1860–1912) from Cuba, a professor in Paris. Venereal diseases, particularly syphilis, were common in the 19th century and Sir James Paget (1814–1889) in 1879 noted that 48% of the total outpatient attendance in his hospital was due to syphilis. The term 'genitourinary medicine' was promoted by Sir William Osler (1849–1919) during his evidence to the Royal Commission on Venereal Diseases in 1914, and the practice of venereology as a specialty started after the report by the commission in 1916. The Medical Society for Venereal Diseases in London was established in 1922 and the *British Journal of Venereal Diseases*, which became *Genitourinary Medicine* in 1985. The field became firmly established in England around 1970. The first professorial chair was established at the Middlesex Hospital Medical School in 1978, with M.W. Adler as professor. *See venereal disease, syphilis, AIDS.*

Gennari, Francesco (1750–1797) *See cerebral cortex.*

Gennerich, Wilhelm (b 1877) German naval surgeon and dermatologist who studied neurosyphilis. He introduced treatment of neurosyphilis by intraspinal injections of arsphenamine or salvarsan, and designed a special device for forcing the salvarsanized cerebrospinal fluid into the brain in 1914.

Genotype [Greek: *genos*, descent + *typos*, image] Concept introduced to genetics by a Danish professor of genetics at Copenhagen, Ludwig Wilhelm Johanssen (1857–1927), in 1909. He proposed the concept of phenotype or visible expression of the genotype.

Gentamycin Antibiotic developed by Marvin Joseph Weinstein (b 1916) and co-workers in 1963.

Gentian Violet Shown to be an antiseptic by American physician, John Woolman Churchman (1877–1937), in 1912.

Genus [Latin: *genus*, race] The Latin names *genus* and *species* were used in the system of classification of organisms by Carl Linnaeus (1707–1778).

Geoffroy Saint-Hilaire, Etienne (1772–1844) French zoologist and a rival to George Léopold Chrétien Cuvier (1769–1832) at the Jardin des Plantes. He proposed the law of development stating that organs do not arise or disappear suddenly during evolution and that one organ can grow at the expense of another. He was professor of zoology at the Museum of Natural History in Paris, and made a comparative study of embryonic forms in which he explained vestigial structures. One of his other main interests was the study of teratology in animals. He published *Philosophie Anatomique* (1818) and other works.

Geoffroy, Stephen Francis (1672–1731) Professor of medicine and chemistry in Paris. He published a history of materia medica.

Geogeny [Greek: *geos*, earth + *genos*, descent] Study of the origin of the Earth as part of the solar system. Commenced by René Descartes (1596–1650) who considered that it originated as a glowing mass, like the sun. In *Principles of Philosophy* published in 1644 he described the formation of layers of the Earth. Athanasius Kircher (1601–1680) in *Subterranean World* (1665) postulated that volcanoes and thermal springs fed by the sea existed under the Earth's surface. English clergyman, Thomas Burnet (1635–1715) of Yorkshire, in *Sacred Theory of the Earth*, published in 1681, suggested that it was a chaotic mixture of oil, water and sand. The theory that it was originally an incandescent mass which cooled and contracted with the formation of an outer crust was proposed by Gottfried Wilhelm Leibniz (1646–1716) in *Acta Eruditorum* published in 1697. The principle of gravitation was used by Isaac Newton (1642–1727) to explain the origin in 1692. *See Earth.*

Geography [Greek: *geos*, earth + *graphein*, to write] A geographical map was made by Anaximander of Miletus in 568 BC. Dicaearchus (355–285 BC), a pupil of Aristotle, gave a physical description of the world accompanied by a map, and drew parallels of latitude across it. A survey of the counties of England and Wales was carried out by Christopher Saxton (1542–1611) from Sowood, Yorkshire in 1579. His atlas was the first national map of any country to be published. The Royal Geographical Society of London was established in 1830. Geography was applied to understand disease on a worldwide scale by Leonhard Ludwig Finke (1747–1828) in 1792.

Geology [Greek: *geos*, earth + *logos*, discourse] Science of the structure and origin of the Earth that originated during the time of Pythagoras (500 BC). He observed the physical changes in the land and its eruptions. The first book on physical geology, *De Ortu et Causis Subterraneorum*, was published by a physician, George Agricola (1494–1555) in 1546. The first work on fossils was produced by another physician, Conrad Gesner (1516–1565). James Hutton (1726–1797), a physician in Edinburgh, published *The Theory of the Earth* in 1785. Horace B. de Saussure (1740–1799) of Geneva introduced the word into scientific nomenclature. One of the greatest geologists of the 19th century was Leopold von Buch (1774–1853), who produced the first geological map of Germany in 1824. The International Union of Geological Sciences was founded in 1878, and held its first meeting in Paris in 1878. Scottish-born geologist, William Maclure (1763–1840) from Ayr, is regarded as the father of geology in America. His *Observations on the Geology of United States* (1817) was one of the first books on the subject in America. Another American pioneer was James Hall (1811–1898) who was the first President of the Geological Society of America. He published 13 volumes (1847–1894) on the paleontology of New York State.

George III *See acute intermittent porphyria.*

Georgi, Walter (1889–1920) A bacteriologist in Frankfurt. He devised a serological test for the diagnosis of syphilis with Hans Sachs (1877–1945) in 1919.

Geothermal Energy Hot springs have been used since ancient times as therapeutic baths. Geothermal energy was used by a Frenchman, François de Larderelle, at his village near Tuscany in 1818. This village, Laderelle, was chosen as a pilot station for production of geothermal energy by Giovanni Conti in 1903. It was converted to electrical energy at this site and was used to light four lamps.

Geraghty, John Timothy (1876–1924) *See phenol sulfonaphthalein test.*

Gerard, John (1545–1607) A famous surgeon, herbalist and botanist from Cheshire, who settled in London. He had a large botanical garden and wrote *Herbal or General History of Plants* in 1597.

Gerard, Louis (1733–1819) French physician and botanist who did research on the natural affinities of plants.

Geraghty, John Timothy (1876–1924) American surgeon from Baltimore who described a new method of perineal prostatectomy in 1922.

Geratology [Greek: *geras*, old age + *logos*, discourse] *See geriatrics.*

Gerbezius, Marcus (1658–1718) Physician in Slovenia who described syncopal attack related to temporary cardiac arrest or standstill in 1692.

Gerdy, Pierre Nicholas (1797–1856) French surgeon in Paris who gave original descriptions of several anatomical structures including: ligamentum of axilla (Gerdy ligment), a specific area of the sagittal fontanel (Gerdy fontanelle) and the tubercle on the lateral tuberosity of the tibia (Gerdy tubercle).

Gerhard, William Wood (1809–1872) American physician who graduated from Pennsylvania. He gave an early, clear clinicopathological description of typhoid in 1837. He made an accurate study of tuberculous meningitis in 1834.

Gerhardt, Carl Jacob Christian Adolf (1833–1902) Professor at Jena (1861), Würzburg (1872) and Berlin (1885). His main interests were pediatrics and laryngology, and he published several works in these fields. He described bilateral adductor paralysis of the larynx (Gerhardt syndrome) in 1863. He devised a test (Gerhardt test) for detection of ketones.

Gerhardt, Charles Frederic (1816–1856) Chemist from Strasbourg who studied at Leipzig and was professor of chemistry first at Montpellier in 1841, and at Paris in 1848. He gave the name 'phenol' to carbolic acid, proposed the concept of the chemical radical and prepared acetanilide in 1852. He also classified organic compounds.

Geriatrics [Greek: *geras*, old age + *iatrecia*, medical treatment] The term 'gerocomice' to denote care in old age was used from the Middle Ages to the 17th century. The value of diet and exercise was stressed by the Roman physician, Galen (129–200) in his treatise on old age. London physician, John Smith (1630–1679) from Buckinghamshire, gave an account of infirmities in old age in *King Solomon's Portraiture of Old Age*, published in 1666. French chemist and gerontologist from Angers, Michel Eugene Chevereul (1786–1889), was a pioneer in psychogeriatrics. The current term was used by a Vienna-born American physician, Ignaz Leo Nascher (1863–1944) in the *New York Medical Journal* in 1909. The first book related to therapeutics in old age, *The Cure of Old Age,* was written by Roger Bacon in AD 1200. The earliest treatise on how to maintain health in old age was published by a Venetian, Luigi Conaro (1467–1566) in 1558. Leonardus Lessius (1554–1623) of Antwerp, in *Hygiafticon, feu vera Ratio Valetidunis bonae vitae* or The True Method of Preserving Life and Health to Extreme Old Age, praised sober life as the principal means of preserving health. In 1724 Sir John Floyer (1649–1734), an eminent English physician who introduced the pulse watch (1707), wrote *Medicina Geronomica,* which laid the foundation for modern geriatrics. *Practical Treatise on the Domestic Management and Most Important Diseases of Advanced Life,* was published by G.E. Day of America in 1849. The first course was inaugurated at the Salpêtrière by the French neurologist, Jean Marie Charcot (1825–1893), in 1867. A book on the history of health in old age was published by German physician, Carl Friedrich Canstatt (1807–1850) of Erlangen in 1839. *Geriatrics: The Disease of Old Age and Their Treatment,* was published in 1914 by Nascher, who is considered as the founder of the specialty in America. A large-scale geriatric study of a psychological nature, *Senescence,* was published by Stanley Granville Hall (1846–1924) in 1922. A pioneer of geriatrics in England was Majorie Warren who worked at the Isleworth Infirmary, which became West Middlesex County Hospital in 1935. She observed the inadequacy and inappropriateness of medical care for the elderly and made attempts to improve it. The American Geriatrics Society was founded in 1942. The importance of falls in old people was stressed by J.H. Sheldon in *Social Medicine for Old Age,* published in 1948. It was established as a specialty in the United Kingdom in 1948 with the appointment of four consultant geriatricians. *See old age, psychogeriatrics.*

Gerlach, Joseph (1820–1896) Professor of anatomy and physiology at Erlangen who introduced carmine as a tissue stain in histology. He described the lymphatic follicles in the mucous membrane of the Eustachian tube, and the mucosal fold near the orifice of the appendix (Gerlach valve).

Gerlier, Felix (1840–1914) Swiss physician who described endemic paralytic vertigo (Gerlier disease), which affected farm workers and stablemen in Switzerland. A similar condition was known as 'kubiasagari' in Japan.

Germ Layers [Latin: *germen*, bud] The concept of embryonic development of organs from different germ layers was proposed in 1828 by Carl Ernst von Baer (1792–1876), a professor at St Petersburg who is considered the founder of embryology. They were classified into ectoderm, endoderm and mesoderm by Robert Remak (1815–1865) in 1845.

Germ Plasm [Latin: *germen*, bud; Greek: *plasmein*, to mold] The aggregate of self-propagating hereditary materials transmitted to the offspring through germ cells. Described and named by German biologist, August Friedrich Leopold Weismann (1834–1914) of Jena, in 1892.

Germ Theory of Disease The dogma of spontaneous generation existed unquestioned up to the 16th century when Fracastorus (1478–1553), a physician in Vienna, proposed a different cause in his treatise *Contagium Vivum* published in 1546. An early attempt to view microscopic organisms in blood in plague was made by Athanasius Kircher (1601–1680), a Jesuit priest, in 1658. He described what he saw as 'worms' of plague in *Scrutium Pestis*. Infection by germs as a cause of disease was proposed by Nicholas Andry (1658–1742) in 1701. Proof that disease is associated with microorganisms was provided by Agostino Bassi (1773–1856) of Lodi, with his work on silkworms in 1835. Oliver Wendell Holmes (1809–1894) wrote *On the Contagiousness of Puerperal Fever* presented to the Boston Medical Society in 1842. Ignaz Semmelweiss (1818–1865) in Vienna demonstrated in 1847 that mortality due to puerperal fever could be reduced from 18% to less than 2% if students and doctors washed their hands before attending patients. His findings were ignored and he was ridiculed and persecuted. The theory was firmly established by Louis Pasteur (1822–1895) who showed the presence of living cells in fermentation. Robert Koch (1843–1910), a German bacteriologist, isolated the anthrax bacillus in 1876. The mycobacterium causing leprosy was isolated by a Norwegian physician, Gerhard Henrik Armauer Hansen (1841–1912) in 1874; gonococcal bacteria by Albert Ludwig Sigmund Neisser (1855–1916)

in 1879; staphylococcus by Alexander Ogston (1844–1929) in 1881; tubercle bacillus by Koch in 1882; and streptococcus of erysipelas by Friedrich Fehleisen (1854–1924) in 1888. A demonstration of a filterable virus as a cause of disease was shown in the tobacco plant by Dmitri Iosifovich Ivanovski (1864–1920), a Russian botanist, in 1892. He extracted the sap of the plant and passed it thorough a filter to clear it of bacteria and showed that the sap was still capable of producing the disease.

German Measles Experimental proof that rubella is caused by a virus was provided by Alfred Fabian Hess (1875–1933) of Germany in 1914. Successful transmission of rubella in children using filtered nasal washings was shown by Y. Hiro and S. Tasaka in 1938. Congenital defects and cataracts in infants following infection in the mother during early pregnancy were reported by Australian ophthalmologist, Sir Gregg Norman McAlister (1892–1966), in 1941. The rubella virus was isolated by Thomas Huckle Weller (b 1915) and Allen Frankelin Neva (b 1922) in 1962.

Germanin *See Bayer 205.*

Germinal Vesicles Shown in the ova of birds by Johannes Evangelista Purkinje (1787–1869) in 1825.

Gerocomice *See geriatrics.*

Gerontology [Greek: *geron*, old man + *logos*, discourse] *See geriatrics.*

Gerontoxon [Greek: *geron*, old man + *toxon*, bow] A synonym for arcus senilis. *See arcus senilis.*

Gerota, Dumitru (1867–1939) Professor of experimental surgery at the University of Bucharest, who introduced lymphatic injection to visualize lymph glands. He also described the perirenal fascia.

Gerster, Arpad Geyza Charles (1848–1923) American medical historian and surgeon who described the use of gold plate to cover cranial defects in 1895. He published *On the Hippocratic Doctrine of the Injuries of the Cranium* in 1902.

Geschickter, Charles Freeborn (b 1901) *See gynecomastia.*

Gesell, Arnold Lucius (1880–1961) A pioneer in child psychiatry, from Alma, Wisconsin. He did extensive work on normal development in childhood while he was professor of child hygiene at the Yale School of Medicine from 1915 to 1948. The present Clinic of Child Development at Yale School of Medicine was founded by him in 1911 as Yale Psychological Clinic.

Gesner, Conrad (1516–1565) Physician in Zurich who gained fame in Europe as a naturalist. His *Hortorum*

Germaniae Descripto Historia Animalium (1551–1621), published in five volumes, earned him the name of 'the modern Pliny'.

Gessard, Carle (b 1850) French physician who isolated *Pseudomonas pyocynae* bacillus in 1882.

Ghon Focus A calcified area of the lung, shown on chest X-ray, and due to healed primary tuberculosis. Described by Austrian pathologist, Anton Ghon (1866–1936), professor of pathology at Vienna, in 1910. He died of tuberculous pericarditis.

Ghosts A treatise dealing with delusions, hallucinations and illusions was written by Ludwig Lavator (1527–1586) in 1570. An English treatise of a similar nature *Phantasmata, Illusions and Fanaticisms,* with case histories of apparitions and illusions, was published by Richard Robert Madden (1798–1886), a physician in Mayfair, London, in 1857.

Giacomo, Carlo (1840–1898) Professor of anatomy and neurologist in Turin. He gave original descriptions of several neuroanatomical structures.

Giant Cell Arteritis *See temporal arteritis.*

Giant Urticaria *See angioneurotic edema.*

Giants Those described in folk tales and mythology may have been of pituitary origin. The famous Irish giant, Cornelius Magrath (1742–1768), was 6 feet 9 inches (2 meters) tall at the age of 16 years, and his skull later showed the presence of a large pituitary fossa. A Chinese giant from Fychon, Chang-Woo-Goo, measured 8 feet 2 inches (2.5 meters) in 1865. An extreme case due to an overactive anterior pituitary was noted in a schoolboy giant, Robert Wadlow of Illinois. He was five years old when he reached a height of 5 feet 4 inches (1.6 meters). He died at 22 years in 1940, having reached a height of 8 feet 10 inches (2.6 meters). Gigantism in relation to acromegaly was studied by Harvey Cushing (1869–1939) of Johns Hopkins Hospital in 1910.

Gianturco, Cesare (b 1905) A radiologist at Mayo Clinic, Rochester, Minnesota who pioneered the use of cinematography in the study of the gastrointestinal tract, with Walter Clements Alvarez (b 1884) in 1932.

Giardia lamblia Protozoan parasite identified by Antoni van Leeuwenhoek (1632–1723), who noted the organism in his own stools in 1681. It is named after a French biologist and parasitologist, Alfred Giard (1846–1908), and a German physician, Vilem Dusan Lambl (1824–1895).

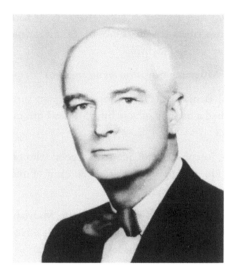

John Heysham Gibbon (1903–1973), Courtesy of the National Library of Medicine

Gibbon, John Heysham (1903–1973) American cardiovascular surgeon who used the heart–lung bypass machine on animals in 1939. He employed the first pump oxygenator in humans during cardiac surgery in 1954.

Gibbon, Quinton (1813–1894) American surgeon who described a large inguinal hernia associated with hydrocele (Gibbon hernia).

Gibbons, William London practitioner who was physician to Queen Anne (1664–1714) following the dismissal of John Radcliffe (1650–1714).

Gibbs, Owen Stanley (b 1898) Scottish physician in Edinburgh who demonstrated the production of acetylcholine on stimulation of the chorda tympani nerve, in 1932.

Gibbs, Josiah Willard (1839–1903) Considered the founder of physical chemistry. He was born in New Haven, Connecticut and graduated from Yale, where he was made professor in 1871. He applied the principles of thermodynamics to chemistry and proposed the ionic theory of the Gibbs–Donnan equilibrium.

Gibbs–Donnan Equilibrium Related to the movement of ions across a membrane. Proposed by American physical chemist, Josiah Willard Gibbs (1839–1903), and studied experimentally by Ceylon-born Irish chemist, Frederick George Donnan (1870–1956).

Gibert, Camile Melchior (1797–1866) French dermatologist in Paris who gave a complete description of pityriasis versicolor (Gibert disease) in 1860.

Gibney, Virgil Pendelton (1847–1927) New York surgeon who described painful fibrositis of the spinal muscles (Gibney perispondylitis).

Gibson Murmur *See patent ductus arteriosus.*

Gibson, Benjamin (1784–1812) Manchester surgeon who described a method of couching for newborn infants with cataract.

Gibson, Joseph (d 1739) Scottish surgeon who practiced in Leith. He was appointed to the first chair of midwifery in Britain, at Edinburgh, in 1726.

Gibson, William (1788–1868) Baltimore, Maryland surgeon who tied the common iliac artery in 1812. He devised a bandage for fracture of the lower jaw in 1824.

Giemsa, Berthhold Gustav Carl (1867–1948) Pharmacist in Hamburg who devised a method (Giemsa stain) for staining blood cells in 1890. He was also a pioneer in chemo-therapy.

Gierke, Hans Paul Bernard (1847–1886) Born in Germany, he was appointed professor of surgery at Tokyo, Japan in 1876. He returned to Germany in 1882 and became professor of physiology at Breslau. He described tractus solitarius of the medulla in 1885.

Gierke, Edgar Otto Konrad von (1877–1945) *See von Gierke disease.*

Giffard, William (d 1731) English obstetrician who recognized and described a case of extrauterine pregnancy. He documented the first use of obstetric forceps in 1726.

Gifford Reflex Constriction of the pupils occurring when the orbicularis oculi muscle is contracted with open eyelids. Described by American ophthalmologist, Harold Gifford (1858–1929) of Milwaukee. He also described lid lag seen in hyperthyroidism.

Gigli, Leonardo (1863–1908) Italian gynecologist who graduated from the University of Florence in 1889. He devised the operation (Gigli operation) of sectioning the pubis in cases of difficult labor. The wire saw which he devised for pubiotomy was also named after him.

Gilbert Disease A benign condition, with intermittent jaundice and normal liver functions, due to a defect in glucuronyl transferase. Described by French physician, Nicolas Augustin Gilbert (1858–1927) in 1901.

Gilbert, Francis Hilary (1757–1800) French veterinary surgeon who dedicated his life to cultivation and management of sheep.

Gilbert, Bennet Judson (b 1898) *See gynecomastia.*

Gilbert, Nicolas Augustine (1858–1927) French hematologist in Paris who described a form of congenital hemolytic anemia, currently known as Gilbert disease in 1901.

Gilbert, William (1544–1603) Born in Colchester, he was physician to the Queen. In 1600 he noticed that substances apart from amber produced electricity. He conducted some of the earliest scientific experiments on electricity and his *De Magnete, Magneticis que Corporibus, te de Magno Magnette Tellure, Physiologia Nova,* was the first major scientific work on it to be published in England. He also introduced the term 'electrics' from which Sir Thomas Browne (1605–1682) derived the term 'electricity' in 1646.

Gilbertus, Anglicus (1180–1250) English medical writer who criticized methods of treatment of diseases by monks. He wrote *Compendium Medicinae* or *Laura Anglica .* He mentioned sublimation and distillation and the use of red light in treatment of smallpox.

Gilbert–Behçet Syndrome *See Behçet syndrome.*

Gilchrist, Ebenezer (1707–1774) Physician in Dumfries, Scotland. He studied medicine in Edinburgh, London and Paris before he returned to his home where he practiced until his death.

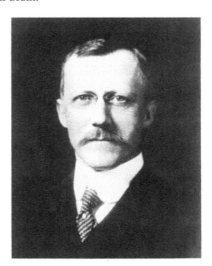

Thomas Casper Gilchrist (1862–1927). Courtesy of the National Library of Medicine

Gilchrist, Thomas Casper (1862–1927) Worked at the Johns Hopkins University and described chronic granulomatous lesions of the skin associated with bony lesions, caused by a fungus (*Blastomyces dermatidis*) in 1897. The disease was found to be exclusive to North America and was named North American blastomycosis.

Gilford, Hastings (1861–1941) English surgeon from

Reading, Berkshire. He described mixed premature and immature development and named it progeria in 1897. *See gastric ulcer.*

Gilles de la Tourette, Georges Edouard Albert Brutus (1855–1909) French neurologist who described the syndrome of echolalia, coprolalia, and chorea in children, in 1885.

Gillespie, James Donaldson (1823–1891) Surgeon at the Edinburgh School of Medicine and Surgery. He designed an operation for excision of the wrist.

Gillette, Eugene Pauline (1836–1886) Surgeon and son of Matthieu Gillette, a pathologist in Paris. He described the longitudinal fibers of the esophagus around the posterior pharynx (suspensory ligament of the esophagus) in 1872.

Gilliam, David Todd (1844–1923) American gynecologist from Columbus, Ohio, who designed an operation for retrodisplacement of the uterus by fixing it to the sheath of the rectus abdominis muscle with the help of the round ligament.

Gillies, Sir Harold Delf (1882–1960) Plastic surgeon from New Zealand who introduced the use of a tubed pedicle in plastic surgery of the face, in 1917. He described his own method of operation for cleft palate in 1921. He devised several surgical instruments named after him (Gillies forceps, Gillies needle-holder).

Gilmer, Thomas Lewis (1849–1931) Dentist in Chicago who devised a splint (Gilmer splint) for treating fracture of the mandible.

Gimbernat, Manuel Louis Antonio don (1734–1816) Surgeon from Barcelona who was appointed surgeon to King Carlos III. He attended William Hunter's lectures in London and described the operation for strangulated femoral hernia in 1793. The ligamentum lacunare he described in 1793 bears his name.

Gingili Oil Sesame oil, mentioned in ancient Sanskrit, Hebrew, Egyptian, Greek and Roman literature. It is referred to as *semsent* in the Ebers papyrus and the term *tila* appears in Ayurvedic literature. *Sesamum indicum,* the plant from which the seeds for the oil are obtained, is indigenous to India. It was cultivated in Cyprus, Egypt and Sicily during the Middle Ages. A picture is given in *Hortus Medicus et Philosophicus* written by a physician and botanist, Joachim Camirarius (1530–1598) of Nuremburg, in 1568.

Ginseng The most celebrated drug in the Chinese materia medica, obtained from the plant genus *Panax*, belonging to the order Araliaceae. Owing to the belief that it revitalized

the elderly and the debilitated, and that it also served as an aphrodisiac, it reached a high market value during the 19th century and fetched as much as $400 per ounce.

Giordano, Davide (1864–1937) Italian surgeon in Venice who described the sphincter (Giordano sphincter) at the opening of the common bile duct into the duodenum.

Giovanni Disease A defect in the development of the hair follicles. Described by a Turin dermatologist, Sebastiano Giovanni (1851–1920) in 1887.

Giraldés, Joachim Albin Cardozo (1808–1875) Portuguese surgeon who was professor of surgery at Paris. He described paradidymis.

Girard Remedy A remedy for seasickness, consisting of a mixture of atropine sulfate and strychnine. Prepared by American naval surgeon, Alfred Conrad Girard (1850–1916), in 1906.

Girard, Charles (1850–1916) French surgeon who performed the first successful hind-quarter amputation in 1895.

Girdlestone Operation An operation for arthrodesis of the hip. Named after the British orthopedic surgeon Gathorne Robert Girdlestone (1881–1950), a graduate of St Thomas' Hospital and an orthopedic surgeon at the Wingfield–Morris Orthopedic Hospital, later the Nuffield Orthopedic Center. He also described an operation for spinal fixation in cases of Pott disease in 1931. He was the first professor at the Orthopedic Center at the Radcliffe Infirmary, Oxford, in 1937.

Girdlestone, Thomas (1758–1822) He initially served as an army doctor, before he settled in Great Yarmouth to practice medicine. He translated the *Odes of Anacreon* into English verse.

Glacial Period The person who proposed the theory of ice ages in 1832 was A. Bernardi, a teacher in a forestry school in The Netherlands. Four years later the naturalist and glaciologist, Jean Louis Rodolphe Agassiz (1807–1873) of Switzerland, traveled to the Alps with the geologist, Johann von Charpentier (d 1855) and formulated the glacial theory which he presented to the Geological Society of London in 1840. His *Etudes sur les Glaciers* was published in the same year. Credibility was given by William Buckland (1784–1856), President of the Geological Society. Agassiz settled in Massachusetts in 1846 and in 1865 unearthed evidence of an ice age in one of the hottest places in the world, equatorial Brazil. Another important study in America on the glacial period was done by Thomas Crowder Chamberlain from

Illinois, chair of geology at Beloit from 1873 to 1882, who published *Our Glacial Drift* around 1880. Joseph Prestwich professor of geology at Oxford from 1874 to 1888, was an authority on the quaternary or recent ice age. *See ice age.*

Gland Term used in the modern anatomical and physiological sense by Thomas Wharton in *Adenographia: sive glandularum totius corporis descriptio,* published in 1656.

Glanders A primary disease of horses but fatal in humans. A complete account was given by a veterinarian, Philibert Chabert (1734–1814) of Paris, in 1782. John Elliotson (1791–1868) showed its communicability to man in 1830. It was also shown to be contagious by Pierre François Olive Rayer (1793–1867) in 1837. The causative organism, *Pfiefferella mallei,* was identified by Friedrich August Johannes Löffler (1852–1915) in 1882. German bacteriologist, Johann Wilhelm Schultz (1839–1920) of the Berlin Veterinary School succeeded in cultivating the organism from a horse dying of glanders in 1886. It was eradicated from England in 1928.

Glandular Fever [Latin: *glans,* acorn or pellet] Infectious mononucleosis was described as 'glandular fever' by Moscow pediatrician, Feodorovich Filatov (1847–1902) in 1887. Emil Pfeiffer (1846–1921), gave a classic description as 'Drusenfieber' in 1889. The characteristic blood changes were observed by Wilhelm Türk (1871–1916) in 1907, and H.L. Tidy and E.C. Daniel also described these blood findings in 1923. The presence of heterophilic antibodies in infectious mononucleosis was shown by John Rodman Paul (1893–1971) and Walls Willard Bunnel (b 1902) in 1932. *See Paul–Bunnel test.*

Glanzmann Syndrome (Syn. Hereditary hemorrhagic thrombasthenia) Hereditary hemorrhagic tendency associated with abnormal morphology and function of the platelets. Described by Swiss pediatrician, Eduard Glanzmann (1887–1959), in 1918.

Glaser, Johann Heinrich (1629–1675) Professor of Greek, anatomy and botany at the University of Basel, who described the petrotympanic fissure in 1680.

Glasgow Royal Infirmary Founded by two professors, Jardine and Stevenson at a meeting held on 5 June 1787. James Adam was chosen as architect and the foundation stone was laid at the site of the old palace of the Bishop of Glasgow in 1792. It opened on 8 December 1794, with 150 patients. David Dale of Ayrshire, a Scottish industrialist and philanthropist, was one of the first directors.

Glasgow University Founded by Bishop William Turnbull

in 1451. The first mention of it is found in a letter written by James II in 1453. The first physician to be mentioned as Doctor in Medicinis was Andre de Garleis in 1469.

Glass Blower's Cataract The German surgeon, Lorenz Heister (1683–1758), noted the relationship between heat and cataract formation in 1739. Its occurrence due to heat was further studied by W. Meyerhofer in 1886. Alfred Greenwood, the secretary of the Glass Bottle Makers of Yorkshire, who himself was partly blind, noticed the increased frequency of cataracts in glass blowers in 1891. The incidence was studied by Thomas Morrison Legge (1863–1932), the first inspector of factories in England, in 1907.

Glauber, John Rudolph (1604–1668) Born in Carlstadt, he was the last of the German alchemists. He discovered a neutral purgative salt, sodium sulfate, which is known as Glauber salt. He also produced sulfuric acid and nitric acid. Glauber prepared several secret remedies that were held in high esteem. The apothecaries during his time displayed wooden figures of Glauber outside, as a symbol of their profession. He published a work on chemistry.

Glaucoma [Greek: *glaucum,* sea green] Around AD 600, Aetius of Amida in the Byzantine Empire divided glaucoma into two categories: 'the first arises from dryness and concretion of the crystalline humor, and is a sea-green color; the second is caused by the humor near the pupil becoming congealed and dry'. Hippocrates (460–377 BC) recommended cautery, and Rhazes (850–932) considered it incurable when the pupils became insensitive to light. Oribasius (AD 326–403) used the juice of wild carrots and germander to treat it, and Paul of Aegina (625–690) advocated bleeding, purging and bitter cucumber. Iridectomy was introduced by Albrecht von Graefe (1828–1870) in 1855. The value of physostimine was demonstrated by Ludwig Laqueur (1839–1909) in 1876 and a new operation, sclerocorneal trepanning, was designed by Robert Henry Elliot (1864-1936) in 1909.

Gleet A continued discharge from the urethra or genital organs after acute symptoms of gonorrhea have ceased. John Hunter (1728–1793) prescribed turpentine, balsam and catharides as treatment.

Glemin, John George (1709–1755) German physician and botanist at Tübingen who published *Flora Siberica.*

Glenard Syndrome The downward displacement of the viscera (enteroptosis) in association with neurasthenia. Described by French physician, Frantz Glenard (1848–1920), in 1885.

Glenny, Alexander Thomas (1882–1965) British bacteriologist who prepared alum-precipitated tetanus toxoid for immunization in 1930.

Gley, M.E. Eugene (1857–1930) *See parathyroid gland.*

Glioma The vascularity of malignant gliomas was shown by Howard Henry Tooth (1856–1925) in 1912. Useful classification was given by Harvey Williams Cushing (1869–1939) and Percival Bailey (1892–1973) in 1926. A series of 113 cases of multiple gliomas from the literature, including his own cases, were presented by C.B. Courville in 1936. H.J. Scherer in 1940 estimated that 40% of gliomas were multiple. A useful classification based on cytology was proposed by Spanish histologist, Pio del Rio-Hortega, in 1941.

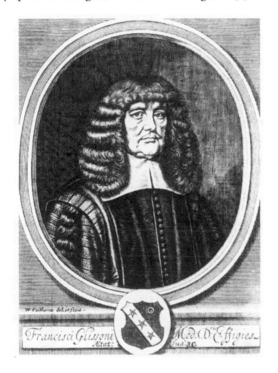

Francis Glisson (1607–1677). Courtesy of the National Library of Medicine

Glisson, Francis (1607–1677) Physician and anatomist from Dorset who was Regius professor of physick at Cambridge in 1636. He was a founder of the Royal Society, and in 1651 he described rickets, known in Europe as morbus Anglicus or English disease. He also described the fibrous capsule of the liver which now bears his name.

Globulin Term for a group of proteins that are sparingly soluble in water, but soluble in salt solutions. Based on the proposal of the British Physiological Society (1907) and the American Physiological Society (1908). *See gamma globulin.*

Glomerular Filtration [Latin: *glomus*, ball] The ancient Greek physicians explained the function of the kidneys on the basis of a filter. This view was opposed by Galen (129–200), who thought that the blood did not circulate through the kidney; and proposed a hypothesis of 'attraction', by which waste products were attracted to the kidney. In 1842 William Bowman (1816–1892), an English physician at King's College London, proposed that urine formation occurred by glomerular filtration and tubular secretion. He also discovered the capsule for filtration which now bears his name. A year later, Carl Friedrich Wilhelm Ludwig (1816–1895) of Leipzig proposed that the glomerulus filtered water as well as solids, and that the water was reabsorbed in the tubules, leaving a greater concentration of solids in the urine. Around the same time, Rudolph Peter Heidenhain (1834–1897) opposed Ludwig's theory and claimed that substances such as urea and uric acid were secreted into the tubules. The resorption of water and salts in the tubules was demonstrated by Arthur Robertson Cushny (1866–1926) in 1917. An attempt to measure glomerular filtration was made by Danish physiologist, Poul Rehberg (1895–1985), in 1926.

Glomerular Nephritis The autoimmune nature of the condition was suggested in 1905 by Bela Schick (1877–1967), an Austrian pediatrician who worked in New York. He assumed this on the basis of an interval of 10–21 days which he observed between an attack of scarlet fever and the onset of nephritis. M. Masugi produced changes in rat kidney similar to glomerular nephritis by injecting them with anti-rat kidney serum in 1933. His study gave further support for the autoimmune theory of glomerular nephritis. The presence of circulating antibodies against kidney was shown using complement fixation reactions by K. Lange (b 1906) and colleagues. Arthur M. Fishberg (b 1898), an associate in medicine at Mount Sinai Hospital, New York, classified nephritis into various forms including focal glomerular nephritis and acute interstitial nephritis, in 1931.

Glomerulus [Latin: *glomus*, ball] *See glomerular filtration, capillary basement membrane, juxtaglomerular apparatus.*

Glossopharyngeal Nerve [Greek: *glossa*, tongue + *pharynx*, gullet] Described by Gabriele Falloppio (1523–1562), a pupil of Andreas Vesalius (1515–1564). Johannes Ehrenritter (d 1790), a Viennese anatomist, described the ganglion of the glossopharyngeal nerve in 1790. The tympanic branch is named after Ludwig Levin Jacobson (1783–1843), a Danish anatomist from Copenhagen, who described it around 1820.

Gloves Originally used as a status symbol and ceremoniously given for bestowing land and wealth during the Middle

Ages. The discovery of rubber and vulcanization made it possible for them to be mass produced cheaply in the latter part of the 19th century. The use of rubber gloves in surgery was suggested by British physician, Thomas Watson, in 1843. One of the first to use them in surgery in Europe was Johann von Mikulicz-Radecki (1850–1905) of Poland. Cotton gloves were replaced with rubber gloves by New York surgeon, William Halsted (1852–1922), in 1894. Boston obstetrician, Horatio Robinson Storer (1830–1922), was also one of the first to wear rubber gloves in surgery.

Glucagon [Greek: *glykys*, sweet] A hormone in extract of pancreas which causes a rise in blood sugar. Discovered by John R. Murlin and C.P. Kimball at the University of Rochester in 1923.

Gluck, Themistokles (1853–1942) German surgeon who devised an improved technique for laryngectomy in 1899.

Glucose [Greek: *glykys*, sweet] The plant sugars, fructose, glucose and sucrose, were identified by Joseph Louis Proust (1754–1826), a professor in Madrid in 1808. Glucose was produced by treating starch with sulfuric acid by German chemist, Gottlieb Sigismond Kirchhoff (1764–1833) in 1811. French chemist, Michel Chevreul (1786–1889), showed that the sugar in diabetic urine was glucose in 1815. Glucose was synthesized by Emil Fischer (1852–1919) in 1887. The metabolic pathway in the formation of glucose was elucidated through radioactive tracer methods by an American chemist of Russian origin, Melvin Calvin (b 1911) of Minnesota around 1950. *See blood glucose.*

Glucose Estimation *See blood glucose.*

Glucose-1-Phosphate A key intermediate of glycogen metabolism, identified by American biochemist, physician and Nobel Prize winner, Carl Ferdinand Cori (1896–1984) from Prague, in 1937.

Glucose-1-Phosphate Kinase The enzyme and its product, glucose-1-6-bisphosphate, were discovered by a Paris-born Argentinian biochemist, Luis Frederico Leloir (b 1906) in 1949. He was educated in Buenos Aires and Cambridge, and set up his own research institute in Argentina where he carried out his studies on diabetes, glucose metabolism and the adrenal gland. He was awarded the Nobel Prize for Chemistry for his work on energy storage mechanisms involved in the production of glycogen in 1970.

Glucose Tolerance Test London pathologist, Hugh MacLean (1879–1957), described a test in 1921. Urinary response to glucose load was studied by Chicago physician, William David Sansum (b 1880) in 1916. American physician, Russel Morse Wilder (1885–1952) studied D-glucose tolerance in health and disease in 1917. A one-hour test with two doses was devised by Detroit pathologist, Sylvester Emanuel Gould (b 1900) in 1937. Response to intravenous glucose load was studied by Samuel Soskin (b 1904) of Chicago in 1943.

Glutamic Acid Amino acid isolated by Ritthausen in 1866.

Glutathione A hydrogen carrier in cellular respiration, isolated in 1921 by Frederick Gowland Hopkins (1851–1947) of Cambridge University.

Glutathione Reductase Deficiency Cause of hemolytic anemia. Described by H.D. Waller, G.W. Lohr and Zysno Gerok in 1965.

Gluteal Muscles [Greek: *gloutos*, rump] The term *gloutos* was used by Hippocrates (460–377 BC) to refer to any rounded eminence. It was later confined to the muscles of the buttocks.

Gluten [Latin: *gluten*, glue] The protein component of grain, including wheat, was initially known as the 'vegetoanimal principle'. It was discovered by James Beccaria (1682–1766) a physician in Bologna.

Gluten-Sensitive Enteropathy *See celiac disease.*

Glyceraldehyde Phosphate Dehydrogenase An enzyme crystallized from rabbit muscle by Theresa Gerti Cori (1896–1957) and colleagues in 1948.

Glycerin Discovered by a Swedish apothecary and chemist, Carl Wilhelm Scheele (1742–1786), who called it 'sweet principle of fats' in 1779. Its nature was further elucidated by Michel Eugene Chevreul (1786–1889) in 1823.

Glycerol *See glycerin.*

Glyceryl Trinitrate Nitroglycerin, introduced as treatment for angina by William Murell (1853–1912) of University College, London, in 1879.

Glycine Amino acid isolated from a hydrosylate of gelatin by Henri Braconnet who named it 'sugar of gelatin' in 1820. Named by Jons Jakob Berzelius (1779–1848) in 1848.

Glycogen [Greek: *glykys*, sweet + *genan*, to produce] Claude Bernard (1813–1878), during his experiments in 1857, noted that the liver produced a starch-like substance which he named 'glycogen'. He also demonstrated the breakdown of glycogen to dextrose. A breakdown product, glucose-1-phosphate, was identified by American biochemist and physician, Carl Ferdinand Cori (1896–1984) from Prague in

1937. He shared the Nobel Prize in Physiology or Medicine in 1947 with his wife.

Glycogen Storage Disease *See von Gierke disease.*

Glycolysis [Greek: *glykys*, sweet + *lyein*, loosen] Breakdown of glucose. *See Krebs cycle.*

Glycosuria [Greek: *glykys*, sweet + *oureon*, urine] The yeast test for detection of sugar in urine was devised by Francis Home (1719–1813) in 1780. The sweet taste of urine was shown to be due to sugar by Matthew Dobson (1713–1784) of Liverpool in 1776. In 1815, French chemist, Michel Chevreul (1786–1889), showed that the sugar was glucose. The Maume test for detecting sugar in urine – adding stannous chloride to give a brown color – was devised by French chemist, Edme Joules Maume (b 1818), around 1850. English physician, Frederick William Pavy (1829–1911), one of the earliest workers on carbohydrate metabolism and diabetes, correlated hyperglycemia and glycosuria in 1862. The occurrence on removing the pancreas was demonstrated by Joseph von Mering (1848–1909) and Oskar Minowski (1858–1931) in 1889. The association between lesions of the islets of Langerhans and glycosuria was suggested by William George MacCallum (1874–1944), a Canadian-born pathologist who worked at Johns Hopkins University. The appearance of glycosuria in animals that had experimentally-induced lesions in the floor of the fourth ventricle was shown by Claude Bernard (1813–1878) in 1855. Glycosuria during increased epinephrine (adrenaline) secretion was noted by F. Blum in 1893. Glycosuria and phosphaturia in familial cystinosis were observed by Emil Aberhalden (1877–1950) in 1903 and described by Guido Fanconi of Zurich in 1936. The Benedict test for detecting sugar in blood and urine was devised by Stanley Rossiter Benedict (1884–1936) in 1931. *See diabetes.*

Glynn, Ernest Edward (1873–1929) English physician who studied phagocytic properties of leukocytes in 1910.

Glynn, Robert (1719–1800) Born in Cambridge, he practiced as a physician for a short time in Richmond, Surrey. He wrote *The Day of Judgment: a Political Essay* in 1757.

Gmelin Test A test for bile pigments devised by German chemist and professor of medicine and chemistry at Heidelberg, Leopold Gmelin (1788–1853).

Gmelin, Johann Frederick (1748–1805) Physician from Tübingen who was professor of chemistry at Göttingen. He wrote *A History of Chemistry,* and discovered several mineral and vegetable dyes.

Gmelin, Johann Georg (1709–1755) A naturalist who graduated in medicine at the age of 18 years, and became professor of chemistry at the age of 22. He published several botanical works which were banned in Russia, owing to his opposition to the establishment. He was appointed professor of chemistry and medicine at Tübingen in 1747.

Gmelin, Leopold (1788–1853) German chemist and son of Johann Frederick Gmelin (1748–1805). He was professor of medicine and chemistry at Heidelberg, where he discovered potassium ferricyanide (Gmelin salt) in 1822. He coined the terms 'ester' and 'ketone' in organic chemistry.

Gnosticism [Greek: *gnosis*, knowledge] An early Christian belief that god had revealed a secret key to the universe to a chosen soul and if man could rediscover it his soul would be free of fate.

Goclenius, Rodolphus (1572–1621) German physician in Würtemberg in Swabia, who published a treatise on the cure of wounds by magnetism. He collected materials from previous and contemporary philosophers, historians and physicians and published a treatise on preserving health, *De Vite Proroganda* in 1608.

Goddard, Jonathan (1617–1674) English physician from Greenwich who formulated the volatile liquid remedy called Goddard drops. It was known as 'Gutta Anglicanae' in France. The secret of Goddard powder was later bought by Charles II for £5000. Goddard also constructed the first telescope in England.

Godlee, Sir John Rickman (1849–1925) British surgeon at the Brompton Hospital, who successfully removed a cerebral tumor on 25 November 1884. He pioneered treatment of liver abscess by drainage through a needle, in 1890.

Godman, John Davidson (1794–1830) American physician from Maryland who described the continuation of the pretracheal fascia into the thorax, in 1824.

Goethe, Johann Wolfgang (1749–1832) German scientist and poet, and pioneer in the study of evolution. He used the term 'morphology' in 1817.

Goeze, John Augustus Ephraim (1731–1786) German clergyman and naturalist, born in Ascherleben. He was educated at Halle and became a minister at Quilenberg. He made several microscopic discoveries including the discovery of the beef tapeworm, *Taenia saginata*, in 1782. His work on entomology was printed in four parts from 1771 to 1781. He also published a history of Germany in 1782.

Goiter *See thyroid goiter.*

Gold [Sanskrit: *jval*, to shine] One of the earliest metals to be identified, owing to its glittering nature in river beds and soil. It was popular in Egypt as early as 3500 BC before the time of the first dynasty. Pliny (AD 23–79) wrote a chapter on it around AD 50, in which he described its properties and uses. During the 19th and early 20th centuries it was used as treatment for a variety of illnesses. It was introduced as treatment for rheumatic disorders by Jacques Forestier (b 1890) of Paris in 1925, and as cure for tuberculosis in Denmark around 1930s. Several physicians in England continued to use gold therapy for asthma up to the 1940s. It is still used in treatment of rheumatoid arthritis.

Gold Amalgam A preparation of gold in mercury described by Roman architect, Markus Vitruvius Pollio, around AD 27.

Gold Leaf Electroscope Invented by Abraham Bennett (1750–1799), an English physicist and clergyman, in 1789.

Gold Therapy *See gold.*

Goldberger, Joseph (1874–1929) Born in Hungary, he emigrated to America as a child, and graduated in medicine from the Bellevue Hospital Medical School in 1895. He joined the US Public Health Service in 1899 and pioneered studies on the cause of pellagra in 1920. He demonstrated that it was due to a deficiency in diet, in 1926.

Goldblatt, Harry (1891–1977) American experimental pathologist who made a detailed study of hypertension by clamping the renal arteries in animals.

Goldflam, Samuel Vulfovich (1852–1932) Neurologist in Warsaw who described myasthenia gravis in 1893. It was earlier described by Wilhelm Heinrich Erb (1840–1921) in 1879 and is known as Erb–Goldflam syndrome.

Gold-Headed Cane Originally a cane carried by John Radcliffe (1650–1714) while he was president of the Royal College of Physicians. He handed it down to his successor, Richard Mead (1673–1754), from whom it was passed to each successive president of the College over the next 120 years. Matthew Baillie (1761–1823) was the last holder of the cane before it was presented to Sir Henry Halford (1766–1844) by Baillie's widow in 1825. Halford presented it to the Royal College to be exhibited in its premises. A book about it and its holders, *The Gold-headed Cane,* was published in 1827, followed by editions in 1828, 1884, 1915 and 1923.

Golding, Benjamin (1793–1863) British physician who founded Charing Cross Hospital in 1818.

Goldmann, Edwin Ellen (1862–1913) Surgeon in Freiburg who described a two-stage operation for removal of pharyngeal diverticulum in 1909.

Goldscheider Disease *See epidermolysis bullosa.*

Goldschmidt, Richard Benedikt (1878–1958) Geneticist who was director of the Kaiser Wilhelm Institute, Berlin. He emigrated to America in 1934 and became professor of zoology at the University of California, where he conducted experiments on geographical and environmental influence on genes and mutation.

Goldsmith, Oliver (1728–1774) A poet and novelist from Dublin. He was supposed to have graduated in medicine, although the source of his medical degree remains obscure. He obtained his BA at Trinity College in 1749 and proceeded to France. He returned destitute to England in 1758 and worked as a druggist's assistant before setting himself up as a physician in Southwark. He presented himself for examination of the Royal College of Surgeons, wearing a borrowed suit in 1758, but failed. He portrayed himself as 'Oliver Smith MB' in his first book *The Traveller,* published in 1764. Oxford University gave him an MB in 1769 as it was believed that he already had a medical degree from Dublin.

Goldstein, Eugene (1850–1930) *See cathode ray.*

Goldstein, Joseph Leonhard (b 1940) Molecular biologist from southern California, who graduated in medicine from the University of Texas in 1966. His main contribution was to the study of familial cholesterolemia and he showed the missing receptor sites for low-density lipoprotein cholesterol in the liver of patients with this. He was awarded the Nobel Prize for Physiology or Medicine in 1985.

Goldthwait Operation Realignment of patella for recurrent dislocation. Described in 1899 by Joel Ernest Goldthwait (1866–1961), an orthopedic surgeon at Massachusetts General Hospital.

Golgi Bodies or Apparatus Reticular formations within the cytoplasm of the cell. Discovered around 1898 by Camillo Golgi (1844–1926), professor of histology at Pavia.

Golgi, Camillo (1844–1926) Italian histologist who graduated in medicine from the University of Pavia in 1865, and became director of the clinic for the incurable at Abbiategrasso, where he pioneered a method of staining nervous tissue. With his method of depositing metallic salts within cell structures, he was able to identify and name the 'axon' and 'dendrites' of the nervous system. He was professor of anatomy at Pavia in 1876, and described the tactile end-organs known as Golgi corpuscles, in 1878.

Goll, Friedrich (1829–1903) Neuroanatomist from Zurich who was a contemporary of Rudolph Virchow (1821–1902), Albrecht Rudolf von Kollicker (1817–1905) and Claude Bernard (1813–1878). He described fasciculus gracilis of the posterior column of the spinal cord in 1868, and wrote a paper on *Minute Anatomy of the Spinal Cord of Man* in 1860.

Goltz, Friedrich Leopold (1834–1902) German physiologist who made important studies on decerebrate animals in 1869. He pioneered work on vestibular disturbances and vertigo in 1870.

Gombault, François Alexis Albert (1844–1904) Neuropathologist in Paris who gave original descriptions of several tracts in the spinal cord in his *Etude sur la Sclerose Laterale Amyotrophique* in 1877.

Gomes, Bernadino Antonio (1768–1823) Spanish chemist who obtained an active substance from cinchona bark and named it cinchonino in 1810.

Gonadotropic Hormone [Greek: *gone*, birth + *trephein*, to nourish] Bernard Zondek (1891–1966) and Selmar Ascheim (1878–1965) of Germany demonstrated the presence of a gonad-stimulating hormone in the anterior pituitary in 1926 and named it gonadotropin or prolan. This was confirmed by Phillip Edward Smith (1884–1970) in 1927. The two different secretory components of the anterior pituitary – the follicle stimulating hormone and luteinizing hormone – were separated by H.L. Fevold, Frederick Lee Hishaw (b 1891) of Wisconsin and S.L. Leonard in 1931. Their method was further refined by Z. Wallen-Lawrence in 1934.

Gonin, Jules (1870–1935) Swiss ophthalmic surgeon who devised a method of operative treatment for detachment of the retina in 1927.

Gonioscopy [Greek: *gonia*, angle + *skopein*, to look] Visualization of the recesses of the anterior chamber of the eye, normally not seen with a slit lamp. Devised by New York ophthalmologist, Manuel Uribe y Tronchoso (b 1867) in 1925.

Gonococcus [Greek: *gone*, offspring + *kokkos*, berry] The causative organism of gonorrhea (*Neisseria gonorrhoeae*), discovered in 1879 by Albert Neisser (1855–1916), while he was a 24-year-old assistant in the dermatological clinic of Oscar Simon at the University of Breslau.

Gonorrhea [Greek: *gone*, offspring + *rhein*, to flow] The disease was confused with syphilis by most workers up to the 18th century. Benjamin Bell (1749–1806), a student of John Hunter (1728–1793) and one of the first surgeons at the Edinburgh Royal Infirmary, differentiated between the two diseases in 1793. The causative organism of gonorrhea, the

gonococcus (*Neisseria gonorrhoeae*) was discovered by Albert Neisser (1855–1916), an assistant at the dermatological clinic in the University of Breslau in 1879. It was grown in culture by Leo Leistikow (1847–1917) in 1882. *See genitourinary medicine, venereal disease.*

Gooch Splint A flexible splint made of leather for treatment of fractures. Devised by English surgeon, Benjamin Gooch (1700–1776) of Norfolk. A description is given in his *Cases and Practical Remarks in Surgery*, published in 1758.

Good, James Mason (1764–1827) A physician and poet, born in Epping in Essex. He obtained his medical diploma from Aberdeen, and started practicing in 1820. His lectures at the Surrey Institute were published as *The Book of Nature* a year before his death. Another of his works *The Study of Medicine*, was published during the last year of his life.

Goodall, Alexander (b 1876) English physician who demonstrated the moderate effectiveness of marmite (autolyzed yeast) in treatment of pernicious anemia in, 1932.

Goodall, Edward Wilberforce (1861–1938) London physician and medical historian who described a mild attack of fever and fleeting rash in infections such as measles.

Goodell Sign Softening of the cervix occurring as a sign of pregnancy. Described by American gynecologist, William Goodell (1829–1894).

Goodenough, Florence Laura (b 1886) American psychologist who devised a test in 1926, called Draw-a-Man, which was used to estimate a child's projected image of adults and itself.

Goodhart, Sir James Frederick (1845–1916) The son of a general practitioner from London. He graduated from Aberdeen and became a physician to Guy's Hospital. He wrote *Student's Guide to Diseases of Children* in 1885, which ran to ten editions by 1913.

Goodman and Gilman Textbook of pharmacology, written by Louis S. Goodman, professor of pharmacology at the University of Utah Medical School, and Alfred Gilman, in the 1940s.

Goodpasture Syndrome Associated with acute nephritis and hemoptysis. Described in an 18-year-old male by American virologist, Ernest William Goodpasture (1886–1960), in 1919.

Goodpasture, Ernest William (1886–1960) American virologist who demonstrated the susceptibility of the chorioallantoic membrane of the chick embryo to fowl pox, in 1931. This formed the basis for study of viruses in culture. He also isolated the mumps virus in 1934. *See Goodpasture syndrome.*

Goodsir, John (1814–1867) Born in Anstruther, Scotland to a family of three generations of doctors. He studied anatomy under Robert Knox (1791–1862) and was a contemporary of James Young Simpson (1811–1870). He published a treatise on the development of teeth in 1839 and was professor of anatomy at Edinburgh in 1846. He was a conservator of the Museum of the Royal College of Surgeons, Edinburgh.

Goormaghtigh, Norbet (b 1890) *See juxtaglomerular apparatus.*

Gordon, Alexander (1752–1799) Obstetrician in Aberdeen who proposed the contagious nature of puerperal fever, and advocated disinfection of clothes of the midwife and doctor attending the mother, in 1795.

Gordon, Alexander James (d 1872) Born in Middlesex, he graduated from Edinburgh in 1814, and was elected physician to the London Hospital in 1828. He founded and edited *The Quarterly Journal of Foreign Medicine and Surgery.*

Gordon, Alfred (1874–1953) American neurologist in Philadelphia who described the extensor plantar response produced by squeezing the calf muscles (Gordon reflex) in cases of pyramidal tract lesions.

Gordon, Andrew (1712–1751) Born in Aberdeen, he was professor of philosophy at the Scots Monastery of the Benedictines at Erfurt. He wrote *Phenomena Electricitasis Exposita, Physica Experimentalis Elementa* and other works on philosophy and science. He used a cylinder instead of a globe in electrical apparatus.

Gordon, Bernard de   Scottish professor who taught at Montpellier from 1285 to 1297. He wrote *Lilium Mediciane* from 1305 to 1307. He was the first medical writer to mention the word 'spectacles'. His other works include: *De Phlebotomia, De Urinis, De Pulsibus* and *De Regime Sanitatis.*

Gordon, Mervyn Henry (1872–1953) British bacteriologist and virologist who pioneered studies on virology. He described a precipitin test for differentiating between smallpox and chickenpox. He published an important study of the viruses of vaccinia and variola in 1925.

Gordon-Taylor, Sir William (1878–1960) British surgeon who designed the one-stage hind-quarter operative amputation in 1935.

Gorer, Peter Alfred (1907–1961) British geneticist who pioneered transplantation genetics and established the concept of transplantation immunity in 1937.

Gorgas, William Crawford (1854–1920) American army surgeon from Mobile, Alabama who graduated in medicine from Bellevue Hospital Medical College, New York in 1879. After graduation he joined the military and was sent to Havana in 1898 to eradicate yellow fever. His methods of improved sanitation resulted in virtual eradication of malaria and yellow fever in Cuba.

Gorget A 16th-century instrument used in lithotomy to cut the prostate gland and the bladder.

Gorham, Lemuel Whittington (b 1885) American physician from Albany, New York who studied the relationship of cardiac pain to coronary occlusion in 1938.

Gorilla The word *gorullai* was used by the navigator, Hanno, in *Periplus,* written in 400 BC to denote a race of 'hairy people'. It was described by an English sailor, Andrew Battel, in 1590. An early account was given by the French explorer, Paul Belloni du Chaillou (1835–1903) in Africa and who wrote *Explorations and Adventures in Equatorial Africa.* A summary of the knowledge was given to the Royal Society by Richard Owen (1804–1892) in 1859, and his *Memoir on the Gorilla* was published in 1865.

Gorreus, John de (d 1572)   Protestant physician who was persecuted for his religion in France. He published a translation of Nicander.

Gorrie, John (1803–1855) American physician who introduced various methods of cooling for patients with fever.

Gorter, John (1689–1762) Born in Holland, he graduated from Leiden and became imperial physician at St Petersburg. He published numerous works on medicine.

Gosselin Fracture V-shaped fracture of distal tibia. Described by French surgeon, Lèon Athanese Gosselin (1815–1887), in 1866.

Göttingen University Founded in Germany in 1737.

Gottstein, Jacob (1832–1895) Otorhinologist from Breslau who described the protoplasmic projections of the lateral cells of the cochlear canal in 1872.

Gougerot, Henri (1881–1955) French dermatologist in Paris who gave a complete description of sporotrichosis (with Charles Lucien de Beurmann) in 1912.

Goulard Lotion Aqua Goulardi, a remedy made of lead and rectified spirit for dressing infected wounds. Prepared by French surgeon Thomas Goulard (d 1784) in 1760.

Goulstonian Lectures Established by Theodore Goulston, an English physician from Northamptonshire. He died in

1632, bequeathing £200 for an annual pathological lecture to be held at the Royal College of Physicians.

Goundou A disease that causes deforming bony growths in African children. Described as *Horned Men in Africa* by MacAlister (1882) and J.J. Lamprey (1887). It was shown to be due to osteoplastic periostitis by Albert John Chalmers (1870–1920) in 1900.

Goupil, James (d 1564) Physician in Paris who edited several Greek medical works.

Gouraud, Vincent Ollivier (1772–1845) French surgeon in Tours who wrote a treatise on inguinal hernia.

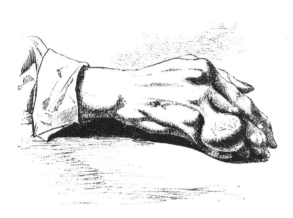

Gout involving the hand. Sir Alfred Baring Garrod, *A Treatise on Gout and Rheumatic Gout* (1876). Longmans, London

Gout [Latin: *gutta*, drop] The present term is derived from the belief that humor or fluid dropped into the joint, causing disease. Hippocratic writings from 500 BC reveal that it was known to Greek physicians. Pliny (AD 23–79) referred to it as 'podagrae morbus'. Dominican doctor, Radulphus, in the 13th century, referred to it as *cum gutta quam podagram vel arthriticam*. Colchicum or meadow saffron, known as 'ephemerum' to the ancients, was recommended as treatment by Arab physicians around AD 1000. Thomas Sydenham (1624–1689), the father of medicine in England, wrote *Tractus de Podagra et de Hydrope* in 1683. His description was based on his own experience of gout. George Cheyne (1671–1743), a Scottish physician who moved to London, published *An Essay on Method of Treating the Gout*. Another authority was Charles Scudamore (1778–1849), physician to Prince Leopold, who published *A Treatise on the Nature and Cure of Gout and Gravel, with General Observations on Morbid State of Digestive Organs*. Sir Alfred Baring Garrod (1819–1907), physician to the Queen and consulting physician to King's College London discovered the presence of excess uric acid in blood of patients with gout. He introduced the thread test for uric acid and differentiated it from rheumatoid arthritis. Lithium carbonate, used as a solvent for bladder calculi by Ure in 1843, was recommended as treatment by Garrod in 1859, and 'Lithia tablets' became over-the-counter treatment around 1867. Allopurinol, for treatment of gout, was developed by George H. Hitchings while he was research director at the Burroughs Wellcome Laboratories in New York in 1943.

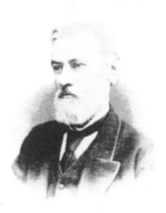

William Richard Gowers (1845–1915). Courtesy of the National Library of Medicine

Gowers, William Richard (1845–1915) An eminent London neurologist who studied medicine at University College Hospital, where he later became professor of clinical medicine. He gave the name 'knee jerk' to the tendon reflex of the knee and introduced the colorimetric method of estimation of hemoglobin. He published *Pseudo-hypertrophic Muscular Paralysis* in 1879, later known as Gowers Disease. He wrote *Epilepsy and other Chronic Convulsive Diseases*, in 1881. He also wrote one of the most important works on neurology of his era, *Diseases of the Nervous System*, in 1886, and a second volume appeared a few years later.

Goyrand, Jean Gaspard Blaise (1803–1866) French surgeon in Paris who described a type of inguinal hernia which protruded into a partial sac.

Graaf, Regnier de (1641–1673) An eminent Dutch physician who studied under Franciscus Sylvius (1614–1672). He was one of the first to experiment on the pancreas and published a treatise on pancreatic juice in 1664. He described the egg-containing follicle, known as the Graafian follicle, and coined the term 'ovary'.

Graafian Follicle [Latin: *folliculus*, little bag] A structure or sac which appears on the surface of the ovary, described by

Regnier de Graaf (1641–1673) of Holland in 1672. The mammalian ovum within the follicle was discovered by Carl Ernst von Baer (1792–1876) in 1827.

Grace, William Gilbert (1848–1915) A physician and famous cricketer from Bristol. He made over 126 test centuries, the highest of which was 400 runs.

Gradenigo Syndrome Associated with acute otitis media followed by abducens nerve or internal rectus palsy. Described by Italian otorhinologist, Giuseppe Gradenigo (1859–1926), in 1904.

Gradenigo Test A test for hearing devised by Italian otorhinologist, Giuseppe Gradenigo (1859–1926), in 1894.

Graefe, Carl Ferdinand von (1787–1840) Professor of surgery in Berlin who founded modern plastic surgery. He developed rhinoplasty and blepharoplasty and published the first book on rhinoplasty in 1818.

Graefe, Friedrich Wilhelm Ernst Albrecht von (1828–1870) Eye surgeon from Berlin who introduced modern surgical ophthalmology. He founded *Archiv für Ophthalmologie* in 1854 and introduced iridectomy in 1855 in treatment of glaucoma and iritis, and as part of the cataract operation. He performed an operation for strabismus in 1857 and introduced the linear method of cataract extraction in 1868. He described the stationary nature of the eyelid or lid lag sign of the eye in thyrotoxicosis, known as 'von Graefe sign'. He designed operations for squint, glaucoma, cataract, conical cornea and other eye conditions.

Graeupner, Salo (1861–1916) German physician who was probably the first to experimentally demonstrate that blood pressure falls during exercise in a weak heart.

Grafenberg, Ernst (1881–1957) Jewish gynecologist in Germany and a pioneer in the study of intrauterine contraception. He studied the cyclic changes in pH of vaginal fluid and devised a coiled silver wire as an intrauterine contraceptive device. He escaped the Nazi regime and went to the United States where he worked at the Margaret Sanger Research Bureau in New York.

Graham Steell Murmur Heard over the pulmonary artery in early diastole, due to pulmonary hypertension resulting from mitral stenosis. Described in 1888 by Graham Steell (1851–1942), a physician at the Manchester Royal Infirmary. His father, John Steell, was a Scottish sculptor who made the statue of Scottish poet, Sir Walter Scott (1771–1832) in Princes Street in Edinburgh.

Graham, Evarts Ambrose (1883–1957) Professor of surgery at Washington University, St Louis. He developed cholecystography and was the first to perform total pneumonectomy. He associated tobacco smoking with lung cancer.

Graham, Georges Sellers (1879–1942) American pathologist from Albany, New York who devised a stain (Graham benzidine stain) consisting of peroxidase and benzidine.

Graham, James (1745–1794) A quack doctor from Edinburgh who set up the Temple of Health and Hymen at Pall Mall. He practiced various forms of alternative therapies, one of which was a mud bath. His premises were seized in 1782 because of debt. He later became insane and died in penury in Edinburgh.

Graham, Thomas (1805–1869) Scottish chemist, born in Glasgow. He studied chemistry in his home town and at Edinburgh. He became a professor at Anderson's College in 1830 and proposed the law of diffusion of gases in 1831. He moved to London as professor of chemistry at University College in 1837 and was appointed first President of the Chemical Society in 1841. He founded colloid chemistry with his work on liquids in 1849, and conducted the first experiments on dialysis. He published *Liquid Diffusion Applied to Analysis* in 1861.

Graham-Little, Sir Ernest Gordon (1867–1950) A politician and a physician who opposed the formation of the National Health Service and its socialist aspects. He represented the London medical graduates in the Senate and promoted the admission of women as external students. He was Chairman of the Medical Parliamentary Committee in 1943.

Graindorge, Andrew (1616–1676) A physician and philosopher from Normandy and an Epicurean. He wrote a curious treatise on fire, light and colors.

Grainger, James (1724–1767) Poet and physician from Berwick. He studied surgery in Edinburgh and took his degree in 1748. He wrote *Historia Febris Anomale Batavae* in 1746. *A Treatise on the Common West India Diseases,* was written during his practice in the West Indies, where he spent the last years of his life. He also published ballads and poems.

Grainger, Richard Dugard (1801–1865) British neurologist who demonstrated the role of gray matter in the spinal cord in reflex activity, in 1837.

Gram Stain A stain for bacteria discovered by Hans Christian Joachim Gram (1853–1938), a Danish physician in Copenhagen, while he was working on methods for double-staining kidney sections in 1883. He incidentally noted that certain bacteria, after undergoing double-staining, could not be decolorized by alcohol. This provided one of the most useful methods of staining bacteria. He was appointed professor of medicine at Copenhagen in 1900. *See stains.*

Gram, B. Hans German physician who took homeopathy across the Atlantic in 1825. He settled in New York and continued to popularize Christian Friedrich Samuel Hahnemann's (1755–1843) work in America.

Grancher, Jacques Joseph (1843–1907) French physician who specialized in chest diseases. He advocated boarding out of children (to healthy families in the country) from tuberculous households. He described several auscultatory physical signs in chest disease.

Grand Mal [Latin: *morbus major*; French: *grand mal*] Hippocratic physicians called epilepsy the 'great disease'.

Grandidier, Johann Ludwig (b 1810) *See hemophilia.*

Granger, Amedee (1879–1939) American radiologist in New Orleans who described a line (Granger line) seen on skull X-ray which represents the superior surface of the sphenoid bone where the optic groove lies.

Grant, Ronald Thompson (1892–1989) A physician from Guy's Hospital who, with Sir Thomas Lewis (1881–1945) in 1924, studied the release and effect of histamine-like substances on the skin secondary to injury.

Granville, Augusto Bozzi (1782–1872) *See gynecology.*

Grasp Reflex The first description was given by Spanish neurologist, J.A.R. Barraquer (1855–1928) of Barcelona, in 1921. His son, L. Barraquer, connected the reflex with lesions of the frontal lobe. *See frontal lobe.*

Grasset, Joseph (1849–1918) Neurologist in Montpellier. He described the drawing of the head to the side in cases of unilateral cerebral lesions producing flaccid hemiplegia (Grasset law). In spastic hemiplegia he observed that the head was turned to the spastic side.

Grassi, Giovanni Battista (1854–1925) Italian parasitologist who established fecal diagnosis of hookworm disease in 1878, before which time it was diagnosed only at postmortem.

Gratarolus, William (1510–1562) Italian physician from Bergamo who practiced at Padua and later in Basel. He published *De Literatorum et eorum qui magistratum gerunt, confervanda valetudine* in 1550, in which he named eating, drinking, labor, sleep and concubinage as important factors affecting health. He also wrote voluminously on other subjects in medicine.

Gratiolet, Louis Pierre (1815–1865) Physician who became a professor of zoology in Paris. He described the occipital visual pathway in 1858.

Graunt, John (1620–1674) Born in London, he was a fellow of the Royal Society, and one of the managers of the New River Company. He is known for the first work on death rates and mortality, *Natural and Political Observations Upon the Bills of Mortality,* published in 1662.

Graves, Robert James (1796–1853) Born in Dublin, he was one of the most important physicians in Irish medicine. He gave an accurate account of exophthalmic goiter, now known as Graves disease, in 1835. His most important work, *Clinical Lectures on the Practice of Medicine,* was published in 1848. He also gave original descriptions of pinpoint pupils in pontine hemorrhage, scleroderma and angioneurotic edema.

Graves, William Phillips (1870–1933) American gynecologist who devised an operation for uterine malposition in 1923.

Graves Disease (Syn. Basedow disease, Parry disease) Exophthalmic goiter. Caleb Hillier Parry (1755–1822), a Bath physician, gave a detailed account in 1786 and published eight more cases. An account of three more cases was given by Robert James Graves (1796–1853), a Dublin physician, in 1835. Carl Adolph Basedow (1799–1854), at Merseberg, near Leipzig, described four more cases in 1840, and it was known as Basedow disease in Germany. *See antithyroid drugs.*

Gravity [Latin: *gravis,* heavy] Considered by the Greeks to be an innate power. Roman philosopher, Lucius Annaeus Seneca (d AD 65) spoke of the moon attracting the waters by this power. The astronomer, Johannes Kepler (1571–1630) investigated it in 1615, and Robert Hooke (1635–1703) proposed a system of gravitation in 1674. The principles were demonstrated by Galileo Galilei (1564–1642) in Florence in 1633. The laws were formulated by Isaac Newton (1642–1727) in 1670 and published in 1687.

Grawitz, Paul Albert (1850–1932) German surgeon and pathologist from Pomerania, who did early work on the origin of hypernephroma (Grawitz tumor) in 1884.

Gray Matter First interpreted as the active and functioning part of the brain by German physician, Franz Joseph Gall (1758–1828) around 1800. Before this time most anatomists relied on the theory of animal spirits proposed by Galen (129–200), to explain the function of the brain. Its role in the spinal cord in reflex activity was shown by Richard Dugard Grainger (1801–1865), a British neurologist, in 1837.

Gray, Asa (1810–1888) Physician in Bridgewater, New York, who gave up medicine for botany. He was professor of natural history at Harvard in 1842, and published over 700 works on botany.

Gray, Henry (1827–1861) Fellow of the Royal College of Surgeons and lecturer in anatomy at St George's Hospital Medical School. He immortalized his name with his *Anatomy, Descriptive and Surgical,* first published in 1858 and popularly known as *Gray's Anatomy.*

Gray, John Edward (1800–1875) London physician who gave up medicine for botany and zoology. He wrote *The Natural Arrangement of British Plants* (1821), *Handbook of British Water Weeds* (1864) and other works.

Gray, Samuel Frederick (1766–1828) Pharmacologist from London who practiced as a pharmaceutical chemist from 1797 in Walsall, Staffordshire. He returned to London in 1800 and published *Supplement to the Pharmacopoeia* in 1818.

Gray, Stephen (1666–1736) Born in London, he was one of the earliest experimenters on electricity. In 1728 he followed up discoveries made by William Gilbert (1544–1603) and demonstrated the flow of electricity from one object to another. He also described a microscope in 1696 which used a water droplet.

Great Ormond Street Hospital for Sick Children Founded in 1852, at the former premises of Sir Richard Mead (1673–1754), by London physician Charles West (1816–1898). He graduated in medicine from Berlin and studied midwifery in Dublin. On his return to London he was physician at the Infirmary for Women and Children at Waterloo Road and lectured on midwifery at the Middlesex Hospital and St Bartholomew's Hospital. After the foundation of the Hospital for Sick Children, he served there as a physician for 23 years.

Great Windmill Street School of Anatomy Founded by William Hunter (1718–1783) in London in 1768. It contained one of the best museums of pathology, and a famous anatomy theater which was attended by many eminent anatomists including Sir Charles Bell (1774–1842), Benjamin Brodie (1783–1862) and John Hunter (1728–1793). *See anatomy, private schools.*

Greef, Carl Richard (1850–1932) Ophthalmologist in Berlin who described a type of intracellular body (Prowazek–Greef body) found in trachomatous secretions. He also published a history of ophthalmology in 1921.

Greek in Medicine Medical and scientific works written in Greek, such as those of Euclid (c 300 BC), Hippocrates (460–377 BC), Aulus Cornelius Celsus (25 BC–AD 50),

Ptolemy (d 285 BC) and Paul of Aegina (625–690), were preserved through their translation into Arabic around the 9th century, mainly through the efforts of the Abbasides dynasty which ruled the Eastern Caliphate of Baghdad. Some treatises of Galen (129–200) in Greek would have been lost forever if it were not for Arabic translations. The study of Greek was revived in Western Europe around 1450 and introduced into Oxford in 1491 by William Grocyn (b 1444) from Bristol. Francis Adams (1796–1861), a Scottish surgeon from Banchory, made valuable English translations of the Greek medical classics of Hippocrates and Paul of Aegina in 1844.

Greek Medicine According to Greek legend, Aesculapius, the ancient Greek god of medicine was the son of Apollo and Coronis. Amongst the hundreds of temples built to him, the chief was built around 600 BC in Epidaurus. The priests glorified and personified Aesculapius and practiced medicine, mysticism and magic. This later gave way to physical medicine with baths in mineral springs, massage, blood letting and therapeutics such as iron, milk and honey. The two main Greek schools of medicine around 600 BC were at Cnidos and Cos. At Cnidos, each disease was studied and a specific remedy was sought, while at Cos, disease was treated generally as a derangement of normal health and reliance was placed on natural remedies. Up to the time of Hippocrates (460–377 BC), the father of modern medicine who trained at Cos, much Greek medicine was derived from Egyptian medicine of earlier origin. His teachings were held in high esteem, by Plato (428–348 BC) and Aristotle (384–322 BC), who referred to him as 'the eminent medical authority'.

Green, Horace (1802–1866) American laryngologist from Vermont who wrote one of the early treatises in America on chronic laryngitis and bronchitis in 1846.

Green, John (1835–1913) American ophthalmologist in St Louis who described a method for surgical correction of entropion.

Green, Joseph Harry (1791–1863) English surgeon who performed a thyroidectomy in 1829.

Green-Armytage Forceps Used for controlling hemorrhage from the uterus during Cesarean section. Devised by London gynecologist, Vivian Bartley Green-Armytage (1882–1961) who served in the Indian Medical Service.

Greene, Charles Lyman (1863–1929) American physician from Minnesota who described the physical sign of cardiac borders being displaced during respiration in cases of pleural effusion.

Greenfield Disease A fatal familial condition characterized by progressive loss of motor power with seizures, blindness, nystagmus and mental deterioration in children. Described by London neuropathologist, Joseph Goodwin Greenfield (b 1884) in 1933.

Greenfield, William Smith (1846–1919) London surgeon who described giant cells in Hodgkin disease in 1878.

Greenhill, Thomas (1681–1740) London surgeon who practiced in Bloomsbury. He published *The Art of Embalming*.

Greenhill, William Alexander (1814–1894) Physician who translated the Latin works of Thomas Sydenham (1624–1689) and in 1845 anonymously published *Anecdota Sydenhamiana, Medical Notes and Observations by Thomas Sydenham* mostly from Sydenham's manuscripts in the Bodleian Library.

Greenhow, Edward Headlam (1814–1888) *See vagabond's disease.*

Greenwich Hospital Erected on the site of the previous royal residence of Edward I (1239–1307). Henry VIII (1491–1546) and his daughters were born here and Charles II (1630–1685) intended to build a new palace at the same site but died before he could complete it. It was converted into a hospital for seamen by William III (1650–1703) and Mary in 1694, and new buildings were added two years later. The estates of the English Jacobite, Earl of Derwentwater (b 1689), who was beheaded in 1716, were bestowed upon it and contributed to its expansion. By 1705 it housed 100 disabled seamen. Its chapel and the great dining hall were destroyed by fire in 1779 and it was rebuilt to accommodate over 2000 men in 1853. It was made an infirmary in 1865, with a portion made a hospital for seamen in 1867.

Greenwood, Major (1854–1917) London practitioner who wrote poems and studied law. He was Deputy Coroner of Northeast London.

Greenwood, Major (1880–1949) Professor of medical statistics and epidemiology at the London School of Hygiene and Tropical Medicine. He wrote *Epidemics and crowd diseases: an introduction to the history of epidemiology* in 1935.

Gregg, Alan (1890–1957) American physician and director at the Rockefeller Foundation who introduced the term 'molecular biology'.

Gregg, Sir Norman McAlister (1892–1966) Australian ophthalmologist from Sydney University who specialized for some time in London. The increased risk of congenital heart disease and congenital cataracts in children of women who contracted rubella during their first trimester of pregnancy was pointed out by him in 1941. This led to a vaccination program against rubella for pregnant women, and he was knighted in 1953. The triad – cataract, congenital heart defects and deafness – in children born to mothers with rubella is named after him (Gregg triad).

Gregory, James (1638–1675) A celebrated mathematician from Aberdeen. He wrote *Optica Promota, feu abdita Radiorum Reflexorum and Refractorum Mysteria, Geometrice Enucleata*, on his reflecting telescope in 1668. While in Padua he published a work on the hyperbola and circle. He became professor of mathematics at St Andrews in 1668, and a year before his death he moved to Edinburgh as professor in mathematics. He was the first of 16 professors in his family.

Gregory, James, the Elder (d 1755) Son of James Gregory (1638–1675) who was mediciner at King's College, Aberdeen in 1725.

Gregory, James (1758–1822) Professor of medicine at Edinburgh who wrote *Conspectus Medicinae Theoreticae* and *Philosophical and Literary Essays*.

Gregory, John (1724–1773) Physician from Aberdeen and son of James Gregory, professor of physick at King's College Aberdeen. He wrote *On the Duties and Offices of the Physician, Elements of Practice of Physic* and *Father's Legacy to his Daughters*.

Greig, David Middleton (1864–1936) Scottish lecturer in clinical surgery at the Medical School of St Andrews. He described hypertelorism as a separate entity in 1924.

Greisofulvin Secondary metabolite of *Penicillium greisofulvum* found by Harold Raistrick (1890–1971), a biochemist in Oxford in 1939. Its effect on fungal hyphae was demonstrated by Grove in 1946 and it was tried successfully on animals. Its first success against fungal infection in humans was recorded by James Clark Gentles at Kings College Hospital, London in 1958. It was marketed in England as Grisovin in 1959.

Gresham College Founded in London in 1575 by Sir Thomas Gresham (1519–1579), the founder of the Royal Exchange. When he died, he left a portion of his property to establish lectures in divinity, astronomy, geometry, civil law and physick. These commenced at Gresham's house in 1597. The founders of the Royal Society used the college as a meeting place in 1645. The buildings were demolished and an excise office was erected at the site in 1768, and the lectures were moved to a room over the Royal Exchange. A new building was erected in Basinghall Street and opened for lectures in 1843.

Grevin, James (1538–1570) French physician and poet who attended Margaret of France, Duchess of Savoy.

Grew, Nehemiah (1641–1712) English physician, born in Atherstone and educated at Cambridge. He practiced medicine in Coventry and London and became a botanist and comparative anatomist. He described the cell structure of plants in 1687, and discovered differences between stem and other tissue. He illustrated the sexes of plants. He wrote: *The Anatomy of Plants* (1682), *Comparative Anatomy of the Stomach and Guts* (1681), *A Catalogue of Rarities Belonging to the Royal Society* and *Cosmologia Sacra*. He extracted the green pigment, chlorophyll, from leaves.

Griesinger, Wilhelm (1817–1868) Born in Stuttgart, he succeeded Moritz Heinrich Romberg (1795–1873) as professor of psychiatry and neurology at the University of Berlin. He was a voluminous writer and produced a textbook of mental diseases before he was 30 years old. He founded the Society of Medical Psychology. The syndrome of pseudohypertrophic infantile muscular dystrophy is named after him.

Griffith Mixture Rose water, ferrous sulfate, potassium carbonate and glucose, for treatment of iron deficiency anemia. Prepared by Philadelphia physician, Robert Eglesfeld Griffith (1798–1850).

Griffith, Frederick (1879–1941) London bacteriologist who differentiated the antigenic types of pyogenic streptococci on the basis of agglutination in 1934.

Grignard, François Auguste Victor (1871–1935) French professor of chemistry at Lyons and Nobel Prize winner in Chemistry in 1912. He discovered a method of synthesizing organometallic compounds (Grignard reaction).

Grijns, Gerrit (1865–1944) Dutch physician who succeeded Christian Eijkman (1858–1930) as director of the Research Institute in Batavia (Java). He advanced work on beriberi started by his predecessor.

Grimaldi, Francesco Maria (1618–1683) Italian physicist at Bologna who discovered diffraction of light. He became professor of mathematics at Bologna in 1648 and postulated the wave theory of light.

Grindall, Richard (1716–1797) Born in Ware, he was an apprentice to Thomas Goodman, surgeon to George II. He became a surgeon at the London Hospital in 1750 and

was the first member of the hospital to receive a court appointment in 1789.

Grissaunt, William English physician, astronomer and mathematician in the 14th century. He was suspected of witchcraft in England and moved to France where he dedicated the rest of his life to the study of medicine. His son became Pope Urban V.

Griswold Splint Formerly used for major fractures of tibia and fibula. Devised by American surgeon, Retig Arnold Griswold (b 1898) of Louisville, in 1934.

Gritti, Rocco (1828–1920) Italian surgeon in Milan who described a method of supracondylar amputation of the femur while retaining the patella, in 1857.

Grocco Triangle The paravertebral triangle, where dullness occurs due to pleural effusion on the opposite side. Named after Italian physician, Pietro Grocco (1856–1916), who described it in 1902.

Groddeck, Georg Walter (1866–1934) German psychiatrist who proposed an emotional role for hysterical conversion symptoms and chronic organic disease. His concept on psychosomatic diseases was preceded by that of Carl Gustav Carus (1789–1868) 50 years earlier.

Gross, Robert Edward (1905–1988) American cardiothoracic surgeon in Boston. He performed the first successful surgical closure of a patent ductus arteriosus in a 7-year-old girl in 1938. With Charles Anthony Hufnagel (1916–1989), he operated on a patient with coarctation in 1945, and demonstrated the success of the procedure by operating on 60 more such patients by 1949. He had some impressive results with his surgical technique for treating atrial septal defect in 1952. A large series of 146 cases of congenital biliary atresia treated by surgery was presented by him in 1953.

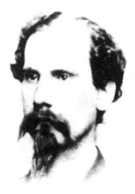

Samuel David Gross (1805–1884). Courtesy of the National Library of Medicine

Gross, Samuel David (1805–1884) American surgeon who was professor of pathological anatomy at Cincinnati Medical School. He wrote on strangulation in 1836, published *Elements of Pathological Anatomy* in 1839, and the first systematic treatise on foreign bodies in the air passages in 1854.

Gross, Samuel Weissel (1837–1889) American surgeon who wrote the first comprehensive treatise on bone sarcoma in 1879.

Grosseteste, Robert Bishop of Lincoln between 1240 and 1244. He made a Latin translation of *Ethics* from Aristotle's (384–322 BC) original Greek text.

Group Therapy Concept started by J.H. Pratt in 1905 with organization of educational meetings to boost the morale of tuberculous patients at the Boston Dispensary. Alfred Adler (1876–1958), around 1919 in Vienna, interviewed children in the presence of their teachers and parents. This method of group therapy was advanced by one of his followers, Rudolph Dreikurs, around 1920. Edward W. Lazell was a pioneer at St Elizabeth's Hospital in Washington in 1919. Family therapy in psychiatry was introduced by John Bell, and counseling and psychotherapy for married couples was started by Clarence Oberndorf in 1934. His initial work went unnoticed until revived by Bela Mittleman in the 1950s.

Grove, Robert (1634–1696) Physician who became Bishop of Chichester. He was the first (and probably the only) bishop of the Church of England to perform vivisection. He demonstrated the effects of the heart from mechanical stimulation. He published his findings in *Carmen de Sanguinis Circuita*.

Grove, Sir William E. Robert (1811–1896) English judge and scientist who devised a new form of voltaic cell that was named after him. He gave an early account of the principle of conservation of energy in *The Correlation of Physical Forces*, published in 1846.

Growth Hormone In 1910 Bernhard Ashner (1883–1960) demonstrated the presence of a substance that influenced growth in the anterior pituitary gland. Herbert McLean Evans (1882–1971) of California showed a growth promoting substance in the pituitary in 1921. American biologist, Joseph Abraham Long (b 1879), identified an active portion of the extract in the same year. Pituitary extracts and implants were shown to restore growth and also sometimes produce gigantism by Phillip Edward Smith (b 1884) of California in 1930. The relationship between acromegaly and an increase in plasma growth hormone levels was demonstrated by Laurence Wilkie Kinsell (1907–1968) in

1948. Choh Hao Li (b 1913) and co-workers obtained a pure extract from anterior pituitary in 1945, but interest in it as a therapeutic agent came only in the 1950s. In 1956 E. Knobil and R. Wolf showed that monkey growth hormone was metabolically active when given to other monkeys. The different properties of extracts from human and beef pituitary were studied by Choh Hao Li and H. Papkoff in 1956. A year later M.S. Raben separated a potent fraction of the hormone from the pituitaries of monkeys and humans. The marked metabolic effects of this on human subjects with hypopituitarism was observed by J.C. Beck in 1957. A year later, Raben reported a marked stimulation of growth in a 17-year-old pituitary dwarf who was treated for 10 months. The Medical Research Council of Britain conducted a short trial in 1959 but their findings were not conclusive. Synthesis was achieved by Choh Hao Li in 1970, and it was genetically engineered in 1985.

Gruber, Max von (1853–1927) Austrian professor of bacteriology. He observed macroscopic agglutination while working with Edward Herbert Durham (1866–1945) on diagnostic reactions of serum from typhoid patients in 1894. *See agglutination.*

Gruber Test A test for hearing using a tuning fork. Devised by Austrian otorhinologist, Joseph Gruber (1827–1900). He was professor at the Clinic for Ear Disease in Vienna in 1873.

Gruber, Wenzel Leopold (1814–1890) Professor of anatomy at St Petersburg. He described several anomalies of muscles.

Gruby, David (1810–1898) Eminent mycologist, the son of a farmer in Hungary. He obtained his medical doctorate in Vienna in 1839 and started a private research laboratory in pathology in Paris in 1841. He published six papers on ringworm and thrush from 1841 to 1844, and proposed the genus *Trypanosoma* after discovering the protozoan in the blood of frogs in 1844. He demonstrated the transmission of microfilaria infection by blood transfusion, developed photomicrography and invented a collapsible hospital tent and a wheeled stretcher. In the later stages of his career he became famous and treated many celebrities. He became eccentric and refused to believe in the germ cause of many diseases, or in vaccination. After his death, 15,000 microscopic preparations and 2000 photomicrographs were found in his possession.

Gruter, Peter (d 1634) Physician from Amsterdam who practiced in Flanders. He wrote *A Century of Latin Letters* in 1609.

Grynfeltt Triangle The superior lumbar triangle through which lumbar hernia occur. Described by a gynecologist in

Montpellier, Joseph Casimir Grynfeltt (1840–1913).

Guaiacum A resin obtained from the tree *Guajacum officinale*, which is indigenous to the West Indies. It has been used for centuries as a treatment for syphilis. The beneficial effects were noted in Europe by Benvenuto Cellini (1500–1570) of Florence, Italy in 1560. The wood was used as a cure for various ailments. The resin was introduced into the *London Pharmacopoeia* in 1677.

Guanethidine A sympathetic ganglion-blocking drug, prepared by Robert Mull in 1959. It was evaluated by Robert Maxwell and introduced as an antihypertensive by Irwin Heinly Page (b 1901) and H.P. Dunstan in America in 1959. It was replaced by safer antihypertensives around 1969.

Guanine [Quechua: *huano*, dung] A purine base originally isolated from the excrement or guano of certain seabirds in 1844.

Guarnieri, Giuseppe (1856–1914) Italian pathologist in Pisa who worked to identify the supposed parasites of variola and vaccinia. The inclusion bodies (Guarnieri bodies) in cells of lesions from these conditions were named after him.

Gubler, Adolphe Marie (1821–1879) *See Millard–Gubler syndrome.*

Gudden, Johannes Bernhard (1824–1886) Neuroanatomist from Munich. He was professor of psychiatry in Zurich in 1869 and described the tract connecting the medial geniculate bodies and inferior corpora quadrigemina of the opposite side in 1870.

Guericke, Otto (1602–1686) The mayor of Magdeburg in Germany and an eminent scientist. He invented an air pump in 1650, the earliest device to generate electrical charges, a weather glass and other ingenious devices. He wrote several treatises on experimental philosophy. His air pump made the study of properties of gases possible.

Guérin, Alphonse François Marie (1817–1895) Professor of surgery at the Hôtel Dieu, Paris who described the terminal portion of the male urethra in 1849.

Guérin, Camille (1872–1961) French bacteriologist who produced the first antituberculous vaccine, Bacille–Calmette–Guérin (BCG). *See* BCG.

Guettard, Jean Etienne (1715–1786) French physician and botanist who showed that some parts of Europe were previously submerged in the sea. He discovered certain mountains in France that were former volcanoes and published his findings in 1752.

Guidi, Guido (1500–1567) Vidianus of Florence was professor of medicine at the University of Pisa. He described the nerve of the pterygoid and its artery and other anatomical structures, some of which bear his name.

Guillain–Barré Syndrome An acute ascending form of demyelinating motor neuropathy, described by French neurologists, Georges Guillain (1876–1971) and Jean Alexander Barré (1880–1967) in 1916.

Guillaume, Charles Edouard (1861–1938) Swiss physicist and Nobel Prize winner in 1920. He produced an alloy of nickel and steel, Invar, which is scarcely affected by temperature change, and was useful in making precision science instruments.

Guillaume, Jacques (1550–1613) Ambroise Paré's pupil, an oculist and an obstetrician. He recommended podalic version and practiced Cesarean section in a dead mother to save the child. His *L'Heureux Accouchment des Femmes* was published in 1609. He also wrote the first French book on ophthalmology, *Traites des Maladies de l'oeil*, in 1585.

Guillemin, Roger Charles Louis (b 1924) French physiologist who graduated in medicine from Lyons in 1949. He was appointed to the chair of physiology at the Baylor School of Medicine, Houston in 1963. He identified the structure of thyrotropin releasing hormone and growth hormone releasing hormone, for which he shared the Nobel Prize with Andrew Victor Schally (b 1926) in 1977.

Guillotine, Joseph Ignace (1738–1814) Physician in Paris who proposed a machine for quick and painless execution by decapitation in 1789. In 1791 a law was passed that everyone condemned to death should be decapitated, and his machine was adopted. *See capital punishment.*

Guinea Worm *See Dracunculus medinensis.*

Guinon, Georges (1859–1929) French physician in Paris who described Gilles de la Tourette syndrome in 1886. The first description was given by Gilles de la Tourette in 1885.

Guldberg, Maximillian (1836–1902) Norwegian chemist from Oslo who proposed the law of mass action in 1865 relating to the speed of a reaction and the concentration of reactants.

Gull, Sir William Withey (1860–1890) Physician at Guy's Hospital, London who described the cretinoid state in the adult (Gull disease) or myxedema (in a woman). He gave a clear description of arteriosclerotic atrophy of the kidney, with Henry Gawen Sutton (1837–1891).

Gullstrand, Alvar (1862–1930) Swedish professor of ophthalmology, born in Landskrona and graduated in medicine from Uppsala in 1888. He obtained his PhD on astigmatism in 1890, and was appointed director of the Stockholm Eye Clinic in 1892. In 1903 he invented the slit lamp which made microscopic study of the living eye possible. The Nobel Prize for Physiology or Medicine was awarded to him in 1911.

Gunde-Shapur *See Jundeshapur.*

Gunn, Robert Marcus (1850–1909) London ophthalmologist who described unilateral ptosis of the eyelid and exaggerated opening of the eye related to jaw movements (jaw-winking phenomenon, or Gunn syndrome) in 1883. The white dots seen in the fundus of the eye in the region of the macula are named after him.

Gunning Splint Used for fracture of the mandible. Devised by American dentist, Thomas Brian Gunning (1813–1889), in 1867.

Gunn Ligament Y-shaped iliofemoral ligament of the hip joint. Described by American surgeon, Moses Gunn (1822–1887) in 1853. Henry Jacob Bigelow (1816–1890) described it in 1869.

Gunshot Wounds The first authors on the subject were Pfolsprudnt (1460), Hieronymus Brunschwygk (b 1452), whose *Buch der Chirirgia* was published in 1497, and Hans von Gersdorf, who published *Feldbuch der Wundarsney* in 1517. Study and treatment remained in the domain of army surgeons, and Ambroise Paré and Dominique Jean Larrey (1766–1842) were two of the most famous army surgeons to write on the subject. Treatment for gunshot wounds up to the 16th century was to pour boiling oil on them. An early work by Antonio Ferri in 1514 advised chopping off the limb with a hatchet followed by application of red-hot iron to the stump. Paré used conservative measures such as dressings and ligatures. *Fifty Strange and Wonderful Cures of Gunshot Wounds* was published by Mattheus Gottfried Purmann (1649–1711), a surgeon in the Brandenburg army in 1693. Thomas Gale (1507–1587), a surgeon to the army of Henry VIII in 1544, was the first Englishman to write on injuries caused by gunpowder projectiles. *A Treatise on Blood, Inflammation, and Gunshot Wounds* was published by John Hunter (1728–1793).

Gunz, Justus Gottfried (1714–1755) Professor of anatomy at Leipzig who discovered the anastomosis between the epigastric and the mammary arteries in 1734.

Gurlt, Ernest Julius (1825–1899) German professor of surgery in Berlin and a medical historian who wrote *Geschichte der Chirurgie* in 1898, one of the best works on the history of surgery.

Gurney, Sir Goldsworthy (1793–1895) Born in Treator, near Padstow in Cornwall, he practiced as a surgeon at Wadebridge before moving to London in 1820. He invented an oxyhydrogen blowpipe, a powerful light from lime and magnesium known as Drummond's light, a steam jet, and the Gurney stove. He introduced lighting to the House of Commons and designed its ventilatory system in 1852. He made the journey by steam locomotive, at a speed of 15 miles per hour, from London to Bath in 1829.

Gussenbauer, Carl (1842–1903) German surgeon at Liège and Prague and an assistant of Theodor Billroth (1829–1894). He devised an internal metal splint (Gussenbauer clamp) for approximating the bones in an ununited fracture. He also demonstrated a method of excision of the pylorus (with Alexander Winiwarter) in 1876. He gave a description of the first removal of a tumor in the bladder (performed by Billroth) in 1875.

Gusserow, Adolf Ludwig Sigismund (1836–1906) German obstetrician who described pernicious anemia in pregnancy in 1871.

Gutenberg, Johannes Gensfleisch (1397–1468) Born in Mainz, he was a pioneer of movable-type printing in Europe. He worked in Strasburg in partnership with a moneylender and printer, John Fust, in 1450. Together they printed the famous Latin Bible in 1456, but after a legal battle they split up. Gutenberg established another press in 1463 and the knowledge and art of printing spread through Europe. *See printing.*

Guthrie, George James (1785–1856) London surgeon who worked in America and in the Peninsular War, and is considered an outstanding military surgeon. He founded the Royal Westminster Ophthalmic Hospital in 1816 and was appointed surgeon to the Westminster Hospital in 1827. He wrote: *On Gunshot Wounds of the Extremities* (1816), *On the Anatomy and Diseases of the Neck of the Bladder* (1834), *The Operative Surgery of the Eye* (1823) and other treatises.

Guthrie, Samuel (1782–1848) American physician from Bloomfield, Massachusetts, who studied at the College of Surgeons and Physicians, New York. After serving in the Army Medical Corps, he practiced in Sacketts Harbor, New York. In 1831 he discovered a method of making chloroform by distilling chloride of lime with alcohol in a copper container.

Gutta Serena A term used by Actuarius to denote amaurosis or a kind of blindness. *See amaurosis.*

Guttmann Sign A bruit heard over the thyroid in hyperthyroidism. Described by German physician, P. Guttmann (1834–1893).

Guttmann, Sir Ludwig (1899–1980) Director of neurology at the Jewish Hospital in Breslau from 1933 to 1939. He emigrated to England and became a research assistant to the Department of Surgery at Oxford. Guttmann established the Stoke Mandeville Hospital in Buckinghamshire in 1944 for treating spinal injuries.

Guy, Thomas (1644–1724) The founder of Guy's Hospital. He was the son of a coal-dealer from Horsleydown, Southwark and a bookseller but made most of his fortune by selling seaman's tickets during Queen Anne's wars. Besides Guy's Hospital, he also erected an almshouse at Tamworth. *See Guy's Hospital.*

Guy, William (1859–1950) Physician from Kent and pioneer of modern dentistry in Britain. He was a founder of the dental school at Edinburgh, and he helped to regulate the practice of dentistry in Britain.

Guy, William Augustus (1810–1885) Born in Chichester, in 1831 he won the Fothergillian Medal for an essay on asthma. He was professor of forensic medicine at Kings College in 1838, and wrote *Principles of Forensic Medicine* in 1844. Another interest was statistics, and he was secretary of the Statistical Society from 1843 to 1868. He edited the *Journal of the Statistical Society* and *Hooper's Vade Mecum.*

Guy's Hospital Founded in 1721 by Thomas Guy (1644–1722), a bookseller from Southwark. The hospital building was commenced in the grounds of St Thomas' premises at the south end of London Bridge in 1707. The present hospital in Southwark was completed after the death of Guy, with funds left by him.

Guynon, Edme Gilles (1706–1786) French scientist and postmaster at Versailles who made the first attempt at catheterization of the Eustachian tube via the oral route in 1724.

Guynon, Jean Casimir Felix (1831–1920) Professor of surgical pathology at Paris. He described the internal os of the uterus and the canal formed by its prolongation, in 1858.

Guyot, Arnold (1807–1884) American geologist of Swiss origin. He emigrated to America in 1848, and was professor of geology at Princeton in 1854. He published *Earth and Man* in 1849.

Gwathmey, James Taylor (1865–1944) Anesthetist in New York. He introduced a new technique for rectal anesthesia using a mixture of ether and olive oil in 1913. This method overcame the problem of celitis caused by ether.

Gwine, Matthew (d 1627) Physician of Welsh descent, born in London. He graduated from Oxford. He became professor of physick at Gresham College, and was physician to the Tower of London in 1605. His works include: *Orations, Letters on Chemical and Magical Secrets,* and a comedy, *Vertumnus,* performed before the King.

Gye, William Ewart (1884–1952) British pathologist and director of the Imperial Cancer Research Fund Laboratories. He advanced the theory that an ultramicroscopic virus combined with an intrinsic chemical factor contributed to development of Rous sarcoma.

Gymnasium [Greek: *gymbos,* naked] Place where ancient Greeks performed public exercises, and philosophers and poets repeated their compositions. Frederick Ludwig Jahn (1778–1852), a physical educationist from Prussia, the father of modern gymnastics, founded the first modern gymnasium in Berlin in 1811. A further revival was brought about by a Swede, Per Henrick Ling (1776–1839), who established an institute for training teachers in gymnastics at Stockholm in 1813.

Gymnastics *See gymnasium.*

Gynandromorph [Greek: *gyne,* woman + *andros,* man + *morphe,* form] An individual containing both male and female genetic elements. Described and named by R. Goldschmidt in 1915.

Gynecology [Greek: *gyne* or *gyne,* woman + *logos,* discourse] Soranus of Ephesus (AD 98–138), who practiced in Alexandria and later in Rome during the reign of Hadrian and Trajan, is regarded as the founder of obstetrics and gynecology. His *De Morbis Mulierium* remained a standard work for 15 centuries. It became a specialty only in the 18th century. Previously, many surgeons dealt with the gynecological problems. Ambroise Paré (1510–1590), the celebrated French surgeon of the Renaissance, attempted to treat vesico-vaginal fistula, and wrote treatises related to gynecology. Caspar Bauhin (1560–1624), professor of anatomy and medicine at Basel, also wrote important treatises. Various structures of the female genital tract, such as the oviducts or Fallopian tubes (discovered by Gabriele Falloppio in 1561), Graafian follicles (discovered by Regnier de Graaf in 1672), and the vulvovaginal glands (discovered by Caspar Bartholin in 1677) were described during this period. The first ovariotomy was performed at Danville,

Kentucky by Ephraim McDowell (1771–1830) of Virginia in 1809. The procedure was introduced into England by Charles Clay (1801–1893) of Manchester and Sir Thomas Spencer Wells (1818–1897). James Marion Sims (1813–1883) of South Carolina was one of the first to establish gynecology as a specialty, around 1840. He pioneered surgery in treatment of vesico-vaginal fistula, and designed the first vaginal speculum. His device developed into the Sims duck-billed speculum. The Women's Hospital in New York was founded by Sims in 1853, and the uterine sound was invented by him in 1843. Myomectomy as treatment for fibroids of the uterus was performed by Washington Lemuel Atlee (1808–1878) in 1844. Uterine myoma was surgically removed by Italian surgeon, Augosto Granville Bozzi (1782–1872), in 1827, but without success. Successful abdominal hysterectomy was performed by American surgeon, Walter Burnham (1808–1883) in 1853, and another American surgeon, Gilman Kimball (1804–1892), performed the second in 1855. Wells performed his first hysterectomy for myoma in 1861. An early American classic, *A Practical Treatise on the Diseases of Women*, was published by Theodore Thomas Gaillard (1832–1903) of Edisto island South Carolina in 1868, who was the first to perform vaginal ovariotomy in 1870. A radical form of hysterectomy for carcinoma was performed by an American gynecologist, John Goodrich Clark (1867–1927) of Indiana in 1895. Abdominal hysterectomy was introduced as treatment of cancer by German surgeon, Wilhelm Alexander Freund (1833–1918) in 1913. The Wertheim radical pan-hysterectomy for cervical cancer was devised by an Austrian gynecologist, Ernest Wertheim (1864–1920) in 1898. Enucleation of uterine fibroids by a vaginal route was devised by Vincenz Czerny (1842–1915), professor of surgery at Freiburg, in 1881. Recognition of the role of hormonal factors in the female reproductive cycle by Eugene Steinach (1861–1944) in 1911, Edgar Allen (1892–1943) and Edward Adelbert Doisy (b 1893) in 1923, Bernhard Zondek (b 1891) in 1927, and Adolf Friedrich Johann Butenandt (b 1903) in 1929, led to better understanding and treatment. Study of exfoliative cytology related to normal cyclical changes of the vaginal epithelium by Nicholas George Papanicolau (1883–1962) in 1917 led to mass screening for cervical cancer.

Gynecomastia Paul of Aegina (625–690) described a condition in which males underwent a feminization, concentrated on the breast. He advised amputation of the breast and cautery as treatment. Anterior pituitary-like hormones and estrin were shown to produce gynecomastia by Baltimore pathologist, Charles Freeborn Geschickter (b 1901) in 1934. Its association with testicular

tumors was demonstrated by Bennet Judson Gilbert (b 1898) in 1940.

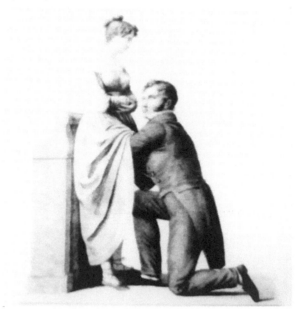

How to conduct a vaginal examination. P. Maygrier, *Nouvelles Demonstrations d' Acchouchement,* (1822). Bechet, Paris.

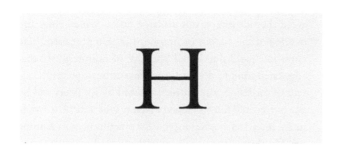

H Antigen Proteus bacillus in normal flagellated form grows as a thin spreading film on nutrient agar, resembling mist produced by breathing on glass. The antigen of this bacillus was named 'H' denoting the 'breatH' form, by Edmund Weil (1880–1922) and Arthur Felix (1887–1956) in 1917.

H Substance Similar to histamine, causes anaphylaxis symptom complex. Demonstrated by Sir Thomas Lewis (1881–1945) and Ronald Thompson Grant (1892–1989) in 1924 in their paper, *Vascular Reactions of the Skin to Injury*.

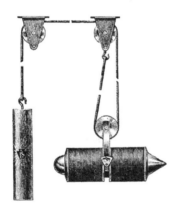

Haab's magnet. L.W. Fox, *Diseases of the Eye* (1904). Appleton and Co, New York

Haab, Otto (1850–1931) Swiss ophthalmologist who described a method of extracting foreign metal particles from the eye with the use of a magnet. He published a series of atlases on ophthalmoscopy.

Habena Surgical restraining bandage used to bring the edges of a wound together without stitching. A frenum or restricting fibrous bandage.

Haberling, Wilhelm Gustav Moritz (1871–1940) German medical historian who prepared a second edition of Ernst Gurlt's (1825–1899) *Biographisches Lexicon* in 1929. He also wrote a history of German medicine.

Habicot, Nicholas (d 1624) French Surgeon who wrote a treatise on plague in the 16th century.

Hacker, Viktor von (1852–1933) Surgeon in Vienna who devised an operation for hypospadias. He described a method for gastrostomy in 1886.

Haden, Russel Landram (1888–1952) Physician and hematologist from Kansas City who described an acid hematin method for estimating hemoglobin. The peculiar target cell, with a bull's eye appearance. The cell anemias were first observed by Haden and F.D. Evans in 1937. These cells were named target cells by A.M. Barrett in 1938.

Hadra, Berthhold Ernest (1842–1903) Orthopedic surgeon from Germany who emigrated to Texas. He performed the first spinal fusion using a silver wire to fix the 6th and 7th cervical vertebrae in 1891.

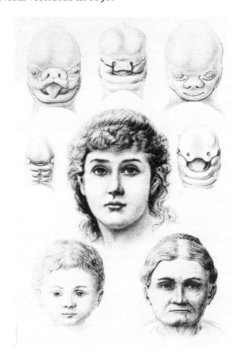

Development of the face. Ernst Haeckel, *The Evolution of Man* (1903). Watts and Co., London

Haeckel, Ernst (1834–1919) Regarded as the founder of modern morphology. Born in Potsdam, and studied medicine at Würzberg, Berlin and Vienna. He quit medicine to become professor of zoology at Jena in 1862, and published *General Morphology* in 1866. His other publications include *Natural History of Creation* (1868), and *Anthropogeny or the Evolution of Man* (1874) on human embryology. The terms 'ontogeny', 'phylogeny' and 'ecology' were coined by him. His Phyletic Museum in Jena contains the most illustrative collection of evolution and development in the world. Haeckel introduced Darwinism into Germany.

Haen, Anton de (1704–1776) Physician who perfected clinical teaching. Born in the Hague and studied under Herman Boerhaave (1668–1738). He became professor of medicine at Vienna in 1756. His *Ratio medendi* (1758–1779), a series of 15 volumes, contained comprehensive case reports and autopsy findings.

Haesser, Heinrich (1811–1885) German physician who wrote an important work on history of medicine: *Lehrbuch der Geschichte der Medicin und der Epidemischen Krankheiten*.

Haffkine, Waldemar Mordecai Wolfe (1860–1930) Pioneer in vaccination against cholera (*Vibrio cholerae*). Pupil of Metchinikoff (1845–1916), born in Odessa, Russia. Between 1889 and 1893 he worked as assistant to Louis Pasteur (1822–1895). He inoculated himself with heat-killed cultures of virulent strains of cholera during his research in 1892, and traveled to India in 1893, where he inoculated nearly 40,000 persons over a period of 29 months. He became a naturalized British citizen in 1899. *See Mulkowal Disaster.*

Hagedorn, Hans Christian (1888–1971) Danish physician at the Steno Memorial Hospital in Copenhagen who started the first large-scale manufacture of insulin (with August Schack Krogh) by establishing the non-profit Nordisk Insulin Laboratory in 1922. *See Insulin.*

Hagedorn, Werner (1831–1894) Surgeon at Magdeburg who pioneered surgical repair of unilateral cleft lip. He devised a curved and flattened surgical suture needle (Hagedorn needle).

Hageman Factor Factor XII. Named after a patient who was a train driver and who had a prolonged clotting time but with no bleeding manifestations.

Hagner, Francis Randall (1873–1940) American urologist from Washington who designed an inflatable rubber bag which could be placed in the urethra to arrest bleeding during prostatectomy. He also devised an operation for acute epididymitis (Hagner operation) which involved making multiple punctures to pockets of pus in the epididymis following incision of the tunica vaginalis testis.

Hahn, Eugene (1841–1902) German surgeon from Berlin who devised an operation for movable kidney in 1881 and a modified cannula with a sponge for use in endotracheal anesthesia.

Hahnemann, Samuel Christian Friedrich (1755–1843) Founder of homeopathy. Born at Meissen in Germany and studied medicine in Leipzig and Vienna, before he obtained his medical degree from Erlangen in 1779. He wanted to avoid the side effects due to large doses of medicines and developed the system of homeopathy. He postulated 'like cures like', and developed 'the law of infinitesimals' that advocated minute doses of medicine as treatment. His system of medicine was strongly resisted by his peers and he was persecuted for his views between 1798 and 1810. Eventually his system was adopted by practitioners in Europe and North America and he was elected as honorary member of the Medical Society of the County of New York in 1832, and settled in Paris in 1835. The Hahnemann Hospital at Bloomsbury Square, London, opened in 1850.

Haig Fergusson Forceps These have a pelvic and cephalic curve and axis traction handle fitting on to the handles of the blades. They were designed by a Scottish obstetrician, James Haig Fergusson (1862–1934) of Edinburgh.

Hailey–Hailey Disease Familial benign chronic pemphigus. Described by two dermatologists from Atlanta, Georgia, William Howard Hailey (1898–1967) and Hugh Edward Hailey (b 1909) in 1939.

Hair [Anglo-Saxon: *haer*, hair] Hippocrates (460–377 BC) believed that the shape of the body revealed the personality, and Aristotle (384–322 BC) studied the nose, limbs, hair and other parts of the body to characterize people. Paul of Aegina (AD 625–690) recommended fig leaves to stimulate hair growth in skin or scalp affected by burns. One of the earliest classification of human races according to the nature of hair was published by Franz Pruner-Bey (1808–1882) of Paris in 1865. The inner layer of the root sheath of the hair follicle (Huxley Layer) in human hair was discovered by Thomas Henry Huxley (1825–1895) while a medical student at Charing Cross Hospital, London. *See depilatories, dyeing of hair.*

Haldane, John Burdon Sanderson (1892–1964) Son of Scottish physiologist, John Scott Haldane (1860–1936) and sister of Naomi Mitchison. Professor of genetics and biochemistry at the University of London. He described the heat cramps caused by excessive salt loss in hot surroundings amongst mine workers, in 1925. He also researched underwater respiratory physiology and submarine safety during World War ll. He was a committed Marxist but left the communist party in 1956 and emigrated to India in 1957. A biography, *Portrait of Haldane,* was written by Eric Ashby (1904–1992), a botanist, in 1974.

Haldane, John Scott (1860–1936) Eminent Scottish respiratory physiologist, father of John B.S. Haldane, educated at the Universities of Edinburgh and Jena, and Fellow of New College, Oxford. He investigated deaths in a colliery explosion in South Wales in 1896, concluding that the 52 men who died succumbed to carbon monoxide poisoning. It was mainly though his work that the physiological mechanism and toxic effects of carbon monoxide were made known towards the end of the 19th century. He also described silicosis, gas warfare, submarine living, hookworm infection causing anemia in miners, and popularized the use of oxygen therapy during World War l. He examined blood gases and produced his first respiratory gas analyzer in 1898. He also discovered the role of ferricyanide in releasing oxygen from oxyhemoglobin. His work culminated in his book, *Respiration*, published in 1922.

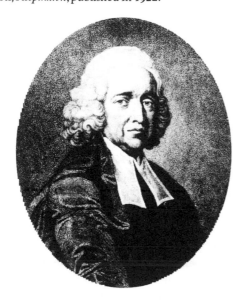

Stephen Hales (1677–1761). Courtesy of the National Library of Medicine

Hales, Stephen (1677–1761) Clergyman and experimental physiologist. Born near Canterbury and educated at Corpus Christi College, Cambridge. He became perpetual curate of Teddington, Middlesex in 1709. He was the first person to measure blood pressure by inserting a copper tube into the femoral artery of a horse, and observing the rise of the blood in a glass tube. He published his findings on circulation and blood pressure in his treatise, *Haemastaticks,* in 1733. His work on plant physiology, *Vegetable Staticks,* was to provide the foundation for this subject. He was elected FRS in 1718 and Member of the French Academy in 1753 and there is a monument to him in Westminster Abbey.

Halford, Sir Henry (1766–1844) Graduated from Oxford and was appointed physician to the Middlesex Hospital in 1793. In the same year he became physician extraordinary to George III and continued in his post as royal physician up to the time of Queen Victoria.

Hall, Granville Stanley (1844–1924) American pioneer in child psychology at Clark University. He founded the journal, *Pedagogical Seminary,* in 1891 for publication of studies on children.

Hall, John (1575–1635) Bedfordshire physician and William Shakespeare's son-in-law. He graduated from Cambridge and took his MA in 1597 before studying at Montpellier in France. He returned in 1600 to start a medical practice at Stratford-upon-Avon and married Shakespeare's daughter, Susanna, in 1607. His gravestone is placed next to Shakespeare's at Stratford-upon-Avon.

Hall, Marshall (1790–1857) British neurophysiologist, born in Basford, Nottinghamshire, and obtained his MD from Edinburgh University in 1812. He returned to Nottingham in 1817, and was appointed physician to the General Hospital in 1825. Hall made the first clear distinction between capillaries and arterioles in 1831. He also pioneered studies on artificial respiration and developed his own method of artificial respiration in 1855. He is mostly known for his work on the nervous system and reflex activity of the medulla and spinal cord.

Hall, Maurice Crowther (1881–1939) *See antihelmintics.*

Hall Sign Diastolic shock transmitted to the trachea due to aortic aneurysm in the thorax was described by the American physician, Josiah Newhall Hall (1859–1939) of Colorado.

Hallé, Jean Noel (1754–1822) French physiologist, natural philosopher and chair of the hygiene committee of the Royal Academy of Medicine. He succeeded Jean-Nicholas Corvisart (1755–1821) in Paris.

Halle, John (1529–1568) Distinguished surgeon from Maidstone who published an edition of Lanfranc's (d. *c* 1315) *Chirugia Magna* in 1565.

Haller, Albrecht von (1708–1777) Eminent Swiss anatomist, physiologist, botanist and poet. After his studies at Tübingen he became a student of Herman Boerhaave (1668–1738) at Leiden and obtained his medical degree in 1727. He was appointed the first professor of anatomy, surgery and botany at the University of Göttingen in 1736, and made it one of the finest institutes in Europe. He described several anatomical structures, particularly related to mechanical automatism of heart muscle function. He wrote voluminously on anatomy, physiology, botany and other subjects. His most important medical works were: *Primae Lineae Physiologiae* and *Elementa Physiologiae Corporis Humanae* (eight volumes).

Hallervorden, Julius (1882–1965) Director of Kaiser Wilhelm Institute of Psychiatry at Berlin. He exploited the euthanasia program of the Nazis to collect the brains of victims for his neuropathological research. He described a congenital neurological condition known as Hallervorden–Spatz disease, with Hugo Spatz (1888–1969).

Halley, Edmond (1656–1742) English astronomer and mathematician, born in Shoreditch. He succeeded John Flamsteed (1646–1719), becoming the second Astronomer Royal in 1720. His *Breslau Tables of Mortality*, published in 1693, was an important early contribution to the field of vital statistics and became the foundation for life insurance and annuities. He was the first to detect the acceleration of the moon's mean motion. He also studied the parabolic orbits ascribed to the comets by Sir Isaac Newton (1642–1727), and applied it to a comet (Halley's Comet) which he observed in 1682.

Halliburton, William Dobinson (1860–1931) Professor of physiology at King's College, London and pioneer of biochemistry in England. He wrote *The Essentials of Chemical Physiology* in 1892. Halliburton was also the first to study the chemical composition of cerebrospinal fluid.

Halliday, Sir Andrew (1781–1839) Graduated in medicine from Edinburgh and was physician to William IV. He published several works on travel and politics. His medical works include two treatises on emphysema and on the state of lunatic asylums.

Hallipeau, François Henri (1842–1919) French dermatologist who described a variant of Neumann pemphigus vegetans (Hallipeau disease) in 1889, among many other conditions. His thesis was on diseases of the spinal cord and he later published on diffuse myelitis and bulbar palsy. He became interested in dermatology in his 40s and published *Practical Treatise on Dermatology* in 1900.

Hallucination [Latin: *alucinor,* to wander in mind] One of the first treatises on the subject of delusions, hallucinations and illusions was written by Ludwig Lavator (1527–1586) in 1570. A description of the condition was given by William Perkins (1558–1602), a theologian at Christ's College, Cambridge in his work *A discourse of the damned art of the witchcraft.* Although he attributed the condition to the devil, his statement of the symptoms was accurate: 'An illusion of the outward senses, is awoke of the devil, where he makes the man to thinke that he heareth, seeth, feeleth, or toucheth such things as indeede he doth not'. A complete clinical description of hallucinations was given by Jean Etienne Dominique Esquirol (1772–1840) in 1838.

Hallucinations were thought for a long time to be a sign of insanity until Alexandre J.F. Brierre de Boismont (1798–1881) attempted to treat them with drugs, baths and psychotherapy.

Hallucinogen [Latin: *alucinor,* to wander in mind; Greek: *gen,* producing] The hallucinogenic effects of lysergic acid, an active ingredient of *Psilocybe* fungus was accidentally discovered by the Swiss chemist A. Hoffmann in 1943 when he sniffed the substance in the laboratory and experienced the effects. Robert Hooke (1635–1703) described the hallucinogenic properties of *Cannabis sativa,* called 'bangue' by the Portuguese and 'gange' by the Moors, in 1689. Another hallucinogenic compound, mescaline, is obtained from Mexican peyote cactus (*Lophophora williamsii*) and distilled liquor from agave (*Agave americana*) while ancient Mexican sculptures show mushroom worship and their knowledge of hallucinogenic properties. A description of the effects was given by an American neurologist, Silas Weir Mitchell (1829–1914) in 1896. *See LSD-25.*

Halothane [Greek: *hals,* salt; French: *méthyle,* black formation] Fluorinated hydrocarbon, first synthesized by C.W. Suckling of Imperial Chemical Industries in 1956. In the same year, J. Raventos used the compound to induce anesthesia in animals. Abnormality of cardiac rhythm and hypotension induced by halothane was demonstrated independently by Michael William Johnston and Raventos, later in the same year. The compound came to be accepted as a regular anesthetic in the early 1960s. Secondary drug sensitivity of halothane in anesthesia was recognized as the cause of hepatotoxicity by C. Trey and co-workers in 1968.

Halstead, William Stewart (1852–1922) Foundation professor of surgery at the Johns Hopkins Medical School. In 1892 he performed the first successful ligation of the subclavian artery in America; pioneered circular sutures for intestines in 1887; devised an operation for radical cure of inguinal hernia in 1889; introduced the use of rubber gloves in surgery in 1894; used cocaine for local anesthesia in 1885; and did experimental transplantation of parathyroid glands in animals, published in 1909. During his meticulous experiments on cocaine, he self-experimented and became addicted but overcame his habit, and returned to the practice of surgery.

Haly Abbas (AD 930–944) Also known as Ali ibn al Abbas, a native of Ahwaz in southwest Persia who became a famous physician 50 years after Rhazes (850–932). His principal work *Kamil al-sina'a al-tibbiya* (or *Libri Pantechni*) contained 400,000 words and was divided into 20 tracts of which the first ten dealt with theory of medicine, and the second ten with its practice. The first three chapters of the first tract contains discussions on the writings of other physicians. *Kamil* remained as a standard of medicine until it was replaced by *Canon of Medicine* of Avicenna (AD 980–1037).

Ham Test Demonstrates hemolysis of red cells after their incubation with acidified serum. It is used in diagnosis of paroxysmal nocturnal hemoglobinuria and was devised by American physicians, G. C. Ham and H. M. Horack in 1941.

Hamilton, Alice (1869–1970) First female professor at Harvard Medical School (1919) and a pioneer of occupational medicine in America. She wrote a treatise on lead poisoning in 1910 and *Industrial Poisons in the United States* and *Industrial Toxicology* in 1934.

Hamilton, Frank Hastings (1813–1886) Born in Wilmington, Vermont, he was a pioneer in plastic and orthopedic surgery in America. He served as an army physician before he became professor of surgery at Bellevue Hospital. He practiced skin grafting for ulcers in 1854, and published *Deformities after Fractures* in 1855 and an important treatise on fractures and dislocations in 1860.

Hamman Disease Spontaneous mediastinal emphysema. Described by Baltimore surgeon, Louis Virgil Hamman (1877–1946).

Hamman Sign Crunching systolic sound noted over sternal edge in mediastinal emphysema. Described by Baltimore surgeon, Louis Virgil Hamman (1877–1946).

Hamman–Rich Syndrome Syndrome of diffuse interstitial pulmonary fibrosis leading to dyspnoea and clubbing was reported by an American physician, Louis Virgil Hamman (1877–1946) of Baltimore, and American pathologist, Arnold R. Rich (1893–1968) of Alabama, at the Johns Hopkins Hospital in 1944. The first description of the condition in England was given by A. G. Heppleston in 1951. A survey of all previous publications on the disease with additional cases was published by E. H. Rubin and R. Lubliner in 1957.

Hammarsten, Olof (1841–1932) *See blood coagulation.*

Hammer, Adam (1818–1878) Born in Mingalsheim, Baden and graduated in medicine from Heidelberg in 1842. He emigrated to America in 1848 and became professor of surgery at St Louis. He was one of the reformers of medical education in America and started the Humboldt Institute for teaching medicine in German. *See coronary artery disease.*

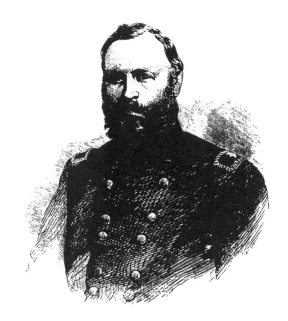

William Alexander Hammond (1828–1900)

Hammond, William Alexander (1828–1900) Surgeon General in the United States Army. In 1857 he produced a report, *Experimental Researches Relative to the Nutritive Value and Physiological Effects of Albumin, Starch, and Gum When Singly and Exclusively Used as Foods,* for which he received a prize from the American Medical Academy. He wrote *Physiological Memoirs* in 1863, a collection of essays on physiological and clinical subjects. He was court-marshaled in 1864 but later reinstated. He also wrote the first monograph in America on neurology, *Diseases of the Nervous System,* in 1871, in which he described athetosis (Hammond disease). He was a founder of the American and New York Neurological Societies.

Hammurabi (1945–1905 BC) King of Babylon who is referred to in the Bible as a contemporary of Abraham. His law code was inscribed on a huge stone monument excavated at Susa by French archaeologist, J. de Morgan in 1897. These cuneiform inscriptions contained a code of conduct for all walks of life and were translated by R. F. Harper of Chicago in 1904. They include rules and regulations for the practice of physicians, set fees for their practice, and prescribed punishment for their failure, e.g.: 'If a man destroy the eye of another man, they shall destroy his eye'.

Hamusco, Johannes Valverdus de (b c 1550) Spanish medical writer in the 16th century who traveled to Scotland. He wrote a book on preservation of health entitled *De animi et corporis sanitate ad Hieronumum Verallum Cardinalem.*

Hancock, Henry (1809–1880) *See appendicitis.*

Hand–Schüller–Christian Disease Condition characterized by a triad of defects in membranous bone, exophthalmos and polyuria. First described by American pediatrician, Alfred Hand (1868–1949) in 1893. Arthur Schüller (1874–1957), a Viennese radiologist, described a further two cases in 1915. A more detail account of this syndrome was given by American physician, Henry Asbury Christian (1876–1951) from Virginia in 1919.

Hand A classic treatise entitled *The Hand its Mechanisms and Vital Endowments,* one of the Bridgewater treatises, was written by the Scottish neurologist Sir Charles Bell (1774–1842). The first comprehensive treatise on hand surgery was published by Allen Buckner Kanavel (1874–1938) in 1912, and it was established as a specialty by Sterling Bunnell (1882–1957) of America who published *Surgery of the Hand* in 1944. In 1963 the Chinese became the first to successfully reimplant a completely severed hand.

Handley, William Sampson (1872–1962) Hunterian professor of surgery at the Royal College of Surgeons and surgeon to the Samaritan Free Hospital for Women. He was a pioneer in surgery for cancer of the breast and wrote *Cancer of the Breast and its Operative Treatment* in 1906.

Hanger, Franklin McCue, Jr (1894–1971) New York physician who devised the cephalin–cholesterol flocculation test for liver function in 1938.

Hanging Said to have been used for the first time in 1241, in England, on William Marise, a nobleman's son during the reign of King Henry III. A classic treatise on the differentiation between murder and suicide due to hanging was published by Antoine Louis (1723–1792) of Paris in 1763. *See capital punishment.*

Hanot, Victor Charles (1844–1896) French physician who described the condition of cholangiolytic biliary cirrhosis (Hanot disease) in 1875. He concentrated on disease of the liver and published on clinical pathological aspects, from hemochromatosis to hepatic malignancy.

Hanover, Adolph (1814–1894) A pupil of Johannes Müller (1801–1858) in Berlin. His work *On the Anatomy, Physiology and Pathology of the* Eye, in Danish, was published in 1846. Hanover also wrote extensively on helminthology.

Hansen Bacillus *Mycobacterium leprae*, causative organism of leprosy, was discovered in 1873 by Norwegian bacteriologist, Gerhard Henrik Armauer Hansen (1841–1912). Aniline dyes were first used to stain the bacillus by Albert Neisser (1855–1916) in 1879. Hansen devoted his life to the etiology, epidemiology, prevention and management of leprosy.

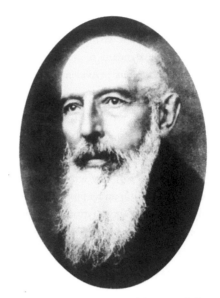

Gerhard Hansen (1841–1912). Courtesy of the National Library of Medicine

Haploid [Greek: *haplos*, simple + *eidos*, appearance] The number of chromosomes in gametic cells (i.e. sperm and ova). Discovered by the Belgian cytologist, Edouard Louis-Hane van Beneden (1846–1910) in 1883.

Harden, Sir Arthur (1865–1940) English physical chemist, born in Manchester, UK, and became head of biochemistry at the Jenner (later Lister) Institute from 1897. He made several discoveries on fermentation of sugars by bacteria. The phosphorylation of sugar, the first step in fermentation, was discovered by him in 1905, and he also isolated glucose-6-phosphate and fructose-6-phosphate, key intermediates in sugar metabolism. He published *Alcoholic Fermentation* in 1911, and shared the Nobel Prize for Chemistry with Hans von Euler-Chelpin (1873–1964) in 1929.

Harder, Johann Jacob (1656–1711) Professor of anatomy and botany at Basel who described the accessory lachrymal gland in the orbit in 1694. He wrote *Prodomus Physiologicus* and several other medical works.

Hardy, Louis Phillipe Alfred (1811–1893) Physician in Paris who described the sign where aphonia occurred in early stages of gangrene of the lung.

Hardy, William Bate (1864-1934) Demonstrated that fixatives used in cytology affect the appearance of the cytoplasm in microscopy. *See isoelectric point.*

Hare, Edward Selleck (1812–1838) English surgeon at Stafford who gave an early description of signs due to a cervical sympathetic lesion (Horner syndrome) in 1838.

Hare Lip Treatment of the condition by freshened edges and special sutures was described by Flemish surgeon,

Jan Yperman (1295–1351). Ambroise Paré (1510–1590) of France practiced surgery for hare lip during the Renaissance period. Hendrik van Roonhuyze (b 1625) also operatively treated the condition in Holland. The pioneers in surgical correction of hare lip were Samuel Sharp (1700–1778) of Guy's Hospital, London and Benjamin Bell (1763–1820) of Edinburgh, and Lorenz Heister (1683–1758) of Germany. The Scottish surgeon, Sir William Fergusson (1808–1877), is said to have performed over 400 operations for hare lip.

Harley, George (1829–1896) Scottish physician who studied intermittent hematuria (1865), later known as paroxysmal nocturnal hematuria or Harley disease. He noted the presence of iron in urine (uribiliogen) and that it was a breakdown product of red blood cells. He was the first to demonstrate on an experimental basis that curare was an antidote to strychnine. He also showed that respired oxygen formed a complex with blood (hemoglobin) and this research led to his election as FRS.

Harman, Nathaniel Bishop (1869–1945) London ophthalmologist who designed special prismatic spectacles for use by the surgeon during ophthalmic surgery and the Bishop Harman diaphragm test for visual images.

Harrington, Charles Robert (1897–1972) Chemist from north Wales who studied protein metabolism at the Royal Infirmary, Edinburgh, and pathological chemistry at University College, London. He elucidated the structure and the empirical formula of tetraiodothyronin and its precursor l-tyrosine in 1926, naming his newly synthesized compound, thyroxin. George Barger (1878–1939), in 1927, synthesized a preparation of thyroxin and determined the full structure. He wrote *The Thyroid Gland: its Chemistry and Physiology* , published in 1933.

Harris, Henry Albert (b 1886) Professor of anatomy at Cambridge, before moving to Khartoum. He described the transverse lines near the epiphysis in the long bones in 1924. His publications include: *The Growth of Long Bones* (1924) and *Bone Growth in Health and Disease* (1933).

Harris, Henry Fauntleroy (1867–1926) American physician who prepared a histological stain from logwood that is known as Harris hemotoxylin. He also published a treatise on pellagra in 1919.

Harris, Walter (1647–1732) Royal physician to William III. Educated at Winchester School and Oxford and Cambridge Universities. He wrote a book on the diseases of children, *A Full View of All the Diseases Incident to Children* (1698).

Harris, Wilfred (1869–1960) Neurologist at St Mary's Hospital, London, was the first to perform alcohol injection of Gasserian ganglion through the foramen ovale for treatment of trigeminal neuralgia. He later became the director of the department of neurology at St Mary's, the first English neurology department to be formed for the purpose of undergraduate teaching. Harris wrote *Neuritis and Neuralgia* in 1926.

Harris Band Hepatoduodenal band consisting of a fold of peritoneum from the gall bladder to the cystic duct across the transverse colon. Described by Chicago surgeon, Malcolm La Salle Harris (1862–1936).

Harrison, John (1718–1753) Born in Deptford, London, he was apprenticed at the age of 14 years to James Ferme at the Barber–Surgeons Hall. He was one of the founders of the London Hospital in 1740, and became its first surgeon. One of the wards at the London Hospital is named after him.

Harrison, Ross Granville (1870–1959) Born in Pennsylvania, he graduated in zoology from Johns Hopkins University in 1894, and became professor of comparative anatomy at Yale University in 1907. He introduced the hanging drop method of tissue culture, and in 1907 demonstrated the growth of nerve fiber from cells outside the organism for the first time. The hanging drop method has proved useful not only in embryology but also in virology, oncology and genetics.

Harrison Sulcus Groove in the thorax extending from the xiphisternum to the axillae in rickets. Described by Edwin Harrison (1766–1838), a physician from Lancashire, in 1798. He also wrote a book on spinal disease.

Hart, Ernest (1836–1898) Graduated from St George's Hospital and became dean at St Mary's Hospital in 1863. He was appointed editor of the *British Medical Journal* in 1866 and served in this post for over 30 years.

Hartley, David (1704–1757) English physician from Halifax. Graduated from Jesus College Cambridge and studied psychology in relation to physiology. His *Observations on Man, His Frame, His Duty and His Expectations,* published in 1749, was the first book in English to use the term, psychology.

Hartline, Haldan Keffer (1903–1983) American physiologist, graduated in medicine from Johns Hopkins Medical School in 1927. Pioneered neurophysiology of vision, for which he shared the Nobel Prize in Physiology or Medicine with Ragnar Granit (b 1900) and George Wald (b 1906) in 1967.

Hartman, Frank Alexander (1883–1971) Professor of physiology at Ohio University who introduced adrenocortical extract as treatment for Addison disease in 1927.

Hartmann, Arthur (1849–1931) *See Hartmann curette, audiometer.*

Hartmann, Henri Albert Charles Antoine (1860–1952) Professor of surgery at Paris. The outpouch of the gall bladder near the its junction with the cystic duct (Hartmann pouch) was described by him in 1891. *See Hartmann operation.*

Hartmann Solution Lactated physiological Ringer solu- tion for intravenous administration. Formulated by American pediatrician, Alexis Frank Hartmann (1898–1964) of St Louis.

Hartmann Curette Used in adenoidectomy and devised by German otorhinologist, Arthur Hartmann (1849–1931) of Berlin. He also devised the first audiometer in 1878.

Hartmann Fossa Inferior ileocecal recess, named after Berlin anatomist, Robert Hartmann (1831–1893).

Hartmann Operation Involves removal of upper rectum or sigmoid for cancer together with closure of the rectal stump and establishment of colostomy. Described by French surgeon, Henri Hartmann (1860–1952) of Paris in 1909.

Hartmann Pouch *See Hartmann, Henri.*

Hartnup Disease Autosomal recessive disease with skin rash, aminoaciduria, pellagra and cerebellar features. First described as *Hereditary pellagra-like rash with temporary cerebellar ataxia and bizarre biochemical features* by D.N. Baron and colleagues in 1956. Charles Dent and co-workers in England used the new technique of electrophoresis to diagnose a new metabolic aspect in 1956. The name was derived from that of the first family diagnosed.

Hartridge, Hamilton (1886–1976) London physiologist who devised a spectroscope (Hartridge reversion spectroscope) which gave two spectra of the same solution. He also proposed the Hartridge cluster theory for color vision, a modification of Young's theory. He published on the velocity of displacement of oxygen by carbon monoxide in hemoglobin with John Worsley Francis Roughton (1899–1972) in 1923.

Harvard College Based at Cambridge, Massachusetts. Founded in 1636 and takes its name from an English-born American colonial clergyman, John Harvard (1607–1638) who bequeathed his library of over 300 volumes and a sum of £779 in 1638. He was born in Southwark, London and went to preach at Charleston, Massachusetts in 1637.

Harvard Medical School Third medical school established in America. Planned by John Warren (1753–1815), a self-taught army surgeon in 1783. Started in the basement of Harvard College. Warren became the first professor of anatomy and surgery in the medical school and pioneered several medical procedures. He taught at the Boston Military Hospital, later the Massachusetts General Hospital, a teaching hospital to the medical school established in 1821. The curriculum at Harvard was improved in 1871 by one of its presidents, Charles W. Eliot who raised the entrance requirements and extended the length of its curriculum to three years. Harvard Medical School moved to its present site through the efforts of John Collins Warren (1842–1927), a grandson of its founder, and Henry Pickering Bowditch (1840–1911). The dormitory for the medical students was also built mainly through the efforts of Collins Warren.

Harvey, Gideon (1637–1700) Physician from Surrey who graduated from Exeter College Oxford in 1655, and became physician to Charles II and the Tower of London in 1689. He wrote several medical treatises. When he died, his post, *Medicus Regius ad Turrim,* was succeeded to by his son of the same name. He published a treatise on consumption and hypochondrical melancholy in 1672.

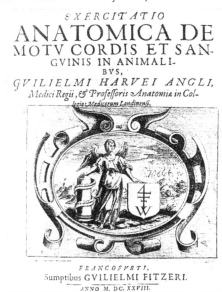

Frontispiece from Harvey's masterpiece of 1628. Courtesy of the National Library of Medicine

Harvey, William (1578–1657) Born in Folkstone, Kent, he became the greatest name in English medicine through his discovery of the circulation of blood. This was published as *Exercitatio Anatomica de Motu Cordis et Sanguinis in Animalibus* (An Anatomical Exercise on the Motion of the Heart and Blood in Animals) in 1628. He graduated from Caius

College Cambridge and proceeded to Padua in order to study anatomy and physiology under Hieronymus Fabricius ab Aquapendente (1537–1619). He obtained his diploma as a doctor of physick at Padua in 1602, and returned to England in the same year. On his return he was appointed physician at St Bartholomew's Hospital in 1609, and physician to James I in 1618, and later physician to Charles I (from 1640). His book on animal reproduction, *Exercitationes de Generatione Animalium,* was published in 1651. Harvey refused to accept the presidency of Royal College of Physicians in 1654 and died three years later, and was buried at Hempstead Church.

Hashimoto Thyroiditis Autoimmune condition of lymphoid infiltration of the thyroid gland was first described in 1912 under the term 'struma lymphamatosa' by the Japanese surgeon, Hakaru Hashimoto (1881–1934). Hashimoto belonged to a family of five generations of medical practitioners in Midau, Nishitsuge and was one of the first medical graduates of the Kyushu University (1907). The presence of autoantibodies to thyroid tissue in rabbits was shown by Ernest Witebsky (1901–1969) and Noel Richard Rose in 1956. The presence of similar antibodies in those with autoimmunc thyroiditis was demonstrated in the same year by Ivan Maurice Roitt (b 1927) and co-workers.

Hashish (*Syn.* ganga, marihuana) Extract of the plant *Cannabis sativa.* Known for over two thousand years in India for its mystic power. A certain murderous Mohammedan sect used hashish as an intoxicant in the 11th century during the time of Crusades. The term *assassin* takes its origin from the word *hashish. See cannabis*

Haskin, Howard Davis (1871–1933) American surgeon from Portland, Oregon who devised a test for urinary proteins using acetic acid and sodium chloride as reagents.

Haslam, John (1764–1844) Superintendent of the Bethlem Mental Asylum from 1795 to 1816. He regularly examined the brains of the insane at autopsy, and recorded the changes in the brain due to syphilis.

Hasner, Joseph Ritter von Artha (1819–1892) Professor of ophthalmology at Prague. In 1850 he described the valve at the lower end of the naso-lachrymal duct.

Hassall, Arthur Hill (1817–1894) English physician from Teddington who described the concentric corpuscles of the thymus. He published the first English textbook on microscopic anatomy, *The Microscopical Anatomy of the Human Body in Health and Disease* in 1846. Hassall spent his last few years on the Isle of Wight. He is remembered eponymously for Hassall corpuscles.

Hassall Corpuscles *See Hassall, Arthur.*

Hasselbalch, Karl A. (1874–1962) Danish biochemist and physician. He did pioneering work on blood pH and, with Nils Bohr (b 1922) and August Krogh (1874–1946), showed that the affinity of blood for oxygen varied with carbon dioxide pressure *See Henderson–Hasselbalch equation.*

Hamilton, Frank Hastings (1813–1886) Professor of surgery at Bellevue Hospital Buffalo, New York, and among the first to treat ulcers by skin grafting.

Hastings, Sir Charles (1794–1866) English physician who founded the British Medical Association at a meeting of fifty medical practitioners convened by him at the Worcester Royal Infirmary in 1832.

Hatter Shakes Also known as Danbury shakes. *See mercury.*

Haudek, Martin (1880–1931) Radiologist in Vienna who described the protrusion of contrast medium into the ulcer crater (Haudek sign) in cases of gastric ulcer.

Haverhill Fever Erythemia athriticum epidemicum caused by *Streptobacillus moniliformis.* A type of rat bite fever first described by Parker and Hudson during an epidemic at Haverhill, Massachusetts in 1926. Edwin Hemphill Place also gave a description of the disease in the same year.

Havers, Clopton (1650–1702) London physician and anatomist who first described the interconnected spaces (Haversian canals) in the compact tissue of the bone in his treatise *Osteologia Nova, or some observations of the Bones and the Parts belonging to them, with the manner of their accretion and nutrition,* published in 1691.

Haversian Canals *See Havers, Clopton.*

Haworth, Sir Walter Norman (1833–1950) English chemist from Chorley who studied under William Perkin at Manchester in 1903, and moved to Imperial College, London in 1911. He was appointed to the chair of organic chemistry at Birmingham in 1925, and elucidated the structure of Vitamin C, naming it ascorbic acid.

Hay Fever First described by Leonardo Botallo under the name of 'summer catarrh' in 1564. John Bostock (1773–1846) gave a modern detailed description between 1819 and 1828. Pollen was identified as the cause by John Elliotson (1791–1868) in 1832 and Charles Harrison Blackley (1820–1900), a Manchester physician, was first to demonstrate that it could be produced by applying pollen to the eyes. He published his work on hay-asthma, *Experimental Researches on the Causes and Nature of Catarrhus Aestivus* in 1873. An oral form of crude epinephrine extract was first used in the treatment by Solomon Solis-Cohen (b 1857) of Jefferson Medical College in 1898. The first attempt to give protection and desensitization by injecting an extract of pollen was made by Leonard Noon (1878–1913) in 1911. The presence of a higher concentration of IgE antibodies in the serum of patients with hay fever and asthma was demonstrated by Kimishige Ishizaka and his co-workers in Denver in 1970 and their findings contributed immensely to further research into the pathogenesis of immediate hypersensitivity reactions.

Hay, Matthew (1855–1932) Succeeded Francis Ogston (1803–1887) as professor of forensic medicine at the University of Aberdeen and held the chair until 1926. He devised the sulfur test (Hay test) for detecting bile in urine.

Hayem, Georges (1841–1933) Professor of clinical medicine and materia medica at the University of Paris. Described chronic interstitial hepatitis in 1874, and gave the first accurate account of blood platelets in 1878. Hayem also identified the early stage of red cells during regeneration (hematoblasts) in 1877, and acquired hemolytic anemia in 1898, the latter known as Hayem–Widal disease.

Hayem–Widal Disease Acquired hemolytic anemia, first described by Georges Hayem in 1898. The disease was later described by George Widal (1862–1929) in 1907.

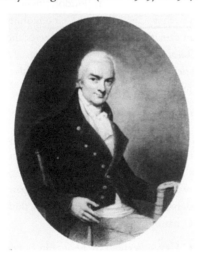

John Haygarth (1740–1827). Courtesy of the National Library of Medicine

Haygarth, John (1740–1827) English physician at Chester Infirmary and later at Bath, and an early epidemiologist. He published the first monograph on acute rheumatism in 1805. The subcutaneous nodules (Haygarth nodes) of the joints in rheumatoid arthritis were named after him.

Head, Sir Henry (1861–1940) London neurologist who studied medicine at the London Hospital and later became consulting physician. He further studied in Cambridge followed by postgraduate training at the Universities of Halle and Prague. He mapped the cutaneous areas of the sensory nerve roots related to visceral organs in 1893. An important book on speech defects, *Aphasia and Kindred Disorders of Speech,* was published by him in 1926. He was knighted in 1927 and spent his retirement in Berkshire.

Head The first book devoted entirely to anatomy of the head *Anatomia Capitis Humani,* with 11 woodcuts, was written by Johan Dryander (1500–1560) in 1536. Another of the early English treatises, *A Treatise de Merborum Capitis Effentis et Prognosticis,* dealing with cerebral and mental affections as well as diseases of the eyes, nose, throat and mouth was published by a physician Robert Bayfield (1630–1690) of Norwich in 1663.

Head Injuries Lanfranc (d *c* 1315) of Paris first described concussion of the brain in his *Chirurgia Magna* in 1296. He also gave a classic description of symptoms following fracture of the skull. The first monograph on the treatment of head injuries, *Tractus de fractura calve sive cranei,* was written by Jacopo Berengario da Carpi (1470–1530), an Italian anatomist from Bologna, in 1518. A comprehensive scientific account of the condition has been given by Percivall Pott (1714–1788) in *Injuries of the Head from External Violence* in 1760. Intracranial infection as a result of head injury was recognized in 1824 by Sir Astley Cooper (1768–1841), surgeon to George lV, but he did not differentiate between meningitis and encephalitis. The effects of concussion in head injury were described by Wilfred Trotter (1872–1939) in 1924. During World War ll, Sir Hugh Cairns (1896–1952), a distinguished Australian surgeon who had worked with Harvey Cushing (1869–1939) in Boston, was appointed as an advisor on head injuries to the Ministry of Health in Britain.

Heaf Gun Method for subcutaneous inoculation using atomized fluid injected under pressure. Devised by British physician, Frederick Rowland George Heaf (1895–1973), who studied medicine at Cambridge University and St Thomas' Hospital and was professor at the University of Wales in 1949.

Healde, Thomas (d 1789) Physician at Witham in Essex before he moved to London in 1767. He delivered the Goulstonian lecture (1763), the Harveian oration (1765), the Croonian lectures (1770, 1784, 1785, 1786), and the Lumelian lecture (1786). He was appointed physician to the London Hospital in 1770. His publications include: *The Use of Oleum Asphalti* (1769), and *The New Pharmacopoeia of the R.C. Physic* (1788).

Hearing The first accurate description of the inner and middle ear, semicircular canals, scalar vestibli and tympanum was given by Gabriele Falloppio (1532–1562) in 1561. The first monograph on the ear was written in 1573 by Volcher Coiter (1534–1576). The apparatus of the middle ear, including the cochlea and the semicircular canals, were further described in 1645 by Cecilio Foli (1615–1660). The first comparative study of the organs of hearing in man and other animals was made by Antonio Scarpa (1752–1832) in 1772. The mechanism of hearing based on resonance, previously mentioned by Albrecht von Haller (1708–1777), was further analyzed and explained by Hermann von Helm-holtz (1821–1894) in 1863. *See audiology, resonance theory, ear.*

Hearst Papyrus Egyptian papyrus of similar content and date to that of the Ebers Papyrus. It was discovered at Derel-Ballas in 1899 and is now at the University of California.

Heart [Anglo-Saxon: *heorte*; Sanskrit: *hardi*; Greek: *kardia*] Recognized as central to life since prehistoric times. The Cro-Magnon cave paintings at Pindel in southern France done about 40,000 years ago, shows the heart as the seat of life. Their belief is reflected in the drawings of a mammoth with a heart at its center. The Ebers Papyrus (*c* 3000 BC) shows the heart as a vital organ with the brain having a lesser role. Empedocles (500–430 BC) of Agrigento in Sicily considered the heart to be the center of the system of blood vessels through which blood was distributed to other parts of the body. The heart was first studied on an anatomical basis by Erasistratus (b 300 BC) and Herophilus (fl 300 BC). One of the earliest accurate anatomical drawings, including valves, was that of Leonardo Da Vinci (1452–1519). Andreas Vesalius (1514–1564) gave a good description of gross anatomical structures in 1543. The first extensive treatise with a review of ancient and medieval theories was written by Ippolito Francesco Albertini (1662–1738) of Italy. William Harvey (1578–1657) described mechanisms of function in his treatise on circulation, published in 1628. The muscular nature was first described by Danish anatomist, Niels Stenson (1638–1686) in *De Musculis et Glandulis Observationum Specimen,* published in 1664. Some of the modern English physicians who concentrated on heart diseases include: William Stokes, Peter Mere Latham, Robert Adams, James Mackenzie, Sir Thomas Lewis and Paul Wood. *See cardiology.*

Heart Beat Ability of the heart to beat without being attached to the body through nerves was observed by the Greek physician, Galen (AD 129–200) who has commented that 'the power to produce pulsation lies in the heart itself'. The Dutch anatomist, Volcher Coiter (1534–1576), demonstrated this in the excised heart of a kitten. William Harvey

(1578–1657) recognized that the heart beat originated in the auricles. The German physiologist, Johannes Müller (1801–1858) was one of the first to observe that the stopped heart beat could be restarted by passing a weak electric current through it.

Heart Block First observation that the heart beat originates from the auricles and later spreads to the ventricles was made by William Harvey (1578–1657) during his work on circulation of the blood. He also noted that the ventricle of the dying heart responded with an increasing period of inactivity to the auricles. This was probably the first observation and description of heart block, although the condition was mentioned in 1602 by Ercole Sassonia (1551–1607). The first report of syncope due to cardiac arrest or heart block was given by Marcus Gerbezius (1658–1718) in 1692. The same condition was described as 'epilepsy with slow pulse' by Giovanni Morgagni (1682–1771) in 1761. The first British physician to give a specific account was Thomas Spence (1769–1842) of Edinburgh. His paper, *History of a Case in Which There Took Place a Remarkable Slowness of the Pulse,* was published in 1793. The first classical description of heart block associated with syncopy was given by Robert Adams (1791–1875) of Dublin in 1827. William Stokes (1804–1878), another eminent Irish physician, also gave an account of heart block with syncopal attacks in 1846, and the condition was later named Stokes–Adams syndrome. The term 'block' was introduced into cardiology in 1883 by Walter Holbrook Gaskell (1847–1914) who did experimental work on tortoises and discovered the correlation between atrioventricular conduction, and the change in the structure of fibers between the atria and ventricles. Joseph Erlanger (1874–1965), an American physiologist at Johns Hopkins demonstrated various degrees of heart block, showing that it was caused by lesions in the bundle of His. Wilhelm His (1831–1904) was the first to experimentally induce heart block. Endocardial electrode pacing in heart block was first tried in animals by John C. Callaghan and Wilfred C. Bigelow in 1951. Paul Maurice Zoll (b 1911) applied external cardiac pacing for the first time in ventricular standstill in two patients in 1952. F. Furman and G. Robinson introduced intracardiac right ventricular pacing in 1958, and the first generator implant for cardiac pacing was done at Karolinska Hospital in Sweden in October 1958.

Heart Size Measurement with X-rays or fluoroscopy was first made in 1896 by Francis Henry Williams (1852–1936).

Heart Sounds *See cardiac sounds.*

Heart Transplant *See cardiac transplant.*

Heart Valves *See artificial valves, mitral valve, aortic valve, tricuspid valve.*

Heart–Lung Machine Developed by American surgeon, John Gibbon (1903–1971). The machine took the patient's blood to be oxygenated and carbon dioxide removed outside of the body. The blood was passed over thin stainless steel screens in an atmosphere of oxygen. It was first used in an 18-year-old girl in an operation to repair a hole in her heart. *See cardiac surgery.*

Heat [Anglo-Saxon: *haetu*, heat] Considered to be one of the properties of the animal body by Aristotle (384–322 BC). Francis Bacon (1561–1626) described heat as a mode of motion, and Robert Hooke (1635–1703) considered it to be a ceaseless motion of particles. Production of heat by mechanical motion was described by English–American scientist, Count Benjamin Thompson Rumford (1753–1814) who observed it in 1796 during the boring of canon. He deduced that there was a relationship between work done and amount of heat generated. German physician, Julius Robert von Mayer (1814-1878) first related mechanical work directly to heat in 1842. He also proposed the law of conservation of energy and explicitly applied it to both living and non-living things. Sadi Carnot (1796–1832) established the science of thermodynamics with his discovery of the mechanical equivalent of heat in 1824, although his initial paper on the subject, *Réflexions sur la Puissance mortrice du feu,* remained unnoticed for over 10 years until reinterpreted by Émile Claypeyron (1799–1864) in 1835. The mechanical equivalent of heat was measured accurately James Prescott Joule (1818–1889) in 1843. *See thermodynamics.*

Heating Lighting a fire to provide warmth has been practiced since prehistoric times. Underfloor central heating existed in ancient Rome. The first use of steam for heating was pioneered with the steam engine, invented in 1784 by James Watt (1736–1819) to heat his office. An elaborate method for warming and ventilating public theaters was invented by the Marquess of Chabanne in 1819. Neil Arnott (1788–1874), an English inventor and physician wrote a treatise on the subject in 1838. A commission on ventilation and warming was appointed in England in 1859.

Heat Cramp First described by Sir Charles Blagden (1748–1820) in experiments published in 1775. Another description was given by Boston physician, David Linn Edsall (1869–1945). John Scott Haldane (1860–1936) noted it to be common amongst mine workers, due to excessive salt loss where temperature varied between 98 and 102 degrees Fahrenheit.

Heat Stroke *See sunstroke.*

Heavy Chain Disease (HCD) Associated with a variant of a paraprotein type accompanied by leukopenia, thrombocytopenia and lymphadenopathy. First described by Berlin-born American physician, E. C. Franklin (1929–1982) and co-workers in the *American Journal of Medicine* in 1964. Franklin graduated from the New York University School of Medicine in 1950 and became a professor there in 1968. The first case of free alpha-chain (heavy chain of IgA) was noted by Seligman and co-workers in 1968 in the serum of a young Arab patient who had marked plasma infiltration of the gut wall. The patients with this disease also have steatorrhea, weight loss and finger clubbing. It was first known as Mediterranean lymphoma as it was thought to be restricted to Arabs and Jews, but has now been detected in other races.

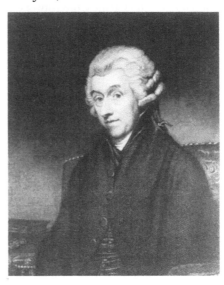

William Heberden the Elder (1710–1801). Courtesy of the National Library of Medicine

Heberden, William, the Elder (1710–1801) London physician, educated at St John's College, Cambridge, member of the Royal College of Physicians, Goulstonian and Croonian lecturer and Harveian orator by the age of 40. He described angina pectoris (1768), acute rheumatic fever, association of renal stones with urinary tract infection, and night blindness (1767). He also observed the nodes in the fingers in patients with osteoarthritis (Heberden nodes) and differentiated it from rheumatic gout in 1802.

Heberden, William, the Younger (1767–1845) Physician to St George's Hospital in 1793. Publisher of his father's *Commentaries* in 1802. He wrote a work in Latin on pediatrics in 1804.

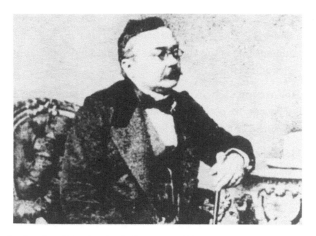

Ferdinand von Hebra (1816–1880). Courtesy of the National Library of Medicine

Hebra, Ferdinand Ritter von (1816–1880) Viennese dermatologist who founded the histologic approach to dermatology with his classification of skin diseases, *Atlas of Skin Diseases,* in 1845. He studied scabies in detail and demonstrated growth of ringworm fungus on the epidermis. His unfinished masterpiece, *On Diseases of the Skin,* was completed by one of his pupils and son-in-law, Moritz Kaposi (1837– 1902) and translated into English by the New Sydenham Society between 1866 and 1880.

Hebrew Medicine *See Jewish medicine.*

Hecker, Justus Friedrich Karl (1795–1850) German medical historian who published a monograph on the great epidemics of the Middle Ages.

Heerfordt Syndrome (Syn: Waldenström uveoparotitis) A form of sarcoidosis involving the parotid glands. Described by Danish ophthalmologist, Christian Fredrick Heerfordt (1872–1953) in 1909.

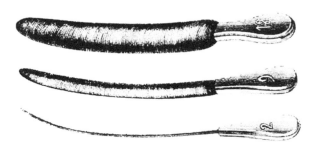

Hegar dilators form his book, *Die Operativ Gynäkologie* (1881). Reproduced with permission of Ferdinand Enke, Stuttgart

Hegar Dilators Curved metal cervical dilators, first described by M. Tchoudowski who had seen them in use in Germany at Hegar's clinic, in 1879. Alfred Hegar (1820–1914) published an account of the dilators in his textbook on operative gynecology in 1881.

Hegar Sign Early sign of pregnancy where the softness and flexibility of the cervix could be felt on digital examination. Described by Alfred Hegar (1830–1914), a professor of obstetrics at Freiburg in 1864.

Hegira *See Higra.*

Heidelberg man A jaw of a primitive man, probably older than Neanderthal man, was found at Mauer in Heidelberg in 1907. The remains of other extinct animals such as *Eliphas antiquus,* a Etruscan rhinoceros found in the same strata have helped to establish the antiquity of Heidelberg man who is supposed to have lived during the Moustrian or middle Paleolithic period about 60,000 years ago.

Heidelberg University The oldest continuously surviving university in Germany, founded in 1386.

Heidelberger, Charles (1920–1983) Professor of oncology at Wisconsin who pioneered research on anticancer agents. He introduced Flurouracil as a tumor inhibitory compound in 1957.

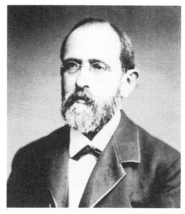

Rudolph Peter Heinrich Heidenhaim (1834–1897). Courtesy of the National Library of Medicine

Heidenhain, Rudolph Peter Heinrich (1834–1897) German professor of physiology and histology at the University of Breslau. In collaboration with Ivan Pavlov (1849–1936), he described the parietal and central cells of the gastric secretory glands in 1888. The Heidenhain cells are named after him.

Heilbrunn Site of the oldest medicinal spring in Bavaria. Rediscovered by monks in 1509 and became medicinally important. The waters contain significant quantities of iodine.

Heine, Jacob von (1800–1879) German orthopedist, one of the first to describe infantile paralysis or poliomyelitis in 1840. He considered it to result from a spinal lesion and as atrophic myasthenia from inactivity.

Hein, Johann Georg (1770–1838) Orthopedic mechanic from Würzburg who invented many instruments. Well respected by surgeons of his period and awarded a doctorate (non-medical) by the University of Jena in 1823. The Hein Orthopedic Institute at Würzburg, founded in 1816, is named after him.

Heine–Medin Disease *See acute anterior infantile poliomyelitis.*

Heine, Leopold (1870–1940) Ophthalmologist at Kiel who designed an operation for glaucoma (Heine operation) where the ciliary body is separated from the sclera using a spatula.

Heineke, Walther Hermann (1834–1901) Surgeon in Erlangen who devised an operation for pyloroplasty (Heineke–Mikulicz operation) involving a longitudinal incision of the pylorus followed by a transverse suture.

Heinz Bodies Small deep purple, irregular bodies seen within red blood cells after staining with crystal violet. First observed in 1906 by Robert Heinz (1865–1924), professor of pharmacology and toxicology at Erlangen in Germany. Characteristic of glucose-6-phosphate dehydrogenase deficiency.

Heister, Lorenz (1683–1758) Regarded as the founder of scientific surgery in Germany. Educated at Giessen, Leiden and Amsterdam Universities. He introduced the spinal brace and was the first to describe appendicitis. The first cancer surgeon operating on salivary gland tumors, and also described thyroid cancer. He established the term 'tracheotomy' for incision of the wind pipe and performed the first surgical correction of club foot.

Heister Valves Spiral folds of mucous membrane in the neck of the gall bladder and the cystic duct. First described by the German surgeon, Lorenz Heister, in 1717.

Held, Hans (1866–1917) Prussian professor of anatomy at Leipzig who described the decussation of certain specific acoustic nerve fibers in the lateral fillet (a lemniscus in the trapezoid body) in 1891.

Helen House First hospice for children in England, opened at Oxford in 1982. *See Hospice.*

Helicobacter pylori Helical, microaerophilic bacterium. Produces urease and is associated with gastroduodenal diseases such as peptic ulcer. *See Campylobacter pylori.*

Helie, Louis Theodore (1804–1867) Professor of anatomy and gynecologist at Paris who described the superficial musculature of the uterus in 1865. Also founded the famous anatomical museum at Paris.

Helioscope [Greek: *helios*, sun+*skopein*, to look] Special telescope to observe the sun without affecting the eye. Invented by Christopher Scheiner in 1625.

Heliotherapy [Greek: *helios*, sun + *therapeia*, medical treatment] Treatment of diseases by exposure to sunlight. Johann Wolfgang Döbereiner (1780–1849) developed a lamp for light therapy in 1816. Arthur Henry Downes (1851–1938) and Thomas Porter Blunt, writing in the *Proceedings of the Royal Society* in 1877, showed that these actinic rays killed bacteria. Danish physician, Niels Ryberg Finson (1860–1904) demonstrated the bactericidal effects of sunlight, and developed a new method of treating lupus vulgaris with ultraviolet light in 1890. Sunlight therapy for children with bone disease and tuberculosis was first introduced by Sir Henry Gauvain. The ultraviolet rays were later artificially produced using mercury lamps as treatment in conditions such as arthritis, strains and sprains. *See actinotherapy.*

Helium [Greek: *helios*, sun] Originally discovered as a yellow line in the spectra of the sun by the Danish astronomer, M. Janssen, in 1868. Thought to be due to a new element, and hypothetically named helium by Sir Joseph Norman Lockyer (1836–1920) and Sir Edward Frankland (1825–1899). Helium gas was identified by Sir William Crookes (1832–1919) in 1895, and found to be a disintegration product of radium by Sir William Ramsay (1852–1916) and Frederick Soddy (1877–1965) in 1903. It was first liquefied by Dutch physicist, Kamerlingh-Onnes (b 1853) in 1908, and solidified by Keesome in 1926. Around 1930 helium was used as a diluent, particularly with oxygen in anesthesia.

Hellebore [*Helleborus*, Greek: *eleio*, to injure + *boros*, eaten] The roots of several species of this poisonous plant have been used since ancient times as a remedy. Pliny (AD 23–79) recommended it as a purgative and treatment for hydrophobia, while Hippocrates (460–377 BC) used it as a cleansing agent for ulcers. Paul of Aegina (AD 625–690) recommended its use for melancholy. The active ingredient (helleborin) from the black hellebore root (*Helleborus niger*) was obtained by A. Husemann in 1864.

Heller, Arnold Ludwig (1840–1913) Anatomist at Kiel, appointed to the chair of pathological anatomy in 1872. He described the arterial plexus in the intestinal wall in 1872, and syphilitic aortitis, a cause of aortic aneurysm, in 1899.

Heller, Hans (1905–1974) Austrian endocrinologist who graduated from Prague. One of the founders of the journal, *General and Comparative Endocrinology.* He was also instrumental in forming the European Society for Comparative Endocrinology in 1965, to which he was elected first president.

Heller, Johan Florenze (1813–1871) Austrian physician in Vienna who devised the nitric acid test for detecting protein in urine. He also designed a form of hydroelectric bath (Heller bath) and wrote an important work on urinary calculi in 1860.

Helmholtz, Hermann Ludwig Ferdinand von (1821–1894) Born in Potsdam of mixed German and French ancestry, he trained under Johannes Müller and Gustav Magnus, before becoming a surgeon in the Prussian Army. Also professor of physiology at Königsberg, professor of anatomy and physiology at Bonn in 1855, and chair of physics at Berlin in 1871. He developed the method of obtaining electromyograms of the muscles in 1851, and did pioneering work on muscle energy around 1850. In 1851 Helmholtz invented an ophthalmoscope independently of Charles Babbage (1792–1871). He was also the first to explain the mechanism of accommodation of the eye, brought about by contraction of ciliary muscles effecting a change in curvature of the anterior surface of the lens, and also studied perception of color.

Helminthology [Greek: *helmins,* worm + *logos,* discourse] Intestinal parasitic worms were known to ancient physicians, and Hippocrates (460–377 BC) divided them into round lumbricae (*Ascaris*), and broad lumbricae (tapeworms in the genus *Taenia*). The symptoms of hookworm disease, also called 'Egyptian chlorosis' or anchylostomiasis, were familiar to the ancient Egyptians. An historic review was presented by Robert Thompson Leiper (1881–1969) in his essay *Landmarks in Medical Helminthology* published in 1929. *See Echinococcus, Anchylostoma duodenale, hydatid disease.*

Helmont, Johannes Baptista van (1577–1644) Born in Brussels and studied philosophy and theology at the University of Louvain before changing to medicine. He settled on his estate at Vilvorde near Brussels in 1609 and concentrated on chemistry, which formed the basis for iatrochemistry. Helmont studied gases, and coined the word *gas* from the Greek term for chaos. He also described centrum tendinosum of the diaphragm in 1644. His *Ortus medicinae vel Opera et Opuscula Omnia* was published posthumously by his son in 1648.

Helmont, Franciscus Mercurius van (1618–1699) Born in

The Netherlands, he was a peripatetic physician and philosopher, and son of Johannes Baptista van Helmont. He promoted treatment for insanity by ducking in water, first introduced by his father. His work on the influence of mind in causing and curing diseases was published at Amsterdam in 1692.

Helsinki Declaration Following the Nuremberg trials of war criminals, including physicians who conducted inhuman experiments on the inmates of the Nazi concentration camps, the Nuremberg Code was established. It lays down ten standards to which physicians are expected to conform when carrying out research on humans and was implemented in 1947. The next most important document on human experimentation, the Declaration of Helsinki was derived from the Nuremberg Code, and accepted by the World Medical Assembly in Helsinki in 1964. The Helsinki Declaration contained further guidelines on biomedical research involving human subjects. *See informed consent, ethics of human experimentation.*

Helvetius, Adrian (1661–1727) Dutch physician who settled in Paris in 1684, establishing a successful and fashionable practice. He obtained ipecacuanha (*Cephaelis ipecacuanha*) from a merchant named Garnier in Paris and used it successfully to treat bloody flux (dysentery) in 1680. Helvetius used the root as the basis of a patent remedy and Louis XIV granted him the sole right to sell it. In 1688 the French government paid Helvetius 1000 louis d'or for the formula which they then made public.

Helvetius, Johannes Claude Adrian (1715–1771) Son of Adrian Helvetius and comparative anatomist in Paris. Described the supporting muscular fibers of the antrum of the stomach.

Helvig, Hans Christian Saxtroph (1847–1901) Psychiatrist and director of the Institute for the Insane in Odense, who described the tractus-olivospinalis of the nervous system in 1887.

Helwig, G. John Otto (d 1698) Physician in the 17th century who was created a baronet by Charles II.

Hemacytometer [Greek: *haima,* blood + *kytos,* cell + *metron,* measure] Instrument for determining the number of blood cells in a given volume, first devised by Karl Vierdort (1818–1884) in 1852. His original method involved counting the number of red blood cells in a line, after the blood was allowed to dry on a slide. English scientist William Cramer (b 1878) improved this method using a capillary cell, and Pierre-Carl Potain (1825–1901) and Louis Charles Malassez (1842–1909) used a capillary tube and a microscope eye piece ruled in squares to count the blood cells. Georges Hayem (1841–1930) of Paris added a volumetric aspect to the method with his apparatus in 1870. The instrument was improved by Sir William Gowers (1845–1915) and was named hematocytometer in 1877.

Hematemesis [Greek: *haima*, blood + *emew*, to vomit] Vomiting of blood due to gastric ulcer was first described in 1859 by William Brinton (1823-1867), physician at St. Thomas' Hospital. *See esophageal rupture.*

Hematin [Greek: *haima*, blood] Complex organic substance in blood contributing to color and containing heme, in which iron is in the Fe^{+3} form. Demonstrated by William Charles Wells (1757–1817), a physician at St Thomas' Hospital in 1797. First used as an indicator for detection of blood in forensic medicine by Teichmann in 1853.

Hematobium [Greek: *haima*, blood + *bios*, life] *See Schistosoma hematobium.*

Hematoblast [Greek: *haima*, blood + *blastos*, bud] Early unidentified stage of development of red blood cells, first identified by Georges Hayem (1841–1930), professor of clinical medicine at the University of Paris.

Hematocele [Greek: *haima*, blood + *cele*, tumor] Condition of swelling of scrotum or spermatic cord due to a collection of blood was described by Celsus (25 BC–AD 50) in 10 AD, and Paul of Aegina (AD 625–690). The first modern surgical description of the condition was given by Percivall Pott (1714–1788), around 1750.

Hematology [Greek: *haima*, blood + *logos*, study] Science of blood founded by Paul Ehrlich (1854–1915) of Germany, who made great contributions to the field with his staining methods. He used aniline dyes to stain white blood cells in 1877, and introduced the method of differential blood cell count in 1879. He identified reticulocytes in 1881 and gave a description of aplastic anemia in 1888. Ehrlich also differentiated between lymphocytic and myelogenous leukemia in 1891. The method of enumerating red blood cells was devised by Karl Vierdort (1818–1884) in 1852. The discovery of blood platelets was made by Alfred Donné (1801–1878) in 1842. Others who gave a description of blood platelets include Georges Hayem (1841–1930) and Sir William Osler (1849–1919). An early comprehensive review of hematology during the 19th century was given by Rud Limbeck of Vienna in his work *Clinical Pathology of Blood* published in 1901. The polymorphs were differentiated into five different groups according to their nuclear configuration by German physician, Joseph Arneth (1873–1955) in 1904. Sternal needle puncture for study of bone marrow was first described by Carly Paul Seyfarth (b 1890) of Germany in 1923. The use of needle puncture in hemopoietic diseases was popularized by Mikhail J. Arinkin (1876–1948) of Germany in 1927. A classification of anemias based on red cell morphology was proposed by Canadian physician, Maxwell Myer Wintrobe (b 1901) in 1930. His classification proposed four groups of anemias: macrocytic, normocytic, simple microcytic, and chronic microcytic. With the discovery of ABO blood groups by Karl Landsteiner (1868–1943) in 1900, blood transfusion became one of the important fields in hematology.

Hematuria [Greek: *haima*, blood + *ouron*, urine] The Arabian physician, Rhazes of Persia (850–932) was one of the first to propose hematuria as a symptom of urinary tract disease. Richard Bright (1789–1858) of Guy's Hospital recognized hematuria as a symptom of nephritis in 1827. George Harley (1829–1896) described a peculiar condition of intermittent hematuria in 1865, later known as paroxysmal nocturnal hematuria, or Harley disease. The focal glomerular lesions in the kidney, caused by minute bacterial emboli were first observed by German physician, Max Hermann Loehlein (1877-1921) in 1910.

Heme Part of the hemoglobin molecule, first synthesized by American biochemist, David Shemin from New York in 1911. Further work on the structure and nature of hemin was done by Shemin and D. Rittenberg in 1946.

Hemin Chloride of ferric protoporphyrin or hematin in blood, first used as an indicator for detection of blood in forensic medicine by German histologist, Ludwig Teichmann (1823–1895) in 1853. He treated the blood sample or material with acetic acid and sodium chloride in order to reveal the formation of hemin in positive cases. This was used in legal medicine for over a century.

Hemlock (*Conium maculatum*) Mentioned in Greek literature dating back to 400 BC. Medicinal effects were known to the ancients and Dioscorides (AD 40–90) recommended it in his *De Materia Medica* as a soothing ointment. The famous hemlock potion by which Greek criminals were put to death was essentially composed of the juice. The effects of hemlock as a poison in the official execution of Socrates (c 469–399 BC), were described by Plato (428–347 BC) in *Phaedo*: 'Socrates after swallowing the poison cup walked about for a short time as he was directed by the executioner; when he felt a sense of heaviness in his limbs he laid down on his back; his feet and legs fast lost their sensibility and became stiff and cold; and the state gradually extended towards the heart, when he died convulsed'. The effect was also described by Nicander in 100 BC who advocated undiluted wine as a remedy for poisoning by the plant. The Abbess Hildegard in the 12th century recommended it for treatment of swellings, and it remained in the pharmacopoeia for centuries. Johannes Storch (1681–1751) was responsible for popularizing its use in medicine as a narcotic. The poisonous nature of the plant was found to be due to the alkaloids, coniine, methyl coniine, conicene and conhydrine. Giescke isolated coniine in 1827, it was incidentally the first alkaloid to be synthesized.

Hemochromatosis [Greek: *haima*, blood + *chroma*, color + *osis*, condition] Excessive accumulation of iron from a disorder of iron metabolism. *See bronze diabetes.*

Hemodialysis [Greek: *haima*, blood + *dia*, through + *luein*, to loosen] Filtration of the blood through a semipermeable membrane. *See artificial kidney.*

Hemaglobin [Greek: *haima*, blood; Latin: *globus*, ball] Complex organic substance, hematin, which contributed to the color of blood was first shown by William Charles Wells (1757–1817) in 1797. The discovery of iron in the blood was made by Vincenzo Menghini (1704–1759) in 1746, and the presence of hemoglobin was demonstrated by Otto Funke (1828–1879) in 1851. The first quantitative estimation was done by Hermann Welcher in 1854. The fact that oxygen could be removed by the use of reducing agents was demonstrated by Sir William Stokes (1804–1878) in 1863. Hemoglobin was obtained in crystalline form and given its present name by Ernst Felix Emanuel Hoppe-Seyler (1825– 1895) of Germany in 1864. The ability of hemoglobin to combine reversibly with oxygen, thus enabling it to act as a transport agent of the gas from air to the tissues was shown by Hoppe-Seyler and Barcroft (1872–1947) of England in 1928 in the latter's monograph, *The Respiratory Function of the Blood.* Its formation from porphyrin and precursor substances within the red cells of the bone marrow was first shown by B. R. Burmeister of Leipzig in 1936. Amino acids of hemoglobin were determined by Austrian-born British biochemist, Max Ferdinand Perutz (b 1914), who became director of Medical Research Council for Molecular Biology in London in 1964. Double Nobel Prize winner, Linus Pauling (b 1901), discovered the alpha-helix in the hemoglobin molecule.

Hemaglobinometer [Greek: *haima*, blood; Latin: *globus*, a ball + *meter*, measure] Instrument for determining hemoglobin in blood. One of the first compared blood color with a standard color and was devised by Sir William Richard Gowers (1845–1915) in 1878. Another was designed by John Scott Haldane (1860–1936) in 1901. The spectrophotometric method was developed by G. E. Davis and C. Sheard in 1927, and the first photoelectric hemoglobinometer was

made by C. Sheard and Arthur H. Sanford (b 1889) in 1929.

Hemaglobinopathy [Greek: *haima*, blood; Latin: *globus*, ball; Greek *pathos*, suffering] Pathological condition caused by abnormal hemoglobin. One of the important inherited forms, leading to state of severe anemia with the presence of sickle-shaped red blood cells, was first recognized by James Bryan Herrick (1861–1954) of America in 1910. The name sickle cell anemia was given to the condition by Verne Rheem Mason (b 1889) in 1922. The first genetic study of sickle cell anemia was done by Clyde Graeme Guthrie (b 1880) and John Gardiner Huck (b 1891) of Johns Hopkins in 1923. The structural variant of hemoglobin responsible for this disease was identified by Linus Carl Pauling (b 1901), an American molecular biologist and chemist, in 1949. The substitution of the amino acid valine for glutamic acid in the hemoglobin of patients with sickle cell anemia was described by Vernon Martin Ingram (b 1924) of England in 1957. Another form of hemoglobinopathy, beta thalassemia associated with bone changes, splenomegaly, and severe anemia in infancy or early childhood, was first des-cribed by Thomas Benton Cooley (1871–1945) and P. Lee in 1925. The hereditary nature of thalassemia was demonstrated by J. Caminopetros in 1938.

Hemoltytic Anemia [Greek: *haima*, blood + *luein*, to loosen] First described by William Dameshek (1900–1969) and K. Singer in 1941. Hemoglobinopathy forms an important group of hemolytic anemias.

Hemolytic Streptococcus *See beta hemolytic streptococci.*

Hemolytic Uremic Syndrome Associated with renal failure, hemolysis and thrombocytopenia. First described by Swiss pediatrician, C. Gasser and co-workers at the University of Zurich in 1955.

Hemopericardium [Greek: *haima*, blood + *peri*, around + *kardia*, heart] Blood in the pericardial sac. One of the first instances of cardiac tamponade was described by Berlin physician, Edmund Rose (1836–1914).

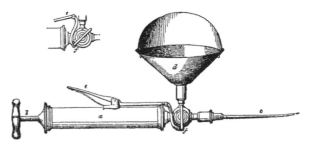

Syringe and apparatus used for blood transfusion by Samuel Armstrong Lane in 1839. *The Lancet* (1841)

Hemophilia [Greek: *haima*, blood + *philos*, loving] Inherited disorder of blood coagulation. The earliest description was given by Spanish physician, Albucasis, around AD 970. A specific description with the observation that females transmit the condition but remain unaffected, was given by John Conrad Otto (1774–1844) of New Jersey in 1803. The immunity of the females was further studied and confirmed by Christian Friedrich Nasse (1778–1851) in 1820. The name 'hemophilia' was given by Johann Schonlein (1793–1864) in 1828. Samuel Armstrong Lane (1802-1892), surgeon at St George's Hospital, gave the first account of a successful blood transfusion in 1839 to an 11-year-old boy who had a bleeding diathesis, probably hemophilia. James Blundell (1790–1877) wrote on the procedure. This is the first record of blood transfusion to a hemophiliac and his article was published in *The Lancet* of 1840. A full clinical description was given by Johann Ludwig Grandidier (b 1810) of Leipzig in 1855. The role of antihemophilic globulin or factor VIII was demonstrated by Arthur Jackson Patek (b 1904) and Francis Henry Laskey Taylor (1900–1959) in 1937.

Hemophilus ducreyii [Greek: *haima*, blood + *philos*, loving] Causative organism of chancroid lesions. Discovered by Italian dermatologist, Augusto Ducrey (1860–1940) in 1888.

Hemophilus influenzae [Greek: *haima*, blood + *philos*, loving] Bacillus first isolated in 1892 and described by Richard Friedrich Johannes Pfeiffer (1858–1945), a Polish bacteriologist. The organism was named 'influenzae' due to Pfeiffer's belief that it was the causative organism of influenza (now known to be of viral origin) whereas the bacillus is actually responsible for complications. The generic name *Hemophilus* was given to the bacteria by the American Committee of Nomenclature in 1920.

Hemopoiesis [Greek: *haima*, blood + *poesis*, making] Process of formation and development of blood cells. *See bone marrow aspiration, bone marrow biopsy, bone marrow transplant, hematology.*

Hemoptysis [Greek: *haima*, blood + *ptysis*, spitting] Spitting of blood. Hippocrates mentioned the condition. Aretaeus was the first to describe the symptoms, pointing out the various causes and treatment. The term was mentioned by Pliny (AD 23–79) who recommended the juice of henbane (*Hyoscyamus niger*) in treatment.

Hemorrhage [Greek: *haima*, blood + *rhegymi*, to burst forth] Escape of blood through vessels. Aulus Cornelius Celsus (25 BC–AD 50) recommended the application of a sponge soaked in cold water combined with hard pressure in order to stop bleeding. He also advocated ligature if these measures failed. Galen (AD 129–200) wrote extensively on the subject and advocated the application of digital pressure on the bleeding vessel to encourage the formation of a clot. Cobwebs were used in the treatment of bleeding or hemorrhage and Shakespeare in *A Midsummer Night's Dream* referred to their use for treatment of a cut finger. English soldiers during the battle of Crecy in 1346 carried boxes of spiders' web as first aid equipment. In most parts of the world cautery or a hot iron was advocated to control bleeding up to the 16th century. Muscle tendons were used by the Masai tribe to ligate bleeding vessels.

Hemorrhagic Disease of the Newborn The first series of infants suffering from this condition was provided by R.S. Beveridge in 1928. The reduced level of prothrombin in the blood of newborn infants was first demonstrated by Kenneth M. Brinkhouse, Harry Pratt Smith (b 1895), and Emory D. Warner (b 1905) in 1937. The use of vitamin K in treatment was first demonstrated by Hugh Roland Butt (b 1910) and Albert Markely Snell (1896–1960) of Mayo Clinic in 1938.

Hemorrhagic Nephritis *See embolic nephritis.*

Hemorrhoids [Greek: *haima*, blood + *rrhoos*, to flow] Swollen mass of dilated veins in anal tissue. Ligature was recommended as treatment in Hippocrates treatise, *On Hemorrhoids*, and by Celsus (25 BC–AD 50), while Aetius of Amida, around AD 600, recommended their excision. One of the early modern works was written by George Ernst Stahl (1660–1734) of Bavaria in 1729.

Henbane (*Hyoscyamus niger*) Used as a medicine by ancient Greek physicians such as Dioscorides and Celsus to induce sleep and allay pain. In mythology the dead in Hades were crowned with henbane as they wandered beside the river Styx. Benedictus Crispus (AD 681), archbishop of Milan named it 'symphonica' or 'hyocyasmus'. According to an American medical observer, John Josselyn in *New England's Rarities Discovered*, the plant was naturalized in North America before 1672. It is referred to as 'henbell' in the Anglo-Saxon works on medicine in the 11th century. It was omitted from the London Pharmacopoeia in 1746 on the recommendation of Johannes Storch (1681–1751) who initially used it in the treatment of epilepsy, nervous and convulsive diseases. It was reintroduced in 1809.

Hench, Philip Showalter (1896–1965) Born and educated in Pittsburgh. While professor of medicine at Minnesota University in 1948, he noticed that conditions such as surgery, pregnancy and starvation which stimulated the adrenal cortex also improved rheumatoid arthritis. He deduced that cortical hormones could be tested for anti-rheumatoid activity, and obtained a few grams of cortisone from Edward Calvin Kendall (1886–1972) to conduct his trial. The dramatic effect of cortisone on certain cases of rheumatoid arthritis, published by Hench and co-workers in 1949, established the place of cortisone in the treatment of rheumatoid arthritis. Hench, Kendall and Reichstein were awarded the Nobel Prize for Physiology or Medicine in 1950 for their work on suprarenal hormones.

Henderson, Lawrence Joseph (1878–1942) Born in Lin, Massachusetts and educated at Harvard and Strasbourg. Developed nomograms to calculate pH values of blood, known as the Henderson–Hasselbalch equation. Karl Hasselbalch (1874–1962) was a Danish biochemist who showed that the affinity of blood for oxygen varied with the pressure of carbon dioxide. Henderson's monograph, *Blood, a Study in General Physiology*, is considered a classic.

Henderson, Melvin Starkey (1883–1954) Born in Rochester, Minnesota, he was an orthopedic surgeon who described the presence of osteocartilagenous bodies in the joints (synovial chondromatosis) in 1918. This condition (Henderson– Jones syndrome) was earlier described by gynecologist and surgeon, Paul Friedrich Reichel (1858–1934) of Chemnitz in 1900. Another orthopedic surgeon, Hugh Toland Jones (b 1892) of Los Angeles, gave an account of the condition in 1924.

Henderson, William (1810–1872) Succeeded John Thompson (1765–1846) as professor of pathology at Edinburgh Medical School in 1842. He wrote a treatise on the skin disease, molluscum contagiosum, in 1841 in which he described the inclusion bodies. He was one of the first to differentiate typhus from relapsing fever in 1844.

Henderson, Yandall (1873–1944) American physiologist from New Haven who made physiological observations (with J.S. Haldane, 1860–1936) on adaptation to low barometric pressure on Pike's Peak, Colorado. Wrote a treatise on decompression sickness in aviation in 1917. He also devised the test for anesthetic risk (Henderson test) where the patient was asked to take a deep breath and hold it as long as possible.

Henderson–Hasselbalch Equation For calculation of pH value of blood was proposed by American biochemist at Harvard, Lawrence Joseph Henderson (1879–1942) and Danish biochemist, Karl A. Hasselbalch (1874–1962).

Henderson–Jones Syndrome *See Henderson, Melvin Starkey.*

Henke, Philip Jakob Wilhelm (1834–1896) Artist and anatomist who was appointed professor of anatomy at Tübingen in 1896. Henke triangle in the inguinal region was described by him in 1879.

Henle, Friedrich Gustave Jacob (1809–1885) One of the greatest German anatomists and histologists, born to Jewish parents in Nuremberg and trained under Johannes Müller (1801–1858) at Bonn. He made the following important contributions: discovery of smooth muscle in the middle coat of smaller arteries (Henle elastic membrane); description of columnar and ciliated epithelial cells; discovery of external sphincter of the bladder (Henle sphincter) and the loop shaped tubules of the kidney (Henle tubules or Henle loop); and identification of many important structures of the brain. He was also the first to demonstrate that urinary casts originated in the kidney, in 1844.

Henle Loop Looped portion of the uriniferous tubule described by German histologist, Friedrich Gustave Jacob Henle, in 1841.

Henna [Arabic: *hinna*, henna] Dried, powdered leaves of the plant, *Lawsonia inermis*, are used as hair dye. Cultivated in Sidjilmasa in the southeastern province of Morocco in the 12th century. Leaves were used to treat jaundice, leprosy, smallpox and skin affections. The Egyptians prepared an oil from it to make limbs supple.

Henoch, Eduard Heinrich (1820–1910) Pupil of Johann Lucas Schönlein (1793–1864) and pioneer of pediatrics in Germany. He was born, educated and worked in Berlin. His book *Lectures on Diseases of Children, A Handbook for Physicians and Students*, published in 1882, is said to have initiated the modern concept of pediatrics. He described Henoch–Schönlein purpurea in 1863.

Henoch–Schönlein Purpura Purpuric eruption without thrombocytopenia. First described by Johann Lucas Schönlein (1793–1864) in 1837. Heinrich Henoch, a pupil of Schönlein, gave a classic description of the disease, including its renal involvement, in 1863.

Henry I (876–936) He and his wife, Queen Maud, founded St Giles Hospital for lepers at Holborn in London. He established four other hospitals: Hospital of St John the Evangelist at Cirencester, Hospital of Holy Innocents near Lincoln, St Bartholomew Hospital at Oxford, and Hospital of St Mary Magdalen at Newcastle-on-Tyne.

Henry II (1132–1189) Introduced regulations to control public stews in England in 1161. Credited with the King's Touch for cure of scrofula.

Henry VI (1421–1471) Revived the practice of King's Touch for cure of scrofula and issued figures of golden angels as touch pieces. Chartered the Guild of Barbers of Ireland in 1446.

Henry VIII (1491–1546) Founded the regius professorship of medicine at Cambridge in 1546 and gave charter to the Royal College of Physicians in 1518.

Henry, Arnold Kirkpatrick (1886–1962) Dublin surgeon who later moved to London. Described an operation in 1938 for femoral hernia through a midline extraperitoneal approach. Also devised the posterior approach (Henry ganglionectomy) for excision of thoracic sympathetic ganglia and the sympathetic trunk.

Henry, William (1774–1836) Manchester physician and chemist who in 1803 proposed the law that the mass of a gas dissolved in a liquid is directly proportional to the pressure (Henry Law). He studied at Edinburgh University, was elected FRS in 1809, and awarded the Copley Medal in the same year.

Henschel, August (1790–1856) Professor of medicine at Breslau and medical historian. He edited *The Janus* from 1846 to 1851, the first journal devoted to the history of medicine.

Hensen, Christian Andreas Viktor (1835–1924) German physiologist and pioneer in the study of hearing whose father was director of the local school for the deaf and dumb. Born in Kiel, he studied medicine at Würzburg and then Berlin, and became professor of physiology at Kiel in 1868. He studied the morphology of the cochlea, describing the Hensen duct and Hensen supporting cells. He also wrote two studies on hearing which were published in 1880 and 1902. Hensen was a keen marine biologist and gave the name 'plankton' to microscopic marine flora.

Hensing, Friedrich Wilhelm (1719–1745) Professor of anatomy at the University of Giessen who wrote *De Peritonaeo* when he was only 23 years old. The phrenicocolic ligament of the spleen is mentioned for the first time in this treatise.

Heparin [Greek: *hepar*, liver] Anticoagulant compound first isolated from dog liver in 1916 by Jay McLean (1890–1957) of America, while still a student. A similar substance from brain, heart and liver tissue was accidentally isolated by William Henry Howell (1860–1945) in 1919. He was studying thromboplastic substances and named the new compound 'heparin' since it was first isolated from liver. It was used as an anticoagulant in 1938 by Canadian physician Charles Herbert Best (1899–1978), of insulin fame. An

important article, *Heparin: A Review of its Chemistry, Physiology, and Clinical Applications*, was presented by M. F. Mason in the *Journal of Surgery* in 1939. The loss of bone substance leading to spontaneous fractures secondary to long-term therapy with heparin was first shown by G.C. Griffith (b 1898) and colleagues in 1965.

Hepatitis B (HBV) Virus responsible for serum hepatitis was first shown to be present in some batches of human pooled serum by Frederick Ogden MacCallum and Dennis John Bauer (b 1914) in 1944. They demonstrated this by injecting the serum into human volunteers. MacCallum first referred to the virus as B, in order to compare it with the virus of infectious hepatitis (virus A). A previously unknown lipoprotein was detected in 1964 in the serum of Australian Aborigines by Baruch Samuel Blumberg (b 1925), an American biochemist and Nobel Prize winner from New York, while he was looking for genetic markers for hepatitis in the sera of people belonging to different races. This new lipoprotein was named Australia Antigen and Blumberg developed a vaccine, now in widespread use. Four years later Alfred M. Prince of New York Blood Center observed the same lipoprotein in patients with hepatitis B and renamed it, hepatitis B surface antigen. The first clinical trials for prevention of hepatitis B with vaccine produced from yeast commenced in 1984. The genetic code for the B surface antigen was discovered in 1981, and led to the production of the first genetically engineered vaccine approved by the US Food and Drugs Administration in 1986.

Hepatitis [Greek: *hepar*, liver + *itis*, inflammation] *See viral hepatitis.*

Hepatolenticular Degeneration Familial liver disease accompanied by cirrhosis and involuntary movements, caused by a disorder in copper metabolism. First described by Friedrich Theodor von Frerichs (1819–1885) in 1860. Samuel A. K. Wilson (1877–1937) described it in 1912 and it is sometimes known as Kinnier Wilson disease. *See subcortical dementia.*

Hepatorenal Syndrome [Greek: *hepar*, liver; Latin: *renalis*, kidney] Association of liver pathology with changes in the kidney in cases of infectious jaundice was first observed by German physician, Emanuel Aufrecht (1844–1933). One of the first accounts was given by S.S. Lichtman and A.R. Sohval in *Clinical disorders with associated hepatic and renal manifestations with especial reference to so-called, hepatorenal syndrome*, in 1937. A review of the subject was given by A.O. Wilensky in 1939.

Heraclides of Tarentum Physician from the school of

Herophilus who lived around 75 BC. He wrote a work on dietetics in dialogue form entitled *Symposium*. He left behind five books on pharmacology and two treatises each on external and internal disorders.

Heraclitus of Ephesus (540–475 BC) Philosopher who proposed that fire and water were fundamental to the balance of the world which was in a state of perpetual flux. He explained breathing as a regular alternation between the proportions of elements within an organ. He is said to have left Ephesus and lived in the mountains on herbs and roots, up to the age of 60. He was known as the weeping philosopher due to his habit of weeping at the follies of his fellow men.

Herbal Medicine [Latin: *herba*; a seed plant without woody stem] First form of remedy used by primitive medical men and witch doctors. A Chinese herbal drug *Ma Huang*, now known to contain the nerve stimulant ephedrine was used 5000 years ago. The Chinese Emperor Shen Nung (2800 BC) listed 365 herbal remedies in his great herbal, *Pen Tsoa*. Galen (129–200 BC) proposed 347 herbs for treatment of diseases. Australian Aborigines were familiar with various herbal remedies, including purgatives, emetics, narcotics, aphrodisiacs, and aromatics. By at least 400 BC, Susruta, the Brahmin physician described over 1000 diseases and 700 medicinal herbs in the *Susruta Samitha*. Dioscorides (*c* AD 40–90), a Greek physician of Anarzaba who lived during the reign of Nero, described over 600 plants in his five books on materia medica. Nicholas Praepositus of Salerno wrote *Antidotarium*, a book mainly on herbal treatment in the 12th century. Aztecs in central America practiced a high standard of medicine combined with a full array of herbal remedies before the Spanish conquest in the sixteenth century. Their city, Tenochtitlan, known as Mexico City today, had pharmacies which listed over 1000 herbal medicines. The most well-known British herbalist, Nicholas Culpepper (1616–1654), was also a physician and astrologer and wrote his *Herbal* in 1649, which ran into numerous editions over two centuries. The transition from herbal medicine to scientific pharmacology started with the discovery of alkaloid extracts from plants in the 19th century. The alkaloids cinchona and quinine were extracted from Peruvian bark (*Cinchona succirubra*) by P.J. Pelletier (1788–1842) and J.B. Caventou (1793–1877) of Paris in 1820, as well as opium. Ephedrine, one of the earliest known alkaloids was extracted from *Ephedra vulgaris* by Nagajosi Nagai (1844–1929) in 1887.

Herbart, Johann Friedrich (1776–1844) Psychologist from Oldenburg who trained in Jena. Pioneer in the application

of psychology to education, and professor of philosophy at Göttingen in 1803. He wrote, *The Aesthetic Presentation of the Universe, the Chief Aim of Education,* followed by *Science of Education, Outlines of Educational Doctrine* and several other works.

Hereditary Cerebellar Ataxia [Latin: *cerebrum*, brain; Greek *a + taxis*, order] Disease of late childhood involving lack of coordination. First described by Pierre Marie (1853–1940) of Paris in 1893.

Hereditary Disease [Latin: *hereditas*, inheritance] The first scientific study was done by British physician, Joseph Adams (1756–1818) and described in *A Treatise on the Supposed Hereditary Properties of Diseases* (1814). Genes were first suggested to be carriers of heredity in 1902 by Cannon (1871–1945) and Walter Stanborough Sutton (1877–1916), both American physicians. The first person to point out the heritable nature of specific diseases such as alkaptonu-ria was Archibald Garrod (1857–1936), a physician at St Bartholomew's Hospital and the Hospital for Sick Children at Great Ormond Street. In 1902 he observed the frequency of alkaptonuria in the progeny of a first cousin by marriage and proposed that the defect was inherited according to Mendel's laws. The first implantation of a human gene for hereditary disease, into mice, was performed by Rudolf Jaenisch and co-workers in 1988. Their achievement opened possibilities for genetic engineering.

Hereditary Hemorrhagic Thrombasthenia [Greek: *haima*, blood + *rhegnymi*, to burst forth + *thrombos*, clot + *asthenia*, weakness] Recurrent bleeding due to defective blood platelets. *See Glanzmann syndrome.*

Heredity [Latin: *hereditas*, inheritance] Term introduced by Herbert Spencer (1820–1903) in 1863. Gregor Mendel's (1822–1884) work on hybridization and the laws of genetics (1865), went unnoticed for over 35 years until William Bateson (1861–1920) translated it as *Mendel's Principles of Heredity* (1902). Sir Francis Galton (1822–1911), founded the science of eugenics and published *Hereditary Genius* (1869) and *Natural Inheritance* (1889) and endowed a chair in eugenics at London University. Germ plasm was named and described by German biologist, August Friedrich Leopold Weismann (1834–1914) of Jena in 1892. Weismann also proposed that it was present in chromosomes. These were shown to be paired by Walter Stanborough Sutton (1877–1916) of New York, who also suggested that they were carriers of heredity. Sex-linked inheritance was demonstrated by the American, Thomas Hunt Morgan (1866–1945), working on *Drosophila* fly in 1910. The first scientific study on the hereditary nature of disease was done by Joseph Adams (1756–1818) in 1814.

The terms 'haploid' and 'diploid' to describe halving and doubling of chromosome numbers were given by German botanist, Eduard Adolf Strasburger (1844–1912) in 1884. The ultimate proof for the chromosome theory of heredity was provided by American geneticist, Barbara McClintock (1902–1992) of Connecticut, through her experiments on maize. *See chromosomes, genetics, hereditary disease.*

Hering, Heinrich Ewald Jr (1866–1948) Born in Vienna and educated in Prague where he became professor of general and experimental pathology. Just before World War 1 he became director of the Institute of Pathological Physiology at Cologne. He studied physiology and pathology of the heart and great vessels and was the first (1903) to describe the irregular pulse as auricular fibrillation. He described the branch of the glossopharyngeal nerve to the carotid sinus and body and its function in 1924.

Hering, Karl Ewald Konstantin (1834–1918) Father of H.E. Hering and German physiologist at Leipzig. Described Hering–Breuer reflex in 1868 while working with Breuer.

Hering–Breuer Reflex Neurogenic reflex arising in the lung and controlling the rate and depth of respiration via the vagus nerve. Described by Austrian psychiatrist, Josef Breuer (1842–1925) and Karl Ewald Hering (1834–1918) in 1868.

Herman, George Ernest (1849–1914) Eminent gynecologist and obstetrician from Kilwarlin, Ireland who worked at the London Hospital.

Herman, John (1738–1800) Strasburg physician, appointed as professor of pathology in 1782 and in 1784 he was appointed professor of materia medica. He published several works on botany, medicine, surgery, and philosophy.

Herman, Paul (1646–1695) Physician to the Dutch East India Company settlers in Sri Lanka. His *Museum Zeylanicum* was used by Linnaeus (1707–1778) in his publication on taxonomy of the flora of Sri Lanka. He returned to Europe and served as professor of botany at Leiden.

Hermaphrodite [Greek: *Hermaphroditus,* son of Hermes and Aphrodite] He was courted by a nymph who failed to win his affections. The nymph eventually appealed to the gods who intervened and united them while retaining the characteristics of each of their sexes.

Hermes Trismegistus Ancient priest and philosopher in Egypt, considered as the father of the mystic sciences of the Alexandrian School and alchemy. The details of his life are not known.

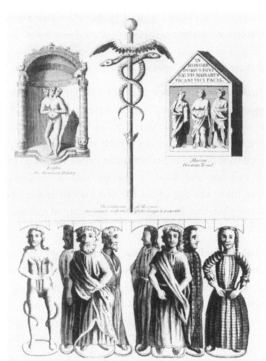

Caduceus of Hermes. Thomas Maurice, *Indian Antiquities* (1794). W. Richardson, London

Hernia Humoralis Condition caused by swelling of the testis usually following gonorrhea, described by John Hunter (1728–1793).

Hernia Term first used by Aulus Cornelius Celsus (25 BC–AD 50) to denote a protrusion of part of the gut through an abnormal opening in the abdominal cavity or wall. Herniotomy for strangulated hernia was first performed in 1556 by French Huguenot surgeon, Pierre Franco (c. 1500–1561) from Provence. One of the early scientific monographs, *Traite des Hernies,* was written by the Italian anatomist Antonio Scarpa (1752–1832) in 1814. Astley Cooper (1768–1841) and Percivall Pott (1714–1788) also wrote comprehensively on the subject. *See femoral hernia.*

Hero (c 100 BC) Scientist in Alexandria who constructed a surveying instrument called a dioptra, as well as inventing a steam turbine. The latter was rediscovered 2100 years later by Swedish Engineer, de Laval. The concept of the air thermometer was also proposed by Hero.

Heroin Derived from poppy, *Papaver somniferum.* Alkaloid obtained from morphine, diacetyl-morphine, formerly used for cough relief, now known as highly narcotic, was described by Heinrich Dreser of the Bayer Chemical Works in Germany in 1898. He named the compound 'heroin' to highlight its heroic discovery.

Herophilus (355–280 BC) Born in Chalcedon in Asia Minor, he studied medicine under Praxagorus of Cos, and rose to fame as a teacher and physician in Alexandria. He was a pioneer in the study of anatomy during the Hellenistic period and wrote a three volume anatomy treatise. He also wrote a book on eyes titled *Periophthalmon*, and another on midwifery. Herophilus was one of the first to describe the brain including its ventricles and meninges and to understand the connection between brain and nerves. He distinguished between veins and arteries, noting that only arteries contained a pulse.

Herpes Genitalis [Greek: *herpein*, to creep] One of the first descriptions was given by Thomas Bateman (1778–1821), surgeon and dermatologist from Whitby, Yorkshire in *A Practical Synopsis of Cutaneous Diseases*, published in 1813. The recurrent nature of the disease was pointed out by another Yorkshireman, Sir Jonathan Hutchinson (1828–1913) in 1887.

Herpes Zoster [Greek: *herpein*, to creep] Caused by varicella zoster virus. The first suggestion that herpes zoster was spread along a nerve was made by Richard Bright (1789–1858) in 1831. Jonathan Hutchison (1778–1821) later thought that the disease was caused by arsenic. The involvement of the Gasserian ganglion in herpes zoster of the face was described by Friederich von Barensprung (1822–1864) in 1861. The occurrence of chicken pox following exposure to cases of herpes zoster was first observed by Janos von Bókay (1858–1937) of Germany in 1892. The virus from the human skin in herpes lesions was grown on the chorioallantois membrane of chicks by Ernest Goodpasture (1886–1960) and Anderson in 1921.

Herrick, James Bryan (1861–1954) Physician and cardiologist, born in Oakpark, Illinois and obtained his MD from Rush Medical College in 1888. He described the clinical features of sudden coronary artery occlusion in 1912. He also gave the first description of sickle-cell anemia in 1910.

Herring, Percy Theodore (1872–1967) Succeeded James Bell Pettigrew (1834–1908) as professor of physiology at St Andrew's University in 1908. He showed the spinal origin of cervical sympathetic nerves in 1903. Herring bodies in the posterior lobe of the hypophysis, thought to be derived from the basophilic cells of the anterior lobe, were named after him.

Hershey, Alfred Day (b 1908) American virologist, born at Owosso, Michigan. Pioneer in the study of the bacteriophage, and set up the Phage Group with Salavador Luria (1912–1991) and Max Delbrück (1906–1981) for using the viral infective agent as an experimental tool. His work with Martha Chase in the early 1950s was one of the first to suggest that DNA was a genetic material rather than protein, using experimentally labeling protein and DNA of phage particles with different markers. In 1969 Hershey, Luria and Delbrück shared the Nobel Prize for Physiology or Medicine.

Herter, Christian Archibald (1865–1910) Born in Glenville, Connecticut, he was a metabolist and pathologist in New York. He described infantilism due to chronic intestinal infection (Herter disease) in 1908. He published studies of experimental myelitis (1889) and chemical pathology (1902). Founder of the *Journal of Biological Chemistry* (1905). He was invited to be the first director of the Rockefeller Institute of Medical Research but was unable to take up the position as he was suffering from myasthenia gravis.

Hertwig, Carl Wilhelm Theodor Richard (1850–1937) Embryologist at Jena who proposed the coelom theory with Oscar Wilhelm August Hertwig (1849–1922) in 1881. He also described the skew deviation of the eyes seen in acute cerebellar lesions (Hertwig–Magendie syndrome).

Hertwig, Oscar Wilhelm August (1849–1922) Professor of anatomy in Jena and Berlin. In 1886 he described the cells at the roots of teeth responsible for the formation of enamel. He also demonstrated that fusion of the nuclei of ovum and spermatozoa was essential for fertilization. He studied nuclear transmission of hereditary characteristics and effects of radioactivity on germ cells.

Hertz (Hurst), Sir Arthur Frederick (1879–1944) Physician at Guy's Hospital who wrote *The Sensibility of Alimentary Canal* in 1911. In 1922 he described 'dumping syndrome' following gastroenterostomy.

Herxheimer Reaction Karl Herxheimer (1861–1944) was a German dermatologist. He died of dysentery and starvation in a Nazi concentration camp. *See Jarsich–Herxheimer reaction.*

Hery, Thierry de (1500–1559) French physician who wrote a treatise on syphilis (1552) in which he recommended guaiacum from resin of the *Guaiacum* tree to be taken internally, or mercury for injection or fumigation.

Heschel, Richard Ladislaus (1824–1881) Professor of anatomy at Olmutz who described the transverse gyri of temporal lobes in 1855.

Hess Test Used to detect capillary fragility with the help of sphygmomanometer cuff to raise venous pressure. Devised by New York physician, Alfred Fabian Hess (1875–1933).

He divided his time between the Rockefeller Institute and the Babies Hospital at Bellevue. He showed that rubella was caused by a virus and wrote books on scurvy and rickets.

Hess, Walther Rudolf (1881–1973) Swiss physiologist who graduated from Zurich in 1906. After giving up his initial career in ophthalmology in 1917, he became director of the Physiology Institute at Zurich where he researched hemodynamics. He commenced studies on the brain in 1925, and was the first to apply small electrodes to various parts of the brain in order to study its functions. By stimulating the hypothalamus he demonstrated that it caused changes in temperature, sleep, sexual arousal and emotional states. He shared the Nobel Prize for Physiology or Medicine with Egas Moniz (1874–1955) for his work on the brain control mechanisms, in 1949.

Hesse, Walther (1846–1911) German bacteriologist at Berlin who studied the biological nature and content of air. His wife, Fanny Eilshemius Hesse, introduced agar as a better alternative to gelatin, for culturing bacteria in the laboratory, in 1883.

Hesselbach Triangle Anatomical area bounded by the inferior epigastric artery, the margin of the rectus abdominis, and the inguinal ligament. First described by Franz Casper Hesselbach (1759–1816), professor of surgery at Würzburg in 1806.

Heterozygote [Greek: *heteros*, other + *zygoos*, yoked] Having different allelic genes at one or more locus. Described and named by William Bateson (1861–1926) in 1902.

Hetrazan or diethylcarbamazine Drug effective against filarial infection. Discovered by Reginald Irving Hewitt in 1947.

Heubner–Herter Disease Infantile celiac disease. *See Heubner, J.O.L., Herter, C.A.*

Heubner, Johan Otto Leonhard (1843–1926) German professor of pediatrics at Berlin and Leipzig. He investigated infant nutrition and warned against prolonged sterilization of milk. He isolated meningococci from cerebrospinal fluid in 1896. He described syphilitic endarteritis of cerebral vessels and the infantile form of idiopathic steatorrhoea.

Heurnius, John (1543–1601) Born in Utrecht, professor of medicine at Leiden. He wrote commentaries on the works of Hippocrates.

Heurteloup, Charles Louis Stanislaus (1793–1864) French surgeon in Paris who designed a lithotrite in 1833.

Hevesy, Georg Charles von (1885–1966) Hungarian chemist and, later, professor of chemistry at Stockholm (during World War ll). He pioneered work on radioisotopes with Bohr (1885–1962) and Rutherford (1871–1937). He demonstrated, using lead and phosphorus tracers, that body tissues such as bone existed in a dynamic state giving up and taking in atoms. Hevesy's research led to the application of radioisotopes in medicine and he was awarded the Nobel Prize for Chemistry in 1943.

Hevin, Prudent (1715–1789) Surgeon in Paris who wrote *Pathologie Chirugica* and a memoir on strange substances in the esophagus.

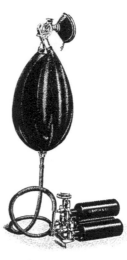

Hewitt's anesthetic apparatus for gas and oxygen. C. C. Choyce, *A System Of Surgery* (1923). Cassell and Co., London

Hewitt, Sir Frederick William (1857–1916) A pioneer in anesthetics. Educated at the Merchant Taylor's School and Christ College, Cambridge. He graduated from St George's Hospital and served as physician to the Charing Cross Hospital, National Dental Hospital and the London Hospital. He designed the first portable apparatus for administering a mixture of nitrous oxide and oxygen for dental and other short operations, in 1886. He returned to St George's Hospital as an anesthetist in 1902 and designed a dental prop and an airway in 1906. In 1893 he wrote *Anaesthetics and their Administration.*

Hewson, William (1739–1774) British hematologist who showed the role of fibrinogen in clotting of blood in 1771. He found that leukocytes first arise from lymphatic glands and the thymus. He isolated coaguable lymph from blood, defined many properties of erythrocytes and recommended paracentesis of air for correction of pneumothorax.

Hey Groves, Ernest William (1871–1944) Born in Bristol and qualified from St Bartholomew's hospital in 1895. After a brief period as a general practitioner in Bristol, he became general surgeon to the infirmary there in 1903. He practiced orthopedic surgery and wrote *Methods and Results of Transplantation of Bone in Repair of Defects caused by Injury or Disease*, which earned him the Jacksonian Prize of the Royal College of Surgeons in 1916. He founded the *British Journal of Surgery* in 1913, and was professor of surgery at Bristol in 1922.

Hey, William (1736–1819) Contemporary of John Hunter (1728–1793) at St George's Hospital. He returned to his home in Leeds in 1759 where he practiced as a surgeon and founded the Medical School. He was one of the founders of Leeds Infirmary. He gave the first description of the falciform ligament (Hey ligament) of the saphenous opening in 1803.

Heymans, Corneille Jean François (1892–1968) French–Belgian physiologist who served as the director of the Institute of Pharmacology and Therapeutics in Gent. He developed the experimental method of cross circulation in anesthetized dogs, and proved that the aorta and carotid arteries had specialized cells which responded to changes in blood pressure and blood chemicals. He was awarded the Nobel Prize in Physiology or Medicine in 1938 for his work.

Hiatus Hernia [Latin: *hiare*, to gape] A description, *Account of a Remarkable Misplacement of the Stomach*, was published by Richard Bright (1789–1858) in the *Guy's Hospital Reports* of 1836. An account of *Thoracic Stomach* was given by C.G. Lyons in 1930. Extensive studies were done by S.W. Harrington in America in 1940, and he presented the largest series of 430 patients who underwent surgical treatment. The transformation of the mucosa of the esophagus into columnar epithelium due to esophagitis was first described by Norman R. Barret (1903–1979) in 1950 and known as Barret epithelium.

Hibbs, Russel Aubra (1869–1933) Born in Kentucky, he was an orthopedic surgeon at the New York Orthopedic Hospital. He described the first spinal fusion operation in 1911 and also designed a frame (Hibbs frame) used for application of plaster in the treatment of spinal scoliosis.

Hiccup [French: *hocquet*, hicket] The Greeks considered hiccup to be a convulsive sob, and Plato (*c* 428–348 BC) and others described treatment. Hippocrates (*c* 460–377 BC) advised gargling with water and tickling the nose to induce sneezing in order to stop the hiccup. According to Galen (AD 129–200) it is caused by irritation of the stomach leading to its violent reaction, and he suggested sneezing as a cure. Aetius, around AD 600, considered inflammation of

the stomach and its surrounding parts as the cause, and prescribed emetics and opium. Venesection was recommended as a cure by Alexander of Trailles (AD 325–400), and many other Arab physicians. The old English term for hiccup, 'yex', means 'a sob'. It was also known as drunkard's cough and the present name came into use in the 17th century.

Hickman, Henry Hill (1800–1830) Pioneer in anesthesia, educated at Edinburgh University and practiced at Ludlow. He studied effects of inhaling carbon dioxide which enabled him to perform painless surgery on animals. He printed the first work on anesthesia in the form of *A Letter on Suspended Animation* addressed to the president of the Royal Society, Thomas Andrew Knight. Hickman's efforts to publicize his discovery, both in England and France, were ignored and he died disappointed at the age of 29.

Hicks, John Braxton (1823–1897) Obstetrician at Guy's Hospital and pioneer of midwifery. Described a combined method of internal and external podalic version in 1860. He was elected FRS in 1861. *See Braxton Hicks sign.*

Hieroglyphics System of writing from ancient Egypt using pictograms. Thought to have been invented by Athotes in 2112 BC. Pythagorus (*c* 600 BC) was the last of the ancient Greek philosophers to use them. One of the first attempts to decipher hieroglyphics was made by Jean François Champollion (1790–1832), the French founder of Egyptology. Most of the Egyptian history and culture was contained in his *Precis du Systeme Hieroglyphigue* of 1824.

Higginson Syringe A nozzle, rubber reservoir and pump used for giving enemas. Devised by Alfred Higginson (1808–1884) from Stockport who became surgeon to Liverpool Southern Hospital in 1857. He retired in 1867.

Highmore, Nathaniel (1613–1685) Born in Hampshire, and graduated in medicine from Oxford in 1641, before practicing in Dorset. The maxillary antrum (illustrated in drawings by Leonardo Da Vinci) was described by Highmore (antrum of Highmore) in 1651. He wrote *Corporis Humani Disquisitio Anatomicae* and several other works.

Higra The period of prophet Mohammed's flight from Mecca to Medina in AD 622 and beginning of the Mohammedan calendar. AD 640 is sometimes quoted as the start of the Mohammedan period when the Arabs burned the second library of Alexandria. Legend states that the library of Greek papyri was used by them to fuel 4,000 baths in Alexandria for a period of six months. Most of the Arab influence in medicine came after this date and lasted until about AD 1200.

Dictionary of the History of Medicine

Hilar Dance Radiological sign in chest X-ray described by C. Pezzi of America in 1925.

Hilar Lymphadenopathy [Latin: small bit + *lympha*, clear spring water; Greek. *aden*, gland + *pathos*, suffering] Later proved to be due to sarcoidosis and other causes and first described by the German, Sven Löfgren, in 1946.

Hildegard of Bingen (1098–1175) Medieval abbess from Boekelheim in Germany. She wrote several medical works including, *Physica*, describing use of plant, mineral, and animal material as medicine. She was one of the first to mention the itch-mite as a cause of scabies.

Hildenbrand, Johann Valentin von (1763–1818) Physician who gave a classic description of typhus (Hildenbrand disease) in 1810.

Hill, Archibald Vivien (1886–1977) Physiologist and early biophysicist, born in Bristol and became professor of physiology at University College London in 1923. In 1911 he measured the heat produced in a contracting or recovering muscle related to lactic acid production, using a sensitive thermocouple. He attempted to measure heat produced by a nerve in 1912, and succeeded in 1926, giving an explanation of transmission of nerve impulses based on physico-chemical equations. He served as secretary on many committees of the Royal Society, as a member of the Academic Assistance Council, and as MP for Cambridge University. Hill shared the Nobel Prize for Medicine or Physiology with Otto Fritz Meyerhof (1884–1951) in 1922. *See Hill–Meyerhof theory.*

Hill, Austin Bradford (1897–1991) Epidemiologist and statistician employed by the British Medical Research Council to gather data on occupational health and vaccine trials. His seminal work was on the relation between smoking and lung cancer.

Hill, Sir John (1716–1775) British writer and botanist from Peterborough, UK who compiled the first British flora. He set up an apothecary shop at St Martin's Lane in London, and practiced as a physician. He wrote voluminously on natural history, philosophy, medicine, astronomy and geology, including: *An Account of all those English Plants which are remarkable for their Virtues and of the Drugs which are produced by Vegetables of other Countries.*

Hill, Leonard Erskin (1866–1952) British physiologist who worked on respiratory physiology of caisson disease in 1915 at the London Hospital. Early member of the Medical Research Council (1920).

Hillary, William (1700–1763) British physician and meteorologist. He studied with Boerhaave (1668–1738) at Leiden, graduating with a dissertation on intermittent fevers. He practiced in Ripon, Bath, London and Bridgetown (Barbados). On his return from Barbados, he published *Observations on the Changes of the Air and the Concomitant Epidemical Diseases, in the Island of Barbados* which included descriptions of lead intoxication, infectious hepatitis and tropical sprue.

Hill–Meyerhof Theory Changes in cytoplasm of muscle during contraction was proposed by Archibald Vivien Hill (1886–1977) and Otto Meyerhof (1884–1951) around 1912.

Hilton, John (1804–1878) Born in Essex, performed the first operation for internal strangulation of the small intestines at Guy's Hospital in 1847. He described the nematode, *Trichinella spiralis*, and suggested its involvement in trichinosis and its parasitic nature in 1833. He published *On the Influence of Mechanical and Physiological Rest on the Treatment of Accidents and Surgical Diseases* in 1863, which became a surgical classic and continued through several editions until 1950. The white line of the anal canal described by him is known as the Hilton line.

Hilton Line *See Hilton, John.*

Himley, Karl Gustav (1772–1837) Professor of ophthalmology at Vienna. He designed an operation for iridodialysis and used hyoscyamine to dilate the pupil before the removal of the lens. He established clinical teaching in ophthalmology and founded the first journal devoted to ophthalmology with Johann Adam Schmidt (1759–1809) in 1801.

Hind–Quarter Operation Amputation of the lower limb including a part of the pelvis. First performed successfully by French surgeon, Charles Girard (1850–1916) in 1895. A new technique was described by Sir Alfred Gordon-Taylor (1874–1960) and Philip Wiles (1899–1967) of England in 1935.

Hindu Medicine *See Ayurvedic medicine.*

Hines and Brown Test Cold pressor test for detecting individuals who are susceptible to hypertension. Involves immersion of an extremity in ice water for 1 to 3 minutes causing an increase in systolic and diastolic blood pressure by 15 mmHg. Devised by two American physicians in Rochester, Minnesota, Edgar Alphonso Hines (1906–1978) and George E. Brown (1885–1935) in 1932.

Hines, Edgar Alphonso (1906–1978) American physician at the Mayo Clinic. Born in South Carolina, studied at the Medical College there and pursued graduate studies at the Mayo School. Specialized in peripheral vascular disease and hypertension. Introduced the drug thiocyanate for treatment of migraine.

Hinshelwood, Cyril Norman (1897–1967) London chemist who received his education at Balliol College, Oxford following World War l. In 1956 he shared the Nobel Prize for Chemistry with Nikolai Seminov (1896–1986) for his work on chemical kinetics of bacterial cells. He wrote *The Chemical Kinetics of the Bacterial Cell* (1946) and *Growth Function and Regulation in Bacterial Cells* (1966). He was elected FRS in 1929 and knighted in 1948.

Hinshelwood, James (1859–1919) *See dyslexia.*

Hinton, James (1827–1875) First aural surgeon to be appointed to Guy's Hospital in London. He performed the first operation for mastoiditis in England in 1868 and wrote *The Mystery of Pain* and *The Questions of Aural Surgery* in 1874.

Hip Joint Dominique Jean Larrey (1766–1842), one of the greatest military surgeons in history, performed three amputations at the hip joint: two in Egypt and one in France, around 1790. Walter Brashear (1776–1860) of Maryland was the first to perform amputation at the hip in the United States in 1806. The next successful amputation in America was carried out by Valentine Mott (1785–1865) of New York in 1827. The first osteotomy in United States for ankylosis of the hip joint was performed by John Rhea Barton (1794–1871), of Lancaster USA in 1826. The complete resection of the hip joint with creation of an artificial joint was first performed by Lewis Albert Sayre (1820–1900), an orthopedic surgeon from New Jersey in 1863. First total replacement with an artificial hip joint made of steel was developed by English surgeon, Philip Wiles (1899–1967), at the Middlesex Hospital, in 1938. An artificial femoral head for arthroplasty of the hip joint was devised by Jean and Robert Judet in 1950. Total hip replacement was performed by British orthopedic surgeon Sir John Charnley (1911–1982) of Manchester Royal Infirmary in 1961. As the long term results of a series of Charnley's artificial joints made of Teflon were unsatisfactory, Charnley started using polythene from 1962. A single assembly total prosthesis for hip replacement was first introduced by Canadian surgeon, James Ennis Bateman (b 1915) of Toronto in 1974. He also holds the honor of being the first orthopedic surgeon from Canada to obtain certification by the American Board of Orthopedics (1948). Subtrochanteric osteotomy as treatment for osteoarthritis of the hip joint was introduced by an orthopedic professor at Liverpool, T.P.C. McMurray (1887–1947), founder of the first military orthopedic center at Alder Hey in Liverpool.

Hip Replacement *See hip joint.*

Hippel, Arthur von (1841–1917) *See keratoplasty.*

Hippel, Eugen von (1867–1939) Ophthalmologist in Göttingen, Germany who gave the first description of angio-matosis of the retina (Hippel disease) in 1895.

Hippel–Lindau Disease Retinal angioma (von Hippel disease) with cerebellar angioma (Lindau disease).

Hippocampus [Greek: *hippocampus*, seahorse] Mythical Greek beast, harnessed to the chariot of Neptune. It's upper body resembled a horse and the lower half that of a dragon. Pliny (AD 23–79) used the name to refer to the sea horse. Julius Caesar Arantius (1530–1589) in 1567 was the first to apply the term hippocampus to a specific part of the brain due to its physical resemblance. Objections to the application of the term to that part of the brain were raised over the next three centuries, and in 1732 Benjamin Winslow proposed the term *cornu arietis* due its resemblance to ram's horn. A French surgeon, René Jacques Croissant de Garengeot (1688–1759) named it *cornu ammonis* in honor of the Egyptian god in 1742, and Carl W. Mayer (1795–1868) suggested *pes hippopotami* in 1799. The term hippocampus was officially adapted by Nomina Anatomica at Basel in 1895.

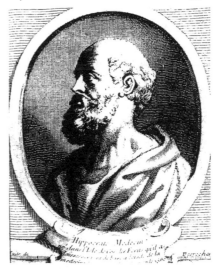

Hippocrates. Courtesy of the National Library of Medicine

Hippocrates (*c* 460–377 BC) Father of medicine, considered a direct descendant of Aesculapius. Born on the Greek island of Cos and tutored by Democritus of Abdera, and Gorgias of Leontini. First person to deliver the practice of medicine from superstition, sorcery and magic, and set it on a course of scientific thinking and observation. He taught and explained medicine in a rational manner. He diagnosed and treated fractures and dislocations, defined many physical signs including succussion splash, and advocated interventions such as paracentesis abdominis and paracentesis thoracis. Plato described Hippocrates as 'a professional trainer of medical students'. Several of Hippocrates' works still exist, some genuine and the others by his followers. His genuine works are believed to be: *The Prognostics, On Airs, etc. Acute Diseases, Book of Aphorisms, Epidemics I and III, On Articulations, On Fractures, On the Instruments of Reduction, On Ancient Medicine, On the Surgery, On Ulcers, On Fistulae, On Hemorrhoids* and *On the Sacred Disease.*

Hippocrates of Chios (460 BC) Born on the Ionian Island of Chios, a contemporary of Socrates, and founder of mathematical school at Athens. One of the first known specialists in mathematics, and solved many complex mathematical problems. He also compiled a work on *Elements of Geometry.* Not to be confused with Hippocrates of Cos.

Hippocratic Facies *See Facies Hippocratica.*

Hippocratic Oath The traditional obligation which Hippocrates (*c* 460–377 BC) imposed on his pupils, but has no traceable definite date of origin. Francis Adams (1796–1861) in his translation of Hippocratic works (1849) ranked the oath as an original treatise.

Hippuran [Greek: *hippos*, horse + *ouron*, urine] Agent in urography, introduced by Moses Swick in 1933.

Hippuric Acid Synthesis Test Benzoic acid combines with glycol in the kidney to form hippuric acid. This was used to test for renal functions by Emile Achard (1860–1944) and Chapelle of Paris in 1920.

Hippuric Acid [Greek: *hippos*, horse + *ouron*, urine] First obtained from horse urine, hence the name.

Hirsch, August (1817–1894) Professor of medicine at the University of Berlin and a medical historian. His *Handbuch der historisch-geographischen Pathologie* (1860–1864) was translated into English by Charles Creighton and published by the New Sydenham Society 1883.

Hirschberg, Julius (1843–1925) Berlin ophthalmologist who translated the work of Aetius of Amida on ophthalmology into German in 1899. He introduced the use of an electromagnet for removing foreign bodies from the eye in 1885. He also designed a test (Hirschberg test) for measuring the angle of squint.

Hirschfeld, Ludwig Moritz (1816–1876) Polish professor of anatomy at Warsaw who described the lingual branch of the facial nerve (Hirschfeld nerve) and the posterior renal sympathetic ganglion in 1866.

Hirschfeld Disease Acute rapidly progressive form of diabetes mellitus first described by German physician, Felix Hirschfeld (b 1863), in 1890.

Hirschfeld Nerve Communicating branch of the facial nerve with the glossopharyngeal nerve is named after Warsaw anatomist, Ludwig Moritz Hirschfeld (1816–1876).

Hirschsprung Disease Congenital megacolon. Danish pediatrician, Harald Hirschsprung (1830–1916) first described this in 1888 in two patients presenting with obstinate constipation and distended abdomen. Autopsy results noted enlargement of the transverse and descending colon. In 1920, A. Dalla Valle, reported the condition in two brothers in whom he found that the ganglion cells of the myenteric plexus were absent in the distal part of the dilated colon. An ingenious surgical method of recto-sigmoidectomy as treatment for the condition was devised by Orvar Swenson (b 1909) of Boston in 1948.

Hirshfield, Magnus (1868–1935) Professor of psychiatry in Berlin who is regarded as the father of medicial sexology. He promoted a medicial approach to sexual problems and founded the Institute of Sexual Sciences in Berlin. In *Sexual Anomalies and Perversions* he dealt with problems such as homosexuality, sadism and murder in a scientific manner.

Hirst Test Used to detect viruses or their corresponding antibodies. Devised by New York physician, George Keble Hirst (b 1909) in 1941. The test showed that influenza virus from an infected allantoic chick embryo agglutinated red blood cells of fowls and certain mammals.

Hirudin [Latin: *hirudo*, leech] Antithrombic substance present in salivary glands of the leech (*Hirudo*) and found to have anticoagulant properties by J. B. Haycraft in 1883. Sir Edward Mellanby (1884–1955) studied it in 1909 and showed that it contained both antithrombin and antithromboplastin. John Jacob Abel (1857–1938) of Johns Hopkins University used the leech to prevent clotting of blood during his experiments on artificial kidneys in 1910, but this method was abandoned as thousands of leeches had to be collected to produce a significant amount of anticoagulant. The anticoagulant substance in hirudin was isolated by F. Markwardt in 1957.

His, Wilhelm, Jr (1863–1934) Born in Basel but moved to Leipzig as a child. German physician, director of the first medical clinic at the Charité in Berlin in 1907. He became a German citizen and served in the army in World War 1 where he described trench fever (calling it Volhynia fever, after the district where it was observed). He had a long-standing interest in gout and diet. He described the atrioventricular bundle which conducts impulses to the heart in 1893 which bears his name.

His, Wilhelm, Sr (1831–1904) Professor of anatomy and embryologist at Basel and Leipzig. He described the special formative cells of blood vessels in 1868. He developed the microtome for cutting very thin sections of tissues in 1866, and also described the formation of allantois in the embryo. His other contributions to histology and embryology included the structure of the thymus, lymph glands, a treatise, *On the Tissues and Spaces of the Body,* and *Anatomy of the Human Embryo.*

Histamine [Greek: *histos,* tissue + *ammoniakos,* resinous gum] Depressor of amine, stimulant of gastric secretions, constrictor of bronchial smooth muscle and vasodilator. First synthesized by Adolf Windhaus (1876–1959) in 1907. A British chemist, George Barger (1878–1939) isolated histamine from ergot during his work with Henry Dale (1875–1968) in 1910. Sir Thomas Lewis (1881–1945) of University College Hospital, and Ronald Thompson Grant (1892–1989), a physician at Guy's Hospital, were the first to study the release and effect of histamine-like substances on the skin, secondary to injury in 1924. *See antihistamine.*

Histidine [Greek: *histos,* tissue] Amino acid, first isolated from protamine of sturgeon sperm by Albrecht Kossel (1853–1927), professor of physiology at Marburg in 1896, and recipient of the Nobel Prize for Physiology or Medicine in 1901.

Histocompatibility [Greek: *histos,* tissue] Antigens were demonstrated on an experimental basis by Clarence Cook Little (1888–1971), an American geneticist in 1916. The term 'histocompatibility genes' was introduced by American geneticist, George Davis Snell (b 1903) of Massachusetts during his research on the tissue transplant rejection reaction in mice in 1938. Its role in transplantation was demonstrated in 1958 by Jean Dausset (b 1916), a French immunologist from Toulouse. Dausset's discovery of the first definite antigen was responsible for the development of the procedure of tissue typing in organ transplantation. Sir Walter Fred Bodmer (b 1936), a German-born English geneticist was another well known pioneer in the study of HLA histocompatibility. The three dimensional structure of the major protein was elucidated by Jack Stromminger and Don Willy in 1987, and their understanding of the HLA molecule raised the possibility of manipulating the immune system.

Histology [Greek: *histos,* tissue + *logos,* treatise] Marcello Malpighi (1628–1694) founded the field of histology with his discoveries and description of several microscopic structures including capillaries and the epidermis. The term was coined by A.F.J.H. Meyer in 1819. The earliest histopathological study of the tissues was done (without the benefit of a microscope) by Marie François Xavier Bichat (1771–1802) of Paris in 1800. Histology was defined as 'the science of the minute structure of the organs of the animals and plants' by John Thomas Quekett (1815–1861) in 1852. The earliest book on the subject *Allgemeine Anatomia* was published by Friedrich Jacob Henley (1809–1885) in 1841. The first textbook in English was *The Microscopic Anatomy of the Human Body in Health and Disease,* published by Arthur Hill Hassall (1817–1894) in 1846. Rudolph Albert von Kollicker (1817–1905) published a further textbook, *Manual of Human Histology,* in 1852. A Czech professor of physiology at Breslau, Jan E. Purkinje (1787–1869) made his laboratory 'a cradle of histology' with several important contributions. Other notable pioneers include: Theodor Schwann (1810–1882); William Bowman (1816–1892); Edward Sharpey-Schafer (1850–1935); Salomon Stricker (1834–1898); Karl Wilhelm von Kupffer (1829–1902); Domenico Majocchi (1849–1929) and Ludwig Aschoff (1866–1942).

Histoplasma capsulatum [Greek: *histos,* tissue + *plasmein,* to mold] Fungus and causative agent of histoplasmosis. Described by American, Samuel T. Darling (1872–1925) during his service at Panama Canal zone in 1905. The fungal nature of the disease was demonstrated by W.A. de Monbreun of America in 1934.

Histoplasmosis [Greek: *histos,* tissue + *plasmein,* to mold] Infectious agent caused by inhalation of fungal spores. The first case caused by the fungus, *Histoplasma capsulatum,* was recognized at postmortem in 1905. The nature and extent of distribution of the disease was not fully known until 30 years later when the first case in the USA was diagnosed in an infant at Tennessee by Katherine Dodd (b 1892) of Vanderbilt University, Nashville. An outbreak of pneumonia due to histoplasma infection from a storm cellar occurred in Oklahoma in 1944. Although only 17 cases were recorded worldwide up to 1945, by 1960 nearly 1000 deaths have been attributed to it in America alone. The causative fungus was first isolated from soil by Chester Emmons (b 1900) in 1949.

History [Greek: *historia,* inquiry] Study of the past. Aristotle (384–322 BC) used the word in his *Historia Animalium* to mean inquiry about animals.

Hitchings, George Herbert (b 1905) American biochemist, born in Washington state and educated at the Universities of Washington and Harvard. Discovered the folic acid antagonist 2-aminopurine in 1948, the anti-malarial pyrimethamine in 1952, the anti-leukemia drug 6-mercatopurine, and the immunosuppressant azathioprine. His lab also produced the anti-AIDS drug zidovudine. He shared the Nobel Prize for Physiology or Medicine in 1988 with Sir James Black (b 1924) and Gertrude Elion (b 1918). *See oncology.*

Hittorf, Johann Wilhelm (1824–1914) German physicist and chemist. Worked on ion migration during electrolysis and determined transport numbers for electrolytes. *See Crooke's tube, radiology, X-rays, electrolysis.*

Hitzig, Julius Eduard (1838–1907) German neurologist and psychiatrist at Berlin who experimented on stimulation of the brain using dogs, and showed that stimulation of the motor cortex produced movements on the opposite side of the body. His work, published with Gustav Theodor Fritsch (1838–1891) in 1870, established neurophysiology. He was appointed professor of psychiatry at Halle in 1881, and became director of the psychiatric clinic in 1885.

HIV Human immunodeficiency virus.

HLA *See histocompatibility.*

Hoagland, Mahlon Bush (b 1921) Boston biochemist who studied medicine at Harvard, Copenhagen and Cambridge. Worked on cancer, liver regeneration and growth control. Confirmed Francis Crick's (b 1916) 'adaptor hypothesis' that protein synthesis requires an oligonucleotide carrier for each amino acid identified by an RNA transcript of the DNA codon.

Hoboken, Nicholas von (1632–1678) Qualified in medicine from Utrecht in 1662 before he became the professor of anatomy at Harderwick in 1672. He described the vessels of the umbilical cord which formed valve-like projections, in 1669.

Hoche, Alfred Erich (1865–1943) Professor of psychiatry at Strasburg in 1899. He described the septo-marginal tract in the region of the spinal cord in 1896.

Hochenegg, Julius von (1859–1940) Surgeon in Vienna who described an operation for removal of a malignant rectum through the sacral route.

HOCM *See hypertrophic cardiomyopathy.*

Hodge, Hugh Lenox (1796–1873) Born in Philadelphia and educated at the College of New Jersey (now Princeton University). He received his medical degree from the University of Pennsylvania in 1818. After establishing his practice in Philadelphia he took up obstetrics in 1832. He wrote *Diseases Peculiar to Women* (1860) in which he discussed displacement of the uterus and advocated use of

pessaries for its correction. He also designed a pessary (Hodge pessary) for holding the uterus in an antiverted position after manual correction.

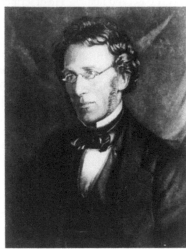

Hugh Lenox Hodge (1796–1873). Courtesy of the National Library of Medicine

Hodgen Splint Made of metal and used for treatment of fracture of the femoral shaft. Designed by a surgeon, John Thompson Hodgen (1826–1882) of St Louis, Missouri.

Hodges, Nathaniel (1629–1688) English physician who graduated from Christ Church College Oxford. He remained in London as a physician during the plague epidemic and gave an historical account, *Loimologia, or an Historical Account of the Plague in London in 1665.* This contained clinical symptoms, means of prevention and modes of treatment.

Hodgkin, Sir Alan Lloyd (b 1914) British physiologist, born in Banbury and educated at Cambridge, where he spent his whole career. Conducted research into nerve impulses in collaboration with Sir Andrew Huxley (b 1917), with whom he shared the Nobel Prize in 1963, together with Sir John Carew Eccles (b 1903). They described the mechanism by which nerves conduct electrical impulses.

Hodgkin, Dorothy Mary, neé Crowfoot (b 1910) Pioneer in the use of crystallography. Born in Cairo and educated at Somerville College, Oxford and Cambridge. With the use of a computer and X-ray crystallography, she worked out the structure of vitamin B12 in 1956, the molecular structure of penicillin in 1949, and made a detailed analysis of cholesterol. She was the third woman to receive a Nobel Prize – for Chemistry – in 1964.

Hodgkin, Thomas (1798–1866) Born in Tottenham, and graduated in medicine from Edinburgh in 1823. After studying further under Laënnec (1781–1826) in France and then Italy, he established his practice at London and was appointed demonstrator in pathology at Guy's Hospital. He introduced the stethoscope to England. The neoplastic disease (Hodgkin disease) accompanied by painless enlargement of the lymph nodes was described by him in 1832. Hodgkin also gave an account of aortic valve insufficiency in 1829, five years before Sir Dominic Corrigan (1802–1880).

Hodgkin Disease A form of (usually) fatal neoplastic disease accompanied by painless enlargement of the lymph nodes. First described by Thomas Hodgkin (1798–1866) in *On Some Morbid Appearances of the Absorbent Glands and Spleen* in 1832. The condition was named Hodgkin disease by Sir Samuel Wilks (1824–1911) in 1865. The presence of giant cells in the lymphatic glands was first noted by Theodor Langhans (1839–1915) of Germany in 1872 and Viennese pathologist, Karl Sternberg (1872–1935) in 1898. It was differentiated from lymphosarcoma by Julius Dreshfeld (1845–1907) in 1892. Rene Gilbert demonstrated a significant prolonged response to radiotherapy in patients in 1939.

Hodgson, Joseph (1788–1869) British surgeon born in Penrith and studied medicine at St Bartholomew's Hospital. He spent much of his working life in Birmingham and helped found the Birmingham Eye Infirmary. In 1815 he published *A Treatise on the Diseases of Arteries and Veins, Containing the Pathology and Treatment of Aneurysms and Wounded Arteries.*

Hofbaur Cells Histiocytes from the connective tissue of chorionic villus were described by a gynecologist from Vienna, Isford Isfred Hofbaur (1879–1961). He emigrated to the United States in 1924 and joined Johns Hopkins, later moving to Cincinnati, Ohio in 1931. Hofbaur was the first to use the extract of posterior pituitary for uterine inertia during labor.

Hoffa, Albert (1859–1908) South African-born German surgeon who designed the Hoffa method of operative treatment for congenital dislocation of the hip in 1890. Also remembered for Hoffa disease, solitary traumatic lipoma of the knee. He worked in Würzburg and Berlin and founded the first journal of orthopedic surgery.

Hoffer, Gustav (b 1887) Otorhinologist from Vienna who became professor at the University of Graz in 1932. His main research was on innervation and surgery of the larynx. He described the depressor nerve of the cardiac plexus, a branch of the superior laryngeal nerve.

Hoffmann, Caspar (1572–1648) German physician from Gotha who became professor of medicine at Altorf.

Leading authority on Galen and published a commentary of his work in 1625.

Hoffmann, Christopher Ludwig (1721–1807) Born at Rheda, Westphalia and served as physician to the Bishop of Münster and electors of Cologne.

Hoffmann, Erich (1868–1959) German dermatologist and syphilologist who worked with Fritz Schaudinn (1871–1906), a protozoologist, and prepared the serum for the historic discovery of *Treponema pallidum* in 1905.

Hoffmann, Friedrich (1660–1742) Eminent physician born in Halle and educated in Jena. He visited England in 1684 and established contact with various scientific men including Robert Boyle. On his return to Halle he was appointed professor of medicine. He published *Systema Medicinae Rationalis, Medicina Consultoria* and numerous other works.

Hoffmann, Johann (1857–1919) German neurologist at Heidelberg. Remembered for Hoffmann finger reflex – flicking the ring finger causes flexion of the forefinger and thumb. *See Werdnig–Hoffmann syndrome.*

Hoffmann, Mauricius (1621–1698) Professor of surgery at Altdorf who described the pancreatic duct in 1661. He gave an account of the perineal muscle under the name 'compressor hemispherius' in 1674.

Hofmeister, Franz von (1867–1926) Surgeon in Stuttgart who described a method of partial gastrectomy where end-to-end anastomosis of the gastric remnant with the jejunum is made with the remnant being partly closed and used as a valve.

Holden, Luther (d 1905) Demonstrator in anatomy at St Bartholomew's Hospital. He described the crease line caused by flexion of the hip (Holden line) in 1877. He published *Human Osteology, Comprising a Description of Bones* in 1855, and *Landmarks Medical and Surgical* in 1877.

Holl, Moritz (1852–1920) Physician from Vienna who practiced surgery at Innsbruck. In 1896 he described the intercrural ligament found in front of the urinary meatus of the female.

Holland, Sir Henry (1788–1873) British physician who attended Queen Victoria and Prince Albert. He published *Medical Notes and Reflections* and several other works.

Holland, Philemon (1552–1637) Physician from Chelmsford, graduated from Cambridge and settled in Coventry. Master at the free school and published a translation of Pliny's *Natural History*, and several other works.

Holley, Robert William (b 1922) American biochemist, born in Urbana, Illinois. Member of the team which first synthesized penicillin in the 1940s. Together with Seymour Benzer (b 1921) he identified two leucyl transfer RNAs and proposed that they may form the basis for degeneracy of the amino acid code suggested by Crick. Holley shared the 1968 Nobel Prize for Physiology or Medicine.

Holloway Sanatorium *See Thomas Holloway.*

Holloway, Thomas (1800c1883) Born at Devonport and received his education at Penzance. In 1836 he came to London and opened a business in Broad Street selling ointments and pills. After several serious setbacks, he finally became successful, with an income of over 50,000 pounds a year. He attended a public meeting on the issues of the mentally ill at the Freemason Hall presided over by Lord Ashley Cooper in 1861 and was moved by the plight of the insane to offer his wealth to establish a sanatorium. He employed the most eminent architects of his time, including Sir Matthew Digby Wyatt and Donaldson to build it in Flemish style. The first brick for the building at Virginia Waters, near London, was laid by Holloway in 1873 and it was completed in 1884.

Holmes, Oliver Wendell (1809–1894) Physician who preceded Semmelweis in proposing the contagious nature of puerperal fever. His paper *On the Contagiousness of Puerperal fever* presented to the Boston Medical Society in 1842, raised violent opposition. Despite this, he reiterated his views with another paper *Puerperal Fever as a Private Pestilence* in 1855. In 1846 he gave the name anesthesia to what was previously called suspended animation or etherisation. Holmes is equally known for his literary works.

Holmes–Adie Syndrome Gordon M. Holmes (1876–1965) described 19 cases of females with *partial irridoplegia associated with other diseases of the nervous system* in 1931. He also introduced the term 'tonic pupils' for the condition. An independent account of this syndrome, *Pseudo-Argyll Robertson pupils with absent tendon reflexes* was given by William John Adie (1886–1935) in the same year.

Holmes, Sir Gordon Morgan (1876–1965) Premier London clinical neurologist who was born in Dublin and educated at Trinity College. He described primary progressive cerebellar degeneration and gave an account of the function of the thalamus and its relationship to the cerebral cortex (with Sir Henry Head, 1861–1940) in 1911. He reported a case of virilism successfully treated by removal of a suprarenal tumor in 1925. He had a life-long association with the National Hospital for Nervous Diseases. He served as consulting neurologist to the British Army during World War 1 and afterwards wrote *The Spinal Injuries of Warfare*. He also

wrote *The Examination of the Nervous System*. See *Holmes–Adie syndrome.*

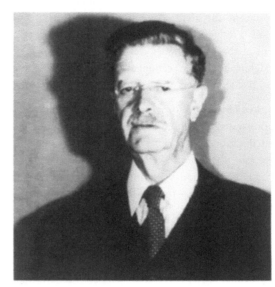

Gordon Holmes (1876–1965). Courtesy of the National Library of Medicine

Holmes Operation Operation for excision of the calcaneum was described by London surgeon, Timothy Holmes (1825–1907).

Holmgren, Alarik Frithiof (1831–1897) Physiologist at Uppsala University in Sweden, and a pioneer in the application of electrophysiology to study visual systems and the first to demonstrate retinal action currents. He devised the electroretinogram in 1865 and also developed the Holmgren test for color blindness.

Holmgren, Emile Algot (1866–1922) Professor of histology at the Royal Institute in Stockholm who described the canaliculi found within cell protoplasm in 1902.

Holt, Luther Emmet (1855–1924) American physician and a pioneer in the field of pediatrics in America. He isolated heparin (with W. H. Howell) in 1918.

Homans Sign Pain elicited in the calf on dorsiflexion of the foot in cases of deep vein thrombosis of the leg. Described by American surgeon, John Homans (1877–1954) of Johns Hopkins University who worked with Harvey Cushing (1869–1939). Homans initially worked on hypophysectomy but later changed to study peripheral vascular disease. He moved to Harvard and wrote *Textbook on Surgery*.

Home, Francis (1719–1813) Edinburgh physician who pioneered experimental inoculation against measles in 1759 and was a forerunner of the experimental approach to medicine. He was the first professor of materia medica (1768).

His work on measles, croup, diabetes and many other areas is contained in *Medical Facts and Experiments*.

Home, Sir Everard (1756–1832) A pupil of John Hunter, whose sister he married in 1771. He was surgeon at St George's Hospital, and described the median lobe of the prostate in 1806. He was a founder member of the 'assistant society' to the Royal Society which was known as the Society for the Improvement of Animal Chemistry. He published *Lectures on Comparative Anatomy, Practical Observations* and several other works.

Homeopathy [Greek: *homoios*, similar + *pathos*, suffering] In an effort to avoid side effects due to large doses of medicines, the system of homeopathy, was developed by Samuel Hahnemann (1755–1843). He postulated 'like cures like' and 'the law of infinitesimals' which advocated the use of minute doses of medicine as treatment.

Homeostasis [Greek: *homoios*, similar + *stasis*, standing] Concept of an equilibrium within the body despite changes in external environment was developed by Claude Bernard (1818–1878) in 1855. The term was coined by American physiologist, Walter Bradford Cannon (1871–1945) of Harvard University, in his *Wisdom of the Body* published in 1932.

Homo sapiens [Latin: *homo*, man + *sapiens*, wisdom] *Homo sapiens*, or modern man, followed Neanderthal man who is supposed to have lived about 25,000 years ago. However, findings of fossils in a cave in Israel by French and Israeli scientists in 1988 have suggested that modern *Homo sapiens* are at least 92,000 years old.

Homocystinuria [Greek: *homos*, similar + *kystis*, bladder + *oureon*, urine] First described as a separate entity by N.A.J. Carson and D.W. Neill in 1962. During their work they noted the metabolic abnormality in a series of backward individuals in Northern Ireland. Homocystine was first identified in urine of patients with this condition by T. Gerritsen and co-workers in the same year.

Homology [Greek: *homos*, similar + *logos*, speech] Study of similarity of structures in the same or different organisms due to their relationship of descent or development. It was described and named by Sir Richard Owen (1804–1892) in 1840.

Homonymous Hemianopia [Greek: *homos*, similar + *nomos*, name + *hemi*, half + *opsis*, sight] First demonstrated by experimental unilateral ablation of the occipital cortex in monkeys by Sharpey-Schafer (1850–1935) in 1888.

Homosexuality [Greek: *homos*, similar; Latin: *sexus*, sex] Sexual and other forms of love between two persons of the same sex has been practiced from ancient times. Homosexuality amongst the ancient Greeks and Romans was endemic. Polycrates, the Tyrant of Samos, erected a statue of his lover, a beautiful boy named Bathyllus. Sir Alexander Morrison (1779–1866), physician to the Bethlem Hospital, considered the condition to be a mental disease. John Gideon Millingen (1782–1862) physician to Middlesex Pauper Lunatic Asylum at Hanwell pointed out the guilt complex of the monomaniac which led to suicidal attempts. The word was first used by Hungarian physician, Bankert, in a small booklet in 1869. Carl Heinrich Ulrichs wrote several books on homosexuality in 1850, and coined the term 'uranism' to denote it. *See lesbianism*.

Homozygote [Greek: *homos*, similar + *zygotos*, yolk] Zygote developed from the union of gametes identical in quality, quantity and arrangement of their genes. First described and named by William Bateson (1861–1926) in 1902.

Hook Worm Disease Caused by a parasitic intestinal nematode. *See Ancylostoma duodenale*.

Hooke, Robert (1635–1703) Pioneer microscopist, born at Freshwater on the Isle of Wight. He became the first curator of experiments at the Royal Society of London, and first to demonstrate artificial respiration in 1667. He kept animals alive by blowing air through their lungs with bellows. The first description of the compound microscope was given by Hooke in 1667, and he was the first to adopt the term 'cell' to denote compartments which he observed in cork tissue under the microscope in 1665. He wrote one of the masterpieces of the age, *Micrographia, or Philosophical Descriptions of Minute Bodies made by Magnifying Glasses, with Observations and Inquiries thereupon*, published in 1655. He also designed the Bethlem Hospital at Moorfields which opened in 1676.

Hoover, Charles Franklin (1865–1927) Born in Cleveland, graduated from Harvard. A physician who investigated pulmonary and hepatic disease and the ventilatory functions of the diaphragm. He described Hoover sign where pressure on one leg caused slight lifting movement of the other leg in cases of paralysis of lower limbs. This sign was also used to distinguish organic hemiplegia from malingering or hysteria.

Hope, James (1801–1841) Born in Cheshire, he spent 5 years in Edinburgh studying medicine, followed by a year at St Bartholomew's Hospital and a period in Paris studying with Chromel. While in Paris he learned about auscultation and pathological anatomy. On his return to England he took up a position at St George's Hospital in London. He was elected to the Royal Society at 31 for his monograph on cardiac disease and morbid anatomy. His best known work was *A Treatise on the Diseases of the Heart and Great Vessels*, in which he described what is now known as Hope murmur. He died from tuberculosis at the early age of 40.

Hope, John (1725–1786) Edinburgh naturalist and physician. Director of the Botanical Gardens and a professor of botany in his native city.

Hope Murmur Apical systolic murmur of mitral incompetence. Described by James Hope (1801–1841).

Hopkins, Sir Frederick Gowland (1861–1947) Born in Eastbourne, he is widely regarded as the father of British biochemistry. He was a self-taught chemist who matriculated in technical chemistry from University College, London at the age of 20. He then studied medicine at Guy's Hospital and worked there with Garrod for 15 years. He moved to Cambridge University in 1898 to teach and research chemical physiology, later becoming chair of biochemistry. The first amino acid, tryptophane, was discovered by him and Sydney William Cole (1877–1952) in 1901. The additional dietary factors required to maintain health were first observed by Hopkins in 1906, and named 'accessory food factors'. Glutathione, an oxygen carrier and hydrogen acceptor in cellular respiration, was isolated by him in 1921. He also studied the effects of lactic acid accumulation in muscle fatigue, precipitation of uric acid with ammonium chloride and, together with Eijkman (1858–1930), he was awarded the Nobel Prize for Biochemistry in 1929 for his work on vitamins.

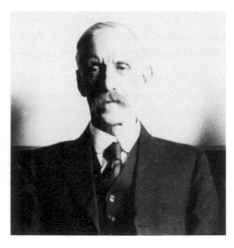

Sir Frederick Gowland Hopkins (1861–1947). Courtesy of the National Library of Medicine

Hopkins, Lemuel (1750–1801) American physician and satirist from Waterbury, Connecticut. He received his training in the form of an apprenticeship but was later awarded an honorary degree from Yale. He introduced the antiphlogistic regimen in the treatment of febrile diseases. He had a familial history of tuberculosis and spent much time studying and treating this. He was also an early advocate of fresh air, wholesome food and exercise.

Hoppe, Hermann Henry (1867–1929) American neurologist, born of German-American parents in Cincinnati. He described myasthenia gravis in 1892. After obtaining his degree in Ohio, he went to study with von Recklinghausen (1833–1910) in Strasburg and Oppenheim (1858–1919) in Berlin before returning to Cincinnati in 1892 and later becoming professor of the Neurology Department.

Hoppe–Seyler, Ernst Felix Emanuel (1825–1895) German physiological chemist who received his medical training in Halle, Leipzig and Berlin. He worked with Virchow (1821–1902) in Berlin and later moved to Tübingen. He obtained hemoglobin in a crystalline form in 1864, and showed that oxygen is released and that hemin is the hydrochlorate of hematin. He quantified the volume of oxygen bound to hemoglobin. He also named it. He wrote a four-volume *Textbook on Physiological Chemistry* which became the standard for its time. He studied blood, urine and bile pigments and isolated cholesterol and lecithin from blood. He was appointed professor of physiological chemistry at Strasburg in 1872 and founded the first biochemical journal *Zeitschrift für physiologische chemie* in 1877.

Hormone Replacement Therapy (HRT) The effect of estrogen therapy in preventing atherosclerosis and osteoporosis in postmenopausal women was first pointed out by Morris E. Davis in 1965. In 1938 Edward Dodds (1899–1973) discovered stilboestrol, a non-steroid estrogen which revolutionized HRT. In the 1920s transplanted ape testicles were used to rejuvenate aging men. Later, antrosterone was discovered and used therapeutically. This was followed by testosterone in 1935.

Hormone Treatment in Cancer *See Huggins, Charles Brenton.*

Hormones [Greek: *hormon*, to rouse] Théophile de Bordeu (1722–1776), a physician from Bern, was the first to suggest that the internal secretions of testis and ovary had remote and overall effect on the organism in his *Recherches sur Glandes* published in 1746. Albrecht von Haller (1708–1777), also of Bern, described thyroid, thymus and spleen as glands without ducts, pouring special substances into the blood. The first evidence of a humoral substance which produced an effect on a site or organ remote to its origin was presented by Arnold Berthhold (1801–1863) in 1849. He transplanted testis to a rooster which previously had its testis removed and demonstrated normal resumption of male sexual characteristics. In 1889, Brown-Séquard (1817–1863) quoted an elderly man who improved his health and vigor by self-injecting testicular extracts. Oliver (1860–1915) and Sharpey-Schafer (1866–1927) in 1894 showed that injections of adrenal extracts elevated blood pressure. Bayliss (1860–1924) and Starling (1866–1927), in their legendary works of 1902, obtained a substance from the intestinal mucous membrane which had an action on the pancreas. They named it 'secretin' and coined the term 'hormone', to denote other similar substances. Insulin, discovered by Banting (1891–1941) and Best (1899–1978), was the first genetically engineered hormone to be commercially marketed in the 1970s and it was followed by growth hormone in 1985. *See ductless glands, internal secretions.*

Horne, Johannes van (1621–1670) Son of John Heurnius, professor of surgery in Amsterdam. He published *Observationes anatomico-medicae* in 1664, in which he gave one of the earliest descriptions of the thoracic duct.

Horner, William Elmonds (1793–1853) Born in Warrenton, Virginia, he was professor of anatomy at the University of Pennsylvania. He described the small muscles at the internal commisure of the eyelids (muscle of Horner) in 1824. He prepared the first treatise in America on pathological anatomy, *A Treatise on Pathological Anatomy*, in 1829.

Horner Syndrome Condition of ophthalmoplegia, meiosis, enophthalmos, and anhidrosis due to a lesion interrupting the cervical sympathetic pathway. First described by Claude Bernard (1813–1878) of Paris in 1863. Johann Friedrich Horner (1832–1886), professor of neurology at Zurich, described ptosis and other features of the syndrome in 1869.

Horoscope [Greek: *hora,* hour + *skopos,* observer]

Horse The first work on anatomy of the horse was published by Carlo Ruini (1530–1598) in 1598. It was the first monograph on a single species other than man. It contained a description of the lesser (pulmonary) circulation and laid the foundation for modern veterinary medicine. The first book in England on the anatomy of the horse was written by Andrew Snape in 1683. Another accurate and original work on equine anatomy was published by George Stubbs (1724–1806) in 1744.

Horsley, Sir Victor Alexander Haden (1857–1916) Founder of neurosurgery in Britain. Born in London and received his medical degree from University College. In 1886 he proved that myxedema and cretinism are due to thyroid deficiency. Horsley also performed the first successful hypophysectomy in dogs in the same year, localized the cerebral functions, and produced the stereotactic apparatus for the accurate location of electrodes in the brain in 1908. The first successful removal of a spinal tumor was performed by him in 1887. Horsley was a great enemy of alcohol which led to the publication of *Alcohol and the Human Body.*

Horsley Wax A mixture of beeswax and almond oil having antiseptic properties and used for controlling hemorrhage from skull bones during brain surgery. Introduced by the English neurosurgeon, Sir Victor Horsley (1857–1916).

Hortega, Pio del Rio (1882–1945) Spanish neuroanatomist who graduated from Vallodid University with a thesis on tumors of nerve tissue. He moved to Madrid and worked in Cajal's (1852–1934) lab, improving staining techniques and describing centrosomes of ganglion cells, microglia and oligodendroglia. On publishing his results he came into disfavor with Cajal and was dismissed. During the Spanish Civil War he worked in Madrid, Paris and Oxford before finally settling in Buenos Aires. *See neuroglia.*

Horton Hospital In Banbury, was founded in 1872 from the legacy of Mary Ann Horton. It initially started with two wards, each with six beds, and later expanded into four wards with a total of 120 beds during World War ll. It was modernized during the mid-20th century.

Horton Disease Described by Bayard T. Horton (b 1895) of the Mayo Clinic, although should be attributed to M. Schmitt (1863–1949) who gave the original description. *See temporal arteritis.*

Horton Syndrome Headache caused by histamine. Described by American physician, Bayard Taylor Horton (b 1895).

Horus Mythical son of the Egyptian deities Isis and Osiris. Horus is considered the Egyptian equivalent of Apollo, founder of the healing arts or medicine. He fought with Set, the demon of evil and lost an eye which was replaced by miraculous means. The symbol Rx is said to represent the eye of Horus and was first used as an amulet 5000 years ago by the Egyptians. The symbol has served as the 'recipe' sign for medical prescriptions throughout the ages.

Hosack, David (1769–1835) American physician who founded the Elgin Botanic Garden in New York. He edited the *American Medical and Philosophical Register* from 1810–1814.

Hospice [Latin: *hospes,* receiver of guests] Movement which cares for the dying through pain control and dedicated nursing. Founded by Dame Cecily Mary Saunders (b 1918) from Barnet in north London. She trained at St Thomas' Hospital and the Nightingale School of Nursing and founded the St Christopher's Hospice in 1967. She received the BMA Gold medal for her work in 1987 and has published several books including *Care of the Dying* (1960) and *Management of the Terminal Disease* (1978). The Helen House, the first hospice for children in England, was opened at Oxford in 1982.

Hospital [Latin: *hospes*, receiver of guests] *See infirmaries and early hospitals.*

Hôtel Dieu or 'house of God's charity', founded in Lyons by King Childebert in AD 542. This remained an institute of excellence in caring for the sick for over a thousand years. Hôtel Dieu of Paris was founded in AD 651 by Landry, Bishop of Paris. The oldest Canadian hospital is Hôtel Dieu of Montreal, founded by a French woman, Jean Mance in 1644.

Hotz, Ferdinand Carl (1843–1909) German ophthalmologist in Chicago who described an operation for entropion.

Houel, Nicholas (1520–1585) Philanthropic industrialist from Paris who wrote *A Treatise on Plague* and *Theriacum Mithridates* which were published in 1573. He also founded an orphanage and the School of Pharmacy in Paris.

Hounsfield, Sir Godfrey Newbold (b 1919) Inventor of the CAT (computerized tomography) scanner. Born in Newark, and educated at the City and Guilds College and Faraday House College, London. After serving as a radar engineer during World War ll, he joined Thorn–EMI, and became director of medical systems research in 1972. He developed the CAT scanner for which he shared the Nobel Prize in Physiology or Medicine with Allan Cormack (b 1924) in 1979.

Houssay, Bernardo Alberto (1887–1971) Argentinian physiologist, twice dismissed from his post by government regimes, whose work on the pituitary gland contributed to the understanding of feedback mechanisms involved in endocrinology, particularly in relation to insulin. He shared the Nobel Prize for Physiology or Medicine with Carl (1896–1984) and Gerty Cori (1896–1957) in 1947.

Houston, John (1802–1845) Dublin surgeon, graduated from Edinburgh University in 1826 and became surgeon at the new City of Dublin Hospital. He introduced the use of the microscope to Dublin and published many papers on cancer. He described sphincter ani tertius (Houston valves) of the rectum in 1830.

How, William (1619–1656) London physician and botanist educated at the Merchant Taylor's School and graduate of St John's College, Oxford. He wrote several works on botany.

Howard, Benjamin Douglas (1840–1900) New York physician who described a method of artificial respiration where the patient is kept in a supine position with a roll of cloth beneath the thorax and the head below the level of thorax.

Howarth, Walter Goldie (1879–1962) London otorhinologist who devised an operation for frontal sinusitis in 1921 where the anterior wall of the sinus was left intact to preserve the cosmetic appearance.

Howe, Samuel Gridley (1801–1876) Pioneer in education of the blind. Born in Boston and obtained his medical degree from Harvard Medical School in 1824. He later traveled to Edinburgh and worked with James Gall in developing an embossed alphabet for the blind. On his return to Boston he established a printing press at the Massachusetts Asylum for the Blind. Howe also pioneered the method of educating blind children which utilized their sense of touch.

Howell, William Henry (1860–1945) Professor of physiology at Johns Hopkins University. He discovered and isolated heparin, an anticoagulant, from liver in 1912 and named it in 1919. He was the first to observe that blood pressure fell significantly during sleep. He also named thromboplastin, the tissue factor noticed in clotting. *See also Howell–Jolly bodies.*

Howell–Jolly Bodies Globular nuclear remnants in the erythrocytes from peripheral blood. Described by William Henry Howell (1860–1945) in 1905. Later described by Justin Marie Jolly (1870–1953), a professor of histopathology at the College of France, in 1923.

Howship, John (1781–1841) Surgeon to St George's and Charing Cross Hospitals in London. He suffered from osteomyelitis of the tibia which led him to study diseases of bone. He published *On the Natural and Diseased state of the Bones* in 1820. Remembered in Howship lacuna, osteoblast accumulation on the bone surface causing depressions and Howship–Romberg sign, pain on inner aspect of the thigh.

Hoyer, Heinrich (1834–1907) Polish professor of embryology, histology and anatomy at Warsaw. He described the communications between small arteries and small veins without the intervention of the capillaries (Hoyer canals) in 1877.

Huatu (AD 115–205) Famous Chinese surgeon who used cannabis and other narcotics as anesthetics during his operations, including laparotomy and excision of the spleen. *See Chinese medicine.*

Huang Ti Ancient Chinese writer on medicine who lived around 2637 BC. *Nuy-kin*, an extant work attributed to him, was probably written during the Christian era under his name by an unknown author. *See Chinese medicine.*

Hubel, David Hunter (b 1926) Canadian-born American neurophysiologist who graduated in medicine from McGill University in Montreal. He was drafted into the US Army and worked at the Walter Reed Army Research Institute on electrical activity of the brain. Later he moved to the Johns Hopkins and then to Harvard. His main study was cortical perception of visual stimulus, for which he shared the Nobel Prize for Physiology or Medicine with American neuroscientist, Roger Wolcott Sperry (b 1913) of Connecticut in 1981.

Huber, John Jacob (1707–1778) Professor of anatomy at Göttingen who described the aberrant ganglion on the posterior root of the first cervical nerve in 1741.

Huber, Robert (b 1937) German biophysicist, director of the Max Planck Institute for Biochemistry at Martinsried. Works on X-ray crystallography of biological macromolecules. Examined active and inactive crystalline phosphorylase, elucidated the antibody structure of the 'light chain' of the antigen binding site that had been proposed by Rodney Porter, analyzed the interaction between trypsin and trypsin inhibitor and studied glutathione peroxidase. Shared the Nobel Prize for Chemistry in 1988 with Johann Deisen- hofer and Hartmut Michel (b 1948).

Hubrecht, Ambrosius Arnold Willem (1853–1915) Comparative anatomist at Leiden who described a thickening at the site of first formation of the primitive streak in 1905. This structure, known as protocordal knot, was previously described by von Hensen (1835–1924) of Kiel in 1882.

Huchard, Henri (1844–1910) French physician in Paris and pioneer in the study of cardiovascular disease, particularly circulation and arteriosclerosis. Described continued hypertension as a cause of athersclerosis in 1887 (Huchard disease). He was probably the first to use the term Stokes–Adam disease for symptoms of bradycardia. He published a monograph on diseases of the heart in 3 volumes (1899–1903).

Hudson, William (1734–1793) Apothecary at Haymarket, London, born and educated in Kendal. He was *praefector horti* at the Chelsea Physic Garden (1765–1767). He adopted Linnaean nomenclature for classification of plants and published the *Flora Anglica* in 1762.

Hueck, Alexander Friedrich (1802–1842) Professor of anatomy at the University of Dorpat. He described ligamentum pectinatum iridis in 1841.

Huefland, Christoph Wilhelm (1762–1836) Physician to the King of Prussia. He published a famous book on personal hygiene in 1797 and a treatise on the art of prolonging life. Both books were translated and published in several European languages.

Hugenin, Gustav (1841–1920) Professor of psychiatry at Zurich. He described a system of levels for motor and sensory neurons in 1879.

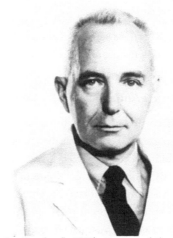

Charles Brenton Huggins (b 1901). Courtesy of the National Library of Medicine

Huggins, Charles Brenton (b 1901) Canadian-born American surgeon from Nova Scotia. Pioneer in hormonal treatment of cancer and investigation of the biochemistry and physiology of the male urinogenital tract. He was appointed professor of surgery at Chicago University in 1936, and was made head of the Ben May Laboratory for Cancer Re-search in 1951. In 1941 he noted that serum levels of acid phosphatase in metastatic carcinoma of the prostate could be further elevated by administering androgens, and could be diminished by giving estrogenic substances. Estrogens were first shown to be effective in the treatment of prostatic carcinoma by Huggins and Clarence Vernaud Hodges (b 1914) in the same year. Huggins also pioneered the use of hormones in breast cancer. He shared the Nobel Prize for Physiology or Medicine with F.S. Rous (1879–1970) in 1966 for their research into cancer.

Hughes, Charles H. (1839–1916) American neurologist, born in St Louis, Missouri. Helped found the Marion-Sims Medical College in St Louis and became professor of psychiatry and neurology there. Founded the *Journal of Neurology and Psychiatry*. Remembered in the Hughes reflex, downward movement of the penis when the glans or prepuce are pulled upwards.

Hughes Syndrome *See antiphospholipid syndrome.*

Huguier, Pierre Charles (1804–1874) French gynecologist and anatomist at Paris who wrote several treatises on surgery. Invented one of the first uterine sounds and described lymphogranuloma venereum involving the perineum. Hugier disease is leiomyoma. The canal from which the cauda tymphani emerges in the petrotymphanic fissure is named after him.

Huhner Test *See post-coital test.*

Huldschinsky, Kurt (1883–1941) German physician who demonstrated the effectiveness of ultraviolet radiation in curing rickets in 1919.

Human Leucocyte Antigen (HLA) *See histocompatibility.*

Human Sacrifice In ancient Egypt the victim was called Apis and was regarded as a god. Sacrifice to the gods is said to have been introduced into Greece by Phroneus, King or Argos in 1773 BC. Human sacrifice seems to have originated from the Chaldeans. Caesar sacrificed two soldiers on the alter in the Campus Martinus in 46 BC and Augustus is said to have sacrificed a maiden named Gregoria. In Mexico the priest of Quetzalcoatl made an image of the god from meal with infant's blood and distributed the body to be eaten after the sacrifice. Khonds of Central India practiced human sacrifice as late as the 17th century. The feast of human sacrifice amongst Maribos, a tribe of West Africa, called *meseletso oa mabele* meaning boiling of the corn, was used to ensure fertility of the soil. In Fiji flesh from the sacrifice could only be eaten by old men and priests. Human sacrifices were not uncommon in northern Europe, and the Yarl of Orkney is recorded to have sacrificed the son of the King of Norway to Odin in 893. In Sweden king Donald was sacrificed to Odin in order to end a famine.

Human Tissue Act British Act passed in 1961 to regulate procedures for obtaining tissues from cadavers for transplant. It specifies that consent must be obtained from next of kin, or a coroner, before tissue is removed.

Humerus, Raphael Bienvenu Sabatier (1732–1811) Paris surgeon and one of the first to recommend resection of the head of the humerus. The first recorded such procedure in England was performed by Charles White (1728–1813) in 1770. Excision of the humeral head was performed in a case of tuberculosis of the shoulder joint by James Syme (1799–1870) in 1826. Wiring ununited fractures of the humerus was first done in 1827 by John Kearny Rodgers (1793–1851) of New York, who also successfully tied the internal iliac artery in 1824.

Humoralism [Greek: *umor*, fluid or juice] System which considers illness to be the result of some disturbance in the body. It stresses the integration of mental and physical processes and the effects of diet, lifestyle and environment. It developed in Greece from the fourth century BC and, by the second century AD, it had spread throughout the Roman Empire and extended to the Arab nations and the Indian subcontinent. A theory incorporating the four elements of earth, air, water, and fire was proposed by Empedocles of Acragas (*c* 492–432 BC). Hippocrates (460–377 BC) applied the four qualities of humors, blood, phlegm, black bile, and yellow bile in the body to medicine and explained disease as imbalance in humors. Galen (AD 129–200) combined the four elements with the four humors and it continues to influence some medical practices even today.

Humphry, Sir George Murray (1820–1896) Born in Suffolk and studied medicine at St Bartholomew's Hospital where he obtained a gold medal in anatomy and physiology. He was surgeon at the Addenbrooke's Hospital in Cambridge and remained there for fifty years. He moved to Downing College Cambridge in 1847 and gained his MD in 1859 and was elected professor of human anatomy in 1866. He founded the *Journal of Anatomy and Physiology* and wrote on subjects as diverse as the skeleton, coagulation of blood, myology and a treatise on old age. He described the posterior cruciate ligament of the knee joint (Humphry ligament) in 1858.

Hunain ibn Ishäq (Abu Zain Hunanin ibd Ishak Al Ibadi) (AD 809–873) Arab Nestorian Christian physician and theologian from southern Iraq who translated important Greek works into Arabic. He was known to western Latin writers as Johannitius. He translated the Old Testament into Arabic and wrote an *Isagoge*, *Ten Treatises on the Eye* and *Medical Questions and Answers*.

Hunger An admirable analysis of the sensation of hunger was published by N. Tiedemann of Darmstadt in 1836. In his treatise he described the two components, the feeling of emptiness of the stomach, and general malaise and weakness. W. Nicolai of Berlin wrote the next important treatise in 1892. G.H. Roger of Paris in his *Alimentation et Digestion* (1907) has quoted the graphic description of hunger and starvation by an Italian magistrate Antonio Vitali under the First Republic who starved to death to escape execution after being condemned to death. Increased bowel sounds over the pylorus on auscultation at the sight of food, especially if it is delayed, was described by G. Glucksmann in 1911. The German naturalist and traveler, Baron Alexander von Humboldt (1769–1859) of Berlin described how the Otomacs living on the banks of the Orinoco ate baked bolus of earth in order to satisfy hunger pangs during the floods when food was scarce.

Hunner, Guy L.R. (1868–1957) American surgeon and gynecologist. One of the first students at the Johns Hopkins Medical School. Worked with Howard A. Kelly (1858–1943) at the Johns Hopkins and later went into private practice in Baltimore. Described the Hunner ulcer, a chronic vesical ulcer at the vertex of the bladder.

Hunt, Harriet Kezia (1805–1877) First woman medical practitioner in America, who practiced with her sister Sarah in Boston. Her application to attend lectures at Harvard Medical School in 1847 was refused despite the support of Oliver Wendell Holmes (1809–1894). She later obtained an honorary medical degree from the Female Medical College of Pennsylvania in 1853.

Hunt, James Ramsay (1872–1937) American neurologist, graduated from the University of Pennsylvania in 1893 and was made professor of neurology at Columbia in 1931. In 1914 he described fresh cerebral softening in people with carotid artery lesions which led to recognition of cerebrovascular disease from extracerebral vascular involvement. He described a rare form of Parkinsonism due to degeneration of globus pallidus, which occurred before the third decade, in 1917. Ramsay Hunt syndrome is geniculate neuralgia, Hunt atrophy is wasting of small muscles in hands without sensory loss and the Hunt tremor is a striocerebellar tremor.

Hunt, Reid (1870–1948) Pharmacologist, born in Martinsville, Ohio and worked in New York and Baltimore. He served as the head of pharmacological division of the Hygienic Laboratory of United States Public Health Service. He studied the role of iodine in the activity of thyroid extract and devised a method of assaying thyroid preparations in 1909. He was made professor of pharmacology at Harvard University in 1913.

Hunt Syndrome *See Ramsay Hunt syndrome.*

Hunter, Charles (1872–1955) Described gargoylism, a hereditary disease due to a disturbance of mucopolysacccharide metabolism in two brothers, in 1917. He was later professor of medicine at the University of Manitoba.

Hunter, John (1728–1793) Leading Scottish surgeon of his era and founder of surgical pathology. Born at Long Calderwood near Glasgow, youngest of ten children. He moved to London and assisted his brother, William Hunter (1718–1783), at his school of anatomy at Great Windmill Street between 1748 and 1759. He then studied surgery at St George's and St Bartholomew's Hospitals and was later appointed Surgeon-Extraordinary to George III at St George's. He collected plant and animal specimens (living and dead) to illustrate his comparative anatomy and developed his own unique museum (now known as the Hunterian Museum) which contains over 13,000 specimens. His investigations were wide-ranging and included embryology, venereal disease and dentistry. In 1767 John inoculated himself with pus from a patient with gonorrhea in order to determine if the same cause existed for syphilis and gonorrhea. Unfortunately the patient had both syphilis and gonorrhea so he maintained that both diseases had the same infectious agent. His later illness is thought to have been due to cerebral syphilis. He developed a technique for tying off arterial aneurysms, differentiated between hard (Hunterian) chancre and chancroid ulcer, and described, shock phlebitis, and pyemia in his epoch making work, *A Treatise on Blood, Inflammation and Gun-shot Wounds* published in 1794.

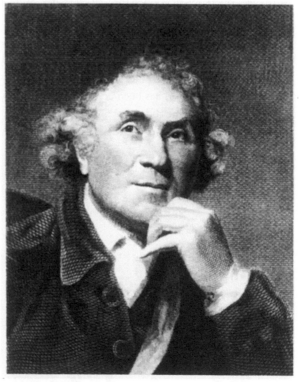

John Hunter (1728–1793). From the title page of his *A Treatise on the Blood, Inflammation and Gun-shot Wounds* (1794)

Hunter, William (1718–1783) Born at Long Calderwood

near Glasgow, and elder brother of John Hunter. He entered the University of Glasgow when he was 14 to study divinity but changed to medicine at the inspiration of William Cullen (1710–1790). He moved to London and worked with William Smellie (1697–1763), a leading obstetrician, and the anatomist James Douglas (1675–1742) and was a surgeon's pupil at St George's Hospital. He succeeded Samuel Sharp (1700–1778) at Guy's as lecturer to the Society of Surgeons in Covent Garden in 1746. Hunter built a private lecture theater, dissecting room and a museum at his residence in Great Windmill Street in 1770. He was appointed accoucheur to Queen Charlotte, and wrote one of the most important illustrated books on gynecology, *The Anatomy of the Human Gravid Uterus* in 1774. In 1794, after his death, a companion volume, *An Anatomical Description of the Human Gravid Uterus and its Contents* was published.

Hunter Canal Subsartorial canal described by John Hunter in 1786.

Hunter–Hurler Syndrome *See gargoylism.*

Hunter Chancre Elevated papule in the penis or vulva seen in primary syphilis. Described by John Hunter. Hunter inoculated himself with the material taken from a patient with the chancre and developed the first two stages. Hunter published his work *On Venereal Diseases* in 1786.

Hunterian Lecture Established from the funds presented by Matthew Baillie (1761–1823) and Everard Home (1756–1832) in memory of John Hunter in 1814. From the time of its inception the oration has been conducted annually by famous men in medicine and science.

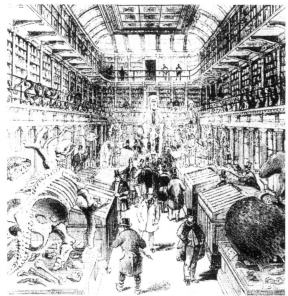

Hunterian Museum. Courtesy of the National Library of Medicine

Hunterian Museum When John Hunter died in 1793 his executors, Matthew Baillie and Everard Home, had to sell some of his prized possessions to maintain Hunter's vast museum of natural history, medicine and other curiosities. A sum of 15,000 pounds was voted by parliament to buy Hunter's museum which was relocated to Lincoln's Inn Fields in 1806. The museum was first offered to the Royal College of Surgeons who declined and then entrusted to the College of Surgeons by the Government in 1800. William Clift was appointed as the first conservator of the museum and he was succeeded by Sir Richard Owen (1804–1892) in 1842. The Hunterian Museum at Glasgow was presented by John's brother William Hunter who died in 1783. William's museum of pictures, manuscripts, geology, coins, archeology and anatomical specimens was transferred to Glasgow in 1807.

Huntington Chorea/Disease Rare familial disease accompanied by progressive involuntary movements, ataxia, and mental deterioration was brought to North America by two Suffolk immigrants in 1630. George Huntington (1850–1916), an American physician, observed this condition in a mother and a daughter while he was traveling in Long Island and described it in 1872. The first genetic marker for Huntington chorea was discovered by James F. Gusella in 1983.

Hurdon, Elizabeth (1869–1941) First director of the Marie Curie Hospital in London, and later an associate in gynecology at the Johns Hopkins University, Baltimore. She was a pioneer in the study of pathology of cancer of the uterus and its treatment by radiation. She published *Vermiform Appendix and its Diseases* with Howard Atwood Kelly (1858–1943) in 1905. Her work, *Cancer of the Uterus*, was published posthumously in 1942.

Hurler Syndrome Gargoylism, a hereditary disease due to a disturbance of mucopolysaccharide metabolism was first described in two brothers by Charles Hunter (1872–1955) in 1917. Further features of the disease, including corneal opacity and mental retardation in two infants, was observed by pediatrician, Gertrude Hurler of Germany in 1919.

Hurst (Hertz), Sir Fredrick Arthur (1879–1944) Physician at Guy's Hospital who first described dumping syndrome after gastrectomy.

Huscheke, Emil (1797–1858) Professor of anatomy at the University of Jena. He described the prominent lower margin (Huschke valve) of the lachrymal duct at its junction with the lachrymal sac in 1854.

Hutchinson, John (1811–1861) British respiratory

physiologist who invented the spirometer.

Hutchinson, Sir Jonathan (1828–1913) Born into a Quaker family in Selby, Yorkshire. Studied at St Bartholomew's Hospital under James Paget (1814–1899) before returning to York for graduate studies at the County Hospital. He returned to London and became surgeon at the London Hospital. At the age of 51 he was appointed professor of surgery at the Royal College of Surgeons. He had wide-ranging interests including, surgery, internal medicine, dermatology, ophthalmology, neurology, syphilology and pathology. He described the peg-shaped incisor teeth in congenital syphilis (Hutchinson teeth) in 1861. He prepared an *Atlas of Skin Diseases* which contains a description of Hutchinson–Boeck disease. Hutchinson founded the New Sydenham Society and was a prolific writer and also published one volume per year of his ten-volume *Archives of Surgery* between 1889 to 1899.

Hutchinson, Sir Robert (1871–1960) Physician at the Hospital for Sick Children at Great Ormond Street. He was the first to isolate a globulin in 1896 which was later named thyroglobulin. He described suprarenal sarcoma of children which led to secondary growths in the skull, in 1907.

Hutchinson Teeth *See Hutchinson, Sir Jonathan.*

Hutchinson Triad Interstitial keratitis, deafness, and pegged incisor teeth in congenital syphilis was described by Jonathan Hutchinson in 1858.

Hutton, James (1726–1797) Edinburgh graduate in medicine who also graduated from Leiden in 1749. He later gave up medicine and took to geology to which he devoted the rest of his career. His most important work *The Theory of Earth* was published in 1785.

Huxam, John (1692–1768) Physician from Devon who studied medicine under Boerhaave at Leiden before returning to England and establishing a practice at Plymouth in 1717. His important treatises include *An Essay on Fevers* (1739), *On the malignant, ulcerous sore throat* (1750), and *Dissertation on the Devonshire Colic* (1758). He advised the use of fresh vegetables and fruits for the prevention of scurvy in his essay *The Method of Preserving the Health of Seamen in Long Cruises.*

Huxley, Sir Andrew Fielding (b 1917) Grandson of Thomas Henry Huxley. He studied natural sciences and physiology at Cambridge and undertook neurophysiological research with Alan Hodgkin (b 1914). Together, they deduced a physico-chemical explanation for conduction of impulses in nerve fibers. In 1950 he worked on muscle contraction and relaxation, proposing the 'sliding filament' theory. He

shared the Nobel Prize for Physiology or Medicine with Hodgkin and Sir John Carew Eccles (b 1903) in 1963.

Huxley, Thomas Henry (1825–1895) Born at Ealing, Middlesex and studied medicine at Charing Cross Hospital, London. His career in biology started with his expedition as assistant surgeon on HMS *Rattlesnake* in the South Seas. He discovered the inner layer of the root sheath of the hair follicle (Huxley layer) in human hair when he was only 19 years old. He was also an anthropologist who advocated Darwin's theory of evolution and refuted Owen's theory of the vertebrate skull. He was also an expert on paleontology and published *Physiography* and *The Crayfish* along with several other treatises. He invented the term 'agnostic' to describe his theological and philosophical views. The evolutionist and humanist, Sir Julian Sorell Huxley (1887–1975) and Sir Andrew Fielding Huxley (b 1917) were his grandsons.

Huygens, Christiaan (1629–1693) Dutch astronomer and physicist from the Hague. At the age of 16 he studied law at Leiden and graduated in mathematics from the University of Breda. He and his brother constructed a twelve-foot telescope in 1656 with which he discovered the rings and the sixth satellite of Saturn, Titan. He published *The System of Saturn* or *Systema Saturnium* in 1659, and made several other important contributions to astronomy. Huygens while at Accademia del Cimento, invented a bifilar pendulum based on the work of Galileo and patented by him in 1657. He described the mechanism of the pendulum clock in *Horologium Oscillatorium*, published in 1673. The undulatory theory of light and polarization were proposed by him in *Treatise on Light*, published in 1690.

Hyaluronidase Enzyme which aids in the absorption of fluid injected into subcutaneous and intramuscular tissues. It was first isolated from testicular extract by Mayer and Palmer in 1934. A full description of it was given by F. Duran Reynals in 1929.

Hybridization [Latin: *hybrida*, offspring of a tame sow and a wild boar] One of the early works was that of Laur who published a treatise *Concerning the hybrid of the Pea and the Vetch* in 1850. Gregor Mendel's (1822–1884) research led to his epoch-making laws of genetics in 1865. In 1856, Vilmorin (1816-1860), a Frenchman and cultivator, independently applied the principles of genetics to plant breeding with success. The significance of Vilmorin's research was realized only a quarter of a century following his death, and his work was published in 1886.

Hydatid Disease [Greek: *hydatis*, a drop of water] The *Taenia* genus of cestodes includes most of the tapeworms and has

Dictionary of the History of Medicine

been known since the time of Hippocrates (460–377 BC) who called them broad lumbrici. The beef tapeworm, *Taenia saginata,* was first described by John Augustus Ephraim Goeze (1731–1786) a German clergyman and a naturalist from Halle. The term *Echinococcus* was first used for the common vesicular hydatid of many species by Karl Asmund Rudolphi (1771–1832) in 1808. Carl Theodor Ernest von Siebold demonstrated that dogs could be experimentally infected with *Taenia* in 1854. The first complete life history and morphology of *Echinococcus* was given by Rudolph Leuckart in 1860. Bernhard Naunyn (1839–1925) demonstrated that the minute tapeworm *Echinococcus hominis* was the mature or adult state of the hydatid cyst in 1864. A complete review of hydatid disease has been given by Albert Neisser (1855–1916) of Berlin in his treatise *Die Echinococcenkrankheit* (1877).

Hydatidiform Mole [Greek: *hydratis,* a drop of water] Vesicular mole. Aetius of Amida observed the condition in the 6th century. The earliest descriptions were given, independently by a Parisian midwife, Marie Ann Victorie Boivin in 1827, and Alfred Velpeau (1795–1867) in his *Treatise on Diseases of the Breast and Mammary Region* in 1854. The incidence of one chorioepithelioma to every 20 cases of mole was estimated by H. J. Stander in 1936.

Hyderabad Commission *See chloroform.*

Hydragyriasis Archaic term for mercurial poisoning.

Hydragyrum Cyanatum Preparation of mercuric cyanide, was introduced as treatment for syphilis into German pharmacopoeia in the 18th century.

Hydrargyria Peculiar eruption due to use of mercury in the 16th and 17th centuries.

Hydroa Term used by Hippocrates to denote a sweat-eruption of the skin.

Hydroadentitis [Greek: *hydor,* water + *aden,* gland + *itis,* inflammation] Infection of the sweat gland accompanied by collection of fluid or pus. First described by Pierre Antoine Ernest Bazin (1807–1878) of France around 1850.

Hydrocardia [Greek: *hydor,* water + *kardia,* heart] *See pericardial effusion.*

Hydrocephalus [Greek: *hydor,* water + *kephale,* head] Excessive accumulation of fluid causing dilation of the cerebral ventricles and raising intercranial pressure. Ancient physicians were familiar with the existence of water on the brain, and Hippocrates (460–377 BC) is supposed to have tapped the ventricles. John Freind (1625–1728) of Croton,

Northamptonshire was one of the earliest to give a description to the Royal Society in 1699. Robert Whytt (1714–1766), an eminent neurologist from Edinburgh wrote a treatise on the subject, *Observation on Dropsy of the Brain.* He described all acute brain disease under acute hydrocephalus. The specific condition of acute hydrocephalus was described by John Cheyne (1777–1836) in 1808. Two cases, treated by withdrawal of cerebrospinal fluid were reported by Heinrich Iranius Quincke (1842–1922) of Germany in 1891. Sir Hugh Cairns (1896–1952), a British neurologist was the first to describe hydrocephalus following obstruction of the flow of cerebrospinal fluid secondary to tuberculous meningitis, in 1949.

Hydrocoel [Greek: *hydor,* water + *koilos,* hollow] Described by Paul of Aegina (625–690) as 'inert fluid collected about the parts which enveloped the scrotum'. He also detailed the anatomical relationship of the fluid to the scrotum, and advocated incision as treatment. Incision had been used earlier by Celsus (25 BC–AD 50). The early modern writers on the subject were few and include Alexander Monro, Samuel Sharp, and Percivall Pott (1714–1788).

Hydrodiascope Device consisting of a small chamber filled with saline solution to be applied to the eye through the palpebral fissure. Invented by Ferdinand Siegrist (1865–1946) of Switzerland in 1897. Its purpose was to fit various spherical lenses through the window on its anterior chamber to correct distance or reading vision. *See contact lenses.*

Hydrogen [Greek: *hydro,* water + *gennan,* to produce] First described as 'combustible air' by Paracelsus (1493–1541). Its properties were described by Henry Cavendish (1731–1810) who named it 'inflammable air' in 1766. Antoine Laurent Lavoisier (1743–1794) published *Elementary Treatise on Chemistry* in 1789, describing the properties of hydrogen, nitrogen and oxygen in the air, and that water, previously considered an element, was actually made up of hydrogen and oxygen. The production of water by combining hydrogen with oxygen was demonstrated by Watts in 1781. The structure of atomic hydrogen, consisting of a single massively charged central nucleus of protons with a single electron traveling around it, was first demonstrated by Danish physicist and Nobel Prize winner, Niels Henrick David Bohr (1885–1962) in 1926. So-called heavy hydrogen (deuterium) was discovered by an associate of Bohr and fellow Nobel Prize winner, Harold Clayton Urey (1893–1981) of Indiana together with Ferdinand Brickwebbe and George Murphy in 1934.

Hydrogen Peroxide Strong disinfectant compound

accidentally discovered by French chemist, Louis Jacques (1777–1857) in 1819.

Hydrometer Instrument to measure the specific gravity of liquids. Probably discovered by Archimedes (*c* 287–212 BC). It is mentioned in the letters of Bishop Synesius to Hypatia (*c* AD 370–415), and Robert Boyle (1627–1691) described one in 1675.

Hydronephrosis in Pregnancy Severe dilatation of the upper urinary tract during pregnancy was first shown at postmortem by Jean Cruveilhier (1791–1874), professor of pathological anatomy at Paris, in 1842.

Hydropathy [Greek: *hydor*, water + *pathos*, suffering] A method of treatment of diseases using water. Mentioned by Hippocrates (460–377 BC) and revived by Johann Sigmund Hahn (1664–1742) of Silesia, Scottish physician, James Currie (1756–1805), and Vincenz Priessnitz (1799–1851) of Austria. *See baths.*

Hydrophobia [Greek: *hydor*, water + *phobos*, fear] Aristotle was one of the first to mention hydrophobia, calling it *lytta* (Greek: madness) *cynanche* (Greek: *kyon*, dog) and podagra. He believed that it affected all animals except man. Celsus (25 BC–AD 50) thought that bites of all animals were dangerous due to the presence of a virus. Pliny (AD 23–79) recommended hellebore as treatment. Alexandrian physician, Andreas of Caryste also wrote on the subject. The best account amongst the ancients was given by Caelius Aurelianus of Numidia in the 5th century. His treatise states that the disease could be transmitted not only by the bite of the rabid dog but also from contact with it or from its secretions. Galen (129–200) gave several preparations as treatment. In Belgium, around AD 800 , the shrine of St Hubert in the Ardennes became a place of pilgrimage for cure of hydrophobia. In England the disease prevailed in 1734 and 1735, and in 1752 several mad dogs were still reported around St James, London and were ordered to be shot. *See rabies.*

Hydrops Articuli Archaic term for effusion into the joint.

Hydrotherapy [Greek: *hydor*, water + *therapeia*, attendant] The first chair of hydrotherapy was created in Vienna in 1881 for William Winternitz (1835–1917). He published a popular treatise on the subject in 1880 and opened the first modern hydrotherapeutic clinic at Kaltenleutgeben in 1893. *See baths.*

Hydroxyproline Amino acid first isolated from gelatin by Emil Fischer (1852–1919) in 1902.

Hygeia Second daughter of Aesculapius. Deity for health and prevention of disease.

Hygiene [Greek: *hygeia*, goddess of health] The art of preserving health through cleanliness and sanitation has been practiced since earliest times. Excavations at Mohanjadaro and Harappa in the Indus Valley by Sir John Hubert Marshall in the 1920s has revealed a system of sanitation and hygiene which existed 5000 years ago and is comparable to modern methods. Hippocrates in his treatise *On Airs, Waters, and Places* insisted on the duty of the physicians to study the effect of all these elements on health.

Hygrometer [Greek: *hygros*, moist + *metron*, measure] Instrument for measuring moisture in the atmosphere. First made at the Accademia del Cimento in the 17th century. Robert Hook (1635–1703) constructed a hygrometer using the beard of wild oat in 1655. Further instruments were invented by French mathematician, Guillaume Amontons (1663–1705) in 1698. Horace Bénédict de Saussure (1740–1799) and many others have constructed variations to study weather.

Hymen [Greek: *hymen*, membrane] Greek god of marriage. Term was originally used to denote any membrane and Vesalius (1514–1564) was the first to restrict it to the female genital membrane.

Hymenolepes nana Helminth parasite of man. Discovered by Theodor Bilharz (1825–1862) in Cairo in 1875 and cause of schistosomiasis (Bilharzia), transmitted through water snails. One year later it was described by von Siebold who named it *Taenia nana*.

Hyoscine Antispasmodic, hypnotic and mild diuretic. Part of the hyoscyamine molecule obtained from henbane, also known as scopolamine. It was first isolated in an impure state by P. L. Geiger (1785–1836) and Hermann Hesse in 1833 and Hohn isolated it in 1871 from seeds. A more refined process of extracting hyoscyamine was devised by Thibaut in 1875. A pure form was isolated by Albert Ladenburg in 1881. It was used as a premedication for anesthetic by Schneiderlinn in 1900.

Hypatia (*c*AD 370–415) Greek philosopher and mathematician who taught in Alexandria. She was the daughter of Theon and was renowned for her beauty and learning.

Hypercalcemia [Greek: *hyper* above; Latin: *calx*, lime] The occurrence during alkali therapy for peptic ulcer was first recognized by C. L. Cope in 1949. Elevation of serum calcium in sarcoidosis was first noted by G. T. Harrell (b 1908) and S. Fisher (b 1915) in 1939. Idiopathic hypercalcemia of infants was first described by R. Lightwood and W. R. Payne of England in 1952. *See parathyroid.*

Hyperemesis Gravidarum [Greek: *hyper* above + *emesis*, vomiting; Latin: *gravidus*, heavy] Paul of Aegina (625–690) in AD 650 wrote of the symptoms of vomiting, salivation, and loathing of food during pregnancy, and advised pomegranate, knot grass and other herbs. One of the early modern classic descriptions was given by Paul du Bois (1795–1871), surgeon-in-chief at the Maternité Hospital in Paris, in 1852.

Hyperinsulinism [Greek: *hyper*, above; Latin: *insula*, island] Term first used by Seale Harris of America in 1933 to denote a condition of abnormally low blood sugar levels with symptoms similar to insulin reaction in non-diabetic patients. A pathological basis was established by Russell M. Wilder (1885–1959) and colleagues at the Mayo Clinic in 1927 who found carcinoma of the pancreas in some patients. Finney performed the first successful surgical resection of pancreas in 1928. The first method of estimating endogenous insulin in microquantities by radioimmunoassay was introduced by Nobel Prize winner, Rosalyn Yalow (neé Sussman) (b 1921) and Solomon Berson (1918–1972) in 1960. More recently the state of hyperinsulinism has been recognized as a risk factor for cardiovascular disease.

Hypernephroma [Greek: *hyper*, above + *nephros*, kidney] German surgeon, Paul Albert Grawitz (1850–1932), was one of the first to study the origin and nature of hypernephroma (Grawitz tumor) in 1884.

Hyperparathyroidism [Greek: *hyper*, above + *para*, beside + *thyreos*, oblong shield] *See parathyroid, osteitis fibrosa cystica.*

Hyperphosphatemia [Greek: *hyper*, above + *phos*, light + *haima*, blood] The rise of phosphate levels in the blood of patients with renal failure was first observed by Greenwald in 1915.

Hyperpituitarism [Greek: *hyper*, above + *pituita*, phlegm] *See acromegaly.*

Hypertelorism [Greek: *hyper*, above + *tele*, far off + *horizo*, to separate] Abnormal distance between two paired organs, as in ocular hypertelorism or cranio-facial dystosis. The first account was given by Octave Crouzon (1874–1938) of Paris in 1912. It was described as a separate entity by David Middleton Greig (1864–1936) of Edinburgh in 1924.

Hypertension [Greek: *hyper*, above; Latin: *tensio*, tension] *See essential hypertension, renal hypertension.*

Hypertensive Retinopathy [Greek: *hyper*, above; Latin: *tensio*, tension + *rete*, net; Greek: *pathos*, suffering]

Disturbance of vision in hypertension was first noted by Richard Bright (1789–1858) in 1836. First observed anatomically by Ludwig Turck (1810–1868), an Austrian physician and neurologist, in 1850. The condition was referred to as albuminuric retinitis in the *Archives of Ophthalmology*, by Richard Liebreich (1830–1917) of Germany in 1859. The ophthalmoscopic description of the condition was first given by Heymann in 1858. The 'silver wire' appearance of the thickened arteries on ophthalmoscopy in hypertension was described by Sir William Richard Gowers (1845–1915) in 1876.

Hyperthyroidism [Greek: *hyper*, above + *thyreon*, oval shield] *See Graves disease.*

Hypertrophic Cardiomyopathy [Greek: *hyper*, above + *trophe*, nourishment+ *kardia*, heart + *mys*, muscle + *pathos*, disease] Also called hypertrophic obstructive cardiomyopathy (HOCM). First described by Alexander Schmincke (1877–1953) of Germany in 1907. W. Evans described the familial occurrence of the disease in 1949. The condition was recognized during surgery and described by cardiac surgeon, Lord Russell Brock (1903–1980), of Guy's Hospital in 1957. A pathological description of the condition was given by D. Teare in 1958, and it was named obstructive cardiomyopathy by J. F. Goodwin and colleagues in 1960.

Hypertrophic Pyloric Stenosis [Greek: *hyper*, above + *trophe*, nourishment; Latin: *pyloros*, gatekeeper; Greek: *stenosis*, narrowing] *See pyloric stenosis.*

Hypertrophy of the Heart An account of the condition including its clinical signs was given by Walter Hayle Walshe in 1851.

Hypervitaminosis D [Greek: *hyper*, above; Latin: *vita*, life + *amine* + *osis*, condition] Associated with metastatic calcification and renal calculi following high intake of irradiated ergosterol in experimental animals. First demonstrated independently by Pfannensteil, and Kreitmer in 1928.

Hypnosis [Greek: *hypnos*, sleep + *osis*, condition] *See hypnotism.*

Hypnotism [Greek: *hypnos*, sleep] The ancients were aware that snakes could be hypnotized with sound and fowls were also susceptible. This phenomenon was revived by Hehl, a Jesuit from Vienna in 1774. His friend, Franz Anton Mesmer (1734–1815) demonstrated the art of hypnosis in Vienna in 1776, and called it animal magnetism in the belief that the hypnosis was due to an effect similar to that of a magnet. John Elliotson (1791–1868), a professor of surgery at the University of London, revived and promoted mesmerism but, due to the opposition from his peers, he had to resign in order to promote its practice. James Braid (1795–1860), a Manchester surgeon, rediscovered the hypnotic phenomena and came to be regarded as the initiator of the scientific study of animal magnetism. Braid substituted the word 'hypnotism' for mesmerism. Hypnosis was used as a form of therapy by the French neurologist, Jean Charcot (1825–1893) in 1885 and Sigmund Freud (1856–1939) learned the method from him. Josef Breuer (1842–1925), a contemporary of Freud, was the first to employ the phenomenon in psychiatry. In his initial interviews with a patient Anna O (pseudonym) he used hypnosis to bring out her experiences which coincided with her symptoms. He called this method 'talking cure' and Freud conceived his idea of psychoanalysis from this method.

Hypocalcemia [Greek: *hypo*, under + Latin: *calcx*, lime] *See hypoparathyroidism*.

Hypodermic Injection [Greek: *hypo*, under + *derma*, skin] Sir Christopher Wren (1632–1723) inaugurated the first intravenous administration of drugs by injecting opium and crocus into the veins of dogs with the help of a quill and a bladder in 1656. In 1662 Johann Daniel Major (1634–1693), professor at Kiel, used the same method to inject drugs to man. His treatise, *Prodomus Inventae a se Chirurgiae Infusoriae*, was published in 1664. The first self-experimentation on intravenous drugs was done by Enoch Hale of West Hampton, Massachusetts who graduated from Harvard. He self injected with castor oil in 1821, and was awarded the Boyleston prize for self-experiment.

Hypodermic Needle The first hypodermic tubular needle and syringe were constructed by Charles Gabriel Pravaz (1791–1853) of Lyons in 1851 and Sir William Fergusson (1808–1877) of Scotland around 1852, and the device was developed to give intravenous injections by a Scottish physician, Alexander Wood (1817–1884) in 1855.

Hypogammaglobulinemia [Greek: *hypo*, under + *gamma*; Latin: *globulus*, globe] An X-linked form was first described in a boy of eight years with recurrent pneumonia and septicemia by O. C. Brunton in 1952.

Hypohyperparathyroidism [Greek: *hypo*, under + *hyper*, over + *para*, beside + *thyreon*, oval shield] Term coined to describe a condition of hypocalcemia, hyperphosphatemia and radiological bone changes in a girl patient by J.M. Costello and C.E. Dent in 1963.

Hypoparathyroidism [Greek: *hypo*, under + *para*, beside + *thyreon*, oval shield] The clinical signs of tetany and laryngeal stridor were first described in 1815 by John Clarke (1761–

1815). Armand Trousseau (1801–1867) described the signs of hypocalcemia in 1864, and Frantisek Chvostek (1835–1884) demonstrated the facial nerve irritability (Chvostek sign) in 1878. Tetany was demonstrated in post-thyroidectomy patients by Weiss of Vienna in 1880. The condition was experimentally produced by Moritz Schiff (1823–1896) (1884) and Victor Horsley (1857–1916) in 1885. The chemical basis of parathyroid deficiency was demonstrated by William George MacCallum (1874–1944) of Johns Hopkins and Carl Voegtlin (1879–1960) in 1908.

Hypophosphatasia [Greek: *hypo*, under + *phos*, light] Hereditary disorder resembling rickets. First described by Chown of Winnipeg in 1935. Rathburn noticed a low alkaline phosphatase activity in this condition and named it in 1960.

Hypothalamus [Greek: *hypo*, under + *thalamos*, bedchamber] Regulation of temperature was one of the first functions of the hypothalamus discovered by V.R. Isenschmidt and Ludolph von Krehl (1861–1937) in 1912. They identified tuber cinerium in the caudal part of the diencephalon as a thermoregulatory center, and their findings were confirmed by Isaac Ott (1847–1916) of America in 1914. Obesity and abnormal sexual characters related to hypothalamic lesions were demonstrated in experimental animals by J. Camus and colleagues in 1921. Walter Rudolph Hess (1881–1973), a Swiss physiologist, was the first to apply small electrodes to various parts of the brain in order to study its functions in 1925. Such stimulation demonstrated that it caused changes in temperature, sleep, sexual arousal and emotional state. The structure and function were described by American neuroscientist, Horace Winchell Magoun (1907–1991), dean and professor of psychiatry at the University of California, Los Angeles.

Hypothermia [Greek: *hypo*, under + *therme*, heat] Galen (AD 129–200) reported some of its effects and Alexander of Trailles discussed methods of cooling the body in the sixth century. Interest was revived by Scottish surgeon, James Currie (1756–1805), who gave a presentation on methods of lowering body temperature at the Royal College of Physicians' meeting in London in 1797. The term artificial hibernation, to denote induction of hypothermia, was coined by Walter Simpson (b 1895) and Arthur Herring (b 1875). In 1938 L.W. Smith and Temple Fay, of Philadelphia, investigated treatment of advanced cancer with hypothermia and presented their findings in 1940. Extracorporeal cooling, a method of allowing the blood from a cannulated artery to pass through tubing immersed in a cooling medium and returning it to a vein, was first described by J. Boerema and colleagues in 1951. Donald

Nixon Ross in 1954 suggested withdrawal of blood from the vein instead of the artery, and Lord Claude Russell Brock (1903–1980) in 1956 devised a method to cool the blood via the venous system without cannulating the artery. Induction of hypothermia gained scientific credibility and became very useful when F.J. Lewis and M. Taufic employed it in open heart surgery in 1953. In 1958 Williams and Spencer used hypothermia to treat patients who sustained neurological damage following cardiac arrest. Gastric freezing was employed as treatment for gastric ulcer by O.H. Wagensteen and E.T. Peters. They lowered the body temperature by making the patient swallow a balloon through which a coolant, such as ethyl alcohol, was circulated.

Hypoxanthine Nucleotide first isolated by Scherer in 1850.

Hyrtl, Joseph (1810–1894) Austrian professor of anatomy at Prague in 1837, later professor in Vienna. He published an influential book, *Handbook of Topographical Anatomy*, in 1847.

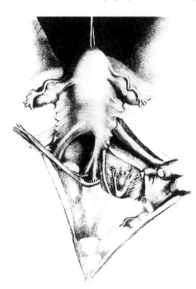

Hysterectomy. Illustration from Wertheim's monograph (1911). Reproduced with permission of Urban and Schwarzenburg, Munich

Hysterectomy [Greek: *hystera*, womb + *ektome*, excision] First surgical uterine removal was by Italian surgeon, Augosto Bozzi Granville, in 1827, but without success. The first successful abdominal hysterectomy was performed by an American surgeon, Walter Burnham in 1853. Sir Spencer Wells (1818–1897) performed his first hysterectomy for myoma in 1861. The first successful vaginal hysterectomy was performed by Sauter of Constance in 1822. The procedure was revived by Czerny in 1879, and later developed by Christian Billroth (1829–1894) and Johann von Mikulicz-Radecki (1850–1905). The development of cancer in the cervical stump following subtotal hysterectomy as a clinical entity was first described by Chrobak in 1896. A radical form of hysterectomy for carcinoma was performed by an American gynecologist, John Goodrich Clark (1867–1927) of Indiana in 1895. Abdominal hysterectomy was introduced as treatment cancer of the uterus by a German surgeon, Wilhelm Alexander Freund (1833–1918) in 1913. The Wertheim radical pan-hysterectomy for cervical cancer was devised by an Austrian gynecologist, Ernest Wertheim (1864–1920) in 1898.

Hysteria [Greek: *hystera*, womb] Term derived from the belief that it occurred only in women due the wanderings of the uterus which lost its moorings in the pelvic cavity. The oldest known amulet to protect against hysteria was found in Egypt and is exhibited at the Museum of Natural History in New York. Silver salts were used commonly for hysteria and epilepsy in England in the 18th century. Golding Bird (1814–1854) used galvanic stimulation on cases of hysteria. The first English book on hysteria, *A Brief Discourse of a Disease Called the Suffocation of the Mother*, was published by London physician, Edward Jorden (1569–1632) in 1603. Jean Charcot (1825–1893) used the term 'grande' for hysterical seizures in 1862, and his pupil Pierre Marie Felix Janet (1859–1947) proposed the theory that hysteria is linked with dissociation and psychic energy. Janet's theory was later described as the first significant concept on the subject by Sigmund Freud (1856–1939). The German psychiatrist, Ernst Kretschmer (1888–1964) used his experiences working with soldiers in World War I as the basis for his book, *Hysteria, Reflex and Instinct.*

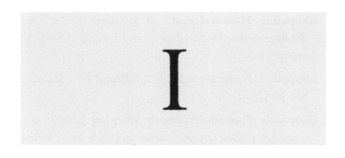

I Kuang Tai Uong Ancient surgeon from Loochoo Island, who practiced in China and was later deified.

Iatraleiptes [Greek: *iatros*, physician + *lipos*, fat] Ancient term for a physician who cures disorders using friction and ointments.

Iatreon [Greek: *iatros*, physician] Art or function of a physician. Hippocrates (460–377 BC) wrote a book on the subject.

Iatrice [Greek: *iatros*, physician] Art of medicine.

Iatrochemical School Sixteenth century school of medicine which considered that health and disease were the result of chemical balances. Paracelsus (1493–1541) was one of the first to use the term iatrochemistry. The first chemistry book dissociated from alchemy, *Tyrocinium chymicum* was written in 1610 by Jean Beguin of France. Iatrochemistry continued under Johannes Baptista van Helmont (1579–1644) and was further developed by German chemist and physician, Johann Rudolf Glauber (1604–1670) and Sylvius de la Boë or Sylvius (1614–1672), another iatrochemist who explained physical functions of the body on a chemical basis. Iatrochemistry was the forerunner of physical and organic chemistry and biochemistry.

Iatrogenic Diseases [Greek: *iatros*, physician + *genos*, offspring] Diseases induced by the physicians have always been present. For example, venesection probably killed more patients than it cured. The advent of iatrochemistry in the 15th century and the use of mercury, arsenic and bromine was a major cause of iatrogenic disease. Sophisticated drugs such as steroids and antibiotics are also iatrogenic.

Iatromathematical School *See iatrophysics.*

Iatrophysics Use of physical laws to explain bodily functions. Founded by Giovanni Borelli (1608–1679), physiologist, physicist and professor of mathematics at Pisa. In his famous book *De motu animalium*, published posthumously, he related movements of animals with laws of mechanics. He studied the mechanics of respiration and suggested that lungs passively followed the expansion of the thorax through contraction of intercostal muscles and that expiration was a process of relaxation. Giorgio Baglivi (1648–1701) regarded the human body as a sort of toolchest. To him teeth were like scissors, the stomach was a bottle, vessels were a system of tubes, and the thorax was a box containing a pair of bellows. Santorio Santorius (1561–1636), professor at Padua, also treated all physiological processes of the body on the basis of laws of physics and mathematics. René Descartes (1596–1650) also contributed to the field.

Iatrophysicus [Greek: *iatros*, physician + *physicus,* natural] One who treats physical subjects in relation to medicine.

Iatrosophist [Greek: *iatros*, physician + *sophos*, skilled] Ancient Greek term for one who practiced and taught medicine.

Ibn Abi Usabi'a or Muwaffaquddin Abdul-Abbas Ahmed ibn Ul-Qasim ibn Abi Usaybia (1203–1269) Probably the first medical historian, born in Damascus and studied medicine there. He moved to Cairo as physician to Emir Azzedin in Sarkar. He wrote the first medical biography containing over 400 medical personalities, *Uyunal-anba fi tabaqat al-attiba* (Pristine Sources of Information on the Classes of Physicians) in 1245 which was later translated into Latin as *Fontes relationum de classibus medicorum* and the manuscripts are in British Museum and at Leiden.

Ibn Jazla or Yahya ibn Isa Ibn Jazla (b AD 1074) Physician born to Christian parents in Baghdad but later converted to Islam. His *Taqwim al-abdan fi tabdir al-insan* (The Proper Assessment of Bodies for the Pursuit of Man's Well-being) was translated by the Jewish writer Farragat, and a Latin version was published in 1532.

Ibn Sina *See Avicenna.*

Ice Age First studied in detail by the Swiss-American geologist and physician, Jean Louis Rodolphe Agassiz (1807–1873). The Great Ice Age occurred in the Pleistocene. Agassiz's work was advanced by James Geike with his standard book on the subject published in 1879. In 1909 Svante August Arrhenius (1859–1927) ascribed the glacial period or ice age to the change in the amount of carbon dioxide in the atmosphere. *See glacial period.*

Ichnology Study of fossilized footprints. First examined by Duncan in 1828 and later by other eminent paleontologists including Sir Richard Owen (1804–1892), Sir Charles Lyell (1797–1875), and Thomas Henry Huxley (1825–1895).

Icterus Term used by ancient Greek and Roman physicians

to describe jaundice. With regard to etymology of the term, Areatus derived it from the name of an animal called ictis. This animal was thought to be a wild ferret by Nicander. Pliny (AD 23-79) in the first century believed that the name was derived from an unknown bird with the name of icterus.

Ichthyology [Greek: *ikhthus*, fish + *logos*, reason] Scientific study of fish. One of the first books was an illustrated monograph of Mediterranean fish by Guillaume Rondelet (1507–1566). Modern writers include Baron Georges L.C. F.D. Cuvier (1769–1832), Sir Richard Owen (1804– 1892), and Jean Louis Rodolphe Agassiz (1807–1873), and Yarrell published a classic work, *British Fishes* (1836–1859). George Brown Goode (1851–1896) of New Albany, Indiana wrote *The Oceanic Ichthyology* (1895) and *American Fishes* (1888)

Ichthyophagous [Greek: *ikhthus*, fish + *phagein*, to eat] Feeding on fish. First described by Herodotus (484– 425 BC).

Ichthyosaur [Greek: *ikhthus,* fish; Latin: *saurus*, lizard] Extinct marine reptile from the Cretaceous or Triassic periods. First fossil was discovered in 1811.

Ichthyosis [Greek: *ikhthus*, fish] Congenital skin disease. *See fish skin disease.*

Id [Latin: *id*, from German: *es*, it] In psychoanalytic theory, the innate, unconscious, primitive aspect of personality, dominated by the pleasure principle. Sigmund Freud's (1856–1939) first work on the general theory of personality, *Ego and the Id*, was published in 1923. He divided the mind into three parts: ego, id, and superego.

Idiocy [Greek: *idiotes*, nonexpert] Profound mental retardation. The first person to study mentally deficient children was Edouard Seguin (1812–1880) of the Bicêtre Hospital in Paris who wrote *Traitment Moral, Hygiene et Education des Idiots et des Autres Enfants Arriers* in 1846. He defined idiocy as an 'infirmity of the nervous system, which has for its effect the abstraction of the whole or part of the organs, and faculties of the child from the normal action of the will'. Desire Magloire Bourneville (1840–1909), a neurologist in Paris, established the first school for defective children in France. The first such school in England was established at Bath in 1846 and later became the Magdalen Hospital. The English physician, John Langdon Down (1828–1909) of Teddington, in his work *Observations of ethnic classification of idiots* (1866), used the term to denote a malady which was essentially different from insanity in both nature and treatment.

Idiopathic Hypercalcemia of Infancy [Greek: *idios*, distinct + *pathos*, disease + *hyper*, above; Latin: *calcx*, lime] *See hypercalcemia.*

Idiopathic Hypercalcemia of Childhood First described by I. McQuarrie in 1954.

Idiopathic Thrombocytopenic Purpura [Greek: *idios*, distinct + pathos, disease + *thrombos*, clot + *kytos*, hollow vessel + *penia*, poverty; Latin: *porphura*, purple]. *See thrombocytopenic purpura.*

Idiot [Greek: *idiotes*, nonexpert] Term originally applied to private citizens in ancient Greece, mainly a country of politicians and statesmen. The modest tastes and leisure habits of these private citizens were thought by many to be due to subnormal intelligence, and the word gradually came to signify low intelligence. The term was first used in medicine in 1866 by John Langdon Down in his book *Observations of ethnic classification of idiots. See idiocy.*

Ileitis [Greek: *eileos*, to roll up + *itis*, inflammation] *See Crohn disease.*

Ileocecal Valve [Greek: *eileos*, to roll up; Latin: *caecus*, blind gut] First described by Spanish anatomist Andreas Lacuna (1499–1516).

Ileus [Greek: *eileos*, to roll up] A form of intestinal obstruction. The condition due to impacted feces is mentioned in a Hippocratic treatise. Gastromesenteric ileus with distension of the duodenum proximal to the root of mesentery was first noticed by Karl von Rokitansky (1804–1878). A classical description of the condition was given by Charles Hilton Fagge (1838–1883) in 1869.

Iliad Epic poem by the Greek poet Homer (*c* 800 BC) about the siege of Troy around 1200 BC. It contains descriptions and treatment of war wounds, diseases and many of the customs of the ancient Greeks. It also contains references to the Greek god of medicine Aesculapius. The two sons of Aesculapius, Machaon and Podalirius are described as physicians and commanders of ships who were skilled in extracting weapons, attending to wounds and applying soothing drugs. *See arrow wounds.*

Illegitimate Children Children born out of wedlock were considered illegitimate in England until the early 19th century. The attempts to make them legitimate in 1236 failed due to protests by the barons. Women who tried to conceal the birth of their children were deemed guilty of murder in 1624, and in Scotland illegitimate children could not dispose of their movable assets until 1836. An act passed in 1845 improved their rights and status.

Imbecile [Latin: *imbecullus*, feeble] *See idiocy.*

Imbibition Pressure [Latin: *imbibere*, to drink] Pressure at which protoplasm absorbs water causing the cell to distend. Principle unknowingly employed by the ancient Egyptians to dislodge huge blocks of stone.

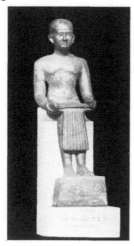

Imhotep, the Egyptian God of medicine. R.C. Macfie, *The Romance of Medicine* (1907). Cassell, London

Imhotep (*I-em-hetep*, He who cometh in peace) (*c* 2650 BC) Egyptian physician, architect and astrologer during the third dynasty. He designed the first pyramid at Saqqara. He was deified as the Egyptian god of healing.

Immune Compromise [Latin: *imunis*, free] Various conditions such as diabetes, blood disorders, and medications have been established as leading to the immune compromised state. Armand Trousseau (1801–1867) observed that candidosis occurred on the previously inflamed mucocutaneous membranes. Acquired immune deficiency syndrome (AIDS) is another example. *See AIDS, agammaglobulinemia.*

Immunoelectrophoresis [Latin: *imunis*, free; Greek: *elektron*, amber + *phoros*, bearing] Separation of immune proteins based on rate of migration in an applied electrical field with the addition of antisera. Electrophoresis was first used by Swedish biochemist and Nobel Prize winner, Arne Wilhelm Tiselius (1902–1971) to determine diffusion constants of proteins. He identified serum proteins and showed that antibodies are globulins. Further advances were made by Pierre Grabar (1898–1986) and Curtis A. Williams in 1953.

Immunoflouorescence [Latin: *imunis*, free + *fluere*, to flow + *escentia*, begin to exhibit] Any immunohistochemical method using a fluorescent labeled antibody. The technique was developed by Albert Hewett Coons (1912–1978) and

Melvin Kaplan (b 1920) in 1941 and contributed to understanding of antigen–antibody reactions both *in vitro* and *in vivo*. *See immunoglobulins.*

Immunogenetics [Latin: *imunis*, free; Greek: *gennan*, to produce] Term coined in 1936 by M. Robert Irwin (1897–1987) to link genetics and immunology.

Immunoglobulins [Latin: *imunis*, free + *globulus*, globule] Arne Wilhelm Tiselius (1902–1971) used electrophoresis to analyze blood proteins and identified globulins, which are antibodies. The structure of human immunoglobulin (IgG) antibody molecules was first determined by New York biochemist and Nobel Prize winner, Gerald Maurice Edelman (b 1929) at the Rockefeller Institute in 1959. His work, together with Rodney Robert Porter (1917–1985) in England, helped establish the typical Y-shaped structure of human immunoglobulin IgG. Porter, professor of biochemistry at Oxford, was the first to propose a symmetrical four-chain structure.

Immunology [Latin: *imunis*, free + *logos*, discourse] The branch of biomedicine concerned with the response of an organism to antigenic challenge. The origins have been attributed to both the Greeks and Chinese. Edward Jenner (1749–1823) and his introduction of smallpox vaccination must be the earliest accredited milestone. While Louis Pasteur's (1822–1895) work on the anthrax bacillus showing that it could be attenuated so as to confer immunity without producing the disease was the beginning of the rise of immunology. The theories of cellular (Pasteur's followers) and humoral (Robert Koch's followers) immunity constituted a period of debate in the latter years of the nineteenth century. Russian zoologist Elie Metchnikoff (1845–1916) was a supporter of the cellular theory and in 1884 he proposed a new theory of the protective influence of inflammation. In 1890 Emil Behring (1854–1917) and Shibasaburo Kitasato (1852–1931) demonstrated the first successful clinical use of diphtheria antitoxin and proposed the word 'alexin' for the substance which was later renamed 'complement'. Behring's work was further advanced in 1895 by Nobel Prize winner, Jules Jean Baptiste Vincent Bordet (1870–1961) of Belgium, and Octave Genou (1875–1959) who discovered the complement fixation (Bordet 'alexin') test and showed that antibody–antigen reactions could be measured. The chemical interaction between cells, antibodies and antigens and quantitation of toxin were deduced by Paul Ehrlich (1854–1915). He and Metchnikoff shared the Nobel Prize for Physiology or Medicine in 1908 for their contributions to immunity and serum therapy. The bactericidal properties of noncellular blood were demonstrated by an American scientist, George Henry Falkiner Nuttall (1862–1937) while he was working towards his PhD at Göttingen in 1888. The first example of experimental induction of autoimmune disease was given by Thomas M. Rivers and Francis F. Schwentker of the Rockefeller Institute in 1940. They produced autoimmune encephalitis in animals by injecting the animal's own brain tissue. The concept of autoimmune disease was put forward by Ernest Witebsky (1901–1969) from Germany who emigrated to America in 1934 and proposed the *Postulate of Autoimmune Diseases* around 1942. The first large study of chemical specificity in immunology *The Specificity of Serological Reactions* was published by Karl Landsteiner (1868–1943) in 1936. Hemolytic anemia was one of the first autoimmune diseases to be observed in humans by William Dameshek (1900–1969) in 1940. *See immunoglobulins, histocompatibility.*

Immunosuppressive Agents [Latin: *imunis*, free + *supressus*, to suppress] Prevention of the immune response. Whole body irradiation was the first such therapy available before the introduction of mercaptopurine and azothioprine in 1962. A sophisticated isolation technique to minimize infection during total body radiation was devised by M.F.A. Woodruff in 1964. Steriods (prednisolone) were first used to suppress acute rejection during organ transplantation in 1965. Antilymphocytic serum was used to prolong survival of transplanted tissues by M.F.A. Woodruff and N. Anderson in 1963.

Imperforate Anus [Latin: *imperforatus*, not open] First description given by Soranus of Ephesus (AD 98–138) in the first century. Paul of Aegina (AD 625–690) recommended rupture of the membrane with fingers. Haly Abbas (d AD 944) advised incision and introduction of a lead pipe to maintain the passage. Several operations to create an artificial anus were described in the 19th century. *See artificial anus.*

Imperiale, John Baptist (1568–1603) Italian physician born in Vincenza. He studied at Bologna and Verona before becoming professor of physick and philosophy at Padua. He published *Exercitationum Exoticarum*.

Imperiale, John (1602–1653) Physician and son of John Baptist Imperiale. Professor of physick at Padua who wrote *Musaeum Physicum, sive de Humano Excercitationum* in 1640.

Impotence [Latin: *in*, not + *potentia*, power] The Ayurveda recommended use of testicular tissue as treatment. Paul of Aegina (AD 625–690) has suggested physical measures, such as rubbing various ointments from seeds of bastard saffron, pepper, or rocket on the genital parts. As a psychological

measure he advocated sexually stimulating books. Avicenna (980–1037) found that diabetes could be a cause. Preparations of testicles of sheep, pig and other animals have been mentioned as treatment in the Chinese book *Pen Tshoo*. A long list of other aphrodisiacs have been recommended by the ancients, including: nettle, lupin, asparagus, parsley, cress, beans and cinnamon. *See aphrodisiacs.*

Imuran *See azothioprine.*

In vitro Fertilization Pioneer work was done by English gynecologist and obstetrician, Patrick Christopher Steptoe (1913–1988) who worked with physiologist, Robert Geoffrey Edwards (b 1925) and achieved the first birth of a test tube baby in 1978.

Inappropriate ADH Syndrome (SIADH) Hypoosmolarity of serum with high urine osmolarity due to inappropriate secretion of antidiuretic hormone (ADH). First described in 1957 by William B. Schwartz of America.

Inborn Errors of Metabolism Genetically determined biochemical disorder producing a metabolic block that may be fatal. First shown by Archibald Garrod (1857–1935) of St Bartholomew's Hospital and the Hospital for Sick Children at Great Ormond Street. In 1902 he observed the frequency of alkaptonuria in the progeny of marriages between first cousins and proposed that the defect was inherited according to Mendel's laws. In his Croonian lectures delivered to the Royal College of Physicians in 1908, he added albinism, pentosuria and cystinuria to the list of inherited or inborn errors of metabolism. Phenylketonuria was described by G.A. Jervis and R.J. Block in 1940. Another inborn error of metabolism – homocystinuria – was formerly confused with Marfan syndrome. The first description of the disease as a separate entity was given by N.A.J. Carson and D.W. Neill in 1962. They noted the metabolic abnormality in a series of backward individuals. Homocystine was first identified in the urine of patients with this condition by T. Gerritsen and co-workers in the same year.

Inca The center of Inca civilization in Peru, the City of the Sun or the Golden city of Cuzco was established by the Inca prince, Manco Capac around AD 1000. This civilization which equaled that of the Mayans of Yucatan lasted for nearly 500 years until the invasion of the Spaniards in 1532. Incas practiced embalming and the mummies of their rulers were prepared in a sitting posture and preserved in the Sun Temple at Cuzco. They regarded disease as sent from the gods and resorted to prayer, fasting and religious rituals. Their materia medica contained quinine and coca, and their physicians practiced venesection.

Incantation [Latin: *incantare*, enchant] Ritual chanting of charms or spells practiced by many primitive races to drive out the devils or evil spirits which cause disease. Babylonian clay tablets have revealed the practice of exorcisms and incantations practiced by the Assipu priests and Babylonian physicians to relieve pain. Some African medicine-men made their living by writing prayers and incantations on a board and selling the water which was used to wash them. The Athara veda and rig veda systems of medicine of the Indian Brahmins originally contained a mixture of incantations, herbals and witchcraft. Aetius of Amida (AD 502–575), the first Christian physician of note, employed charms and incantations in preparing his remedies and treating his patients. *See temple medicine, Babylonian medicine.*

Incest [Latin: *incestus*, unchaste] Sexual intercourse between closely related persons. Practiced by ancients Egyptians, Iranians and other races to preserve the bloodline and dynasty. Cleopatra was married to her brother Ptolemy. Incest is prohibited by the Incest Acts of Scotland (1867) and England (1908).

Incisors [Latin: *incidere*, to cut into] Any of the four anterior teeth in the jaw. Teeth were first classified into molars, bicuspids, cuspids and incisors by John Hunter (1728–1793) in *A Practical Treatise on the Diseases of the Teeth* published in 1778.

Inclusion Bodies [Latin: *inclusio*, to shut] First observed by Stanislaus Joseph von Prowazek (1875–1915) in 1907, he postulated that they were collections of virus enveloped by material deposited from an infected cell. Herpes inclusions within the nucleus of cells in man and animals were discovered by Benjamin Lipschutz (1878–1921) in 1920 and by A. Luger in 1921.

Incontinence Galen (AD 129–200) remarked that incontinence is caused by injury of the spinal marrow either through violence or application of cold. According to Avicenna (980–1037) it is occasioned by relaxation of the muscles (sphincter vesicae), or weakness of the bladder. Haly Abbas (930–994), an Arabian physician, considered the cause to be enervation of sphincter vesicae and loss of the retentive faculty of the bladder. These basic mechanisms have been confirmed as some of the main causes of incontinence.

Incubus [Latin: Nightmare] Described by Thomas Willis (1621–1675) as a due to ailment of digestion. Symptoms described by him during sleep include heaviness in the chest, tightness in the throat, and inability to talk.

Incunabulum Book printed from movable type before 1501. One of the earliest known medical incunabula titled *Agregator de Medicinis Simplicibus* of Giacomo de Dondis (1298–1359) was published later in 1470. One of the earliest incunabula with pictorial representation is that of Mondino de Luzzi completed in 1316 and printed at Padua in 1487. Some of the other illustrated or graphic incunabula include: *Fasiculus Medicinae* (1491) of Johannes de Ketham, *Philosophiae naturalis compendium* (1499) of Johanes Peyligk, *Conciliator* (1496) of Peter of Abano, and *Antropologium* (1501) of Magnus Hundt.

Incurables Despite lack of knowledge and facilities, few diseases were considered incurable even by the ancients. Leprosy was considered incurable because of its chronic nature, deformity and social impact. The first Royal Hospital for incurables in England was founded by a physician, Andrew Reed at Carlshalton Surrey in 1850.

Indian hemp *See Cannabis indica.*

Indian medicine *See Ayurvedic medicine.*

Indians of North America The tribes (e.g. Dakota, Navaho, Apache, Crow, Ojibwa) of North American Indians had some variations in their practice of medicine which consisted of drugs, herbs and religious rituals. Like most other early races elsewhere in the world they believed that diseases were sent by gods and they resorted to a number of deities to drive out disease. Terawa, the creator or the great spirit, was the lord of the Earth. The next important deity was his wife, followed by other gods of winds, clouds, lightning and thunder. Their medicine man was often a survivor of an almost fatal accident or chosen through a miraculous dream. Others who became medicine men were chosen at a young age and had to undergo long periods of training. Blackfoot Indians had to undergo a form of training called seven tents of medicine, each tent or stage of one year's duration. Medicine men, who had to have a supernatural power wore masks, charms and necklaces, held effigies and played an important role in most ceremonies asking the gods for rain, grain or victory in war. Their medicine included willow bark, the source of salicylic acid, podophyllin, wintergreen and sarsaparilla. They treated snake bites with incision and suction. They used bone needles for suturing, and splints made of raw hide for fractures. John Josselyn described various diseases affecting Indians in 1674. One of the earliest modern account on the diseases of the North American Indians was written by Benjamin Rush (1745–1813) in 1774.

Indium Metallic element used in semiconductor research. Radioactive isotopes are used in nuclear medicine. Discovered by Ferdinand Reich (1799–1882) German professor of physics at Freiburg and Hieronymous Theodor Richter (1824–1898) of Dresden in 1863.

Induction Current Discovered by Michael Faraday (1791–1867) who first published his findings in *Experimental Researches* in 1831. His discovery played an important part in the development of electrotherapy.

Induction of Labor Some tribes of the American Indians had a horseman ride towards a full-term pregnant woman threatening to trample her in order to induce labor. In Greece, around the time of Hippocrates, the woman was repeatedly lifted and dropped on a couch to hasten labor. Another ancient Greek method involved tying the woman to a couch and turning it upright, repeatedly striking it on the ground. With the development of midwifery these practices were abandoned. A systematic account of various operative methods used in the more recent past was given by an English obstetrician, Robert Barnes (1817–1907) in 1861. These include: puncture of the amniotic sac, use of ergot, separation of the membranes, introduction of a sound and tapping the sac, introducing a flexible catheter into the sac and leaving it *in situ*, dilation of the cervix, introducing a calf bladder into the vagina and distending it with water, use of air pessary, use of galvanism, application of sinnapisms to the breast, use of cupping-glasses, injection of carbonic acid into vagina, warm douche to the vaginal portion of the uterus, employment of intra-uterine injections, direct uterine douche, and several other means.

Indus Valley Civilization The excavations carried out at Mohanjadaro and Harappa in the Indus valley in the 1920s by English archeologist, Sir John Hubert Marshall (1876–1958) have provided evidence for an advanced civilization which existed around 2500 BC or perhaps earlier. The brick-built cities had an advanced system of sanitation and hygiene. Drains were used to carry sewage into tanks from where it was hygienically disposed.

Industrial Chemistry One of the first treatises, *Pirotechnica*, was written by Italian, Vanocchio Biringuccio (1460–1539) of Sienna in 1540. He set out the economic advantages of large-scale chemical production. The first modern scientific book, *Chemistry applied to the Arts* was published by French statesman and chemist, Jean Antoine Claude Chaptal (1756–1832) of Nogaret in 1807. The discovery of aniline in coal tar by August Wilhelm von Hoffmann (1818–1892) working at the College of Chemistry in London, led to the establishment of a dyestuffs industry and production of benzene and other hydrocarbons on a commercial scale.

Industrial Disease *See occupational disease.*

Industrial Medicine Charles Turner Thackrah (1795–1833), a Yorkshire-born physician who practiced at Leeds, is regarded as the founder of industrial medicine in England. In 1831 he published the first treatise on the subject in England, *The Effects of the Principle Arts, Trades and Professions, and of Civic States and Habits of Living, on Health and Longevity, with Suggestions for the Removal of the Agents which produce Disease and shorten the Duration of Life. See occupational disease.*

Industrial Schools Act Made provision for education and care of vagrant, destitute and disorderly children and was enacted in 1857. Two further acts on it were passed in 1861 and 1866. By 1864 47 such schools were established in England.

Inebriety [Latin: *in*, intensive + *ebrietas*, drunkenness] *See drunkenness, alcohol, addiction.*

Inert Gas [Latin: *iners*, inactive] *See argon, helium, krypton, xenon.*

Infancy [Latin: *in*, negative + *fans*, speaking] *See breast feeding, pediatrics.*

Infant Feeding *See breast feeding.*

Infant Mortality Rates up to the 18th century in England and Europe were appalling. Out of the 31,951 children admitted to the Paris Foundling Hospital from 1771 to 1777, 80% died. In Ireland, out of 10,272 children admitted to the Dublin Foundling Asylum from 1775 to 1796, 99.6% died. In England the average infant mortality rate from 1791 to 1801 was 437 per 1000 births. An improvement of 50% on these figures were achieved in England over the next 50 years. The trend continued until a strong lobby, including Samuel Johnson, prevailed to enact the Parish Poor Infants Act in 1767. Despite these efforts, in 1875 the rate in England and Wales was still 158 per 1000. In the United States only half of all the children in the mid-19th century reached their fifth year.

Infant Welfare Movement Originated by Pierre Budin (1846–1907) chief at the Charité Hospital in Paris in 1892. He organized the first 'consultation de nourrissons' for screening babies one month after delivery. Nathan Straus (1848–1931), a New York philanthropist, set up a system of milk feeding stations in Manhattan. The milk depot meant for infants in England was set up by F. Drew Harris at St Helen's in 1899. The first International Congress devoted entirely to child welfare was held at Paris in 1905.

Infanticide [Latin: *infans*, infant + *caedere*, to kill] In 1532 Charles V introduced a code for magistrates to call for medical evidence in cases of assault, infanticide and pretended pregnancies. Jan Swammerdam (1637–1680) of Holland made the observation during postmortem that the lungs of an infant born alive would float in water while that of a still-birth infant would sink. He described his postmortem findings on dead infants in *Tractus de Respiratione* in 1667. His observations were first used medico-legally by Johann Schreyer in 1690 to free a girl accused of infanticide. William Hunter's essay on the signs of murder in bastard children in 1783, was the most important English contribution on the subject. Paul Broudal (1837–1906) of Paris wrote another important monograph on the subject in 1897. The Infant Life Preservation Act of the UK, which made the destruction of children at or before birth punishable with penal servitude for life, was passed in 1925. The Infanticide Act is only applicable to the mother and was passed in 1938.

Infantile Paralysis The term was first coined by German orthopedic surgeon, Jacob von Heine (1799–1879) in 1840. *See acute anterior poliomyelitis.*

Infantilism Characteristics of childhood persist into adult life. First used by Paul Joseph Lorain (1827–1875) of Paris in 1871 to denote idiopathic arrest of growth in connection with tuberculosis. It was adapted to hypopituitarism by Ettore Levi from Florence, in 1908.

Infection [Latin: *in*, + *facere*, to do] *See germ theory of disease.*

Infectious Disease Notification Act British act first enacted by the local body at Bolton in 1877. This was followed by similar Local Acts in other towns. Infectious diseases became notifiable throughout the country with the Infectious Diseases Act of 1889.

Infectious Mononucleosis First described by Nils Fedorovich Filatov (1847–1902) in 1887. Emil Pfeiffer (1846–1921) gave a classic description in 1889, calling it 'drusenfieber'. The characteristic blood changes were first observed by Wilhelm Turk in 1907, while H.L. Tidy and E.C. Daniel gave further details in 1923. The presence of heterophilic antibodies was first demonstrated by two American physicians, John Rodman Paul (1893–1971) and Walls Willard Bunnel (1902–1966) in 1932. Caused by the Epstein-Barr virus, also called glandular fever, Filatov disease, kissing disease and Pfeiffer disease.

Inferior Carotid Ganglion [Latin: *inferius*, beneath; Greek: *karos*, deep sleep + *ganglions*, knot] Found in the cavernous plexus. First described in 1744 by Kasimir Christoph Schmiedel (1716–1792), professor of anatomy and botany at Erlangen.

Inferior Laryngeal Nerve [Latin: *inferus*, beneath + *laryngis*, larynx] Discovered by Marinus, Roman physician around AD 100.

Inferiority Complex [Latin: *inferus*, beneath + *complexus*, entwined] Mechanisms involved in overcoming this psychological state were described by psychoanalyst, Alfred Adler (1870–1937) of Vienna in 1907 in *Study of Organ Inferiority and its Psychical Compensation.*

Infibulation [Latin: *infibulare*, to buckle together] A method of fastening of the sexual organs to prevent coitus. The first mention of it in English language is made in Bulwer's *Anthropometamorphosis* written in 1650, where buttoning of the prepuce of the male with a metal button is described. The method has also been described by Aulus Cornelius Celsus (25 BC–AD 50) for use on males to preserve their voice and health. Vogel in 1786 suggested infibulation as a remedy for masturbation. Effective mechanical prevention for masturbation was also described by J.L. Milton in his *Spermatorrhoea* in 1880.

Infirmaries [Latin: *infirmus*, not strong] Hospitals to care for the sick. Established by religious orders during the 6th century to care for the infirm, pilgrims, wayfarers and the destitute using simple medicinal herbs grown in monastic gardens. During the medieval period Christians built institutions called 'nosokomea' for the sick, and 'gerocomeia' for the aged. The first Christian hospital was in Edessa in Western Mesopotamia, built by St Ephrem around AD 372. Nestorius, the Bishop of Constantinople in AD 431 established the Nestorian order, and founded two hospitals which developed into a school of medicine. Fabiola, a Roman lady, devoted her entire life to working for the poor sick and built the first Christian hospital in Rome around AD 390. The first of the Hôtel Dieu or 'house of God's charity' was founded in Lyons by king Childebert in AD 542. The Hôtel Dieu of Paris was founded in AD 651 by Landry, bishop of Paris. The first Moslem hospital was established by Caliph Walid at Baghdad in AD 707. One of the earliest hospitals in Cairo, the El-Nazuri Hospital, was founded in AD 874. The oldest hospital in Scotland, the *Soltray* or *Soltar*, was founded by Malcolm IV in Midlothian in 1164. *See Edinburgh Royal Infirmary, Glasgow Royal Infirmary.*

Inflammation [Latin: *inflammatio*, to set on fire] Aulus Cornelius Celsus (25 BC–AD 50) established the four cardinal signs of inflammation: heat, pain, redness and swelling. These are still used in diagnosis. Epoch-making studies on blood and inflammation were done by John Hunter (1728–1793), founder of surgical pathology in Britain. William Addison (1802–1881) from Malvern published his work on blood and inflammation in seven sections in *the Transactions of the Provincial Medical and Surgical Association* in 1843. He gave the first description of leucocytosis and diapedesis of blood cells. His theory on the role of white blood cells in inflammation and suppuration was advanced by Julius Cohnheim (1839–1884) in 1867.

Influenza [Italian: *influenza*] Thomas Willis (1621–1673) and Thomas Sydenham (1624–1689) described it. The term was first used to denote a characteristic illness found in northern Italy. It was previously known as epidemic catarrhal fever and many outbreaks occurred in England between 1729 and 1847. The name was first used in England by John Huxam (1692–1768). One of the worst epidemics occurred in 1918–1919, killing about 30 million people worldwide. The influenza of swine was first shown to be due to a virus by an American virologist, Richard Edwin Shope (1901–1966), and first cultured by Australian immunologist, Sir Frank Macfarlane Burnet (1899–1985) in 1935. The influenza B virus was isolated independently by Thomas Francis (1900–1969) and Thomas Pleines Magill (b 1903), in 1940.

Informed Consent The first directive was issued to prisons by the Prussian Minister of Interior in 1891 for use of tuberculin to treat tuberculosis. He specified that it should not be given against the person's will. Albert Neisser (1855–1916), the discoverer of the gonococcus and a professor of venereology at Breslau, in his search for prevention of syphilis injected the serum of syphilitic patients to patients who were admitted for other medical conditions without informing them in 1898. Some of these patients developed syphilis and Neisser explained it on the basis that they contracted syphilis through prostitution and that his serum was not effective. He was investigated by the public prosecutor and fined by the Royal Disciplinary Court. Following the publicity of this case, Albert Moll collected over 600 instances of unethical research in *Physicians Ethics*. He advocated the procedure of informed consent for human experimentation.

Infrared Radiation [Latin: *infra*, below + *radiare*, to furnish with spokes] Discovered by Sir Frederick William Herschel (1738–1822) in 1800. In his experiments he passed light through a prism and set up thermometers beyond the red end of the spectrum to demonstrate the heating effect of infrared.

Infusoria [Latin: *in*, into + *fundere*, to pour into] Former name for Ciliophora. Anton van Leeuwenhoek (1632–1723), a Dutch maker of lenses and a early microscopist, described the microscopical forms as 'animalcules' in 1683. An important work on infusorial animalculae was

published by Christian Gottfried Ehrenberg (1795–1876) of Berlin in 1838, and a valuable summary on the subject is given in Andrew Pritchard's *Infusoria*, published in 1861.

Ingenhousz, Jan (1730–1799) Physician, botanist and chemist from Breda, who settled in Britain. He visited England to learn the method of inoculation for smallpox and inoculated members of the Austrian imperial family. He was the first person to generate static electricity by pressing a leather pad against a revolving disc. He published several works on medicine, botany and chemistry. Following Joseph Priestley's (1733–1804) discovery in 1771 that plants give off oxygen, Ingenhousz showed that oxygen fixed is proportional to light intensity. This was expounded in *Experiments upon vegetables, discovering their great power of purifying the common air in the sunshine and of injuring it in the shade and at night* published in 1779.

Ingrassias, Giovanni Filippo (1510–1580) Sicilian physician who graduated from Padua in 1537 and became a professor of medicine and anatomy at Palermo. He published a guide for jurists on medico-legal matters in 1578 which included discussions on torture, deformity, frigidity and the duration of pregnancy. He did some original work on the ear and described the stapes.

Inguinal Hernia [Latin: *inguen*, groin + hernia] An early treatise on the surgical treatment was written by Sir Astley Paston Cooper (1768–1841) in 1807. A surgical method for radical cure was described by Sir William Macewen (1848–1924) in 1886 and two further such methods were used by Eduardo Bassini (1844–1924) of Padua in 1887, and William S. Halsted (1852–1922) of Johns Hopkins Hospital in 1889.

Inhalational Anesthesia [Latin: *inhalatio*, to breath in] Herodotus (*c* 484 BC) mentioned the Scythians who inhaled vapors of cannabis. The effect of inhalation of gases was studied by Sir Humphry Davy (1778–1829) in 1796. The first demonstration of painless surgery in animals using carbon dioxide anesthesia was performed by Henry Hill Hickman (1800–1830) around 1821 and published as *A Letter on Suspended Animation* in 1824. Boston surgeon J. C. Warren (1778–1856) used ether in 1846 while nitrous oxide was given by dentist, Horace Wells (1818–1897) from Hartford, Connecticut in 1844. Chloroform was first successfully used on a woman in labor by James Y. Simpson (1811–1870) of Edinburgh in 1847. Thomas Joseph Clover introduced an inhaler for administering ether and chloroform in 1876. A mixture of chloroform, ether and absolute alcohol was suggested by George Harley (1829–1886) and found to be safer than chloroform by the Royal Medical and Chirugical Society in 1884. Frederick

William Hewitt (1857–1916), anesthetist to Charing Cross and London Hospitals designed the first portable apparatus for administering a mixture of nitrous oxide and oxygen for dental and other minor operations in 1886. *See anesthesia, chloroform, endotracheal anesthesia, ether.*

Inhibitory Nerve [Latin: *inhibere*, to restrain] *See vagus.*

Injection [Latin: *injectio*, to throw in] *See hypodermic injection.*

Injury Potential   First demonstrated by Emil du Bois-Reymond (1818–1896), a German scientist of French ancestry, professor of physiology at the University of Berlin in 1840. He showed that if one end of a muscle was killed by any agent, the dead portion became negative in relation to the preserved or living end.

Innominate Artery [Latin: *innominatus*, nameless] Abraham Colles (1773–1843), professor of surgery at Dublin, is supposed to have been the first to successfully tie the innominate artery in 1811.

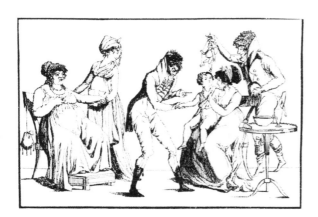

A caricature on Inoculation (1800). *Curiosités Médico-Artistiques* (1907). Albin Michel, Paris

Inoculation [Latin: *in*, into + *oculus*, a bud] Practiced in India for smallpox since ancient times. Giacomo Pylarini (1659–1718), an Italian physician inoculated three children with smallpox material. Lady Mary Wortley Montagu (1689–1762), the wife of British ambassador to Constantinople, introduced the method, inoculating her five-year-old daughter in the presence of seven physicians in 1718. King George I became interested in the procedure, and he had it tried on six condemned criminals on death row in 1721. The next trial was done on eleven children from charity schools, and finding it a success King George's two grandchildren were inoculated. In America the material taken from the pustule of a person with smallpox was used to inoculate his son by a Boston physician, Zabdiel Boyston (1680–1766) in 1721. This was the first instance of smallpox inoculation in America. The first book in America, which dealt with smallpox vaccination was written in the same year by Benjamin Colman (1673–1747) of Boston. Benjamin Jesty (1731–1816) from Yetminster, England, introduced the method of inoculation with the material taken from a cowpox sore in the udder and, using a stocking needle, successfully inoculated his wife and two sons. Edward Jenner (1749–1823), a physician in Berkeley, Gloucestershire, noted that dairymaids contaminated with cowpox were immune to smallpox and published his findings in 1798. The wide dissemination of his papers led to his cowpox vaccine being shipped to the United States on pieces of fabric soaked in the virus and sealed into glass vials. Benjamin Waterhouse (1754–1846) of Harvard first used this vaccine and sent some to Thomas Jefferson who vaccinated his family, servants, friends and neighbors.

Inosinic Acid   First nucleotide to be isolated from meat extract by Justus von Liebig (1803–1873) in 1847.

Inotropics [Greek: *inos*, fiber + *trepein*, influence] Affecting the energy of muscle contraction. The action of adrenaline was first described by R. Eliot in 1905 in the *Journal of Physiology*, but its use was limited by its tendency to induce arrhythmias. Effect of dopamine was first presented by L.I. Goldberg in 1972. The selective action of dobutamine on the heart in increasing its contractility was demonstrated by R.R. Tuttle and J. Mills in 1975.

Insanity [Latin: *in*, not + *sanus*, sound] Mentioned in the Hippocratic Corpus as 'mania' and 'melancholia'. During medieval and earlier times, the insane were subjected to harsh treatment. Caelius Aurelianus in the fifth century AD was one of the first to advise a humane and rational approach to insanity. The Arabs, around AD 1000, considered the insane to be divinely inspired and treated them more kindly. Felix Platter (1536–1614) and Richard Napier (1559–1634) included biological and socio-environmental factors in their writings. Reginald Scott (1538–1599) of England suggested insanity in those involved in witchcraft. John Locke (1632–1704), David Hartley (1705–1757) and William Cullen (1710–1790) incorporated physical and psychological theory into their treatises. Thomas Arnold (1742–1816) wrote an early treatise on its history and nature in 1758. Philippe Pinel (1745–1826), a neuropsychiatrist at Paris, was one of the first to follow Cullen's work and to call it an illness, unchain the patients, and treat them humanely. The eminent English psychiatrist Henry Maudsley (1835–1918) of Britain maintained that insanity was fundamentally a bodily disease in *The Physiology and Pathology of Human Mind* published in 1867. *See asylum.*

Institute of Medical History (Institut für Geschichte der Medizin) Established at Leipzig in 1905 through funds left by the widow of a tutor in medical history at Vienna and Leipzig, Theodor Puschmann (1844–1899). Karl Sudhoff (1853–1938) of Frankfurt-am-Main, a self-taught scholar in medical history served as its first director.

Institute of Medical History Formed in 1929 at the Johns Hopkins University through the benefaction of the Rockefeller Foundation. William Henry Welch (1850–1934) was appointed as its first professor of medical history and Fielding Hudson Garrison (1870–1935) became its first librarian.

Insulin Antibodies Discovered by New York biophysicist and Nobel Prize winner, Rosalyn Yalow neé Sussman (b 1921) and Solomon Berson (1918–1972).

Insulin Secreting Tumor of Pancreas In 1924 Seale Harris noted spontaneous hyperinsulinism in four patients but did not connect it with tumors of the pancreas. Severe spontaneous hypoglycemia was noted in a surgeon by Russel Morse Wilder (1885–1959), F.N. Allen and M.H. Power in 1927. Adenoma of the islets of Langerhans was noted in this patient during the operation. Another similar case was noted by W.V. McClelnahan and G.W. Morris in 1928. The first large series of 62 patients was presented by an American surgeon and pathologist at Columbia University, Allen Oldfather Whipple (b 1881) and Virginia Franz (1896–1967) in 1935.

Insulin Shock Treatment Used as treatment for schizophrenia by Manfred Joshua Sakel (1900–1957) in 1929.

Insulin Tolerance Test Used for the diagnosis of hypopituitarism where glucose levels fail to return to pre-injection levels of insulin after two hours. First devised by R. Fraser, Fuller Albright (1900–1969), and P.H. Smith in 1941.

Insulin [Latin: *insula*, island] The role of pancreas was first demonstrated in 1889 by Joseph von Mering (1849–1908) and Oskar Minkowski (1858–1931) of Strasbourg who removed the pancreas in a dog and found that it developed glycosuria. This substance was first called 'isletin' and the name 'insulin' was given by Sir Edward Albert Sharpey-Schafer (1850–1935) in 1916. It was first isolated by Canadians, Frederick Banting (1891–1941) and Charles Herbert Best (1899–1978), under the direction of John James Rickard Macleod (1876–1935) in 1922. Bertram James Collip (1892–1965) a chemist from Alberta, obtained a purified extract of insulin in 1923. The first person to receive insulin treatment in America was Jim Havens, the son of the president of Eastman Kodak Company, in 1922.

It was soon realized that diabetic patients needed frequent insulin injections to maintain normal blood glucose levels. An insulin combined with protamine from salmon roe (to prolong effect) was first prepared by Hans Christian Hagedorn (1888–1971) at the Steno Memorial Hospital in Copenhagen in 1935. The possibility of a single injection to last for a whole day was brought within reach by D.A. Scott and Albert Fisher who added zinc to form a relatively insoluble protamine zinc insulin in 1936. A neutral protamine insulin called isophane insulin, which contained less protamine and unmodified zinc insulin, was introduced by Hagedorn in 1945. The sequence of amino acids in the protein chain of insulin was deduced by Frederick Sanger (b 1918), an English biochemist and Nobel Prize winner, in the 1940s and the difference in the sequence of amino acids of insulin from pig, sheep, horse and whale was worked out by him in the early 1950s. The first trials on ultralente, lente and semilente long-acting insulin preparations in zinc suspensions were conducted by Knud Hallas-Moller (b 1914) and colleagues in 1951. Insulin was the first genetically engineered hormone to be approved by the FDA, and marketed by Eli Lilly in 1982. *See Zuelzer, Georg Ludwig.*

Intal The plant *Ammi visnaga* has been used for centuries in the treatment of asthma, and the crude extract of its seeds was known as khellin. Cromoglycic acid, the active ingredient, was purified in 1967 and given its current name. It is widely used in treatment of asthma as a prophylactic. It was introduced as a vasodilator in the treatment of angina by G.V. Anrep, a pupil of Ivan Pavlov (1849–1936), and Ernest Starling (1866–1927) but proved ineffective.

Intelligence Quotient William Stern (1871–1938) was the first to suggest the concept. This measure was obtained by dividing the mental age of the child by the chronological age and remained constant. Lewis M. Terman (1877–1956) of Stanford University renamed the test intelligence quotient (IQ) and modified it. In his calculation the chronological age is divided by mental age and multiplied by 100.

Intelligence Tests Alfred Binet (1857–1911), a French experimental psychologist pioneered the study of intelligence. He carried out ingenious experiments on his two daughters and published *L'Etude Experimentale de l'Intelligence* in 1895. The Binet–Simon test was devised in 1905, together with Theodore Simon (1873–1961) of Paris. It was introduced into the United States by Henry H. Goddard at the Training School in Vineland, New Jersey in 1910. A test for adults was devised by New York psychologist, David Wechsler (b 1896). Tests using numerical measures were developed by Edward Lee Thorndyke (1874–1949) of Massachusetts in 1926. *See intelligence quotient.*

Interatrial Septal Defect [Latin: *inter*, between + *atria*, ante-chamber] *See foramen ovale.*

Interferon Glycoprotein with antiviral activity. Discovered by a Scottish virologist, Alick Isaacs (1921–1967) of Glasgow and Jean Lindemann in 1957. The successful cloning of the human interferon gene and production of interferon in bacteria was achieved by Charles Weissmann (b 1931) from the University of Zurich in 1980.

Intermittent Catherization Used in urology by J. Lapides and co-workers in 1972.

Intermittent Claudication First described by J. Bouley in 1831. He gave a description of lameness due to arterial disease in a horse after exercise. Sir Benjamin Brodie (1783–1862) gave a description of the condition in humans in 1846. The symptom of intermittent claudication was related to arterial disease by Wilhelm Heinrich Erb (1840–1921). George W. Pickering (1904–1982) and P. Rothschild also studied the condition in detail, and Sir Thomas Lewis (1881–1945) devoted one chapter to intermittent claudication in his *Clinical Science* published in 1934.

Internal Cartoid Artery Aneurysm Large aneurysm of the internal carotid artery eroding the sella and producing signs of bitemporal hemianopia, similar to that seen in a pituitary tumor. Reported by Byrom Bramwell (1847–1931) of Edinburgh in 1887. The first successful modern surgical operation was performed by Norman M. Dott (1897–1973), also of Edinburgh, in 1933. *See intracranial aneurysm.*

Internal Cartoid Artery Thrombosis Four cases were diagnosed using carotid angiography by Portuguese Nobel Prize winner, Egaz Moniz (1874–1955) and Almeida Lima in 1937. Another case was diagnosed with the use of angiography by H.R.I.Wolfe in 1948.

Internal Secretions *See ductless glands, hormones.*

International Congress The first in science, the International Chemical Congress, was organized in 1860 by German professor of chemistry, Friedrich August Kekulé von Stradonitz (1829–1896) in Bonn. The first International Medical Congress was held at Paris in 1867 and London in 1881. The first International Physiology Congress was held at Basel in 1889, mainly through the efforts of British physiologist, Sir Michael Foster (1836–1907). The first International Congress devoted entirely to child welfare

was held in Paris in 1905, and the first European Congress of Pediatric Urology was held in 1961.

International Red Cross *See Red Cross Society.*

International Society for Human and Animal Mycology (ISHAM) Founded in Paris. First president in 1953 was P. Redaelli of Milan.

Interstitial Pulmonary Fibrosis *See Hamman–Rich syndrome.*

Interventricular Septal Defect [Latin: *inter*, between + *ventriculum*, ventricle] *See ventricular septal defect.*

Intervertebral Disc Prolapse [Latin: *inter*, between + *vertebra*] One of the earliest treatises on sciatica was given by Domenico Cotugno (1736–1822) of Naples in 1770. The first report of the rupture of the intervertebral disc was given by Theodore Kocher (1841–1917) in 1896. Its occurrence following trauma was shown independently by George Stevensen Middleton (1854–1928) and John Hammond Teacher (1869–1930) of Britain, and Joel E. Goldthwait (1867–1961) of Boston in 1911. A case of sciatica due to rupture of the intervertebral disc was also described by Middleton in 1911. Brachial neuritis due to lateral herniation of the cervical intervertebral disc was first described by B. Stooky in 1940, and later by Ralph Eustace Semmes (b 1886) of Memphis, in 1943. Chymopapain was first used to dissolve the nucleus pulposus of the intervertebral disc by Lyman W. Smith of North Western Medical School, Chicago in 1963. *See sciatica.*

Intestinal Anastomosis The first recorded case of suturing, after complete division of the intestines was achieved by Karl A. Ramdohr of Halle in 1780. An important early monograph on the subject, *An Inquiry into the Processes of Nature in Repairing of the Intestines*, was published by Benjamin Travers (1783–1858), surgeon at St Thomas' Hospital in 1812. Jacques Gilles Thomas Maisonneuve of France established a communication to bypass (but unsuccessful) bowel obstruction around 1845 in two patients. The subject was revived by Hacken in 1863 and advanced by Nicholas Senn (1844–1908) in 1887, professor of surgery who specialized in intestinal surgery at Rush Medical College, Chicago. Catgut for suturing was introduced by New York surgeon Robert Abbe (1851–1928) in 1889.

Intestinal Resection Two feet of gangrenous bowel were resected from a strangulated hernia for the first time by Karl A. Ramdohr of Halle in 1727. Following a rupture of the cecum, Arnaud de Ronsil, surgeon at the Academy of

Surgery in Paris successfully excised the cecum, and part of the colon and ileum in 1732. A carcinomatous growth of the sigmoid flexure was removed, together with three inches of normal gut, by Jean François Reybard (1790–1863) in 1843. In 1888 McArdle presented a series of 26 excisions following gangrenous hernia and, in 1890 Theodor Billroth (1829–1894) reported 140 resections of stomach and intestines which he performed.

Intestinal Tuberculosis Auguste Chauveau (1827–1917) of Paris was the first to demonstrate experimentally, in 1868, in animals that swallowing tubercular matter led to ulceration in the intestines. Tuberculous cavities in the lungs as a source of intestinal lesions was noted independently by Theodor Albrecht Edwin Klebs (1834–1913), and F. Mosler of Germany in 1873.

Intracardiac Thrombus *See cardiac thrombus.*

Intracranial Tumors One of the early modern monographs on the subject was written by Byrom Bramwell (1847–1931), a physician to the Edinburgh Royal Infirmary in 1888. *See brain tumors.*

Intracranial Aneurysm The first suggestion that aneurysms could occur in cerebral vessels was made by Swiss physician Johann Jacob Wepfer (1620–1695). It was noted as a cause of apoplexy by another Swiss physician, Johann Brunner (1633–1727). The occurrence of bilateral intracranial aneurysms was shown by Sir Gilbert Blane (1749–1834) in 1800. The first suggestion that subarachnoid hemorrhage is related to aneurysm was made by William Gull (1816–1890) of Guy's Hospital in 1859. An excellent case of a rupture of an aneurysm at the bifurcation of the middle cerebral artery was reported by Sir William Osler (1849–1919) in 1877. A. Eppinger was the first to suggest a congenital defect in the arterial wall as a basis for the development of intracranial aneurysms in 1887. Sir Charles Putnam Symonds (1890–1978), a neurologist to Guy's Hospital and the National Hospital for Nervous Diseases in Queen's Square, reviewed 124 cases of subarachnoid hemorrhage in 1923 and concluded that the rupture was the commonest cause. Sir Victor Horsley (1857–1916) first used ligation outside the cavernous sinus in 1885. The first planned surgery to prevent rupture was performed by Wilfred Trotter (1872–1939) in 1924. Sir Astley Paston Cooper (1768–1852) unsuccessfully ligated the artery for treatment of carotid aneurysm in 1805. On his second attempt in 1808 the patient lived for 13 years. Another carotid artery ligation for berry aneurysm was performed by Benjamin Travers (1783–1858) in 1811. C. Pilz in 1863 collected a series of 600 carotid ligations out of which 43%

died. The first successful modern surgical technique for the treatment of an intracranial aneurysm in the internal carotid artery was that of Norman M. Dott (1897–1973) of Edinburgh in 1933.

Intraocular Pressure *See tonometer, glaucoma.*

Intrauterine Death A radiological method for diagnosis was devised independently by two Americans, D.A. Horner and Alfred Baker Spalding (1874–1942) in 1922. Their method was based on the appearance of the skull of the dead fetus upon X-ray.

Intrauterine Device (IUD) The earliest was made of silkworm gut bound by spiral metal wire and was described by German physician, Richard Richter, in 1909. A similar device was proposed independently by Karl Pust of Jena in 1923. The forerunner of modern IUD was devised by a German gynecologist, Ernest Grafenberg (1881–1957) in 1930. Another inert device was introduced by Jack Lippes in 1961.

Intravenous Anesthesia Chloroform and ether were first used as intravenous anesthetics by L. Burkhardt in 1909. Intravenous paraldehyde was introduced by H. Noel and Henry Sessions Souttar (b 1875), in 1913, and magnesium sulfate was used by C.H. Peck in 1916. The first intravenous barbiturate to be used for anesthesia was sodium amytal which was synthesized by Irvine Heinly Page (b 1901) in 1923. It was used as an anesthetic by Leon Grotius Zerfas (b 1897) and J.T.C. MacCallum of Indianapolis in 1929. Nembutal was introduced in the same year by J.S Lundy (1894–1973) of the Mayo Clinic. Barbiturates were also used by P. Fredet and R. Perlis in 1934, and Lundy introduced intravenous thiopentone in the same year. The first clinical use of the arrow poison, curare, was by the American H.R. Griffiths (1894–1985) and derivatives of this were made by the Swiss Nobel Prize winner, Daniel Bovet (1907–1992). *See intravenous medications.*

Intravenous Fluids Intravenous saline was first used as treatment for circulatory collapse following cholera by Thomas Atchison Latta in 1832.

Intravenous Local Anesthesia Injection of a local anesthetic into a vein of a limb, using a tourniquet was introduced by August Karl Gustav Bier (1861–1949) of Kiel in 1909.

Intravenous Medication Sir Christopher Wren (1632–1723) inaugurated the intravenous administration of drugs by injecting opium and *Crocus metallorum* into veins of dogs using a quill and a bladder in 1656. In 1662 Johann Daniel

Major (1634–1693) used the same method in man. Various other substances such as snail water, amber and cinnamon, were used in the 17th century. The first self-experimentation on intravenous drugs was done by a physician, Enoch Hale from West Hampton, Massachusetts who graduated from Harvard. In 1821 he self injected with castor oil using a primitive needle and was awarded the Boyleston prize for self-experiment. The first hypodermic needle was developed by Scottish physician, Alexander Wood (1817–1884) in 1852.

Intrinsic Factor [Latin: *intrinsecus*, inward] Antibodies in patients with pernicious anemia was first demonstrated by M. Schwartz in 1950.

Introvert [Latin: *intro*, within + *vertere*, to turn] Psychological type first described by Carl Gustav Jung (1875–1961) in 1923. In *Psychological Types* he described an introvert as one who directed his libido inwards and orientated himself towards the environment from the subjective point of view, adapting reality to his own subjective needs.

Intubation Armand Trousseau (1801–1867) of the Hôtel Dieu, Paris was a pioneer, and one of the first to perform a tracheostomy in 1851. Intubation of the upper laryngeal orifice and trachea through the mouth was first performed by William Macewen (1848–1924), a surgeon from Glasgow, in 1878. Intubation of the larynx in cases of laryngeal stenosis and croup was first performed by Joseph P. O'Dwyer (1841–1898) of Cleveland Ohio, in 1885. *See endotracheal intubation, inhalational anesthesia.*

Intussusception [Latin: *intus*, within + *suscipere*, to receive] Defined by John Hunter (1728–1793) as a 'disease produced by the passing of one portion of the intestine into another, and commonly from the upper passing into the lower part'. The first successful operation in an adult was performed by Cornelius Henrick Velse of Holland in 1742. It was described in greater detail in the late 18th century by George Langastaff of Edinburgh and Matthew Baillie (1761–1823), a nephew of John Hunter, in *Morbid Anatomy* published in 1793. Another successful case of abdominal surgery was performed by Sir Jonathan Hutchinson (1828–1913) in 1874.

Inulin Clearance Method Used to estimate glomerular filtration of the kidney. First introduced by Danish physiologist, Poul Brandt Rehberg (1895–1985) in 1926 and further refined by Alf Sven Alving (b 1902) and Frank Benjamin Miller (b 1907) in 1940.

Inversion of Uterus [Latin: *inversio*, to turn around] Two cases were described by William Lowder (d 1801), an English obstetrician, in 1766. Two more cases caused by the midwives pulling on the cord were described in 1783 by William Perfect, a male midwife from Kent. A case of fatal hemorrhage due to a midwife using force to extract the placenta was described in *The Lancet* in 1861. An effective treatment for this often fatal condition was proposed by James Vincent O'Sullivan in 1945. It consisted of the application of hydraulic pressure through a vaginal douche to return the uterus to its normal position.

Invertase [Latin: *invertere*, to turn around] Catalytic enzyme obtained commercially from yeast. Breaks sucrose into glucose and fructose. Eduard Buchner (1860–1917) prepared the first extract from yeast and named it 'zymase' in 1897.

Involuntary Action [Latin: *in*, against + *voluntas*, will] *See reflex action.*

Iodine [Greek: *ioeides*, violet-like] Seaweed and sponges have been used for centuries to treat a swollen thyroid gland. Iodine was first prepared from seaweed by Bernard Courtois (1777–1838), a manufacturer of nitre in 1811. Straub from near Bern was the first to suggest that the active ingredient in the seaweed was iodine in 1819. François Coindet (1774–1834), a physician in Geneva, was the first to treat cases of goiter with iodine in 1820. Deficiency of iodine was shown to be the principal cause of goiter in 1918 by David Marine (1880–1976) from Cleveland Ohio and Jean François Coindet (1774–1834). Iodine was also found to be effective as an antifungal agent by William Dick (1793–1866), an eminent veterinary surgeon at Edinburgh who used potassium iodide for actinomycosis in cattle in 1839. In 1923 Henry Plummer (1874–1936) of the Mayo Clinic used iodine preoperatively in cases of toxic goiter. Radioactive iodine was first used to prove that thyroid gland contained iodine by Herbert M. Evans (1882–1971) in 1940 and was introduced as treatment for Graves disease by Saul Hertz (b 1905) and A. Roberts in 1942.

Iodism [Greek: *ioeides*, violet-like] Caused by chronic iodine poisoning, with an acute reaction involving the mucous membranes. First described by Boinet in *Iodotherapie* published in 1865.

Iodoform Greenish-yellow compound, CHI_3 used as a topical anti-infective. Discovered by George Simon Serullas (1774–1832) in 1822, and recommended as a general remedy by Bouchardat in 1840.

Iodothyronine [Greek: *ioeides*, violet-like + *thyreos*, shield] First active agent in extract of thyroid gland. Discovered by German chemist, Eugen Baumann (b 1845), in 1896.

Ion [Greek: *ion*, going] Term was first used in the study of electricity by Michael Faraday (1791–1867).

Ipecacuanha Dried rhizome of *Cephalis ipecacuanha* or *C. acuminata*. Used as a cure for chronic dysentery by the ancient Indians and Chinese. Called 'Igpecaya' by a Portuguese friar who lived in Brazil in 1570. Two kinds are described in *Natural History of Brazil* written by Willem Piso or Guillame le Pois (1611–1678) in 1648. The substance was introduced into Europe from South America by a traveler named Legras in 1672. The Dutch physician Adrian Helvetius (1661–1727) used it successfully to treat dysentery in 1680.

Iridectomy [Greek: *iris*, rainbow + *ektemein*, to cut out] According to Antonio Scarpa (1747–1832), William Cheseldon (1688–1752) was the first to perform partial section of the iris to create an artificial pupil in cases of chronic iritis. The procedure was revived as treatment for iritis, glaucoma and iridochoroiditis by Swiss ophthalmologist, Albrecht von Graefe (1828–1870) in 1855.

Iridium [Greek: *iris*, rainbow] Rare element was discovered by an English chemist, Smithson Tennant (1761–1815) of Selby in 1804.

Iris [Greek: *iris*, rainbow] The contractile property of the iris was discovered by a Venetian monk and physiologist, Pietro Sarpi (1552–1623). The inflammation of the anterior portion of uveal tunic or iris was named 'iritis' by Johann Adam Schmidt (1759–1809) of Germany in 1801. The effect of circulation upon the movements of iris was studied by Adolf Kussmaul (1822–1902) in 1856.

Irish Sisters of Charity Roman Catholic order that reorganized hospital nursing in English speaking countries. Founded by Mother Mary Aikenhead (1787–1858) of Dublin in 1815.

Irish Sisters of Mercy Roman Catholic order that assists the deprived. Founded by Mother McAuley (1787–1841), a wealthy Dublin woman. She also established a house of shelter for destitute young women in her town. A hospital – the Mater Misericordiae Hospital of Dublin – was established in 1860.

Iron Deficiency Anemia 'Chlorosis' first described in young women by Johannes Lange (1485–1565) in 1554, probably referring to iron deficiency anemia. It was previously known as: icterrius amanterium, morbus virginius and cachexia virginium. Hippocrates (460–377 BC) described a condition similar to chlorosis in his book on diseases of virgins. Danish physician, Knud Heldge Faber (1862–1956) described the findings of microcytic hypochromic, acholorhydria and glossitis associated with chronic iron deficiency anemia (Faber syndrome) in 1909. *See iron therapy.*

Iron Lung Device to assist respiration by placing the patient in a chamber where alternate compression and decompression occur. Invented by Philip Drinker (1894–1972) of Harvard University in 1927. The American firm, Warren E. Collins, was the first to manufacture it, and it was initially used in treatment of respiratory failure following poliomyelitis.

Iron Therapy Melampus, believed by the Greeks to have been the first to practice medicine, advised his patient, Iphiclus to take the rust from a knife and drink it for ten days. This was the first documented prescription of iron to a patient. Its use as a remedy in chlorosis or morbus virginius and other conditions is mentioned by Hippocrates (460–377 BC), Dioscorides (AD 40–90), Abbess Hildegard (1098–1178), Paracelsus (1493–1541), and several other important personalities in medicine. Thomas Sydenham (1624–1689) recommended treatment of anemia with iron filings in wine. Iron was first found in blood by Vincenzo Menghini (1704–1759) in 1746, and the coloring matter in the blood was shown to be a complex of iron by William Charles Wells (1757–1817) in 1797. Quevenne's iron, a finely powdered form of reduced metallic iron, was introduced as a remedy by French physician, Theodore Auguste Quevenne (1805–1855). Aitkin's pill, a remedy consisting of reduced iron, quinine, strychnine and arsenic, was introduced by Scottish physician, Sir William Aitkin (1825–1892). A condition where iron is deposited in the liver, skin and other organs leading to pigmentation, cirrhosis and diabetes, was first described by Armand Trousseau (1801–1867) in 1865 and shown to be an inborn error of metabolism by J. H. Sheldon in 1927. Iron was shown to be an important component of red blood cells by American physician and Nobel Prize winner, George Hoyt Whipple (1878–1976) in 1925. One of the first studies on the absorption of iron using radioactive iron was done by Paul Francis Hahn (1908–1967) and co-workers in 1943. The intravenous use of iron for anemia was introduced by Abraham Joseph Nissim in 1947.

Iron The earliest sources of iron known to man were meteorites and lodestone. Meteorites containing iron were worshipped during prehistoric times. They were known as thunderbolts from the skies, and a reference to them is made in the Holy Writ of Joshua in 1400 BC. The dark reddish brown substance was known as a metal to the Egyptians in 4000 BC, but it came into general use only around 1350 BC.

Iron objects were also found in the tomb of Tutankhamun who ruled around 1360 BC. The Iron Age followed the Bronze Age and reached China around 600 BC. Homer (*c* 800 BC) wrote of it, and Pliny referred to the fatal use of iron weapons in wars, murders and robberies. Iron as a utility metal was known in Britain at least two centuries before the arrival of Romans. Iron coins were introduced from Gaul, and Britons used iron bars as currency. Cast iron was be made in Britain around AD 1300. The first industrial treatise on iron, *L 'art de convertir le fer forge en acier* (The art of converting iron into steel), was published by Rene de Reaumur in 1722. The symbol Fe for iron or ferrum in Latin was assigned to the metal by Jöns Jacob Berzelius (1779–1848), a Swedish physician and chemist in 1826. *See iron therapy, lodestone.*

Irritability [Latin: *irritare*, to provoke] The concept of sensitivity to nerve impulse and resulting irritability of tissues was first proposed by Albrecht von Haller (1708–1777), the eminent Swiss physician in 1752.

Irritable Bowel Syndrome Or spastic colon. One of the first descriptions was given in 1928 by John Alfred Ryle (1889–1950), a physician at Guy's Hospital.

Irvine, William (1743–1787) Physician and chemist who assisted Joseph Black (1728–1799) with his experiments on latent heat. Irvine was the first lecturer of materia medica at Glasgow in 1766.

Isaacs, Alick (1921–1967) Scottish virologist, born in Glasgow and studied medicine there. After doing research later at Melbourne he became the chief of the virology division of the National Institute for Research in 1961. He discovered interferon, a protein capable of interfering with the multiplication of viruses, with Jean Lindemann in 1957.

Isaacs, Charles Edward (1811–1860) Surgeon to Brooklyn City Hospital, King's County Hospital, and Blackwell's Island Hospital. He introduced dye experiments in the study of kidneys and defined the functions of Bowman capsule and Malpighian tubules.

Isabella Queen of Spain, one of the first to organize a modern system of care for the wounded in the army during the 15th century. In 1489 she sent tents and medicines, along with physicians and surgeons to the battle site at the siege of Granada to attend the wounded. She often visited the campsite, called the Queen's Hospital, and had over 400 wagons to transport the wounded and equipment. These wagons were called 'ambulancias', the first use of the name for mobile medical care.

Isambert Disease Tuberculous ulceration of the larynx and pharynx was described by French physician, E. Isambert (1827–1876).

Ischemic Heart Disease [Greek: *ischein*, to suppress] *See coronary artery disease, cholesterol, coronary artery bypass graft, angina pectoris, cardiac enzymes, coronary care unit.*

Isidorus (AD 595–635) Bishop at Seville who published a great cyclopaedia *Etimologiarum libri XX* which became one of the most popular works on science, medicine and theology during medieval times.

Isihara Test *See color blindness.*

Isis Healing goddess of the Egyptians, wife of Osiris and mother of Horus, guardian of health. Under the Roman empire, the practice of invoking her magical cures extended almost to the entire western world.

Isis An influential journal of biology and science founded by a German naturalist, Lorenz Oken in 1813. An international review on history of science, ISIS, was founded by George Sarton in 1927. Sarton was a graduate from the University of Ghent and was appointed professor of history of science at Harvard in 1940.

Isletin Original term for antidiabetic substance from the pancreas before it was re-named insulin by Sir Edward Albert Sharpey-Schafer (1850–1935). *See insulin.*

Islets of Langerhans Islets in the pancreas which are quite distinct from acinar tissue were first identified by Paul Wilhelm Heinrich Langerhans (1847–1888) of Berlin in 1869. Gustav-Édouard Laguesse (1861–1927) of Lille (1893) and Diamare (1899) independently demonstrated that the function of these islets was concerned with internal secretions controlling carbohydrate metabolism. In 1903, Eugene Lindsay Opie (1873–1971), an American pathologist, suggested that an antidiabetic substance was present in the islets of Langerhans. The alpha and beta cells in the islets of Langerhans were identified independently by M.A. Lane (1907), and R.R. Bensley (1911) in America. The name insulin was given to the active extract of the pancreas by Sir Edward Albert Sharpey-Schafer (1850–1935) on the basis that it came from the islets of Langerhans.

Isoelectric Point [Greek: *isos*, equal + *elektron*, amber] First demonstrated by W.B. Hardy (1864–1934) in 1899 using denatured egg albumin which moved towards the cathode in acid solutions and towards the anode in alkaline solutions. The pH value at which it did not move was defined as the isoelectric point by a German-born American biochemist, Leonor Michaelis (1875–1949) in

1910. The knowledge of isoelectric point was later found to be useful for characterization, isolation and purification of proteins.

Isoenzymes [Greek: *isos*, equal + *en*, in + *zyme*, leaven] Term to denote molecules with different physical properties but similar enzymatic properties. Proposed by Clement L. Markert in 1963. The isoenzyme variations in man was studied by Lars Beckman (b 1928) in 1966. *See diagnostic enzymology.*

Isoleucine Amino acid was first isolated from beet sugar molasses by Felix Ehrlich in 1903.

Isomerism [Greek: *isos*, equal + *meros*, part] Compounds with identical chemical composition but different structure and properties. First observed by Justus von Liebig (1803–1873) in 1824. The term was coined by Jöns Jacob Berzelius (1779–1848) in 1830. The study of isomerism was revived by a German-born Swiss chemist and Nobel Prize winner, Alfred Werner (1866–1919), professor at Zurich.

Isomers [Greek: *isos*, equal + *meros*, part] *See stereochemistry.*

Isomorphism [Greek: *isos*, equal + *morphe*, form] The phenomenon where compounds with similar chemical composition exist in similar crystalline form. Discovered and named by a German physical chemist, Eilhardt Mitscherlich (1794–1863) in 1819. The capacity of some elements to occur in two distinct forms – dimorphism – was also first noted by Mitscherlich.

Isoniazid (isonicotinic acid hydrazide) First prepared by Hans Meyer in 1912. The antituberculous properties of the compound were demonstrated independently in 1952 by four groups: Bernstein and colleagues, Edward Heinrich Robitzeg (1912–1984), Steenken and Wolinskine of America, and Nobel Prize winner, Gerhard Johannes Paul Domagk (1895–1964) of Germany.

Isotonic Solutions [Greek: *isos*, equal + *tonos*, tone] Solutions in which body cells can be bathed without net flow of solutes in either direction. First prepared by Sydney Ringer (1835–1910) in 1882, and later by Locke in 1900. *See Ringer solution.*

Isotopes [Greek: *isos*, equal + *topos*, place] Elements which have identical atomic numbers but different atomic weights. Term coined in 1913 by Nobel Prize winner, Frederick Soddy (1877–1965). Isotopes of neon exist as two forms and were first described by another Nobel Prize winner, Sir Joseph John Thomson (1856–1940). Later followed by a third Nobel Prize winner, Francis William Aston (1877–1945), who made a significant contribution in 1919 by designing a mass spectrograph for separation. The therapeutic use of radioactive isotopes was demonstrated by John Hundale Lawrence (b 1904) in 1939. Radioactive iodine was used to study thyroid disease by M.P. Kelsey and co-workers in 1949 and introduced as treatment for thyrotoxicosis by G.W. Blomfield and co-workers in 1951. A new method of assessing several aspects of kidney functions with radioisotopes was introduced by C.C. Winter and G.V. Taplin in 1955. Estimation of renal blood flow using albumin I-131 isotope was first performed by L. Perskey in 1957. *See nuclear medicine.*

Israel, James Adolf (1848–1926) Urologist from Berlin who discovered the fungus *Actinomyces israelii* in 1878.

Itai–Itai disease [Japanese: *itai–itai*, ouch–ouch] Peculiar bone disease resembling osteomalacia. Noted in 1939 amongst people living near heavily polluted rivers containing cadmium and other metals in Japan.

Itard, Jean Marie Gaspard (1774-1838) Parisian otorhinologist who wrote one of the first modern textbooks on the ear in 1821. He also devised a catheter for the Eustachian tube.

Itch Mite [Anglo-Saxon: *gictha*, an itch or a scab] *See Acarus scabiei.*

Ivanovski, Dmitri Iosofovich (1864–1920) Russian botanist who investigated tobacco mosaic disease in 1892. He extracted sap and passed it thorough a bacterial filter and showed that filtered sap was still capable of producing the disease. This was the first demonstration of a filterable virus. He did not realize the significance and the phenomenon was rediscovered by M. W. Beijerinck in 1898.

Ivemark syndrome Congenital condition of agenesis of the spleen, situs inversus and cardiac abnormalities. First described by Björn Ivemark (b 1925) of Uppsala in 1955.

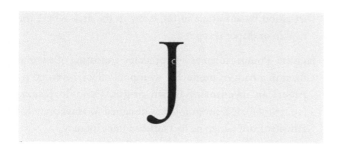

J

Jaboulay, Mathieu (1860–1913) French neurosurgeon from Lyons. He performed the first sympathetectomy for relief of vascular disease in 1900. He performed the interpelvi-abdominal amputation, and introduced the procedure of gastroduodenostomy in 1892.

Jaccoud Disease Form of arthritis of hands and fingers occurring in patients with rheumatic fever. Described by French professor of pathology at Paris, Sigismond Jaccoud (1830–1913), in 1869. He also described the prominence of the aorta in the suprasternal notch (Jaccoud sign) in aortic dilation, febrile meningitis in patients with tuberculous meningitis (Jaccoud dissociated fever) and progressive periarticular fibrosis in recurrent rheumatic fever or lupus erythematosus (Jaccoud arthritis).

Jackson, Chevalier (1865–1958) *See bronchoscopy, endotracheal intubation.*

Jackson, Charles Thomas (1805–1880) Chemist and physician from Harvard, who suggested the use of ether as anesthesia to his pupil William Thomas Green Morton (1819–1868). His claim to the discovery of ether anesthesia over Morton was unsuccessful.

Jackson, James Jr (1810–1834) Son of a prominent Boston physician of the same name at the Massachusetts Hospital. He wrote a treatise on cholera and described the prolonged expiratory sound in phthisis.

Jackson, Jabez North (1868–1935) Professor of anatomy at Kansas. He described the peritoneal attachment of the cecum and the ascending colon to the right abdominal wall (Jackson membrane) producing obstruction of the bowel, in 1913.

Jackson, James (1777–1868) Boston physician trained under Astley Cooper (1768–1841) at St Thomas' Hospital, London. He was appointed as the first physician to Massachusetts General Hospital in 1810, and wrote a book on practice of physick in 1825. He published one of the earliest accounts of alcoholic neuritis in 1822. *See Massachusetts General Hospital.*

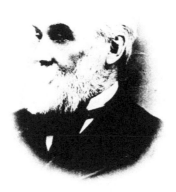

John Hughlings Jackson (1834–1911). Courtesy of the National Library of Medicine

Jackson, John Hughlings (1834–1911) British neurologist born in Providence Green, Yorkshire. He graduated in medicine from St Bartholomew's Hospital in 1856 and worked in York before he returned to London in 1859. He received his MD in 1860, and was made assistant physician to the London Hospital in 1863. He became physician to the National Hospital for the Paralyzed and Epileptic in 1867 and retained the post until 1906. Jackson established the use of the ophthalmoscope in brain disease and made valuable contributions to studies on aphasia. In 1864 he proposed that areas which caused specific isolated movements existed in the cortex and also described the unilateral localized form of epilepsy (Jacksonian convulsion, epilepsy and seizure). The temporal lobe as a center for olfactory and gustatory sensations was demonstrated by him in 1889. A tumor in the right temporosphenoidal area causing olfactory seizures was described by Jackson in 1890. He was also the first to observe the abnormal sensation of smell and taste in a patient with temporal lobe tumor.

Jacksonian Seizures *See Jackson, John Hughlings.*

Jacobaeus, Hans Christian (1879–1937) Stockholm surgeon who used a modified cystoscope to perform cautery division of pleural adhesions in 1916. His work led directly to the development of the thoracoscope and other similar instruments to view the interior of the body.

Jacob, François (b 1920) French biochemist who worked at the Pasteur Institute in Paris. He examined the nutritional requirements of *Escherichia coli* and its production of galactosidase in response to feeding with lactose. This led him to postulate gene regulation and to formulate the 'operon' theory, structural genes which encode for a protein and regulator genes which control them by producing a 'repressor' molecule which binds to the DNA operator. He shared the Nobel Prize with André Michel Lwoff (b 1902) and Jacques Lucien Monod (1910–1976) for this work.

Jacob Membrane Layer of the retina containing rods and cones was first described by Irish ophthalmic surgeon, Arthur Jacob (1790–1874) in 1819.

Jacobi, Abraham (1830–1919) Born in Germany but emigrated to New York and regarded as the father of pediatrics in America. He married Mary Putnam (1842–1906), one of the first women physicians, and advocated the education of women in medicine. He was elected as the first president of the American Medical Association and established the first pediatric clinic at New York in 1862.

Jacobius, Oliger (1650–1701) Danish physician and professor of physick at Copenhagen. He wrote *Compendium Institutionium Medicarum, de Ranis et Lacertis* and several other works in medicine.

Jacobson, Julius (1828–1889) Ophthalmologist from Königsberg who used a scleral flap incision for cataract operations in 1863. He also described syphilitic retinopathy.

Jacobson, Ludwig Levin (1783–1843) Anatomist and physician from Copenhagen who described: the tymphanic branch of the glossopharyngeal nerve (Jacobson nerve), the canaliculus tymphanicus (Jacobson canal); and the vomeronasal organ (Jacobson organ).

Jacobson Nerve Tymphanitic branch of the glossopharyngeal nerve discovered in 1818 by Ludwig Leven Jacobson (1783–1843).

Jacobus, Psychristus (AD 457–474) Physician in Constantinople in the fifth century.

Jacod Triad Optic atrophy, ophthalmoplegia and trigeminal neuralgia caused by a space-occupying lesion in the petrosphenoid space. Described by French neurologist, Maurice Jacod (b 1880) in 1921.

Jacquemet Recess Peritoneal pouch between the liver and gallbladder. First described by French anatomist, Marcel Jacquemet (1872–1903) of Marseilles in 1897.

Jacques Catheter The first soft rubber urethral catheter was invented by a production manager James Archibald Jacques (1815–1878) at the rubber mill of William Warne and Company at Barking, Essex in England.

Jacquet, Leonard Marie Lucien (1860–1914) Paris dermatologist who in 1889 described a rash (Jacquet disease) due to irritation by ammonia in the urine in the area where the napkin or diaper is applied.

Jacuzzi Popular form of hydrotherapy consisting of a pump fixed in a bath to produce a whirlpool effect. Invented by American inventor of Italian origin, Candido Jacuzzi (1903–1986). His invention was designed to ameliorate his arthritis, from which he had suffered since infancy.

Jadassohn, Josef (1879–1921) Dermatologist from Breslau. He gave a description of maculo-papular erythroderma (Jadassohn disease). Jadassohn nevus, a plaque-like lesion of the skin which contains excess sebaceous glands, was described by him.

Jaeger Test Test for near vision devised by Viennese ophthalmologist, Edouard Jaeger von Jastthal (1818–1884), in 1854. He also designed operations for cataract, entropion and ectropion. He published an atlas of ophthalmology in 1869.

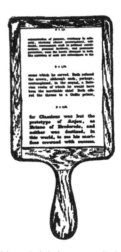

Jaeger Test. W.A. Fisher, *Ophthalmoscopy, Retinoscopy and Refraction* (1928). F.A. Davis & Co., Philadelphia

Jaffe, Max (1841–1911) Biochemist from Königsberg who introduced several biochemical techniques including those for detection of urobilin in urine (1868) and in the intestines (1871); detection of creatinine (1886); and isolation of indican in urine (1877).

Jaffna Moss (Ceylon Moss, *Alga Ceylanica*) A light purple seaweed used by the ancient Chinese and inhabitants of the Indian subcontinent. It was brought to the notice of European physicians by O'Shaughnessy who mentioned it in the *Indian Medical Journal* of Calcutta in 1834.

Jake Also called Jamaican Ginger paralysis due to poisoning by tri-ortho cresyl phosphate. First reported in America in 1931.

Jakob–Creutzfeld Disease *See Creutzfeld–Jakob disease.*

Jaksch, Rudolph von (1855–1947) Physician in Prague who described pseudo-leukemia, or acute hemolytic anemia, in children (von Jaksch anemia) in 1889. He was also one of the first to investigate the presence of acetone bodies in the urine in 1885.

James Mackenzie Institute Promotes clinical research by general practitioners to improve guidelines for treatment of common diseases. Founded as the Institute of Clinical Research at St Andrew's in 1918 by British physician and cardiologist, Sir James Mackenzie (1853–1925).

James IV (1473–1513) King of Scotland who took a great interest in medicine and performed some operations under the guidance of surgeons. He also practiced bleeding.

James VI (1566–1625) King of Scotland, the only monarch to have written a treatise related to psychiatry. He work, *Demonologie, in forme of a dialogue* on the existence of witch-craft and its evils, was published in 1597.

James, Robert (1703–1776) Physician from Kinverstone in Staffordshire. He published a *Medical Dictionary* in three volumes in 1743, and the *Practice of Physic* in two volumes. He invented the James fever powder which remained a popular secret remedy for over two centuries.

James, William (1842–1910) Eminent psychologist, born in New York and graduated in medicine from Harvard University, where he later taught anatomy and physiology from 1872 to 1878. He later became the professor of psychology at Harvard and wrote the *Principles of Psychology*, which took him twelve years to prepare. It was first published in 1890 and came to be considered a classic. He was also the first to teach psychology in America and his *Textbook of Psychology* was published in 1892. His most famous doctrine was the theory of emotion proposed in 1884, which explained emotional experience in terms of bodily accompaniments.

James–Lange Theory Theory of emotions. Independently developed by Danish psychologist, Carl Georg Lange (1834–1900) and William James (1842–1910), professor of psychology at Harvard University.

Janet, Pierre Marie Felix (1859–1947) Professor of psychiatry at the College de France and a contemporary of Jean Charcot (1825–1893). He proposed the concept of psy-choasthenia in 1903, where psychological weakness or asthenia followed shock, fatigue or constitutional weakness.

Janeway, Theodore Caldwell (1872–1917) Son of the emi-nent American physician, Edward Gamaliel Janeway (1841–1911) of New Brunswick, New Jersey. He served as professor of medicine at the Johns Hopkins University from 1914 to 1917 and published *Clinical Study of Blood Pressure* in 1904.

Janeway Lesions Nodular hemorrhagic spots on the palms of the hands and soles of feet of patients with subacute bacterial endocarditis. First described in 1899 by American physician, Edward Gamaliel Janeway (1841–1911) of New Jersey. He succeeded Austin Flint (1812–1886) as professor of medicine at Bellevue Hospital, New York and established the first infectious disease hospital in New York at Manhattan.

Jansen Syndrome Congenital metaphyseal dysostosis consisting of mental retardation, dwarfism, metaphyseal widening of all bones. Described by a Dutch orthopedic surgeon, Murk Jansen (1867–1935) in 1934.

Janus Damescenus *See Mesue, Senior.*

Japanese Fever *See aka mushi.*

Jarisch–Herxheimer Reaction Acute exacerbation of syphi-litic lesions within 6 to 10 hours of treatment. Usually of short duration. First described in 1895 by Austrian derma-tologist, Adolf Jarisch (1850–1902) of Vienna. He wrote an influential German book, *Textbook of Skin Diseases*. The same reaction was described in 1902 by a German derma-tologist Karl Herxheimer (1861–1944), who died in a Nazi concentration camp.

Jarjavay Ligaments [Latin: *ligamentum*, bandage] Utero-sacral and utero-recto-sacral ligaments of the broad ligament. Described in 1852 by French physician, Jean François Jarjavay (1815–1868), of Dordogne.

Jarvik, Robert American prostheticist who pioneered arti-ficial hearts. One of his models, the Jarvik-7, the 70th to be made by him, was implanted in a retired dentist named Barney Clark by Willem J. Kolff and William de Vries in 1982. Clark was kept alive with his artificial heart for 112 hours.

Jarvis, William Chapman (1855–1895) Laryngologist from New York who devised a wire snare (Jarvis snare) for removing polypi in the nose and throat in 1881.

Jaundice [French: *jaune*, yellow] Described by Paul of Aegina (AD 625–690) as a diffusion of bile over the whole body, sometimes black and sometimes yellow. He also stated that jaundice could be induced by drinking certain deleterious substances, one of the early instances of recognition of drug-induced jaundice. Hippocrates (460–377 BC) laid down a prognostic rule, when the liver was hard it is a bad symptom. His rule still remains valid in jaundice due to cirrhotic liver. Aretaeus of Cappadocia (AD 81–138) insisted that there were other causes such as spleen, stomach, kidneys and colon. Theophilus of Edessa (d AD 785) said that some cases arose from obstruction of the ductus choledochus. Most ancient physicians recommended conservative measures: Paul of Aegina advocated bleeding and various herbal decoctions, Hippocrates advised refraining from fatty food and regular baths for three days, Aetius recommended bleeding and purging, Haly Abbas (d AD 944) advised tepid baths and fumes of vinegar to remove yellowness of the eyes and a special remedy – a draught containing lentils, fennel and the urine of a boy not come to puberty.

Java Man The teeth, calvarium and femur of a primitive man were discovered by Marie Eugene Dubois (1858–1940), a surgeon in the Dutch army, while he was stationed in Java in 1893. His finding was later acclaimed as the missing link in the evolution of man. Java man was later named *Pithecanthropus erectus*. The British anthropologist, Sir Arthur Keith (1866–1955) has estimated him to be 350,000 years old.

Jaw German surgeon, Carl Ferdinand von Graefe (1787–1840), professor of surgery at Berlin, was the first to excise the jaw. The procedure was performed by Guillaume Dupuytren (1777–1835) for the first time in France in 1812 on a man of 39 years with a tumor. Almost the entire upper jaw was removed in a case of osteosarcoma of the superior maxillary bone by David Rodgers (1799–1877) of America. Partial excision of the lower jaw in a case of osteosarcoma was carried out by another American, Valentine Mott (1785–1865) in 1822. James Marion Sims (1813–1883) excised both the upper and lower jaws of a patient in 1837.

Jeanselme, Antoine Edouard (1858–1935) Paris dermatologist who described pityriasis versicolor and published a history of syphilis in 1931.

Jebb, John (1736–1786) Physician and clergyman from London who published several works on theology, politics and medicine.

Jeffreys, Alec John (b 1950) English molecular biologist, born in Oxford and educated at Merton College, Oxford. He spent most of his career at the University of Leicester and was made professor of genetics in 1987. He became Wolfson research professor of the Royal Society in 1991. He developed the technique of DNA fingerprinting, now widely used in forensic medicine. *See genetic fingerprinting.*

Jeffries, John (1744–1819) American physician from Boston who was educated at the University of Cambridge. After

practicing in Boston as an army physician he became the surgeon-general to the British army in India before he settled in London in 1780. Jeffries also studied atmospheric temperature and made two aerial voyages in a balloon for this purpose.

Jeghers, Harold Jos (b 1904) American physician and professor of medicine at Tufts Medical School in Boston and later at the New Jersey College of Medicine and Dentistry. *See Peutz–Jeghers syndrome.*

Jehovah's Witnesses Religious sect founded by American, Charles Taze Russell (1852–1916) of Pittsburgh in 1872. They oppose blood transfusion on the basis of their scriptures.

Jejunostomy [Latin: *jejunus*, empty; Greek: *stomoun*, to cut] *See duodenal ulcer.*

Jejunum [Latin: *jejunus*, empty] So called because it was supposed to empty after death.

Jellinek Sign Pigmentation of the upper eyelid in cases of exophthalmic thyrotoxicosis was described by Viennese physician, Stefan Jellinek (b 1871) in 1932.

Jena Nomina Anatomica Terminology introduced in 1933 by a committee of German anatomists in Jena.

Jendrassik, Ernst (1858–1921) Budapest physician who, in 1885, described the reinforcement of the knee jerk reflex by pulling the two hands against each other.

Jenner, Louis Leopold (1866–1904) London physician who introduced a new staining preparation consisting of methylene blue and eosin for fixing and staining blood films in 1899.

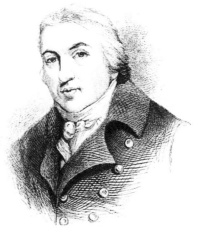

Edward Jenner (1749–1823). Courtesy of the National Library of Medicine

Jenner, Edward (1749–1823) English physician from Berkeley, Gloucestershire who introduced vaccination against smallpox. He was apprenticed to a surgeon at Sodbury near Bristol, before he went to London to study under John Hunter (1728–1793) in 1770. He started his practice at Berkeley in 1773 where he began investigating the immunity of milkmaids (previously exposed to cowpox) to smallpox. His publications include *An Inquiry into the Causes and Effects of the Variolae Vaccinae* (1798), *On the Natural History of Cuckoo* and another paper in the *Philosophical Transactions of the Royal Society*. *See inoculation.*

Jenner, Sir William (1815–1898) English physician from Chatham who graduated from the University of London, worked at the London Fever Hospital and appointed professor in 1848. He differentiated between typhus and typhoid fever in 1851. He found that patients suffering from typhoid tended to be younger, around 22, whereas typhus affected all ages.

Jensen, Carl Oluf (1864–1934) Veterinary pathologist in Copenhagen who, in 1903, demonstrated the inoculability of cancer by transmitting sarcoma through 40 generations of rats.

Jensen Sulcus Sulcus intermedius primus of the cerebral cortex was first described in 1871 by Julius Jensen (1841–1891), director of the Allenburg Institute of Mental Diseases.

Jerne, Niels Kai (b 1911) London-born Danish immunologist and founding director of the Basel Institute of Immunology in 1969. He explained the development of T-lymphocytes in the thymus and formed the network theory of the relationship of interacting lymphocytes and antibodies. He shared the Nobel Prize for Physiology or Medicine in 1984 with Cesar Milstein (b 1927) and George Köhler (b 1946).

Jerusalem Hospital The first hospital is supposed to have been built in 150 BC, by John Hircanus from the Maccabees family, in order to care for pilgrims who visited the Temple of Solomon. Around AD 400 several other hospitals were built to care for pilgrims to the Holy Sepulcher. In 1048 some rich sea merchants at Amalfi, a seaport near Naples, began to build a further hospital for these pilgrims. It was arranged in two sections, one dedicated to St John the Almoner and the other to St Mary Magdalene. During the Crusades the Christians founded a hospital dedicated to providing shelter and care for the wounded. The providers and protectors of the Hospital of St John later organized themselves into the famous Knights Hospitalers, an order recognized by Pope Paschal II in 1113.

Jesty, Benjamin (1731–1816) Introduced the method of inoculation with cowpox to protect against smallpox in England. He obtained the cowpox material from the sore in the udder of a cow and, using a stocking needle, he successfully inoculated his wife and two sons. *See inoculation.*

Jesu Haly or Isa ibn Ali Arab oculist in Baghdad and a pupil of Johannitius (Hunayn ibn Ishaq) (AD 809–873). He wrote an original work in three parts on eye disease which was translated into Latin under the title *Liber memorialis ophthalmicorum*. The first part contained anatomy and physiology of the eye, and the second dealt with external diseases of the eye.

Jesuit Bark *See cinchona bark.*

Jewish Medicine The standard source of information is the Old Testament. Moses advocated a high standard of hygiene and personal cleanliness and laid down rules for consumption of food. Preventive medicine played an important role amongst the Jews and they isolated the sick, supervised slaughtering of animals, had burial laws, and practiced sexual hygiene. Circumcision was performed on all boys using flint instruments during the time of Moses. Jews performed amputations, surgically treated imperforate anus, and made artificial limbs and crutches. The Hebrew priests also served as physicians until the Jewish king Asa (950–875 BC) separated the roles of physicians and priests during his regime. Their earliest recordings of human anatomy is found in The Talmud, the law book. However as Jews did not permit human dissections, most of their anatomical knowledge was derived through inspection of meat at slaughterhouses. A materia medica, or *Antidotarium*, the oldest known medical work in Hebrew containing descriptions of over 120 remedies was written in 946 by a Jewish physician, Sabbatai ben Abraham (AD 913–970) from Otranto in southern Italy. He also wrote on astrology and described the doctrine of macrocosm and microcosm. During the Mohammedan era the Jews occupied positions as court physicians in Spain. When they were banished in 1412 they were well received at the School of Salerno in Italy. The Council of Vienna forbade them to practice medicine in 1267 and the Church of Rome also curtailed their work in the 15th century. *See Talmud.*

Jewitt Nail-plate An implant for fixing hip fractures, invented in 1941 by Eugene Lyon Jewitt (b 1900), American orthopedic surgeon from Orlando, Florida.

Jex-Blake, Sophia Louisa (1840–1912) Pioneer of medical education for women and pupil of Elizabeth Blackwell (1821–1910) in New York. She continued her medical education in Edinburgh, against considerable opposition, and graduated in 1869. She founded schools of medicine for women in London (1874) and Edinburgh (1886).

Jiwaka Physician to the Lord Buddha around 400 BC.

Johannes de Ketham Also known as Johann von Kirch-heim. German physician in the 15th century who published the first book illustrated with woodcuts on medicine, *Fasciculus Medicinae*, in 1491.

Jodrell, Sir Paul (d 1803) Middlesex physician to the Nawab of Arcot in India in 1787, and died at Madras. He wrote *Illustrations of Euriphedes* (1781) and was also the author of 6 plays which were published under the title *Select Dramatic Pieces* in 1787.

Joffroy Sign Failure to wrinkle the forehead when asked to bend the head and look up, seen in thyrotoxicosis. First described by French neurologist, Alexis Joffroy (1844–1908). Together with Jean Charcot (1825–1893), he showed that the anterior horn cells were damaged in poliomyelitis.

Johannitius *See Hunayn ibn Ishaq.*

Johannsen, Wilhelm Ludwig (1857–1927) Danish botanist and geneticist from Copenhagen who first coined the term 'gene' to denote the unit of heredity. The concepts of 'geno-type' and 'phenotype' were introduced into genetics by him in 1902. His influential work *Elements of Heredity* was published in 1909.

John of Gaddesdon (1280–1361) English physician who graduated from Montpellier. He wrote *Rosa Angelica* which, besides medical advice, also contains a mixture of superstition and absurdities. John is depicted as the 'Doctor of Physick' by Chaucer in his *Canterbury Tales*.

Johns Hopkins University and Hospital Founded in Bal-timore in 1876 from the bequest of Johns Hopkins (1795–1873), a businessman from Maryland. He designed his bequest in 1867 to establish a university and a hospital supervised by a board of trustees. John Shaw Billings (1838–1913), an army medical officer, was chosen to plan and build the hospital which took over 14 years to com-plete. Daniel C. Gilman was elected first president to the university in 1875. The foundation professors were William Welch (1850–1934) in pathology, William Osler (1849–1919) in medicine, W.S. Halstead (1852–1922) in surgery and Franklin Mall (1862–1917) in anatomy.

Johnson, Thomas (d 1644) Apothecary from Selby, Yorkshire in the 17th century who practiced as a herbalist in London. Johnson's publications include *Iter in Agrum Canturarium*, and *Ericetum Hamstedianum*, which were the first catalogues of local plants published in England. He served in the Royal army in the Civil War and died from a wound received at the siege of Basinghouse in 1644.

Johnson, Frank Bacchus (b 1919) Born in Washington, DC, he became resident in pathology at the Jersey City Medical Center in 1945, later moving to the Howard University as acting pathologist and director of the clinical laboratories. In 1990 he was appointed chief of the Division of Chemical Pathology, Department of Toxicology at the Armed Forces Institute of Pathology in Washington. *See Dubin–Johnson syndrome.*

Johnson, Frank Chamblis (1894–1934) American pediatrician. *See Stevens–Johnson syndrome.*

Johnston, Arthur (1587–1641) Physician from Aberdeen who graduated from Padua. He was appointed physician to Charles I and wrote several literary works.

Johnstone, James (1730–1802) Physician from Annan in Dumfries. He graduated from Edinburgh and practiced first at Kidderminster and later at Worcester. He published *Medical Essays and Observations, those disquisitions relating to the Nervous System* and several other papers.

Johnstone, John (1768–1836) Physician and a son of James Johnstone who practiced medicine at Worcester. He gradu-ated from Merton College, Oxford and worked in Birmingham. He wrote several papers on medical subjects.

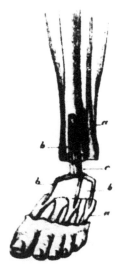

Joint replacement of ankle with ivory and metal prongs. T. Gluck *Arch. Kiln. Chir.* 41 (1891)

Joint Replacement Pioneered by Rumanian-born sur-geon, Themistokles Gluck (1853–1942) who was professor of surgery at Bucharest. He commenced his work on a prosthesis for joints around 1885 and started using intramedullary nails and an ivory intramedullary peg in 1890. He inserted a hinged ivory knee joint prosthesis in the same year and also used various prosthesis for ankle, elbow and hip joints. Parisian surgeon, Jules Emile Pean (1830–1898) was another pioneer in the field who used platinum and rubber prosthesis for tuberculosis of the shoulder joint in 1894. In 1961 John Charnley (1911–1982) of Manchester published a paper on low friction arthroplasty using a metal femoral head, neck and stem and a plastic acetabular cup. This formed the basis for modern joint replacement surgery. *See artificial hip joint.*

Joliot-Curie, Irene (1897–1956) Daughter of Marie and Pierre Curie (1867–1934, 1859–1906). She served as a radiographer in military hospitals during World War 1, before joining her mother at the Radium Institute in Paris in 1918. She made the first artificial radioisotope (of phosphorus) by bombarding aluminum with alpha particles, with her husband Frédéric Joliot (1900–1958) in 1933. They were jointly awarded the Nobel Prize for Chemistry in 1935. She died from leukemia induced by long periods of exposure to radioactivity.

Jolly, Justin Maric Jules (1870 -1953) *See Howell–Jolly bodies.*

Joly, John Swift (1876–1943) London urologist who devised an irrigating urethroscope, also used for cystoscopy.

Joly, John (1857–1933) Irish geologist and physicist, born at Offaly, King's County, and entered Trinity College Dublin in 1876, where he became a professor of geology and mineralogy in 1897. He was a pioneer in the study of radioactivity in geology. He also pioneered radiotherapy for cancer using radium emanation-filled needles. he was also a pioneer of color photography.

Jones, Arthur Rocyn (1883–1972) Welsh bone setter and a graduate of University College London. He was a consultant at the Royal National Orthopaedic Hospital and a founder member of the British Orthopaedic Association in 1918.

Jones, Cecil Price (1863–1943) Pioneer in hematology. He graduated from Guy's Hospital in 1889 and worked in the pathological department there. His first set of papers on the diameters of red blood cells was published in 1910. This work led to the establishment of normal values of red cell size and hemoglobin concentration.

Jones, Henry Bence (1814–1873) *See Bence-Jones proteins.*

Jones, Inigo (1572–1652) Celebrated London architect and the reviver of classical architecture in England. He was a friend and patient of William Harvey (1578–1658).

Jones, Sir Robert (1858–1933) Orthopedic surgeon and student of Hugh Owen Thomas, the founder of modern orthopedic surgery in England. Jones advocated active surgical intervention in orthopedics and pioneered bone grafting and other reconstructive procedures.

Jones, Thomas Wharton (1808–1891) British ophthalmologist who designed an operation for ectropion. He published *A manual of the principles and practice of ophthalmic medicine and surgery* in 1847.

Jones, Walter Born in Barking, elected surgeon extraordinary to the London Hospital in 1746. He inherited the Manor of Wyfield through his wife, Ann Bamber, who was his master-surgeon's daughter.

Jonnesco, Thoma (1860–1926) Professor of surgery at Bucharest who described the retro-duodenal fossa (Jonnesco fossa or fold) in 1889. He also did an operation for removal of the cervical ganglia of the sympathetic trunk (Jonnesco operation).

Jonstonus, Johannes Polish physician in the 17th century who wrote a treatise in 1661 on preserving health in old age, *Idea Hygieines resensita.*

Jorden, Edward (1569–1632) London physician who graduated from Padua. He was the first English physician to contend that mental disease was the underlying cause of so-called possession and witchcraft. His work *A brief discourse of a disease called the suffocation of the mother,* published in 1603, was the first English book on hysteria.

Jorgensen, Alfred (1848–1925) Danish pioneer in the field of fermentology who introduced a method of making pure cultures of yeast in 1884.

Josnia Legendary king of Scotland who lived during 200 BC, said to have learned medicine from the physicians in Ireland. He held physicians in high esteem and is believed to have written a treatise on medicinal herbs.

Joule, James Prescott (1818–1889) Discoverer of the law of the conservation of energy. Born in Salford to a family of brewers. He started his study and research on electricity and electromagnetism in a room at his family home and became a self taught chemist and physicist. His earliest invention, an electromagnetic engine was made when he was only 19 years of age. Joule was the first to establish a definite relationship between electrical conductance and resistance in 1840. He also established the unit of static electricity on the basis of quantity needed to decompose 9 grams of water, and in 1843 calculated the mechanical energy as that required to warm a pound of water by one degree.

Joule-Thomson Effect A gas becomes cooler on expansion. First described by James Prescott Joule (1818–1889) and William Thomson, Lord Kelvin (1824–1907) in 1852.

Journal of Bone and Joint Surgery Started as the *Transactions of the American Orthopedic Association* in 1889 and was renamed *American Journal of Orthopedic Surgery* in 1903. It became *The Journal of Orthopaedic Surgery* to accommodate British colleagues in 1919. Its title was changed again to *Journal of Bone and Joint Surgery* in 1922.

Journal of Comparative Pathology and Therapeutics Founded by medical graduate and veterinary surgeon, McFadyean in 1888. He graduated from Edinburgh Veterinary School in 1876 and obtained his medical degree in 1882. McFaydean moved to London and became principal of the London Veterinary School in 1894. He edited the journal for 52 years.

Journal of Natural Philosophy, Chemistry and Arts Founded by London chemist, William Nicholson (1758–1815) in 1793.

Journal of Neurology and Psychopathology Founded by a British–American neurologist, Samuel Alexander Kinnier Wilson (1877–1937) of the National Hospital, Queen's Square, London in 1920.

Journal of Physiology Founded in 1878 by Michael Foster (1836–1907), professor of physiology at Cambridge. It began as a collection of papers from his laboratory which had been published as *Publications from the Cambridge Physiological Laboratory*. Early volumes contained original research papers and up-to-date bibliography. The *American Journal of Physiology* first appeared in 1898, followed by the *Journal of General Physiology* started by Jacques Loeb (1859–1924) in 1918 and the *Journal of Applied Physiology* in 1948.

Journals in Medicine The first medical journal in England, *Medicina Curiosa*, was published in 1684, but after two issues in the same year it ceased to exist. *Acta Medicorum Berolinensium* in Latin, was the first medical journal to be published in Germany in 1717. Also in Germany, Johann Reil (1759–1813) started the *Archiv für die Physiologie* in 1795. Many medical journals followed in the next 100 years most of which were extinct by 1900. *Annals of Medicine*, Edinburgh, was one of the earliest British medical journals to be published, in 1796. In 1805 it became the *Edinburgh Medical and Surgical Journal* and continued until 1855, when it combined with *Monthly Journal of Medicine* to become the *Edinburgh Medical Journal*. The *American Journal of Obstetrics* was the first specialized journal to be published in America in 1868. Its name was later changed to *American Journal of Obstetrics and*

Gynecology in 1920. The *Journal of Physiology* in England was founded by Michael Foster, professor of physiology at Cambridge in 1878. The *Australian Medical Journal* was first published in 1846 in Sydney. After an year it was discontinued and a journal with the same title was commenced in Melbourne in 1854. It continued under different titles for the next 54 years and merged into *Medical Journal of Australia* in 1914. *See British Medical Journal, American medical journals.*

Judaeus, Isaac (AD 855–955) Egyptian-born Jewish physician and a contemporary of Rhazes (*c* 850–932). His treatises were the first Arab medical work to be translated into Latin, and remained some of the best medical works available during the Middle Ages.

Julius Caesar (102–44 BC) Roman emperor and the first to initiate a complete survey of the Roman Empire, continued by his successor Augustus. The project was completed by Vipsanious Agrippa, the son-in-law of Augustus, in 20 BC.

Jundeshapur (Gunde-Shapur) In Persia, was the seat of the Mohammedan school of medicine, founded by Sasanian Shapur I after he defeated Emperor Valerian and sacked Antioch. He named the new city Veh-az-Andev-i-Shapur, which meant 'Shapur is better than Antioch'. This name was later condensed in Arabic to Gunde-Shapur. The Nestorian Christian physicians were said to have been expelled from Edessa and moved to Jundeshapur, the great university established by Chosroes Anushirvan of Persia.

Jung, Carl Gustav (1875–1961) Psychoanalyst, trained in Switzerland and Paris. He was a psychiatrist at the Burgholzli public mental hospital in Zurich and a colleague of Swiss psychiatrist, Eugen Bleuler (1857–1939). He met Sigmund Freud (1856–1929) in 1907 who entrusted him with the presidency of the newly formed psychoanalytic association in 1908. Jung later broke with Freud in 1912, over the question of whether sexuality was central to personality, and formed the School of Analytical Psychology. He based his work on mental association methods and developed a word association test which was used to explore the unconscious and describe 'complexes' in the patient. Self-realization was central to Jung's treatment methods.

Jung, Joachium (1587–1657) Physician from Lubeck who gave up his practice to study mathematics and botany. He did some important work in botany while he was a director at a school in Hamburg during the last 20 years of his life, but failed to publish it. His works, *Doxoscopiae* and *Isagoge phytoscopia*, were published by one of his pupils after his death. These revealed a valuable system of botany on which Linnaeus and others later based their work. Jung founded

Societas Ereneutica, one of the earliest scientific societies to be formed in Berlin.

Jungius, Joachim (1587–1657) *See Jung, Joachium.*

Junior Red Cross A resolution to organize the youth of the country into the Red Cross Society was passed by the General Council of the League of Red Cross Societies in 1915. The Junior Red Cross Society came into effect a few years after the resolution.

Junius, Adrian (1512–1575) Physician from Holland who graduated from Paris. He came to London and was appointed physician to the Duke of Norfolk. He published a Greek and Latin Lexicon which was condemned by the Vatican as it was dedicated to Edward VI.

Junker Inhaler For use of chloroform or methylene as anesthesia. Introduced in 1867 by German surgeon, Ferdinand Ethelbert Junker (1828–1901) of the Samaritan Hospital, London.

evidence in cases of assault, infanticide, pretended pregnancies, simulated diseases and poisoning. The first work on the subject, *Constituto Criminalis Cardina,* was published in Germany in 1553.

Jurrasic Period An era of 200 million year-old life forms. Derives its name from the Jura mountains where German geologists first found evidence for its existence.

Justinian Plague An epidemic of plague which occurred during the reign of the Emperor Justinian (AD 527–565) in AD 541. The outbreak lasted for over 60 years and spread throughout Europe.

Juxtaglomerular Apparatus [Latin: *juxta,* close + *glomerare,* to form into a ball) Structure continuous with the afferent arteriole at its entrance to the glomerulus. First described by Norbert Goormaghtigh (b 1890) and H. Handovsky of Germany in 1938 and the function was identified in the early 1950s.

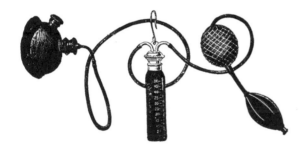

Chloroform inhaler designed by Ferdinand Ethelbert Junker (1828–1901). C.C. Choyce, *A System of Surgery* (1923). Cassell & Co, London

Jurin, James (1684–1750) Graduated from Trinity College Cambridge and became a physician at Guy's Hospital. He published *Physico-Mathematical Dissertations, an Essay upon distinct and indistinct vision* and several other works. While secretary to the Royal Society, he published a paper on smallpox, 'To give a plain Proof from Experience and Matters of Fact that the Small Pox procured by Inoculation (even by the Accounts of those oppose the Practice) is far less Dangerous than the same Distemper has been for many years in the Natural Way', one of the earliest statistical evaluations of immunization.

Jurisprudence In medicine or forensic medicine it is a relatively new specialty, dating back to 1507 when the Bishop of Bamberg introduced a penal code requiring the production of medical evidence in certain cases. In 1532, Charles V introduced a code for magistrates to call for medical

Kaempfer, Englebrecht (1651–1716) *See Kampfer, Englebert.*

Kaes, Theodor (1852–1913) Neurologist from Friedrichs-berg, Germany, who described a new layer in the cerebral cortex, the Kaes–Bekhterev layer, in 1907. Together with Vladimir Mikhailovitch Bekhterev (1857–1927), Russian neurologist.

Kahlbaum, Karl (1828–1899) German psychiatrist who was amongst the first to group symptoms and relate them to definite disease patterns, such as general paresis and schizo-phrenia. He introduced the terms 'symptoms complex', 'cyclothymia' and 'catatonia' to psychiatry.

Kahler, Otto (1849–1893) German physician and professor of medicine at the University of Prague and later at Vienna. Together with Arnold Pick (1867–1926) he described the course of the posterior nerve roots that enter the posterior columns so that fibers at higher levels medially displace those from lower levels – Kahler–Pick Law. *See multiple myeloma (Kahler disease).*

Kahn Test Diagnostic precipitin test, similar to Wassermann test for diagnosis of syphilis, devised by Reuben Leon Khan (b 1887), a bacteriologist at the University of Michigan School of Medicine, in 1922.

Kahun Papyrus Egyptian papyrus written around 2150–1900 BC. Found at Kahun, southwest of Cairo, by British archaeologist, Sir Flinders Petri (1853–1942) in 1889. It mainly deals with gynecology and veterinary medicine.

Kaiserwerth Institute Nursing institute founded in 1833 by a Protestant pastor, Theodor Fliedner (1800–1864) and his wife Frederike at Kaiserwerth on the Rhine. Florence Nightingale trained there for a short period before she established her nursing school in England.

Kala Azar [Hindu: black fever] Also known as Sirkari disease, Burdwan fever, Dum Dum fever, visceral leishmaniasis. The earliest mention of this disease was by John James Clarke (1827–1895) in 1869 who later described it in the *Assam Sanitary Report* of 1880. Thomas Benjamin Brisco also gave a full account of the disease in the Proceedings of the Bengal Medical Department in 1870. During these times the dis-ease was considered to be a form of malaria. Some peculiar inclusions in the spleen of a soldier who died at Dum Dum, near Calcutta, were found by Sir William Boog Leishman (1865–1926) in 1900. However Leishman mistakenly associ-ated these bodies with trypanosomiasis. Similar bodies were found by Charles Donovan (1863–1951) in the spleens of patients at autopsy in 1903 and he subsequently also identi-fied the same bodies in the splenic blood of live patients. Similar bodies in cases of kala azar were demonstrated by Leonard Rogers (1868–1962) in 1904. These bodies were later identified as protozoa and named Leishman–Donovan bodies (LD Bodies) while the protozoan was named *Leishmania donovani.* The death rate in India amongst the sufferers of leishmaniasis was almost 90% until antimony was introduced in 1913 as treatment.

Kallikrein Serine protease, a proteolytic enzyme found in blood plasma, lymph, urine, saliva and exocrine secretions. First isolated from urine in 1926 by Emil Karl Frey (b 1888) and H. Kraut. The same substance was observed during drainage of a large pancreatic cyst by Frey in 1929.

Kamasutra [Sanskrit: *kama,* love, desire + *sutra,* thread] Trea-tise from the fourth to seventh century, probably written by Hindu physician, Vatsyayana Malanaga, which laid down rules according to Hindu law for erotic love and marriage.

Kamen, Martin David (b 1913) Canadian-born American biochemist and professor of biochemistry at the University of California, San Diego. He was a pioneer in the isolation and application of radioisotopes in biology. He confirmed Cornelis van Niel's (b 1898) results that oxygen produced in photosynthesis is from water and not carbon dioxide. He studied nitrogen fixation and molybdenum, the role of iron in porphyrin metabolism, calcium exchange in squamous cell carcinoma and elucidated the structure of many cytochromes. He published *Radioactive Tracers in Biology* in 1947 and *Primary Processes in Photosynthesis* in 1963.

Kamerlingh Onnes, Heike (1853–1926) Born in Grönin-gen, he was professor of physics at Leiden. He discovered superconductivity of metals and obtained liquid helium in 1908. He was awarded the Nobel Prize for Physics in 1913.

Kampfer, Englebert (1651–1716) Born in Westphalia, Ger-many, he traveled as a physician to Persia (1683–1685), India (1690), and Japan (1690–1692). His unpublished manu-scripts were purchased by Sir Hans Sloane in 1753 and were presented to the British Museum. Kampfer's *History of Japan and Siam* was published in English in 1727.

Kanavel Sign Point of maximal tenderness in infections of the tendon sheath. Found in the palm, proximal to the base of the little finger and first described by American surgeon, Alan Buchner Kanavel (1874–1938) of Kansas, professor of surgery at North Western University Medical School.

Kant, Immanuel (1724–1804) German philosopher, born in Königsberg in Prussia where he remained throughout his life. He was appointed professor of logic and metaphysics in 1770. His early publications were in the natural sciences, particularly geophysics and astronomy, in which he predicted the existence of Uranus. His greatest philosophical works were *Critique of Pure Reason*(1781), *Critique of Practical Reason* (1788) and *Critique of Judgment* (1790).

Kantor String Sign Constriction of the terminal ileum seen during barium meal follow through radiological studies in cases of Crohn disease. It was first described by John Leonard Kantor (1890–1947), a gastroenterologist at the Presbyterian Hospital, New York.

Kaposi Sarcoma Pigmented sarcoma of the skin, first described in 1872 by one of Ferdinand von Hebra's (1818–1880) pupils (and his son-in-law), Moritz Kaposi (1837–1902). He was a Viennese dermatologist born in Hungary.

Karrer, Paul (1889–1971) Swiss biochemist, born in Moscow, who studied chemistry under Alfred Werner (1866–1919) at Zurich. He joined Paul Ehrlich (1854–1915) at Frankfurt in 1912, before he returned to Zurich where he succeeded Werner as professor. He identified the structure of many vitamins including carotene in vitamin A, riboflavin (vitamin B2), vitamins E and K. He shared the Nobel Prize for Chemistry with Norman Haworth (1883–1950) for their work on vitamin C and biotin, in 1937.

Kartagener Syndrome Hereditary disorder involving bronchiectasis with transposition of the viscera. Described by Swiss physician, Manes Kartagener (1897–1975), in 1935.

Karyokinensis [Greek: *karyon*, nut + *kinesis*, movement] Splitting of chromosomes within the nucleus. The process was first described by a German biologist, Walther Flemming (1843–1905), in 1882.

Kashevaro-Rudneya, Varvara Aleksandrovna (1844–1899) First Russian woman to qualify as a doctor of medicine.

Kast Syndrome Chondroma associated with cavernous hemangiomas and skin pigmentation. Described by German physician, Alfred Kast (1856–1903).

Katayama Test Test for carbon monoxide in blood that uses ammonium sulfide and acetic acid as reagents. Devised by a Tokyo physician, Kunioshi Katayama (1855–1931).

Katz, Sir Bernard (b 1911) German-born British neurophysiologist who left Germany in 1935, joined Archibald Hill (1886–1977) at University College, London and moved to the Kanematsu Institute at Sydney in 1938 to work with Sir John Carew Eccles (b 1903) and Stephen Kuffler (1913–1980). In 1946 he returned to University College and worked on the chemical mechanism of neurotransmission, particularly acetylcholine. He shared the Nobel Prize in 1970 with Ulf Svante von Euler (1905–1983) and Julius Axelrod (b 1912) for his work on electrical impulse transmission from nerves to muscles. Katz published *Electrical Excitation of Nerve* in 1939. *See neurotransmitters.*

Kaufmann, Eduard (1860–1931) *See achondroplasia.*

Kawasaki Disease Mucocutaneous lymph node syndrome. First described by Tomisaku Kawasaki, a Japanese pediatrician working at the Red Cross Medical Center in 1967. The disease is also known as infantile polyarteritis nodosa.

Kay-Shuttleworth, Sir James Phillips (1804–1871) Physician from Rochdale who was appointed in 1837 by the Poor Law Commission to investigate typhus mortality in London. He was also a reformer of English education and instrumental in establishing a system of government inspection of the schools, and founded his own teacher training college at Battersea which later became St John's College.

Kayser-Fleischer Ring Ring of brown pigments seen in the outer border of iris in hepatolenticular degeneration or Wilson disease. Described by two German ophthalmologists, Bernard Kayser (1869–1954) and Bruno Fleischer (1874–1965).

Keats, John (1795–1821) English poet and son of a livery-stable keeper in London. He was educated at Enfield and studied medicine for a year at Guy's Hospital. He suffered from phthiasis of the lung and died at the age of 26 years.

Keen, William (1837–1932) America's first brain surgeon. He was born in Philadelphia and graduated from Jefferson Medical College where he became professor of surgery in 1889. He successfully removed a meningioma in 1888, and tapped the ventricles in 1889. He published a *System of Surgery* in eight volumes from 1906 to 1921.

Keetley, Charles Robert Bell (1848–1909) *See orchidopexy.*

Keetley-Torek operation Correction of undescended testis by implanting temporarily into the subcutaneous tissue of the thigh. It was described independently by London surgeon, Charles Robert Bell Keetley (1848–1909), and New York surgeon, Franz J.A. Torek (1861–1938).

Kehr Sign Pain in the left shoulder in cases of splenic rupture due to diaphragmatic irritations from free blood in the peritoneum. Described by German surgeon, Hans Kehr (1862–1916).

Keilin, David (1887–1963) British biochemist, son of a Polish businessman and born in Moscow. After his education in Warsaw and Paris, he joined Cambridge University where he became Director of the Molteno Institute in 1931. He investigated cytochromes a, b and c and cytochrome oxidase, hydrogen acceptors in cellular respiration.

Keir, James (1735–1820) Scottish chemist and industrialist who studied medicine at Edinburgh University, where he met and befriended Erasmus Darwin (1731–1802). In 1776 he published a translation of Pierre Macquer's (1718–1784) *Dictionary of Chemistry*. He was also an influential member of the Lunar Society.

Keith, Sir Arthur (1866–1955) Anatomist and anthropologist from Aberdeen who studied medicine at Marischal College. He discovered the sino-atrial node of the heart in 1907 while working with Martin Flack (1882–1931). He was appointed Curator of the Museum at the Royal College of Surgeons in 1908 and made many contributions to surgical pathology and anatomy, including 14 cases of esophageal atresia. Some of his many publications include: *The Antiquity of Man* (1915), *Human Embryology and Morphology* (1902), and *Engines of the Human Body*.

Keith, Thomas (1827–1895) Assistant to Scottish obstetrician and pioneer of anesthesia, Sir James Young Simpson (1811–1870) in Edinburgh. He devised a clamp for ovariotomy and published his results in 1865.

Kekule von Stradonitz, Friedrich August (1829–1896) German chemist, born in Darmstadt and educated at Giessen. He proposed that molecules consist of atoms linked together by bonds according to their valence. He considered that carbon had a valence of 4 and that it could be linked in chains. In 1865 he proposed the 6-carbon ring structure for benzene.

Keller Operation Correction of hallux valgus through arthroplasty of the first metatarsophalangeal joint. Described by Connecticut surgeon, William L. Keller (1874–1959).

Kelly, Adam Brown (1865–1941) Otorhinologist from Victoria Infirmary in Glasgow. *See Plummer–Vinson syndrome*

Kelly, Howard Atwood (1858–1943) American gynecologist and surgeon from Camden, New Jersey who became the first professor of gynecology at Johns Hopkins Medical School in 1889. He was one of the first to employ radium in the treatment of cancer and he published *Operative Gynecology* (1898), and *Medical Gynecology* in 1908. Kelly also developed an air cystoscope, and several surgical instruments.

Kelly Proctoscope Designed by Howard Atwood Kelly (1858–1943) of Johns Hopkins University.

Kelly-Paterson syndrome *See Plummer–Vinson syndrome.*

Keloid [Greek: *kelis*, blemish + *eidos*, form] Elevated, irregular scar caused by excessive collagen produced during connective tissue repair. First mentioned by Retz in 1790, and an accurate description of the lesion was given by Jean Louis Marc Alibert (1768–1837) in 1810. Keloid from hypertrophy of a scar was described by Caesar Henry Hawkins (1798–1884) in 1833.

Kelvin, William Thomson, 1st Baron of Largs (1824–1907) British natural philosopher, born in Belfast and accompanied his father to Glasgow in 1832, where he was professor of mathematics. He and his elder brother James (1822–1892) were professors of natural philosophy and engineering, respectively, in the same university during the time of their father's professorship and he held his chair for 47 years. He invented the galvanometer and the first electric transatlantic submarine cable (1857), improved the compass and proposed the second law of dynamics with Rudolf Clausius (1822–1888) in 1848. He made numerous other important contributions and published over 600 papers. He was the first scientist in the House of Lords in 1892.

Kendall, Edward Calvin (1886–1972) Biochemist, born in South Norwalk, Connecticut. He joined the Mayo Clinic, Rochester in 1914 as professor and head of biochemistry. In December of the same year he isolated thyroxin, a pure extract from the thyroid gland, which he further described in 1917. He further isolated cortisone and 29 related steroids from the adrenal cortex and pioneered their uses in treatment of rheumatoid arthritis and rheumatic fever, with Philip Showalter Hench (1896–1965) in 1948. Kendall, Hench and Tadeus Reichstein (b 1897) were awarded the Nobel Prize for Physiology or Medicine in 1950.

Kendrew, Sir John Cowdery (b 1917) British molecular biologist, born in Oxford and educated at Trinity College, Cambridge. He was co-founder with Max Ferdinand Perutz (b 1914) of the Medical Research Council Unit for Molecular Biology at Cambridge. Using X-ray crystallography, he elucidated the structure of myoglobin between 1957 and 1959. In 1962 he received the Nobel Prize for Chemistry, jointly with Perutz. *See myoglobin.*

Kenealy, Arabella (d 1938) Graduate of the London School of Medicine for women who practiced in London from 1888 to 1894. She wrote *D. Janet of Harley Street* in 1893, *The Failure of Vivisection and Feminism,* and *Sex-extinction,* in addition to fifteen novels.

Kennedy, Robert Foster (1884–1952)Irish neurologist who graduated from the Royal University of Ireland in 1906, and worked at the National Hospital at Queen's Square, London. He was invited to join the recently established New York Neurological Institute in 1910. During World War l he worked close to the front and was the first to describe shell shock as a form of hysteria. On his return to the US there was an encephalitis outbreak, this led him to describe Foster Kennedy syndrome in 1923 in a paper entitled, 'Epilepsy and the convulsive state'. It consists of unilateral optic atrophy with contralateral papilledema and anosmia in cases of frontal lobe tumor. He became professor of neurology at Cornell University, and in 1940 was elected President of the American Neurological Association.

Kenny, Elizabeth (1886–1952) Pioneer of nursing in Australia. She started her nursing in the bush country in Australia and later established clinics for providing physical therapy to polio victims in several parts of the world, including Britain and America.

Kent, Albert Frank Stanley (1863–1958) English physiologist from Torrey, Wiltshire who graduated in natural sciences from Magdalen College, Oxford in 1886. He helped to found the X-ray department at St Thomas' Hospital. He was the first professor of physiology at University College, Bristol (1899) and campaigned for it to become a university in 1909. He did much research on the mammalian heart, and in 1893 described the specialized band of cardiac connective tissue at the atrioventricular junction, now known as the Bundle of His but also as the Bundle of Kent.

Kepler, Johannes (1571–1630) German astronomer born in Weilerstadt near Würtemberg. He entered the University of Tübingen in 1589, obtained his master's degree in theology in 1591 and took the post of professor of mathematics at Graz in 1594. One of his duties was to prepare weather almanacs which encouraged his interest in astronomy. He succeeded Tycho Brahe (1546–1601) as imperial mathematician to Emperor Rudolf ll in Prague. While there Kepler made many discoveries. He published *Astronomia Nova* in 1609, in which he showed that planets do not move around the Sun in perfect circles but in ellipses and stated what are now known as Kepler's First and Second Laws of planetary motion. This broke with the 2000-year-old tradition on planetary motion. His third law was published in 1619 in *De Harmonica Mundi, On Celestial Harmonies.*

Keratitis [Greek: *kera,* horn + *itis,* inflammation] Inflammation of the cornea which has many different causes. The term was coined by James Wardrop (1782–1869), a surgeon from Edinburgh in 1808. He practiced as an ophthalmic surgeon in Edinburgh before moving to London in 1818 as surgeon-extraordinary to Prince Regent.

Keratoconus [Greek: *kera,* horn + *conus,* cone] Also known as conical cornea. The first description was given by Albrecht von Graefe (1828–1870) in 1868. He is considered the founder of ophthalmology and creator of modern eye surgery.

Keratoplasty [Greek: *kera,* horn + *plastikos,* to build up] Corneal grafting or plastic surgery of the cornea. The procedure was first described by Arthur von Hippel (1841–1917) of Germany in 1888. The first successful corneal transplantation was done by Eduard Conrad Zirm (1863–1944) in 1906, and further developed by Anton Elschnig (1863–1939) of New York in 1930. A new method was introduced by Ramon Castroviejo (1904–1987) in 1932. *See corneal grafts.*

Kerckring, Theodorus (1640–1693) German-born anatomist at Amsterdam who described a separate center (Kerckring ossicle) of ossification at the posterior margin of the foramen magnum.

Kerley Lines Horizontal lines seen on a chest X-ray, in the lower zones of the lungs in cases of cardiac failure. Described by British radiologist, Sir Peter J. Kerley (1900–1978), of Cambridge.

Kernicterus [Anglo-Saxon: *cyrnel,* a grain; Latin: *icterus,* jaundice] Johannes Orth (1847–1923) of Germany, around 1875, noted that the brain of infants dying with jaundice was yellow at autopsy. In 1904, Christian Georg Schmorl (1861–1932) studied these findings in more detail and noted that certain areas of the brain, such as the basal ganglia were more intensely colored and he named the condition kernicterus. The symptoms due to involvement of basal ganglia were observed by L. Guthrie in 1914.

Kernig, Vladimir Michalovich (1840–1917) Russian neurologist who received his medical education in Estonia. He served as the director of the Obuchovosky Hospital in St Petersburg from 1865 to 1911. The Kernig sign, flexion of the thigh at the hip and extension of leg causes pain and spasm in the hamstrings in cases of meningitis or encephalitis, was first described by him in 1909. Kernig was also a pioneer in the education of women in Russia.

Kernig Sign *See Kernig, Vladimir Michalovich.*

Keroselene Product of distillation of coal tar extracted by W.B. Merril of Boston. It was tried as an anesthetic in 1861.

Kerosene [Greek: *keros*, wax] Colorless volatile liquid obtained from petroleum and given its present name by Abraham Gesner in 1852. It was used for control of malaria by spreading it over ponds in the early 1900s. The American army physician, William C. Gorgas (1845–1920) used it to control yellow fever in Havana in 1901.

Kerr, Robert (1755–1814) Surgeon from Roxburgh in Scotland who initially studied medicine at Edinburgh University He wrote books on many subjects including: *A History of Scotland during the reign of Robert Bruce, Lavoisier's Elements of Chemistry, Lacepede's History of Quadrupeds and Serpants*, and *Theory of the Earth.*

Ketoacidosis *See acetones, acidosis, Kussmaul.*

Ketone [German: *keton*, acetone] The term was introduced into organic chemistry by Leopold Gmelin (1788–1853), professor and director of the Chemical Institute at Heidelberg. He also introduced the term 'ester', developed the Gmelin test for presence of bile pigments and wrote a ten-volume handbook of chemistry. *See acetone, acidosis.*

Ketosteroid Excretion The measure of 17-ketosteroid levels in the urine was introduced as a diagnostic test for hypopituitarism by R. Fraser and P.H. Smith in 1941.

Kettlewell, Henry Bernard David (1907–1979) English geneticist and entomologist, born in Howden, Yorkshire and studied medicine at Gonville and Caius College, Cambridge and St Bartholomew's Hospital, London. Best known for his study of industrial melanism in the peppered moth in response to atmospheric pollution.

Key, Charles Aston (1793–1849) British surgeon who performed successful ligations for aneurysms of the subclavian artery (1823) and external iliac artery (1822). He described a surgical method for relieving strangulated inguinal hernia (1833) and also designed a lateral operation for lithotomy with a straight staff.

Key, Ernst Axle Henrik (1832–1901) Swedish professor of pathological anatomy at Stockholm who was one of the first to describe the sensory nerve endings (Key bulb).

Khepera Green stone amulet which signified the essence of life in ancient Egypt at the time of the first dynasty around 3400 BC. The stone was placed over the body before burial in the belief that it would enable the dead person to eat and drink again. *See amulet.*

Khorana, Har Gobind (b 1922) Indian-born American biochemist who was born in Raipur, Pakistan. After studying at the Punjab University, he obtained his PhD in organic chemistry from Liverpool University and then moved to Vancouver as Head of the Department of Organic Chemistry (1952–1960). He determined the sequence of nucleic acids in each of the 20 amino acids of the human body. He was appointed professor of biology and chemistry at the Massachusetts Institute of Technology in 1970. He was also one of the first to artificially synthesize a gene, from yeast and also from *Escherichia coli*. He shared the Nobel Prize for Physiology or Medicine in 1968.

Kidd, Frank Seymour (1878–1934) London urologist who designed an operating cystoscope (Kidd cystoscope) with an electrode for diathermy of bladder tumors.

Kidney One of the earliest illustrations of the structure of the kidney was given by Eustachio (1520–1574) in 1564. A classic description of the gross anatomy of the kidney was provided by Lorenzo Bellini (1643–1704), who discovered the renal excretory ducts around 1662. The uriniferous tubules, or the Malpighian bodies, were discovered by Marcello Malpighi (1628–1694) in 1666. William Bowman (1816–1892), an English physician at King's College, proposed the idea that urine formation consisted of glomerular filtration and tubular secretion in 1842. Bowman also discovered the capsule responsible for filtration which now bears his name. The concept that urine formation in the kidneys was a simple process of filtration brought about by the hydrostatic pressure of the blood, was proposed in 1843 by Carl Friedrich Wilhelm Ludwig (1816–1895) who was an experimental physiologist and professor at Zurich. *See nephrology, renal transplantation, glomerular filtration, artificial kidney.*

Kidney Function The mechanical theory of kidney secretion was proposed by Carl Friedrich Wilhelm Ludwig (1816–1895) in 1843. The secretory theory for renal function was put forward by Rudolf Peter Heinrich Heidenhain (1834–1897) in 1874. William Bowman's (1816–1892) theory in 1842 was based on the anatomical concept of tubules and glomeruli. Arthur Robertson Cushney (1866–1926) explained the functions based on both secretory and mechanical theories in 1917. Glomerular filtration in man was first measured by Poul Brandt Rehberg (1895–1985) in 1926. The ability of vertebrate kidney to secrete foreign substances was demonstrated by Eli Kennerley Marshall (1889–1966) in 1929. *See renal function.*

Kidney Transplant *See renal transplantation.*

Kielland, Christian Casper Gabriel (1871–1941) Norwegian obstetrician and gynecologist. He was born in Zululand

443

and received his medical degree from Oslo in 1899. While working as an obstetrician at the University Clinic in 1910, he designed his own obstetric forceps and demonstrated them at the Copenhagen Rigshospital. He published the description of his forceps in 1916.

Kielland Forceps *See Kielland, Christian.*

Kienböck, Robert (1871–1953) Austrian radiologist from Vienna who described acute atrophy of bone in inflammatory conditions (Kienböck atrophy) in 1901, and traumatic osteomalacia (Kienböck disease) in 1910.

Kiernan, Francis (1800–1874) London surgeon who described the interlobular spaces (Kiernan spaces) of the liver in 1833.

Kiesselbach, Wilhelm (1839–1902) German otorhinologist from Erlangen who described the site of common hemorrhage in the nasal septum (Kiesselbach area) in 1884.

Kilian, Hermann Friedrich (1800–1863) German gynecologist who graduated from Edinburgh and became professor of gynecology at Bonn. He described the level of promontory of the sacrum (Kilian line) in 1834. The importance of spondylolisthetic pelvis in pregnancy was demonstrated by him on a specimen called 'Prague pelvis' in 1853.

Killian Operation Radical treatment for diseased frontal air sinuses through an incision in the eyebrow was described by Berlin otolaryngologist, Gustav Killian (1860–1921), in 1903. The lowest muscle of the inferior constrictor muscles of the pharynx (Killian bundle) is named after him.

Kilmainham Hospital Situated in Dublin, it was founded by Arthur, Earl of Granard for aged and disabled soldiers. He served as Marshall-General of the army in Ireland in 1675.

Kilogram [Greek: *chilioi*, thousand] Established as an official unit of weight by the Bureau of Weights and Measures at the Pavilion de Bretail near Paris in 1875. The standard bar which contains a platinum–iridium alloy remains unchanged as the standard weight.

Kimmelsteil–Wilson Lesion Peculiar spherical masses in the central portion of glomerular globules were described in 1936 (intercapillary glomerular sclerosis) in 8 patients with diabetes by German-American pathologist, Paul Kimmelsteil (1900–1970), and English physician, Clifford Wilson (b1906). The same workers also observed albuminuria, edema and hypertension characteristic of nephritic syndrome in the same patients.

Kindergarten [German: children's garden] System of education for children founded by Friedrich Wilhelm August Froebel (1782–1852) of Germany who believed that children should be happy. The first such school was opened by him in 1837 in Blankenburg. The basic concept of education from infancy to manhood was proposed by a pioneer in educational reforms, John Amos Comenius (1592–1671) of Moravia, who wrote the first book on kindergarten, *School of Infancy.* The concept was popularized in Germany and introduced into England in 1851. The American pioneer was Bessie Locke (1865–1952) of Arlington, Massachusetts. She helped to establish over 3000 kindergarten schools in America serving over a million children.

Kinetic Theory of Gases [Greek: *kinein*, to move] Built upon the discovery of Brownian movements in cells by Scottish botanist, Robert Brown (1773–1858) in 1827. The impact of the molecules on the walls of the container under pressure was demonstrated by Swiss mathematician, Daniel Bernoulli (1700–1782), in 1738. The concept of kinetic theory of gases was revived by Scottish engineer and philosopher, John James Waterson (1811–1833), and further advanced by a Viennese mathematical physicist, Ludwig Boltzman (1844–1906), and Josiah Willard Gibbs (1839–1903), a theoretical physicist from New Haven, Connecticut who introduced the idea of chemical potential. Their work was followed by that of Krönig and Rudolf Julius Emmanuel Clausius (1822–1888) (who introduced the term entropy) in 1857. Scottish physicist, James Clerk Maxwell's (1831–1879) discovery of the law of distribution of velocities among gas molecules in 1866 led to a significant advance in the subject.

King, Albert Freeman Africanus (1841–1914) American physician who was one of the first to associate transmission of malaria with the mosquito, in 1883. He was born in Oxfordshire, England and emigrated to America in 1861. He graduated from the University of Pennsylvania and practiced in Washington DC, where he attended president Abraham Lincoln immediately after his assassination. His *Manual of Obstetrics* published in 1882 ran into 11 editions.

King, Edmund (1629–1709) London physician to Charles II who published a paper on dissection of the brain in relation to the pineal gland in 1686.

King, John (c 1800) Surgeon from Edisto Island, South Carolina who performed an operation for abdominal pregnancy in 1816, saving both mother and the child. He wrote the first book on ectopic pregnancy, *An Analysis of the subject of Extra-uterine Foetation, and of the retroversion of the Gravid Uterus* in 1818.

King, Thomas Wilkinson (1809–1847) Physician from Dover

who practiced in London. He succeeded Thomas Hodgkin (1798–1866) as curator of the museum and lecturer in anatomy at Guy's Hospital. He described the muscular band of the heart extending from the ventricular septum to the base of the anterior papillary muscle. He also described the colloid of thyroid gland.

King and Armstrong Method Used to estimate serum alkaline phosphate. Devised in 1934 by Toronto biochemist, Earl Judson King (1901–1962), and Canadian physician, Arthur Rily Armstrong (b 1904) of Hamilton, Ontario.

Kingsley, Norman William (1823–1913) American dentist and a pioneer in maxillofacial surgery. He designed several devices for use in fracture of the upper jaw (Kingsley oral bars) and fractured maxilla (Kingsley splint).

King Edward VII Two days before his coronation King Edward VII developed appendicitis which was diagnosed and successfully operated on by Sir Frederick Treves (1853–1923), surgeon at the London Hospital. The anesthesia was given by Sir Frederick William Hewitt (1857–1916), anesthetist to the Charing Cross and the London Hospital, and inventor of the first portable apparatus for administering a mixture of nitrous oxide and oxygen.

King George III The earliest symptomology of acute intermittent porphyria has been constructed from manuscripts related to the treatment of King George III (1738–1820). The King's illness was originally thought to be primarily psychiatric but a careful retrospective analysis of the symptoms from the period 1765 to 1810 has strongly suggested that it was acute porphyria.

King's College Medical School (New York) The second medical school in North America, established in 1768. It was renamed Columbia Presbyterian Hospital after independence from Britain and revived in 1792 by Samuel Bard (1742–1821), its dean and professor of physick. It was rebuilt by the College of Physicians and Surgeons of the University of New York in 1807.

King's College Medical Society, London Took its origins from the King's College Medical and Scientific Society, founded in 1833. In 1908 it became the King's College Medical Society, and was renamed Listerian Society of King's College Hospital in 1912.

King's College (London) It was incorporated in 1829 and opened in 1831. It amalgamated with the University of London in 1837. The King's College Hospital at Denmark Hill was established in 1839.

King's Evil or scrofula It was believed that it could be cured

by the King's touch. In 1058 Edward the Confessor used this method as a cure, and Charles I touched over 92,000 persons for the same purpose. A classic essay on the subject titled *Of the Cure of the Evill by the King's Touch* was written by a London physician, Richard Wiseman (1622–1676). The practice continued until 1714 until George I abolished it after the death of Queen Anne.

Kinnier Wilson Disease *See Wilson disease.*

Kinsey, Alfred Charles (1894–1956) American sexologist and zoologist from New Jersey. He conducted over 18,500 interviews and published *Sexual Behavior in the Human Male* in 1948, followed by *Sexual Behavior in the Human Female* in 1953. He founded the Institute for Sex Research while he was professor of zoology at Indiana in 1942.

Kipp Apparatus Used for continuous production of gases such as carbon dioxide and hydrogen sulfide in the laboratory was designed by a Dutch chemist, Petrus Jacobus Kipp (1808–1864) from Utrecht. A representation of his apparatus appears on the coat of arms of the Dutch Chemical Society.

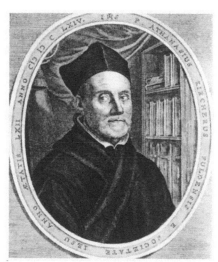

Athanasius Kircher, (1601–1680). Wiliam Stirling, *Some Apostles of Physiology* (1902). Waterlow & Sons, London

Kircher, Athanasius (1601–1680) Jesuit priest and a scientist from Geissen in Germany. In 1635 he was made professor of mathematics at the Collegium Romanum in Rome by Pope Urban VI. He was the earliest to attempt to view microscopic organisms in 1658, using a primitive microscope which he constructed. He examined blood from plague victims, and described what he saw as 'worms' of plague in *Scrutium Pestis*. It is probable that what he saw were only pus cells or red cells as his microscope was only capable of a magnification of x 32. Some of his other publications include: *Oedipus Aegyptiacus, Ars Magnesia, Organon*

Mathematicum, Musurgia Universalis, and *Mundus Subterraneus.* Kircher also did experiments on magnets and published *Magnes sive de arte magnetica* in 1640.

Kirchhoff, Gustav Robert (1824–1887) German physicist from Königsberg who served as professor at Heidelberg (1854–1875) and Berlin (1875–1886). He invented the spectroscope in 1859 with Robert Wilhelm Bunsen (1811–1899), and was the first to measure electrical resistance in absolute terms in 1849

Kirkland, Thomas (1721–1798) Physician from Leicestershire who wrote: *An inquiry into the state of Medical Surgery, Observations on Pott's remarks on Fractures, A Treatise on Childbed Fevers, Thoughts on Amputation,* and *Commentary on Apoplectic and Paralytic Affections.*

Kirmisson, Edouard (1848–1927) Surgeon from Paris who described the operation (Kirmisson operation) where the tendo calcaneous is transplanted to the peroneus longus muscle. He also published an important work on diseases of the locomotor apparatus in 1890.

Kirschner Wire Used for stabilization of bone fragments and joint immobilization. It was devised by German professor of surgery, Martin Kirschner (1879–1942) at Heidelberg in 1909.

Kirstein, Alfred (1863–1922) Laryngologist in Berlin who described the first direct laryngoscope in 1895.

Kirstenius, Peter (1577–1640) Professor of medicine at Uppsala in Sweden. He was also a linguist who knew 25 languages and wrote many medical works in oriental languages.

Kitasato, Baron Shibasaburo (1852–1931) Japanese bacteriologist who graduated from Imperial University of Tokyo in 1883. He worked under Robert Koch (1843–1910) in Berlin and developed the antitoxin to the diphtheria organism in 1891. He founded a Japanese Institute for Infectious Diseases. Together with Emil von Behring (1854–1917), he discovered antitoxic immunity in 1890 which led to development of treatments and immunization for tetanus and diphtheria. He isolated the causative organism of bubonic plague, *Pasteurella pestis,* in 1894, independently of Alexandre Yersin (1863–1943).

Kitchener School of Medicine Founded in 1923 for men at Khartoum in the Sudan. It was renamed University College of Khartoum in 1950.

Kitchener, William (1775–1827) Physician and son of a wealthy coal merchant from London. He was educated at Eton and practiced in London. His main interest was gastronomy and he published *The Cook's Oracle.* His other works include: *The Art of Invigorating and Prolonging Life, The Economy of the Eyes,* and the *Traveller's Oracle.*

Kjeldahl Method Used to measure total nitrogen inorganic compounds. It was designed by Danish chemist Johan Gustav Christoffer Kjeldahl (1849–1900) of Copenhagen.

Kjelland Forceps Used for rotation in deep transverse arrest during labor. They were devised by Norwegian obstetrician, Christian Kjelland (1871–1941) in 1915.

Klaproth, Martin Heinrich (1743–1817) German analytical chemist and mineralogist who became the first professor of chemistry at the University of Berlin in 1810. He discovered and named six elements including: strontium, uranium, zirconium and tellurium. He published *A Mineralogical System, Chemical Essays* and *Dictionary of Chemistry.*

Klebs, Theodor Albrecht Edwin (1834–1913) German bacteriologist who, in 1873, pointed out the tuberculous cavities in the lungs as a source of intestinal tuberculosis. The peculiar property of acid fastness of the tuberculous bacilli was demonstrated by Klebs (1896), and *Corynebacterium diphtheriae* (Klebs–Löffler bacillus) was discovered by him and Friedrich Löffler (1852–1915) in 1883. Klebs disease, glomerulonephritis, was named after him.

Klebsiella pneumoniae A genus of gram-negative bacillus first isolated from a series of patients with pneumonia by Karl Freidlander (1847–1887) in 1882 and named Freidlander bacillus. Theodor Albrecht Edwin Klebs (1834–1913) independently discovered the organism in 1883.

Kleptomania [Greek: *kleptein,* to steal + *mania,* madness] Saint Augustine (AD 354) in his *Confessions* admitted to stealing and displayed a remarkable insight into the psychology of stealing and kleptomania. Most forms of compulsive disorders including kleptomania were studied by Jean Etienne Dominique Esquirol (1772–1840).

Klinefelter Syndrome Also known as XXY syndrome, consisting of gynecomastia, azoospermia with increased levels of follicle-stimulating hormone in male. Described by American professor of medicine at the Johns Hopkins Medical School, Harry Fitch Klinefelter (b 1912) and coworkers, in 1942. The condition was shown to be due to a sex chromosomal defect, by P.A. Jacobs and J.A. Strong in 1959.

Klippel–Feil Syndrome Incomplete development, fusion or absence of the first cervical vertebra. Described by French neurologists at the Sâlpetrière Hospital in Paris, Maurice Klippel (1858–1942) and Andre Feil (b 1884) in 1912.

Klotz, Oscar (1878–1936) Born in Preston, Ontario, he was a

Canadian pioneer in the study of fatty acids and arteriosclerosis. He published *Concerning the pathology of some arterial diseases* in 1925.

Klumpke Paralysis The first description of atrophy and paralysis of the muscles related to a lesion in the brachial plexus, eighth cervical nerve, and the first thoracic nerve was given by Augusta Dejerine-Klumpke (1859–1927) of Paris in 1885.

Knapp, Hermann Arnold Jakob (1832–1911) Born in Dauborn, Hesse–Nassau, he was a leading ophthalmologist in New York who designed several operations for squint, pterygium, and cataract. He founded the *Archives of Ophthalmology and Otology* in 1869, and wrote a treatise on curvature of the cornea in 1859.

Knee Injury [Anglo-Saxon: *cneow*, knee] Surgery for displaced semilunar cartilage of the knee was first performed on a 30-year-old miner by Thomas Annandale (1838–1909) from Newcastle-upon-Tyne in 1884. The replacement of lateral ligaments with artificial ligaments in cases of knee injury was first performed by Frederick Jay Cotton (1869–1938), a surgeon at Newport, Rhode Island in 1934.

Knee Jerk [Anglo-Saxon: *cneow*, knee] The term was coined by Sir William Gowers (1845–1915) to denote the involuntary tendon reflex of the knee. The physical sign was called 'patellar tendon reflex' by Wilhelm Erb (1840–1921). It was named 'knee phenomenon' by Karl Westphal (1833–1890). Erb also demonstrated the loss of knee jerk, in syphilis of the spinal cord. The reinforcement of the reflex was described independently by Silas Weir Mitchell (1829–1914), and Morris J. Lewis in 1886. Sir Charles Sherrington (1857–1952) in 1893 demonstrated that knee jerk was an innate phenomenon, thus establishing it as a genuine reflex.

Knee Joint [Anglo-Saxon: *cneow*, knee] The first amputation of the knee joint in America was performed by Nathan Smith (1762–1829), a surgeon from Connecticut in 1825. One of the first English monographs on the surgery of the knee joint, *Excision of the Knee Joint,* was published by a surgeon Richard James Mackenzie (1821–1854) of Edinburgh Royal Infirmary. Another important treatise on the surgical diseases of the knee joint was written by Peter Charles Price (1832–1864) from London in 1865. Surgery for displaced semilunar cartilage of the knee was first performed on a 30-year-old miner by Thomas Annandale (1838–1909) from Newcastle-upon-Tyne in 1884. The method of positive pressure arthrodesis as treatment for tuberculosis of the knee joint was introduced in 1932 by John Albert Key (1890–1955), an orthopedic surgeon at Harvard. *See knee*

injury, knee transplantation.

Knee Transplantation [Anglo-Saxon: *cneow*, knee] Knee and other joint transplantation from cadavers as treatment for advanced joint disease was first performed by Eric Lexer (1867–1937), a surgeon from Königsberg, Germany in 1907 who became a pioneer of plastic surgery during World War I.

Knighton, Sir William (d 1836) He entered the medical profession as an apothecary in Tavistock. Later he moved to London and obtained his medical diploma as an accoucheur and physician and was appointed physician and private secretary to George IV.

Knoop, Franz (1875–1946) Physiologist from Freiburg who described the formation of acetoacetic acid and ß-hydroxybutyric acid in the liver (ß-oxidation theory) for catabolized fats in 1905.

Knopf, Sigard Adolphus (1857–1940) New York physician and a pioneer in the study and treatment of tuberculosis in America. He promoted the method (Knopf treatment) of breathing using diaphragmatic muscles rather than intercostal muscles in cases of apical lobe tuberculosis.

Knowles Pins Used for fixing fractures of the femoral neck. Devised by American orthopedic surgeon from Iowa, Frederick Knowles (1888–1973).

Knox, Robert (1791–1862) Scottish anatomist who was born in and graduated from Edinburgh in 1814. He joined the army as a surgeon and was wounded during the battle of Waterloo. He later returned to Edinburgh to lecture in anatomy. His alleged involvement in the Burke and Hare murders for dissection contributed to his decline as a brilliant comparative anatomist. He served as pathologist to the London Cancer Hospital towards the declining stages of his career and died at Hackney.

Kobelt Venous Plexus Formed by the veins of the bulb of the vestibule below the clitoris. It is named after German anatomist, George Ludwig Kobelt (1804–1857) of Freiburg.

Kober, George Martin (b 1850) One of the first in America to point out that flies are carriers of disease in his report on typhoid fever in the district of Columbia in 1895. He was also a pioneer in industrial hygiene in America and published several works on industrial pollution in 1908–1916.

Koberle, Eugene (1858–1915) *See fibroid.*

Koch, Heinrich Hermann Robert (1843–1910) German physician and pioneer in bacteriology, educated at the University of Göttingen and member of the Imperial Board of Health, German Cholera Commission and professor of hygiene and bacteriology at the University of Berlin. In 1876 he showed that rod-shaped organisms could be isolated from anthrax lesions, cultured in the laboratory and were capable of infecting experimental animals. He devised a staining and fixing method for bacteria in 1877, developed methods of producing pure cultures, and introduced nutrient agar for culture in 1881. The tubercle bacillus was discovered by him in 1882, which was responsible for one in seven deaths in Europe at this time. He proposed four criteria (Koch postulates) necessary to ascertain that an organism is responsible for a particular disease. In 1905 he was awarded the Nobel Prize for Physiology or Medicine.

Kocher, Emil Theodor (1841–1917) Swiss professor of surgery from Bern. He demonstrated the function of the thyroid and developed surgical treatments for disorders of the thyroid, including tumors and goiter. By the time of his death, Kocher had performed over 2000 thyroid operations with a mortality rate of just over 4%. He isolated one of the thyroid hormones and used it in replacement therapy. He pioneered methods of brain and spinal cord surgery and an operation for reduction of subluxation of the shoulder joint. Kocher was one of the first surgeons to be honored with the Nobel Prize for Physiology or Medicine in 1909. His *Operative Surgery*, published in 1894, ran into many editions and was translated into several languages.

Koch Triangle Part of the wall of the right atrium which overlies the atrioventricular node is named after Berlin cardiologist and pathologist, Walter Karl Koch (b 1880).

Koebner Phenomenon Lesions develop along the lines of mechanical irritation of skin, especially in cases of psoriasis. Described by a German dermatologist at Breslau, Heinrich Koebner (1838–1904), in 1876.

Koeberlé, Eugene (1828–1915) French surgeon and gynecologist who introduced ovariotomy in France. He modified the artery forceps and included a locking device (Koeberlé forceps) in 1865.

Köhler, Georges Jean Franz (b 1946) German immunochemist from Munich. After receiving his degree from the University of Freiburg, he went to work with Cesar Milstein (b 1927) at the Medical Research Council Laboratory in Cambridge, UK. Here he discovered how to make hybridomas, cells with an infinite lifespan which can produce monoclonal antibodies. In 1984 he became one of three directors of the Max Planck Institute of Immune Biology at Freiburg. His major research was on structural

mutants of immunoglobulins and formation of hybridomas. He shared the Nobel Prize in 1984 with Cesar Milstein and Niels Kai Jerne (b 1911) for his pioneering work .

Kohler, Wolfgang (1887–1967) German psychologist who studied the underlying principle of motion pictures, where the viewer filled in the short visual gaps that took place between the separate pictures which made up the film. This perception of illusory continuity was further studied using Gestalt theory.

Köhler Disease (Syn: metatarsal head osteochondritis) Aseptic necrosis of the navicular bone. Described by German radiologist from Wiesbaden, Alban Köhler (1874–1947), in 1908. The disease is also named after an American surgeon, Albert Henry Freiberg (1868–1940) of Cincinnati, Ohio, who described it in 1926.

Kolbe, Adolph Wilhelm Hermann (1818–1884) Born in Elliehausen near Göttingen in Germany. He was an eminent chemist and one of the founders of organic chemistry. He developed electrolysis for preparation of alkanes.

Kolff, Willem Johan (b 1911) Dutch-born American physician and pioneer of the artificial kidney. He was born in Leiden, and received his medical degree in 1946 from Gröningen University. He constructed the first rotating drum artificial kidney in wartime Holland with off-the-shelf components, and treated his first patient in 1943. He emigrated to America in 1950 and continued to develop the artificial kidney and a heart–lung machine at the Cleveland Clinic. *See artificial kidney.*

Kolle, Wilhelm (1868–1935) He introduced heat-killed phenolized vaccine for cholera in 1896. He was a serologist at Bern in Switzerland and Frankfurt in Germany. He prepared several other vaccines against cholera, typhoid and plague which are named after him.

Koller, Carl (1857–1944) Ophthalmologist from Bohemia who was the first to demonstrate the local anesthetic effect of cocaine on the eye in 1884. After his disappointment with the progress of his career in Vienna, he emigrated to New York in 1888.

Köllicker, Rudolph Albert von (1817–1905) Swiss anatomist, embryologist and a pioneer in the field of histology. He described the structure of tissues and cells, and published the standard textbook on the subject, *Manual of Human Histology,* in 1852.

Koplik Spots Diagnostic sign in measles described by a New York pediatrician, Henry Koplik (1858–1927) in the *Archives of Pediatrics* of New York in 1898. Koplik graduated from Columbia University in 1881 and did postgraduate work in Berlin, Prague and Vienna. He then served as pediatrician to Mount Sinai Hospital in New York for 25 years. He started the first sterilized milk depot for infants in the USA and was a founder of the American Pediatric Society. His work, *The Diseases of Infancy and Childhood,* was published in 1902. This sign was, however, described earlier by a pediatrician from Moscow, Feodorovich Filatov (1847–1902).

Kopernik, Mikolaj (1473–1543) *See Copernicus, Nicolaus.*

Koranyi, Baron Alex von (1866–1944) *See benzene.*

Kornberg, Arthur (b 1918) American biochemist from Brooklyn, New York who graduated in medicine from Rochester University. He became the head of the microbiology department at Washington University in 1953, and professor at Stanford University in 1959. He discovered the enzyme, DNA polymerase, and showed that synthesis required a DNA template and base-pairing to produce the helical strands of opposite polarity suggested in the Crick and Watson molecular model. He was awarded the Nobel Prize in 1959, together with Severo Ochoa (b 1905), for this work. He also worked out the synthetic pathways of the coenzymes, nicotinamide adenine dinucleotide (NAD) and flavine adenine dinucleotide (FAD).

Kornberg, Sir Hans Leo (b 1928) German-born British biochemist who worked mainly on microbial metabolism. He discovered the glyoxylate cycle of fatty acid metabolism used by plants, fungi and microorganisms. He was elected FRS in 1965, knighted in 1978 and has been Chairman of the Royal Commission on Environmental Pollution and a trustee of both the Nuffield and Wellcome trusts.

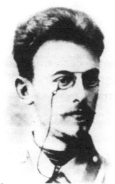

Nikolai Sergeivich Korotkov, (1874–1920). Comroe, J., *Exploring the Heart,* first edition. Norton, New York, with permission

Korotkoff, Nicolai Sergeivich (1874–1920) *See Korotkov.*

Korotkov, Nikolai Sergeivich (1874–1920) Russian physician who devised a method of measuring diastolic blood pressure by applying the stethoscope to the brachial artery during the deflation of the cuff of the sphygmomanometer. *See diastolic blood pressure.*

Korsakoff psychosis *See Korsakov syndrome.*

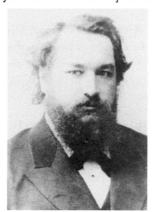

Sergei Korsakov (1854–1900). Courtesy of the National Library of Medicine

Korsakov Syndrome Condition of polyneuritis, confabulation and memory gaps due to excessive alcohol intake. First described by Swedish physician, Magnus Huss (1807–1890) in his book, *Alcoholismus Chronicus,* published in 1852. A classic description of the syndrome was given by the Russian neuropsychiatrist, Sergei Segeivich Korsakov (1854–1900), in 1887. The beneficial effect of vitamin B1 or thiamin in the condition was first observed by K.M. Bowman and colleagues in 1939.

Kossel, Albrecht (1853–1927) Swiss-born German physiological chemist, professor of physiology and director of the Physiological Institute at Marburg. He separated protein and nucleic acid and showed that the latter was rich in phosphorus and made up of the four DNA bases, adenine, thymine, cytosine, and guanine. He also discovered histidine in spermatozoa in 1896. He was awarded the Nobel Prize for Physiology or Medicine in 1910. His son, Walther Kossel (1888–1956), was an atomic physicist at Kiel and Danzig, who proposed the physical theory of chemical valence.

Kosterlitz, Hans Walter (b 1903) German biochemist educated at Heidelberg, Freiburg and Berlin Universities. He served as a radiologist under Wilhelm His in Berlin, before moving to Aberdeen University in 1933 where did research on carbohydrates under Macleod. He then moved on to research on the effects of opioids on the autonomic nervous system and gastrointestinal motility. He was made professor of pharmacology in 1968 and worked with John Hughes (b 1942) on naturally occurring opiates, discovering the action of two enkephalins.

Kraepelin, Emil (1856–1926) German experimental psychiatrist, father of descriptive psychiatry, who introduced the term 'dementia praecox' to psychiatry in 1901. He also introduced the term 'paranoia' to denote a state of extreme suspiciousness, in 1888.

Krafft-Ebing, Richard (1840–1902) German forensic psychiatrist and a pioneer in the field of sexual pathology. He defined and named many sexual deviations, such as masochism and sadism, in his *Psychopathia Sexualis* published in 1876.

Kraske, Paul (1851–1930) Surgeon from Freiburg described an operation (Kraske operation) for carcinoma of the rectum, where the surgical approach is gained by excision of the sacrum and coccyx.

Krause Operation For trigeminal neuralgia, involving extradural excision of the gasserian ganglion, was described by Berlin surgeon, Fedor Victor Krause (1857–1937).

Krause, Karl Friedrich Theodor (1797–1868) Professor of anatomy at Hannover in Germany, who described several anatomical structures which bear his name.

Krause, Wilhelm Johann Friedrich (1833–1909) Professor of anatomy at Göttingen in Germany. He described the septa which divide the sarcomeres within muscles (Krause membrane) and several other structures which bear his name.

Krause bulb Sensory nerve end organ, first described by Wilhelm J.F. Krause (1833–1910) in 1860.

Krebs Cycle The citric acid cycle in which energy is produced during the metabolism of glucose, was first described by Sir Hans Adolf Krebs (1900–1982), while he was at Sheffield University in 1937. *See citric acid cycle.*

Krebs, Sir Hans Adolf (1900–1982) German-born British biochemist, the discoverer of Krebs cycle, was born in Hildesheim. He assisted Otto Warburg at the Kaiser Wilhelm Institute of Cell Pathology, Berlin. He emigrated to England in 1934 and worked with Frederick Gowland Hopkins on redox reactions. He was made professor of biochemistry at Sheffield in 1945, and later at Oxford in 1954. He first described the urea cycle in which carbon dioxide and ammonia form urea in the presence of liver slices and catalytic amounts of ornithine and citrulline. This led on to his elucidation of the citric acid cycle. He also discovered purine synthesis in birds and utilization of ketone bodies in starved rat heart muscle. Krebs shared the Nobel Prize for Physiology or Medicine with an American biochemist, Fritz Albert Lipman (1899–1986) in 1953.

Kreidl, Alois (1864–1928) Austrian physiologist, one of the first to study the hypothalamus, together with Johan Karplus (1866–1936) in 1909.

Krogh, August Schack (1874–1949) Danish physiologist who graduated from Copenhagen University and spent the rest of his working life there. He was a pioneer in the study of the human capillary system. He demonstrated that the capillaries are under nervous, hormonal and chemical control, and that the greater the activity of the tissue the greater is the proportion of capillaries that are dilated. He was awarded the Nobel Prize in 1920. His work, *The Anatomy and Physiology of Capillaries,* was published in 1922.

Kronecker, Karl Hugo (1839–1914) German physiologist who described the swallowing reflex involved in the act of deglutition in 1880. He also described a cardio-inhibitory center (Kronecker center).

Kronig, Claus Ludwig Theodore Bernhard (1863–1913) *See antiseptics.*

Kuffler, Stephen William (1913–1980) American neurobiologist who was born in Hungary, educated in Vienna and worked in the Kanematsu Institute in Sydney with Sir Bernard Katz (b 1911) and Sir John Carew Eccles (b 1903) before moving to the Johns Hopkins School of Medicine in 1945. He studied mechanisms of synaptic transmission, retinal physiology, and electrophysiology of glial cells.

Krukenberg, Adolph (1816–1877) Born in Halle, he was professor of anatomy at Brunswick and described the central vein (Krukenberg vein) of the hepatic lobule in 1843.

Krukenberg Amputation Method used to allow the stump to retain some function. Described in 1917 by a German orthopedic surgeon, Hermann Krukenberg (b 1863), brother of the pathologist, Friedrich Ernst Krukenberg (1871–1946).

Krukenberg Tumor Fibrosarcoma of the ovary, first described by the pathologist, Friedrich Ernst Krukenberg (1871–1946) of Germany in 1896.

Krypton [Greek: *kryptos*, hidden] Inert gas discovered by Nobel Prize winner, Sir William Ramsay (1852–1916) and Morris William Travers (1872–1961) in 1898.

Kuhlmann Test Modified form of Binet–Simon test for intelligence, devised by American psychologist, Frederick Kuhlmann (1876–1941).

Kuhn, Richard (1900–1967) German biochemist, born in Vienna, who studied at Vienna and Munich Universities. He served as the director of the Kaiser Wilhelm Institute for

Medical Research in Heidelberg in 1929. His main interest was study of enzymes and vitamins and he isolated riboflavin, or vitamin B2, from several sources for the first time in 1933 and was awarded the Nobel Prize for Chemistry in 1938.

Kühne, Wilhelm (1837–1900) German biochemist and physiologist who studied under Rudolph Virchow (1821–1902) and Claude Bernard (1813–1878). He coined the term 'enzyme' (Greek for 'in yeast') in 1878 to denote ferments and other organic substances which activate chemical reactions. He also demonstrated the visual purple in the retina which was later called 'rhodopsin' and which is bleached by light and restored in darkness.

Kühne Spindle Neuromuscular organ described in 1862 by Wilhelm Kühne (1837–1900) professor of physiology at Heidelberg.

Kulchitsky, Nicolai (1856–1925) Russian anatomist and histologist who described the cells in the intestinal epithelium between the crypts of Lieberkuhn (Kulchitsky cells) in 1897.

Kümmell Disease A form of traumatic spondylitis due to a fracture of the vertebra. Described by German surgeon Hermann Kümmell (1852–1937) in 1892. He was the first professor of surgery at Hamburg University.

Kunckle, John (1630–1703) Eminent chemist from Sleswick. He made several discoveries in chemistry and also extracted phosphorus from urine.

Kundrat Disease A form of lymphosarcoma arising from groups of lymph nodes, without leukemic features or involvement of the spleen. It was described by Viennese pathologist, Hans Kundrat (1845–1893) in 1893.

Küntscher Nail Used for intramedullary fixation of fractures of the femur and tibia. It was devised by a German surgical professor at Kiel, Gerhard Küntscher (1902–1972).

Kuntz, Albert (1859–1957) Professor of histology at St Louis University, Kentucky. He described the gray ramus running from the second thoracic ganglion to the first thoracic nerve in 1927.

Kupffer Cells Stellate cells with phagocytic properties found in the lining (endothelium) of the capillaries of the liver. They were described by Karl Wilhelm von Kupffer (1829– 1902), professor of anatomy at Königsberg, in 1876.

Kuru [Papua New Guinea: laughing death] A form of spongiform encephalopathy found amongst the Fore tribe of a very isolated area of the Eastern Highlands of Papua New Guinea who were cannibals. Anthropologists, Robert Glasse and Shirley Lindenbaum, had observed that mortuary ceremonies involved the eating of the deceased's brain and this proved to be the route of transmission of the disease. It was elucidated by American virologist, Daniel Carleton Gajdusek (b 1924) and Zigas in 1957. He demonstrated the importance of slow viruses in chronic diseases of the central nervous system which earned him the Nobel Prize for Medicine in 1966. His work led to other studies on bovine spongiform encephalopathy (mad cow disease), scrapie, and Creutzfeldt–Jakob disease, all caused by slow viruses.

Kussmaul, Adolf (1822–1902) German professor of surgery at Heidelberg, who made the first attempt at gastroesophagoscopy in 1869. He also studied the effect of circulation upon the movements of the iris in 1856, and in 1874 he noted the presence of acetone in blood and acetonemia as a cause of diabetic coma. He described 'air hunger' during acidosis (Kussmaul respiration), two cases of ascending neuropathy, later known as acute infective polyneuritis (1859), periarteritis nodosa (1866), progressive bulbar palsy (1873), and pulsus paradoxus (1873).

Kveim Test Intradermal diagnostic skin test for sarcoidosis using a saline suspension of sarcoid tissue. It was devised by R.H. Williams and D.A. Nickelson in 1935. Norwegian pathologist from Copenhagen, Morten Ansgar Kveim (b 1892) gave a comprehensive evaluation of the test in 1941 and it was named after him.

Kwashiorkor [Ghanaian: 'displaced child' or disease suffered by a child displaced from the breast] Severe protein malnutrition in children leading to retarded growth, edema, pathologic changes in the liver, mental apathy. It is responsible for a large proportion of deaths in the under five year olds and is thought to be related to marasmus. It was described by British pediatrician, Cicely Williams (1893–1992), in 1933.

Kymograph [Greek: *kyma*, wave + *graphein*, to write] Device to measure pressure, muscle movements and other parameters in experimental physiology. The principle and use of it was first suggested by the English physician, Thomas Young (1773–1829), in 1807. The apparatus was first constructed and used by Carl Frederick Ludwig (1816–1895) of Germany in 1849. It consisted of smoked paper fixed on a rotating drum on which recordings were made with a stylus.

Kyotai or Kawagata Type of hard condom made of thin leather which was formerly used by the Japanese for contraception.

Kyphosis [Greek: *kyphosis*, humpback] A cause of necrosis of the epiphyses of the vertebrae leading to deformity in the thoracic spine (Scheurmann disease). It was first described by Danish radiologist, Holger Werfel Scheurmann (1877–1967), in 1921.

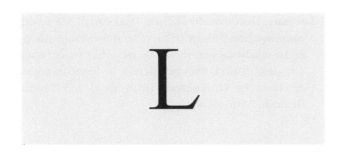

La Mettrie, Julian Offray de (1709–1751) Controversial French physician who proposed the materialistic philosophy that the ultimate goal of life is enjoyment of pleasure, soul perished with the body, and virtue was enlightened by self-interest. His book, *L'Histoire naturelle de l'ame* (1745) was publicly burnt and he had to take refuge in Berlin under the protection of Frederick the II of Prussia.

Labarraque Solution Popular disinfectant up to the early 1900s was prepared by French chemist and pioneer in occupational diseases, Antoine Germain Labarraque (1777–1850).

Labat Syringe Glass and metal device for locking the needle with a finger hold, devised by a French surgeon in Paris, Louis Gaston Labat (1877–1934). He also perfected the method of infiltration of the nerve to produce nerve block for anesthesia.

Labbe, Ernest Marcel (1870–1939) French physiologist from Paris who was the first to give a full description of chromoffin cell tumors of the adrenal medulla in 1922.

Labbé, Léon (1832–1916) Paris surgeon who developed the practice of pre-anesthetic medication in 1872. The Labbé triangle between the inferior border of the liver and lower border of the 9th costal cartilage is named after him. *See Labbé vein.*

Labbé Vein Inferior anastomotic vein connecting the superficial middle cerebral vein and the transverse sinus of the dura mater, named after Paris surgeon, Léon Labbé (1832–1916).

Labium Minus [Latin: *labium*, lip + *minus*, least] Part of the external female genitalia, known to the Greeks as nymphae or pterygomata (wings).

Laborde, Jean Baptiste Vincent (1830–1903) Paris physiologist who described a form of artificial respiration with intermittent traction of the tongue in 1897.

Labor Laws The first act to control labor in England, known as the Statutes of Labourers, was passed in 1349. It allowed the landlord to force his men to work and brand them with hot iron if they refused to do so. Their wages were also controlled and heavy punishment was meted out to those who disobeyed. *See Factory Acts.*

Labor Many methods of accelerating labor have been practiced by different races in the past. The Ebers papyrus mentions the application of peppermint to the woman's posterior. Early Christians considered the pain of childbirth to be due to carnal sin. Paul of Aegina (AD 625–690), in his third book, gave an excellent scientific account of the causes and treatment of a difficult labor. The obstetric chair, mentioned in the Old Testament, was in continuous use for thousands of years until the French obstetrician, François Mauriceau (1637–1709) replaced it in the 17th century. The first work in England on labor was written by William Harvey (1578–1657), *De Partu* in his *Exercitationes de generatione animalium* published in 1651. The mechanism of labor was first explained by Sir Fielding Ould (1710–1789) of Galway, Ireland in his *Treatise on Midwifery* published in 1742. When chloroform was first tried as an inhalational anesthetic in labor by James Young Simpson (1811–1870) in 1847, objections were raised on religious grounds that a woman should be allowed to suffer pain. The debate on the use of chloroform in labor came to an end when John Snow (1813–1858) of Soho, London successfully administered chloroform to Queen Victoria during delivery of Prince Leopold in 1853. Blair William Bell (1871–1936), a Liverpool obstetrician, was the first to use oxytocin in labor in 1909. *See induction of labor.*

Labrinudi Operation Anterior wedge tarsectomy with triple fusion for drop foot. Described by an orthopedic surgeon at Guy's Hospital, Constantine Lambrinudi (1890–1943) in 1927.

Labyrinth [Greek: *labyrinthos*, structure with connecting passages] The membranous labyrinth of the ear, including the semicircular canals, vestibule and cochlea, was discovered by Antonio Scarpa (1747–1832) in 1772. A Viennese otologist, Robert Bárány (1876–1936) was the first to study the labyrinthine function of the ear, and he devised the Bárány caloric test for labyrinthine function in 1906. *See hearing.*

Lacassagne, Antoine Marcellin (1884–1971) Born in France, he demonstrated the carcinogenicity of estrogens in mice by injecting them with folliculin which led to development of breast carcinomas, in 1932. He also devised a method for treatment of carcinoma in the neck of the uterus using radium.

Lachrymal Duct [Latin: *lacrimae*, tear] A screw to compress the lachrymal sac was invented by Hieronymus Fabricus ab Aquapendente (1537–1619) in the 16th century. Dominique Anel (1679–1730) of Toulouse was the first to catheterize the lachrymal duct in 1712. Sir William Blizard (1743–1835) proposed injection with mercury to overcome obstruction in 1780. Radiographic visualization with the use of bismuth was first described by James Ewing (1866–1943) in 1909. His technique was improved by Aurel von Szily (1847–1926) in 1920 and D. M. Campbell in 1924.

Lachrymator Gas *See gas warfare.*

Lacnunga Book of recipes for medications written during the Anglo-Saxon period, around the tenth century. About 200 prescriptions, remedies and charms are included in it. *See Anglo-Saxon medicine.*

Lacock, Thomas (1812–1876) Professor of medicine at Edinburgh who made several contributions to neurology. He wrote: *A Treatise on Nervous Diseases of Women, comprising an inquiry into the Nature, Causes, and Treatment of Spinal and Hysterical Disorders* (1840), *Lectures on the Principles and Methods of Medical Observation and research* (1856) and *Mind and Brain* (1860).

Lacquer Poisoning Lacquer originated in China and Japan and was obtained from *Rhus vernicifera*, known to the Japanese as *urushi-no-ki*. A disease caused by contact and inhalation of vapor of lacquer in China was first described by du Halde in 1736, and later by P. Incarville in 1760. The condition was described in Japan by A. Gortz in 1876. Englishman, Stuart Eldridge, gave an account of it in 1878.

Lactation [Latin: *lactatio*, to suck milk] *See breast milk.*

Lacteals *See lymphatic system.*

Lactic Acid [Latin: *lac*, milk] Discovered by Swedish chemist, Carl Wilhelm Scheele (1742–1786) in 1780. It was found in opium liquors produced during the manufacture of morphine by T. Smith and H. Smith in 1860. They named it lactic acid and exhibited it at the London International Exhibition of 1862. Sir Walter Morley Fletcher (1873–1933) and Sir Frederick Gowland Hopkins (1861–1947) were the first to demonstrate that lactic acid appeared in the muscle after exercise in 1907. Otto Fritz Meyerhof (1884–1951) at the University of Kiel identified glycogen breakdown as the source of lactic acid in 1920 and demonstrated that the process was anaerobic. A quantitative microchemical method of measuring lactic acid was devised by Bruno Mendel and I. Goldscheider in 1925.

Lactate Dehyrogenase First crystallized in 1940 from extract of beef heart by F.B. Straub.

Lacteals Discovered by G. Aselli (1581–1625). The French anatomist, Jean Pecquet (1627–1674) showed their passage to the subclavian vein via the thoracic duct while he was a student in 1647. Intestinal lacteals or lymphatics were described by O. Rudbeck (1639–1702) and Thomas Bartholin (1616–1680).

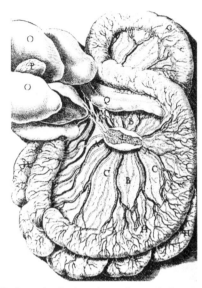

Gaspar Aselli's figure showing lacteals pressing on the liver. *De lactibus, sive lacteis venis, quarto vasorum mesaraicorum genere, novo invento dissertatio* (1627). Milan

Lactobacillus acidophilus The so-called 'lactic acid bacteria' were first studied by Louis Pasteur (1822–1895) in 1857, and extensively investigated by Orla-Jensen between 1900–1930. The first group of *Lactobacillus* was isolated from fermented milk by Kern in 1881. A similar organism was observed in vaginal secretions of pregnant women by German obstetrician, Albert Siegmund Gustav Döderlein (1860–1941) in 1892. It was isolated from feces of breast-fed infants by Ernst Moro (1874–1951) of Germany in 1900 and he named it 'acidophilus'.

Ladd, George Trumbell (1842–1921) American psychologist and professor of philosophy at Yale. He studied the relationship between the nervous system and mental phenomena and published *Elements of Physiological Psychology* in 1887.

Ladd–Franklin Theory On evolution of color vision, proposed by American psychologist, Christine Ladd-Franklin (1847–1930) of Baltimore.

Ladd, William Edwards (1880–1967) American professor of pediatric surgery at Harvard Medical School. He described the persistent peritoneal band (transduodenal band of Ladd) which caused intestinal obstruction, in 1932.

Laënnec, Réne Théophile Hyacinthe (1781–1826) French physician, pupil of Jean Nicholas Corvisart (1755–1821) and Guillaume Dupuytren (1777–1835). He became an army physician in 1799, and was made editor of the *Journal de Medicine* in 1814. He was appointed chief physician to the Necker Hospital in Paris in 1816, where he invented the stethoscope in 1819. He introduced basic vocabulary to describe heart and lung sounds in *Traite de l'auscultatione meditate* published in 1819. He also coined the term 'cirrhosis' [Greek: *kirrhos*, tawny colored] to describe the yellowish or tawny appearance of a hard shrunken liver (Laënnec portal cirrhosis). He died of tuberculosis. *See auscultation.*

Laënnec Cirrhosis *See Laënnec, Réne Théophile.*

Lagnesis [Greek: *lagneia*, lust] A synonym for uncontrollable sexual desire or nymphomania. *See nymphomania.*

Lagrange, Pierre Félix (1857–1928) French ophthalmologist from Bordeaux who devised a drainage procedure (cyclodialysis) for glaucoma in 1907.

Lahey Clinic Started in 1923 by Boston surgeon, Frank Howard Lahey (1880–1953). Its original medical staff at Back Bay consisted of only four physicians and it moved to a new site at 605 Commonwealth Avenue in 1926. The new seven-story Lahey Clinic Medical Center was opened in Burlington in 1970. It is of international repute and currently has over 70 branches in New England alone.

Lahey, Frank Howard (1880–1953) Founder of the Lahey Clinic, born to parents of Irish origin in Haverhill, Massachusetts. He did his undergraduate study at Harvard University and trained in surgery at the Boston City Hospital. After working on the staff of Harvard and Tufts Medical Schools he opened his own clinic at 638 Beacon Street. He served as the chairman of the Navy's Medical Consultant Board during World War ll. *See Lahey Clinic.*

Laidlaw–Green Hypothesis Postulates that viruses arose from larger microorganisms due to their redundant parasitic mode of life, was proposed independently by Sir Patrick Playfair Laidlaw (1881–1940) of Cambridge and R.P. Green in 1938.

Lake Dwellings At the close of the Stone Age in Europe, around 1800 BC, several lake dwellings existed where man erected his dwellings on wooden poles to protect himself from wild animals. The Paenonian Civilization on lake Prasias was described by Herodotus in 450 BC. The remains of ancient civilizations on many of the Swiss lakes were uncovered by Keller in 1855, and evidence for several other such settlements were subsequently unearthed in Germany,

Italy and Scandinavia. Robert Munro, a physician from Ross-shire who worked on the subject published *Ancient Scottish lake Dwellings* (1882), and *The Lake Dwellings of Europe* (1890).

Lamarck, Jean Baptiste Pierre Antoine Monet de (1774–1829) Born at Bazentin in France, at 19 he joined the army and was later a bank clerk in Paris where he studied botany and medicine. He was appointed keeper of the Royal Garden and later, keeper of invertebrates at the Natural History Museum. He postulated the theory of organic evolution, that species must adapt to survive environmental changes, and proposed that function precedes and creates structure. His *Philosophie Zoologique*, on the origin of species, was published in 1809. He also made the original distinction between vertebrates and invertebrates which was published between 1815–1822 in his *Natural History of the Invertebrates*. He proposed the law of use and disuse, suggesting that organs which are not used would atrophy. He introduced the term 'biology' in its current sense.

Lamalle, Antoine Joseph Jobert de (1799–1867) French surgeon who published a surgical work on the intestinal canal in 1829. He described a plastic surgical operation for closure of vesicovaginal fistula and wrote a treatise on the subject in 1852.

Lamblia A protozoan parasite (*Giardia lamblia*) of the small intestine. It is named after a Prague physician, Vitem Dusan Lambl (1824–1895) who discovered the organism in 1860.

Lamson, George Henry (d 1881) Medical practitioner from Bournemouth who was tried and sentenced to death in 1881 for poisoning his brother-in-law, Percy Malcolm John, with aconite.

Lancefield Group A classification of pathogenic hemolytic streptococci based on serology and pathogenicity. Proposed by a bacteriologist from the Rockefeller Institute in New York, Rebecca Craighill Lancefield (1895–1981) in 1933.

Lancet The longest running weekly medical journal to have survived without change of name. It was founded in 1823 by Thomas Wakley (1795–1862) who was also its first editor.

Lancisi, Giovanni Maria (1654–1720) Professor of anatomy and physician to several Popes, including Clement Xl who gave him the anatomical works of Eustachio (1520–1574) on engraved copper plates that had remained unpublished in the Papal library. He edited and published them in 1714, with the help of Giovanni Battista Morgagni (1682–1771). Lancisi was also an epidemiologist, describing epidemics of influenza and malaria and even suggesting that malaria was transmitted by the mosquito and that drainage of the local swamps would reduce infection. He attempted to classify cardiac diseases and is eponomously remembered in the Lancisi sign, a 'V' wave in the jugular venous pulse. He left his library of over 20,000 volumes to the Hospital of the Holy Ghost.

Landolt Ring Incomplete circle used to test for visual acuity. Devised by French ophthalmologist of Swiss origin, Edmond Landolt (1846–1926).

Landouzy–Dejerine Dystrophy A hereditary form of facio-scapulo-humeral muscular dystrophy transmitted by an autosomal dominant trait. First described by Louis Theophil Joseph Landouzy (1845–1917) and Joseph Jules Dejerine (1849–1917) in 1884.

Landry Paralysis Acute febrile polyneuritis. Two cases of acute ascending paralysis were described by Adolf Kussmaul (1822–1902) in 1859. French physician, Jean Baptiste Octave Landry (1826–1865), described the condition later in the same year and the disease was named after him.

Landsteiner, Karl (1868–1943) American pathologist who was born in Vienna. He received his medical degree in 1891 then studied chemistry with Emil Fischer (1852–1919). In 1900 he discovered isoagglutinins in human blood and in the following year he published a paper on specific blood groups, so making blood transfusion a safer option. He was appointed to the chair of pathology at the University of Vienna in 1909 and demonstrated transmission of poliomyelitis by intraspinal injection and later isolated the virus. He emigrated to America in 1922 where he joined the Rockefeller Institute in New York. During his work with Brooklyn physician, Alexander S. Wiener, he discovered the rhesus (Rh) factor in 1940. His *The Specificity of Serological Reactions*, published in 1936, was the first large-scale study of chemical specificity in immunology. He was the first American to win the Nobel Prize (1930), for his discovery of blood groups.

Lane, Clayton Arbuthnot (1868–1949) British physician and parasitologist who worked in India. He devised a flotation technique for examination of the feces for helminthic ova.

Lane, Sir William Arbuthnot (1856–1943) Born in Fort George, Inverness-shire. He was a surgeon at Guy's Hospital who, in 1883 treated empyema in a child by resecting a rib, in 1897 he devised an operation for cleft palate, and in 1893 he introduced internal fixation for fractured long bones. He was a great believer in inner cleanliness and thought that the body's waste products would poison it. He therefore freely advocated use of paraffin oil as a preventative! He devised the Lane tissue forceps

Lanercost Priory Near Carlisle, on the Scottish border, it served as a hospital for Edward I when he was taken ill in 1307 during his battle with Robert Bruce.

Lanfranc (1290–1296) Italian surgeon from Milan who wrote a system of surgery, *Chirurgia Magna*, which was completed in 1296. An English version was published by an English surgeon, John Halle (1529–1568) from Maidstone in 1565. Lanfranc was the first to describe concussion of the brain. He also wrote on cancer of the breast.

Lange Test For cerebrospinal fluid using gold chloride to detect various forms of cerebrospinal syphilis. Devised by Carl Friedrich August Lange (1883–1953) of Berlin in 1913.

Langenbeck, Bernhard Rudolf Konrad von (1810–1887) Professor of surgery at Berlin who first observed candidosis in 1839 and also operated on cleft palate. He described the Langenbeck triangle – an area over the head of the femur between the pyriformis and the gluteus medius.

Langenbeck, Conrad Johann Martin (1776–1851) Professor of surgery at Göttingen who described the superficial nerve of the scapula (Langenbeck nerve) in 1803.

Langenbuch, Carl Johann August (1846–1901) First to successfully remove a gall bladder in 1882. He also performed duodenostomy in 1879.

Langendorf, Oskar (1853–1908) Professor of physiology at Rostock who described the principal cells of the thyroid (Langendorf cells) in 1889.

Langerhans, Paul (1847–1888) German pathologist who was born in Berlin and became professor of anatomy at Freiburg in 1871. He described the islets in the pancreas which produce insulin in 1869 while studying for his doctorate in the Berlin Pathological Institute, these cells are distinct from the acinar tissue. *See islets of Langerhans.*

Langerhans Cells Epidermal cells involved in the immune response in contact dermatitis. The cells contain tubular granules whose function is unknown. They were discovered by Paul Langerhans (1847–1888) in 1868.

Langhans Layer A cytotrophoblast which covers the chorionic villi beneath the syncytial layer. Described by German pathologist and anatomist, Theodor Langhans (1839–1915) in 1870, while working in Bern. He also described the multinucleated foreign body giant cell (Langhans cell).

Langley, John Newport (1852–1925) Neurophysiologist from Newbury, Berkshire who studied mathematics and natural sciences at Cambridge. He coined the terms 'preganglionic' and 'postganglionic' during his work on the sympathetic nervous system while he was professor at Cambridge. He introduced the term 'autonomic' in 1898. Langley was also the founder-owner of the *Journal of Physiology* which he edited from 1894 until his death. The first part of his book *The Autonomic Nervous System* was published in 1921, but part two was never realized.

Langton, Christopher (1521–1578) London physician who wrote on madness and affections of the mind. He published *An introduction into phisyke, wyth an universal dyet* (1550) and several other works.

Lanolin [Latin: *lana*, wool + *oleum*, oil] Fat from sheep's wool purified by A. Rey of Berlin in 1864. It was known as 'oesypus' to the ancients who used it as a remedy and a cosmetic.

Lanz Line Joins the two anterior superior iliac spines. Described by Swiss surgeon, Otto Lanz (1865–1935), professor of surgery at Amsterdam in 1908.

Lao-Tsu Celebrated Chinese philosopher around 600 BC who was the founder of Taoism and author of the *Tao-te-Ching* (Way of Life).

Laparoscopy [Greek: *lapara*, flank + *skopein*, to examine] An endoscopic method of examining the peritoneal cavity. A cytoscope was first experimentally used on dogs for this purpose by Dresden surgeon, G. Kelling, in 1900. He called the procedure celioscopy. Hans Christian Jacobius (1879–1937) developed it independently by using a Nitz cystoscope in 1910. The first laparoscopic pictures were published by R. Korbsch in 1927. H. Kalk developed his own laparoscope with a wide angle lens in 1929 and used the instrument to perform liver biopsies in 1935.

Laplace, Pierre Simon (1749–1827) French mathematician and astronomer from Beaumont-en-Auge in Normandy who served as professor of mathematics at the École Militaire in Paris. He proposed the Laplace law in mathematics, and the barometric formula in physics. He proved the stability of the solar system in 1773. His *Theorie analitique des probabiliti*, published in 1812, was one of the early works on vital statistics. His other important work, *Systeme du Monde*, was published in 1796.

Lardner, Dionysius (1793–1859) Prolific Irish scientific writer from Dublin who served as professor of natural philosophy and astronomy at University College, London. He edited the *Lardner's Cabinet Cyclopedia* (1829–1849) in 133 volumes, *Lardner's Natural Philosophy* (1858), *Common Things Explained* (1856) and several other encyclopedic works.

Largactil *See chlorpromazine.*

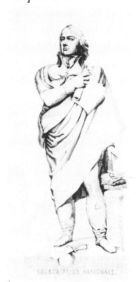

Dominique Jean Larrey (1766–1842). Courtesy of the National Library of Medicine

Larrey, Dominique Jean (1766–1842) Born in Paris, he was one of the greatest military surgeons in history who dedicated his life to soldiers in the field. While working in the École de Médecine Militaire, he introduced the 'flying ambulances' to provide first aid for the wounded. These were either two or four wheeled carts drawn by horses. He wrote a five volumes *Memoires de Chirugie Militaire* in 1812. Larrey performed the first three amputations at the hip joint: two in Egypt and one in France, around 1760. The occurrence of trench foot due to prolonged exposure of feet to water was first described by him in 1812. Larrey sign is pain in the sacroiliac region on sitting.

Lartet, Edouard Arman Isidore Hippolyte (1801–1871) French paleontologist who discovered the fossil jaw bone of the ape, later named *Pliopithecus* in 1836 in Tertiary formations near Gers. This contradicted the prevailing thinking that fossils of men and apes did not exist. His son Louis Lartet (1840–1899) was also an eminent paleontologist.

Laryngectomy [Latin: *larynx*, upper part of wind pipe; Greek: *ektome*, to excise] The first complete excision of the larynx was performed in a case of stenosis of the larynx (due to syphilis) by Patrick Heron Watson (1832–1907) in 1866, but the patient died after three weeks. The second was done as treatment for carcinoma by Berlin surgeon, Theodor Billroth (1829–1894) in 1873, the patient survived for seven months until his carcinoma recurred. From 1873 the operation was more common and the first large series of 90 cases was presented by Jacob da Silva Solis-Cohen (1838–1927) in 1884.

Laryngismus Stridulus [Greek: *laryngismos*, whooping] An original description of the spasm of the larynx was given by Scottish physician, John Millar (1733–1805) in 1769. *A Essay on Laryngismus Stridulus* was published later by Hugh Ley (1790–1837) of Abingdon, Berkshire, a physician at the Middlesex Hospital.

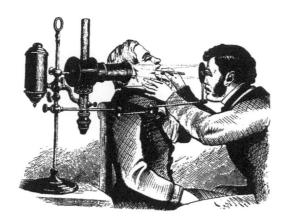

Large laryngoscope and student lamp. J.W. MacDonald, *A Clinical Text Book of Surgical Diagnosis and Treatment* (1898). Rebman, London

Laryngoscope [Latin: *larynx*, upper part of wind pipe; Greek: *skopein*, to examine] Endoscope for direct visual examination of the larynx, invented by Benjamin Babington (1794–1866) in 1829, another was designed by London surgeon, John Avery in 1846. A modern instrument was designed by Manuel Garcia (1810–1868), a Spanish music teacher in London in 1855. Ludwig Türck (1797–1887), an Austrian neurologist and laryngologist from Vienna, designed a laryngoscope in 1857, Czech physician Johann Czermak (1828–1873) devised another in 1862. The first direct vision laryngoscope was invented by Alfred Kirstein (1863–1942), Nuffield professor of anesthesia at Oxford in 1895. Robert Reynolds Macintosh (b 1897) described his curved laryngoscope in 1943.

Laryngotomy [Latin: *larynx*, upper part of wind pipe; Greek: *tome*, cutting] Mentioned but not practiced by Areteaus in the first century. A detailed description has been left by Paul of Aegina in the 7th century.

Larynx [Latin: *larynx*, upper part of wind pipe] The first monograph on diseases of the larynx was written by Giovanni Battista Codronchi (1547–1628) of Italy in 1597. Hieronymus Fabricus ab Aquapendente (1537–1619) gave a full account of the larynx as a vocal organ in *De Larynge vocis organo* in 1600. The removal of a laryngeal polyp was first done by Charles Henry Ehrmann (1792–1878) of Paris in

1844. A laryngoscope was used to remove a tumor by Viktor von Bruns (1812–1883) in 1865. A successful operation for cancer of the larynx was performed by Jacob da Silva Solis-Cohen (1838–1927) in 1867. Sir Morell Mackenzie (1853–1925), the father of British laryngology published an important monograph, *Essay on Growth in the Larynx* in 1871. *See laryngoscope, laryngectomy.*

Laser Therapy *See laser.*

Laser The Light Amplification by Stimulated Electromagnetic Radiation (LASER) was first described by Arthur Leonard Schawlow (b 1921) in 1958. The concept of the emission of radiation stimulated by photons was first proposed by Albert Einstein (1879–1955) in 1917. His theory was developed in 1951 into microwave amplification with the use of stimulated electromagnetic radiation (MASER) by American physicist and Nobel laureate, Charles Hard Townes (b 1915) of Greenville, South Carolina. The use of semiconductors in lasers was proposed by a Russian physicist, Nikolai Gennadiyevich (b 1922) in 1955. The first effective ruby laser was invented in 1960 by American physicist, Theodore Harold Maiman (b 1927) of Los Angeles, and the gas laser was invented by A. Javan in the following year. Further work was done by French scientist, Alfred Kastler (b 1902) who was awarded the Nobel Prize in 1966. The use of lasers in medicine was made possible with the invention of a microlaser of 2.5 microns in diameter, by a Frenchman, Marcel Bessis, in 1962. The first surgical operation in ophthalmology with the use of Nelas laser was done in 1964 by an American, H. Vernon Ingram (b 1924). The Bistoury laser was developed by a group of Americans: D.R. Herriott, E.I. Gorden, H.A.S. Hale and W. Gromnos from the Bell Telephone company in 1967. The argon laser used in ophthalmology was developed in 1978 by a Frenchman, Gabriel J. Coscas. Lasers were used for the first time to clean up clogged arteries in 1985. *See free electron laser.*

Lasègue Disease Persecution mania was described by French physician from Paris, Ernest Charles Lasègue (1816–1883). He was a favorite pupil of Armand Trousseau (1801–1867) and became his Chef de Clinique from 1852 to 1854.

Lassa Fever Cardiac and renal involvement with pneumonia due to a virus, named after Lassa in Nigeria where the disease was first described in 1959.

Lassar Paste Acetylsalicylic acid and zinc oxide, formulated by German dermatologist, Oskar Lassar (1849–1908).

Latah Disease Form of neurosis or jumping disease, found in Southeast Asia. Described by George Gilles de la Tourette

(1857–1904) in 1884. The patients affected showed involuntary movements and made incoherent sounds and obscene expressions. *See coprolalia.*

Latarget, Andre (1876–1947) French professor of anatomy at Lyon who described the anterior gastric nerves which are used for selective vagotomy

Latent Heat [Greek: *latens*, hidden] The principle was discovered in 1762 by Joseph Black (1728–1799), a Scottish physician and chemist from Edinburgh. A standard method of determining the latent heat of steam was invented by the French chemist and politician, Marcellin Berthelot (1827–1907).

Lateral Rectus Muscle, Muscle of the eye ball, once known as 'musculus amatorius' [Latin: *amor*, love] as it is involved in sidelong glances seen in lovers.

Latex [Latin: fluid] On his second visit to South America Columbus noted that the people amused themselves by bouncing a ball made of vegetable gum. The Spanish named the tree from which the gum was obtained as 'latex', meaning milk. In 1730 French explorers of the Amazon identified the source of rubber, the *Hevea* tree. Rubber was introduced into England for erasing pencil marks by Joseph Priestley (1733–1804) in 1780. Condoms, previously made of dry sheep gut, came into large scale use with the introduction of vulcanization in 1844, independently by Goodyear in America and Hancock in England. Latex or rubber gloves were first introduced for aseptic technique in surgery by William Halstead (1852–1922), foundation American surgeon at Johns Hopkins Hospital. He made bronze casts of his hand upon which the first surgical gloves were molded in 1890. Improved latex condoms were introduced in 1930.

Latham, John (1740–1837) Naturalist and physician from Eltham in Kent. He published *A General History of Birds* (1821–1828) in 10 volumes, *Heald's Pharmacopoeia, improved*, *A General Synopsis of Birds*, and several other works.

Latham, John (1760–1843) Born in Gawsworth, Chester and practiced as a physician in Manchester before he moved to London and was elected president of the Royal College of Physicians in 1814. Latham's published works include *Facts and Opinions concerning Diabetes* and several contributions to *Medical Transactions*.

Latham, Peter Mere (1789–1875) Physician at St Bartholomew's Hospital from 1824 to 1841. He gave a classical description of the symptoms of coronary thrombosis in 1856 and was one of the earliest to advocate auscultation in England. He described the area of dullness over the precordium (Latham circle) in *Lectures on the Diseases of the Heart* published in 1845.

Lathyrism Condition due to poisoning by seeds of *Lathyrus*, known since the time of Hippocrates (460–377). His description stated, 'At Ainos those men and women who continually fed on pulse were attacked by weakness in both legs which remained permanent, even those who lived on peas suffered from pain in the knees'. A further description from India and some parts of Africa was given by Sir Henry William Sleeman (1788–1856) in 1844. *See fabism.*

Latin Classified under the Aryan group of languages by Max Muller, professor of comparative philology at Oxford in *Science of Language* (1861). Latin was introduced into England by Adelmus in the 7th century. It was used in law in England, but largely replaced by English during the reign of King Henry III. Its use in religious worship was discontinued in 1558, and in law in 1731. Latin ceased to be spoken in Italy in AD 581. The earliest translation of Hippocrates (460–377 BC) into Latin was done by François Rabelais (1490–1553).

Laubry, Charles (1872–1941) Parisian cardiologist who pioneered the radiological method of studying the heart and blood vessels by injecting radio-opaque substances into the blood. His work on the subject, *Radiologie Clinique du Coeur et des Gros Vaisseaux*, was published in 1939.

Laughing Gas *See nitrous oxide.*

Laurence–Moon–Biedl Syndrome Hereditary autosomal recessive disease manifesting as retinitis pigmentosa, mental retardation, polydactyly, and hypogonadism was first described by London ophthalmologist, John Zachariah Laurence (1830–1874), and American ophthalmologist, Robert Charles Moon (1844–1914) of Philadelphia in 1866. The condition was redescribed by Hungarian physician, Arthur Biedl (1869–1933) in 1922.

Laurentius, Andreas (1550–1609) Physician to Henry IV who moved from Montpellier to Paris. He published *Historia Anatomica Humani Corporis* in 1602. His work on melancholy was published in French in 1597 and translated into English by Richard Surphlet in 1599.

Lavator, Johann Gaspar *See Lavetor.*

Laveran, Charles Louis Alphonse (1845–1922) French parasitologist and professor of military medicine and epidemic diseases at the Military College of Val de Grace from 1874 to 1878. He studied malaria at Algiers and in 1880 discovered the causative organism, a protozoan parasite – *Plasmodium* – while he was professor of pathological anatomy at the University of Rome, and the toxoplasma in 1900. Laveran was awarded the Nobel Prize for his work on malariology in 1907.

Lavetor, Johann Gasper (1741–1801) Physiognomist from Zurich who became a pastor at his local church of St Peter. He published *Treatise on physiognomy* in 1772 and several other works. He died from a wound which he received when the French took Zurich in 1799.

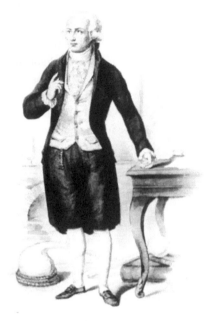

Antoine Laurent Lavoisier (1743–1794). Courtesy of the National Library of Medicine

Lavoisier, Antoine Laurent (1743–1794) Founder of modern chemistry, born in Paris to a wealthy lawyer's family. He first qualified as a lawyer in 1764, but gave up to study science. In 1789, he defined an element as 'a substance that cannot be split into a simpler form by any means'. He investigated 'dephologisticated air' in 1774, previously described by Joseph Priestley (1733–1804). He named it the 'acidifying principle' [Greek: *oxygine*] from which the present name 'oxygen' is derived. Lavoisier and Pierre Simon Laplace (1749–1827) proved that respiration is a process of combustion. His important work, *Traite Elementaire de chimie,* was published in 1789. He was an advisory member of 'Ferme-General' which collected taxes before the French revolution. He was guillotined during the revolution for his involvement with the Ferme and other government affairs.

Law of Conservation of Energy First suggested in 1748 by Russian scientist, Mikhail Vasilievich Lomonosov (1711–1765) from St Petersburg Academy of Sciences. The relationship between heat and work was published in 1842

by Julius Robert von Mayer (1814–1878), a physician and physicist at Heilbronn, Bavaria, who explicitly applied his theory to both living and nonliving things. James Prescott Joule (1818–1889), a natural philosopher from Salford, conducting a long series of experiments on heat, starting in 1839, and demonstrated the relationship between work done and heat generated in 1847.

Law of Constant Proportions Joseph Louis Proust (1754–1826), French analytical chemist, born in Angers, France and later director of the Royal Laboratories at Madrid, was the first to show that the proportions of the constituents of any chemical compound are always the same, regardless of the method used in its preparation. His finding formed the basis for the law of constant proportions.

Law of Equivalent Proportions Discovered by German chemist, Jeremias Benjamin Richter (1762–1807) of Silesia, a pupil of Kant at Königsberg. He analyzed chemical compounds to determine the proportions mathematically, which he called 'stoichiometry'. The full significance was realized after the atomic theory of John Dalton (1766–1844), an English chemist from Cockermouth, later provided an explanation in 1803.

Law of Mass The influence of reactant concentration on rate of reaction. Proposed by Norwegian chemist and professor at Oslo, Peter Waage (1833–1900) and his brother-in-law, Cato Guldberg (1836–1902), in 1864.

Law of Octaves John Alexander Reina Newlands (1837–1898), an English chemist from London, was the first to arrange the elements in order of their atomic weights and to recognize similarity between every eighth element. His Law of Octaves, proposed in 1864, was a forerunner of the periodic table.

Lawrence, Thomas (1711–1783) Born in Westminster, grandson of another Thomas Lawrence who was physician to Queen Anne and three other sovereigns. He qualified in medicine from Oxford in 1740, and practiced at Essex Street in The Strand in London. He published *De Hydrope* (1756), *De Natura Musculorum Praelectiones* and *Praelectiones Medicae* in 1759. He was elected president of the Royal College of Physicians in 1767, and continued to be re-elected for the next six consecutive years.

Lawrence, Sir William (1783–1867) Surgeon at St Bartholomew's Hospital and a pupil of John Abernethy (1764–1831). He served as president of the Royal College of Surgeons from 1846 to 1855 and was appointed surgeon to Queen Victoria in 1858. In 1819 he wrote *Lectures on Physiology,*

Zoology, and the Natural History of Man in which he suggested that a superior breed of man could be obtained by selection.

Laxative [Latin: *laxativus*, to unloosen] Hippocrates (460–377 BC) recommended gentle purgatives for preservation of health. Galen (AD 129–200) wrote two treatises on the use of purgatives but denounced their use in good health. Aetius in his 7th book recommended plantain, parsley and bitter almonds as laxatives. Paul of Aegina (625–690) in AD 650 also recommended parsley and wormwood as purgatives. Oribasius (AD 325–400) described the use of laxatives fully in his eighth book, written around AD 380. *See aperients.*

Lazear, Jesse William (1866–1900) Baltimore doctor in Walter Reed's (1851–1902) medical team. He was sent to Havana to investigate an outbreak of yellow fever in 1900 where he deliberately allowed a mosquito to bite him in order to investigate the cause. He died within 12 days, at the age of 34 years. His supreme self-sacrifice helped to establish the mosquito as a transmitter of yellow fever.

LD Bodies Leishman–Donovan bodies. Peculiar staining bodies found in the spleen of a soldier who died of Dum Dum fever (kala azar). They were first noted in 1900 by Sir William Boog Leishman (1865–1926) at autopsy, he mistakenly associated them with trypanosomiasis. Charles Donovan (1863–1951) found the same bodies in 1903 in the spleen of patients at autopsy, and also identified them in spleenic blood of live patients. Similar bodies were found in blood by Felix Jacob Marchand (1846–1928) in the same year and later identified as protozoal parasites.

Le Boë, Franciscus de Sylvius (1614–1672) French Huguenot from Hanau. He graduated in medicine from Basel in 1637 and practiced at Amsterdam before being appointed professor of medicine at Leiden in 1658. He founded the iatrochemical school which explained the physiological conditions of the body on a chemical basis. He also described the aqueduct of Sylvius and the lateral cerebral fissure (fissure of Sylvius) in 1660. He published *Disputationes medicae* (1663) and *Praxeos medicae idea nova* (1671). *See iatrochemistry.*

L-Dopa A current mainline drug for treatment of Parkinson disease. Its clinical effectiveness in patients with post-encephalitic parkinsonism was demonstrated by British neurologist, Oliver Sacks (b 1933) around 1960. It became a standard drug in the treatment of Parkinson disease in 1967.

L E Cells The diagnostic presence of L E cells in acute disseminated systemic lupus erythematosus was discovered by Malcolm MacCallum Hargraves (b 1903) in 1948. *See systemic lupus erythematosus.*

Le Veen Shunt Used to relieve ascites by draining the ascitic fluid into the great veins via an implanted valved conduit. It was devised by Harry H. Le Veen (b 1914), an American gastroenterologist at Veterans Administration Hospital, Brooklyn.

Lead Encephalopaphy In 1836 Augustin Grisolle (1811–1869) of Paris studied 29 cases of the condition and divided them into convulsive, comatosed and delirious states. Optic atrophy due to lead poisoning was described by Jonathan Hutchinson (18128–1913) in 1873. In 1945 C.P. MacCord reported 12 men who died or committed suicide due to encephalopathy after working with lead in Detroit car factories.

Lead Neuritis Saturnine palsy. *See lead poisoning.*

Lead Palsy Various clinical types of lead palsy, including wrist drop, were first described in detail by Guillaume B.A. Duchenne (1806–1875) in 1872.

Lead Poisoning Poisoning due to lead in food products was mentioned by Hippocrates (460–377 BC), Pliny (23–79), and several other philosophers and medical men of ancient times. Vitruvius, a celebrated Roman architect who lived during the time of Julius Caesar and Augustus, was the first to point out the problems of using lead pipes for water. Eathius in the 16th century noted that certain wines produced colic, and the cause of the illness was identified in 1757 as lead poisoning from the storage vessels coated with lead dioxide. George Baker (1722–1809), a physician from Devonshire, discovered (1767) that lead in cider presses caused a similar disease, previously known as Devonshire colic. Various other sources such as cooking utensils, earthenware, old timber coated with lead paint that was used as firewood, lead pipes in public houses, dyes used in coloring food and tea imported in lead-lined chests, have all been found to cause lead poisoning. The first elaborate scientific study of modern times was done by L. Tanquerel des Planches of Paris who reviewed 1200 cases of lead poisoning in 1839. A treatise on *The Action of Water upon Lead* was published in 1842 by Robert Christison, (1797–1881) professor of materia medica at the University of Edinburgh. Other contributors include: A. Grissole of Paris, on lead encephalitis and blue line of the gums (1836), Réne Théophile Hyacinthe Laënnec (1781–1826) on anemia (1831), Guillaume Duchenne (1807–1875) on lead palsy (1872), and Sir Jonathan Hutchinson (1828–1913) on amaurosis (1873). Polyneuritis due to lead was described by Ernst Julius Remak (1849–1911) of Berlin in 1878. The toxic accumulation of lead in the bones was shown by A. Gusserow in 1861 and by E. Heubel of Berlin in 1871. More

461

recent studies were done by Thomas Oliver and Thomas Morrison Legge (1863–1932) in England during the late 19th century. Legge also wrote an important treatise with K.W. Goadby, *Lead poisoning and lead Absorption*, in 1912. The British Public Health Act of 1925 contained a section on preservatives, and prohibited the use of compound lead for food coloring. One of the first recorded successful treatments of lead encephalopathy with the use of a powerful chelating agent, EDTA (ethylene diamine tetraacetic acid), was given to an 18-month-old baby in 1955 by James B. Sidbury (b1922).

Lead Metal used by the ancient Hebrews and Egyptians as early as 4000 BC, and a lead figure from 3800 BC can be found in the British Museum. The hanging garden of Babylon had pans made of lead, and lead pipes have been found in the ruins of Rome and Pompeii. Theophrastus described the preparation of lead oxide by treating lead with vinegar in 300 BC. *See lead poisoning.*

Leake, John (1729–1792) Eminent physician from Cumberland in England who founded the lying-in-hospital at Westminster in 1765. He published several books on midwifery and gynecology, and introduced a modified delivery bed for women in labor.

Leber Optic Atrophy A sex-linked recessive trait occurring mostly in adolescent males. It was first described in 1871 by Theodor von Leber (1840–1917), professor of ophthalmology at Heidelberg. He also described the plexiform veins of the iris associated with the ciliary processes (Leber venous plexus) in 1866.

Leblanc, Nicolas (1742–1806) French physician and a chemist, well known for invention of the Leblanc process. A simple and cheap method of producing soda or sodium bicarbonate from salt and sulfuric acid.

Leclerc, Nicholas Gabriel (1726–1798) Born in Franche Compte in France, in 1757 he became the first physician to be appointed to the forces of the Emperor of Germany. He returned to France in 1777, and published *Historie Physique morale, civili et politique de la Russie* and several medical works.

Lectures [Latin: *lectura*, commentary] Formal lectures in physick was instituted by Thomas Linacre (1460–1524) in 1502. Clinical lectures at the patient's bedside was initiated in England by Sir Benjamin Brodie (1783–1862) in 1813.

Lederberg, Joshua (b 1925) American geneticist, born in Montclair, New Jersey and studied biology at Columbia University, before becoming a professor at Wisconsin in 1947. In 1952 he coined the term 'plasmid' to describe the process of transduction where a small non-integral piece of deoxyribonucleic acid was transferred between bacteria. This became the basis of genetic engineering, and he shared the Nobel Prize for Physiology or Medicine with Edward Lawrie Tatum (1909–1975) and George Wells Beadle (1903–1989) in 1958.

Lederer Anemia Rare form of severe acute hemolytic anemia of unknown cause, associated with leucocytosis, enlarged spleen, reticulocytosis and pyrexia. It was described by Max Lederer (1855–1925) in 1925.

Lee, Rebecca First black American woman to receive an MD in 1864 from New England Female Medical College.

Lee, Robert (1793–1877) Physician to the Lying-in-Hospital in London, and lecturer at St George's Hospital. He described the sympathetic ganglion of the cervix uteri (Lee ganglion) in 1842.

Leech Book of Bald The earliest known Saxon medical manuscript. It was written around the tenth century by a physician named Bald or Cild of a monastic background. It contains herbal remedies, charms and incantations and includes many practices used by earlier Greeks and Romans.

Leech Anglo-Saxon term for a doctor during the Middle Ages.

Leeches (Syn: hirudines, sanguisuga medicinalis) Used in medicine to induce bleeding. A large leech was capable of drawing 12 grams or 2 drachms of blood. The active anticoagulant substance, hirudine, in the leech was identified by J.B. Haycraft in 1891. *See hirudin.*

Leeds School of Anatomy This was opened by Charles Turner Thackrah (1795–1833) a Yorkshire-born physician who practiced at Leeds. It later developed into the present Leeds University School of Medicine.

Leeuwenhoek, Antoni van (1632–1723) Pioneer microscopist, was born in Delft, Holland and learned the art of making lenses in Amsterdam. On his return to Delft in 1652, he developed an interest in microscopy. He announced the discovery of protozoa in 1677 in the *Philosophical Transactions*. He was the first to distinguish bacteria and he published his drawings in the same journal in 1683. He is esteemed as the first protozoologist and bacteriologist. He also observed canals in bone in 1675, later called the Haversian canals. Following his death, his 248 microscopes were auctioned by his daughter Maria.

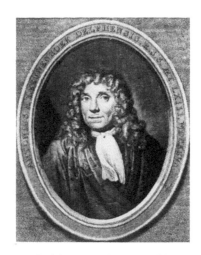

Antoni van Leeuwenhoek (1632–1723). Courtesy of the National Library of Medicine

Left Ventriculography The visualization of opacified cardiac chambers by injecting contrast material through peripheral veins was first described by George Porter Robb (b 1898) and Israel Steinberg (b 1902) of America in 1939. The first truly quantitative study of left ventricular function by this method was done by R.F. Rushmer and N.Thal in 1951. *See angiocardiography.*

Legal Medicine *See forensic medicine.*

Legal Test Use of sodium hydroxide, sodium nitroprusside and hydrochloric acid to determine acetonuria. It was devised by German physician, Emmo Legal (1859–1922).

Legallois, Julien Jean Cesar (1775–1814) Physician and physiologist from Cherneix, Brittany, in France. He was one of the earliest to demonstrate the respiratory center in the medulla oblongata in 1812.

Legg–Calvé–Perthes Disease Osteochondritis deformans, consisting of femoral osteochondrosis leading to tenderness and muscular spasm of the hip. Described independently by American orthopedic surgeon Arthur Thornton Legg (1874–1939) of Harvard Medical School in 1908, French orthopedic surgeon, Jacques Calvé (1895–1954) and Georg Clemens Perthes (1869–1927) professor of surgery at Tübingen in 1910.

Legge, Morison Thomas, Sir (1863–1932) Born in Hong Kong and came to England with his father who took up an appointment as professor of Chinese at Oxford. Legge studied at St Bartholomew's Hospital, and concentrated on public health in Europe. He was appointed first medical inspector of factories and he wrote, *Public Health in European Capitals* in 1896. Together with K.W. Goadby, he also wrote

another important treatise *Lead poisoning and lead Absorption* in 1912.

Legionnaires' Disease The first recorded outbreak occurred in 1976 in Philadelphia during an American Legion Convention. The first scientific account of the epidemic was given by David William Fraser in 1977 who named the bacterium *Legionella.*

Leighton, Alexander (1568–1644) Clergyman and physician from Edinburgh and professor of moral philosophy at Edinburgh University. He moved to London and wrote *Zion's Plea* and *The Looking Glass of the Holy War.* The latter book led to his imprisonment and a sentence in the pillory, his ears being cut off and a whipping. He remained imprisoned for eleven years and died insane.

Leiomyosarcoma [Greek: *leios,* smooth + *myos,* muscle + *sarcoma,* a fleshy excrescence] *See esophageal rupture.*

Leipzig University Famous institution in south Germany, founded in 1409.

Leishman, Sir William Boog (1865–1926) Scottish bacteriologist, born in Glasgow and obtained his MD in 1886. He joined the Army and served in India from 1890 to 1897. On his return he helped in the development of an anti-typhoid vaccine which was used on troops during World War 1. He became director of the Army Medical Services in 1923. In 1900 he discovered the peculiar staining bodies in the spleen in kala azar leading to the disease being named leishmaniasis. He also pioneered the use of vaccines. *See LD bodies, kala azar.*

Leishman Stain Used to detect parasites in blood films. Devised by Scottish parasitologist, Sir William Boog Leishman (1865–1926).

Leishman, William (1833–1894) Professor of midwifery at Glasgow and editor of *Glasgow Medical Journal* in 1862. His chief work, *A System of Midwifery,* published in 1870, remained the standard textbook until it reached its fourth edition in 1888.

Leishman–Donovan Bodies *See LD bodies.*

Leishmaniasis *See kala azar.*

Leloir, Luis Frederico (b 1906) French-born Argentinian biochemist, educated in Buenos Aires and Cambridge. He set up his own research institute in 1947 and worked on diabetes and the adrenals. He noted the proteolytic action of renin from kidneys leading to production of angiotensin, discovered glucose-1-phosphate kinase, that glucose 1,6-bisphosphate acts as a coenzyme and linked the reactions to production of glycogen. He shared the Nobel Prize for Chemistry with Carl Cori (1896–1984) in 1970. *See glucose-1-phosphate kinase, renin.*

Lémery, Louis (1708–1743) Physician and son of French chemist Nicholas Lémery (1645–1715). He served as physician to the Queen of Spain and wrote several medical treatises.

Lémery, Nicholas (1645–1715) Eminent French chemist and pharmacist from Rouen in Normandy. As a Protestant, he was driven out of Paris in 1683 by religious persecution and converted to Roman Catholicism in 1685 after Protestants were denied all legal rights under the Edict of Nantes. He published the first textbook of chemistry, *Cours de Chymie* (1675) which ran into 31 editions by 1756 in many European languages, *Universal Pharmacopoeia* and *A Treatise on Drugs.*

Lennox–Gastaut Syndrome Myoclonic and akinetic seizures in children with a petit mal type of EEG. Described independently by French neurologist, Henri Gastaut (b 1915) in 1957, and American neurologist, William G. Lennox (1884–1960) in 1960.

Lens [Latin: lentil] The Ancients knew how to construct lenses, and a convex lens made of rock crystal was discovered by Layard in the ruins of Nimrud and later by Sir David Brewster (1781–1868). The oldest convex lens in existence is from Crete and dates back to the Minoan civilization around 1000 BC. The Greeks used lenses to create fire around 424 BC. Alhazen's work in AD 1000, *Kitab Al-Manazir* (Book of Optics), had sections on refraction, reflection, and the study of lenses. It formed the basis for the invention of spectacles, telescopes and the microscope. Roger Bacon (1214–1294), and Robert Grosseteste (1175–1253), Bishop of Lincoln, were among the first in England to experiment with lenses. One of the first compound microscopes made of several convergent lenses was constructed around 1590 by Zacharias Jansen, a spectacle maker from Middelburg in Holland. Franciscus Cornelis Donders (1818–1889), a Dutch ophthalmologist and physiologist at Utrecht, introduced the use of prismatic and cylindrical lenses in the production of spectacles around 1850. *See convex lenses, concave lenses.*

Leonardo Da Vinci (1452–1519) From Vinci in the valley of Arno, south of Florence in Italy, was an artist, inventor, engineer and anatomist. He attempted to grasp the fundamentals of human anatomy and physiology and was the first to illustrate anatomical structures of the heart. His drawings of the human heart showed valves and the aortic root. He

was also the first to draw the frontal and maxillary sinuses. William Hunter (1861–1937) referred to Da Vinci as 'the greatest anatomist of his epoch'. Da Vinci did the first design of a flying machine around 1500, and his inventive power is displayed in his illustrations of water gear wheels, cranks, paddle wheels, mining devices and many other instruments which came into use much later.

Leoniceno, Niccolò (1428–1524) Born in Lonigo in Italy. He was a physician who studied medicine in Padua where he later became professor. He translated the works of Hippocrates (460–377 BC) and Galen (129–200) into Latin and pointed out botanical mistakes in Pliny's (AD 23–79) *Natural History.* He published a treatise on syphilis (1497) in which he suggested that the disease was known to Hippocrates and the ancients.

Leprosy [Greek: *lepros*, rough, scaly] Considered an antisocial disease amongst all civilizations since ancient times. The earliest records date from the time of the exodus of the Israelites from Egypt. Aristotle (384–322 BC) was one of the first Greeks to give a description. Leprosy was introduced into Greece around 300 BC and conveyed to Italy by the troops of Pompeii returning from Egypt in the first century BC. It spread to Spain around AD 700 and reached England in AD 950. It became prevalent during the Middle Ages in England and over 400 hospitals were established to accommodate lepers. It died out in the 18th century and the last case in Great Britain was reported in Shetland in 1798. In the Scandinavian countries leprosy lingered until the end of the 19th century. Despite its antiquity the first medical treatise was written in 1848 by Cornelius Daniel Danielsson (1815–1894) and Carl Wilhelm Boeck (1808–1875). Rudolph Virchow (1821–1902) described the condition in 1874 and the causative organism, *Bacillus leprae* (Hansen bacillus), was discovered by Armauer Hansen (1841–1912) in 1874.

Leptospira icterohemorrhagiae *See Weil disease.*

Leptospirosis [Greek: *leptos*, slender + *speira*, coil] *See Weil disease.*

Leriche Syndrome Impotence caused by thrombotic occlusion at the bifurcation of the aorta. Described by René Henri Marie Leriche (1879–1955), French professor of surgery at Lyons (1920) and Strasbourg (1927) in 1940.

Lesbianism [Greek: *Lesbios*] (Syn, amor lesbicus, Sapphism, Phoenician love, tribadism) Sexual love between women. Derives its name from the Greek poetess Sappho who lived on the island of Lesbos, around 700 BC. An ancient Greek festival, known as Callistea of the lesbians where the fairest was awarded a prize, was held in the temple of Juno around 300 BC.

Lesch–Nyhan Syndrome Familial disorder consisting of hyperuricemia, choreoathetosis, mental retardation, cerebral palsy and compulsive self mutilation. Described in 1964 by New York pediatrician, Michael Lesch (b 1939), and a physician at the University of California, William L. Nyhan Jr (b 1926).

Leslie, Sir John (1766–1832) Scottish physicist and natural philosopher from Largs, Fife in Scotland. He entered St Andrews University at the age of 13 but transferred to study divinity at Edinburgh before changing to science. He published *Experimental Inquiry into the Nature and Propagation of Heat* in 1804, which earned him the Royal Society Rumford Medal in 1805.

Letterer–Siwe Disease Disorder of infancy with skin infiltrates, splenomegaly and bone tumors affecting the reticuloendothelial system. Described in 1924 by German pathologist, Erich Letterer (b 1895) from Frankfurt. Other manifestations of the disease, including hepatosplenomegaly, were described in 1933 by Swedish pediatrician, Sture August Siwe (1897–1966).

Lettsom, John Coakley (1744–1815) British Quaker physician, born on the island of Little Vandyke, near Tortola, in the Virgin Islands. He graduated from St Thomas' Hospital and practiced for a short time in Tortola before returning to London where he became a successful practitioner. He was a philanthropist and founded the Medical Society of London (1773), General Dispensary at Aldersgate (1770) and the Royal Sea Bathing Hospital at Margate in 1779. He published *Hints on Beneficence, Temperance and Medical Science.*

Leuce or albinism [Greek: *leukos*, white] Aristotle (384–322 BC) was the first to mention it as a disease in which all the hairs of the body turn white. It was previously called 'snow-white leprosy' by the ancient Jews. Moses mentioned the condition in the Old Testament and distinguished it from 'alphos' and 'melas'. It was defined as 'a change of skin to a white color by a viscid and glutinous phlegm' by Paul of Aegina (625–690). He also pointed out that 'alphos' was similar to leuce, except that it produced a deep color change in the skin. Aulus Cornelius Celsus (25 BC–AD 50) described a variety of vitiligo which resembled leuce. Arabian physicians called it 'morphoea alba', a name also used by Guy de Chauliac (1300–1367).

Leucine [Greek: *leukos*, white] Amino acid, first isolated from cheese by Louis Joseph Proust (1754–1826) in 1819. Braconnot isolated the pure form from wool in 1820.

Leucippus of Abdera Greek philosopher who lived around 600 BC. He originated the concept of the atomic system which was disseminated by his pupil, Democritus. *See atomic structure.*

Leuckart, Karl Georg Friedrich Rudolf (1822–1898) German zoologist, born in Helmstadt and educated at Göttingen, before becoming professor of zoology at Giessen in 1850. He described the lifecycles of many parasites including a complete life history and morphology of *Echinococcus* in 1860. He also described mature *Trichinella spiralis* and several other parasites in *Parasites of Man* (1863–1876).

Leuco–Erythroblastic Anemia Condition where younger red blood cells and nucleated forms are found in the peripheral blood, with a shift of erythopoiesis to the left. Described by Janet M. Vaughan of England in 1936.

Leucocythemia The first blood disease to be scientifically described by Edinburgh physician, John Hughes Bennett (1812–1875) in 1845. *See leukemia.*

Leucopenia [Greek: *leukos*, white + *penia*, poverty] The first fatal case was described by Philip King Brown (1869–1940) and William Ophuls (1871–1933) of America in 1901.

Leucotomy [Greek: *leukos*, white + *tome*, cutting] The stereotactic method was introduced by Desmond Hamilton Kelly and co-workers in 1973. *See prefrontal leucotomy.*

Leukemia [Greek: *leukos*, white + *haima*, blood] Term used for the cellular disorder of blood was first coined by Rudolph Virchow (1821–1902) in 1845, and the first description was given by John Hughes Bennett (1812–1875) in the same year. Bennett later published a monograph on leucocythemia in 1852 in which he showed the microscopic blood picture in leukemia. Radioactive isotopes were employed for the first time in the treatment by John Hundale Lawrence (b 1904) and co-workers in 1939. *See bone marrow transplant, chronic myeloid leukemia.*

Leukocyte Count German physician, Joseph Arneth (1873–1955) differentiated polymorphs into five groups according to their nuclear configuration in 1904. He also described a method of counting cells in each group in order to assess the bone marrow response to toxemia and infection. This method, which was initially called the Arneth count, was later renamed the polynuclear count by William Edmond Cooke (1881–1939) and Eric Ponder in 1914. Another system was devised by Austrian hematologist, Victor Schilling (1883–1960) in 1929.

Leukocytes [Greek: *leucos*, white + *kytos*, hollow] First noted as arising from the lymphatic glands and the thymus in 1774 by British hematologist, William Hewson (1739–1774). The production of leukocytes and their role in inflammation was described by Thomas Addison (1793–1860) in 1843. The term 'leucocytosis' for the process of formation of leukocytes was coined by Rudolph Virchow (1821–1902) in 1858. The first case of complete disappearance of polymorphonuclear leukocytes (agranulocytosis) from the blood was described by Werner Shultz (1878–1947) in 1907.

Levaditi, Constantin (1874–1953) Rumanian bacteriologist who worked in Paris. He devised a method of staining *Treponema pallidum* in 1906. *See bismuth.*

Levene, Phoebus Aaron Theodor (1869–1940) American biochemist and founder member of the Rockefeller Institute in New York (1905). He was born in Sasar, Russia and studied medicine at St Petersburg before he emigrated to America in 1892. He was a pioneer in the study of nucleic acids and he established the nature of sugars in RNA and DNA around 1928.

Leventhal, Michael Leo (1901–1971) Graduate of Rush Medical College, Chicago, in 1925. He served as a US Army physician during World War II. On his return he practiced obstetrics. *See Stein–Leventhal syndrome.*

Levine, Samuel A. (1891–1966) Cardiologist and professor of medicine at Harvard Medical School. He attempted thyroidectomy as treatment for angina, together with Herman Ludwig Blumgart (1895–1977) in 1933. In 1923 he and Elliot Carr Cutler (1888–1947) did the first successful mitral valve section in treatment of mitral stenosis. He described Lown–Ganong–Levine Syndrome, a condition with shortened PR interval and normal QRS on ECG associated with paroxysmal tachycardia, in 1952.

Levinus Lemnius (b 1505) Born in Zealand, he was a physician who took holy orders after the loss of his wife. He wrote several treatises on morality and physick.

Lewes, George Henry (1817–1878) London author of: *Studies in Animal Life* (1862), *Problems of Life and Mind* (1874), and *Aristotle* (1864). The translation of one of his works on physiology into Russian is said to have inspired Ivan Petrovich Pavlov (1849–1936).

Lewinshon, Abraham (1888–1955) Studied at Northwestern Medical School and was a pioneer in pediatrics. He wrote *Cerebrospinal Fluid in Health and Disease* in 1919.

Lewis, Gilbert Newton (1875–1946) American physical chemist, educated at the University of Nebraska and Harvard. He worked in Leipzig and Göttingen before taking up a post at the University of California, Berkeley.

He wrote *Thermodynamics and the Free Energy of Chemical Substances, Valence and the Structure of Atoms and Molecules* in 1923. *See acid–base theory, valence.*

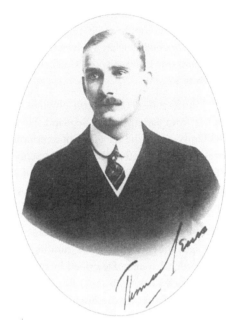

Sir Thomas Lewis (1881–1945)

Lewis, Sir Thomas (1881–1945) Eminent Welsh physiologist and cardiologist, born in Cardiff, and received his preclinical training there at the University College. He moved to University College Hospital, London in 1902 and later became chief of the department of research. He was a pioneer in application of the electrocardiographic method for examination of the heart. He performed a series of investigations on normal hearts between 1909 and 1916 which led to the explanation of the QRST complexes as a sequential spread of electrical excitation over the different parts of the atria and ventricles. He also described 'effort syndrome', a condition earlier noted in 1871 amongst soldiers in the American civil war by Da Costa from Philadelphia. Einthoven's (1860–1927) string galvanometer was improved by Lewis who added two strings instead of a conventional single string, making it possible to record different leads. He postulated a histamine-like substance (H substance) as a cause of anaphylaxis in 1924. Some of his important publications include: *Clinical Electrocardiography* (1917), *Harvian Oration on Clinical Sciences* (1933), *Diseases of the Heart* (1933), *Clinical Science* (1934), *Vascular Disorders of the Limb*, and *Clinical Disorders of the Heart Beat*.

Lewis, Timothy Richard (1841–1886) British parasitologist who identified the larval nematode of filariasis and named it *Filaria sanguinis hominis* in 1872. The first demonstration of a trypanosome (*Trypanosoma lewisi*) infecting a mammalian species, the rat, was given by him in 1879 while he was in Calcutta. *See filariasis, African trypanosomiasis.*

Lewis, W. Lee (1879–1943) American chemist. *See lewisite.*

Lewisite Poisonous arsenic compound used in gas warfare. First produced from acetylene and arsenic chloride by Belgian-born American chemist, Julius Arthur Niewland (1878–1936), who realized its deadly nature and discontinued his research. It was later developed into a weapon for use in World War 1 by W. Lee Lewis (1879–1943) of North Western University in America and named Lewisite in his honor. *See gas warfare.*

Lewontin, Richard Charles (b 1929) American geneticist from New York who developed the subject of population genetics. His main research area is explaining the distribution of variation within and among natural populations. In 1974 he published *The Genetic Basis of Evolutionary Change* which was a synthesis of his views. He introduced gel electrophoresis to assess variation in protein sequences.

Ley, Hugh (1790–1837) Born in Abingdon, Berkshire, he graduated in medicine from Edinburgh, before becoming a physician at the Middlesex Hospital. In 1835 he was appointed to the obstetric chair at St Bartholomew's Hospital. He wrote *Essay on Laryngismus Stridulus* and several other papers.

Leyden, John (1775–1811) Physician, poet and oriental scholar, born to a farming family in Denham, Roxburgh in 1775. He graduated from Edinburgh University and assisted Sir Walter Scott in making illustrations for *Minstrelsy of the Scottish Border* in 1801. Leyden served as surgeon in Madras and Calcutta and devoted his time to the study of oriental literature. His *Poetical Remains* was published in 1819.

Leyden The University of Leiden was inaugurated by Prince William in 1575. Gerard de Bondt or Bontius (1592–1631) was its first professor of medicine. The first English student to obtain a medical degree there was John James in 1568. It later became a center of medical learning and produced many eminent medical men throughout the world.

Leyden, Ernst Victor von (1832–1910) German physician who worked on tabes and poliomyelitis. He established sanatoria for treatment of tuberculosis. First to describe fatty infiltration of the heart in 1882. He gave a comprehensive account of coronary heart disease in 1884 and also described a form of muscular dystrophy known as 'Leyden paralysis'.

Leydig Cell Interstitial cells of the testis, first described in

1850 by Franz von Leydig (1821–1908), professor of histology and comparative anatomist at Würzberg.

Lhermitte Syndrome Internuclear ophthalmoplegia seen in disseminated sclerosis. Described by French neurologist and Clinical Director of the Salpêtrière, Jacques Jean Lhermitte (1877–1959), in 1920.

Liaig Ancient Irish term for a physician which means 'leech' in old English.

Libau, or Libavius, Andreas (1560–1616) German alchemist and physician from Saxony who became the first rector at the Gymnasium Casmirianum in Coberg in 1607. His work, *Alchemia*, is a landmark in the transition stage from alchemy to chemistry.

Libman–Sacks Endocarditis Verrucous endocarditis in systemic lupus. Described in 1923 by two New York physicians, Emanuel Libman (1872–1946) and Benjamin Sacks (1873–1939).

Library [Latin: *libraria*] The earliest known public library was that at Athens, founded by Pisitratus in 540 BC. The library at Alexandria was established by Ptolemy in 284 BC but was destroyed in 47 BC. The Vatican Library was founded by Pope Nicholas V in 1447. Harvard University library was formed in 1638. The libraries in Great Britain were formed in the following order: St Andrews (1411), Glasgow University (1473), Royal College of Physicians (1518), Bodleian, Oxford (1598), Royal Society (1667) and Radcliffe, Oxford (1714).

Librium Tranquilizer, chlordiazepoxide hydrochloride, first synthesized in 1960 by Lowe Randall of America.

Liddel, Duncan (1561–1613) Physician and mathematician from Aberdeen. He traveled to Europe and served as professor of mathematics at Helmstedt where he graduated in medicine in 1596. He returned to Aberdeen and established a successful practice. He published *De Febricus, Ars Medica* and several other works. He bequeathed his books and instruments to Marischal College and a sum of money as bursary for medical students.

Liddell, Edward George Tandy (1895–1981) Neurophysiologist who worked on tendon reflex activity with Nobel Prize winner, Sir Charles Sherrington (1857–1952), at Oxford. Their work was published in 1924 and a more comprehensive book, *Reflex Activity of the Spinal Cord,* was published by Sherrington, Sir John Carew Eccles (b 1930), Creed, Derek Ernest Denny-Brown (1901–1981) and Liddell in 1932.

Liddle Syndrome Defective reabsorption in the distal tubule. First described in 1963 by American endocrinologist from Utah, Grant Winder Liddle (1921–1989) and co-workers.

Lieberkühn Glands Found in the lining of the intestines by Marcello Malpighi (1628–1694) in 1688 and described by Johann Brunner (1635–1727) in 1715. They were named after Johann Nathaniel Lieberkühn (1711–1756), an anatomist at Berlin who further described them in 1745.

Liebig, Justus von (1803–1873) Father of industrial chemistry in Germany, born in Darmstadt. After a childhood of poverty, he was apprenticed as an apothecary at the age of 16. He entered Bonn University and, after graduation, served as assistant at Joseph Gay-Lussac's (1778–1850) laboratory in Paris when he was only 19. He mastered the science of chemistry and began his ascent to fame with the discovery of the structure of fulminic acid. At 23 he was made professor of chemistry at Giessen which, under his direction, became one of the greatest schools of chemistry in the world. Much of the early work on biochemistry was based on his books: *Chemistry in its Application to Agriculture and Physiology* (1840), and *Organic Chemistry in its Application to Physiology and Pathology* (1842).

Lifeboat Invented by Lionel Lukin, a coach builder from Dunmow, Essex. It consisted of a series of airtight chambers to give buoyancy and was patented in 1785. Henry Greathead (1787–1816), a boatbuilder from Richmond, Yorkshire, after hearing of the tragic wreck of the *Adventure* at the mouth of river Tyne in 1789, built an admirable lifeboat in 1789, which was bought by the Duke of Northumberland and presented to the people of North Shields.

Life Expectancy One of the earliest computations on life expectancy was given by John Ward in *Young Mathematician's Guide*, published in 1706. In this he pointed out an earlier work by mathematician and astronomer, Edmond Halley (1656–1742). *See vital statistics.*

Ligature [Latin: *ligatus*, bound] Aulus Cornelius Celsus (25 BC–AD 50) recommended ligature if other measures, such as application of a sponge in cold water combined with pressure by the hand, failed to stop the bleeding. Archigenes was the first to suggest it to stop bleeding during amputation. It was recommended as treatment for hemorrhoids in one of the Hippocratic treatises. Absorbable suture materials made of buckskin were first used as surgical ligatures by American surgeon, Philip Syng Physick (1768–1837) in 1816. Catgut was used in surgery by Sir Astley Cooper (1768–1841) in 1817. Catgut treated with carbolic acid to promote asepsis was introduced by Joseph Lister (1827–1912) in 1869. Catgut was used in 1889 for suturing intestines by New York surgeon, Robert Abbe (1851–1905).

Light One of the earliest proponents of the wave theory of light was Italian physicist, Francesco Maria Grimaldi (1618–1663) of Bologna, around 1638. The speed of light through space was calculated with impressive accuracy from astronomical observations by Danish astronomer Olaus Roemer (1644–1710) in 1695, and by James Bradley (1693–1762) in 1727. Roemer used the time differences of eclipses of the satellites of Jupiter to determine the speed of light at 240,000 kilometers per second. Two important theories – Sir Isaac Newton's (1642–1727) corpuscular theory and Christiaan Huygen's (1629–1693) undulatory theory – were proposed around the same time at the end of 17th century, but Newton's theory came to be accepted. A treatise which differentiated between red and violet rays was written in 1802 by English physician, Thomas Young (1773–1829). Another English physician, William Hyde Wollaston (1766–1828), was the first to notice that the Sun's spectrum was crossed by dark lines in 1802 and Joseph von Fraunhofer (1787–1826) measured their wavelength using wire gratings in 1814. Sir Charles Wheatstone (1802–1875) in 1834 proposed a method of estimating the velocity of light using a rotating mirror, and Jean Foucault (1819–1868) applied a new method for this purpose in 1850. The velocity of light was first calculated, without using astronomical distances or phenomena, by French physicist, Armand Hippolyte Louis Fizeau (1819–1896) in 1849. *See optics.*

Lightning The Greek philosopher Anaxagorus in 435 BC postulated that earthquakes were produced by subterraneous clouds bursting out into lightning which shook the vault that confined them. The practice of hanging the herb, St John's wort, outside the door to protect from lightning persisted for several centuries. Lightning was first shown to be a form of electricity by the American statesman and scientist, Benjamin Franklin (1706–1790), in 1752. The demonstration of atmospheric electricity was achieved by John Canton (1718–1772), a physicist from Stroud, Gloucestershire. John Hunter (1728–1793) in *A Treatise on the Blood, Inflammation and Gunshot wounds*, published in 1794, mentioned that animals killed by electricity or lightning had no blood clots. This was later recognized to be caused by fibrinolysis. Cataracts due to lightning were described in 1864 in a 18-year-old woman by Edwin Theodor Saemisch (1833–1909), an ophthalmologist from Bonn.

Lignac, George Otto Emile (1891–1954) Dutch pediatrician. *See aminoaciduria, cystinosis.*

Lignocaine or lidocaine (Xylocaine) A compound called 'gramine' with local anesthetic properties was noted in the plant, *Hordeum vulgare*, by Hans von Euler in 1932. The same substance, under the name iso-gramine, was synthesized in 1935 by Holger Erdtman, an assistant to von Euler. Lofgren, in 1943, produced xylocaine, a more potent and specific local anesthetic in 1946.

Lillehei, Clarence Walton (b 1918) American pioneer of open-heart surgery. He was born and trained in medicine in Minnesota where he spent most of his career, except for the period 1967–1974 which he spent as professor at Cornell University, New York.

Limb [Anglo-Saxon: *lim*, limb] *See amputation, hand.*

Lime Juice Established as a cure for scurvy in 1747 by naval physician, James Lind (1716–1794). He published his findings in *A Treatise on the Scurvy* in 1753. His observations, however, were not fully used until 1795 when Sir Gilbert Blane (1749–1834), commissioner of the Board of the Care of Sick and Wounded Seamen, issued an order for regular use of lime or lemon juice in the Navy.

Linacre, Thomas (1460–1524) Physician and humanist who founded the Royal College of Physicians in 1518 under charter from King Henry VIII. Linacre served as physician to four successive sovereigns and took religious orders towards the end of his life.

Lind, James (1716–1794) Eminent Scottish naval physician who was born and qualified in medicine in Edinburgh. He introduced lemon juice as prevention and cure for scurvy in 1747. His work, *A Treatise on the Scurvy*, was published in 1753. He also wrote one of the earliest books on tropical medicine, *Essay on Diseases Incident to Europeans in Hot Climates* in 1768. *See lime juice.*

Lindeman, Edward E. (1883–1913) New York surgeon who devised a direct method of transfusing blood through a two-way syringe in 1913.

Linnaean System First systematic classification of plants was done by Swedish botanist and physician, Carl Linnaeus (1707–1778) in his descriptions of 11,800 genera and species of plant. His library and herbarium were purchased after his death by Sir James Edward Smith (1759–1828) who presented them to the Linnaean Society, founded in 1788. Smith also served as the first president of the Linnaean Society and wrote over 3000 botanical articles.

Linnaeus, Carl (1707–1778) Swedish naturalist and physician and founder of scientific nomenclature for plants and animals. He studied in Lund and Uppsala and received his medical degree from Holland in 1735, where he published his system of botanical nomenclature, *Systema Naturae* in 1735, *Fundamenta Botanica* in 1736, *Genera Plantarum* and *Critica Botanica* in 1737. In 1741 he became the professor of medicine and botany at Uppsala University and in 1749 introduced his binomial Latin nomenclature on plants. *See Linnean system.*

Linolenic Acid Initially called vitamin F and found in fish oils and oil seeds, it is essential for formation of prostaglandins. It was isolated by Herbert McLean Evans (1882–1971) and co-workers in 1934. *See essential unsaturated fatty acids.*

Linus Plastica *See Brinton, William.*

Lipid Profile *See cholesterol, lipids.*

Lipid [Greek: *lipos*, fat] Michel Eugène Chevreul (1786–1889), a French chemist and gerontologist, was a pioneer in the study of soap, margarine, olein, stearin and other fatty acids. During his classical studies on animal fats in 1823 he discovered that fat was composed of fatty acids and glycerol. Cholesterol, one of the earliest known sterols, was first described by Chevreul in 1815. An early study on fat absorption and blood lipids was done by American biochemist, Walter Ray Bloor (b 1877) in 1915, and he suggested the term 'lipide' to include true fats and tri-acid fatty esters of glycerol, in 1925. *See cholesterol.*

Lipiodol Iodized oil, first used as a contrast medium in cerebral radiology by J.A. Sicard (1872–1929) and J. Forestier (b 1890) in 1921 and 1929, respectively.

Lipmann, Fritz Albert (1899–1986) American biochemist, born in Königsberg and studied medicine at Berlin before emigrating to America in 1939. He became professor at Harvard Medical School in 1949 and, in 1950, described the formation of citric acid from oxaloacetate and acetate and in 1952 discovered coenzyme A of the respiratory cycle. Lipmann shared the Nobel Prize for Physiology or Medicine in 1953 with Adolf Hans Krebs (1900–1981).

Lippershey, Hans (1571–1619) Dutch optician who discovered that the combination of two separated long and short focus lenses can make distant objects appear closer, i.e. a telescope, or in reverse, a microscope. *See spectacles.*

Lippmann, Gabriel Jonas (1845–1921) French physicist who invented a mercury capillary electrometer, an astatic galvanometer, and a seismograph. His most notable development, for which he received the Nobel Prize for Physics in 1908, was a technique for color photography based on interference phenomena. *See capillary electrometer.*

Liquefaction of Gas The earliest method of liquefying oxygen was the 'cascade process' devised by Marc-Auguste Pictet (1752–1825), a physicist from Geneva. The process was improved by Linde who introduced the regenerative method in 1895. Helium was first liquefied by Dutch physicist, Heike Kamerlingh Onnes (1853–1926) in 1908.

Liquorice Inspissated juice from the plant, *Glycyrrhiza glabra*, has been used since the time of Dioscorides (AD 40–90), and is noted in the writings of Oribasius (325–403). It was commonly used during the Middle Ages for various ailments and was amongst the entries of Wardrobes Accounts of King Henry III in 1264. It was included in the list of drugs of the city of Frankfurt in 1450.

Lisfranc, Jacques (1790–1847) French surgeon who designed an operation for partial removal of the foot, now known by his name. He also advocated the extirpation of the rectum as treatment for cancer in a paper presented to the Academie Royale de Médicine in 1830.

Li Shih-Chen (1518–1593) Celebrated Chinese physician, father of Chinese herbal medicine, who compiled his *Pen Tshao Kang Mu*, or Great Herbal, of 52 volumes between 1552 and 1578. It contains detailed descriptions of 1000 plants and 1000 animals together with 11,000 prescriptions. The book was not confined to pharmacy but included many other natural sciences and demonstrated many advances in Chinese medicine. One such was their use of mercury-silver amalgam to fill teeth which was not introduced into European dentistry until the 19th century. *See Chinese medicine.*

Lissauer Tract Posterior lateral tract (marginal tract) of the spinal cord described by a neurologist from Breslau, Heinrich Lissauer (1861–1891), in 1885.

Lister, Joseph Jackson (1786–1869) Father of Lord Joseph Lister, he was a microscopist and botanist who devised the achromatic lens for the modern microscope.

Lister, Joseph, Lord (1827–1912) English surgeon and founder of the antiseptic system of surgery. He was born in Stoke Newington where his father Joseph Jackson Lister (1786–1869) was a microscopist. He graduated in arts from University College, London in 1847 and obtained his medical degree there in 1852. He became house surgeon to James Syme (1799–1870) at Edinburgh in 1853 and later married his daughter. Lister was appointed professor of

surgery at Glasgow in 1859, during which time he advocated the use of carbolic acid for prevention of infection during surgery. He further experimented on carbolic acid in 1866 and devised a hand-driven spray for use during surgery. The spray was later steam-driven and remained in use for the next two decades. After Syme's resignation Lister succeeded him at Edinburgh in 1869 and the use of catgut treated with carbolic acid to promote asepsis was introduced by him in the same year. He was appointed professor of clinical surgery at King's College London in 1877 and became the first medical man to be elevated to the peerage.

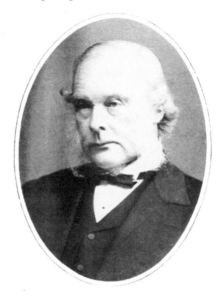

Lord Joseph Lister (1827–1912). Courtesy of the National Library of Medicine

Lister, Martin (1638–1712) Physician from York who proposed the concept of geological maps. He practiced in London and was made a Fellow of the Royal Society in 1671. His most important work, *Historia Animalium Angliae*, was published in 1678.

Liston, Robert (1794–1847) Edinburgh surgeon, one time colleague, relative and friend of James Syme (1799–1870). He presented a dissertation, *Fracture of the Neck of the Femur*, and published a series of 5 cases of aneurysms in 1820. He moved to London as professor of surgery at University College, and performed the first major operation under anesthesia in 1846.

Literary and Philosophical Society of Liverpool Founded by Thomas Stewart Traill (1781–1862) while working at Liverpool from 1803 to 1832. Traill also established the Liverpool Mechanics Institution and the Royal Institution of Liverpool.

Lithia Tablet *See lithium.*

Lithium [Greek: *lithos*, stone] Natural spring waters were recommended as treatment for ill humor in Hippocratic times, and it is now known that these waters contain appreciable amount of lithium salts. Lithium was discovered in 1817 by Johann August Arfvedson (b 1792) of Stockholm, a pupil of Jöns Jacob Berzelius (1779–1848), who isolated it in 1818. Haeddon, around 1900, demonstrated that tobacco contained significant amounts of lithium. Lithium carbonate was used as a solvent for bladder calculi by Ure in 1843. It was recommended as treatment for gout by Sir Archibald Garrod (1857–1936) in 1859, and 'Lithia tablets' became an over-the-counter treatment around 1867. Periodic depression was suspected to be due to uric acid diathesis and Alexander Haig of London used lithium to treat depression in 1892, based on this concept. Danish neurologist, Carl Georg Lange (1834–1900), promoted its use in depression in 1896. The free use of Lithia tablets was denounced in *The Practitioner* in 1907 and deaths due to cardiac failure following its use were noted in 1949. Around the same time Johann Frederick Joseph Cade (b 1912) demonstrated the use of lithium in psychiatry and its use in manic and depressive episodes was established around 1967.

Lithography Art of engraving on stone invented by Bavarian printer, Alois Sennefelder (1771–1834) of Prague in 1796. It was introduced into England in 1801 and popularized by Ackemann of London in 1817.

Lithotomy [Greek: *lithos*, stone + *tome*, cutting] Definitive treatment for urinary stones recognized by Hippocrates (460–377), Galen (AD 129–200) and other ancient physicians. Lithotomists were the earliest group of surgeons to practice and it was well established as a specialty by Hippocratic times. Ammonius, a surgeon of Alexandria, described the method of extraction of stones from the urinary bladder in 240 BC. Frere Jacques (1651–1714) of Paris was an eminent lithotomist who performed over 5000 lithotomies. Pierre Franco was one of the best lithotomists of the 16th century in France, who introduced the suprapubic approach in 1556. William Cheselden (1688–1752) was a well known lithotomist in England and was famous for his speed in performing the operation.

Lithotripter [Greek: *lithos*, stone + *tribein*, to rub] Ultrasonic device to fragment kidney stones without causing bleeding. Invented by two Germans, Eisenberger and Chaussey, in Munich in 1972. The prototype machine was introduced by the German firm, Dornier Medical Systems of Munich in 1980.

Lithotrity [Greek: *lithos*, stone + *tribein*, to rub] Method of bruising the urinary stone with surgical instruments, first practiced by M. Leoroy Etiolles in 1822. Jean Civiale (1792–1867) introduced an instrument in 1826.

Litmus [Dutch: *lakmoes*, an infusion of purple color] Vegetable coloring matter obtained from lichens particularly, *Roccella tinctoria*. Paper dipped in litmus is used to measure acidity or alkalinity in a pH range from 4.5 to 8.3.

Litten Sign Visible depression of the lower part of the sides of the thoracic wall in respiratory effort or distress. Described by German physician, Moritz Litten (1845–1907).

Little, Clarence Cook (1888–1971) American pioneer of cancer genetics. He was born in Brookline, Massachusetts and attended Bussey Institute (an agricultural college attached to Harvard University). While still an undergraduate, he established the first inbred strain of mice. This was an essential stage in our understanding of drug action and transplantation and treatment of cancer. *See organ transplantation.*

Little, Louis Stromeyer (b 1840) Son of William John Little (1810–1894), eminent British orthopedic surgeon. He was born in Finsbury Square in London and named after Louis Stromeyer of Hannover who operated on his father for talipes. He went to Shanghai in 1876 and served as surgeon at the Shanghai General Hospital for 30 years. He was also an astronomer and founded an observatory at Shanghai in which he photographed the transit of Venus.

Little, William John (1810–1894) British orthopedic surgeon and son of a publican in London. He visited Louis Stromeyer at Hannover and was operated on by him for talipes equino-varus. He wrote a monograph on talipes which contained the first description of tenotomy. On his return he settled at Finsbury Square and founded the Orthopedic Institution in 1839, which later became the Royal National Orthopedic Hospital. He pioneered the use of intravenous saline in treatment of cholera. He performed the first subcutaneous heel tenotomy for club foot in 1837 and described a form of cerebral palsy (Little disease) in 1861. His famous work, *On the Deformities of the Human Frame*, was published in 1853. *See cerebral palsy.*

Little Area In the nasal septum, described by James Laurence Little (1836–1885), professor of surgery at Vermont in 1876.

Little Disease *See cerebral palsy.*

Littlejohn, Sir Henry Duncan (1826–1914) Born in Edinburgh, he was appointed first medical officer of health for

Edinburgh in 1862. He was a pioneer in the field of public health and his report on sanitary conditions in Edinburgh in 1865 contributed to a significant improvement in the state of hygiene in the city and led to a fall in death rate.

Littré Glands Found in the mucous membrane of the spongy part of the urethra. First described by Alexis Littré (1658–1726), an anatomist and surgeon from Paris, in 1719.

Litzmann, Carl Conrad Theodor (1815–1890) Born in Gadebusch in Germany and studied at the University of Halle. He was professor of obstetrics at Kiel in 1848 and published a paper on surgical treatment of ectopic pregnancy (1880) and several other works, including a textbook on obstetrics.

Liver Abscess Hippocrates (460–377) has given a detailed account on the diseases of the liver. He directed that they be opened by cautery and stated that they were least dangerous when opened externally. The first cannula to drain a liver abscess was devised by Joseph Fayrer (1824–1907), a surgeon to the East India Company. Treatment by drainage through a needle was pioneered by Rickman John Godlee (1849–1929), a London surgeon at the Brompton Hospital, in 1890. This method was later adopted by several workers, including Godlee, to drain pulmonary cavities.

Liver Biopsy First performed by Italian, Luigi Lucatello (1863–1926) in 1895. Its role as a diagnostic procedure was firmly established by J.H. Dible, J. McMichael and S. Sherlock in 1943. It was used in the diagnosis of sarcoidosis by J.G. Scadding and Sherlock in 1948. The first laparoscopic liver biopsy was performed by H. Kalk in 1929.

Liver Extract The ancients unknowingly used raw liver as a cure for anemia and other diseases. The first potent liver extract for oral administration in anemia was prepared by William Parry Murphy (1892–1987), George Richards Minot (1885–1950), and co-workers in 1927. This followed the work of George Hoyt Whipple (1878–1976) on feeding raw liver to anemic dogs. Murphy, Minot and Whipple shared the Nobel Prize for Physiology or Medicine in 1934. Oral preparations of raw liver, such as 'extractum hepatis siccum' and 'extractum hepatis liquidum', were included in the pharmacopoeia until the late 1940s. Intravenous use of liver extract for treatment of anemia was introduced by American physician, William Bosworth Castle (b 1899) and Francis Henry Laskey Taylor (1900–1959) in 1929. *See pernicious anemia.*

Liver [Anglo-Saxon: *lifere*, liver] According to ancient Greek physicians it is the seat of natural power and the grand organ of sanguification. Galen (129–200) and Avicenna

(980–1037) ascribed its function as drawing chyle from the stomach. Hippocrates (460–377) described three varieties of liver disease due to bilious fever. Aretaeus (81–138) advocated venesection and the use of wormwood and diuretics for acute hepatitis.

Liverpool Medical Institution Founded by a Quaker, John Rutter (1762–1838), a physician who graduated from Edinburgh in 1786. Rutter also founded the Liverpool Athenaeum.

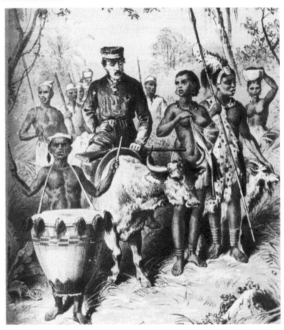

Livingstone weak from fever, being escorted by natives. *The Life and Explorations of David Livingstone* (1875). Adam & Co., London

Livingstone, David (1813–1873) Famous African explorer and doctor, born in Blantyre, Scotland. He attended the Theological School in Glasgow and became a member of the London Missionary Society in 1839. He attended medical lectures at Charing Cross Hospital and obtained his licentiate in medicine. He made his first journey to Africa in 1841, which lasted 15 years. During his travels he observed ancient medical practices of the peoples and described the disease of cattle caused by the bite of the tsetse fly. On his return to England he published *Missionary Travels* in 1857 in which he has given an illustration of the tsetse fly. His second trip to Africa took nearly 5 years and on his return he wrote *The Zambezi and its Tributaries* in 1864. He traveled to Africa one year later and died at Chitambo's Village, Ilala on 1 May 1873.

Lizars, John (1787–1860) Professor of surgery at Edinburgh. The surgical lines of the buttocks (Lizars lines) were described by him in 1838.

Loa Loa [Native Angolan word] Also known as the African eye worm, *Dracunculus oculi*, a filarial worm (*Filaria diurna*). Mongin, a French surgeon in the West Indies, gave the first description in 1770, followed by Bajon in Cayenne in 1768. Africans at this time were already aware of the relation between mango flies and the eye worm. Guyot of Paris observed and studied the parasite in 1838. The larval form in the eye was studied by Patrick Mason (1844–1922) in 1891.

Lobar Pneumonia The infectious nature of lobar pneumonia was described by Austrian physician, Theodor von Jürgensen (1840–1907), in 1874. Theodor Edwin Klebs (1834–1913) came to the same conclusion a year later and the bacteria in lobar pneumonia were first observed by Carl Joseph Eberth (1835–1926) in 1880. Similar bacteria were isolated from patients with lobar pneumonia by Carl Friedlander (1847–1887) in 1882. The presence of pneumococcal cocci in pairs was noted by C. Talmon around the same time. The occurrence of arterial anoxemia in cases of lobar pneumonia was first shown by Alvin Leroy Barach (1895–1977) and M.N. Woodwell in 1921 and their work formed the basis for oxygen therapy in pneumonia. *See pneumococcal vaccine, quellung reaction.*

Lobectomy *See frontal lobectomy.*

Lobectomy of Lung Removal of a lobe of the lung. Partial lobectomy as treatment for tuberculosis was first done by David Lowson (1850–1907) in 1893. Theodore Tuffier (1857–1929) of Paris demonstrated a cure for tuberculosis by removing the lung apex in 1897. The surgical principles for a one stage lobectomy were described by Harold Brunn (1874–1950) in 1929. Lung resection for treatment of carcinoma of the lung was pioneered by Evarts Ambrose Graham (1883–1957) in Washington in 1932.

L'Obel, Matthias de (1538–1616) Flemish physician and botanist, born in Lille and studied medicine at Montpellier. He served as physician to William the Silent before he came to England under the patronage of Elizabeth I. He was made superintendent of the medicinal garden of Lord Zouche at Hackney, London. He was later appointed physician to King James VI and I of Scotland and England. L'Obel described a system for classification of plant leaves in his *Stirpium Adversaria Nova* published in 1570. *See Lobelia.*

Lobelia Plant named after the Flemish physician and botanist Matthias de L'Obel (1538–1616) of Lille. It has been known as a medicinal plant for centuries and was introduced into Europe as a tincture in the early 19th century.

Lobotomy [Greek: *lobos*, lobe + *tome*, cutting] A Swiss psychiatrist removed part of the frontal lobe in a psychiatric patient in 1890, but his work was not followed up for ethical reasons. Destruction of frontal lobes was shown to produce character changes by Leonardo Bianchi (1848–1919) in 1920. Excision of the frontal lobe as treatment in a psychiatric patient was first performed by Antonio Egaz Moniz (1874–1955), a Portuguese neurology professor, and Almeida Lima, a Portuguese surgeon in 1935. *See prefrontal leucotomy.*

Lobstein Ganglion Accessory ganglion of the great sympathetic system in connection with the solar plexus. Described by Johann Georg Christian Martin Lobstein (1777–1835), professor of pathology and clinical medicine at Strasburg in 1823. He also described osteogenesis imperfecta (Lobstein syndrome) in 1833. *See osteogenesis imperfecta.*

Lobstein Syndrome Osteogenesis imperfecta, described by Johann George Christian Martin Lobstein (1777–1835), professor of pathology and clinical medicine at Strasburg, in 1833. *See osteogenesis imperfecta.*

Local Anesthesia Ether was used as a local anesthetic in 1854 by Guerard and Didier Dominique Richet (1816–1891) of France who made painless incisions after applying it to the skin. Benjamin Ward Richardson (1828–1896) devised an ether spray for local anesthesia. The anesthetic effect of cocaine on the eye was demonstrated by Carl Koller (1857–1944) of Vienna in 1884. W.C. Burke of Connecticut was the first to inject cocaine into the nerve trunk in 1885. Around the same time, William Halsted (1852–1922), professor of surgery at the Johns Hopkins, also independently discovered the same method. Novocaine was discovered by Alfred Einhorn (1856–1917) around 1912 in Germany and introduced into clinical practice by Heinrich Friedrich Wilhelm Braun (1862–1934), the father of local anesthesia. It was later produced in 1916 under the name 'procaine' in America. Braun also found a method of prolonging the effect of procaine by adding epinephrine in 1897. Giesel introduced tropococaine in 1891 and stovaine was introduced by Ernst Fourneau (1872–1949) in 1904. Lignocaine or lidocaine, with more potent effect, was synthesized by N. Lofgren and B. Lundqvist of Stockholm in 1946. *See anesthesia.*

Lock Hospital Founded in 1746 by William Bromfield (1713–1792), a surgeon at Guy's Hospital in London, to treat venereal diseases.

Lock–Hospital Old term for a venereal and leprosy hospital.

Lockjaw Tetanus is one of the most ancient diseases described. In the *Aphorisms* Hippocrates (460–377) stated that 'those attacked by tetanus die within four days, or if they get through these they recover'. *See tetanus.*

473

Locke, John (1632–1704) English philosopher and physician, born at Wrington, Somerset, and educated at Christchurch College, Oxford, and became personal physician to Anthony Ashley Cooper in 1667. The most celebrated early work on analytic and corpuscular philosophy, *Essay Concerning Human Understanding*, was published by him in 1690 and ran into 17 editions over 50 years. He argued that all knowledge of man came through experience and sensations. His other treatises include: *A Treatise on Civil Government, Thoughts concerning Education* and *Letters on Toleration*.

Lockwood, Charles Barrett (1856–1914) Born in Stockton-on-Tees, he was a surgeon at St Bartholomew's Hospital in London, and founded the Anatomical Society of Great Britain and Ireland in 1887. He described the suspensory ligament of the globe of the eye (Lockwood suspensory ligament) in 1886.

Lockyer, Sir Joseph Norman (1836–1920) English astronomer. Founder (1897) and first editor of the journal, *Nature*. *See spectroscopy, astrophysics.*

Locock, Sir Charles (1799–1875) He graduated from Edinburgh in 1821 and later moved to London where he established an influential practice in midwifery. He attended Queen Victoria during the birth of all her nine children.

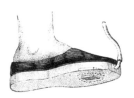

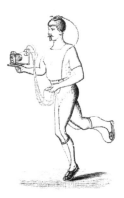

Marey's instrument for recording movements in locomotion. J.G. M' Kendrick, *A Textbook of Physiology* (1889). James Maclehose & Sons, Glasgow

Locomotion Etienne Jules Marey (1830–1904), a French physiologist, was one of the first to study locomotion on a scientific basis, in 1881. He developed an apparatus for recording movements during locomotion and invented a camera that could take rapid pictures. Zoopraxiscope, a forerunner of cinematography was invented and used to study locomotion by photographer, Edward Muybridge (1830–1904) from Kingston-upon-Thames, Surrey in England, who emigrated to California in 1852. He used this method to study the movements of animals and humans at the University of Pennsylvania, and published *Animal Locomotion* in 1887. Christian Wilhelm Braune (1831–1892) of Germany was the first to study and describe locomotion on a mathematical basis, in 1891. Nicholas Berstein (1896–1966), a Russian physiologist made a lifetime study of self-regulated motor systems and cybernetics. His work *On the Construction of Movements* was published in 1947.

Locomotor Ataxia Tabes dorsalis was described as 'locomotor ataxy' by Guillaume Benjamin Amand Duchenne (1806–1875), an eminent neurologist from Paris in 1858. An early description of joint symptoms was given by Sir Thomas Clifford Allbutt (1836–1925) of Dewsbury, England in the same year.

Locusts One of the biblical plagues of Egypt, said to have occurred in 1491 BC. Another epidemic came to Egypt and Libya in 128 BC and 800,000 people were said to have perished. The other major epidemics occurred in Palestine (AD 406), France (837), London (1748), Germany (1749), and Warsaw (1816).

Lodestone [Saxon: *loedan*, to lead] Ore iron with magnetic properties containing oxide. Early Greek miners treated it with awe and Lucretius described it as a wonder stone in 100 BC. Saint Augustine, around AD 400, said that he was thunderstruck to see an iron ring suspended by lodestone. The earliest known treatise, *Epistola de Magnete*, was written by Picard Petrus Perigrinus in 1269. In 1770 Father Hehl, a Jesuit priest and professor of astronomy at Vienna, used it for treatment of diseases and he invented several devices and plates for this purpose.

Lodge, Thomas (d 1635) English physician and poet who wrote *Wounds of Civil War*, and *Looking Glass for London and England*.

Loeb, Jacques (1859–1924) Born in Germany and graduated from Strasburg in 1884. He emigrated to America in 1891 and became the head of experimental biology at the Rockefeller Institute for Medical Research from 1910 to 1924. He founded the theory of 'tropism' in lower animals, proposed the mechanistic conception of life, and achieved artificial parthenogenesis in 1899. His extensive works on physiology of the brain in the same year led to the concept of chain reflexes. He published *Dynamics of Living Matter*

(1906), *Artificial Parthenogenesis and Fertilisation* (1913), and *The Organism as a Whole*.

Loeb, Leo (1869–1959) German-American pathologist who later became professor of pathology at Washington University. During his studies on carcinogenesis in 1900 he experimentally transmitted carcinoma through several generations of animals. He also transmitted cystic sarcoma of mice though 40 generations. In 1911 he demonstrated that the extirpation of corpora lutea of the ovary in guinea pigs accelerated the next ovulation, while extirpation of other parts of the ovary had no effect.

Loeb, Robert Frederick (1895–1973) American physician from Harvard whose main interest was electrolytes in relation to physiology. He designed original experiments in 1933 with G.A. Harrop which showed the importance of sodium in diet of patients with Addison disease. The activity of chloroquine against malarial was first tested by Loeb in 1946.

Loewi, Otto (1873–1961) German pharmacologist and physiologist from Frankfurt who was educated at Strasburg. He worked with Ernest Starling (1866–1927) at University College London in 1904 before becoming a professor at Graz in 1905. In 1921 he demonstrated that a substance liberated from stimulation of the vagus nerve ending, when perfused on to a second heart, was capable of slowing the rate of heart beat. This substance was the first neurotransmitter to be isolated and was later identified as acetylcholine by British physiologist, Sir Henry Hallett Dale (1875–1968). Loewi shared the Nobel Prize with Dale in 1936 for work on chemical transmission. During the Nazi occupation in 1940 Loewi emigrated to America and became professor at New York College of Medicine.

Löffler, Friedrich August Johann (1852–1915) German microbiologist who started his career as a military surgeon and became a professor at Greifswald in 1888. He was the first to culture diphtheria (1884) and discovered the causal organism of glanders. He and Paul Frosch (1860–1928) demonstrated in 1897 that foot and mouth disease in animals was caused by a filterable agent and made a vaccine for it. He was made director of the Koch Institute for Infectious Diseases in Berlin in 1913.

Löffler Endocarditis Rare form of endocarditis associated with eosinophilic infiltration. Described by Wilhelm Löffler (1887–1972) of Switzerland in 1936.

Löffler Syndrome Pulmonary symptoms and eosinophilic infiltration of the lung secondary to helminthic infection. Described by Wilhelm Löffler (1887–1972) of Switzerland in 1935.

Logic Branch of philosophy which deals with the study of ideal method in thought and research, and applies observation, deduction, induction, hypothesis and analysis to experimentation. Aristotle (384–322 BC) was one of the first philosophers to apply logic in understanding nature. Anaximander (610–540 BC), a pupil of Thales (624–545 BC), applied logic to astronomy and geography. Anaximenes (d 500 BC) proposed three forms of matter – gas, solid and liquid – in 450 BC. Anaxagorous (500–428 BC) used logic to show that plants and fishes respired.

Lombard, Etienne (1868–1920) French physician who devised the test for simulated unilateral deafness (Lombard test) in 1910.

London Hospital Established in the East End of London after a meeting of philanthropists at The Feathers Tavern, Cheapside, in 1740. A register of patients was made and they were admitted only once a week. The infirmary moved to Prescott Street, Goodman's Field in 1741 and its first student, Godfrey Webb, entered as apprentice to surgeon John Harrison (1718–1753) in the same year. A lease for new premises at Whitechapel was drawn up in 1752 and the foundation stone laid by Peter Warren in the same year. Admission was only through a letter from the Governor, except in cases of emergency, and the maximum stay was limited to two months in 1755. The outpatients department was opened in 1757 and the first inpatient was admitted in the same year, with 161 beds in place. A charter of incorporation was granted in 1757, and a seal designed by John Ellicot, a famous clockmaker and a member of the committee. The land adjoining the hospital was used as a burial ground for patients from 1758. The annual cost of a bed in 1767 was 17 pounds and 16 shillings. The committee decided in 1769 that physicians at the hospital should hold a diploma of the College of Physicians. The first thermometer was purchased in 1791. The committee decided in 1822 only to admit nurses who could read and write. The east wing was extended in 1840 and special wards were allocated to Jews in 1842. The first microscope was purchased in 1849, and Florence Nightingale (1820–1910) became Life Governor in 1856. The Alexandra wing was opened in 1866 and the Grocer's wing (established by donation of 20,000 pounds by the Grocer's Company) opened in 1876. The first nurse's home was built in 1887 and the dental school was established in 1911.

London Mechanics Institution Founded in 1822 by George Birkbeck, a physician. It became Birkbeck College in 1907 and was later incorporated into London University.

London Pharmacopoeia The first edition was published by the Royal College of Physicians in 1618. It contained remedies such as scorpion, spider webs, snake skin, and woodlice. The second and third editions were published in 1650 and 1677.

London School of Tropical Medicine Established as part of the University of London in 1905. It amalgamated with the School of Hygiene in 1925 to become the London School of Hygiene and Tropical Medicine.

London Society of Anesthetists Founded in 1893.

London University Founded in 1826 and building work commenced in 1827. It opened for lectures in 1828. In 1836 two charters were granted which transformed it into University College and University of London.

Long-Acting Insulin *See insulin.*

Long-Acting Thyroid Stimulator Differs from thyroid stimulating hormone and was first detected in serum of thyrotoxic patients by New Zealand researchers, Duncan Adams and Herbert D. Purves in 1956.

Long Island Society of Anesthetists The first society of anesthetists in America, formed by G. A. F. Erdmann in 1905. In 1911 it combined with a group from Manhattan to form the New York Society and in 1936 it became the American Society.

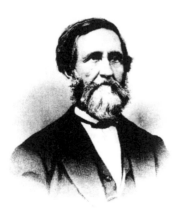

Crawford Williamson Long (1815–1878). Courtesy of the National Library of Medicine

Long, Crawford Williamson (1815–1878) Physician from Danielsville, Georgia was first to recognize the anesthetic property of ether and use it in 1842 in removing a tumor from the neck of a patient named James Venable. Sadly, his failure to report his results denied him the credit for his great discovery. A museum was built on the site of his original surgery in 1957 at Jefferson, Georgia.

Longevity [Latin: *longus*, long + *aevum*, age] Several claims defying the natural life span have been made, most notably the Old Testament claim that Methuselah lived nearly a thousand years. More recently, during the time of Charles I, a man named Golor McCrain from the Hebrides is said to have celebrated 180 Christmases. Thomas Parr, from Shropshire on his 153rd year in good health was brought to London by the Earl of Arundel in 1635. Henry Jenkins of Yorkshire died at the age of 163 in 1670 and was buried at Bolton.

Lonsdale, Dame Kathleen, née Yardley (1903–1971) Irish crystallographer who worked with Sir William Bragg (1862–1942) at University College London and later at the Royal Institution. She was one of the first female fellows of the Royal Society (1945) and was awarded the Society's Davy Medal in 1957. *See X-ray diffraction.*

Loop of Henle *See Henle loop.*

Loose Bodies in Joints The French surgeon Ambroise Paré (1510–1590) mentioned 'a hard polished white body of the size of an almond' which was found in the knee joint of a patient when he made an incision for aqueous aposteme or hydrops articuli in 1558. Similar bodies were also noted by Alexander Monro (1697–1767) of Edinburgh. Giovanni Battista Morgagni (1682–1771) reported similar bodies in the ankle joint. John Hunter (1728–1793) investigated them and concluded that they formed as a result of deposits of coagulated blood on the end of the bones which separated and acquired the nature of the cartilage.

Looser Zones Seen on X-rays and mimicking fractures in osteomalacia. Described by Swiss surgeon from Zurich, Emil Looser (1877–1936).

Lorenz, Adolf (1854–1946) Born in Vienna, he was a leading orthopedic surgeon in Europe who designed an osteotomy operation and a manipulative reduction for congenital dislocation of the hip. He published a treatise on scoliosis in 1884 and performed obturator neurectomy for spastic paraplegia in 1891.

Loreta Operation Method for opening the stomach and performing either a digital or instrumental dilatation of the pyloric or cardiac orifice. First described in 1882 by Pietro Loreta (1831–1889), professor of surgery at Bologna.

Lorica [Latin: breastplate] One of the earliest extant books from the Anglo-Saxon period. Several versions were written, one by Aethelwold, Bishop of Lichfield around AD 820. It is essentially a book of prayer in which several anatomical parts of the human body are mentioned while praying to god for protection.

Loring Ophthalmoscope Incorporates a disk of graduated lenses and a series of introduceable quadrant lenses. Designed by New York ophthalmologist, Edward Greely Loring (1837–1888).

Loschmidt, Johann Josef (1821–1895) Austrian chemist who rose from poverty and bankruptcy to become Chairman of the Physical Chemistry Institute in Vienna in 1875. In 1865 he calculated the number of molecules in one milliliter of an ideal gas under standard conditions, the Loschmidt number.

Loschmidt Number *See Loschmidt, Johann Josef*

Louis, Pierre Charles-Alexandre (1787–1872) Contemporary of Armand Trousseau (1801–1867) and a professional teacher at La Petit Hospital in Paris. He established medical statistics in France during his classic study of typhoid. He stressed the importance of number of subjects in random trials in order to obtain reliable relative mortality figures. The term 'fievre typhoide' for typhoid fever was first used by him in 1829. He was also a leading authority on tuberculosis and described the angle between the manubrium and the body of sternum (angle of Louis). *See statistics.*

Lovit, or Loewit, Moritz (1851–1918) Professor of pathology at Innsbruck. He described the erythroblasts (Lovit cells) and other cellular elements of blood in 1894.

Low Density Lipoprotein Receptors (LDL receptors) The lack of receptors that bind LDL in cells of patients with familial hypercholesterolemia was first noted around 1980 by two American molecular geneticists, Michael Stuart Brown (b 1934) of New York, and Joseph Leonard Goldstein (b 1940) of South Carolina. They were awarded the Nobel Prize for Physiology or Medicine in 1985.

Low, George Carmichael (1872–1952) London physician who demonstrated the chain of transmission of filaria from mosquito to man.

Lowe, Peter (1550–1630) Surgeon from Glasgow who was appointed by King James VI in 1599 as examiner to screen for competence those who wanted to practice surgery at Glasgow. He published *Chyurgerie* based on his surgical experiences in France in 1597. The faculty of Physicians and Surgeons of Glasgow was inaugurated under Peter Lowe in 1599.

Lowe Syndrome Hereditary oculocerebrorenal syndrome associated with cataracts, glaucoma, mental retardation, rickets and dwarfism. First described by Charles W. Lowe (b 1921), Mary Terrey and Elsie A. MacLachlan in 1952.

Lowenstein–Jensen Medium Used to culture *Mycobacterium tuberculosis*. It was prepared by Viennese pathologist, Ernest Lowenstein (b 1878) and Danish bacteriologist, Orla Jensen.

Löwenthal Tract The anterior marginal bundle of the cerebellar tract, first described in 1885 by German physician, Wilhelm Löwenthal (1850–1894).

Lower, Richard (1631–1691) Pioneer of blood transfusion, born in Cornwall and received his MD from Oxford in 1665 where he studied with Thomas Willis (1621–1673). He followed Willis to London and set up in practice there. He and Edmund King (1629–1707) performed the first blood transfusion from the artery of one animal to the vein of another in 1665, and gave the first transfusion of sheep's blood to man in 1667. He recognized the difference between venous and arterial blood and deduced that respiration added something to the blood. Lower also suggested the endocrine nature of the pituitary gland, saying 'fluids from it are poured again into the blood and mixed with it'. He described the prominence between the two venae caval orifices in the atrium in *Tractus de Corde* (Treatise on the Heart) published in 1669.

Lowman, Charles LeRoy (1879–1977) Graduate of the University of Southern California Medical School. He founded the Orthopedic Hospital at Los Angeles in 1922. He devised a bone holding instrument (Lowman clamp).

Lown–Ganong–Levine Syndrome Condition consisting of shortened PR interval and normal QRS on ECG associated with paroxysmal tachycardia. Described in 1952 by three American cardiologists, Bernard Lown (b 1921) of Brigham Hospital, Boston, William F. Ganong (b 1924) of the University of California, San Francisco, and Samuel Albert Levine (1891–1966).

Lowry, Thomas Martin (1874–1936) English chemist from Bradford, West Yorkshire. He studied under Henry Armstrong at the City and Guilds Institute in South Kensington. In 1912 he was appointed the first chemistry professor to a medical school in London, at Guy's Hospital. He redefined the terms 'acid' and 'base'.

LSD-25 Lysergic acid diethylamide is a constituent of the ergot alkaloids. It was first obtained from fungus by Swiss chemists, Albert Hoffmann (b 1906) and Arthur Stroll in 1938. The hallucinogenic property of the compound was described by Hoffmann, who accidentally swallowed it, in 1943. *See hallucinogens.*

Lubbock, Montague (1842–1925) Son of Sir John Lubbock (1834–1913) and a graduate of Guy's Hospital in 1872. He served as physician to Charing Cross Hospital and the West London Hospital. He translated Sigismond Jaccoud's (1830–1913) *The Curability and Treatment of Pulmonary Phthiasis* and Pierre Marie's (1853–1940) *Lectures on Diseases of Spinal Cord*.

Lubbock, Sir John, First Baron Avebury (1834–1913) English politician and biologist, born in London, and educated at Eton. He was instrumental in the introduction of bank holidays in 1871, and the Shop Hours Act of 1889. He was president of the Anthropological Institute and introduced the terms 'Paleolithic' and 'Neolithic' in 1865 to denote the two stages of the Stone Age. He published several works on geology and ethnology including, *Prehistoric Times*, a study of ancient customs and manners (1865, revised in 1913). His work on entomology, *Ants, Bees, and Wasps*, was published in 1882. He was elevated to the peerage in 1900.

Luc, Jean André de (1727–1817) A Swiss mathematician and geologist who settled in England in 1773 and became reader to Queen Charlotte and a friend of George III. He was one of the first to use the term 'geologie', and published *Cosmology and Geology* in 1803.

Luc, Henry (1855–1925) Otorhinologist from Paris who designed several operations for diseases of the maxillary and frontal sinuses.

Lucas–Championnière, Justin Marie Marcellin (1843–1913) French surgeon from Paris who introduced the Listerian system of antiseptic surgery into France in 1876. He also described chronic pseudomembranous bronchitis (Lucas–Championnière disease).

Lucas, Keith (1879–1916) English neurophysiologist, born in Greenwich, and educated at Trinity College, Cambridge. Lecturer and Fellow of Trinity College Cambridge. He described the 'all or none law', that a given stimulus evokes a maximum contraction or no contraction at all in muscles. Together with his pupil, Lord Edgar Douglas Adrian (1889–1977), he showed the same principle in motor nerve fibers. His *The Conduction of the Nervous Impulse* was prepared by Adrian and published posthumously in 1917.

Lucas, Richard Clement (1846–1915) Surgeon at Guy's Hospital, the first to describe the groove made by the chorda tymphani nerve on the spine of sphenoid (Lucas groove) in 1894.

Luciani Triad Hypotonia, ataxia and weakness seen in cerebellar disease. Described by Italian physician, Luigi Luciani (1840–1919) professor of physiology at Sienna, Florence and Rome.

Lucretius (*c* 95–55 BC) Roman poet and philosopher who proposed that disease was spread by 'seeds', some of which are contagious and others not. He wrote *De Natura Rerum* in which he advocated theories on the origin of the universe that had been proposed by Democritus (460–370 BC) and Epicurus.

Ludovicus or Juan Luis Vives (1493–1540) Spanish philosopher from Valencia who settled in Paris. He published *De Subventione Pauperum* in 1525 in which he advocated institutions for the sick and poor to ensure their spiritual and corporeal well-being and to keep them off the streets! His other major work was on psychology and science, *De Anima, De Vita*, published in 1538.

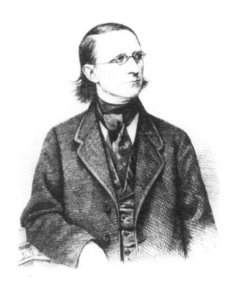

Karl Friedrich Wilhelm Ludwig (1816–1895). Courtesy of the National Library of Medicine

Ludwig, Karl Friedrich Wilhelm (1816–1895) German experimental physiologist, born in Witzenhausen, and studied medicine at Marburg. He taught at Zurich, Vienna and Leipzig and made several important contributions to understanding of blood pressure and heart activity. In 1865 he was involved in the establishment of the Institute of Physiology at Leipzig. His achievements include the invention of the kymograph in 1846 used to measure circulation and respiration; the mercurial blood pump in 1959; a method of perfusion to maintain circulation in an isolated organ in 1965; and the steam gauge in 1867. *See kymograph, Ludwig ganglion*.

Ludwig Angina Cellulitis of the submandibular space usually caused by anaerobic bacteria. It was first observed in Queen Catherine of Würtemberg by Wilhelm Friedrich von Ludwig (1790–1865) in 1836. He was an assistant army surgeon on the Russian front and was imprisoned by the

Russians for two years. On release in 1816 he became professor of surgery and midwifery in Tübingen and personal physician to King Frederick ll.

Ludwig Ganglion A mass of ganglia on the cardiac nerves in the atrial septum. Described by Karl Friedrich Wilhelm Ludwig (1816–1895) in 1862.

Lues Venera Term coined by French physician, Jacques de Bethencourt of Rouen in 1527 to denote syphilis and gonorrhea. The two diseases were differentiated by Benjamin Bell (1749–1806), a surgeon from Glasgow, in his treatise *Gonorrhoea Virulenta and Lues Venera* published in 1793. *See syphilis, genitourinary medicine.*

Lugol Iodine A mixture of 5% iodine and 10% potassium iodide, introduced in 1829 as a treatment for tuberculosis by French physician, Jean Guillaume Auguste Lugol (1786–1851). He was an advocate of drugs, fresh air, cold baths and exercise for treatment of tuberculosis. The solution was found to have little effect in treating tuberculosis but was later used in thyrotoxicosis by Henry S. Plummer (1874–1936). *See iodine.*

Luke, James (1798–1881) Born in Exeter, he was a pupil of John Abernethy (1764–1831) and Sir Astley Cooper (1768–1841). He joined the London Hospital as an anatomy lecturer in 1823 and was appointed surgeon to the hospital in 1849. He served there for 46 years and developed a special interest in surgical treatment of hernias. An operation for femoral hernia was devised by him in 1841.

Lumbar Disc Prolapse *See sciatica.*

Lumbar Puncture [Latin: *lumbus*, loin] One of the first methods of obtaining cerebrospinal fluid was by removing it from the skull. A great advance in the study of cerebrospinal fluid was made by J. Leonard Corning (1855–1923) of New York in 1885. He performed a lumbar puncture between the two spinous processes of two dorsal vertebrae of a dog in order to inject cocaine for experimental purposes. His experiment was the first demonstration of spinal anesthesia. Therapeutic lumbar puncture in man was performed by a London physician, Walter Essex Wynter (1860–1945) in 1889, and later by Heinrich Irenaeus Quincke (1842–1922) in 1891. For the next two years no advances were made and no papers were published. In 1893 Ludwig Lichtheim (1845–1928) revived it as a valuable procedure and two years later Paul Fürbringer (1849–1930) of Berlin reported a series of 107 spinal punctures. From 1896 onwards it became a standard diagnostic and therapeutic technique in neurology. *See cerebrospinal fluid.*

Lumbar Sympathectomy First performed through an anterolateral extraperitoneal approach by René Leriche (1879–1955) of Paris in 1933.

Lumelian Lectureship Public lectures on subjects connected with the human body. Established by Lord Lumley (1534–1609) and Caldwell in 1582–3. William Harvey (1578–1657) became a Lumelian lecturer in 1615.

Lumiere, Marie Louis Nicolas (1862–1954) *See cinematography.*

Lunar Society Institution to promote arts and sciences, formed by Matthew Bolton and Erasmus Darwin (1731–1802) at Birmingham in 1766. Several prominent persons including James Watt (1736–1819), Charles Darwin (1809–1892), Joseph Priestley (1733–1804), Josiah Wedgwood, and William Withering were members and known as 'lunatics'. The society derives its name from the practice of holding meetings nearest to the time of the full moon, so that its members could return home in moonlight.

Lunatics *See Lunar Society.*

Lung Abscess [Anglo-Saxon: *lunge*, lung] The earliest recorded incision and drainage of a lung abscess was done by English physician, Charles Hastings (1794–1866) in 1844. During this procedure, a large left apical lung abscess was approached through an incision in the second intercostal space and drained by insertion of a tube. Karl Friedrich Mosler (1831–1911) of Griefswald aspirated the lung cavities and injected them with iodized solutions in 1873. In 1876 he also advocated opening a lung abscess with dressing forceps. Rickman John Godlee (1859–1925) adopted the use of a cannula in 1884 for draining the lung abscess, this was previously used by Sir Joseph Fayrer (1824–1907) in liver abscesses.

Lung Cancer *See carcinoma of the lung.*

Lung Elasticity *See lung function.*

Lung Fluke *See Paragonimus westermani.*

Lung Function [Anglo-Saxon: *lunge*, lung] The importance of the elastic recoil property of the lung in respiration, the effect of venous return of the blood to the heart, and the production of a negative pleural pressure were first studied in 1820 by James Carson (1772–1843), a physician from Liverpool. The vital capacity of the lung was determined by John Hutchinson (1811–1861), who devised the first spirometer in 1846. The residual elastic tension was measured experimentally by Dutch physician Franciscus Cornelius Donders (1818–1889) in 1853, who connected a manometer to the trachea and carefully opened the thorax. He concluded that it was equivalent to 80 millimeters (3 inches) of water in a healthy person. Henry Hyde Salter (1823–1871) estimated it to be 4 inches of water in dogs in 1865. Max Perls (1843–1881) devised his own manometer in 1869 and conducted over 100 experiments on lung function. French physiologist, Paul Bert (1833–1886), in 1870 performed some ingenious experiments in which he measured the elastic pressure of the lung while he simultaneously opened the chest wall of a dog. The expansion of the lung was studied by Ludwig Traube (1818–1876) of Berlin in 1871. A essay on *Some effects of lung elasticity in Health and Disease* was published by Douglas Powell of the Middlesex and Brompton Hospitals in 1876. The part played by the diaphragm in respiration was studied independently by Traube and Le Gros Clark in 1871, and by G. M. Garland of New York in 1878. Two of the early instruments to measure the chest wall and lung function were the cyrtometer, devised by M. Woillez, and made of jointed whale bone which was used to trace the outline of the chest wall, and the pneumatometer invented by Louis Waldenburg (1837–1881) in 1880. The vitalograph came into use in 1954 and the use of peak flow meter for clinical monitoring of lung functions started around 1960.

Lupoid Hepatitis The term was coined in 1955, following the finding of LE cells in 15% of patients with a specific form of hepatitis, by R. A. Joske and W. E. King. *See active chronic hepatitis, LE cells.*

Lupus Anticoagulant *See antiphospholipid syndrome.*

Lupus Erythematosus [Latin: *lupus*, wolf] The Romans first used the term 'lupus' for cancer because it consumed the body like a wolf. The earliest description of the immunological disease, lupus erythematosus, was given by French dermatologist, Laurent Theodore Biett (1781–1840) of Paris. *See systemic lupus erythematosus.*

Lupus Pernio [Latin: *lupus*, wolf] Skin lesion seen in sarcoidosis, first described by Paris dermatologist, Ernest Besnier (1831–1909) in 1889.

Lupus Vulgaris [Latin: *lupus*, wolf] The ultraviolet treatment for lupus vulgaris was developed by a Danish physician, Niels Ryberg Finsen (1860–1904), in 1890.

Luria, Salvador Edward (1912–1991) American biologist, born in Turin, Italy and graduated from Turin University in 1935. He moved to the Radium Institute in Paris to study radiation techniques in relation to bacterial phages. He emigrated to the USA at the start of World War II and taught at Indiana University. In 1943 he and Max Delbrück (1906–1981) showed that bacteria can mutate and in 1951 he showed that phage genes also mutate, producing different strains. Alfred Day Hershey (b 1908), Delbrück and Luria

formed the Phage Group for genetic investigations. In 1969 they received the Nobel Prize for Physiology or Medicine. *See bacteriophage.*

Luschka Foramen Found at the lateral recesses of the fourth ventricle of the brain. Described by Hubert von Luschka (1820–1875), professor of anatomy at Tübingen in 1855.

Lusk, Graham (1866–1932) Born in Bridgeport, Connecticut, he was a pioneer in the study of nutrition in America. He published a treatise on amino acids (1910) and *The Elements of Science of Nutrition* (1906).

Lusk, William Thompson (1838–1897) New York obstetrician who wrote a treatise on his subject in 1882. The Bandl ring is also known as the Lusk ring. *See Bandl ring.*

Lutembacher Syndrome A congenital condition of atrial septal defect associated with mitral stenosis, first described by René Lutembacher (1884–1968) of Paris in 1916.

Luys, Jules Bernard (1828–1897) Neurologist at the Sâlpetrière in Paris, who did research on hypnosis, hysteria and insanity. In 1877 he was awarded the Légion d'Honneur. He founded *L'Enchéphale*, a journal of nervous diseases. He described hemiballismus caused by lesions in the subthalamic body or the medial nucleus of the thalamus (nucleus of Luys or Luys body lesion) in 1865.

Lycanthropia or lycaon [Greek: *lykos*, wolf + *anthropos*, man] Those suffering with this condition wander in the night, imitating wolves and lingering about sepulchers, according to the description given by Paul of Aegina (625–690). A man in the Gospel of Luke appears to have been affected, and Nebuchadnezzar, King of Assyria, may also have been a sufferer. The Arabians called it 'catubuth' and it was also known as 'melancholia canina'. Early medical treatises on the werewolf include: *Discours de la Lycanthropie* by B. de Chauvincourt in 1599, and *De la Lycothopie* by J. de Nynald, published in 1596. The condition is also mentioned in Burton's *Anatomy of Melancholy*.

Lyceum Peripatetic school of philosophy founded by Aristotle at Athens in 334 BC.

Lyell, Sir Charles (1797–1875) Born at Kinnordy in Scotland, the eldest son of mycologist, Charles Lyell (1767–1849). He initially studied law at Exeter College, Oxford and then took up geology, becoming the professor of geology at King's College in 1831. The first volume of *The Principles of Geology* appeared in 1830 and the other two volumes followed in the next two years. The terms 'Pliocene',

'Miocene' and 'Eosene' were coined by him. His friend and contemporary, Charles Darwin, is supposed to have built his theory of evolution on Lyell's theory of uniformity.

Lying–in–Hospitals The first such hospital in Great Britain was established at Dublin by a physician, Bartholomew Mosse, in 1745. *See maternity hospitals.*

Lymphadenitis [Latin: *lymph*, water; Greek: *aden*, gland] *See struma.*

Lymphangiogram [Latin: *lymph*, water + *angeion*, vessel + *graphe*, writing] The technique of lymphatic injection to visualize glands was introduced by Dumitru Gerota (1867–1939), professor of experimental surgery at the University of Bucharest.

Lymphangioma [Latin: *lymph*, water + *angeion*, vessel] First described by E.F. Hamm (1876–1941) in 1903.

Lymphatic System [Latin: *lymph*, water] The thoracic duct was first observed in the horse by Eustachio (1520–1574) in 1563. In 1622, Gaspar Aselli (1581–1626), professor of anatomy at Milan, noted the milky fluid from the lacteal vessels in a dog when it was killed soon after eating. The receptaculum chyli was first described by Jean Pecquet (1627–1674), a French anatomist, in 1647 and the lymphatic vessels were described by Thomas Bartholin (1616–1680), a physician from Copenhagen in 1652. The technique of injecting the lymphatic system in order to visualize the lymph glands was first demonstrated by Dumitru Gerota (1867–1939), professor of experimental surgery at the University of Bucharest.

Lymphocytic Choriomeningitis [Latin: *lymph*, water; Greek: *kytos*, cell + *chorion*, protective + *meningos*, membrane] The causative virus of St Louis encephalitis (mosquito-carried arbovirus, named after an epidemic in St Louis, USA) and lymphocytic choriomeningitis was identified by Charles Armstrong and Lillie in 1934. They obtained an inoculum from a fatal case and cultivated the virus successfully in monkeys. *See aseptic meningitis.*

Lymphogranuloma Venereum [Latin: *lymph*, water + *granum*, grain] (Syn: climatic bubo, maladie de Nicolas et Favre) Sexually transmitted disease caused by *Chlamydia trachomatis*. First described as a separate disease from syphilis and gonorrhea by John Hunter (1728–1793) in *A Treatise on Venereal Disease* published in 1786. One of the early descriptions was given by William Wallace (1791–1837) of Dublin in his treatise on venereal diseases published in 1833. The first important description was given in 1913 by Maurice Favre (1876–1954), professor of clinical dermatology at

Lyons, along with two other physicians, Joseph Guillaume Marie Nicolas (1868–1960), a French dermatologist and J. Durand (b 1876). The Frei test, an intradermal diagnostic skin test for lymphogranuloma inguinale, was devised by Wilhelm Siegmund Frei (1885–1943) of Germany in 1925. The common etiological factor of lymphogranuloma venereum and climatic bubo was demonstrated by G.M. Findlay in 1933. *See climatic bubo.*

Lymphosarcoma [Latin: *lymph*, water + *sarcoma*, fleshy excrescence] Differentiated from Hodgkin disease by Julius Dreschfield (1845–1907) in 1892. First described by Hans Kundrat (1845–1893), professor of pathological anatomy in Vienna.

Lysine [Greek: *lyein*, to dissolve] Amino acid first isolated from casein by Drechsel in 1889.

Lysosomes Cell organelles discovered in 1915 by English-born Belgian biochemist, Christian René De Duve (b 1917). He graduated in medicine from Louvain in 1945 and became professor of biochemistry there in 1951 and was appointed to the chair of biochemistry at the Rockefeller Institute, New York in 1962. He shared the Nobel Prize in Physiology or Medicine with Albert Claude (1899–1983) and George Emil Palade (b 1912) in 1974. A detailed description was given by Kurt Aterman in 1952.

Lysozyme [Greek: *lysis*, loosening + *zyme*, leaven] Term coined in 1921 by Sir Alexander Fleming (1881–1955) to denote bacteriolytic substances in nasal secretions and tears.

M

MacAlister, Alexander (1844–1919) Dublin surgeon who was appointed professor of anatomy at Cambridge in 1883, a post which he subsequently held for 36 years. He described the crico-trachealis muscle in 1871.

MacBraire, John (d 1841) Born in Halifax, Nova Scotia, and graduated from Edinburgh University in 1824. He founded the lectureship of jurisprudence at the London Hospital Medical School and published *A System of Nosology* (1830), and *An Introductory Lecture on Medical Jurisprudence* in 1832.

MacBride, David (1727–1778) Physician from Ballymony in Antrim, who served as a surgeon in the army before returning to practice in Dublin in 1749. He published *Experimental Essays* (1764) and *Methodical Introduction to the Theory and Practice of Medicine*. The latter book was highly appreciated by William Cullen (1710–1790) and was translated into Latin.

MacCallum, William George (1874–1944) Canadian-born pathologist who worked at the Johns Hopkins University. He demonstrated the use of calcium in the treatment of tetany following parathyroidectomy. He was also the first to suggest the association between lesions of the Islets of Langehans and glycosuria. He studied fertilization of malarial parasites in birds, which led to his discovery of the sexual phase of malarial parasites in humans.

MacCartney, Sir Samuel Halliday (1833–1906) Born in Castle Douglas, he was a physician who graduated from Edinburgh University. He served as director of the Arsenal at Nanking in China for ten years, and most of his career was involved in establishing political and trade relationships between China and England.

MacConkey Agar Used for culture of bacteria. Consists of a mixture of malachite green, bile, dextrose and meat and was invented by English bacteriologist, Alfred Theodore MacConkey (1861–1931) from Liverpool.

Macewen, Sir William (1848–1924) Born on the island of Bute in Scotland, and educated in Glasgow where he rose to regius professor of surgery at Glasgow Royal Infirmary. His interest in surgery was as a result of Joseph Lister's (1827–1912) teaching, and he used Lister's antiseptic techniques. He was also one of the first to successfully operate on brain tumors, abscesses and trauma and he removed a tumor involving the meninges of the brain in 1879. He carried out some of the first bone grafts, developed new proceedures for hernia repair and treated aneurysms with acupuncture. He wrote *On the Growth of Bone,* published in 1912. He was one of the first to intubate the upper laryngeal orifice and trachea through the mouth, using a metal tube in 1878. He was knighted in 1902.

MacFarlane, Robert Gwyn (1907–1987) Hematologist in Oxford who obtained Factor VIII fraction from bovine blood in 1953.

MacFie, Ronald Campbell (1867–1931) Medical graduate from Aberdeen who wrote several works on science and art. His *Romance of Medicine* was published in 1907, and his other books include *Art of Keeping Well, War* and *Quartercentenary Ode.*

MacGillivray, William (1805–1852) Curator of the Royal College of Surgeons in Edinburgh. He was appointed professor of natural history at Aberdeen University in 1841. He commenced *History of British Birds* in 1848 and completed the five volumes in 1852.

MacGregor, Douglas (1906–1964) Pioneer in industrial psychology who graduated from Harvard in 1935. He published *The Human Side of Enterprise* in 1960.

MacGregor, Sir William (1847–1919) Physician from Aberdeen who practiced in the Seychelles, Mauritius and Fiji. Most of his later career was spent as a diplomat and he was made a Privy Councillor in 1914.

Mach, Ernst (1838–1916) Austrian physicist and philosopher who graduated from Vienna and became professor of mathematics at Graz in 1864. He proposed the concept of 'psychophysics' where all knowledge was a conceptual organization of sensory experience and that not so reducible should be rejected. Albert Einstein (1879–1955) credited Mach with a role in helping him to develop his theory of relativity.

Machaon Greek god of medicine, physician and elder of the two sons of Aesculapius.

Macintosh, Charles (1766–1843) Scottish industrial chemist from Glasgow who was a student of Joseph Black (1728–1799). He invented the waterproof 'Macintosh' cloth in 1820, which was of immense use in surgery, nursing and various other fields. He patented the process in 1823 and started making waterproof cloth on a commercial basis with Thomas Hancock in Manchester. Some historians however have credited the Edinburgh surgeon, James Syme (1799–1870) with the invention of this waterproof cloth. Macintosh also introduced the method of Turkey red dying and the manufacture of cudbear. *See rubber, Syme, James.*

Macintosh, Robert Reynolds (b 1897) Born at Timaru, New Zealand, he was an original member of the All-Blacks rugby football team and trained as a fighter pilot. During World War l he was a prisoner of war. After the war he qualified as a surgeon from Guy's Hospital and obtained his FRCS from Edinburgh. He first practiced anesthesia in London and moved to Oxford in 1937 to take up the first Chair for Anesthesia created by Lord Nuffield. Macintosh traveled widely in America, Japan, Egypt, Canada, South America, Europe and other countries to give advice and promote the practice of anesthesia. He published *Essentials of Anaesthesia* in 1940.

MacIntyre, John (1857–1928) Laryngologist at Glasgow Royal Infirmary and a pioneer in clinical radiology. He established the department of radiology at the infirmary, where his initial training as an electrician helped him to construct the first portable X-ray unit before 1900. MacIntyre was also the editor of the *British Journal of Laryngology*, and applied electricity to medicine.

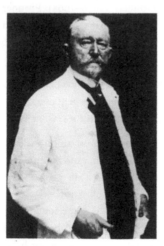

Alwin Mackenrodt (1859–1925). Reproduced with permission from *Zentralblat für Gynäk.* 50:1041, (1926)

Mackenrodt Ligament [Latin: *ligamentum*, bandage] Also called the ligamentum transversum colli of the uterus. It was first described by Alwin Karl Mackenrodt (1859–1925), professor of gynecology at Berlin in 1895.

MacKenzie, Sir James (1853–1925) Regarded as one of the greatest English cardiologists. He was born in Scone,

Scotland and studied medicine at Edinburgh University. He established his practice at Burnley, Lancashire where he developed his own ink polygraph with which he was able to simultaneously record the arterial and venous pulsations during his study on arrhythmias. He was the first to note the loss of effective atrial contraction and named it 'atrial paralysis'. The condition was later re-named 'atrial fibrillation' by Sir Thomas Lewis (1881–1945). MacKenzie also described the functional pathology of cardiac tissue in 1907 and established the use of digitalis in treatment of auricular fibrillation. He published *Diseases of the Heart* (1908), *Principles of Diagnosis and Treatment in Heart Affections* (1916), and *The Future of Medicine* (1919). He was knighted in 1915, and in 1918 he founded the James MacKenzie Institute at St Andrew's to promote clinical research.

MacKenzie, Sir Morell (1853–1925) British laryngologist and surgeon from Leytonstone who became physician to the London Hospital in 1873. He first rose to fame with his publication, *Growths in the Larynx* in 1871 and his magnum opus *Diseases of the Throat and Nose* was published in two volumes between 1880–1884. He presented one of the earliest and largest series on congenital esophageal atresia, consisting of 43 cases, in 1884.

MacKenzie, Richard James (1821–1854) Anatomist and surgeon at the Edinburgh Royal Infirmary. His original contributions to surgery include: *A Successful ligation of Subclavian Artery, Excision of the Knee Joint,* and *Amputation at the Ankle by an Internal Flap.* MacKenzie died of cholera at 33 during his army service in the Crimea.

MacKenzie, Sir Stephen (1844–1909) English physician who described a syndrome of unknown etiology consisting of a feeling of ill health, sensitivity to cold, dyspepsia, and intestinal disorders (MacKenzie syndrome).

MacKenzie, William (1791–1868) Ophthalmologist from Glasgow of international repute. The first specialist eye hospital in Scotland, the Glasgow Eye Infirmary, was founded by him and Monteath in 1824, MacKenzie published *Diseases of the Eye.*

MacKintosh, Sir James (1766–1832) Eminent statesman and lawyer from Inverness who initially qualified in medicine and trained at Leiden. He later took law and practiced at Lincoln's Inn. He subsequently served as an administrator in Bombay, India, where he established a literary society to which he was the first president. On returning to England he took part in many state affairs and brought a motion to amend criminal law in 1818. He published several works on law and history.

Macklin, Alexander Hepburn Born in Melrose, Scotland, he was a medical graduate of Manchester University who joined Shackleton as a medical officer on his Antarctic expedition in 1914. Their ship, *Endurance*, was crushed by ice and sank in the Weddle Sea, but all 28 crew returned safely after a terrible ordeal at sea lasting for over three months. On his return in 1925 he went into general practice in Dundee. In 1947 Macklin was appointed as physician in charge of the student health service at the University of Aberdeen. When he died at the age of 77 years he was still working full time as an orthopedic house officer at Aberdeen.

Maclagan, Sir Andrew Douglas (1812–1900) Leading authority on toxicology and professor of jurisprudence and public health at the University of Edinburgh. He was also a poet, and his collected works, *Nugae Canorae Medicae*, were published in 1850.

Maclean, Hugh (1883–1959) Professor of medicine at the University of London and director of the Medical Clinic at St Thomas' Hospital, who designed the urea concentration test for renal function in 1920. Maclean published *Modern Views on Gastric Digestion* in 1926.

Maclean, John (1771–1814) Physician and son of a surgeon from Glasgow. He emigrated to the United States and became professor of chemistry and natural history at New Jersey College. He published *Lectures on Combustion*.

Macleod, John James Rickard (1876–1935) Scottish professor of physiology from Cluny who graduated from Aberdeen University. He was professor of physiology at the Western Reserve University, Cleveland in 1903, and later appointed to the chair of physiology at Toronto in 1918. He began his research on carbohydrates in 1907, and published a book on diabetes in 1913. His famous, *Physiology and Biochemistry in Modern Medicine*, which ran into 7 editions, was first published in 1918. He employed Frederick Banting (1891–1941) and Charles Best (1899–1978) for experiments on the pancreas in 1921. While he was on holiday in Scotland, Banting and Best succeeded in producing the first extract of pancreas which effectively reduced blood sugar levels in pancreatectomized dogs. Macleod shared the Nobel Prize with Banting for the discovery of insulin in 1923. He returned to Aberdeen as professor of physiology in 1928.

Macleod, John (1782–1820) Physician from Burnhill, Dumbartonshire in Scotland. He made several voyages as a naval surgeon and also served in China. He published *The Voyage of Alceste to the Island of Lewchew*.

Macleod, Roderick (1795–1852) Scottish physician who described a syndrome of effusion into the synovial capsules, bursae, and sheaths in rheumatoid arthritis.

Macleod Syndrome Consisting of abnormal radiotranslucency of one lung with no apparent clinical abnormality was first described by British physician, William Mathieson Macleod (1911–1977) in 1954.

MacNamara, Dame Annie Jean (1899–1968) Australian physician, born in Beechworth, Victoria, and educated at Melbourne University. Her special interest was poliomyelitis and she discovered (together with Sir Frank MacFarlane Burnett, 1899–1985) that there was more than one strain of the virus. This paved the way for development of the Salk vaccine. She also introduced the first iron lung into Australia.

MacNish, Robert (1802–1837) Physician from Glasgow who obtained his master of surgery at the age of 17. He received his medical diploma following his thesis, *Anatomy of Drunkenness*, which was published in 1827. MacNish's other publications include: *Philosophy of Sleep* (1830), *Book of Aphorisms* (1834), and *Introduction to Phrenology* (1835).

Macquer, Pierre Joseph (1718–1784) French chemist and physician who obtained his medical degree from Paris in 1742. He published *Élemens de chyme théorique* and the first dictionary on chemistry, *Dictionnaire de chyme*, in 1766.

Macrocyte [Greek: *makros*, large + *kytos*, cell] Danish physician, Hans Christian Joachim Gram (1853–1938) was one of the first to recognize the occurrence of abnormally large red blood cells, or macrocytes, in cases of pernicious anemia and jaundice due to liver disease.

Macrophage [Greek: *makros*, large + *phagein*, eat] Mononuclear phagocyte arising from bone marrow cell. The term was first coined by Elie Metchnikoff (1845–1916) to denote certain cells with characteristic distribution and staining.

Macula [Latin: *macula*, spot] *See retina.*

MacWilliam, John Alexander (1857–1937) Professor of physiology at the University of Aberdeen who gave the first account of death due to ventricular fibrillation in 1889. He also devised the MacWilliam test for albuminuria, using a saturated solution of salicylsulfonic acid.

MacWilliam Test *See MacWilliam, John Alexander.*

Mad Houses Established for the insane and mentally ill. In London they were mostly privately owned by physicians. A mad house at Clerkenwell Green, one of the first to appear in London in 1674, was owned by James Newton who called himself an expert in madness and melancholy. This was taken over by his son, from whom William Battie took over in 1704. It was later run by John Monroe (1715–1791) and his son and became a boarding school in 1803.

Madden, Richard Robert (1798–1886) Son of a silk manufacturer from Dublin. He graduated as a physician in 1829 and obtained his fellowship of the Royal College of Surgeons in 1855. For a short period he was a newspaper correspondent in Italy before he returned to Curzon Street, Mayfair where he practiced surgery. He became colonial secretary to Western Australia in 1847 and protected the rights of the aborigines. Madden also served in Ireland for a short period. He wrote *Phantasmata, Illusions and Fanaticisms* in 1857, and several other books of varying interest.

Maddox, Ernest Edmund (1860–1933) English ophthalmologist from Bournemouth who devised several visual tests and designed a number of eye instruments.

Madelung, Otto Wilhelm (1846–1926) German surgeon from Gotha, who served as professor at Strasburg. He described congenital dislocation of the wrist.

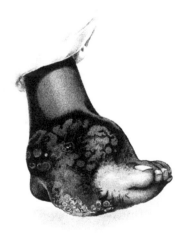

Madura Foot. H. Vandyke Carter, *Mycetoma of Fungus Diseases of India*. Churchill, London

Madura Foot [Madurai: a town in South India] This was described under the name 'padavalmika' (meaning foot-ant-hill) in the *Athara Veda* of the Brahmins written around 1000 BC. It was observed in India by a physician from Westphalia, Englebert Kaempfer (1651–1716), who called it 'perical' (Tamil: *peri*, big + *kal*, leg) in 1712. The first mention as a specific disease is found in Brett's *Surgery of India*, published in 1840. It was also described by George Ballingal (1778–1855) who suggested a parasitic cause in 1818. Eyre gave another account in 1860, and a more detail study was done by Henry Vandyke Carter (1831–1907) in 1874. Jean Hyacinthe Vincent (1862–1950) identified the causative agent and

named it *Streptomyces madurae* in 1894. Various species of actinomyces fungus were shown as a cause of it by E. Pinoy in 1913. The first cure, using neoarsphenamine, was reported by L. C. Audrain in the *Journal of American Association* in 1924.

Maffucci, Angelo (1845–1903) Italian pathologist from Genoa, who was a pioneer in the study of tuberculosis. He isolated the avian tubercle bacillus (*B. gallinaceous*) in 1890. The Maffucci syndrome is endochondromatosis with cutaneous hemangioma.

Magdalen College Founded in 1578 at Oxford. The hospital was later annexed and it was converted to college of 'secular persons studying theology and philosophy'. It was intimately connected with the teaching of medicine and a charter of the old hospital at Oxford is still preserved in its archives.

Magendie, François (1783–1855) Pioneer of pharmacology and founder of experimental physiology. He was professor of pathology at the College of France, and physician to the Hôtel Dieu. He was born in Bordeaux and graduated in medicine from Paris in 1808. He described the mechanism of deglutition and vomiting in 1813, showing the three stages of passage of the food through the mouth, pharynx and esophagus. He also described the functions of the CSF in 1825. The foramen of Magendie of the brain, a canal leading to the fourth ventricle, was described by him in 1828. Magendie came to England in 1831 to study cholera and served on the Committee of Public Health. He founded the first physiology journal, *Journal de Physiologie Expérimentale*. See Bell–Magendie law.

Maggot Dominique Jean Larrey (1766–1842), the legendary French military surgeon, was the first to describe the therapeutic effect of maggots on wounds in 1812. His method was revived by orthopedic surgeon from Baltimore, William Stevenson Baer (1872–1931), who used them to treat chronic osteomyelitis in 1931.

Magic Bullet *See salvarsan, side-chain theory.*

Magill Tube Endotracheal tube used in anesthesia and resuscitation. Devised by Sir Ivan Whiteside Magill (1888–1986), consultant to the Brompton and Westminster Hospitals in London.

Magitot Disease A form of osteoperiostitis of the alveoli of the teeth. First described in 1867 by French dentist, Emile Magitot (1833–1897).

Magnesium Carbonate Probably first used as a medicine by the Count de Palma in Rome. The compound was known to alchemists and is mentioned in Geber's works. It was introduced into the materia medica by Friedrich Hoffmann

(1660–1742). Sulfate of magnesia was discovered in a spring in Epsom, Surrey by a physician, Nehemiah Grew (1641–1712) in 1675. *See Epsom Salt.*

Magnesium Deficiency First noted to be endemic in cattle pastured in fields heavily fertilized with organic nitrates. The disease was called 'grass staggers' or 'grass tetany'. Its cause was later identified to be due to the formation of a complex between insoluble ammonium magnesium phosphate and the fertilizer which impaired the absorption of magnesium. The method to estimate small quantities of magnesium in blood was first devised by A.P. Briggs in 1922. Magnesium deficiency in man is uncommon and the first experimentally induced magnesium depletion in man was reported by M.E. Shils of America in 1964. The symptomatology of the two cases described by him was similar to that of calcium depletion.

Magnesium Element first obtained by Sir Humphry Davy (1778–1829) in 1807. The metal became popular in the 19th century as a source of bright light when burnt. The first photographs of the interior of the pyramids were taken with the help of magnesium lamps in 1865. *See magnesium deficiency.*

Magnet *See electricity, magnetic cure, magnetism.*

Magnetic Cure Aetius of Amida, a Byzantine physician around AD 600, recommended its use for treatment of gout affecting the hands. Paracelsus (1493–1541) and Athanasius Kircher (1601–1680) also recommended it for several diseases. In the 17th century magnetic toothpicks and earpicks were sold as secret remedies for diseases of teeth, ear, and eyes. Hildanus Fabricius (1560–1634) and Giovanni Morgagni (1682–1771) used them to remove foreign bodies made of iron from the eyes. In 1770 Father Hehl, a Jesuit priest and professor of astronomy in Vienna, used a lodestone in treatment of diseases and invented several devices and plates for this purpose. He was a friend of Franz Anton Mesmer (1734–1815), whose work on animal magnetism was probably inspired by Hehl.

Magnetic Resonance Imaging (MRI) The method of molecular beam magnetic resonance was developed to study atomic nuclei by Austrian-American physicist, Isidor Rabi (1898–1988), and German-American physicist Polykarp Kusch (b 1911) in 1937. It was demonstrated by Zurich-born American physicist, Felix Bloch (1905–1983) professor at Stanford University, and Edward Mills Purcell (b 1912) of Illinois, in 1946. It was used for over 40 years to study molecular structure in organic chemistry until it was applied to living tissues by Swedish physicist, Erik Odeblad,

around 1960. English chemist, Sir Rex Edward Richards (b 1922), later vice-chancellor of Oxford University, made a significant contribution to the development of NMR as a diagnostic technique in medicine in the late 1960s. The first image was produced by Paul Lauterbur, professor at the University of Illinois, Chicago in 1973, although the appreciable clinical images of the brain were produced only around 1980. The two dimensional Fourier transformed NMR, of more use in biology and medicine was pioneered by Swiss physical chemist, Richard Robert Ernst (b 1933).

Magnetism Phenomenon exhibited by the lodestone, known to Homer, Aristotle, and Pliny. Greeks obtained lodestone from Asia around 1000 BC. Roger Bacon in the 13th century was acquainted with the property of a needle pointing to the north. Another Englishman, Robert Norman from London also observed the phenomenon in 1576. Gilbert's famous treatise *De Magnete* was published in 1600. The first scientific theory was announced by Réné Descartes (1596–1650) in his *Principia Philosophiae* published in 1644. Artificial magnets were made by Gown Knight in 1756, and electromagnetic induction was discovered by Michael Faraday (1791–1867). The first special observatory to study terrestrial magnetism was established by Carl Friedrich Gauss (1777–1855) at Göttingen in 1834.

Magnus-Levy, Adolf (1865–1955) American physiologist of German origin who pioneered study of the thyroid. In 1895 he administered thyroid extract from animals to humans and found that their basal metabolic rate became elevated. He was a pupil of Bernard Naunym (1839–1925) and studied the role of metabolites in diabetic coma.

Magoun, Horace Winchell (1907–1971) American neuroscientist and pioneer in neuroendocrinology from Philadelphia. His early research was on the structure and function of the hypothalamus in relation to sleep, eating and body temperature. In 1963 he wrote *The Waking Brain* on brain–endocrine interactions. He helped found the Brain Research Institute at UCLA.

Mahavira (*c* AD 850) Great Hindu mathematician from Mysore whose work included a discussion of operations including zero, and treatment of division by zero as having no effect on the dividend. He also gave several verbal problems in arithmetic.

Mahomed, Frederick Akbar (1849–1884) Physician who graduated from Guy's Hospital, and practiced there for most of his career. He was a pioneer in the study of blood pressure in clinical medicine and used his own modified spygmograph for this.

Maida Vale Hospital Founded as the London Infirmary for Epilepsy and Paralysis by Julius Althaus (1831–1900), a physician in 1866. Its original location was at Marylebone, and it moved to its Maida Vale site in 1903.

Maier Sinus A depression in the internal surface of the lachrymal sac. It was described by Rudolph Maier (1824–1888), professor of pathological anatomy at Freiburg, in 1859.

Maier, Rudolph (1824–1888) *See Maier sinus, periarteritis nodosa.*

Maimonides (1135–1204) Also known as Rabbi Moses ben Maimon. He was a Jewish physician from Cordoba and a pupil of Avenzoar (AD 1070). He fled from Spain due to persecution of Jews and, after having lost his fortune, settled in Egypt where he became physician to Saladin (1170–1193), the first sultan of Egypt. His book on diet and personal hygiene, *Tractus de regime sanitatis* (Book of Counsel), was written in the form of letters to the Sultan. Maimonides had an ethical, philosophical and religious approach to medicine, and often quoted from the Bible. He translated the *Canon of Avicenna* into Hebrew and made a collection of the aphorisms of Hippocrates (460–377 BC) and Galen (AD 129–200), *Aphorismen Mosis*. His treatise in 1198 on reptile poison and antidotes was frequently referred to by Western physicians. He also wrote a treatise on asthma, *Tractus contra Passionem Asmatis*, the manuscripts of which are in Madrid.

Maisonneuve, Jules Germain François (1809–1897) French surgeon, eponomously remembered for his amputation, sign and urethrotome. *See gas gangrene, intestinal anastomosis.*

Mal de Rosa A condition now known as pellagra. It was described by Gaspar Casal (1679–1759), a Spanish physician, in 1735.

Maladie de Roger (Roger disease) A defect in the interventricular septum of the heart. Described in 1879 by Henri Louis Roger (1809–1891), a surgeon in Paris.

Malarene A cinchona febrifuge preparation introduced in 1926 as treatment for malaria in Madras, India.

Malaria Inoculation Form of fever therapy for neurological diseases, first suggested by Austrian psychiatrist, Julius Wagner-Jauregg (1857–1940), in 1887 for cases of dementia paralytica. In 1917 he demonstrated the beneficial effects of treating general syphilitic paresis by inoculation with malaria, and his method remained one of the main treatments for syphilis until penicillin was proved to be effective by John F. Mahoney (1889–1957) and co-workers in the US

Public Health Service in 1943.

Malaria The disease dates back to ancient times and the Egyptian word 'Aat' inscribed at the temple of Dendrah is supposed to indicate the annual recurrence of malaria. Periodic fevers were also noted by Hippocrates (460–377 BC), who classified them into quotidian, tertian, subtertian and quartan depending on their periodicity. Malarial epidemics plagued ancient Rome and the illness was familiar to Galen (AD 129–200) and Aulus Cornelius Celsus (25 BC–AD 50). The introduction of cinchona in 1630 by Spanish physician Juan del Vego helped to differentiate malaria from other fevers, although nothing was known of the etiology. Italian physician, Francesco Torti (1658–1741), introduced cinchona into Italy and coined the term 'mal aria' (bad air) for it in 1712. Johann Friedrich Meckel (1781–1833) noticed certain pigments in the cells of the spleen and blood in malaria, and this was confirmed by Rudolph Virchow (1821–1902). Their significance was not recognized until Alphonse Laveran (1845–1922), professor of pathological anatomy at the University of Rome, recognized in 1880 that they represented malarial parasites. Ettore Marchiafava (1847–1935) observed them in 1885 in red blood cells as hemocytozoa, described their life cycle, and a gave the first description of *Plasmodium*. Natives of some countries noticed the relationship of malaria to mosquito bites but this was not scientifically pursued until 1894 when Sir Patrick Manson (1844–1922) proposed the extracorporeal life cycle for the malarial parasite in the mosquito. His suggestion was followed up by Sir Ronald Ross (1857–1932) who demonstrated the presence of the parasite in the *Anopheles* mosquito in 1897. *See cinchona bark, antimalarials.*

Malaria Therapy *See malaria inoculation, artificial fever.*

Malassez Disease Testicular cyst described by French physiologist, Louis Charles Malassez (1842–1909) of Paris in 1875.

Malecot Catheter Large-bore suprapubic urinary catheter designed by French surgeon in Paris, Achille Etienne Malecot (b 1852).

Male Fern Oil from the rhizome of *Dryopteris Felix mas* was used as a vermifuge by Theophrastus (372–287 BC), Dioscorides (AD 40–90) and Pliny (AD 23–79). Valerius Cordus (1515–1544) of Hesse and Daniel Mathieu, an apothecary from Neuchatel, France, used it successfully for treatment of helminthic worms in the 18th century, and his secret formula was purchased by Frederick the Great for an annuity of 30 pounds and title of councilor in 1770.

Male Hormones *See androgens.*

Male Sterility *See post-coital test*

Malformation *See teratology, congenital heart disease.*

Malgaigne, Joseph François (1806–1865) Professor of surgery at Paris who described the superior carotid triangle in 1837. He was also the first to use ether for anesthesia in France.

Malinowski, Bronislaw (1884–1942) Polish anthropologist from Cracow who settled in London. He founded the field of social anthropology and his publications include: *Crime and Custom in Savage Society* (1926), *Sex and Repression in Savage Society* (1927), and *A Scientific Theory of Culture* (1944).

Mall, Franklin Paine (1862–1917) Born in Belle Plaine, Iowa, he was professor of anatomy at Johns Hopkins University and director of embryological studies at the Carnegie Institute. He described the small areas of splenic pulps (Mall lobules) within the spleen in 1898.

Mallory, Franklin Burr (1862–1941) American pathologist from Harvard. He was a pioneer in the study of stains in histology and he devised the Mallory stain for identifying collagen fibers in 1900.

Mallory–Weiss Syndrome Hematemesis due to post-emetic mucosal laceration of the lower esophagus and gastric cardia. First recognized by American professor of pathology at Boston University, Kenneth G. Mallory (b 1900) and American physician, Soma Weiss (1898–1942), in 1929.

Malpighi, Marcello (1628–1694) Founder of microscopical anatomy, born in Bologna, Italy, where he studied philosophy and medicine. He became professor of physick in 1656 at Pisa and moved to Messina in 1662. He described capillary anastomosis in *De Pulmonibus*, published in 1661. The uriniferous tubules or the Malpighian bodies were discovered by him in 1666, and he first observed the ductus epoophori in 1681. He became physician to Pope Innocent XII in 1691 and died in Rome.

Malta Fever (Syn: Mediterranean fever, Neapolitan fever, Rock fever of Gibraltar) Brucellosis was first named Malta Fever as physicians mistakenly thought that it was confined to Malta. Sir David Bruce (1855–1931) isolated the bacteria in 1887 and the organism was named *Brucella* in his honor. *See abortus fever, Bang, Bernhard, brucellosis.*

Malthus, Thomas Robert (1766–1834) Clergyman from Dorking, England and pioneer in economics and statistics. He was a curate at Albury before becoming the first professor of history and political economy at Haileybury College, founded by the East India Company, in 1805. His *Essay on the Principle of Population or A View of its Past and Present Effects* was published anonymously in 1789. In it he suggested checks on population by moral restraint and late marriage. It aroused controversy and led to the formation of the Malthusian League to defend and propagate his ideas. *See statistics.*

Malus, Étienne Louis (1775–1812) Physicist from Paris who served as a military engineer in Napoleon's army from 1796 to 1801. He discovered polarization of light by reflection.

Mammography [Latin: *mamma*, breast; Greek: *grapho*, write] Used to detect breast cancer. Developed by German surgeon, A. Salomen, in 1913.

Mammoth Fossil tusks and a full body of this extinct elephant were found in Siberia between 1765 and 1797. One of the earliest known decorative amulets made from a mammoth's tooth by Neanderthal man, dating back 100,000 years, was found in Hungary. A tooth with an engraving of a mammoth on it was found by Armand Isidore Hippolyte Lartet (1801–1871) in 1860. Half the world's ivory source in the 19th century came from the fossil tusks of mammoths. Georges Cuvier (1769–1832) attributed its extinction to a catastrophic change in climate. In 1977 a baby mammoth which was frozen in ice for over 40,000 years was found in Siberia.

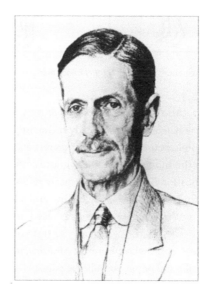

Archibald Donald (1860–1937). Reproduced from *J. Obst & Gynae. Brit. Emp.* 47, 527 (1937)

Manchester Operation For uterine prolapse, involving high amputation of the cervix and repair of the anterior and posterior vaginal walls. Devised by Archibald Donald (1860–1937) of Manchester, and his assistant William Edward Fothergill (1865–1926) of Southampton, in 1890.

Mandelic Acid First used in treatment of urinary tract infections by Max Leonhard Rosenheim (1908–1972) in 1935.

Mandeville, Bernard (1670–1733) Dutch physician from Dorpat who settled in London around 1700. He published *The Virgin Unmasked* (1709), *Hypochondria and Hysteric Passions* (1711), and several other works.

Mandible The first description of the dislocation of the mandible and its treatment by manipulative reduction is found in an Egyptian papyrus (1600 BC) known as the Edwin Smith Papyrus. A specialist book on oral surgery was written by Berchillet Anselme Louis Bernard Jourdain (1734–1816) and describes disease of the mandible in detail.

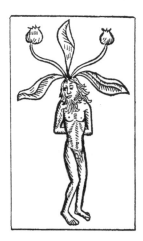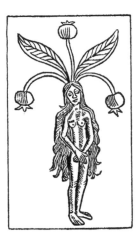

Mandrake. Illustrations from 15th century French manuscript, *Hortus Sanitatus*

Mandrake Also known as *Mandragora* root, in the family Solanaceae. Ancient herbal remedy and an important ingredient in philters used by ancient sorcerers. Its root is said to resemble the human form. Theophrastus called it 'anthropomorphos' for this reason. Shakespeare refers to the root in at least four plays. The Babylonians and Hebrews were familiar with it and a wine was used in surgery by Dioscorides (AD 40–90) during the time of Nero. Aulus Cornelius Celsus, who wrote *De Medicina,* mentioned use of mandrake and poppy for relief of pain.

Manetho (*c* 200 BC) Egyptian priest and a historian at the Alexandrian Museum who recorded the antiquities of Egypt. His works were destroyed by Bishop Eusebius to preserve the traditions and beliefs of the Old Testament.

Manganese Metallic manganese was produced on a large scale by Swedish mineralogist, Johann Gotlieb Gahn (1745–1818). The first record of poisoning by manganese dioxide

during the manufacture of bleaching powder from chlorine was described in five factory workers in France, by J. Couper in 1837. The extrapyramidal syndrome resembling Parkinsonism in manganese poisoning was also observed by Couper in 1821 and later by Rudolf von Jaksch (1855–1947) in 1901.

Mania Described as psychiatric illnesses by physicians of the Hippocratic period. The other groups of major mental illnesses in their classification included epilepsy, melancholia and paranoia. Phillipe Pinel (1745–1826) divided mania into two groups, one with delirium and other without. *See manic-depressive psychosis.*

Manic Depressive Psychosis Aretaeus of Cappadocia (AD 82–138) studied mental illness and concluded that manic and depressive states could occur in the same patient. This was probably the earliest recognition of bipolar illness. Jean Pierre Falret (1794–1870), French psychiatrist, recognized the alternating moods of excitement and depression and named the condition 'de la folie circulare' in 1854. Jules Gabriel François Baillarger (1809–1890) in the 19th century described the same syndrome as 'folie a double forme' and it became known as manic depressive psychosis. Although John Frederick Joseph Cade (b 1912) demonstrated the use of lithium in psychiatry in 1949, its use in preventing manic and depressive episodes was only established around 1967.

Mann, John Dixon (1840–1912) Manchester physician and forensic toxicologist. He described a change in electrical resistance of the skin thought to be associated with certain neuroses.

Manna The sugary sap of the plant, *Fraxinus ornus,* which grows on the Mediterranean coast, from Spain to Smyrna. In summer it trickles from the branches like white honey, and it has been used as a food and gentle laxative since Biblical times. Manna may also be obtained from the tamarisk tree, *Tamarisk gallica* var *mannifera* which, when attacked by the insect, *Coccus manniparus,* bleeds a honey-like substance. However, modern research says that the manna from the Sinai peninsula is actually an exudate from the insects and, furthermore, the biblical manna was a form of fungus. The Bedouins use it as a condiment and it has been used as an alternative to sugar for diabetics. Its content was analyzed by Marcellin Berthelot (1827–1907) in 1861 and it was found to contain 1.5 % water, 55 % cane sugar, 25 % invert sugar, and 20 % dextrin and vegetable mucus.

Mannaberg, Julian (b 1860) Viennese physician who described the accentuation of the second heart sound (Mannaberg sign) in appendicitis and abdominal diseases.

Mannkopf Sign Increase in pulse rate on applying pressure over the site of pain, mainly to distinguish it from simulated pain. Described by German physician, Emil Wilhelm Mannkopf (1836–1918).

Manson, Sir Patrick (1844–1922) Father of tropical medicine in England, born in Fingask, Aberdeen, Scotland. After obtaining his medical degree from Aberdeen University, he worked in Formosa and China (1871) and Hong Kong (1883). He studied the cause of elephantiasis in China and showed that it was caused by a parasite spread by the mosquito, the first disease shown to be transmitted by an insect vector. On his return he established a successful practice in London in 1890 and founded the London School of Tropical Medicine in 1899. Manson proposed the extracorporeal life cycle for the malarial parasite in the mosquito in 1894 and his suggestion was followed up by Sir Ronald Ross (1857–1932) who demonstrated its presence in the *Anopheles* mosquito in 1897. Manson also described the periodicity of filarial parasite and identified the *Anopheles* mosquito as its vector in 1879. Tokelau disease, described in the Philippines by Sir William Dampier (1652–1751) during his voyage around the world in 1686, was first identified as a fungal disease by Manson in 1879. Manson's *Tropical Diseases* was first published in 1898.

Mansur Hospital *See Egyptian medicine.*

Mantoux Test Intradermal tuberculin test for diagnosis of tuberculosis was devised by Austrian pediatrician, Clemens von Pirquet (1874–1929) in 1907. Old tuberculin was applied to the skin with a needle scratch in Pirquet's technique. Subcutaneous injection of a controlled amount of tuberculin for diagnosis of tuberculosis was introduced by a French physician, Charles Mantoux (1877–1947) in 1910. The Heaf gun for use in the tuberculin test was devised by British physician, Frederick R.G. Heaf (b 1895).

Manubrium [Latin: *manubrium*, handle] *See angle of Louis.*

Manz, Wilhelm (1833–1911) Professor of ophthalmology at Freiburg who described epithelial utricles found on the cornea (Manz utricular glands) in 1859.

Maple Bark Disease Also known as maple bark stripper's lung, an allergy caused by spores in the bark of stored timber. Described by Towey and co-workers of Michigan in 1932.

Maple Syrup Disease *See Menkes syndrome.*

Mapp, Sara *See bone setters.*

Marbeck, Roger (1536–1605) Clergyman from Windsor who graduated in medicine from Oxford University in 1573. He was the first registrar of the Royal College of Physicians and served as chief of physicians to Queen Elizabeth.

Marble Bone Disease *See Albers Schönberg.*

Marburg Disease African hemorrhagic fever or green monkey disease, similar to that caused by Ebola virus. Acute febrile illness with a high mortality. Reported from Marburg in Germany in 1967.

Marcacci, Arturo (1854–1915) Professor of physiology at Pavia who described the muscle fibers underlying the areola of the nipple (Marcacci muscles) in 1883.

Marsilio Ficino (1433–1499) Physician who translated Plato. He was born in Florence and became tutor to the sons of Cosmo de Medici. He wrote *Liber de Vita* in 1489, 'for the health of students or those who work in letters'. He called Galen the physician of the body, and Plato the physician of the soul. He published a treatise on health and long life.

Marcet, Alexander (1770–1822) British clinical chemist. He graduated from Edinburgh and practiced in London before he went to Switzerland in 1814. He published *An Essay on the Chemical History of Calculi.* Marcet died while on a short visit to London.

March Albuminuria *See benign albuminuria.*

Marchand, Felix Jacob (1846–1928) German pathologist, born in Halle. In 1872 he used a crude differential rheotome connected to a galvanometer to measure the electrical variation of the frog's heart at given intervals of time. He also gave the first pathological account of carotid body tumors in 1891 while professor of pathology at Giessen. The term 'atherosclerosis' was introduced by him while he was professor at Leipzig in 1904. The abnormal position of suprarenal glands in certain patients was described by him in 1891.

Marchant, Gerard (1850–1903) Born in Toulouse, France, and practiced as a surgeon in Paris. The points or areas of easily detachable connections of the dura mater to the basal, sphenoidal, and occipital bones of the skull (Marchant zone) were described by him in 1881.

Marchi, Vittorio (1851–1908) Anatomist from Florence who described the anterolateral descending tract of the spinal cord (Marchi tract) in 1887.

Marchiafava, Ettore (1847–1935) Italian pathologist who described malarial parasites in red blood cells as 'hemo-cytozoa' in 1885. He gave the first description of *Plasmodium* in 1880.

Marchiafava–Bignami Syndrome A neurological disorder consisting of tremor, convulsions and coma related to alcohol intake, first described by Ettore Marchiafava (1847–1935) and Amico Bignami (1862–1929) in 1903.

Marchiafava–Micheli Syndrome Named after Ettore Marchiafava (1847–1935) and Ferdinando Micheli (1847–1935). *See paroxysmal hemoglobinuria.*

Marcille, Maurice (1871–1941) French surgeon who designed a motor ambulance during World War 1. He also described the triangle in the ilioinguinal region (Marcille triangle), formed by the medial margin of the psoas muscle, lateral border of the vertebral column and the ilio-lumbar vertebral ligament.

Marcille Triangle *See Marcille, Maurice.*

Marcy, Henry Orlando (1837–1924) Born in Otis, Massachusetts, American surgeon who introduced antiseptic sutures in the surgical treatment of hernia in 1878. He wrote an important treatise on hernia and another on surgery of the perineum in 1889.

Marechal, George (1658–1736) Surgeon from Calais who attended Louis XIV for an abscess in his neck and was later appointed as his surgeon.

Marek Disease Herpes virus-induced neoplasm associated with polyneuritis in fowls, first described by Josef Marek (1867–1952) of Germany in 1907.

Marey, Etienne-Jules (1830–1904) French physiologist who obtained the first tracing of the impulse of the heart on the radial artery during the cardiac cycle, using smoke-covered paper on a drum in 1863. A method of obtaining myograms introduced by H. von Helmholtz (1821–1894) in 1851 was improved by Marey around 1870.

Marfan Syndrome A disorder of collagen and elastic tissue. Slender long limbs, ectopia lentis, cardiovascular defects and hypermobility of the joints. Described by Antoine Bernard Jean Marfan (1858–1942), a pediatrician from Paris in 1896. The term 'arachnodactily' was coined by Emile Charles Achard (1860–1944) of Paris to denote the spider-like appearance of the fingers seen in Marfan syndrome in 1902.

Margarine Invented at a competition organized by Napoleon III to find an alternative to butter. Its inventor, a Frenchman, Hippolyte Merge-Mouries (1817–1880) prepared it from melted tallow, butter, milk and vegetable oils in 1868. The modern process was patented by F. Boudet in 1872. Catalytic hydrogenation of oils used for producing it was discovered by Paul Sabatier (1854–1941), French professor of chemistry at the Academy of Sciences, and Jean Baptiste Senderens (1856–1936).

Marggrafe, Andreas Sigismond (1709–1782) German chemist and agricultural scientist who discovered sugar in sugar beet. He identified it from crystals using a microscope, the first time that the microscope had been used for chemical identification. *See beet sugar.*

Mariani Elixir French chemist, Angelo Mariani realized the value of coca in the 18th century and imported it from South America. It was sold under various names such as 'Mariani wine', 'Mariani elixir', 'Mariani tea' and 'Mariani lozenges'.

Mariani Coca *See coca.*

Mariano, Santo de Barletta (1490–1550) Neapolitan surgeon who described the perineal median operation for stone in the bladder in 1535.

Marie, Pierre (1853–1940) Pupil of Jean Charcot (1825–1893) in Paris, he was the first to observe pituitary disorder associated with gigantism in 1886. He described the clinical features in two female patients and named it acromegaly in 1886. He later published a series of 17 cases of acromegaly in 1888, but did not ascribe any cause to the disorder. Marie also described the condition which is now known as ankylosing spondylitis in *La Spondylose rhizomelique* in 1898. This disease is also known as Marie–Strümpell arthritis. The condition of hypertrophic pulmonary osteoarthropathy (Marie–Bamberger disease) was described by him in 1890.

Marihuana *See Cannabis sativa, hashish,*

Marinesco, Georges (1863–1938) Neurologist at Bucharest who described trophic changes in the skin of the hand in cases of syringomyelia. He demonstrated the fatality of removing the pituitary glands in animals in 1895.

Mariotte, Edmé (1620–1684) Born in Burgundy, he was a French prior at the Cloister of Saint Martin, Dijon, before he moved to Paris in 1670. He proposed some important theories on hydromechanics, and investigated the sap pressure in plants which he compared to the circulating blood in animals, in 1676. He was one of the founder members of Academie des Sciences, and the blind spot of the retina was discovered by him in 1668.

Marischal College University of Aberdeen, founded at the site of Greyfriars Monastery by George Keith, the 5th Earl of Marischal in Scotland in 1593. A chair in medicine at the college was created by the 9th Earl in 1700, to which Patrick Chalmers was appointed as first professor. The original building was demolished in 1840, new buildings appeared at Broad Street in 1895.

Marjolin Ulcer Results from breakdown of a cicatrix. It was described by French surgeon, Jean Nicolas Marjolin (1780–1850). Some historians have credited another French physician, R. Majolin (1812–1895), with the first description of the ulcer.

Markam, Sir Robert Clements (1830–1916) Born in Stillingfleet, near York, he was educated at Westminster, and started his career as a clerk in London. He later traveled to South America to study the history of the Incas. During his travels he became interested in Peruvian bark. On his return to London he organized an expedition in 1859 and successfully brought back cinchona plants and seed from Peru which were later used to develop cinchona cultivation in British India and Ceylon. Markam served as president of the Royal Geographical Society from 1893 to 1905.

Marmite Autolyzed yeast product, found to be as effective as liver extract in treatment of tropical nutritional anemia by British biochemist, Lucy Wills in 1931. Also shown to be effective in treatment of macrocytic anemia caused by idiopathic steatorrhoea by J.M.Vaughan and D. Hunter in 1932.

Marmod of Anjou (*c* AD 1123) Medieval writer whose work was amongst the first to bring Arab influence into European medical systems. His *Liber Lapadium* contains descriptions of 60 different stones with medical virtues.

Marriotte, Edmé (1620–1684) French physicist. *See blind spot.*

Marrow [Anglo-Saxon: *mearg,* pith] *See bone marrow.*

Marryat, Thomas (1730–1792) London physician who graduated from Edinburgh University. His *Sentimental Fables for the Ladies* was published at Belfast in 1771 and reprinted at Bristol in 1791.

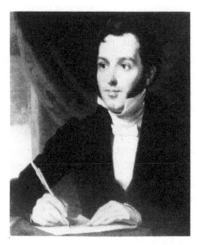

William Marsden (1796–1867)

Marsden, William (1796–1867) London surgeon who founded the Royal Free and Royal Marsden Hospitals (formerly the London Cancer Hospital).

Marsh, James (1789–1846) London chemist and toxicologist who served as assistant to Faraday. He designed the chemical test (Marsh test) used in forensic medicine to distinguish antimony from arsenic.

Marshal, Andrew (1742–1813) Physician from Fife who studied at Glasgow and Edinburgh Universities. His *The Morbid Anatomy of the Brain* was published after his death.

Marshall, Eli Kinnerly (1889–1966) American pharmacologist and physiologist at the Johns Hopkins in Baltimore. He demonstrated the secretory function of the renal convoluted tubule by using phenolsulfonephthalein in 1924. He introduced sulfaguanidine for treatment of bacillary dysentery in 1941.

Marshall, Francis Hugh Adam (1878–1949) Born in High Wycome, Buckinghamshire, he was a pioneer in the physiology of reproduction, who published a classic on the subject in 1910.

Marshall, John (1818–1891) Professor of surgery at University College London who described the vena cava and the associated structures in 1850.

Marston, Robert (1853–1925) Dentist from Leicester, England, who patented the first modern anesthetic injector for regulating the strength of anesthetic vapor in 1898. He published *Anesthetist's Pocket Companion* in 1899.

Martin, Archer John Porter (b 1910) London biochemist educated at Cambridge University, and did research on vitamins at the Lister Institute. He demonstrated the importance of nicotinic acid, aneurin and riboflavin. His most important contribution was the development of partition chromatography for separating amino acids (with Richard Laurence Millington Synge, b 1914) in 1941. He also introduced electrodialysis for deionising protein hydrolysates in 1947, for which he shared the Nobel Prize for Chemistry with Synge in 1952.

Martin, August (1847–1933) Berlin gynecologist who performed an incision of the cervix in a case of difficult delivery due to an unyielding cervix in 1883. He also designed a caliper for pelvimetry.

Martin, Benjamin (1704–1782) Mathematician and optician in London, born at Worplesdon in Surrey. He practiced as an optician and globemaker at Fleet Street and published several mathematical treatises and papers on natural philosophy.

Martin, George (1702–1743) Scottish physician who qualified from Leiden. He accompanied Lord Cathcart to America and died there. He published *Tractus de Similebus, Animalibus, et Animalium Colore* and several other treatises.

Martin, Sir James Ranald (1793–1874) Scottish surgeon who served in India for 44 years and published an early treatise on tropical diseases, *Influence of Tropical Climates on European Constitutions* in 1855. He was a founder of the Royal Victoria Hospital at Netley.

Martindale, William (1840–1902) London pharmacist who first published *Extra Pharmacopoeia* in 1883, and continued through ten editions during his lifetime. He also served as president of the Pharmaceutical Society of Great Britain in 1899.

Martinotti Cells A distinct type of cell in the cerebral cortex, described by Giovanni Martinotti (1857–1928), professor of anatomy at Bologna, in 1888.

Mascagni, Paul (1752–1815) Anatomist from Tuscany in Italy and a professor at Florence. He gave original descriptions of several anatomical structures in his *Historia et Scenographia Vasorum Lymphaticorum corporis humani*.

Maser Microwave Amplification Stimulated Electromagnetic Radiation. *See laser.*

Masochism Leopold von Sacher-Masoch (1836–1895), an Austrian novelist in his *Venus in Furs* described a form of sexual aberration where pleasure was derived through self-infliction of pain. The term was coined by the German psychiatrist Richard Krafft-Ebing (1840–1902) in *Psychopathia Sexualis* published in 1886.

Mason Good, John (1764–1827) Physician and linguist, fluent in 15 languages, who translated the works of Lucretius and published *The Book of Nature* in 3 volumes. He practiced medicine in London around 1820. The manuscripts of his work were published by Samuel Cooper, professor of surgery at London University.

Massachusetts General Hospital Rev John Bartlett, chaplain to the Boston Almshouse, was first to call for establishment of a general hospital (for the mentally ill) in 1810. Five months later James Jackson Jr (1810–1834), son of a Newburyport merchant, and John Collins Warren (1778–1856), son of John Warren first professor of anatomy and surgery at the Harvard Medical School, sent out a letter to prominent citizens of Boston calling for a general hospital in Boston. Their appeal was well received and a charter for incorporation of the Massachusetts General Hospital (MGH) was granted in February in 1811. The first meeting of the corporation, two months later, was attended by James Bowdoin and 55 other prominent Bostonians. Funds were obtained through private subscription and from leasing of Province House (presented by the legislature). The Massachusetts Hospital Life Insurance Company was started in 1818 to provide financial support to the hospital. A leading American architect, Charles Bulfinch, was chosen and the hospital opened its doors to the first inpatient in 1821. Jackson and Warren served as its first physician and surgeon, respectively. By 1823 the building was completed to accommodate 73 beds. The first successful use of anesthesia in surgery with sulfuric ether was demonstrated on October 16 1846. The pathology laboratory was established in 1896. Use of radiology was pioneered in 1896 by Walter J. Dodd who later succumbed to radiation injuries. The first social service anywhere in the world was started at the outpatient department by its outpatient physician, Richard C. Cabot (1868–1939) in 1907. The well-known clinical pathological conferences, still published weekly in the *New England Journal of Medicine*, were started by Cabot and the hospital's pathologist, J. Homer Wright (1869–1928) in 1910. The metabolic ward, known as Mallinckrodt-Ward 4, where Fuller Albright (1900–1969) and other famous men worked, was established in 1925 by James Howard Means (1885–1967), who was chief of medical services.

Massachusetts Institute of Technology (MIT) Founded in 1861 by Erastus Bigham Bigelow (1814–1879) from West Boylston, Massachusetts, an American inventor of looms.

Massage Practiced as therapy for thousands of years. Captain Cook gave an account of its practice by people of Otaheite, New Holland. They used a method called 'toogi-toogi' for relief of muscular fatigue, involving regular percussion for long periods. Amongst Greeks a class of rubbers existed who anointed the bodies of athletes. Massage was also practiced at the Temples of Aesculapius and amongst the ancient Egyptians and Romans. A book on the subject, *Massage as a Mode of Treatment*, was published by William Murrell (1853–1912) who also introduced nitroglycerin therapy for angina in 1876. Another work, *Deep Massage and Manipulation Illustrated*, was published by James Cyrex, chief medical off-icer of physiotherapy at St Thomas' Hospital in 1942. *See aromatherapy.*

Masset Test Used for detection of bile pigments in urine by adding sulfuric acid and potassium nitrite to give a distinctive green color. Devised by French physician, Alfred Auguste Masset (b 1870) in 1895.

Massol Bacillus *Lactobacillus bulgaricus* was described by Swiss bacteriologist, Leon Massol (1837–1909). It was isolated from fermented milk in Bulgaria by Grigoroff in 1909.

Mast Cells The granular nature of some cells in the mesentery of the frog was first observed by Friedrich Daniel von Recklinghausen (1833–1910), a pupil of Rudolph Virchow (1821–1902) in Berlin in 1863. These cells were named 'mast cells' by Paul Ehrlich (1854–1965) in 1863.

Mastectomy [Greek: *mastos*, breast + *ektome*, to cut out] Aulus Cornelius Celsus (25 BC–AD 50) practiced excision of breast cancer while keeping the pectoralis major intact. Leonidas of Alexandria excised breast cancer in AD 180 with the removal of surrounding healthy tissues – a method similar to modern radical mastectomy. The Arabian physician, Rhazes (850–932), was weary of removing cancers of the breast and described a case of breast cancer which occurred on the other side after its removal. Antyllus in AD 300 recommended that advanced cancers should be left as they were inoperable. A modern procedure for removing the breast was described by Johann Schultes (1595–1645) in *Armentarium chirugicum* in 1655. English surgeon and pioneer in the treatment of cancer, Charles Hewitt Moore (1821–1870), was one of the first to insist on removal of the entire breast. Radical mastectomy was introduced by American surgeon, William Stewart Halsted (1852–1922) in 1890.

Mastoidectomy Excision of mastoid bone. *See mastoiditis.*

Mastoiditis [Greek: *mastos*, breast + *oid*, form + *itis*, inflammation] Surgery was first performed by Jean Louis Petit (1674–1750) of Paris around 1720, and a modern method was devised by Anton Friedrich von Tröltsch (1829–1890) of Germany in 1860. The first clear description was given by Friedrich Bezold (1842–1908) in 1877. Mastoidectomy was performed in England by James Hinton of Guy's Hospital, London in 1868. Radical mastoidectomy was introduced by Ernest von Bergmann (1836–1907) of Berlin in 1888.

Matches They were used in fire lighting by Chinese women around AD 577. Chemical matches were made by Chancel of Paris in 1805 of brimstone and asbestos mixed with oil of vitriol. The friction match was made by John Walker (1781–1859), a chemist from Stockton-on-Tees, England in 1827. Phosphorus was used by Arthur Albright of Birmingham in 1845. Necrosis of the jaw (phossy jaw) secondary to white phosphorus exposure in industry was observed in match factories near Vienna in 1844 and described by Karl Thiersch (1822–1895), professor of surgery at Erlangen in 1867. Finland abolished use of white phosphorus in the match industry in 1872, and it was prohibited in England in 1910. *See red phosphorus, phossy jaw.*

Materia Medica Term coined by Dioscorides (AD 40–90) during the early days of the Roman Empire to denote a compilation and description of medical substances taken internally. It has now largely been replaced with the term pharmacopoeia. *See pharmacology.*

Maternity Hospitals The first lying-in hospital in Britain was founded by Bartholomew Mosse (d 1749) in 1745 at Dublin, with only 10 beds at South Great George's Street. Three years later Mosse raised a considerable sum of money through lotteries and bought a site for a 150-bed hospital which developed into the famous Rotunda Hospital. The first in London was founded by Sir Richard Manningham (d 1759) adjoining his house at Jermyn Street in 1739. His unit started with 24 beds and became the General Lying-in Hospital in 1752. In 1791 it came under the patronage of Queen Charlotte and moved to Old Manor House in Lisson Grove where it was re-named Queen Charlotte's Hospital in 1813. The Lying-in Hospital at Westminster was established in 1767 and the British Lying-in Hospital at Brownlow Street, where William Hunter (1718–1783) initially practiced, was founded in 1749.

Mathematical Symbols Signs for addition (+) and subtraction (–) are found in the work of Johannes Widman, published in 1489. An English book, *Whetstone of Witte*, was published by Robert Recorde in 1557 and included the equals sign (=). The symbol for multiplication (x) was introduced by William Oughtred (1575–1660), a clergyman from Eton in *Clavis Mathematica* published in 1631. The symbol for division (÷) was used by J. H. Rahn, a Swiss mathematician in 1659 and π for the ratio of circumference to the diameter of the circle was introduced by William Jones in 1706. The greater than > and lesser than < signs were introduced by Thomas Harriot (1560–1621), a mathematician from Oxford.

Mathematics The Chaldeans who ruled Babylonia from 606 to 539 BC applied mathematics to astronomy. They divided the Zodiac into twelve parts and the celestial equator into 360 degrees. The oldest existing mathematical manuscript by Ahmes in 1650 BC was copied from an earlier manuscript. It was brought to London around the middle of the 19th century by Alexander Henry Rhind (1833–1863), a Scottish Egyptologist, and came to be known as Rhind's papyrus. It is now in the British Museum in London. Thales (640–546 BC), a merchant from the city of Miletus in Asia Minor, was one of the first to devote his time to the study of mathematics. He measured the height of a pyramid by its shadow and developed geometry. Pythagorus, from the island of Samos, was his pupil and introduced geometry as an essential science. Other notable ancient mathematicians include: Euclid (300 BC), Eratosthenes (274–194 BC), Hippocrates of Chios (430 BC) and Archimedes (278–212 BC). Four of the most important Hindu mathematicians were: Aryabhata (AD 475–550) of Benares, Brahmagupta (AD 628) of Ujjain, Mahavira (AD 850) of Mysore, and Bhaskara (AD 1114–1185) of Ujjain. In Britain, Harriot (1560–1621) contributed to algebra, Briggs (1560–1630) and Napier (1550–1677) invented logarithms, and Oughtred (1574–1660) invented the slide rule. The first substantial book on history of mathematics, *Histoire des Mathematiques*, was written by a Frenchman from Lyons, Jean Etienne Montucula (1725–1799) in 1758. *See algebra, arithmetic.*

Mather, Cotton (1663–1728) Born in Boston, son of Increase Mather, president of Harvard College in 1681. Though he was a distinguished clergyman his belief in witchcraft led him to persecute those accused of the practice. He also practiced medicine, and attributed diseases to man's sins. He advocated smallpox inoculation in America, where the first inoculation was done by Zabdiel Boylston (1680–1766), a Boston physician, in 1721. Mather published *The Wonders of the Invisible World, or the Trials of Witches*, a treatise on smallpox vaccination (1722), and 381 other works on a variety of subjects.

Mathijsen, Antoine (1805–1878) Belgian surgeon who introduced plaster-of-Paris into surgery in 1851 and pioneered the use of galvano-cautery.

Matteucci, Carlo (1811–1868) Italian physiologist who, in 1838, showed that current can be made to flow from the cut end of an isolated muscle to its uncut surface, if these points were connected by a galvanometer.

Matthiolus, Pietro Andrea (1500–1577) Born in Sienna, a medical graduate from Padua who practiced in Rome, where he was appointed physician to Maximillian II. He published *Commentary on Dioscorides.*

Mauchart Ligaments [Latin: *ligamentum*, bandage] Found at the neck of the ocular muscles and described by Burkhard David Mauchart (1696–1751), professor of surgery at Tübingen.

Maudsley, Henry (1835–1918) English psychiatrist from Giggleswick in Yorkshire who advocated the idea that insanity is fundamentally a disease of the body. He qualified from University College Hospital and became superintendent of the Royal Lunatic Asylum at Manchester in 1859. Maudsley's *The Pathology and Physiology of the Mind* published in 1867 is considered a classic in English psychiatry. *See Maudsley Hospital.*

Maudsley Hospital Established in 1907 with a fund of 30,000 pounds gifted by Henry Maudsley (1835–1918), a psychiatrist from Yorkshire. A site was bought at Denmark Hill in London in 1911 and building commenced in 1913. After a delay due to the war, it opened in 1923. The Maudsley Hospital and Bethlehem Hospital were amalgamated in 1948 to become the Institute of Psychiatry.

Maugham, William Somerset (1874–1965) Surgeon and writer of Irish origin, born in Paris and qualified from St Thomas' Hospital. He practiced in the London slums and wrote his first novel *Liza of Lambeth* in 1897. His famous book, *Of Human Bondage,* was published in 1915.

Maumené Test Used to detect sugar in urine by adding stanous chloride to give a distinct brown color. Devised by French chemist, Edme Joules Maumené (1818–1891) around 1850.

Mauriac Disease Erythema nodosum syphiliticum was first described by French physician, Pierre Mauriac (1832–1905). Another syndrome of growth retardation, obesity and hepatomegaly in juvenile diabetes was described by him in 1930.

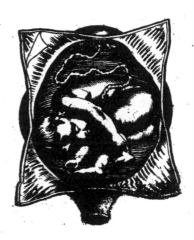

Transverse fetal presentation. From the translation of Mauriceau's work, *The Disease of Women with Child and in Child-bed* by Hugh Chamberlain, the Elder. London

Mauriceau, François (1637–1709) French obstetrician who dispensed with the obstetrical chair that had been used since biblical times and delivered his patients in bed. His *Des Maladies des Femmes Grosses et Accouchees* was translated into English by Hugh Chamberlain in 1693.

Mauthner, Ludwig (1840–1894) Professor of ophthalmology at Vienna who described the membrane surrounding the axis cylinder of the nerve within the sheath of Schwann (Mauthner membrane) in 1860.

Maxilla [Latin: *maxillus*] The maxillary antrum was illustrated in the drawings of Leonardo Da Vinci (1452–1519) and Nathaniel Highmore (1613–1685) gave a description in 1651. The first series of operations was published by William Cowper (1666–1760) in 1707. The successful removal of a tumor of the maxillary sinus was performed by Plaignaud of Paris in 1791, and excision of the superior maxilla was done by Horatio Gates Jameson (1788–1855) of America in 1820.

Two cases of empyema of the maxillary antrum were described by M. Saint Hillaire in 1898.

Maxillary Sinus *See maxilla.*

Maxwell, James Clerk (1831–1879) *See Clerk Maxwell.*

Maxwell, Sir James Crawford (1869–1932) Physician from Dundee who graduated from Edinburgh University. He was appointed Governor and Commander-in-Chief of Northern Rhodesia in 1927.

May, Charles Henry (1861–1943) Chief of the eye clinic of Columbia University and eye surgeon to Mount Sinai Hospital in New York. He designed a simple self-illuminating ophthalmoscope and published *Manual of Diseases of the Eye* (with Claude Worth) in 1906.

Mayan Civilization The first archeological evidence was unearthed by John Lloyd Stephens (1805–1852), a lawyer from New Jersey, and an artist, Fredrick Catherwood (1799–1856), during their exploration of MesoAmerica in 1839. Their work brought the cities of Copan, Quirigua and Palenque in the Yucatan peninsula, dating back to about 300 BC, to light. They practiced human sacrifice, ancestral worship and self-mutilation. Their major city, Teotihuacan, was well planned and remained central until about AD 600. They devised an advanced system of counting and recorded astronomical events using a system of glyphs, and had accurate calendars. It peaked around AD 600 and went into decay around 900, possibly due to the spread of yellow fever. They were replaced by the Aztecs. *See Aztecs.*

Maydl, Karel (1853–1903) Surgeon at Prague and Vienna who performed the first successful colostomy in 1888 and the uretero-intestinal anastomosis with insertion of the extroverted bladder into the rectum for ectopic vesicae in 1894.

Mayer, Julius Robert von (1814–1878) German physicist and a medical practitioner from Heilbron, Bavaria. After obtaining his medical degree in 1838 he traveled to Java as a ship's surgeon in 1840. He was one of the first to propose the laws of the mechanical equivalent of heat in *Bermerkungen uber die krafte der unbelebten Natur* which appeared in the *Annals der Chemie und Pharmacie* in 1846. Mayer attempted suicide in 1850, and spent several years in an asylum. His theory on heat was later recognized as forerunner of the law of conservation of energy.

Mayer Ligament [Latin: *ligamentum*, bandage] A suspensory ligament of the carotid body first described by an anatomy professor at Bonn, M. F. Mayer in 1833.

Mayerne, Sir Theodore Turquet (1573–1661) Successful physician in London who was born in Geneva. He obtained his MD from Montpellier in 1597 and practiced as royal physician at Paris before he came to England in 1616. He was physician to four royals: Henry IV of France, James I, Charles I, and Charles II. He left his magnificent library to the Royal College of Physicians but most of his books, along with other possessions of the college, were destroyed during the Great Fire of London ten years later.

Maynwaring, Everard (1626–1699) Graduated from Dublin and practiced medicine in London. His treatise on protection of long life and detection of its brevity, published in 1664, was an important work on preservation of health.

Mayo, Charles Horace (1865–1939) Son of William Worrall Mayo who emigrated from England to the United States in 1845. After practicing as a chemist in New York City he took his medical degree in 1854 and settled in Rochester, Minnesota. *See Mayo Clinic.*

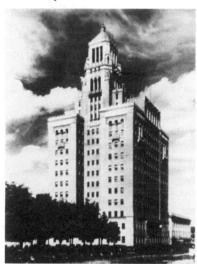

Mayo Clinic. Courtesy of the National Library of Medicine

Mayo Clinic Started with 13 patients and 5 nurses by William Worrall Mayo and his two sons, William James Mayo (1861–1939) and Charles Horace Mayo (1865–1939) in 1889. It developed into the present prestigious Mayo Clinic at Rochester in 1905. The Mayo Foundation for Medical Education and Research was founded by the two brothers in 1917.

Mayo, William James (1861–1939) Surgeon from the Mayo family and one of the reformers of American medicine during the latter part of the 19th century. He devised a new procedure of partial gastrectomy for carcinoma of the pyloric end of the stomach in 1900. He co-founded the famous Mayo Clinic with his brother Charles Horace Mayo (1865–1939) in 1905.

Mayou, Marmaduke Stephen (1876–1934) London ophthalmologist who described the symmetrical changes in the macula in juvenile amaurotic idiocy in 1904.

Mayow, John (1641–1679) English chemist and physiologist who studied medicine at Oxford University and practiced in Bath and London. He observed that the process of combustion involved a chemical union with a substance in the atmosphere. He named this substance 'igneo-aereum', later shown to be oxygen. He also demonstrated the difference between arterial and venous blood in 1668 and is regarded as the first experimenter in respiratory physiology.

McArdle Syndrome Rare form of myopathy due to a deficiency of phosphorylase enzyme in the muscle leading to accumulation of glycogen. Described by London neurologist, Brian McArdle (b 1911) who graduated from Guy's Hospital (1933) in 1959.

McBain, James (1807–1879) Scottish surgeon and naturalist from Kirriemuir, Forfarshire, who did official surveys of the shores and seas of Orkney and Shetland in 1827.

McBurney Incision The abdominal wall is opened during appendectomy, along the layer of muscle fibers, rather than cutting across the fibers. Described by New York surgeon, Charles McBurney (1845–1913) in 1889.

McBurney Point Site of maximum tenderness in the right iliac fossa in appendicitis. Described by New York surgeon, Charles McBurney (1845–1913), in 1889.

McCarrison, Sir Robert (1878–1960) Director of the Nutritional Research Laboratories at Coonoor in India who pioneered studies on nutrition and essential food factors and performed classical research on goiter and iodine deficiency. He described the three-day Chitral fever of the Blue Mountains or Nilgri (6000 feet above sea level) in India. He proved that the sand fly was the cause of phlebotomus fever in 1903.

McCarthy, Daniel Joseph (1874–1965) Urologist in New York who designed a panendoscope, prostatic electrotome and several other endoscopic instruments.

McClellan, George (1796–1847) American surgeon who founded the Jefferson Medical School in 1825 to which he was appointed first professor of surgery.

McClintock, Barbara (b 1902) American botanist and geneticist who discovered the genes in corn move from one area to another and thus affect future plants. She received the Nobel Prize in 1983.

McClintock Sign Pulse rate of over 100, indicative of post partum hemorrhage. Described by an Irish physician, Alfred Henry McClintock (1822–1881).

McClung, Clarence Erwin (1870–1946) American cytologist who suggested in 1902 that accessory chromosomes were determinants of sex.

McCollum, Elmer Verner (1879–1967) American biochemist from Fort Scott, Kansas and assistant professor at the University of Wisconsin when he gave the first description of an accessory food factor and discovered vitamin A in 1913. He was appointed professor of biochemistry at the School of Hygiene at Johns Hopkins University in 1917 and detected the rickets-preventing factor, vitamin D, in cod liver oil in 1922. He published *Chemistry for Medical Students* (1916), *The Newer Knowledge of Nutrition* (1918), *The American Home Diet* (1918), and *A History of Nutrition* (1957).

McCoy, George Walter (1876–1952) Professor of preventative medicine at the medical school of Louisiana State University. He observed tularemia amongst rodents in 1911.

McCrae, John (1872–1915) Physician and poet, born at Guelph, Ontario and educated in Toronto. He joined McGill University as a pathologist in 1899 and later served as an officer in the South African war. His poem *In Flanders Fields* was first published anonymously in *Punch* in December 1915. A volume of his poems with the same title was published by Sir Andrew Macphail in 1919.

McCulloch, John (1773–1835) Geologist and physician from Jersey who graduated from Edinburgh at the age of seventeen. He undertook several scientific surveys of Scotland for the government, and published *System of Geology, and Theory of the Earth* (1831), *A Geological Classification of Rocks* (1821), *The Highlands and Western Isles of Scotland* (1824), and *A Description of the Western Islands of Scotland, including the Isle of Man* (1819). His medical publications include *Malaria* (1827), and *Remittent and Intermittent Diseases* (1829). MacCulloch died during amputation of one of his limbs following an accidental injury which he sustained during a holiday in Cornwall.

McDermott, Walsh (1909–1881) American physician and a founder of the Institute of Medicine of the National Academy of Sciences. He introduced pyrazinamide in combination with isoniazid as first-line treatment for tuberculosis in 1954.

McDougall, Rev Francis Thomas (1817–1886) Born in Sydenham in Kent, he was the only bishop of England to pass examinations and become a Fellow of the Royal

College of Surgeons in 1854. He served as a bishop in Labuan and Sarawak.

McDougall, William (1871–1938) Psychologist from Manchester who was educated at Owen's College. He graduated from St Thomas' Hospital in London and traveled to Borneo where he studied pagan tribes. On his return he established a new tradition of psychology at Oxford and published *Social Psychology* in 1908.

McDowell, Benjamin George (1829–1885) Dublin surgeon at Sir Patrick Dun's Hospital, and physician to the King in Ireland. He was the first to describe the suspensory ligament of the pectoralis major tendon which is named after him.

McDowell, Ephraim (1771–1830) Born in Danville, Kentucky, he was a pioneer in abdominal surgery. He performed the first removal of an ovarian cyst, weighing 22 pounds, without anesthesia in 1809.

McGill, Arthur Ferguson (1846–1890) English surgeon who first performed a suprapubic prostatectomy in 1887.

McGill University First medical school to be established in Canada, founded by James McGill (d 1813) from Glasgow. He studied for a year at Glasgow University and emigrated to Canada before the American Civil War. He settled in Montreal and left his estate to establish a college (McGill University) in the traditions of Glasgow University. Lectures on medicine were first started in 1822 by four physicians who had trained in Edinburgh. Sir William Osler served as professor of medicine for ten years from 1874.

McGraw, H. Theodore (1839–1921) Surgeon at Detroit, Michigan who introduced a new method of ligature for performing intestinal anastomosis.

McGregor, John (1848–1932) Medical graduate of Glasgow University who served as a surgeon in the Indian Medical Service. He published several literary works including: *Luinneagan Luaineach* (1897), a set of poems in Gaelic, *Through the Buffer State* (1896), and *The Legend of Alampra* (1923).

McGrigor, Sir James (1771–1858) Born in Inverness-shire, he was the founder of the Aberdeen Medical Society with James Robertson and ten medical students from Marischal College in 1789. He was appointed surgeon-general of the Army Medical Service in 1815.

McIndoe, Sir Archibald Hector (1900–1960) New Zealand-born London surgeon who described a procedure for reconstruction of the urethra with the use of a dermal graft.

He used skin grafting to establish the relationship between twins who became separated after birth. He also devised an operation for construction of the vagina in cases of its congenital absence in 1938. He developed long curved scissors known as the McIndoe scissors.

McKenzie, Robert Tait (1867–1938) Canadian sculptor and a physician who graduated from McGill University in 1891. He was professor of physical education at the University of Pennsylvania for 27 years and sculptured several athletes for which he was decorated by the King of Sweden at the Olympic games in 1912.

McLean Hospital Rev John Bartlett, the chaplain for the Boston Almshouse, first pointed out the need for a hospital for the mentally ill in Boston in 1810. This led to the formation of the Massachusetts General Hospital, whose trustees established an asylum for the mentally ill in 1816. They purchased a colonial house in Charlestown, designed by Charles Bulfinch, and opened a 60 bed asylum. A country physician, Rufus Wyman, was appointed as its first superintendent in 1818. In 1823 John McLean, a Boston merchant, left $150,000 to the institution and it was renamed McLean Hospital in 1892. The first training school for nurses in a hospital for mentally ill anywhere in the world was established there in 1882. It moved to its present location in 1895.

McMurray, Thomas Porter (1887–1947) First professor of orthopedics in England at Liverpool and founder of the military orthopedic center at Alder Hey in Liverpool. He introduced subtrochanteric osteotomy as treatment for osteoarthritis of the hip joint and described the clinical test (McMurray test) for meniscal tear by rotating the knee.

McNaughten Rules Formulated after the case of Daniel McNaughten who shot and killed Edward Drummond, private secretary to Robert Peel, after mistaking him for Peel. He was tried in 1843 and not found responsible for his actions due to his mental state, and was committed to the Bethlehem Hospital. The matter was taken up in the House of Lords in 1843 and the judges stated that 'to establish a defense on the grounds of insanity, it must be clearly proved that, at the time of the committing of the act, the party accused was laboring under such a defect of reason, from the disease of the mind, as not to know the nature and quality of the act he was doing, or if he did know it, that he did not know he was doing what was wrong'. It established that the accused in any crime was sane until proved otherwise.

MDU (The Medical Defence Union) The longest

established defense organization in Britain, offering protection to members of the medical profession, established in 1885.

Mead, George Herbert (1863–1931) American psychologist from South Hadley Massachusetts. He published *Philosophy of the Present* (1932), and *Mind, Self, and Society* in 1934.

Mead, Richard (1673–1754) Physician and one of the holders of the gold-headed cane of the president of the Royal College of Physicians. He was physician to King George II and wrote a book on diseases in the Bible, *De Morbis Biblicis*. His other publications include: *A Mechanical Account of Poison, Discourse containing Pestilential Contagion* and *Monita Medica.* Westminster Hospital erected a monument in his honor.

Mean Corpuscular Hemoglobin Concentration (MCHC) *See red cell indices.*

Mean Corpuscular Volume (MCV) *See red cell indices.*

Measles Vaccine Developed by American bacteriologist and Nobel Prize winner, John Franklin Enders (1897–1985) of West Hartford, Connecticut in 1962.

Measles The oldest treatise on smallpox and measles, *Liber de variolis et morbillis*, was written by Rhazes (850–932) in 910. He mentioned the *Pandects* written by the Alexandrian physician, Aaron, who appears to have been well acquainted with these two diseases in the 7th century. The term 'variola' was first employed by bishop Marius of Avenches in 570. 'Bothor' is an ancient Arabic term for measles or smallpox. The term 'mesles' was first used by Gilbertus Anglicus in 1595. An accurate description was given by Thomas Sydenham (1624–1689) in *Processus integri* published in 1676. Francis Home (1719–1813), a physician from Edinburgh, pioneered experimental inoculation against measles and demonstrated human transmission in 1759. Kopick spots as a diagnostic sign were described by American pediatrician, Henry Kopick (1858–1927), and by Russian pediatrician, Nils Fedorovich Filatov (1847–1902). The successful cultivation of the virus was achieved by Harry Plotz (1890–1947) of Paris in 1938. *See German measles.*

Measures Many of the names used as units of measurement came from body parts or easily obtainable materials. The oldest preserved standard of length, the foot, derives its origin from the foot of the statue of the ruler of Gudea in the Mesopotamian city of Lagash, in 4000 BC. It measures 10.41 inches and was divided into 16 parts. The inch probably comes from the Latin word 'uncia' for thumb. The ounce was fixed as 640 dry grains of weight by King Henry III. The yard denoted the distance from the tip of the nose to the end of the fingers when the right arm was outstretched. It was

later defined by a Royal decree in England in 1824 as the length of a pendulum placed at Greenwich with a period of one second. The Imperial Standards for measures in Britain was set by a commission in 1758. The carat (Greek: *keration,* horn-like pods) for measurement of diamonds and gold was originally obtained from the average weight of seeds of the carob tree, a native tree of Africa and the southern Mediterranean. When diamonds were first discovered in India the seeds were transported to be used as a measure. The English carat was fixed at 3.1683 grains by the Board of Trade in 1888 and was replaced by the metric carat in 1914. The kilogram was established as an official unit by the Bureau of Weights and Measures at the Pavilion de Bretail near Paris in 1875. It is a standard bar of a platinum-iridium alloy and has remained unchanged up to today. *See metric system.*

Meat Poisoning *See food poisoning.*

Mechnikov, Eliya *See Metchnikoff.*

Meckel, Johan Friedrich, Jr (1781–1833) Professor of anatomy at Halle, regarded as one of the greatest comparative anatomists prior to Johan Muller. The diverticulum of the ileum resulting from the persistence of the yolk sac of the embryo (Meckel diverticulum) was discovered by him in 1809. The cartilage of the first brachial arch (Meckel cartilage) was described by him in 1805.

Meckel, Johann Friedrich, Senior (1724–1774) Professor of anatomy and gynecology at Berlin. He described the sphenopalatine ganglion (Meckel ganglion) and the dural space (Meckel cave) in which the Gasserian ganglion was lodged in 1749.

Medawar, Sir Peter Brian (1915–1987) British immunologist and pioneer in the study of rejection reactions in organ transplantation. He was born in Rio de Janeiro to an English mother and a Lebanese father. He studied zoology at Magdalen College, Oxford and became interested in immunology through his work on skin grafting for burn victims during World War ll. He shared the Nobel Prize in 1960 with Sir Frank Macfarlane Burnet (1899–1985) for his work on immunological tolerance in organ transplantation. He was appointed as director to the National Institute for Medical Research in 1962.

Median Nerve Compression Carpal tunnel syndrome. The Tinel sign, where tapping over the carpal tunnel causes paraesthesia over median nerve distribution of the hand, was described by French neurologist, Jules Tinel (1879– 1952) of Rouen. It was shown in 1947 to be due to pressure on the transverse carpal ligament of the wrist by British neurologist Walter Russel Brain (1895–1966), Baron of Eynsham.

Mediastinum [Latin: *mediastinus*, servant] *See oat cell carcinoma, diaphragm.*

Medical Acts King Hammurabi (1945–1905 BC) of Babylon devised a code of conduct that was inscribed on a huge stone excavated at Susa, east of the Tigris. The inscriptions contained a code of conduct for all walks of life, including rules and regulations for the practice of the physicians, how to set their fees, and prescribed punishments for their failures. The Aquilian Law made physicians and surgeons in Rome accountable for their action and was enacted in 300 BC. The Laws of Manu (200 BC–AD 200) of the Indian Brahmins contain the rules for daily life, and stated that physicians could be punished for improper treatment, that if the cured patient refused to pay the doctor his property should be confiscated and given to the doctor. Brahmin priests, the poor, and friends were exempted from payment of medical fees. Roger, founder of the Christian kingdom of Sicily, declared in 1140 that anyone who desired to practice medicine should present himself before a magistrate and obtain authorization, or otherwise would be imprisoned and have his wealth confiscated. His law led directly to the granting of medical degrees by universities. The edicts controlling education and licensing of medical men in Sicily and southern of Italy were issued by Frederick II in 1224. *See General Medical Council, Anatomy Act.*

Medical and Chirurgical Society of London Founded in 1805 and received a royal charter from King William IV in 1834.

Medical Books *See books on medicine.*

Medical Degree The title of doctor was first conferred by the church. The first degree of doctor for a medical person was conferred at Salerno in the 11th century. The degree of doctor in England was conferred in 1207. The first Bachelor of Medicine degree in America was given to ten men who graduated from the College of Philadelphia in 1768. King's College, New York awarded medical degrees to two more men in 1769.

Medical Dictionaries *See dictionary of medicine.*

Medical Directory The first medical directory, a guide to recognized medical practitioners, was produced by James Yearsley (1805–1869), a London otorhinologist in 1845.

Medical Journals *See Journals in medicine, British Medical Journal, American medical journals, The Lancet, New England Journal of Medicine.*

Medical Jurisprudence *See forensic medicine.*

Medical Murders *See Pritchard, Edward; Crippen, Harvey; Lamson, George.*

Medical Officer of Health Sir Edwin Chadwick (1800–1890), the great sanitary reformer of England, gave his report in 1842 after which the City Sewage Act was passed and the post of medical officer was created in 1848. Sir John Simon (1816–1904) was appointed as the first medical officer in London, and by 1855, others were appointed for most districts. The Association for Medical Officers was formed in 1856. Sir Henry Duncan Littlejohn of Edinburgh was appointed as the first medical officer of health in his town in 1862. He was a pioneer in public health and gave his report on the sanitary conditions of Edinburgh in 1865.

Medical Photography The method of photographing capillary vessels of the eye with the use of a krypton–xenon laser was developed by American electrical engineer and professor at Massachusetts Institute of Technology, Harold Eugene Edgerton (1903–1990) from Nebraska. *See photomicrography.*

Medical Physics Some of the major advancements in medicine include: the compound microscope of Robert Hooke (1635–1703) (1667); the invention of the short-stemmed clinical thermometer by Sir Thomas Clifford Allbutt (1836–1925) (1866); the introduction of sphygmomanometer by Samuel von Basch (1837–1905) (1893); the discovery of X-rays by Röntgen (1895); the development of the electrocardiograph from the string galvanometer of Willem Einthoven (1860–1927) (1903); the invention of a microlaser for use in medicine by Marcel Bessis in 1962; the discovery of computerized axial tomography by Sir Godfrey Newbold Hounsfield (b 1919) and Allan MacLeod Cormack (b 1924) around 1973; and the application of ultrasound to examine the fetus *in utero* by Ian Donald (1979). *See radiotherapy, CAT scanner, laser, ultrasound, X-rays.*

Medical Research Council Following the National Health Insurance Act of 1911, a Medical Research Committee was created in 1913. This developed into the Medical Research Council, which received its Royal charter in 1920.

Medical Social Service *See social services in medicine.*

Medical Society of Edinburgh The oldest medical society in Britain, founded in 1737.

Medical Society of London The oldest medical society in London was founded by physician and philanthropist, John Coakley Lettsom (1744–1815) in 1773. Its original membership was limited to 30 from each of the three groups of physicians, surgeons and apothecaries.

Medical Statistics The first book, *Elements of Medical Statistics*, was published by Francis Bisset Hawkins (1796–1894) in 1829. He defined medical statistics as 'the application of numbers to illustrate the natural history of man in health and disease'. William Farr (1807–1883) proposed a column to record disease or cause of death in the first Registration Act of England. The founder of medical statistics in France was Charles Pierre Alexander Louis (1787–1872), a contemporary of Armand Trousseau (1801–1867). He provided medical statistics on diphtheria, typhoid and yellow fever. A 20th century classic, *Principles of Statistics*, was published by Sir Austin Bradford Hill (1897–1991) in 1939. *Epidemics and crowd diseases: an introduction to the history of epidemiology* (1935) was published by Major Greenwood (1880–1949), professor of medical statistics and epidemiology at the London School of Hygiene and Tropical Medicine in 1935. *See normal distribution curve, statistics.*

Medicare A federally financed insurance system in America for care of those eligible for social security benefits. The amendment of social security laws by President Lyndon Johnson in 1963 paved the way for the program, and it was set up by the Congress in 1965. It became effective in 1966.

Medin, Oskar (1847–1927) Swedish pediatrician. *See acute anterior poliomyelitis.*

Meditation Technique for attaining a state of inner peace and tranquillity, known as 'Nirvana' by Buddhists. First practiced by Gautama Buddha, a Hindu prince who founded Buddhism around 500 BC.

Mediterranean Fever (Syn: abortus fever, brucellosis, undulant fever, Malta fever) Low-grade fever with remissions noted in the Mediterranean region since Hippocratic times. The causative organism, *Micrococcus melitensis*, was discovered by Sir David Bruce (1855–1931) in 1887. Karl Friedrich Meyer and Shaw of America named it 'brucellosis' in 1920 in honor of Sir David Bruce (1855–1931). *See brucellosis.*

Medulla Oblongata [Latin: *medulla*, innermost part + *ob*, over + *longus*, long] Julien Jean Cesar Legallois (1775–1814), a physician and physiologist from Cherneix in Brittany, demonstrated the presence of a respiratory center in the medulla oblongata in 1812. M. J. Pierre Flourens (1794–1867) confirmed it in 1837 by inducing a lesion in the bilateral 'vital nodes' of the respiratory centers leading to asphyxia in experimental animals. Basal ganglia were suggested to be internodes connecting the medulla oblongata and the cerebrum by Thomas Willis (1621–1675) in 1664.

Medullary Sponge Kidney The first case was described in 1938 by G. Lenarduzzi, and the second was reported 10 years later by H. J. Dammermann. The disease was initially known as sponge kidney and a detailed description was given by Cacchi and Ricci in 1949. The term 'medullary' was added to 'sponge kidney' by Di Sieno and Guarechi in 1956.

Megacolon [Greek: *megas*, large + *colon*] *See Hirschsprung disease.*

Megakaryocytes [Greek: *megas*, large + *karyon*, a nut + *kytos*, cell] *See platelets.*

Megaloblastic Anemia [Greek: *megas*, large + *blastos*, bud + *ahaima*, without blood) *See pernicious anemia, anemia.*

Megaloblasts [Greek: *megas*, large + *blastos*, bud] Primitive nucleated blood cells, first described by Paul Ehrlich (1854–1915) around 1881. Further studies were made by J.R. Gilmour in 1941.

Meges of Sidon (*c* 20 BC) Regarded by Aulus Cornelius Celsus (25 BC–AD 50) as a skilled surgeon. He invented several instruments for use in lithotomy.

Méglin Point Point of emergence of the descending palatine nerve from the palato-maxillary canal. Described by French physician, J.A.M. Méglin (1756–1824), an anatomist at Sultz, in 1816.

Meibomian Gland Sebacean follicles between the tarsi and the conjunctiva of the eyelids. Described by German anatomist, Heinrich Meibom (1638–1700), professor of medicine at Helmstadt in 1666 who published *Scriptores rerum Germanicarum*. The gland was described earlier by Guilio Casserius (1561–1616) of Padua in 1609.

Meibom, John Henry (1590–1655) Physician from Helmstadt who published *Life of Maecenas*. His son was Heinrich Meibom (1638–1700).

Meige Disease Form of hereditary edema of the lower limbs, described by French physician, Henri Meige (1866–1940) in 1901. *See Milroy disease.*

Meigs Capillaries Capillary blood vessels in the muscular fibers of the heart, first described by Arthur Vincent Meigs (1850–1912), a lecturer in histology at the University of Philadelphia, in 1899.

Meigs, Charles Delucina (1792–1869) Professor of midwifery at Jefferson Medical College who was the first to recognize embolism as a cause of maternal death in 1849.

Meigs Syndrome Ovarian tumor associated with ascites and pleural effusion, first described in 1937 by American professor of gynecology at Harvard, Joseph Vincent Meigs (1892–1963).

Meiosis [Greek: *meiosis*, diminution] Cell division in sex cells at maturation by means of which each daughter cell receives half the number of chromosomes found in a somatic cell. First observed in 1887 by Belgian cytologist, Edouard Joseph Louis-Marie van Beneden (1846–1910). The process where the nucleus divides twice but the chromosomes only once was first described by J.B. Farmer (1865–1944) and J.E. Moore (b 1892) in 1905.

Meissner Corpuscles Tactile sensory nerve endings, described in 1852 by Georg Meissner (1829–1905) and Rudolf Wagner (1805–1864), professors of physiology at Göttingen, Germany.

Meissner Plexus Found in the submucous layer of the alimentary canal. Described by Georg Meissner (1829–1905), professor of physiology at Göttingen in 1853.

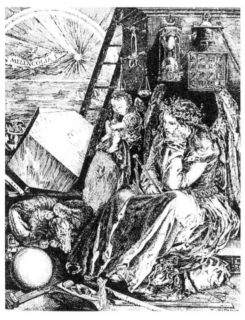

Melancholy. Lucien Nass, *Curiosités Médico-Artistiques* (1907), Albin Michel, Paris

Melancholy [Greek: *melano*, black + *chole*, bile] Black bile from the lower intestines was thought to be the cause of melancholia or depression by Hippocrates (460–377 BC), and he proposed purgatives as treatment. Several centuries later Cicero (143–106 BC) disputed this theory and attributed melancholia to psychological difficulties. Galen (AD 129–200), observed that it sometimes changed into epilepsy. Various treatments from demonology to bezoars, were employed, and precious stones, parts of animal bodies and metals were used by high priests. Paul of Aegina (AD 625–690) defined it 'as a disorder of the intellect without fever, occasioned mostly by a melancholic humor seizing the

understanding'. He recommended the use of hellebore, decoctions, other herbs, and also coitus 'to relieve the mind from cares that beset it'. Bartholomeus Angelicus, Paris professor of theology, wrote a chapter in his book *De Proprietatibus* of 1535. One of the greatest monographs, *Anatomy of Melancholy*, was written by Robert Burton (1577–1640) in 1621. He is said to have suffered from it and gained an insight which contributed to the success of his book, which is supposed to have been inspired by *A Treatise on Melancholy* written in 1586 by Timothy Bright (1551–1616), an English physician. English clergyman, Richard Baxter (1615-1691), published *A discourse Connecting Trouble of Mind and the Disease of Melancholy* in 1691.

Meletius (AD 400) Christian monk from Rome who wrote several works on physiology and anatomy.

Melioidosis [Greek: *melis*, a distemper of asses + *eidos*, resemblance + *osis*, process] A glanders-like disease, first described in 1912 by Alfred Whitmore (1876–1946) and C.S. Krishnaswami. Whitmore was a surgeon in India and he studied further cases in Rangoon, Burma, and isolated a motile Gram negative bacillus from patients. The causative organism was named *Bacillus whitmori*, and the disease was called melioidosis by Sir Ambrose Thomas Stanton (1875–1938) in 1917 and William Fletcher (d 1938) and Stanton published a book in 1921.

Mellanby, Lady May, née Tweedy (1882–1978) Wife of Sir Edward Mellanby (1884–1955), she was a pioneer in nutrition and vitamins A and D related to the development of teeth. She spent her early years in Russia and in 1902 entered Girton College, Cambridge where she was permitted to attend some lectures not normally open to women. She was the first woman to present a paper to the British Orthodontics Society in 1919.

Mellanby, Sir Edward (1884–1955) English pharmacologist and pioneer in the study of vitamins and nutrition. Born in West Hartlepool and educated at Emmanuel College, Cambridge where he began research with Frederick Gowland Hopkins (1861–1947). He moved to London in 1907, graduated in medicine from St Thomas' Hospital Medical School in 1910 and became a physiology demonstrator there. His first paper, on creatine and creatinine, was published in 1908, before his graduation. He was appointed in 1913 as professor of physiology at the King's College for Women, London. He became professor of pharmacology at Sheffield University in 1920 and was elected secretary to the Medical Research Council in 1933. He produced rickets in dogs by maintaining them on a deficient diet and suggested that the missing nutrient factor was a fat-soluble substance, vitamin D. He advocated cod liver oil as a source of vitamin D which led to the elimination of what was then a prevalent disease. His research on vitamin A during embryonic development caused him to suggest that a bleaching process used in wheat flour may lead to serious bone and nerve defects.

Meltzer, Samuel James (1851–1920) American physiologist and pioneer in endotracheal insufflation of ether as anesthesia during thoracic surgery. He also did clinical studies to demonstrate the physiological mechanisms involved in asthma.

Melvill, Thomas (1726–1753) Scottish scientist from Glasgow University who demonstrated the spectra of the luminous gases in 1753.

Membrane Potential The basic theory states that electric forces in muscles and nerves are related to selective permeability of the living membranes to cations and anions. It was proposed by German chemist and Nobel Prize winner, Wilhelm Ostwald (1853–1932) around 1909. Julius Bernstein (1839–1917), a German professor of physiology at Halle who invented a differential rheotome to record the voluntary contractions of the muscle on a time related basis in 1890, proposed the theory to explain electrical properties of muscle in 1912.

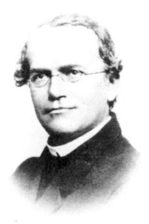

Gregor Mendel (1822–1884). Courtesy of the National Library of Medicine

Mendel, Gregor Johann (1822–1884) Founder of genetics, born near Udrau, a remote village in Moravia. He worked on hybridization of pea plants, while a monk at an Augustinian monastery at Brünn, growing about 30,000 plants which he artificially fertilized to produce specific characteristics. He studied science in Vienna and returned to his monastery, becoming abbot in 1868. As a lone worker he acquired his own microscope and worked laboriously and published his epoch-making work enunciating the laws of genetics. His laws of segregation and of independent

assortment were published in 1865. They went unheeded until English geneticist William Bateson (1861–1926) rediscovered them and wrote *Mendel's Principles of Heredity* published in 1902. *See Mendel's laws.*

Mendel, Lafayette Benedict (1872–1935) American professor at Yale. In 1913 he demonstrated the fat-soluble nature of the accessory nutritional factor, later called 'fat soluble A' by Elmer Verner McCollum (1879–1967) of Wisconsin and N. Simmonds in 1917. *See night blindness.*

Mendel's Laws Discovered by Gregor Mendel (1822–1884), an Augustinian monk, who corresponded with Karl Wilhelm von Nägeli (1817–1891), a contemporary Swiss botanist who gave negative comments. Mendel later published his findings in the local *Brunn Natural History Society Transactions* in 1865. They went unnoticed for 30 years until Hugo de Vries (1848–1935) of The Netherlands, and Erich Tschermak (1871–1962) independently expanded Mendel's work.

Mendeleeff Periodic Table Sequential arrangement of elements according to their atomic weight, devised by the Russian chemist, Dimitri Ivanovich Mendeleeff (1834–1907). The elements show similar characteristics at regular intervals, making it possible to predict their properties even before they were discovered. *See periodic law.*

Mendeleeff, Dmitri Ivanovitch (1834–1907) Russian chemist, born at Tobolsk in Siberia. He was the 14th and youngest child of a schoolteacher. After his father lost his job due to blindness, his mother set up a glass workshop and worked single handedly to support the family and educate the children. He studied at the local school and went to the University of St Petersburg at the age of 16, and later to the University of Heidelberg. He became a professor at St Petersburg Technical Institute in 1863 and the University of St Petersburg in 1866. He published his great work, *Principles of Chemistry*, in 1869 proposing his periodic law which he refined over the next 20 years. This was initially received with some skepticism but, as more elements were discovered and fitted his table, it became accepted. His greatest contribution was in recognizing that some elements still had to be discovered, and that their properties could be predicted, and so he left gaps in his table for them. *See Mendeleeff periodic table.*

Mendelson Syndrome Aspiration of gastric contents during general anesthesia in labor. Described by American obstetrician and gynecologist, Curtis Lester Mendelson (b 1913) in 1946.

Ménétrier Disease Giant gastric hypertrophy with

hypoproteinemia, diarrhea and protein losing enteropathy. Described by French histopathologist, Pierre E. Ménétrier (1859–1935) in 1888.

Menghini, Vincenzo Antonio (1704–1759) Italian physician who demonstrated the presence of iron in blood in 1746.

Menière Syndrome Characterized by episodic vertigo, tinnitus and progressive deafness. Described by French otorhinologist, Prosper Menière (1799–1862) of Paris in 1861. A method of surgical treatment was described by Walter Edward Dandy (1886–1946) of America in 1928. The beneficial effects of betahistidine was described by T.J. Wilmot in 1972.

Meningioma [Greek: *meninx*, membrane + *oma*] Tumor of the meninges, usually next to the dura mater, first called endothelioma by Camille Golgi (1843–1926) in 1869. Harvey Cushing (1869–1939) wrote a monograph in 1938.

Meningitis [Greek: *meninx*, membrane + *itis*, inflammation] *See cerebrospinal fever, aseptic meningitis, tuberculous meningitis.*

Meningococcal Meningitis *See cerebrospinal fever.*

Meningococcus [Greek: *meninx*, membrane + *kokkos*, berry] Gram negative bacterium, *Nesseiria meningitides*, first isolated from six patients with acute cerebrospinal meningitis by Anton Weichselbaum (1845–1920) of Vienna in 1887 and named *Diplococcus intracellularis meningitides*. His observations were confirmed and the organism was established as a the cause of meningitis by von Lingleshiem of Germany in 1905.

Menkes Syndrome Inborn error of leucine and isoleucine metabolism leading to mental deficiency. Described by American pediatrician, John H. Menkes (b 1928), in 1954. Due to the maple syrup odor of the urine, it is also known as maple syrup disease, or, because of the effect on hair, as kinky hair syndrome.

Mensturation [Latin: *mensis*, month + *sturere*, to flow] Rest from physical activity was first suggested by New York gynecologist, Mary Putnam Jacobi (1842–1906) in 1876. She was the first woman to receive a medical doctorate from the University of Paris, and to be admitted to the New York Academy of Science. Premenstrual swelling of the endometrium was first noted by Hans Kundrat and George Englemann in 1873. The normal cyclical changes in the endometrium were first described by two Viennese gynecologists, Ludwig Adler (1876–1958) and Fritz Hitschmann (1870–1926) in 1907. *See premenstrual tension, safe period.*

Mental Deficiency *See idiocy.*

Mental Disease *See psychiatry, psychology, asylum.*

Mental Hospitals *See asylum.*

Mental Hygiene [Latin: *mens*, mind; Greek: *hygieia*, health] Term first used by William Sweetser (1787–1875) in the title of his book published in 1843. It was used in psychiatry by Adolf Meyer (1866–1950) of the New York State Psychiatric Institute. The Connecticut Society of Mental Hygiene was formed in 1908 and the National Committee for Mental Hygiene was set up in 1909. The journal *Mental Hygiene* appeared in 1917.

Mental Quotient *See intelligence quotient.*

Mepacrine Quinacrine hydrochloride, used against malaria in World War ll. *See Atebrine.*

Mephenesin or Mynesin Early tranquilizer and muscle relaxant, discovered in 1946 by F.M. Berger and Bradley of England during their search for a preservative for injections. The muscle relaxing action due to its effect on the nervous system was the first pharmacological property to be noted, hence its use in anesthesia until it was recognized as a tranquilizer.

Meprobamate Tranquilizer first synthesized by F.M. Berger, medical director of the Wallace Laboratories, around 1952.

Meralgia Paresthetica [Greek: *meros*, thigh + *algos*, pain] Affects the external cutaneous nerve of the thigh. Also called Bernhardt disease or Bernhardt–Roth disease. Described by German neurologist, Martin Max Bernhardt (1844–1915) in 1878, and Russian neurologist, Vladimir Karolovich Roth (1848–1916).

Mercaptopurine Antileukemic drug (6–mercaptopurine) produced by two American biochemists, George Herbert Hitchings (b 1905) of Washington and New York biochemist, Gertrude Belle Elion (b 1918) in 1953. Its clinical evaluation in patients was done by Joseph Holland Burchenal (b 1912) and co-workers in the same year.

Mercier, Charles Arthur (1852–1919) Physician to a private asylum in London. He delivered the FitzPatrick lectures on *Astrology in Medicine* in 1913, and in the same year he published a small volume of verses, *The King's Fishing.*

Mercier Bar Transverse curved ridge joining the internal openings of the urethras within the bladder. Described in 1848 by Louis Auguste Mercier (1811–1882), a urinary surgeon from Paris.

Mercurialis, Hieronymus (1530–1606) Professor of medicine at Bologna, Padua and Pisa who wrote the first systematic treatise on skin diseases in 1572. He also wrote the first Italian book on obstetrics in 1586 in which he advocated cesarean section in cases of contracted pelvis. He produced an illustrated book on gymnastics and exercises for health, *De Arte Gymnastica*, in 1569.

Mercury [Latin: *mercurius*] Called quicksilver by Aristotle (384–322 BC) and liquid silver by Dioscorides (AD 40–90). It was used for treatment of syphilis by Paracelsus (1493–1541), and became a common drug for venereal diseases. Gabriele Falloppio (1523–1562) opposed its extensive use for syphilis during the mid-16th century. Mercury injections in the form of diethyl mercury was introduced as treatment for syphilis by P. Hepp of Germany in 1887, but abandoned due to toxicity. *See mercury poisoning.*

Mercury Poisoning Common cause of necrotizing nephrosis. Anuria was first observed by Ulrich von Hutton (1488–1523) in 1519. Mercury poisoning in goldsmiths was described by Bernadini Ramazzini (1633–1714) in his treatise on occupational diseases in 1700. Adolf Kussmaul (1822–1902) described loss of teeth, stomatitis and reddening of the pharynx (Kussmaul sign) in mercurial poisoning. Hatter's shakes or mercurial tremor were observed in workers in industry who constantly dipped hats in mercuric nitrate in the 18th century. Organic mercurial compounds were used in chemical research in 1863, and two research workers at St Bartholomew's Hospital died as a result of their research with dimethyl mercury in 1866. Diethyl mercury injections used as treatment for syphilis in Germany in 1887, were abandoned due to toxicity. Mercurial compounds as fungicidal seed dressings for cereal led to several cases of poisoning. Sodium formaldehyde sulfoxylate was introduced as an antidote by Rosenthal in 1934. *See mercury.*

Merkel Corpuscles Sensory tactile nerve endings first described by Friedrich Sigmund Merkel (1845–1919), professor of anatomy at Göttingen in 1880.

Merkel Fossa Central fossa between the two cavities of the larynx. Described by Carl Ludwig Merkel (1812–1876), professor of laryngology at Leipzig in 1857.

Merriam, Clinton Hart (1885–1942) New York zoologist, naturalist and early conservationist, instrumental in establishing the National Geographical Society (now the Fish and Wildlife Service) in 1888. He devised a system of life zones based on temperature differences in *Life Zones and Crop Zones of the United States* published in 1898.

Merrit, Hiram Houston (1902–1979) Professor of neurology at the College of Physicians and Surgeons in New York. He was editor of the *Archives of Neurology*. He introduced

diphenylhydrantoin (epinutin) as treatment for epilepsy in 1938.

Merry Andrew Another name for Andrew Boorde (b 1490) who lived in the reign of Henry VIII. *See Boorde, Andrew.*

Merseberg Triad Consisting of exophthalmos, goiter and palpitations in hyperthyroidism. Described by Carl Adolph von Basedow (1799–1854), who named it in honor of his home town, Merseberg in Germany.

Mersenne, Marin (1588–1648) French Minim friar and mathematician from Paris. He discovered the law relating to the length and period of oscillation of a pendulum and measured the speed of sound.

Mesenteric Embolism The first diagnosis in a living subject was made by Adolf Kussmaul (1822–1902) in 1864.

Mery, Jean (1645–1722) Surgeon at the Hôtel Dieu at Paris who described the pair of Cowper glands related to the male urethra in 1684. These were later named after William Cowper (1666–1760) who re-described them in 1700.

Mescaline Poisonous alkaloid obtained from the cactus (*Lophophora williamsii*) and used in ancient rituals for its hallucinogenic properties. The first clinical description of its effects was given by American neurologist, Silas Weir Mitchell (1829–1914), in 1896.

Mesmer, Franz Anton (1734–1815) Physician from Mersberg in Swabia who introduced the practice of animal magnetism. His first publication appeared in 1766 and contained a description of the planetary influence from heavenly bodies which diffused through a subtle fluid and acted on the nervous system. Though his theory was scientifically unfounded his method later developed into the practice of hypnotism. *See animal magnetism, mesmerism, hypnosis.*

Mesmerism Animal magnetism, named after its founder, Franz Anton Mesmer (1734–1815) by his friend and philosopher Karl Wolhart. Mesmer published his doctrine in 1766 and called it 'animal magnetism' in the belief that the trance was due to an effect similar to that of a magnet. His method was later developed to produce anesthesia and renamed 'hypnosis' by James Braid (1795–1860), a Manchester surgeon, in 1843. *See animal magnetism, hypnosis.*

Mesoderm [Greek: *mesos*, middle + *derma*, skin] Middle layer of the three primary germ layers of the embryo. The concept of embryonic development of organs from different germ layers was first proposed by Estonian, Karl Ernst Ritter von Baer (1792–1876), professor at St Petersburg in 1828. The germ layers were classified into ectoderm, endoderm and mesoderm by Polish-born German physician, Robert Remak (1815–1865), in 1845.

Mesopotamian Medicine The area between the rivers Tigris and Euphrates, known as Mesopotamia, was the cradle of civilization around 4000 BC. Writing was developed here by the Sumerians around 3000 BC. Mesopotamian doctors attributed disease to sin and sought divine help to reveal them. They regarded the liver as the storage organ of blood and hence the seat of life. They studied livers of animals and made clay models of the organ with markings on them. Their medical practice was chiefly in the hands of three groups of priests. Of them, Asu, was a physician; Ashipu was an exorcist; and Baru predicted the outcome of diseases through divine help. *See Sumerian medicine, Babylonian medicine, Hammurabi.*

Mesothelioma [Greek: *mesos*, middle + *thele*, nipple] *See asbestosis.*

Messenger RNA Ribonucleic acid units which serve as templates for protein synthesis. The existence of messenger RNA was confirmed by François Jacob (b 1920) and Jacques Lucien Monod (1910–1976) of Paris in the *Journal of Molecular Biology* in 1960. The chromosome segment that codes for a single mRNA molecule and regulates transcription and translation of a protein was discovered and named 'operon', by F. Jacob, Sydney Brenner (b 1927), F. Cuzin and Monod in 1963.

Mesue, Jr or Maswijah al–Marindi (d 1015) Born at Marindi on the Euphrates and studied medicine and philosophy at Baghdad. He wrote several medical treatises including one on surgery, *Phlebotomia secundum Damascenum*. The materia medica, *Grabadin*, bearing his name was very popular in the Middle Ages, and was one of the first medical works printed in Venice in 1471.

Mesue, Sr or Yohannan ibn Masawayh (AD 777–857) Arabian physician, known to Latin Europe as Janus Damescenus. He was born at Jundishapur where his father was a pharmacist. His work is mentioned by Rhazes (850–932), and nine editions are in the British Museum. The *Mesue Opera*, illustrated with pictures of medicinal herbs, was printed in Venice in 1603. His other works include: *Aphorisms, Book of Fevers* and *On the Pulse.*

Metabolic Disease [Greek: *meta*, after + *bole*, change] One of the oldest known diseases of metabolism, diabetes, was described and named by Aretaeus (AD 81–138). Santorio Santorius (1561–1636) pioneered scientific study of metabolism in health. His findings, following 30 years of study, were published in *Ars de statica medicina* in 1614. The earliest scientific monograph on diabetes, *Der Diabetes Mellitus*, was written by Bernard Naunym (1839–1925) in 1895. Frederick William Pavy (1829–1911), a physician at Guy's Hospital devoted his career to the study of metabolism of sugars. Sir Archibald Edward Garrod (1857–1936), of St Bartholomew's Hospital, pioneer in the study of inborn errors of metabolism, gave original descriptions of alkaptonuria, cystinuria, and pentosuria. *See metabolism, basal metabolic rate.*

Metabolic Pathway *See citric acid cycle, carbohydrates, Krebs cycle, glucose-1-phosphate kinase, glucose-1-phosphate.*

Metabolism [Greek: *meta*, after or beyond + *bole*, change] The first person to experimentally study metabolism was Sanctorio Sanctorius (1561–1636), a physician from Padua. He designed a balance to calculate the weight of invisible respiration and perspiration. His work was published in *Ars de statica medicina* in 1614, and translated into English by John Quincy (d 1723). He also invented the first clinical thermometer for use in his metabolic studies. The pathway through which food is converted to energy was first demonstrated by German physiologist, Karl von Voit (1831–1908) in 1865, who also developed a test for basal metabolism in 1873. Max Rubner (1854–1932), a physiologist from Munich, was a pioneer in the modern study of metabolic diseases. He demonstrated that the body obtained its energy from fats, carbohydrates and proteins and used the nitrogen from these sources for its vital functions. He measured metabolic changes in the body in 1891 using it as a calorimeter. He also described the specific dynamic action of food.

Metapsychosis Term for various philosophies where theories are not justifiable on logical grounds but verifiable by experiment or observation, was first proposed by Pythagorus in 528 BC. The practice of embalming of dead bodies by the Egyptians is supposed to have resulted from this belief.

Metamorphosis [Greek: *meta*, after + *morphosis*, shaping] Term first used by a London naturalist, Thomas Moufet (1553–1604), in entomology to denote changes of the embryo during its development into an adult.

Metaphase Stage in mitotic cell division during which the undivided centromeres lie on the spindle. Described by German botanist from Bonn, Eduard Adolf Strasburger (1844–1912) in 1880.

Metaphysics [Greek: *meta*, beyond, *phuein*, make grow] Science of abstract reasoning began with Aristotle (384–322

Dictionary of the History of Medicine

BC). Andronicus of Rhodes, a Greek philosopher who lived around 58 BC, introduced the term 'metaphysics' for the science of thought and influences unseen, and incapable of direct recognition by senses. One of the earliest books (of ethics) on metaphysics and psychology was written by Benedict de Spinoza (1632–1677) and published in 1677 after his death. The International Institute of Metaphysics at Paris was founded in 1919.

Metastatic Carcinoma [Greek: *meta*, after + *statikos*, causing to stand] The spread of a tumor by metastasis was first investigated by German anatomist, Wilhelm Gottfried Waldeyer (1837–1921) in 1867.

Metchnikoff, Elie (1845–1916) Immunologist and embryologist, born to Jewish parents in the Ukraine, he attended Kharkov University and received his doctorate from the University of St Petersburg in 1867. After his initial interest in zoology, he studied bacteriology in 1882. He left Russia and, after spending time in Italy and Odessa, in 1887 he became director of the Pasteur Institute in Paris. The *Nature of Man* was one of his first books translated into English by Peter Chalmers Mitchell and published in 1903. While at the Pasteur Institute in Paris, he discovered the phagocytic function of white blood cells and demonstrated their role in combating bacterial invasion. He also successfully transmitted syphilis from man to a higher animal. He advocated eating large quantities of yogurt to promote good health. He did classic studies on antibacterial immunity and was awarded the Nobel Prize for Physiology or Medicine in 1908 (together with Paul Ehrlich, 1854–1915).

Meteorites They were worshipped during prehistoric times and known as thunderbolts from the skies. The dark reddish brown sacred stone, Kaaba at Mecca, is believed to be a meteorite. The largest known meteorite lies at Grootfontein in South West Africa. They contain a mixture of iron and silica in varying proportions. Edmund Halley, Wallis and others studied them.

Methemoglobinemia [Greek: *meta*, after + *haima*, blood; Latin: *globus*, globe] Condition in which oxidation of hemoglobin to the ferric state results in cyanosis, headache, fatigue, nausea, tachycardia, coma and, sometimes death. It may be chemically or drug induced, or be an abnormality in hemoglobin M, or due to a deficiency in cytochrome b5 reductase. It can also be caused by administration of sulfacompounds, and the mechanism of formation of sulfhemoglobin or methemoglobin was shown by L. Snapper in 1925. Methylene blue was first used as treatment for methemoglobinemia by W.B. Wendel in 1939.

Methane Holy phosphorescent light over marshy ground was noticed in 16th century Europe and named, Will-o-the-wisp or Jack-o-Lantern. The inflammability of the air from the marshes was shown to be caused by methane gas by Alessandro Volta (1745–1827) in 1778. Its inflammability was a major threat to mine workers and Sir Humphry Davy invented the miner's lamp in 1816 to overcome this.

Methanol Methyl alcohol toxicity was reported as early as 1855. Its toxicity to the eye was recognized in 1910, but it was still used as an alternative to ethyl alcohol in alcoholic drinks in New York and other places until around 1920.

Methionine Amino acid discovered in 1921 by American pathologist, John Howard Mueller (b 1891) during his research on growth factors for microorganisms.

Methodists An ancient sect or school of medicine, rival to the Hippocratic system, founded by Themison of Laodicea (100 BC), a physician and disciple of Aesculapiades in 50 BC. He explained diseases on the basis of relaxation or contraction of pores in the body. Methodists named acute disease 'status strictus', state of contraction, and chronic disease 'status laxus', state of relaxation.

Methotrexate Developed by Sidney Faber, a cancer scientist in the United States, from aminopterin in 1948 as a folic acid antagonist in treatment of leukemia. Li, Hertz and Donald B. Spencer used it in the treatment of choriocarcinoma in 1956. The use of methotrexate and cyclophosphamide in the treatment of Burkitt lymphoma (a viral cancer) was introduced by Denis Parsons Burkitt (1911–1993) of Enniskillen, Northern Ireland in 1960, while working in Uganda. Chemotherapy with it in metastatic osteosarcoma was pioneered by South African surgeon, Norman Jaffe (b 1933) of Johannesburg in 1972.

Methyl Bromide Non-inflammable gas used for refrigeration, as a fire extinguisher, and fumigant was first noted to cause poisoning by A. Jaquet in 1893. Escape of this gas from refrigerators led to a number of casualties in Europe and America in the 1920s.

Methylene Blue Histological stain for nerve tissue introduced by Paul Ehrlich (1854–1915) in 1885. Also tested by Ehrlich as chemotherapy against the malarial parasite in 1891. It was first used as treatment for methemoglobinemia by W.B. Wendel in 1939.

Metric System In 1790 a committee consisting of Claude Louis Berthollet (1749–1822), Pierre Simon Laplace (1749–1827) and others devised a uniform system for measures. A meter is a distance equal to a ten millionth part of the distance between the poles and the equator. The rest of the metric system was completed in 1799.

Metrodorus of Chios Disciple of Democritus (460–370 BC) and a physician. Hippocrates (460–377 BC) is said to have been one of his pupils.

Metropolitan Ear and Throat Hospital Founded by James Yearsley (1805–1869), a London otorhinologist, in 1838 at Fitzroy Square, London. He described the artificial tympanum, and identified affections of the nose and throat that cause deafness.

Mevalonic Acid Key intermediate in synthesis of steroids and terpenes. Isolated from a yeast byproduct by American biochemist, Karl August Folkers (b 1906) and his team in 1956.

Meyer, Adolf (1866–1950) Psychiatrist and neurologist, born in Niederweiningen in Switzerland. He emigrated to America in 1892 and joined the Johns Hopkins Medical School in 1910 as head of the new Phipps Psychiatric Clinic, where he served until his retirement. He proposed the concept of psychobiology which integrated medicine and psychiatry, and sought to explain mental disorders on the basis of maladjustment.

Meyer, Carl Friedrich (1884–1974) Professor of microbiology at the University of California. In 1920 he introduced the generic term *Brucella* for bacteria which caused Malta fever, in honor of its discoverer Sir David Bruce (1855–1931).

Meyer, Hans Horst (1853–1939) German pharmacologist who suggested in 1899 that the effect of an anesthetic agent is related to its lipid solubility in the nerve tissue.

Meyer, Julius Lothar von (1830–1895) German chemist and medical graduate from Zurich. He was first professor of chemistry at Tübingen University. He demonstrated in 1857 that oxygen combines with hemoglobin during respiration. He demonstrated that atomic volumes were functions of atomic weights, and proposed the periodic table independently of Dimitri Ivanovich Mendeleeff (1834–1907) in 1864. He also suggested that the carbon atoms in benzene formed a ring structure.

Meyer, Viktor (1848–1897) German chemist, born in Berlin, and professor of chemistry at Zurich, Göttingen, and Heidelberg. He coined the term 'stereochemistry' for the study of molecular shapes and devised a method of determining vapor density.

Meyer Cartilage Anterior extremities of the inferior thyroarytenoid ligaments were described by Edmund Victor Meyer (1864–1931), professor of laryngology at Berlin in 1901.

Meyer Glands Found beneath the tongue, in the hypoglossus muscle. Described by Georg Hermann von Meyer (1815–1892), professor of histology at Zurich in 1871.

Meyerhof, Otto Fritz (1884–1951) American biochemist of German origin who trained in medicine at the University of Heidelberg and became the director of Kaiser Wilhelm Institute for Medical Research in Berlin (1924–1929) and Heidelberg (1929–1938). He left Germany in 1938 and, after working in France and Spain, went to the University of Pennsylvania in America in 1940. He worked out the pathway of glucose use in muscle metabolism known as the Embden–Meyerhof cycle. The Hill–Meyerhof theory related to metabolic changes in the cytoplasm of muscle during contraction was proposed by Archibald Vivian Hill (1886–1977) and Meyerhof around 1912. Meyerhof also discovered glycogen as a source of lactic acid in the muscle in 1920. Meyerhof and Hill shared the Nobel Prize in Physiology or Medicine in 1922.

Meynert Decussation On the tracts of tegmenti within the spinal canal, first described by Theodor Herman Meynert (1833–1892), professor of neurology at Vienna in 1869. Meynert also studied cortical cells and identified the five horizontal layers in 1867.

Meynet Nodes Nodules in the capsules of joints or tendons in rheumatic conditions, especially affecting children. Described by French physician, Paul Claude Hyacinthe Meynet (1831–1892) of Lyons.

Michael the Scot (1175–1235) Translator of Arabic and Greek science into Latin. His work on astrology was a major work in Latin. The first Latin versions of the works of Averroes and Aristotelian biology were produced by him.

Michaelis Rhomboid Diamond-shaped area over the posterior aspect of the pelvis bounded by the dimples of the posterior iliac spines, the lines formed by the gluteal muscles, and a groove at the lower end of the spine. Described by Gustav Adolf Michaelis (1798–1848), an obstetrician from Kiel.

Michaelis–Menten Equation The rate at which catalytic reactions take place. Developed by Berlin-born American biochemist, Leonor Michaelis (1875–1945) and American physician, Maude Lenore Menten (1879–1960) in 1913. They worked on rate-controlling steps in enzyme reactions, assuming that substrate combines with enzyme to form an intermediate complex which then breaks down to give the product and the unmodified enzyme. The equation was further modified by John Burdon Sanderson Haldane (1892–1964) to give half maximum velocity.

Micheli, James Bartholomew (1692–1766) Astronomer, physicist and mathematician from Geneva who invented a new form of thermometer.

Micheli, Pier Antonio (1679–1737) Botanist from Florence and a founder of the Society of Natural History of Florence. He was director of the botanical gardens formed by Cosimo de Medici and published an early work on mycology, *Nova Plantarum genera*, in 1729.

Michell, John (1724–1793) English geologist from Nottinghamshire and professor at Cambridge who founded seismology and invented a torsion balance. He published an important treatise on an artificial magnet in 1750.

Michelson, Albert Abraham (1852–1931) American physicist, born in Poland and came to America at the age of four. He studied the velocity of light in 1878 and replaced the rotating mirror with a prism. He invented the echelon grating made of quartz plates capable of producing dispersion of light. He is remembered for the Michelson–Morley experiment to determine ether drift, which paved the way for Einstein's theory of relativity. He was professor of physics at Chicago in 1892 and was the first American to win a Nobel Prize in 1907.

Microangiopathic Hemolytic Anemia [Greek: *micro*, small + *angeion*, vessel + *pathos*, disease] Term coined by William St Claire Symmers (1863–1937) in 1932 to denote the mechanical damage to red blood cells resulting in poikilocytosis or abnormally shaped red cells.

Microbiology [Greek: *micros*, small + *bios*, life + *logos*, discourse] The earliest recorded attempt to view microscopic organisms was made in 1658 by Athanasius Kircher (1601–1680), a Jesuit priest. He examined blood in plague victims in his primitive microscope with a magnification of only 32, and described what he saw as 'worms' of plague in *Scrutium Pestis*. Antoni van Leeuwenhoek (1632–1723), a Dutch lens maker described 'animalcules', mostly protozoan organisms in 1674. He also identified and described bacteria from samples of material taken from his teeth. Modern microbiology was established by Louis Pasteur (1822–1895) with his study of the chemical activities of microorganisms in 1857. The link between microbiology and biochemistry was further strengthened by Russian microbiologist, Sergei N. Winogradsky around 1900. *See bacteriology.*

Microchemistry Technique for measuring concentration of chemicals in small samples of biological fluids was introduced around 1910. The photometer, an instrument which utilized a photocell linked to a sensitive microammeter, for analysis of the chemical constituents in small samples of

blood and urine, was invented by G.E. Davis and C. Sheard of America in 1927. A photoelectric hemoglobinometer was developed by Sheard and A.H. Sanford in 1928.

Microcytic Anemia [Greek: *mikros*, small + *kytos*, cell] A classification of anemias based on red cell morphology was proposed by Maxwell Myer Wintrobe (b 1901) in 1930. He proposed four groups: macrocytic, normocytic, simple microcytic, and chronic microcytic. He also developed the Wintrobe hematocrit to measure the hematocrit and erythrocyte sedimentation rates in a single tube. *See microcytosis.*

Microcytosis [Greek: *mikros*, small + *kytos*, cell] Characterized by the presence of small hemoglobin-containing erythrocytes or microcytes in the blood. Observed by Constant Vanlair (1839–1914) and Jean Baptiste Nicolas Voltaire Masius (1836–1912) of Belgium around 1890. *See iron deficiency anemia.*

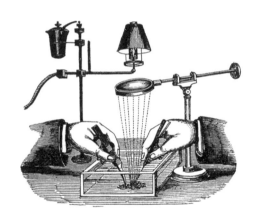

Microdissection. Jabez Hogg, *Microscope, Its History, Construction, and Teaching* (1854). The Illustrated London Library, London

Microdissection First suggested by Johannes E. Purkinje (1787–1869) in 1844, and it was performed with the use of a mechanically controlled needle by H.D. Schmidt in 1859. Chabrey reintroduced the technique in 1877 and micromanipulation in embryology, cancer and genetics was pioneered by Wilhelm Roux (1850–1924), Edmund Beecher Wilson (1856–1939), and Jacques Loeb (1859–1924). The pioneers of instruments were: S.L. Schouten from Holland (1899), C.V. Taylor, Barber and Kyte, from America (1900).

Micron [Greek: *mikros*, small] It represents one millionth of a meter.

Microscope [Greek: *mikros*, small + *skopein*, to view] Term first used in 1625. Cornelius Jacobson Drebble (1570–1633) of Holland in 1621 and Domenico Fontana (1500–1537) from Rome have been credited with its discovery. The

Dutch spectacle maker, Zacharius Jansen and his son appear to have made microscopes before 1590. Athanasius Kircher (1601–1680) of Giessen used 32 magnification to view blood cells in 1658. The first description of the compound microscope was given by Robert Hooke (1635–1703) in 1667, and Eustachio Divini in 1668. Antoni von Leeuwenhoek (1632–1723) ground his own lenses and constructed over 200 microscopes. Phillip Bonnai published an account of two compound microscopes in 1698. Le Pere Cherubin, a French philosopher was the first to view small objects with both eyes in 1677. Benjamin Martin in England improved the microscope and sold pocket versions in 1740. Henry Baker of London improved the microscope in 1763, and recapitulated much of Leeuwenhoek's work in *The Microscope made Easy* published in 1743. A diamond microscope was made by Andrew Pritchard in 1824, who also introduced 'test objects' to compare quality. The Microscopical Society of London was established in 1839. Giovanni Battista Amici (1786–1863) of Florence constructed a reflecting microscope and improved the achromatic objective in 1812. A binocular microscope was constructed by Riddel in 1851. Other early treatises were by: J. Queckett in 1848, W.B. Carpentier in 1856, and Lionel Smith Beale (1828–1906) in 1858. The *Micrographic Dictionary* was published by Griffith and Henfreys in 1856. A spectrum microscope capable of detecting one millionth of a grain of blood was exhibited by Henry Clifton Sorby (1826–1908) in 1865. Ernst Abbe (1840–1905), a partner of Carl Zeiss, modernized the microscope by adding the apochromatic objective and the oil immersion lens in 1878. Abbe also improved phase-contrast microscopy in 1892. The modern phase-contrast technique was introduced by a Dutch physicist, Frits Zernike (1888–1966) in 1935. The ultramicroscope, capable of seeing particles, was invented by Nobel Prize winner, Richard Adolf Zsigmondy (1865–1929) in 1903. *See electron microscope.*

Microscopic Anatomy Marcello Malpighi (1628–1694), a professor at Bologna, discovered capillary circulation in 1661, and is regarded as the father of microscopic anatomy. His work was advanced by French physician, Marie François Xavier Bichat (1771–1802), from Thoitette while he was at the Hôtel Dieu in Paris. The first textbook in English, *The Microscopic Anatomy of the Human Body*, was written by Arthur Hill Hassall (1817–1894) in 1846, followed by Rudolph Albert von Köllicker's (1817–1905) textbook in 1852. Friedrich Gustav Jakob Henle (1809–1885), a German histologist who discovered smooth muscle in the middle coat of smaller arteries, described columnar and ciliated epithelial cells, the external sphincter of the bladder, and the Henle tubules of the kidney.

Microscopical Society of London Established in 1839. *See microscope.*

Microsporum audouinii Species of pathogenic fungus, commonly causes puerperal tinea capitis. Named in honor of French physician, Jean-Victor Audouin (1797–1841) from the Natural History Museum of Paris, by David Gruby (1810–1898) in 1843.

Microtome [Greek: *mikros*, small + *tome*, to cut] First devised by Alexander Brandt in 1870 and further developed in 1880 by Richard Thoma (1847–1923) professor of pathology at Heidelberg.

Micrurgy [Greek: *mikros*, small + *ergon*, work] Term coined in 1920 by Tibor Peterfi (b 1891) of Jena in Germany to denote the technique of micromanipulation. *See microdissection.*

Middle Ages Refers to a period that lasted from the coming of Saxons to the accession of the Tudors. Arab and Jewish doctors of this era include Avicenna (980–1037), Averroes (1126–1198), Maimonides (1135–1204) and Rhazes (850–932). Arnold of Villanova (1234–1311), Hildegard of Bingen (1098–1199), Lanfranchi (d 1315), Henri de Mondeville (1230–1320) and Guy de Chauliac (1300–1370) were notable European doctors. A notable English surgeon was John of Ardane (1306–1390) and Roger Bacon (1214–1294) was a naturalist, scientist and physician.

Middle Lobe Syndrome *See Brock syndrome.*

Middleton, Peter (d 1781) American physician of Scottish origin who performed the first dissection on record in America in 1750, and founded a medical school in New York where he served as professor of physiology from 1767 to 1776. He became governor of King's College, New York in 1775 and published *Historical Inquiries into Ancient and Present State of Medicine* in 1769.

Midgley, Thomas (1889–1944) American inventor from Beaver Falls, Pennsylvania, who was handicapped by childhood polio. He introduced freon as an agent for domestic refrigeration and devised the octane rating for petrol.

Midwifery Women were the only practitioners amongst ancient Hebrews and Egyptians. The first known professional association was formed at Regensburg, Germany in 1452. Louise Bourgeois (1563–1636) of France was the first female midwife to publish a book on obstetrics, *Observationes Diverses sur la Sterilite*, in 1626, followed by Jane Sharp (fl 1670) of England and Justina Dietrich of Prussia. Male midwives appeared in the Renaissance period, and William Harvey (1578–1657) is said to have engaged in obstetric practice in 1603. Elizabeth Cellier (fl 1680), a well respected midwife in England, asked King James ll to provide a hospital for mothers and to educate nurses. Other early famous male midwives include: Ambroise Paré (1510–1590) and François Rousette (1535–1590) of France. Male midwives became fashionable in Europe after the French surgeon, Julian Clement, attended during the labor of Madame de la Valliere, mistress of Louis XIV. *See accoucheur, Midwives Institute.*

Midwives Institute The first attempt in England to establish midwives as a recognized body was made by Mrs Cellier around 1700. She planned a training school and a Royal Hospital but failed to obtain a charter from the king. The Midwives Institute was founded in 1881 with the object of raising the standard of midwifery and the general status of midwives in England. The Central Midwives Board was created following the Midwives Act of 1902. A state midwifery service was established through the Midwives Act of 1936, and the Midwives Institute became the Royal College of Midwives under the patronage of the Queen in 1947. *See midwifery.*

Migraine An accurate clinical description of this form of headache was given by Quaker physician from Yorkshire, John Fothergill (1712–1780) in 1776. Another early description of headache associated with conditions such as allergy and asthma was given by Edward Liveing (1832–1919) of London in 1873. Ergotamine tartarate was first observed to provide relief by Tzanck in 1928, and the therapeutic effect of this drug was explained W G. Lennox of America in 1934.

Mikulicz Syndrome Associated with hypertrophy of the salivary glands and xerostomia. Described by Johann von Mikulicz-Radecki (1850–1905), a Polish surgeon in 1892.

Mikulicz-Radecki, Johann von (1850–1905) German-born Polish professor of surgery at Cracow who was an early advocator of antiseptic surgery and one of the first to use gloves and a mask.

Miles Operation Abdominoperineal resection of the rectum for rectal carcinoma. Devised by English surgeon, William Ernest Miles (1869–1947) in 1908.

Military Medicine *See army medicine and surgery.*

Military Surgery *See army medicine and surgery.*

Milk Alkali Syndrome *See Burnett syndrome.*

Milk Sickness Deaths due to ingestion of cows milk occurred in certain parts of America in the early 19th century. White snake root, used to feed the cows, was later

identified as the cause by American physician from New Jersey, Daniel Drake (1785–1852) in 1840.

Milk Mentioned as a medicine as well as food by Hippocrates (460–377 BC) who realized that it on occasions caused the formation of stones in the bladder. He recommended it for convalescence, and dissuaded its use for those who had flatulence and bloody discharge from the bowels. Galactophagi, a Scythian nation which lived principally on milk, is mentioned in Homer's *Iliad*. Aristotle (384–322 BC) considered milk of the camel, ass, and mare to be of the same consistency. According to Galen (AD 129–200), the thickest and fattest milk is that of the cows, and the least fat milk is from the camel. Dioscorides (AD 40–90) described it as a laxative and flatulent, but nutritious. Paul of Aegina (625–690) recommended it be taken in the morning and to restrain from hard exercise and food until it was digested.

Milkman Fractures Pseudo-fractures seen on X-rays in osteomalacia. Described by American radiologist, Louis Arthur Milkman (1895–1951) of Pennsylvania in 1930. *See Looser zone.*

Millar, John (d 1827) Physician from Glasgow who published *Observations on Tunnels under Navigable Rivers* (1807), and *Guide to Botany* in 1819. He edited the fourth edition of *Britannica.*

Millard–Gubler Syndrome Interference of the vascular blood supply to the pons causing abducens and facial nerve paralysis with contralateral hemiplegia. Described by two French physicians, Adolphe M. Gubler (1821–1879) at Paris in 1856 and re-described by Auguste Louis Jules Millard (1830–1915).

Miller Fisher Syndrome External ophthalmoplegia, ataxia, and areflexia due to a vascular cause. Described by Canadian neurologist, Miller Fisher (b 1910) in 1956.

Miller, Jacques Francis Albert Pierre (b 1931) French-Australian immunologist who graduated from the University of Sydney in 1955. He worked on leukemia in mice and found that the thymus gland is an important control in the immune system.

Miller, James (1818–1853) Graduated from Edinburgh in 1841, and became assistant physician to the London Hospital in 1853. He published *Pathology of Kidney in Scarlet Fever* in 1850.

Mills, Charles Karsner (1845–1931) Early professor of neurology in America, at the University of Pennsylvania. He described unilateral progressive ascending paralysis (Mills disease) in 1900.

Mills Disease Ascending hemiplegia, described by a neurologist, Charles Karsner Mills (1845–1931) of Philadelphia.

Milman, Sir Francis (1742–1821) Physician from Devonshire who practiced in Rome for a brief period before he returned to England as physician to the royal household. He published *Animadversiones de Natura Hydropsis ejesue Curatione,* and *A Treatise on the Source of Scurvy, and Putrid Fever* .

Milne-Edwards, Henri (1800–1885) Naturalist who qualified in medicine from Paris and wrote *Cours Elementaire de Zoologie* in 1834.

Milroy Disease Hereditary form of edema of the legs described by American professor of clinical medicine from Omaha, Nebraska, William Forsyth Milroy (1855–1942) in 1892. It was named after him by Sir William Osler (1849–1919) but had been described by German neurologist, Max Nonne (1861–1939) in 1891 and Henry Meige (1866–1940) of France re-described it in 1901.

Milton Disease Angioneurotic edema. A classic description under the name 'giant urticaria' was given by London dermatologist, John Laws Milton (1820–1898). *See angioneurotic edema.*

Minamata Disease (Syn: Kyko) Mysterious neurological illness which affected Japanese fisherman on the west coast of Kyushu in 1953. It was later identified to be due to contamination of fish by mercurial waste products from a factory.

Miner's Anemia (Syn: miner's cachexia) An epidemic of anemia and cachexia occurred in engineers and laborers who worked in the construction of St Gothard Tunnel in Italy. The intestinal parasite *Anchylostoma* or hook worm was identified as the cause by Italian pathologist Aldo Perroncito (1882–1929) in 1880.

Miner's Disease *See coal miners disease, Caplan syndrome, occupational diseases.*

Miner's Lamp Sir Humphry Davy invented the miner's wire gauze lamp in 1816, making it safer to work in mines. His *On the Safety Lamp for Coal Miners* was published in 1818.

Miner's Nystagmus Affected about 6000 coal workers per annum during the 19th century. The etiology, presenting with oscillatory movements of the eye, was not established and various factors such as exposure to poisonous gases and inadequate illumination were proposed to explain the illness.

Mineral Waters First analyzed by Swedish chemist, Torbern Olof Bergman (1735–1784) who discovered hydrogen sulfide in mineral springs. He was a pioneer in analytical chemistry and he prepared the first artificial mineral water using carbon dioxide in 1778.

Minister of Health The General Board of Health in England evolved into the Ministry of Health in 1917. The post of minister was established through the Ministry of Health Act of England and Wales in 1919. Christopher Addison, Viscount Addison of Stallingborough, an anatomist at St Bartholomew's Hospital, was appointed as the first minister and he held the office from 1918 to 1921. *See Bevan, Aneurin.*

Mink Encephalopathy Form of spongiform encephalopathy of animals first observed in America in 1947. It was described by Hartsough and Burger in 1965.

Minkowski, Oskar (1858–1931) Born in Lithuania, he studied medicine at Königsberg and Strasburg, and became a professor at Breslau in 1909. He established the role of the pancreas in diabetes. *See diabetes, acholuric jaundice.*

Minnitt Apparatus Apparatus to provide an intermittent supply of nitrous oxide and air for obstetric analgesia. Devised by English anesthetist, Robert James Minnitt (1889–1974) of Liverpool in 1934.

Minoan Civilization Investigations on Crete began with Milchhoffer in 1883 who studied objects picked up by shepherds. An excavation was initiated by Halbherr in 1886, and further studies were done by Sir Arthur Evans (1851–1941), curator at the Ashmolean Museum at Oxford who dated it to around 3500 BC. Excavation at the palace of Minos at Knossos revealed a system of water drainage and sewerage, comparable to modern systems. The name 'Minoan' was given due to the legend of King Minos, son of the god Zeus and Europa. Its sudden disappearance around 1400 BC is attributed to eruption of the volcano on the island of Santorini.

Minot, Charles Sedgwick (1852–1914) Professor of comparative anatomy at Harvard who designed a rotary microtome and also studied the placenta in 1891. His theory of cytomorphosis in aging, *The problem of age, growth and death,* was published in 1908.

Minot, George Richards (1885–1950) American physician, born in Boston and qualified from Harvard Medical School where he was later appointed as professor. He demonstrated that some anemias are caused by failure of bone marrow to produce enough red blood cells, and others are caused when blood cells are destroyed too rapidly. During his work with William Parry Murphy (1892–1987) in 1927 he established treatment for pernicious anemia with a raw liver diet. Minot was diabetic and one of the first to benefit from the discovery of insulin. He shared the Nobel Prize for Physiology or Medicine in 1934 with Murphy and George Hoyt Whipple (1878–1976) for his treatment for pernicious anemia.

Miocene Period [Greek: *meio*, less + *cene*, recent] Geological age in Earth's history, identified and named by British geologist, Charles Lyell (1797–1875) in 1833.

Miquel, Pierre (1850–1922) Physician and naturalist from Paris who devoted his life to studying the biology and quality of air. His doctoral thesis *Les Organisemes vivant de l'Atmosphere* was published in 1883.

Misericordia Ambulance brotherhood formed by volunteers in Florence in 1244. They were also known as the Masked Brotherhood and played an important role during the epidemic of plague.

Mistletoe Parasitic plant, *Viscum album*, used for centuries as an aperient, antispasmodic and abortifacient. The Druids venerated it and it was considered a panacea for most illnesses by the ancients. The berry was thought to contain a milky life substance of a powerful deity.

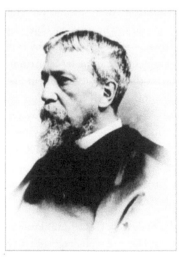

Silas Weir Mitchell (1830–1914). Courtesy of the National Library of Medicine

Mitchell, Silas Weir (1830–1914) Born in Philadelphia, he was a leading American neurologist who described a condition associated with painful feet, erythromelalgia, in 1872. The same disease was mentioned by Robert Graves (1795–1853) in 1848. The knee jerk reflex was demonstrated by Mitchell in 1886. The psychotic properties of mescaline were investigated by him in 1896. Mitchell also wrote several historical novels and poems. His medical publications include: *Injuries of Nerves* (1872), and *Fat and Blood* (1877).

Mite *See Acarus scabiei.*

Mithridatism State of immunity to poisons acquired by taking the poison in small non-lethal doses. Named after the Persian king Mithridates (d 63 BC).

Mithridate General antidote to poison is supposed to have been prepared by Mithridates, King of Pontus around 80 BC.

Mitochondria [Greek: *mitos*, thread + *chondrion*, granule] In 1894 Richard Altmann (1852–1900) devised staining methods which revealed granules in the cell which he thought were independent living constituents. Carl Benda (1857–1933) of Germany identified these and named them mitochondria in 1903. The first electron microscopic study showing cell structures was done by American cytologist, Albert Claude (1899–1983) of Belgian origin, in 1945. He also isolated mitochondria by high speed centrifugation and demonstrated that they were the site of respiration in the cell.

Mitochondrial Antibodies Demonstrated in 98% of the patients with primary biliary cirrhosis, 31% with cryptogenic cirrhosis, and 28% with active chronic hepatitis, by Deborah Doniach (b 1912) in 1966.

Mitosis [Greek: *mitos*, a thread] Process of nuclear division involving the chromosomes, described and named by German biologist, Walther Flemming (1843–1905) in 1882.

Mitral Stenosis [Latin: *mitra*, head band] Described by John Mayow (1640–1679) in 1674. John Hunter (1728–1793) also gave a classic description from mitral and aortic valves preserved in his museum. The pathological state was also described by French anatomist, Raymond de Vieussens (1641–1715) in 1705. The presystolic component of the mitral murmur was described by Sulpice Antoine Fauvel (1813–1884) in 1843 and Walter Hayle Walshe (1812–1892) of University College London in 1851. A murmur in early diastole that can be heard over the pulmonary artery, due to pulmonary hypertension, was described by Graham Steell (1851–1942), a cardiologist from Manchester Royal Infirmary in 1888. Sir Thomas Lauder Brunton (1844–1916), a physician at St Bartholomew's Hospital suggested valvotomy for relief of symptoms in 1902. Elliot Carr Cutler (1888–1947) of the Western Reserve University of Cleveland, Ohio performed the first valvotomy through a transventricular approach in 1923. In 1925 Sir Henry Sessions Souttar (1875–1964) pioneered a valvotomy procedure by introducing his fingers through the left atrium and splitting the mitral commisures.

Mitral Valve Andreas Vesalius (1514–1564) compared the left auriculoventricular valves to an episcopal mitre, and

William Harvey (1578–1657) used the term 'mitral' in relation to valves of the heart. Current terminology was established by William Cheselden (1688–1752) in *Anatomy of Human Body* published in 1713. He has stated that 'Over the entrance of auricles in each ventricle are placed valves to hinder the return of blood when the heart contracts. Those in the right ventricle are termed tricuspides and those in the left, mitrales'. *See mitral stenosis.*

Mitral Valve Prolapse *See systolic click.*

Mitral Valvulotomy *See mitral stenosis, valvulotomy*

Mitscherlich, Eilhard (1794–1863) *See isomorphism.*

Mivart, St George Jackson (1827–1900) Advocate of an alternative theory of evolution. He became an anatomy lecturer at St Mary's Paddington in 1862. He was an evolutionist but he opposed Charles Darwin's (1809–1882) theory of the survival of the fittest, and proposed the concept of neovitalism in which there was an inherent life force in the body which directed development or evolution. He was excommunicated by the Roman Catholic church for his views in 1900.

Mnemonics [Greek: *mneme*, memory] Method to enhance memory, introduced by Simonedes the younger in 477 BC. *Mnemonica* was published by John Willis in 1638, and *Memoria Tecnica* by Grey appeared in 1730.

Moebius, Godfrey (1611–1664) Professor of medicine at Jena who published *Physiological Principles of Medicine* and several other works. His son was also a physician of the same name and published *Synopsis Medicinae Practicae.*

Möbius Sign Incomplete convergence of the eyes in toxic goiter. Described by Paul Julius Möbius (1854–1907) of Leipzig.

Moehsen, John Charles William (1722–1795) Physician to Frederick the Great who wrote several treatises on the history of medicine.

Moffet, Thomas (1553–1604) *See Moufet, Thomas.*

Mohl, Hugo von (1805–1872) German botanist and physician, born in Stuttgart and studied medicine in Tübingen before he became professor of physiology at Bern in 1832. He showed that the sarcode or protoplasm in living cells of animals was the same as that in plant cells in 1846. He also gave a clear description of cell structure and of osmosis.

Moir, David Macbeth (1798–1851) Physician, poet and novelist from Musselburgh, Scotland. He graduated in medicine from Edinburgh University and obtained his diploma as a surgeon in 1816. He wrote the humorous novel, *The Life of Mansie Waunch*, and *Legend of Genevieve* in 1824. Moir also wrote two treatises on cholera and *Outlines of the Ancient History of Medicine* in 1831.

Moissan, Henri (1852–1907) French chemist, born in Paris and qualified there as a pharmacist in 1879. He isolated fluorine in 1866 and was professor of toxicology and inorganic chemistry at the University of Paris. He discovered carborundum and invented a method of producing artificial diamonds. He received the Nobel Prize in 1906.

Molars Teeth were first classified into molars, bicuspids, cuspids and incisors by John Hunter (1728–1793) in *A Practical Treatise on the Diseases of the Teeth* published in 1778.

Molisch Test Test for carbohydrates using α-naphthal and alcohol. Devised by Czech botanist in Calcutta, Hans Molisch (1856–1937).

Moll Glands Ciliary glands described by Jacob Antonius Moll (1832–1914), an ophthalmologist at the Hague, Holland, in 1857.

Moloy, Howard Carman (1903–1953) New York gynecologist who proposed a valuable classification for the female pelvis with William Edgar Caldwell (1880–1943) in 1933.

Molluscum Contagiosum [Latin: *molluscus*, soft] Skin disease characterized by red warty lesions leading to a discharge of caeseous material. Observed by W.G. Tilesius in 1793 and Thomas Bateman (1778–1821) of Whitby, Yorkshire described it in 1813. William Hendersen (1810–1872), professor of pathology at the Edinburgh Medical School wrote a treatise on it in 1841 in which he described the inclusion bodies. A filterable agent as the cause was shown by Max Juliusberg (b 1874) in 1905.

Momberg, Fritz August (1870–1939) Born in Bielefeld, German surgeon who devised a belt for compressing the abdominal aorta in cases of post-partum hemorrhage in 1908.

Monakow Bundle Rubro-spinal tract of the spinal cord, described by Konstantin von Monakow (1853–1930), a Russian neurologist at Zurich in 1885.

Monastic Medicine Ancient Babylonian priests played a key role in curing or attempting to cure diseases. The modern monastic medicine was founded by St Benedict who lived in the sixth century. His work was consolidated by another Benedictine monk and Syrian physician, Cassidorus (490–585) who established two monasteries and collected and translated Greek manuscripts. Saint Augustine, in the fifth century, was one of the greatest introspective psychiatrists, and his *Confessions* is still considered a classic. St Cosmos and St Damian were famous physicians in the 5th century who offered their services free. Monastic schools taught a limited amount of medicine and the physicians were named *physicus*. Constantinius Africanus, a Jew who became a Benedictine monk in the eleventh century, was responsible for translating Hippocratic writings into Latin. He also used the term 'variola' for smallpox. Pope John who died in 1277 is credited with the authorship of the most popular medical recipe book *Thesaurus Pauperum*. There were over 600 monasteries in England during the reign of King Henry III. Oliver Cromwell persuaded Parliament to pass an act which dissolved all the monasteries in Britain. Several important contributors to medicine and science during the past five centuries were men from the clergy. Stephen Hales (1677–1761), a clergyman from Teddington, measured blood pressure. French ecclesiastic, Edmé Mariotte (1620–1684), investigated and explained plant sap pressure and compared it to circulating blood in animals in 1676. The founder of genetics, Gregor Mendel (1822– 1884), was an Augustinian monk.

Mönckeberg Arteriosclerosis Caused by calcification of the medial layer of the arteries. Described by German pathologist, Johann Georg Mönckeberg (1877–1925), professor at Bonn, in 1903.

Monday Dyspnea *See byssinosis.*

Mondeville, Henri de (1260–1320) French surgeon and pupil of Theodoric of Cervia (d 1293). He became surgeon to Philip-le-Bel, King of France, and wrote one of the earliest texts on surgery in Europe. His *Chyrurgia* was edited by Pagel (Berlin, 1889) and by Nicaise (1883) in Paris.

Mondino, de Luzzi (1276–1328) Professor of anatomy at Bologna, who was the first to dissect human bodies during the Middle Ages. Mondino published *Anatomica Omnium humani corporis interiorum membrorum* which remained as a general textbook and dissecting manual for two centuries.

Mondor Disease Superficial thrombophlebitis of the chest wall and the breast. Described in 1951 by Henri Mondor (1885–1962), professor of clinical surgery at the Hospital Sâlpetrière, Paris.

Mongol *See Down syndrome.*

Mongolian Spots Pigmented spots seen on the iris in Down syndrome. Described by Thomas Brushfield of England in 1924.

Moniliasis Fungus responsible for thrush, in the family *Monilia*, as classified by W. Zopf of Breslau in 1890. This led to it being commonly called moniliasis. Pulmonary

moniliasis or 'tea taster's cough' was described by Aldo Castellani (1877–1971) in Sri Lanka in 1927. *See candidosis.*

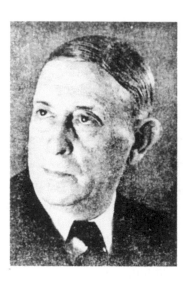

Antonio Caetano de Abreu Freire Egas Moniz (1874–1955). Courtesy of the National Library of Medicine

Moniz, Antonio (Caetano de Abrea Freire) Egas (1874–1955) Portuguese professor of neurology and a diplomat at Lisbon. He introduced a method of radiologically visualizing cerebral circulation by injecting radio-opaque sodium iodide into the carotid artery in 1927. He performed the first frontal lobotomy with Portuguese neurosurgeon, Almeida Lima, on a psychiatric patient in 1935. Moniz was also a deputy in the Portuguese parliament (1903) and its Foreign Minister in 1918.

Monoamine Oxidase Inhibitors (MAOI) The side-effects due to combination of MAOIs with certain foods was recognized in early 1960s and its well known 'cheese reaction' was described by B. Blackwell in 1963. Fatal hepatocellular jaundice following MAOI therapy was first reported by C.M.B. Pare and J.O. Cole in 1964. *See antidepressants.*

Monoclonal Antibodies [Greek: *monos*, alone + *klon*, twig] Produced by an Argentinian-born immunologist, Cesar Milstein (b 1927) while he was at the Medical Research Council Laboratory of Molecular Biology in England in 1975. His pioneering work was done in conjunction with Georges Jean Franz Köhler (b 1946) of Munich and they shared the Nobel Prize with Niels Kai Jerne (b 1911) in 1984. The first monoclonal antibody, OKT3, was approved for therapeutic use by the US Food and Drug Administration in 1986.

Monocytic Leukemia [Greek: *monos*, alone + *kytos*, cell +

leukos, white + *haima*, blood] Described by Hamburg physician Hassan Reschad and V. Schiling-Torgau in 1913. Until 1930 only 16 cases were identified in the literature and William Dameshek (1900–1969) recorded two cases. A critical review with a complete bibliography was given by Otto Naegeli (1871–1938) in 1931.

Monod, Jacques Lucien (1910–1976) French biochemist, born and educated in Paris where he obtained his degree in 1931. He worked at Columbia University on a Rockefeller Fellowship and returned to Paris to work at the Pasteur Institute. He was made professor of molecular biology at College de France in 1967, and continued to work on genetic mechanisms of bacteria. He proposed the operon theory of gene regulation and the concept of messenger RNA with François Jacob (b 1920) in 1963. He shared the Nobel Prize for Physiology or Medicine with André Michel Lwoff (b 1902) in 1968.

Monro, Alexander, Primus (1697–1767) Born in London and studied under William Cheselden (1688–1752). He was later a pupil of Herman Boerhaave (1668–1738) at Leiden, and lectured on anatomy and surgery at Edinburgh in 1717. He was appointed professor of anatomy there in 1721, and played a key role in founding the Edinburgh Royal Infirmary. His influence lasted for 128 years through three generations of his descendants who served as anatomy professors at Edinburgh. He published: *Osteology, or a Treatise on the Anatomy of Bones* (1726), *An Account of the success of Inoculation in Scotland* (1765), *Essay on Comparative Anatomy* (1744), and *Observations Anatomical and Physiological* (1758).

Monro, Alexander, Secundus (1733–1817) Son of Alexander Monro, Primus (1697–1767). He pursued his studies under John Hunter (1728–1793) in London in 1757 and succeeded his father in 1758. He published several treatises: *Observations on the Structure and Function of the Nervous System* (1783), *The Structure and Physiology of Fishes* (1785), *A Description of Bursae Mucosa, Three Treatises on the Brain, Eye, and Ear* (1797), *Observations on the Crural Hernia*, and *Outlines of the Anatomy of the Human Body*. He was succeeded by his son Alexander Monro, Tertius (1773–1859) in 1808. The Monros contributed to the development of Edinburgh University through three generations over a period of 128 years.

Monro, Alexander, Tertius (1773–1859) He succeeded his father as professor of anatomy at Edinburgh in 1808. He published *Elements of the Anatomy of the Human Body* in 1825.

Monro, John *See Monroe, John.*

Monro, Thomas Kirkpatrick (b 1865) Physician to the Glasgow Royal Infirmary, who was made the professor of medicine at the Infirmary in 1913, and served as editor of the *Glasgow Medical Journal*. He published *A Manual of Medicine* and *The Physician as Man of Letters, Science, and Action*.

Monro Foramen The foramen intraventriculare of the brain described by Alexander Monro, Secundus (1733–1817), professor of anatomy at Edinburgh in 1783.

Monroe, John (1715–1791) Physician from Greenwich in Kent who succeeded his father, James Monroe, as physician to the hospitals of Bridewell and Bethlem.

Monsters Learned men such as Athanasius Kircher (1601–1680), the Jesuit priest and scientist; Ambroise Paré (1510–1590), French surgeon to Henry III; Albertus Magnus, Olaus Magnus of Uppsala; Aldrovandus, a naturalist of Bologna; Gesner, a physician and geologist and others believed in superstition and monsters despite their scientific training.

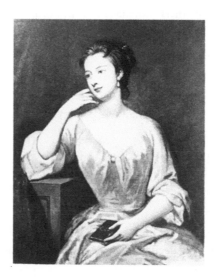

Lady Mary Wortley Montagu (1689–1762). A.R. Ropes, *Lady Wortley Montagu* (1896). Seeley & Co., London

Montagu, Lady Mary Wortley (1689–1762) Eldest daughter of the Duke of Kingston, born at Thoresby in Nottinghamshire. She married Edward Wortley Montagu who later served as British ambassador to Turkey. She introduced inoculation for smallpox into England. In a letter written by her in 1717, she mentioned 'ingrafting' in Turkey, and described the procedure. The method was first tried in England on seven condemned criminals in 1721. Later two members of the royal family were inoculated.

Montanus, John Baptist (1488–1551) Physician from Verona who graduated from Padua, and later served as professor in the same university. He published a Latin translation of Aetius and several other works.

Montessori System of self-education for children through skillfully directed play without formal classes. Founded by Maria Montessori (1876-1952), the first woman medical graduate from Rome. Her work was inspired by Seguin's *Idiocy and its Treatment by Physiological method* which she translated into Italian around 1895. She established four pioneer schools between 1907 and 1908.

Montgomery, William Fetherston (1797–1859) Obstetrician from Dublin, Ireland, who described the sebaceous glands of the areola of the nipple (Montgomery glands) in 1837.

Montpellier The famous medical school was established in the eighth century. It received the status of a Faculty of Medicine from Cardinal Conrad, a representative of Pope Honorius III, in 1180. Guy de Chauliac (1300–1367), father of modern surgery, was a student. He initiated the Order of the Holy Ghost at Montpellier, a movement for nursing lepers and others with infectious diseases in France and the rest of Europe.

Montreal General Hospital The oldest teaching hospital in Canada, established in 1819, and it became a part of McGill University in 1829.

Moon, Robert Charles (1844–1915) *See Laurence–Moon –Biedl syndrome.*

Moon Molars First molars in congenital syphilis, described by a dental surgeon at Guy's Hospital, Henry Moon (1845–1892) in 1876.

Moon, William (1818–1894) Inventor from Kent who became partially blind at the age of four. He was a teacher of the blind and devised an embossed system of reading based on Roman capitals in 1845.

Moore, Austin Talley (1899–1963) Surgeon at the Moore Clinic in Columbia, South Carolina. He designed the Austin Moore prosthesis used as femoral head replacement in hip arthroplasty, in 1957.

Moore, Charles Hewitt (1821–1870) London surgeon who described a method of treating aneurysm by introducing a wire in order to produce coagulation in 1864.

Moore, Francis (1648–1717) Physician and astrologer who practiced at Lambeth. He published *Almanac kalendarium ecclesiasticum* in 1699.

Moore, John (1730–1802) Physician, novelist, and political historian born in Stirling and studied medicine at Glasgow. He traveled and practiced in Europe before settling in London in 1777. He published his experiences of Europe in

A View of Society and Manners in France, Switzerland and Germany in 1799. He followed this with publications on the French revolution, Italy, and a novel *Zeluco*. His only medical treatise was *Medical Sketches*.

Moore, Sir Norman (1847–1922) Physician at St Bartholomew's Hospital and a medical historian. He contributed 469 biographies to *The Dictionary of National Biography*, and was Harveian librarian from 1910 to 1918.

Moore, Stanford (1913–1982) American biochemist, born in Chicago and educated at Vanderbilt University. He joined the Rockefeller Institute in 1939. He invented a column chromatography method for identification and quantification of amino acids from the hydrosylates of proteins and tissues with William Howard Stein (1911–1980) in 1950. They further developed an automated method for RNA base sequence analysis. The amino acid composition of bovine pancreatic ribonuclease was determined by them between 1954 and 1956 and, together with Christian Boehmer Anfinson (b 1916) who studied the structure of the molecule, they shared the Nobel Prize for Chemistry in 1972.

Moore Fracture Fracture of the lower end of the radius with dislocation of the head of the ulna and entrapment of the styloid process within the annular ligaments. Described by American surgeon, Edward Mott Moore (1814–1902).

Moorfields Eye Hospital Established as a special Infirmary to the City of London by John Cunningham Saunders (1773–1810) in 1805. It was later named the Royal London Ophthalmic Hospital. Teaching started in 1811, and it became internationally famous.

Mooser, Herman (1891–1971) *See murine typhus.*

Moral Philosophy Science of ethics dealing with duties and virtues, founded by Socrates (469–399 BC) in 430 BC. Aristotle's theory of goodwill as an essential attribute of mankind, was accepted by most philosophers until John Locke (1632–1704) in 1671 questioned it in *Essay Concerning Human Understanding.* He considered that morals were not an innate feature of man and proposed that they were the outcome of individual experience. Jeremy Collier (1650–1726), a clergyman from Cambridge published *Essays Upon Several Moral Subjects* in three volumes in 1697, and Thomas Cogan (1545–1607), a physician from Northamptonshire, who founded the Royal Humane Society, *The Haven of Health* in 1584. John Abercromby, a physician from Aberdeen applied his medical knowledge and experience to mental and moral philosophy and wrote *Philosophy of Moral Feelings* in 1833.

Morals *See moral philosophy.*

Morax–Axenfeld Bacillus Gram-negative bacterium described as a cause of angular conjunctivitis in man by Swiss ophthalmologist in Paris, Victor Morax (1866–1935) in 1896, and German ophthalmologist Theodor Polykarpos Axenfield (1867–1930) in 1897. It was named *Moraxella lacunata* by André Michael Lwoff (b 1902) in 1939.

Morbus Gallicus *See syphilis.*

Morenheim Space Infra-clavicular fossa. The boundaries were first described by Joseph Jacob Morenheim (1759–1799), professor of surgery at St Petersburg in 1781.

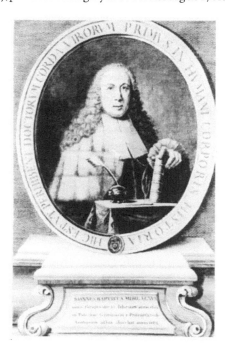

Giovanni Battista Morgagni (1682–1771). Courtesy of the National Library of Medicine

Morgagni, Giovanni Battista (1682–1771) Founder of pathological anatomy, born at Forli in Italy and studied medicine under Antonio Maria Valsalva (1666–1723) and Ippolito Francesco Albertini (1662–1738) in Bologna. He was appointed first professor of anatomy at Padua in 1715 and served there for 59 years. He discovered several anatomical structures which are named after him. He noted syphilitic tumors of the brain, tuberculosis of the kidney, and that paralysis on one side of the body was caused by a lesion in the opposite side of the brain. His most important work, *De Sedibus et Causis Morborum per Anatomen Indagatis*, prepared from over 600 postmortems and written in the form of 70 letters to an anonymous colleague, was published in 1761.

Morgagni Cartilage Cuneiform cartilage of the larynx, described by Giovanni Battista Morgagni (1682–1771) in 1723.

Morgagni Hernia Anterior diaphragmatic hernia, described by Giovanni Battista Morgagni (1682–1771) in 1761.

Morgan, John (1735–1789) Born in Philadelphia, he was a reformer of medical education in America, and founder of the School of Medicine at the University of Pennsylvania. He studied under Alexander Monro (1733–1817) in Edinburgh, and returned to America as first professor of medicine at Philadelphia.

Morgan, Thomas Hunt (1866–1945) Pioneer in modern genetics, born in Lexington, Kentucky and graduated in zoology from the State College, Kentucky in 1886. He obtained his PhD from Johns Hopkins University in 1890, and was appointed professor of physiology at Columbia University in 1904 and at Caltech in 1928. His first book, *Evolution and Adaptation*, was published in 1911. Sex-linked inheritance was established by him while working on the *Drosophila* fly in 1910, for which he received the Nobel Prize in Physiology or Medicine in 1933. His other works include: *The Theory of the Gene* (1926), *Embryology and Genetics* (1933), and *The Mechanism of Mendelian Heredity* (with C.B. Bridges) in 1915.

Morin, John Baptiste (1583–1656) Born in Villefranche, France, he was a physician and professor of mathematics at the University of Paris. His *Astrologia Gallic*, which took thirty years to write, was published after his death.

Morin, Louis (1635–1714) French physician and botanist from Mons, who served as a physician at Hôtel Dieu in Paris.

Morison, James Rutherford (1853–1939) Born in Durham, he was surgeon to the Royal Infirmary at Newcastle-upon-Tyne. He pioneered pelvic surgery for women and published *Abdominal and Pelvic Surgery* in 1925. He also pioneered surgical treatment for gallstones and gastric cancer.

Morison Pouch Hepatorenal pouch, described by James Rutherford Morison (1853–1939) in the *British Medical Journal* of 1894.

Morley, Henry (1822–1894) Physician from King's College London. He gave up medicine and became assistant editor for Dicken's *Household Words*. He was professor of English at London University from 1865 to 1889.

Moro Reflex A startling reflex in infants producing an embracing attitude. Described by a pediatrician in Vienna, Ernst Moro (1874–1951).

Moron [Greek: *moros*, stupid] *See idiocy.*

Morphea [Greek: *morphe*, form] Form of scleroderma, limited plaques or bands in the skin, observed by C. Hilton Fagge (1838–1883) in 1868.

Morpheus Attendant to the Greek god Somnus, who himself was god of sleep. The drug, morphine, was named by its discoverer Friedrich Wilhelm Sertürner (1783–1841), an apothecary's assistant in Westphalia, in 1806.

Morphine A derivative of the opium poppy, *Papaver somniferum*. Friedrich Wilhelm Sertürner (1783–1841), a German pharmacist, crystallized the extract of opium and obtained morphine in 1801. He tried the effects on himself and found that it killed pain and produced deep sleep accompanied by dreams. He named the substance morphine after the Greek god of sleep, Morpheus, in 1806. He announced his discovery in Ludwig Gilbert's journal *Annalen der Physick* in 1806. Sertürner considered it a vegetable alkaloid, and gave a full description in 1817. It was further purified by Pierre Joseph Pelletier (1788–1842) and Bienaimé Caventou (1793–1877). It was first used as a preanesthetic by Lorenzo Bruno of Turin in 1850 and Claude Bernard (1813–1878) in 1869. It was synthesized by Gates and Tscudi in 1952.

Morphology [Greek: *morphe*, form + *logos*, discourse] Introduced into biology in 1817 by Johann Wolfgang von Goethe (1749–1832), a German writer and scientist.

Morquio Syndrome Mucopolysaccharidosis type IV, an autosomal recessive disease leading to dwarfism, waddle gait, and deafness but not mental retardation. Described by Uruguayan pediatrician from Montevideo, Luis Morquio (1867–1935) in 1929.

Morris, Sir Henry (1844–1926) Born in Petworth, Sussex, he was surgeon to the Middlesex Hospital in London, and president of the Royal College of Surgeons from 1906 to 1909. He published *A Treatise on Human Anatomy* in 1893.

Morris, Robert Tuttle (1857–1945) Surgeon in New York who was born in Seymour, Connecticut. He described the point of maximum tenderness (Morris point) in acute appendicitis.

Morrison, Charles (d 1756) Scottish surgeon from Renfrew who discovered electric telegraphy. He described his method of transmitting messages through wires in the *Scots Magazine* in 1753.

Morsher, Harris Peyton (1867–1954) Professor of laryngology at Harvard and chief of laryngological unit at Massachusetts General Hospital. The ethmoidal sinus beneath the bulla ethmoidalis (Morsher cells) was described by him in 1902.

Mortality [Latin: *mors*, death] The practice of recording weekly and yearly burials in the London parishes, called Bills of Mortality, started around 1563. It became more detailed to include the causes of death, especially due to plague. A book on the subject was published by London haberdasher, John Gaunt (1620–1674) in 1662. He also calculated life expectancy from these tables. They became a regular issue, and christenings were also recorded in the parishes as an indication of birth rates. In the year 1649 there were 85,338 burials and 50,465 christenings in London. Sir William Petty observed and studied mortality rates in the 17th century and his work on vital statistics and mortality rates was further advanced by Gregory King (1648–1712). Life tables for life insurance were first published by Edmund Halley in 1693. *See infant mortality rates.*

Morton, Samuel George (1799–1851) Born in Philadelphia and graduated from the University of Edinburgh. He was a craniologist and paleontologist who collected over 1000 skulls and published two important atlases, *Crania Americana* (1839) and *Crania Aegyptiaca* (1844). His *Illustrations of Pulmonary Consumption* appeared in 1834.

Morton, Thomas George (1835–1903) Born in Philadelphia, he carried out the successful removal of an inflamed appendix in 1887. He gave a complete description of metatarsalgia (Morton disease) associated with neuralgia of the lateral plantar nerve in 1876.

Morton, William Thomas Green (1819–1868) He introduced ether inhalation as an anesthetic and administered it in an operation for a neck tumor carried out by Boston surgeon, J.C. Warren (1778–1856) in 1846 at the Massachusetts General Hospital. His claim to the discovery of ether was contested by one of his lecturers, Charles T. Jackson, and Morton failed to establish his claim. *See anesthesia, ether.*

Morvan Disease Form of syringomyelia with trophic changes in the extremities. Described by French physician, Augustin Marie Morvan (1819–1897) from Finesterre.

Mosasaur The skull of a prehistoric reptile, later named mosasaur, was discovered at a stone quarry near the Meuse river in The Netherlands in 1780. It was the first prehistoric reptile identified by George Cuvier (1769-1832) in 1795.

Moschcowitz, Eli (1879–1964) Physician in New York who studied the physiology of blood circulation and wrote *Hypertension of the Pulmonary Circulation* in 1927. He also pioneered psychosomatic medicine.

Moschcowitz Operation Femoral herniotomy through an inguinal route, described by New York surgeon, Alexis Victor Moschcowitz (1865–1933).

Moseley, Benjamin (1739–1819) Physician from Essex who

practiced as a surgeon and apothecary at Kingston in Jamaica before he returned to London in 1785. He served as physician to the Chelsea Hospital and opposed inoculation. Moseley published *Observations on the Dysentery of the West Indies* and *On Coffee and Sugar*.

Moseley, Harry (1887–1915) English physicist, born in Weymouth and graduated from Oxford. He worked under Ernest Rutherford at Manchester University and determined the atomic number of elements using X-ray spectra and crystal diffraction. His work formed the basis for nuclear physics.

Moseley, Henry Nottidge (1844–1891) English naturalist from Wandsworth, London who studied natural science at Oxford and medicine at University College, London. He joined a government expedition to Ceylon in 1871, where he observed a solar eclipse, made spectroscopic measurements, and brought back a collection of plants. He was appointed Linacre professor of human and comparative anatomy at Exeter College, Oxford in 1881, and founded the Marine Biological Association.

Mosquito Transmission of malaria by mosquitoes was mentioned by the Brahmin physician, Susruta in AD 500. Patrick Manson (1844–1922), author of *Tropical Diseases* (1898) identified the *Anopheles* mosquito as a vector for the worm which caused filariasis in 1879 and proposed the existence of an extracorporeal life cycle for the parasite in 1894. Its part in transmission of yellow fever was mentioned by Walter Reed (1851–1902) and Carlos Finlay (1833–1905) in 1900 who discovered the vector. Their hypothesis was tested by Jesse William Lazear (1866–1900), who allowed himself to be bitten while investigating an outbreak of yellow fever in Havana, and died of the disease. Sir Ronald Ross (1857–1932), an Indian Army surgeon, who demonstrated the presence of the parasite in birds in 1897, advocated the extermination of mosquitoes. Adolphe Laveran (1845–1922), a French physician, identified the protozoan in malaria and G.B. Grassi (1854–1925), from Italy, showed that the mosquito was a vector of malaria. *Aedes aegypti* was shown to be the vector in transmission of dengue fever by Thomas Lane Bancroft (1860–1933) in 1906. In the 1940s the insecticide DDT (dichlorodiphenyl trichloroethane) was introduced. *See Aedes aegypti, Anopheles, malaria, yellow fever.*

Mosso, Angelo (1846–1910) Italian physiologist who did one of the earliest studies on the mechanism of apnoea in 1903. His laboratory at Monte Rosa was an important center for the study of high altitude on health.

Mother Theresa *See Theresa of Calcutta.*

Motor Cortex [Latin: *movere*, to move] First suggested by Robert Boyle (1627–1691) in 1691 who recorded the case of a man who developed palsy of the arm and leg following a depressed fracture of the skull. The surgeon who operated found a bone specule impinging on the brain, and the patient fully recovered after its removal. No further study in the field was made for nearly two hundred years until 1864, when Hughlings Jackson (1835–1911) proposed the existence of certain areas in the cortex which caused specific movements. Theodor Fritsch (1838–1891), a military surgeon during the Prussian–Danish war in 1867, while caring for soldiers who sustained brain injury, noted that the stimulation of one side of the brain caused the opposite side to twitch. He later joined Julius Eduard Hitzig (1838–1907), a brilliant neurologist, in experiments on stimulation of the brain in dogs. Their paper, published in 1870, paved the way for neurophysiology. The areas of the motor cortex controlling specific motor functions of the hands and limbs were identified by Sir David Ferrier (1843–1928) in 1873.

Motor Neuron [Latin: *movere*, to move; Greek: *neuron*, nerve] Unit of reflex action, first recognized by Wilhelm His (1831–1904) in 1889, and German anatomist, Heinrich Wilhelm Gottfried von Waldeyer (1836–1921) in 1891. He also suggested the term, neuron. Reaction of a single motor neuron following its activation by a stimulus was demonstrated by Derek Denny-Brown (1901–1981), New Zealand- born neurologist at Oxford in 1929. *See motor unit.*

Motor Unit [Latin: *movere*, to move] Sir Charles Scott Sherrington (1857–1952) used the term in 1925 to denote 'an individual motor nerve fiber together with a bunch of muscle fibers enervated by it'. Louis Doyere (1811–1863), professor of physiology and applied zoology in France, observed the termination of motor nerves in muscles of insects in 1837. *See motor neuron.*

Mott, Valentine (1785–1865) American surgeon who treated an aneurysm of the subclavian artery by tying it within the scleni muscles in 1833. He performed the first successful amputation at the hip joint in America in 1827. He carried out a successful excision of osteosarcoma of the clavicle in 1828.

Moufet, Thomas (1553–1604) Zoologist, poet and physician from Cambridge. After traveling in Europe he established a successful practice in London. He published *De Jure et Praestantia Chemicorum Medicamentorum, Epostelae quinque Medicinales, Nosomantia Hippocratica* and several other works. He completed a valuable work on insects in 1590 which was published after his death by Sir Theodore Mayerne (1573–1675), a medical practitioner in London in 1634.

Mountain Sickness *See altitude sickness.*

Mountcastle, Vernon Benjamin (b 1918) American neurophysiologist, born in Shelbyville, Kentucky and educated at Roanoke College and the Johns Hopkins Medical School, where he became professor of physiology in 1959. He demonstrated that the cells of cerebral cortex in anesthetized cats were able to respond to specific skin stimulation, in the 1950s. This served as an important tool for experimental study of the sensory nervous system.

Moxibustion Chinese treatment where cauterization was performed by applying cone shaped masses of combustible material so as to form a blister.

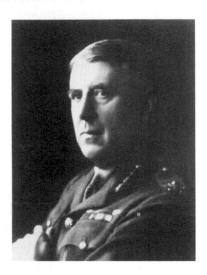

Baron Berkeley George Andrew Moynihan (1865–1936). Courtesy of the National Library of Medicine

Moynihan, Baron Berkeley George Andrew (1865–1936) British surgeon, born in Malta and educated at Leeds. He served at the Leeds Infirmary and did extensive work on surgical pathology of gastric and duodenal ulcers. He identified chronic gastric ulcer as a precursor of gastric carcinoma in 1923 and designed the Monynihan method, a modification of the Pólya operation, for treatment.

MRI *See magnetic resonance imaging.*

Mudge, John (d 1793) Physician from Plymouth who wrote *On the Catarrhous Cough* and improved the reflecting telescope.

Muir, Sir Robert (1864–1959) Born in Balfron, Stirling, he was professor of pathology at the University of Glasgow from 1899 to 1936. He made several important contributions to experimental pathology and immunity.

Mulder, Gerrit Jan (1802–1880) Dutch chemist at Utrecht who coined the term 'protein' for complex substances found in materials such as silk, blood fibrin, egg white and gelatin. His wrote *General Physiological Chemistry*, published between 1844–1851.

Mule Spinner's Cancer The spinning machine used in cotton industry and invented by Samuel Crompton of Bolton, Lancashire in 1779 caused scrotal cancer due to prolonged contact with lubrication oil in the spindles and this was recognized by S. R. Wilson of the Royal Infirmary Manchester in 1906.

Mulkowal Disaster Waldemar Mordecai Wolfe Haffkine (1860–1930) pioneered inoculation against cholera in India in 1892 and conducted an antiplague vaccination program using live vaccine in the village of Mulkowal in India in 1902. Nineteen villagers died of tetanus and Haffkine was blamed. A subsequent commission revealed that it was due to contamination of the vaccine following careless handling and Haffkine was cleared of blame.

Müller, Friedrich Max (1823–1900) He was born in Desau and educated in Leipzig and Berlin. He studied Sanskrit and published an edition of the *Rig-Veda*, the sacred hymns of the Hindus. He emigrated to England in 1846 and became professor of comparative philology at Oxford in 1868. The term 'Aryan' was used by him in *History of Ancient Sanskrit Literature* (1859), to denote the origin of Indo-Iranian languages amongst the Indo-Germanic people of Iran. His popular, *Lectures on the Science of Languages*, was published from 1861 to 1864.

Müller, Heinrich (1820–1864) Professor of anatomy at Würzberg who described several anatomical structures that have been named after him including a muscle and a fiber.

Müller, Hermann Joseph (1890–1967) American geneticist, born in New York City, and educated at Columbia University. He pioneered the study of mutation. He studied under Thomas Hunt Morgan (1866–1945) at Columbia University. He was professor of zoology at the University of Texas in Austin during the 1920s and then moved to St Petersburg to work at the Institute of Genetics, the Institute of Animal Genetics in Edinburgh and became professor of zoology at Indiana University in 1945. He created gene mutations following exposure to X-rays in 1927, for which he was awarded the Nobel Prize in 1946. He campaigned on the dangers of radiation-induced mutations and against nuclear bombs. In *Out of the Night*, published in 1935, he discussed the possibility of sperm banks for genetically improving the human race.

Muller, Johan (1436–1476) Scholar from Königsberg who combined humanism with science. He translated the works of Ptolemy into Latin and founded an observatory at Nüremburg in 1471. He wrote the first systematic treatise on trigonometry, published in 1533 after his death.

Müller, Johannes Peter (1801–1858) German physiologist, born in Köblenz and graduated in medicine from Bonn University 1822, where he was appointed professor of physiology in 1826. He moved to Berlin University as professor of anatomy and physiology in 1833. While working with Rudolph Kölliker (1817–1905), a Swiss physiologist, in 1855, Müller used a crude but ingenious apparatus made of frog skeletal muscle and connected it to the frog's heart, to show that, with each systole, two contractions of the skeletal muscle were produced. This was probably the first demonstration of the electrical nature of the heart. Another of his interests was embryology, and he described the primordial female genital tract or oviduct (Müller duct) in 1830 and showed that blood from the embryo changed color entering and leaving so showing that it respired. In 1840 he proposed the law of specific nerve energies that states that each sensory system will respond in the same way to a stimulus regardless of the nature of the stimulus.

Müller, Paul Hermann (1899–1965) Swiss chemist and inventor of the insecticide, DDT and other pest control compounds. He received the Nobel Prize for Physiology or Medicine in 1948. *See DDT.*

Multiple Myeloma (Syn: Kahler disease, plasmacytoma) The presence of albuminoid protein in urine of some patients was described by Henry Bence Jones (1814–1873) in 1847, and the disease was described as mollities ossium, a bone disorder, by William Macintyre in 1850. The first microscopical study of bone tissue from Macintyre's patient was done by John Darymple (1804–1852) of Dublin in 1846. The term was first used by O. J. von Rustizky in 1883. A full account was given by an Austrian professor of medicine at Prague, Otto Kahler (1849–1893), in 1899. Plasma cells were detected in the blood by Schridde in 1906. Infiltration of the spleen, liver, bone marrow and lymph glands by plasma cells was demonstrated by E. E. Osgood and W.C. Hunter in 1934. Anuria due to precipitation of abnormal proteins in the tubules following contrast injection for urography in patients with myeloma was reported by R.L. Holman in 1939. *See Bence Jones proteins.*

Multiple Sclerosis [Latin: *multus*, many; Greek: *sklerosis*, hardness] A description and illustration of the lesions was given by London pathologist, Robert Hooper (1773–1835) in *The Morbid Anatomy of the Human Brain* published in 1828. It was further described in 1840 by Jean Cruveilhier (1791–1874), professor of pathological anatomy at Paris.

Jean Martin Charcot (1825–1893) noted the lesions in 1868 and an English description was given by W. Moxon in 1875. The occurrence of nystagmus in multiple sclerosis (Uhthoff sign) was described by a German physician and ophthalmologist, Wilhelm Uhthoff (1853–1927) of Breslau. Retro-bulbar neuritis was shown by William John Adie (1886–1935). Internuclear ophthalmoplegia in disseminated sclerosis (Lhermitte syndrome), was described by French neurologist, Jean L. Lhermitte (1877–1959) in 1920.

Mummery, John Howard (1847–1926) Physician and dentist who graduated from University College London. He practiced at Cavendish Square, London and was president of the British Dental Association and Odontological Society. In 1891 he described the fibrillar structures of developing dentine (fibers of Mummery).

Mummy [Arabic: *mum*, wax] Preservation of the body by embalming, common in Egypt, although the oldest known mummies are those of the Chinchorro Indians of Peru from 6000 BC. Powdered mummy was used as a remedy for all illness in Europe during the 16th century. The first Egyptian mummy was brought to England by Captain William Lethieullier in 1722, and an essay on the mummy was published by Alex Gorden in 1737. *See embalming, embalmer.*

Mumps Disease known since ancient times but whose cause was only established in 1914, when Mervyn Henry Gordon (1872–1953) showed it to be caused by a filterable agent. An accurate clinical description of mumps associated with orchitis was given by Robert Hamilton (1721–1793) of Edinburgh in 1790. Ernest William Goodpasture (1886–1960), an American pathologist, and Claud D. Johnson transmitted mumps from monkeys to humans and confirmed the viral etiology in 1934.

Munchausen Syndrome Dramatization of symptoms of an imaginary illness, described by R. Asher in *The Lancet* in 1951. It was named after Baron Hieronymus von Munchausen (1720–1797) who told wildly exaggerated stories of his travels. His experiences were published by Rudolf Erich Raspe in 1785.

Mundinus (1270–1326) Italian professor of anatomy at Bologna (1306–1325) who commenced dissections of the human body in 1315 and gave anatomical demonstrations. His *Anatomia Mundini* or *Anathomia*, published in 1316, remained a popular manual for over 200 years (first print 1478) and 39 editions.

Munk Roll Biographical data on members of the Royal College of Physicians from 1518 up to 1825, including founder members since the College was established by

King Henry. Compiled by William Munk (1816–1898) in 1855. It is continually updated with new members.

Munroe, Robert (1835–1920) Physician from Ross-shire who graduated from Edinburgh University in 1867. He changed to archaeology and published *Ancient Scottish lake Dwellings* (1882), *The Lake Dwellings of Europe* (1890), and *Prehistoric Scotland and Its Place in European Civilization* in 1899.

Munzer, Egmont (1865–1924) Professor of medicine at Prague who described the tract from the internal geniculate body to the lateral part of the pons (Munzer tract) in 1895.

Murchison, Sir Roderick Impey (1792–1871) Born at Tarradale in Ross, he devoted his entire life to geology and pioneered the drift theory to explain deposits of boulder clay. He published *The Silurian System* in 1839. He was knighted in 1846.

Murine Typhus (*Rickettsia typhi*, Syn: flea borne typhus, endemic typhus) Howard Taylor Ricketts (1871–1910), in 1920, named the causative organism *Dermacentroxenus typhi*. Rollo Eugene Dyer (b 1886) and co-workers isolated rickettsia from rat fleas in 1931. In the same year, Hermann Mooser (1891–1971) and Hans Zinsser (1878–1940) obtained the infective agent from rats in Mexico, and the name murine typhus was proposed by Mooser in 1932. The infective agent, a rickettsial organism, was isolated by Mooser in 1928 from the tunica vaginalis of guinea pig after intraperitoneal injection of blood from patients with murine typhus. The species was named *Rickettsia mooseri*, in honor of Ricketts and Mooser.

Murmur Murmurs and heart sounds were described by English physician, James Hope (1801–1841) in 1832. He described the diastolic murmur of mitral stenosis which was later known as the Hope murmur. Walter Hayle Walshe (1812–1892) of University College London gave an account of the presystolic component of mitral murmur in mitral stenosis in 1851. William Tennant Gairdner (1824–1907), regius professor of medicine at Glasgow University, wrote an important treatise on cardiac murmurs in 1861. An exhaustive account of presystolic murmurs was given by Charles Hilton Fagge (1838–1883) of Guy's Hospital in 1871. Austin Flint murmur, an apical mid-diastolic or presystolic functional murmur originating from the mitral valve in patients with aortic stenosis, was first described by Austin Flint (1812–1886) of New York in 1862. A murmur in early diastole, heard over the pulmonary artery, and caused by pulmonary hypertension resulting from mitral stenosis, was described by Graham Steell (1851–1942), a cardiologist

at Manchester Royal Infirmary in 1888. Two separate murmurs heard over the femoral or brachial artery, during diastolic and systolic phase of the heart in cases of aortic insufficiency were described by French physician, Louis Paul Duroziez (1826–1897) in 1861. The mechanism of production of several murmurs was explained by Hermann Ludwig Blumgart (1895–1977) in 1933.

Murphy, John Benjamin (1857–1916) Pioneer in vascular surgery, born in Wisconsin and graduated (1879) from Rush Medical College, Chicago, where he became professor of surgery. He demonstrated in 1896 that severed arteries and veins could be reunited by end to end anastomosis. He was the first surgeon in America to perform artificial pneumothorax. He introduced the continuous method of giving saline (Murphy drip) through the rectum and designed an ingenious device (Murphy button) for effecting intestinal anastomosis.

Murphy Sign Patient is unable to take a deep breath when the examiner exerts digital pressure over the gallbladder in the hypochondrium, in cases of cholecystitis. Described by Chicago surgeon, John Benjamin Murphy (1857–1916).

Murphy, William Parry (1892–1987) American physician, born in Wisconsin, who proved with George Richards Minot (1885–1950), the effect of raw liver in the treatment of pernicious anemia in 1925. He was born in Stoughton, Wisconsin and educated at Harvard Medical School. He shared the Nobel Prize for Physiology or Medicine with Minot and George Hoyt Whipple (1878–1976) in 1934.

Murray, John (d 1820) Scottish physician and chemist at Edinburgh who published *Elements of Chemistry, Elements of Materia Medica and Pharmacy, A System of Chemistry*, and *A System of Materia Medica and Pharmacy*.

Murray, Joseph Edward (b 1919) American surgeon and pioneer in renal transplantation, born in Milford, Massachusetts and graduated from Harvard Medical School in 1943. He and his colleagues performed the first renal transplant between identical twins at Peter Bent Brigham Hospital in Boston in 1954 and non-identical twins in 1961 (using the immunosuppressant drug, azathioprine). Murray shared the Nobel Prize with Donnall Thomas (b 1920) in 1990.

Murrell, Christine (1874–1933) Born in Clapham, London, she was a pioneer of women in medical politics. She studied medicine at the Royal Free Hospital and became a general practitioner in London. She obtained her MD on mental diseases and psychology from the University of London in 1905, and published *Womanhood and Health* in 1923. She was the first woman member to the council of the BMA (1924), and the first woman member of the General Medical Council (1933).

Murrell, William (1853–1912) Born in Wimbledon, and graduated in medicine from University College, London in 1874. His special interest was therapeutics and he introduced nitroglycerin as treatment for angina in 1879. He published *Manual of Pharmacology and Therapeutics* (1896), *What to do in Cases of Poisoning* (1881), *Massage as a Mode of Treatment* (1876), and *Aids to Forensic Medicine and Toxicology* in 1894. *See angina.*

Musa Physician to Emperor Augustus around 20 BC. He is supposed to have prescribed cold baths as treatment for diseases.

Muscle Action Direct measurements of heat evolved during the contraction of a muscle were first made by British Nobel Prize winner, Archibald Vivian Hill (1886–1977) in 1911. ATP (adenosine triphosphate) was shown to be a key factor in supplying energy for muscle contraction in *in vitro* studies by Hungarian biochemist and Nobel Prize winner, Albert von Szent-Györgi (1893–1986) in 1938. He brought the proteins, actin and myosin, together to effect muscle contraction in 1942. He said 'to see actomyosin contract for the first time was one of the most exciting experiences of my scientific career'.

Muscle Contraction *See muscle action.*

Muscle Spindle Stretch afferent is a neuromuscular end organ of the muscle that was studied and named by Wilhelm Kühne (1837–1900) in 1862. The sensory nature of the spindle was proposed by Sir Charles Scott Sherrington (1857–1952) in 1894, and it was described by Angelo Ruffini (1874–1929) who conducted studies between 1892 to 1898. Three different types of discharge, α_1, α_2 and β, from mammalian muscle and tendon spindles were shown by R. Matthews in 1933.

Muscular Dystrophies *See myopathy.*

Museum *See Hunterian museum.*

Musgrave, Samuel, (d 1782) Physician and grandson of William Musgrave (1657–1721), who practiced at Exeter. In 1763 he became politically notorious after charging British ministers with taking bribes to make a disadvantageous settlement with France. He published an edition of Euripides and two dissertations on Grecian mythology.

Musgrave, William (1657–1721) Physician from Charlton in Somerset, educated at Winchester School and New College Oxford, and practiced at Exeter. He wrote several treatises in Latin on gout and four volumes of dissertations on Roman and British antiquities.

Mushroom *See poisonous fungi.*

Music Remedy employed by Daniel Hack Tuke (1827–1895), a lecturer in mental disease at the Charing Cross Hospital, to cure madness, and described in *A Manual of Psychological Medicine*, published in 1858. In 1605 Francis Bacon (1561–1626) wrote 'The poets did well to conjoin music and medicine in Apollo'. Richard Browne, an apothecary from Oakham in Rutland, published the first English book on the medicinal value of music, *A Mechanical essay on singing, musick and dancing demonstrating the alterations they produce in a human body*, in 1727. The powerful effect of music on George III during his last episode of illness was described by Sir Henry Halford (1766–1844) in *On the treatment of insanity, particularly the moral treatment*, published in 1833. According to Etienne Dominique Esquirol (1772–1840) in 1813, music brings peace and composure of mind but it does not bring cure.

Mussel Poisoning *See shellfish.*

Mustard Gas Obtained by Richie in 1854 by mixing chloride with ethyl sulfide. The properties were described by Guthrie in 1860, and Victor Meyer (1848–1897) in 1886 and they found it to be very poisonous. *See gas warfare.*

Mutation [Latin: *mutare*, to change] The modern theory of mutation which proposed that new species arise by a single mutation was advanced in 1890 by Hugo de Vries (1848–1935), professor of botany at Amsterdam in *The Mutations Theory*, published in 1901. Mutation due to radiation effects was established in *Drosophila* fly by Hermann Joseph Müller (1890–1967) of America in 1927 who received the Nobel Prize in 1946. Mutation in mammals due to X-ray exposure was demonstrated by American geneticist, Georg Davis Snell (b 1903) of Massachusetts in 1929. Chemical methods were used by Charlotte Auerbach (b 1899) and J.M. Robson in 1941. The development of cancer from a single cell initiated by mutation of its DNA was shown by Hugh John Foster Cairns (b 1922), a molecular biologist and professor at Harvard School of Public Health.

Mutual Aid Society The first such society in Europe was formed by miners from Goslar in the Harz mountains (Germany), and it received its charter from Friedrich I in 1188. Similar societies to help poor workers were common in Europe in the 13th century.

Myalgic Encephalitis ME syndrome. *See chronic fatigue syndrome.*

Myasthenia Gravis [Greek: *myos*, muscle + *astheneia*, weakness; Latin: *gravis*, heavy] Fatigue, muscular exhaustion or atrophy caused by a disorder in neuromuscular function due to presence of antibodies to acetylcholine receptors. Also called Erb–Goldflamm disease. The first definite account was given by Samuel Wilks (1824–1911) in 1877, and Wilhelm Heinrich Erb (1840–1921) of Berlin and Samuel Goldflamm (1852–1932) of Warsaw described it in 1879. An association between myasthenia and thymus was noted by German pathologist, Karl Weigert (1845–1904) in 1901, and thymectomy as treatment was performed by Ernst Ferdinand Sauerbruch (1875–1951) of Germany in 1912. The similarity between myasthenia gravis and curare poisoning was noted by Hermann Oppenheim (1858–1919) in 1908. Electromyographic studies were done on patients by E.A.B. Pritchard in 1933. Testing the effect of an antidote to curare on myasthenic patients was suggested by Mary Broadfoot Walker (1888–1974) in 1934, and she introduced physostigmine as treatment in the same year. Prostigmin was introduced by Lazar Remen (b 1907) of Germany in 1934. Clinical evaluation of the benefits of thymectomy was done by Alfred Blalock (1899–1964) and colleagues in 1937. A myasthenic reaction associated with small cell carcinoma of the bronchus was described by American neurophysiologists, Edward H. Lambert (b 1915) and Lee M. Eaton (1905–1958) (Eaton–Lambert Syndrome) in 1956.

Mycobacteria [Greek: *mykes*, fungus + *bakterion*, small rod] The leprosy bacillus (*M. leprae*) was the first member of this group discovered by Norwegian bacteriologist, Gerhard Henrik Armauer Hansen (1841–1912) in 1874. The mammalian tubercle (*M. tuberculosis*) was discovered by Robert Koch (1843–1910) in 1882, and the avian type of tubercle bacilli (*M. avium-intracellulare*) was discovered by several workers including Rivolta, Angelo Maffuci (1847–1903), Roger, and Sibley in 1890. The peculiar property of acid fastness of the tuberculous bacillus was noted by Theodor Klebs (1834–1913) in 1896. *See tubercle bacillus.*

Mycology [Greek: *mykes*, fungus + *logos*, discourse] Scientific study of infectious diseases caused by fungi in man and higher animals was initiated in the first half of the 19th century. However, the fungal disease, thrush, was described by Hippocrates (460–377 BC) and Madura foot was described over 3000 years ago in the *Athara-Veda*. Mycology as a branch of medicine was pioneered by David Gruby (1810–1898) of Paris, around 1842. Thereafter it was intensified by several workers including: Johan Lucas Schonlein (1839), M. J. Berkeley (1836), Tilbury Fox (1863), Charles Robin (1853), R.J.A. Sabouraud (1890), E. Bodin (1902), Castellini (1910), and others. It was recognized as a specialty

in America in the early 20th century with the appointment of the first medical mycologist, Chester Emmons.

Mycosis Fungoides The causative organism was discovered in Buenos Aires by Alejandro Posadas, a student of Robert Wernicke, in 1892. The same organism was independently described by Rixford of California in 1896, and named 'coccidioides imitis'.

Mycosis [Greek: *mykes*, fungus] *See fungal disease.*

Mydriasis Dilatation of the pupil. Considered by ancient physicians to be due to congestion in the brain. Aetius of Amida, around AD 600, recommended general and local bleeding, clysters, diet and friction of the extremities as treatment. Avicenna (980–1037) later related it to cephalae and injuries of the head. Haly Abbas (d AD 944) described it but thought it was almost incurable.

Mydriatics Hyoscyamus and belladona were used to dilate the pupils by C. Himley (1772–1837). Belladona was also used by fashionable ladies of Florence to dilate their pupils in order to improve their appearance, and the plant derives its name from this practice. *See belladonna, Atropa belladona.*

Myelin Sheath Observed in nerve tissue by microscopist, Antoni van Leeuwenhoek (1632–1723) in 1677. Myelinated nerve fibers were differentiated from the unsheathed fibers by Christian Gottfried Ehrenberg (1795–1876) of Germany in 1836. Further studies were done by Robert Remak (1815–1865) and Wilhelm His (1831–1904). Carl Weigert (1845–1904) of Frankfurt in 1882 developed a stain for it.

Myecetoma *See Actinomyces madurae, fungal disease.*

Myelocyte [Greek: *myelos*, marrow + *kytos*, hollow] Earliest cell line of white blood cells was observed and described by Charles Austin Doan (b 1896) and co-workers in 1925.

Myelofibrosis [Greek: *myelos*, marrow; Latin: *fibra*, band] Disease of adults, characterized by excessive production of fibrous tissue in the bone marrow. Found by R.A. Hickling in 1937, and by E.A. Gall in 1938.

Myeloma [Greek: *myelos*, marrow] *See multiple myeloma.*

Myeloscopy [Greek: *myelos*, marrow + *skopein*, to view] Procedure for direct visualization of the spinal canal through lumbar puncture. Pioneered by M.D. Burman of America in 1931.

Myenteric Reflex [Greek: *myos*, muscle + *entos*, within; Latin: *reflectare*, to bend back] It effects the propulsion of food or a foreign body in the intestines. Described by American physiologist, Walter Bradford Cannon (1871–1945), in 1912.

Myleran [Greek: *myelos*, marrow] Treatment in chronic myeloid leukemia introduced by D.A.G. Galton and M.Till in 1955.

Myocardial Infarction One of the earliest accounts of coronary thrombosis was given by Peter Mere Latham (1789–1875), a physician at St Bartholomew's Hospital in 1846.The occurrence of myocardial necrosis was described by Henrick Pehr Malsten (1811–1883) and Wilhelm Gustav Johann Duben (1822–1892) in 1859. Symptomatology was given by Karl Weigert (1845–1904) of Germany in 1880. Electrocardiographic changes were described by New York cardiologist, Harold Ensign Bennett Pardee (1886–1972) in 1920. The first study on the value of anticoagulation was done by Irving Sherwood Wright (b 1901) and co-workers in 1948. The syndrome of pericarditis, pleurisy and fever following myocardial infarction or trauma to the heart (Dressler syndrome) was described by William Dressler (1890–1969) of America in 1955. Elevation of serum glutamic oxaloacetic transaminase (SGOT) in acute cases was demonstrated by John Samuel LaDue (1911–1980) and Felix Wroblewski (b 1921) in 1954, and raised levels of lactic dehydrogenase enzyme (LDH) were observed by Wroblewski in 1956. Electrophoresis was first used to characterize serum fractions of LDH enzymes by Vessel and Bearn in 1957. Elevated CPK (creatinine phosphokinase) was observed by J.C. Dreyfus in 1960. Isoenzymes of CPK were recognized by S.B. Rosalki (b 1921) in 1965, and following his work, the heart muscle was found to contain about 30% of one form, MB-CPK (M-muscle, B-brain). The rise of CK-MB or MB-CK levels in the blood is presently established as the most specific indicator of acute myocardial infarction. The concept of a coronary care unit, where the patients are intensively monitored during the early stages of myocardial infarction, was introduced by K.W.G. Brown and H.W. Day in 1963. *See coronary artery disease, coronary artery bypass graft, angina.*

Myocardial Ischemia *See angina, coronary artery disease, myocardial infarction, coronary artery bypass graft, coronary angioplasty.*

Myocarditis [Greek: *myos*, muscle + *kardia*, heart + *itis*, inflammation] Term coined by Joseph Friedrich Sobernheim (1803–1846) of Berlin in 1837. Karl Albert Ludwig Aschoff (1866–1942), a German pathologist, described the characteristic lesion, called Aschoff body, in rheumatic carditis in 1904. A syndrome of fatal myocarditis associated with infiltration of leukocytes, lymphocytes, and multinucleate giant cells, was described by Carl Ludwig Alfred Fiedler (1835–1921) of Germany in 1900. This disease (Fiedler myocarditis) is also known as giant cell or granulomatous myocarditis.

Myoclonus [Greek: *myos*, muscle + *klonus*, turmoil] Clonic spasm of a muscle group in paroxysms in a rare form of epilepsy, myoclonus epilepsy. Described by German physician, Heinrich Unverricht (1853–1912).

Myoglobin [Greek: *myos*, muscle; Latin, *globus*, ball] Crystals of this muscle protein were isolated in 1932 by Swedish biochemist, Axel Hugo Teodor Theorell (1903–1982), director of the Nobel Institute of Biochemistry at Stockholm. He was awarded the Nobel Prize for Physiology or Medicine in 1955 for his work on cytochrome c, oxidation enzymes, the sulfur linkage between heme and protein, vitamin B2, and myoglobin. The structure was discovered using X-ray crystallography by English molecular biologist, Sir John Cowdery Kendrew (b 1917) of Oxford in 1957. He confirmed the alpha-helical structure of the polypeptide chain and was jointly awarded the Nobel Prize for Chemistry, with Max Ferdinand Perutz (b 1914), in 1962.

Myographion [Greek: *myos*, muscle + *graphein*, to record] Instrument for determining the velocity of the nerve current. Invented by Hermann von Helmholtz (1821–1894) in 1850, and improved by Emil Heinrich du Bois-Reymond (1818–1896).

Myonesin *See mephenesin.*

Myopathy [Greek: *myos*, muscle + *pathos*, suffering] Guillaume Benjamin Amand Duchenne . (1806–1875) described a form of progressive muscular atrophy in 1849, and François Amilcar Aran (1817–1861) called it progressive muscular atrophy (PMA) in 1850. Aran's view that it was a primary disease of muscle was shared by Duchenne and Nikolaus Friedrich (1825–1882). Jean Cruveilhier (1791–1874) detailed it in 1853 and it was known as Cruveilhier disease. Wasting of ganglion cells in PMA was described by Jean Martin Charcot (1825–1893) who distinguished it into two types: Aran–Duchenne type, manifesting primarily as muscle wasting, and the other with degeneration of the pyramidal tract of the spinal cord. A peroneal form of muscular atrophy (Charcot–Marie–Tooth disease) was described by Jean Martin Charcot and Pierre Marie (1853–1940) in 1866 and Henry Howard Tooth (1856–1925) later in the same year. Dystrophia myotonica was named by Francisque Deleage (b 1862) of Paris in 1890. An infantile form was described independently by Guido Werdnig (1844–1919), and Johan Hoffmann (1857–1919) in 1891. Oppenheim disease, a form of myopathy in infants, known as amyotonia congenita, was given by Herman Oppenheim (1858–1919) in 1900.

Myopia [Greek: *myein*, to shut + *opsis*, sight] The first book, *The Anomalies of Refraction and Accommodation,* formed the basis for fitting eye glasses for myopia, strabismus, and hypermetropia and was published by Dutch ophthalmologist, Franciscus Cornelius Donders (1818–1889) in 1864.

Myosin *See actomyosin.*

Myositis Ossificans [Greek: *myos*, muscle + *itis*, inflammation; Latin: *osseus*, bony] Condition studied experimentally in animals by Spanish orthopedic surgeon, F. Martin Lagos in 1945. He published his work, *Experimental production of Heterotrophic Bone,* in 1946.

Myotonia Congenita [Greek: *myos*, muscle + *tonos*, tension; Latin: *con*, with; Greek: *gennao*, to produce].

Myotonia Dystrophica *See Curshmann–Batten–Steinert syndrome.*

Myrrh Natural resin extracted from the plant, *Commiphora abyssinica*, used as medicine by the ancient Greeks. Romans used the substance to treat eye and mouth sores, and Egyptians used it for embalming. It was an ingredient of holy oil used in Jewish ceremonials. A bitter wine made from it called 'vinum murratum' was said to have been offered to Christ on the cross by the soldiers. Recent research has shown that it contains analgesic substances. Christian Gottfried Ehrenberg (1795–1876), a German naturalist of Prussian origin and professor at Berlin, who visited Ghizzan in Egypt, brought specimens of the tree to Europe in 1820.

Myxedema [Greek: *myxa*, slime + *oidema*, swelling] Five cases of cretinism in adults were described by Thomas B. Curling (1811–1888) of the London Hospital and Sir William Withey Gull (1816–1890) of Guy's Hospital in 1873. The disease was previously described by J. B. Bramwell in 1869. The term was coined by William Miller Ord (1834–1902) of St Thomas' Hospital in 1877. The term 'cachexia strumpriva' was used in 1883 by Swiss surgeon, Theodor Kocher (1841–1917), to denote myxedema after total removal of the thyroid gland. In the same year, Sir Felix Semon (1848–1921) recognized loss of thyroid function as a common cause of cachexia strumpriva, cretinism, and myxedema. It was treated successfully with injections of glycerin extract of thyroid gland of sheep by George R. Murray (1865–1939) of Newcastle-upon-Tyne in 1891. *See cretinism, thyroid gland.*

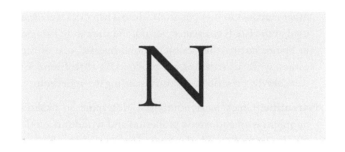

Naboth Follicle Small retention cysts of the mucous glands of the uterine cervix. Described by French surgeon, Guillaume Desnoues, professor of anatomy at Genoa in 1681. Martin Naboth (1675–1721), professor of chemistry at Leipzig in Germany, described the cysts in 1707.

Naegeli, Otto (1871–1938) Hematologist and professor of medicine at Zurich. He described myelomonocytic leukemia, and published *Lehrbuch der Blutkrankheiten und Blutdiagnostik* in 1931.

Nagana Deaths in cattle in Africa following tsetse fly bites, noted by the explorer David Livingstone (1813–1873) in 1857. However, the first mention of a fly disease of African horses, 'nagana', was made by English naval surgeon, John Atkins (1685–1757) in 1734. An accurate description of this disease, known as 'kondee' in Africa, was given by English doctor Thomas Masterman Winterbottom (1765–1859) in 1804. Sir David Bruce (1855–1931) identified a trypanosome, the causative agent of nagana, in the blood of diseased animals in 1894. The same protozoan flagellates were demonstrated in men in Algeria by Gustave Nepvue (1841–1903) in 1890.

Nagel Test Test for color vision performed with a set of cards printed in concentric circles of color. Devised by German physiologist, Willibald Nagel (1870–1911).

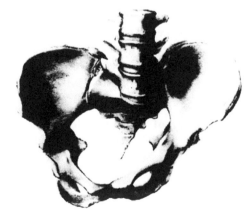

Nägele's illustration of an obliquely contracted pelvis (1839)

Nägele Pelvis Distorted pelvis in which the conjugate diameter takes an oblique direction. Described by German obstetrician, Franz Karl Nägele (1777–1851).

Nageli, Karl Wilhelm von (1817–1891) Swiss botanist from Zurich who became professor of botany at Munich in 1858. He proposed the concept of cell organelles, and differentiated between vegetative and reproductive cell formation.

Nageotte, Jean (1866–1948) French physician who became professor of comparative histology at the College of France in 1912. He worked on nerve grafting and the myelin sheath. *See Babinski–Nageotte syndrome.*

Nail–Patella Syndrome Hereditary disease due to a dominant trait. Described by K. Osterreicher of Germany in 1929. It is characterized by a small or absent patella, anonychia and limitation of movement in the elbow. It was described independently by J. W. Turner of America in 1933.

Nakra Fever *See nasha fever.*

Nalorphine Antagonist to morphine and related substances. Described by McCawley, Hart, and Marsh in 1940, and synthesized by Weijlard and Erickson in 1942. It was first used as an antagonist by Eckenhoff in 1951.

Nansen Fibers Ascending and descending branches of the dorsal spinal nerve roots. Described by Fridtjof Nansen (1861–1930), curator of the Bergen Museum and Arctic explorer, in 1885.

Nanukayami (Syn: Sakushu fever, 7-day fever, akiyami) Leptospirosis with fever and mild jaundice. Caused by a spirochete, *Leptospira interrogans* serogroup *hebdominis,* vectored through the field vole and described by Yutaka Ido (1881–1919), Minor Ito and Hidetsune Wani in 1918.

Napier, John (1550–1617) Scottish mathematician, inventor of logarithms, born at Merchiston Castle, Edinburgh and educated at St Andrew's University, before he began extensive travel in Europe. On his return he was determined to find a shorter and simpler method of calculation and devised a table of logarithms. His *Mirifici Logarithmorum Canonis Descriptio* (Description of the Marvelous Canon of Logarithms) was published in 1614. He devised a calculating machine using a set or rods, Napier bones, in 1617.

Napier Bones Simple device to facilitate multiplication, designed by John Napier (1550–1617) in 1617. He described his method in *Rabdologiae* published in 1617.

Napthalene Obtained from coal tar by London physician and chemist, John Kidd (1776–1851) in 1819. Used as an antiseptic in diarrhea of typhoid fever.

Narceine Alkaloid of opium with narcotic properties, isolated by French pharmacist, Pierre Joseph Pelletier (1788–1842) in 1832.

Narcissism Term to denote a state of excessive and abnormal self love, derived from the legend of Narcissus, son of the Greek river god Cephissus and the nymph Lyriope and loved by the nymph Echo. His indifference to Echo, who adored him, led to her wasting away until she was reduced to only her voice. Narcissus was punished for his act by the gods who made him fall in love with his own reflection in the lake. He jumped into the lake to take hold of his own image and drowned. The gods and goddesses tried to recover his body and found only a flower, which is now named after him. Sigmund Freud (1856-1939) wrote on narcissism in 1914.

Narcolepsy [Greek: *narke*, numbness + *lepsis*, seizure] Recurrent, uncontrollable episodes of sleep. Term coined by French neurologist, Jean Baptiste Edouard Gelineau (1859–1906) of Paris in 1880, and a description of the condition was given by Carl Friedrich Otto Westphal (1833–1890) in 1877. French physicians, Jean Lhermitte (1877–1959) and Auguste Tournay (1878–1969) in 1927, defined it as 'a morbid manifestation which, common to the most varied pathological states, has for its fundamental element an imperious, irresistible need of sleep to which the subject succumbs, however strong may be his determination not to yield to it'. William John Adie (1886–1935), Australian-born English physician and graduate of Edinburgh University, also gave a description.

Narcosis [Greek: *narkotikos*, benumbing] Depression of the function of the CNS marked by stupor and produced by opiod drugs. The lipid theory of narcosis, proposed by Hans Horst Meyer (1853–1939) of Berlin in 1889, explained the action of narcotics through their solubility in lipids. It was further developed by Charles Ernest Overton (1865–1933) in 1901.

Narcotherapy [Greek: *narke*, numbness + *therapeia*, treatment] Method developed in the 1940s of using drugs to enable the patient to express his emotions. Barbiturates were one of the commonest drugs used to treat World War II patients who suffered from trauma.

Narcotics [Greek: *narkotikos*, benumbing] Opium, mandrake and cannabis were known to Egyptians and Greeks, Babylonians and Jews. Mandrake wine was used to perform surgery by Dioscorides (AD 40–90). It was also the most popular anesthetic in the Middle Ages. Hua Tu, a Chinese surgeon in the second century, used cannabis and other narcotics in his operations. Herbal narcotics were less used in the late Renaissance period, and they were banned in France during this period. Chloral hydrate, one of the earliest synthetic sedatives, was produced in 1870. Bromides were heavily prescribed as sedatives during the 19th century.

Narcotine [Greek: *narke*, numbness] Noscapine, an alkaloid of opium with antipyretic properties and without narcotic effects. Isolated by Charles Louis Derosne (1780–1846) in 1803.

Nasha Fever Fever involving mucous membrane of the upper respiratory tract with toxic symptoms, occurred in India, mainly in Bengal. It was described by Fernandez at the Indian Medical Congress in 1894. It is known as 'nakra' fever in other states of India.

Nasmyth Membrane Primary cuticle of dental enamel, described in 1839 by Alexander Nasmyth (d 1847), a Scottish dental surgeon at Hanover Square, London.

Nasogastric Tube [Latin: *nasus*, nose; Greek: *gaster*, stomach] Avenzoar (1092–1162), an Arab surgeon, used a silver tube in feeding patients with a stricture of the gullet. Placing food into the stomach through a tube was called 'gavage', and was revived by Georges Maurice Débove (1845–1920) in 1881. A tube was first used by American physician, Martin Emil Rehfuss (1887–1964), in 1914 to study digestion, by withdrawal of a test meal from the stomach. His tube contained a metal capsule which sometimes caused damage to the gastric mucosa. It was improved by John Alfred Ryle (1889–1950) in 1921 who covered the entire tip with rubber with perforations above the bulb.

Nasopharyngeal Carcinoma [Latin: *nasus*, nose; Greek: *pharyngx*, gullet] *See Trotter syndrome.*

Nasse Law The immunity of females to hemophilia despite their ability to transmit the disease was proposed by Christian Friedrich Nasse (1778–1851) of Germany in 1820.

Nathans, Daniel (b 1928) American microbiologist, born in Wilmington, Delaware and graduated from the University of Delaware. He pioneered the use of restriction enzymes to fragment DNA and made the first genetic map of the SV 40 viral DNA. He shared the 1978 Nobel Prize for Physiology or Medicine with Werner Arber (b 1928).

National Academy of Sciences (NAS) Founded as a private organization dedicated to science and given a charter by the American Congress in 1863. It now has its headquarters in Washington and advises the US government in an official capacity on national matters involving technology and science. The Institute of Medicine of the NAS was founded in 1970.

National Foundation for Infantile Paralysis The first center in the world for research into polio was established in America in 1935. The idea was started in 1932 by the American president Franklin Delano Roosevelt (1882–1945) who himself had suffered from polio which he contracted in 1921. The killed polio virus vaccine was discovered at the Institute by Jonas Salk (1914–1995) in 1953.

National Health Insurance Act The first move towards the British government taking responsibility for the health of the nation was made by enactment of the National Insurance Act of 1911. The Ministry of Health was set up in 1919. The Act only provided medical care to insured workers, but not their families.

National Health Service Following the *Report on Social Insurances and Allied Services* by William Henry Beveridge (1879–1963) in 1942, the British government produced a White Paper in 1944, and the National Health Service Act was passed in 1946 and enacted in 1948. This channeled money into the hospital system. The Family Doctor Charter of 1965 provided financial subsidies to general practitioners. The NHS Act was revised in the 1970s and was superseded by the National Health Service Act of 1977. *See Bevan, Aneurin.*

National Hospital for the Relief of Paralysis, Epilepsy and Allied Disorders First neurological center in the world, started at Queen's Square, London by Louisa Chandler and her sister in 1859, with Jabez S. Ramskill as its first physician. He was followed by Charles Edouard Brown-Sequard (1817–1894) in 1860 and John Hughlings Jackson (1834–1911) in 1862. It is currently known as National Hospital for Neurological Disease, Queen's Square.

National Institute for Medical Research (NIMR) Initially located at Hampstead in 1920 and moved to Mill Hill, London in 1949. As a research establishment, NIMR has made significant contributions in chromatography, protein synthesis, and carbohydrate metabolism. Notable workers at the Institute include: Sir Henry Hallett Dale (1875–1968) and Sir Peter Brian Medawar (1915–1987).

National Library of Medicine Originally started in 1836 by the American Surgeon-General, Lovell. It became the Surgeon-General's Library in the latter half of the 19th century under the leadership of John Shaw Billings (1838–1913) of Indiana who served as an army surgeon during the Civil War and was a founder of the Johns Hopkins Hospital. In 1876 Billing's published a catalogue of authors and subjects in an alphabetical order, and in 1880 he produced the first volume of the index catalogue, which was the most exhaustive bibliography produced at this time. The name of the library changed to Armed Forces Library in 1952, and became the National Library of Medicine in 1956. It is one of the largest medical libraries in the world.

Natural Philosophy A new system of philosophy embracing the entire field of natural science begun by German philosopher and theologian, Friedrich Wilhelm Joseph von Schelling (1775–1854). His work *Erster Entwurf eines Systems der Naturphilosopie* was published in 1797 portrayed the entire world as the creation of all-pervading universal will.

Natural Selection *See evolution theory.*

Naude, Gabriel (1600–1653) French physician from Paris who served as librarian to Cardinal Richelieu, and was later librarian to Queen Christina in Sweden. He published *Bibliographica Politica, On Liberal Studies* and several other works.

Naunyn, Bernard (1839–1925) Professor of clinical medicine first at Dorpat (1859) and then at Bern (1872). He succeeded Adolf Kussmaul (1822–1902) as professor at Strasbourg, and devoted his career to study of metabolism in diabetes and diseases of the liver and pancreas. He introduced the concept of cholangitis and advocated drainage of bile ducts in 1892. Naunyn noted the formation of acid in diabetic coma in 1906 and named it acidosis. His work on diabetes, *Der Diabetes Mellitus*, was published in 1898. He also founded the *Archiv für Experimentale Pathologique und Pharmakologie* and the interdisciplinary periodical, *Mitteilungen aus den Grenzbebieten der Medizin und Chirurgie* in 1896.

Naval Medicine The earliest attempts to provide health care for seamen were made by Sir Francis Drake, Sir John Hawkins and Admiral Howard in the 16th century. They levied a tax of six pence on seamen and formed a body to provide medical care for them. This was probably the first system of health insurance on record. Henry VIII established a permanent medical service at sea with a list of surgeons to attend his Royal Navy. Royal Naval Hospitals were established in England at Portsmouth in 1761 and near Plymouth in 1765. One of the earliest book on naval medicine was *The Surgeons Mate*, written in 1617 by John Woodall (1556–1643), a surgeon with the East India Company. He suggested use of lime juice as a cure for scurvy. Another treatise on conditions affecting seamen was written in 1696 by a navy surgeon from London, William Cockburn (1669–1739). James Lind (1716–1794), first senior physician at the Portsmouth Royal Naval Hospital, conducted controlled trials on the use of lemons and oranges in prevention of scurvy in 1747. Thomas Trotter (1760–1832), another prominent naval physician from the Royal Hospital at Portsmouth and physician to the fleet in 1794, took measures to eradicate scurvy and wrote *Medica Nautica, or an Essay on the Diseases of Seamen,* and a *Review of the Medical Department of British Navy.*

Neanderthal Man Skeletal remains of a primitive man from the Paleolithic period, including a skull (Neanderthal skull), were found at a limestone cave at Neanderthal, near Düsseldorf in 1858 and described by Hermann Schaafhausen (1816–1893). Neanderthal man lived 20 to 50 thousand years ago and was followed by Cro-Magnon or *Homo sapiens,* who had facial and other body features of modern man. The first complete Neanderthal skeleton was assembled by Marcellin Boule (1861–1942), professor at the Natural History Museum in Paris, who published *Les Hommes Fossiles* in 1921. *See Cro-Magnon.*

Neapolitan Fever *See Malta fever.*

Nebuchadnezzar ll (630–562 BC) Chaldean king who rebuilt the Assyrian empire and sacked Jerusalem. He is said to have suffered from a delusion that he was a wolf (lycanthropy). His palace and a temple were unearthed by Sir Henry Rawlinson (1810–1895) of Chadlington, Oxford.

Nebular Hypothesis [Latin: *nebula,* mist] Theory that the universe was formed from a shapeless mass of nebulae and clusters of stars, proposed by Sir William Herschel (1792–1871). Pierre Simon Laplace (1749–1827) proposed a similar hypothesis in 1796, suggesting that the solar system originated from a nebula, a vast cloud of high temperature gas.

Necator americanus A genus of nematode including the species, *N. americanum,* American hookworm, discovered by Allan J. Smith and named by Charles Wardell Stiles (1867–1941) of the US Public Health Service in 1902. The parasite is thought to have been brought to America with slaves from Africa. *See Anchylostoma duodenale.*

Necrobiosis Lipoidica Diabeticorum [Greek: *nekros,* dead + *biosis,* life] Degenerative disease of skin in diabetes, reported by Austrian dermatologist, Maurice Oppenheim (1876–1949) in 1929. Eight cases were recorded at the Mayo Clinic over the next 7 years. Erich Urbach (1893–1946), Czech-born American dermatologist, described it in 1932.

Necrophilia [Greek: *nekros,* dead + *philos,* love] Desire to have sexual intercourse or sexual contact with cadavers. Richard Krafft-Ebing (1840–1902) described a case in 1849 of Sergeant Bertrand, who dug up 15 female bodies. In 1924 Magnus Hirsfield (1868–1935) described the case of a man

who made a secret passage to his wife's tomb in order to have sexual intercourse.

Needham, Joseph (b 1900) English biochemist and historian, born in London and educated at Cambridge where he became a demonstrator in biochemistry (1928–1933) and made a study on differentiation of the fertilized egg. He went on to become Master of Gonville and Caius College (1966–1976) and worked on organizers in amphibian development. He published *Chemical Embryology* (1931), *The Sceptical biologist* (1929), and *A History of Embryology* in 1934. He was head of a British Scientific Mission in China during World War ll, and wrote extensively on Chinese science, including acupuncture.

Neelsen, Friedrich Karl Adolf (1854–1894) Pathologist at Dresden who developed the acid-fast method of staining mycobacteria.

Neftel Disease Hysterical disease in which the patient is unable to sit, stand or walk without experiencing pain and paresthesia of the back and head but can perform any movements while lying down. Described by William Basil Neftel (1830–1906), an American physician of Russian origin.

Negative Numbers Found in algebra and arithmetic by Hindus in the 7th century. The Hindu mathematician Brahmagupta of Ujjain gave rules and signs for their operation.

Negri Bodies Characteristic acidophilic cell inclusion bodies in the pyramidal cells of Ammon's horn, diagnostic for rabies. Observed by Italian pathologist, Adelchi Negri (1876–1912) in 1903. He initially mistook them for parasitic protozoal organisms. *See rabies.*

Neher, Erwin (b 1944) German biophysicist, educated at the Technical University of Munich and the University of Wisconsin. Together with Bert Sakmann (b 1942), he recorded electric currents in single channels of biological membranes and developed the 'patch-clamp' technique for discrete biophysical measurements. He and Sakmann shared the 1991 Nobel Prize for Physiology or Medicine.

Neisser, Albert Ludwig Siegmund (1855–1916) German bacteriologist who discovered the gonorrhea bacterium while a 24-year-old assistant in the dermatological clinic of Oscar Simon at the University of Breslau, in 1879. He succeeded Simon as professor of skin and venereal diseases in 1900. He was censored for using healthy human subjects in syphilis research. He also gave a complete review of hydatid disease *Die Echinococcenkrankheit* in 1877. *See ethics of human experimentation.*

Neisseria gonorrhoeae　Causative bacterium of gonorrhea, named after its discoverer, Albert Ludwig Neisser (1855–1916). *See Neisser, Albert.*

Neisseria meningitidis　Meningococcus bacteria and causative organism in meningitis. Isolated from cerebrospinal fluid of patients by Anton Weichselbaum (1845–1920) in 1887. It was later named *Neisseria meningitidis* after the German bacteriologist, Albert Ludwig Neisser (1855–1916).

Nelaton, Auguste (1807–1873) French surgeon from Paris who graduated in medicine from the University in 1836. He used a rubber urethral catheter in 1860 and introduced electrocautery into surgery. He was professor of surgery at the St Louis Hospital in 1851 and surgeon to Napoleon III in 1867.

Nelaton Line　Line extending from the anterior superior iliac spine to the ischial tubercles in congenital dislocation of the hip. Described by Auguste Nelaton (1807–1873), professor of surgery in Paris in 1844.

Nematology　[Greek: *nema*, thread] *See helminthology.*

Nembutal　Sodium pentobarbital. *See intravenous anesthetics.*

Nemesius　(AD 400) Greek Christian philosopher and Bishop of Emissa. He wrote *De Natura Homonis* in which he discussed the role of bile in digestion, purging of blood, imparting heat to the .body, and the doctrine of pre-existence.

Nencki Test　Use of nitric and nitrous acid to detect indole. Test devised by Polish physician, Marcellus von Nencki (1847–1901).

Neoarsphenamine　Paul Ehrlich (1854–1915) produced neosalvarsan or neoarsphenamine in 1911, which was found to be effective in treatment of relapsing fever, syphilis and trypanosomiasis.

Neolithic Age　[Greek: *neo*, new + *litho*, stone] Name given to the Stone Age by Sir John Lubbock (1834–1913) in 1865. He subdivided it on the basis of stone artifacts into: rough stone instruments or Paleolithic period, and polished stone instruments or Neolithic period.

Neomycin　Antibiotic obtained from *Streptomyces fradiae* by American physicians, Selman Abraham Waksman (1888–1973) or Rutgers University and Hubert Arthur Lechevalier (b 1926) in 1949.

Neon　[Greek: *neos*, new] Inert gas discovered by Sir William Ramsay (1852–1916), and London chemist, Morris William Travers (1872–1961) in 1898.

Neonatology　[Greek: *neos*, new; Latin: *natus*, born] Oxygen therapy was suggested in resuscitation of asphyxiated neonates by François Chaussier in 1780. The Schultz's method for reviving them by inverting and swinging the infant was described German gynecologist, Bernhard Sigmund Schultz (1827–1919). *See Apgar score.*

Neoplasm　[Greek: *neos*, new + *plasma*, molded or formed] *See cancer.*

Neoprotonsil　*See ulcerative colitis.*

Nephrectomy　[Greek: *nephros*, kidney + *ektome*, to cut out] First performed in 1870 as treatment for urinary tract fistula by Gustav von Simon (1824–1876), professor of surgery at Heidelberg. The first nephrectomy for malignant disease of the kidney was done in 1877 by Karl Johann August Langenbuch (1846–1901) of Berlin.

Nephritis　[Greek: *nephros*, kidney + *itis*, inflammation] A classical description of chronic non-suppurative nephritis (Bright disease) was given by Richard Bright (1789–1858) of Guy's Hospital in 1827. The pathological anatomy of Bright disease was provided by Karl Weigert (1845–1904) in 1879. Classification of nephritis, based on the hemorrhagic nature and nephrosclerosis, was proposed by American biochemist, D. D. Van Slyke and colleagues in 1930. American physician Thomas Addis (1881–1949) and Henry Astbury Christian (1876–1951) gave another classifications in 1934. Arthur Maurice Fishberg (1898–1992), associate in medicine at Mount Sinai Hospital, New York, described focal glomerular nephritis and acute interstitial nephritis in 1931. Clinical and histological features were given in 1942 by Sir Arthur William Mickle Ellis (1883–1966), a London physician. *See embolic nephritis, glomerular nephritis.*

Nephrolithotomy　[Greek: *nephros*, kidney + *lithos*, stone + *tome*, to cut] One of the first procedures where the renal stone was removed through a lumbar incision was performed by Sir Henry Morris (1844–1926) of London in 1880. *See lithotomy.*

Nephrology　[Greek: *nephros*, kidney + *logos*, discourse] Dropsy caused by the diseased kidneys was described by Guiliemus da Saliceto (1201–1277) of Italy. The microscopic anatomy of the kidney was given by two Italians, Lorenzo Bellini (1643–1704) and Marcello Malpighi (1628–1694). Albumin and blood in urine of patients with renal dropsy were observed by William Charles Wells (1757–1817), a physician at St Thomas' Hospital in 1812. Richard Bright's (1789–1858) classic description of chronic nephritis in 1827 was one of the earliest to focus on renal disease. The artificial kidney was introduced in the 1930s, and renal biopsy for detection and management of renal diseases appeared in the mid-1950s. *See artificial kidney, kidney, renal transplant, nephritis.*

Nephropexy [Greek: *nephros*, kidney + *pexis*, fixation] Operation to fix a movable kidney was performed by Eugen Hahn (1841–1902) in 1881. A French surgeon of Cuban origin, Joaquín Domínguez Albarrán (1860–1912) developed a further method.

Nephrosis [Greek: *nephros*, kidney + *osis*, disease] Used by Friedrich von Müller (1858–1941) in 1905 to refer to primary degenerative forms of Bright disease and to differentiate it from diseases of an inflammatory nature. His classification was modified by American physicians, Albert Arthur Epstein (1880–1965), F. Volhard (b 1931) and G. Fahr (b 1937) to include amyloid kidney and other conditions in which the renal parenchyma was not primarily involved. *See nephrotic syndrome.*

Nephrostomy [Greek: *nephros*, kidney + *tome*, cut] An operation for treatment of hydronephrosis in a four-year-old boy was performed by Thomas Hillier (1831–1868) in 1865. It was popularized by Joaquín Domínguez Albarrán (1860–1912), a genitourinary surgeon from Cuba and a professor in Paris, in 1895.

Nephrotic Syndrome The association between edema and coagulable substances in urine was first observed by Cotunnius or Domenico Cotugno (1736–1822) in 1770 and in 1827 by Richard Bright (1789–1858). Samuel Wilks (1824–1911) in 1853 showed that a variety of renal conditions could give rise to nephrotic syndrome. The term was introduced by Friedrich von Müller (1858–1941) in 1905.

Neptunium Element heavier than uranium obtained by bombarding uranium with neutrons. Found by two American atomic scientists, Edwin Mattison McMillan (1907–1991) and Philip Hauge Abelson (b 1913).

Nernst Theory The effect of an electric current on the tissues causing a change in concentration of electrolytes in membranes. Put forward by German physicists, Walther Hermann Nernst (1864–1941) and E. H. Riesenfeld in 1902.

Nerve [Greek: *nervus*, nerve] The concept of nerve in neurology was proposed by Aristotle (384–322 BC). Hippocrates (460–377 BC) used the term 'nervus' to refer to whitish fibrous structures such as tendons, nerves, and fascial bands.

Nerve Cell The structure, including the axis cylinder and dendrons was first shown by Otto Friedrich Karl Deiters (1834–1863), a pupil of Rudolph Virchow (1821–1902).

Deiters' work was published two years after his death. *See neuron, axon, myelin sheath.*

Nerve Conduction The involvement of electric currents in nervous stimulus was shown by Emil Heinrich du Bois-Reymond (1818–1896) of Berlin in 1843. In 1846 Johannes Müller (1801–1858) stated that the time taken for transmission of sensation from the periphery to the brain was infinitely small and unmeasurable. Hermann von Helmholtz (1821–1894), of the University of Bonn, measured the speed of nerve conduction in experimental animals in 1852. His study on frogs showed that the maximum velocity was 30 meters per second. Joseph Erlanger (1874–1965) and Herbert Spencer Gasser (1888–1963) received the Nobel Prize for their work on functions of nerve fibers in 1944. Study of nerve transmission was refined by Lord Edgar Douglas Adrian (1889–1977) and New York neurophysiologist, Detlef Wulf Bronk (1887–1975) around 1932. *See neurotransmitters.*

Nerve Regeneration First mentioned by Felice Fontana (1730–1805) in 1767. Experimental studies in animals were done by English surgeon, Joseph Swan (1791–1874), who won the Jacksonian Prize of the Royal College of Surgeons for his treatise *The Treatment of Local Morbid Affections of the Nerves* in 1819. Further experimental work was done by Edmé Felix Alfred Vulpian (1826–1887) of Paris in 1861. The success of nerve suture was demonstrated by Pierre Marie Jean Flourens (1794–1867) of Paris. Sir James Purves Stewart (1869–1949), a neurologist at the Westminster Hospital, and London neurosurgeon, and Sir Charles Alfred Ballance (1865–1936) demonstrated partial recovery of the facial nerve after suturing it to an accessory nerve in 1895.

Nervous System *See brain, neurology.*

Nessler Reagent Test for ammonia used in the analysis of blood, urea and plasma proteins was prepared by a German chemist, Julius Nessler (1827–1905) of Karlsruhe.

Nestorian Medicine The Nestorian order was founded by Nestorius, Syrian Bishop of Constantinople (AD 431) who was excommunicated for suggesting that the Virgin Mary should not be called the Mother of God. He established two hospitals in Edessa in Mesopotamia which developed into a very successful school of medicine. His followers later moved to Persia, devoted their time to medicine and established the famous medical school at Jundeshapur. *See Jundeshapur.*

Nettleship Disease Urticaria pigmentosa, a form of chronic skin disease which leaves brown stains. Described by London dermatologist, Edward Nettleship (1845–1913) in 1869.

Neubauer Artery Deep thyroid artery described by German anatomist, Johann Ernst Neubauer (1742–1777).

Neuburger, Max (1868–1955) Born in Vienna, he was a medical historian who published: a history of the physiology of the nervous system (1897), nutrition (1900), antitoxins (1900), Austrian and Viennese medicine (1918–1922) and an extensive history on medicine (1906–1911).

Neufeld, Fred (1861–1945) German bacteriologist who described bacteriotrophins in 1904. He demonstrated lysis of pneumococci by bile salts.

Neuman, Franz Ernst Christian (1834–1918) Professor of pathological anatomy at Königsberg, who described the semicalcified layer of the matrix (Neuman layer) surrounding dentine in 1863.

Neurasthenia [Greek: *neuron*, nerve + *astheneia*, debility] Jean Antoine Eugene Bouchut (1818–1891) of Paris recognized a state of nervous exhaustion and asthenia which he called 'nervosisme' in 1860. George Miller Beard (1839–1883) introduced the concept of neurasthenia and nervous exhaustion in 1869. *See chronic fatigue syndrome.*

Neurilemma [Greek: *neuron*, nerve + *eilema*, covering] Thin membranous outer covering of the myelin sheath of the nerve fiber (sheath of Schwann) described and named by Theodor Schwann (1810–1882), professor of anatomy and physiology at Liége in 1847.

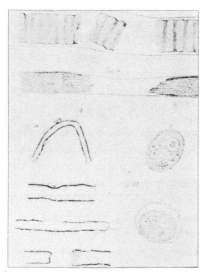

Neurilemma. Theodor Schwann's original figure of muscle and nerve tissue. William Stirling, *Some Apostles of Physiology* (1902). Waterlow & Sons, London

Neurodermatitis [Greek: *neuron*, nerve + *derma*, skin + *itis*, inflammation] Chronic lichenoid itching described by Jean Baptiste Emile Vidal (1825–1893) of Paris in 1886.

Neurofibromatosis [Greek: *neuron*, nerve; Latin: *fibra*, fiber] Familial condition characterized by developmental changes in the nervous system, skin and bones with soft tumors and areas of pigmentation. An early account was given by Robert William Smith (1807–1873), a surgeon from Trinity College, Dublin in 1849. His *Treatise on Pathology, Diagnosis, and Treatment of Neuroma* preceded Friedrich Daniel von Recklinhausen's (1833–1910) description by 33 years. Smith provided life-size illustrations of two cases. A classic description was given by von Recklinghausen in 1882, and the disease was named after him. *See elephant man.*

Neuroglia [Greek: *neuron*, nerve + *glia*, glue] Supporting structure of the nerve tissue described by Rudolph Virchow (1821–1902) in 1854. It was differentiated into microglia and oligodendroglia using silver stain in 1919 by Spanish histologist, Pio del Rio Hortega (1882–1945) of the National Institute for Cancer in Madrid.

Neurohypnology [Greek: *neuron*, nerve + *hypnos*, sleep + *logos*, discourse] Mesmerism was introduced by Franz Anton Mesmer (1734–1815) and renamed 'neurohypnology' and used as anesthesia by a Manchester surgeon, James Braid (1795–1860). He published *Neurohypnology, or the Rationale of Nervous Sleep, Considered in Relation with Animal Magnetism* in 1843. *See hypnotism, animal magnetism.*

Neurology [Greek: *neuron*, nerve + *logos*, discourse] Term coined by Thomas Willis (1621–1675). One of the earliest significant contributions was made by Sir Charles Bell (1774–1842), who differentiated nerves into sensory and motor components in 1811. The first modern treatise, *Lehrbuch der Nerven-Krankheiten*, was written by Moritz Heinrich Romberg (1795–1873) of Berlin in 1840. He gave a clear account of ataxia. Earlier treatises were written by: Robert Whytt (1714–1766) of Edinburgh on tuberculous meningitis in 1768, Domenico Cotugno (1736–1822) of Naples on sciatica in 1770, and James Parkinson (1755–1824) of London on paralysis agitans in 1817. Guillaume Benjamin Duchenne (1806–1875) of Paris described spinal muscular atrophy in 1849, differentiated between various forms of lead palsy, described spinal pathology of anterior poliomyelitis and pseudohypertrophic muscular dystrophy. Jean Martin Charcot (1825–1893) of Paris, a physician at the Hospital of Sâlpetrière described: localization and functions of cerebral diseases (1876), cortical motor centers in man (1893), lesions in muscular atrophy (1886) and peroneal muscular atrophy. Sir William Richard Gowers (1845–1915), a London professor of medicine at University College, gave the name 'knee jerk' to the tendon reflex of the knee, and in 1879 published an important textbook, *Diseases of the Nervous System* and *Pseudo-hypertrophic*

Muscular paralysis (named Gower disease). Cortical areas responsible for specific isolated movements in the body were proposed by John Hughlings Jackson (1835–1911) in 1864, he described the unilateral localized form of epilepsy (Jacksonian fits).

Neuron [Greek: *neuron*, nerve] Any of the conducting cells of the nervous system. Galen (AD 129–200) first used the term in *De Motu Musculorum* (AD 180) as he believed that nerves caused the limbs to nod. German anatomist, Heinrich Waldeyer (1837–1921), revived the term and used it in the modern sense in 1891. The first attempt to classify them in the spinal and other ganglia was made by Alexander Stanislavovich Dogiel (1852–1922), a neurologist and professor of histology at St Petersburg in 1898. *See motor neuron.*

Neurophysiology [Greek: *neuron*, nerve + *physis*, nature + *logos*, discourse] Gustav Theodor Fritsch (1838–1897), a military surgeon during the Prussian-Danish War, noted that stimulation of one side of the brain caused the opposite side to twitch. He later joined with Julius Eduard Hitzig (1838–1907) and did experiments on stimulation of the brain in dogs. Their paper, published in 1870, is considered a classic of neurophysiology. In England, Lord Edgar Douglas Adrian (1889–1977) the founder of British neurophysiology, examined the activity of the nervous system and paved the way for development of the electroencephalogram. *See electroencephalography, electromyography, motor cortex.*

Neurosis William Cullen (1710–1790) used the term in 1769 in *Synopsis Nosologiae Practicae* which divided disease into fevers, neuroses, cachexias and local disorders and classified them into four groups in his *Nosology*. The influence of emotions on the viscera was presented by Sir Thomas Clifford Allbutt (1836–1925) in his Goulstonian lectures in 1884, *On the neuroses of the viscera.* Alfred Adler (1870–1937) of Vienna in 1929 suggested that neurosis is a defect or failure in adjustment to the social environment and arises as a defense to defend the ego. Thomas Arthur Ross (1875–1941), a psychiatrist at Edinburgh, rejected the Freudian hypothesis and psychoanalytic methods and published *Common Neuroses* in 1935.

Neurosurgery Trepanning is the oldest form of neurosurgery and has been practiced since the Neolithic period. Studies by Pierre Paul Broca (1824–1880) in 1876 showed evidence of healing in such skulls which indicate, not only that the procedure must have been performed while they were alive, but also that they survived. Skulls from the pre-Incan period with trephine holes were identified by Muniz in 1894. The practice of trepanning amongst some races from Melanesia and Algeria in the 19th century have

shown that it was used to cure conditions such as epilepsy, head injury, and demonic possession. The first modern scientific work on neuroanatomy was written by Félix Vicq d'Azyr (1748–1794) of Paris in 1786. Surgical treatment of a cerebral abscess by opening the lateral ventricles was performed by William Detmold (1808–1894) of America in 1850. Surgical removal of a brain tumor arising from the dura mater was performed by Sir William Macewen (1848–1924), professor of surgery at the Glasgow Royal Infirmary in 1879. Sir Victor Horsley (1857–1916), founder of neurosurgery in England, removed a tumor of the spinal cord in 1888. Neurosurgery in Europe was advanced by Fedor Krause (1856–1937) of Berlin. Harvey Williams Cushing (1869–1939) was a pioneer of brain surgery in America who devised his own technique for removing intracranial tumors in 1932. *A History of Neurological Surgery* edited by an American neurosurgeon, A.E. Walker (b 1907) of Johns Hopkins, was published in 1951.

Neurosyphilis [Greek: *neuron*, nerve] Niccolò Massa (1485–1569), a professor at Venice, gave an early account in 1539. The late-stage effects of syphilis on the brain were described by Thomas Willis (1621–1675) in *Pathologiae cerebri* in 1667. John Hunter (1728–1793) experimentally inoculated himself with samples taken from a gonorrheal patient and unknowingly contracted syphilis, and symptoms during his later life were probably due to neurosyphilis. Sir Thomas Clouston from Orkney and superintendent at the Royal Morningside Asylum, associated juvenile paresis with congenital syphilis in 1877. Various infective and toxic agents, including leishmania, malarial parasites, spirochetes of relapsing fever and tuberculin, were used to produce shock as treatment at the turn of the 19th century. The colloidal gold test for diagnosis was introduced by Carl Friedrich August Lange (1883–1953) in 1913.

Neurotransmitters Otto Loewi (1873–1961), a German-born American pharmacologist at Strasburg demonstrated in 1921 that a substance liberated from the stimulated vagus nerve ending, when perfused on to a second heart, was capable of slowing heart beat. This substance was the first neurotransmitter to be isolated and was identified as acetylcholine by British physiologist, Sir Henry Hallett Dale (1875–1968), in 1929. The role of acetylcholine in the transmission of nerve impulses was demonstrated by Wilhelm Siegmund Feldberg (b 1900) and Sir John Henry Gaddum (1900–1965) in 1965. The mechanism of its release by nerve impulses was discovered by Sir Bernard Katz (b 1911), a biophysicist at University College, London, in 1969. Noradrenaline was shown to be the main transmitter of sympathetic nerve impulses in 1946 by Swedish pharmacologist, Ulf Svante von Euler (1905–1983), who was awarded the Nobel Prize in 1970. Selective uptake of noradrenaline by sympathetic nerves was demonstrated, with the use of radioactive tracers, by Julius Axel (b 1912) of the American National Institute of Health in 1960.

Neurotrophic Viruses [Greek: *neuron*, nerve + *trophein*, to nourish] Polio was the first virus with primary affinity for nervous tissue discovered by Louis Pasteur (1822–1895) in 1884. Its neurotrophic nature was proved in 1909.

Neutron [Latin: *neuter*, neither] In 1932 English physicist and Nobel Prize winner, Sir James Chadwick (1891–1974) bombarded the element beryllium with alpha particles and obtained a new particle with the same mass as the proton but with no charge. He announced his discovery, which he named 'neutron', at the Cavendish Laboratory in the same year and published it in *Nature* on February 27 1932. The life of a neutron was estimated by Austrian-Swiss physicist and Nobel Prize winner, Wolfgang Pauli (1900–1958).

Neutrophil ([Latin: *neuter*, neither; Greek: *philos*, love] *See leukocytes, leukocyte count*.

New England Journal of Medicine Started as *New England Journal of Medicine and Surgery* in 1812 by two doctors, James Jackson (1777–1868) son of Newburyport merchant, and John Collins Warren (1778–1856), son of John Warren the first professor of anatomy and surgery at Harvard Medical School. It merged with the *Boston Medical Intelligencer* as the *Boston Medical and Surgical Journal* in 1828. Weekly clinical pathological conference proceedings were initiated by Richard C. Cabot (1868–1939) of Massachusetts General Hospital in 1895.

Newlands, John Alexander Reina (1837–1898) London chemist who arranged the elements in order of atomic weight and recognized similarity between every eighth element. His Law of Octaves proposed in 1864 is regarded as a forerunner of the periodic table.

Newman, Sir George (1870–1948) Civil servant and physician from Leominster who was appointed as chief medical officer to the British Ministry of Health in 1919, and published *Hygiene and Public Health* (1917), *Outline of the Practice of Preventive Medicine* (1917), and *Building of a Nation's Health* in 1939.

Newton, Sir Isaac (1642–1727) He was educated at Grantham and entered Trinity College, Cambridge in 1660. He developed his Binomial Theorem at the age of 24 years and three years later became a professor at Cambridge. His work on mechanical principles and the motions of bodies,

Philosophiae naturalis principia mathematica, was edited and published at the expense of Edmund Halley (1656–1742) in 1687. The first book dealt with derivation of the inverse square law, book two deals with motion in a resisting medium. Application of the laws of gravity to motion of the planets is in the third book. He was appointed master of the mint in 1699, a post which he held until his death. His work was written for mathematicians and was interpreted by Voltaire (1694–1778) in 1737

New York Cancer Hospital The first hospital for cancer in the United States was established in 1884. It was renamed the Memorial Hospital in 1899.

New York Hospital for the Diseases of the Skin One of the first three specialist hospitals (Massachusetts Eye and Ear Infirmary in 1824, Boston Lying-in Hospital in 1832) in America was founded in 1836.

NHS *See National Health Service.*

Niacin Nicotinic acid (a B vitamin) was called niacin by the Food and Research Council of the USA in 1942 to distinguish it for the general public who associated the term 'nicotine' with a poisonous substance. *See nicotinic acid.*

Nicandros *See Nikandros.*

Nicholls, Frank (1699–1778) London physician who graduated from Christchurch, Oxford. He married the daughter of Richard Mead (1673–1754), and succeeded Sir Hans Sloane (1660–1753) as physician to George II. Nicholls published *De Anima Medica, De Motu Cordis et Sanguis* and several other works.

Nicholson, William (1758–1815) Physicist and inventor from London who served in India at an early stage of his career and later became an agent of Josiah Wedgwood on the continent. He invented the Nicholson hydrometer while a waterworks engineer at Portsmouth. He constructed the first voltaic pile in England and demonstrated that water could be dissociated by electricity in 1800. He published *Dictionary of Chemistry*, and *Introduction to Natural Philosophy*.

Nickel [Latin: *niccolum*] Isolated by Swedish metallurgist and mineralogist, Axel Frederick Cronstedt (1722–1765) of Turinge in 1751. Nickel carbonyl, developed by Ludwig Mond of Cheshire in 1888, revolutionized the metal industry. Nickel itch or dermatitis in workers who did nickel plating was first described by J. Rambousek in 1908. A 150-fold increase of carcinoma of the ethmoid bone of the nose in nickel refiners in Great Britain was detected by Sir Austin Bradford Hill (b 1897) in 1965.

Nicol Prism Made from Iceland spar and having double refracting properties. Created by a Scottish geologist and physicist, William Nicol (1768–1851) of Edinburgh in 1828. It was a valuable tool for studying polarized light.

Nicolle, Charles Jules Henri (1866–1936) French physician and pupil of Emile Roux (1853–1933) and Elie Metchnikoff (1845–1916) at the Pasteur Institute, born in Rouen and educated in Paris. He became director of the Pasteur Institute in Tunis. He identified the body louse as a transmitter of typhus fever in 1911, for which he was awarded the Nobel Prize for Physiology or Medicine in 1928.

Nicotinamide Adenine Dinucleotide (NAD) Coenzyme and electron carrier being alternatively oxidized and reduced. *See Kornberg, Arthur.*

Nicotinamide Coenzyme discovered in yeast concentrates. Conrad Arnold Elvihjem (1901–1962) and Dodge William Frost demonstrated its growth promoting properties in 1937.

Nicotine The plant *Nicotiana tabacum*, from which the alkaloid nicotine is obtained, is named after Jean Nicot (1530–1600), French ambassador to Portugal, who brought seeds to France for medical use around 1560. The first pure form was prepared by Reimann and Posselt in 1828. *See tobacco.*

Nicotinic Acid The B vitamin niacin is found in yeast, milk and liver. Its efficacy in treatment of pellagra was demonstrated by an American biochemist, Conrad Arnold Elvehjem (1901–1962) of Wisconsin in 1938. The occurrence of encephalopathy in nicotinic acid deficiency was described by N. Jolliffe in 1940.

Niemann–Pick Disease Lipoidosis with anemia, mental retardation, retinal degeneration, hepatosplenomegaly and skin pigmentation caused by a lack of the enzyme sphingomyelinase and a subsequent accumulation of sphyngomyelin. Described by Albert Niemann (1880–1921), a Berlin pediatrician in 1914. It was described in more detail by Ludwig Pick (1868–1944), a German pathologist, in 1926.

Niemeyer Pill Quinine, digitalis and opium preparation sold by German physician, Felix von Niemeyer (1820–1871).

Night Blindness Nyctalopia was recognized in the Ebers papyrus (1600 BC) and liver was recommended as treatment. The Chinese, around the same time, used liver, honey, flying fox dung and tortoise shell as a cure. Hippocrates (460–377 BC) recommended liver of ox dipped in honey. Jacques Guillemeau (1550–1612) in France gave a clear

description and advised liver as treatment, as did Muffet in *Health's Improvement* in 1655. Conjunctival changes due to deficiency in diet was demonstrated in rats by P. Knapp of Germany in 1909. The fat soluble nature of this factor was shown by American biochemists, Thomas Burr Osborne (1859–1929) and Lafayette Benedict Mendel in 1913. Elmer Verner McCollum (1879–1967) and N. Simmonds named the factor 'fat soluble A' in 1917. H. Steenbock (1886–1967) made a connection between vitamin A and carotene, a precursor. Carotene from plants was demonstrated as a cure by Otto Rosenheim (1871–1955) and Jack Cecil Drummond (1891–1952) in 1920. The chemistry, isolation and synthesis of vitamin A was done by Swiss chemist, Paul Karrer (1889–1971) and R. Kuhn (1900–1967) in 1931.

Nightshade *See Atropa belladonna.*

Nightingale, Florence (1820–1910) British nurse who was born in Florence. She trained at the Kaiserswerth Institute, founded by Theodor Fliedner (1800–1864), and became superintendent of a hospital for invalid women in London. She volunteered to serve in the Crimean War and took 38 nurses to Scutari. Her organization and dedication led to a drastic reduction in mortality. She returned to England in 1856 and organized a fund to establish a training institute for nurses at St Thomas' Hospital in 1860. She published *Notes on Nursing* in 1859. *See Nightingale fund.*

Nightingale Fund Started in 1855 by Florence Nightingale to raise funds to establish a training institute for nurses and hospital attendants. The singer Jenny Lind gave a concert at the Exeter Hall and contributed the proceeds to the fund and Queen Victoria gave a valuable jewel. The fund closed in 1857 with a final sum of 44,000 pounds.

Nightmare or Incubus Disorder known as 'ephialtes' to the Greeks. Paul of Aegina (625–690) described it and prescribed black hellebore as treatment. Other ancient physicians, including Aetius of Amida (AD 502–575), Avicenna (980–1037) and Rhazes (850–932) recommended bleeding and purging as treatment. Caelius Aurelianus, around the fourth century, suggested shaving the head as a cure.

Nikandros Kolophonois of Klaros was a physician and poet from Ionia in 200 BC. He described several herbal remedies.

Nineveh Knowledge of ancient Babylonian medicine is mainly derived from 700 medical tablets out of the 12,000 which were found by English archeologist Sir Austen Henry Layard (1817–1894) in 1849 during excavations in Nineveh, the capital of the Assyrian empire. These showed that Babylonian prescriptions included drugs of vegetable and mineral origin. They specialized in having a doctor for every different disease. Amulets, chants and incantations were also used to prevent and cure diseases.

Nirvana Ideal state devoid of all passion achieved by Gautama Buddha, founder of Buddhism. It is said to be attained through meditation and is considered by some workers as the earliest form of psychotherapy.

Nirenberg, Marshall Warren (b 1927) American biochemist from New York who worked at the National Institutes of Health in Bethesda. He worked out the sequence of amino acid codes needed to synthesize a protein. He shared the Nobel Prize for Physiology or Medicine in 1968.

Nisbet Chancre Nodular abscess in the penis following acute lymphangitis of soft chancre was described by English physician, William Nisbet (1859–1882).

Nissl Bodies Chromophil granules in the cytoplasm of nerve cells described by Bavarian neurologist, Franz Nissl (1860–1919) in Munich in 1894.

Nissl Stain Alcohol-based stain for extranuclear RNA in nerve cells devised by Franz Nissl (1860–1919), a neurologist from Munich in 1894.

Nitric Acid [Greek: *nitro*, soda] Also called aqua fortis, prepared by an alchemist and medical missionary in Africa, Raymond Lully (1235–1312) in 1287. Saltpetre was shown to contain nitric acid and potash by Robert Boyle (1627–1691) in 1661. Nitrous acid was discovered by Carl Wilhelm Scheele (1742–1786) in 1774, and Henry Cavendish (1731–1810) demonstrated its nature in 1785. A modern process of making it from ammonia was invented by Friedrich Wilhelm Ostwald (1853–1932), German professor of chemistry at Leipzig.

Nitrite Test To detect urinary tract infection, devised by J. Cruikshank and J. Moyes of England in 1914.

Nitrite The vasodilator effect of nitrites in relieving angina was demonstrated by Sir Lauder Brunton (1844–1916) in 1867. *See glyceryl trinitrate.*

Nitroprusside Discovered by a Scottish chemist, Lord Lyon Playfair (1818–1898) around 1845. Sodium nitroprusside became the most commonly used vasodilator for cardiac failure in the 1970s.

Nitrofurantoin Oral urinary antibacterial compound developed in 1947 from nitrofuran drugs, introduced by M. Dodd in 1946.

Nitrogen Fixing Bacteria The fixation of nitrogen from air by some leguminous plants was first observed by German botanist, Hermann Helriegel (1831–1895) in 1886. His observation was explained by the presence of nitrogen fixing bacteria in roots of certain legumes by Sir Henry Gilbert (1817–1901) at Rothamsted in England in 1893.

Nitrogen Mustard Introduced as treatment of Hodgkin disease by Alfred Gilman (b 1908) and Stanley Frederick Philips (b 1916) in 1946.

Nitrogen [Greek: *nitron*, niter + *gennan*, to produce] Obtained from air by Daniel Rutherford (1749–1819), a pupil of Joseph Black (1728–1799) at the University of Edinburgh in 1772. In 1784 Henry Cavendish (1731–1810) demonstrated that it was capable of combining with oxygen to form oxides in the presence of an electric arc. Its compressibility to 430 atmospheres was shown by French physicist, Émile Hilaire Amagat (1841–1915). *See air.*

Nitroglycerine Prepared by Italian chemist, Ascanio Sobrero (1812–1888) of Turin, in 1847. Alfred Nobel (1833–1896) of Sweden used it as an explosive in 1863. It was introduced as treatment for angina by William Murrell (1853–1912) in 1879.

Nitrosomonas Soil bacterium that converts ammonia to nitrite. Discovered by Russian microbiologist, Sergi N. Winogradsky, in 1890.

Nitrous Oxide Discovered by British chemist, Joseph Priestley (1733–1804), in 1776. Sir Humphry Davy (1778–1829) of Penzance experimented on the inhalational effects in 1796. The induction of anesthesia by inhalation of nitrous oxide was demonstrated by Boston dentist, Horace Wells (1815–1848) in 1844 and was introduced on a commercial basis by 1868 but involved a cumbersome apparatus to make the gas. The firms of Coxeter and son and Barth in Britain overcame this difficulty by devising a method of liquefying the gas, and supplied it on a commercial scale. Their method provided readily available nitrous oxide in smaller cylinders, and popularized its use in anesthesia. Its use in dentistry was revived in 1863 by Gardner Quincy Colton (1814–1894), a lecturer in chemistry, who first used the gas with Horace Wells at Boston in 1844. It was used to relieve labor pains by Stanislaw Klikovich (1853–1910) of Russia in 1880, and a machine for self-administration in obstetrics was devised by Arthur E. Guedel (1883–1956) in 1910.

Nitze, Max (1848–1906) Berlin pioneer in the field of urology who invented the modern electrically-lit cystoscope in 1879.

NMR or nuclear magnetic resonance. *See magnetic resonance imaging (MRI).*

Nobel, Alfred Bernhard (1833–1896) Inventor of dynamite and originator of the Nobel Prize. He was born in Stockholm and provided with private tutors by his father, an architect and an inventor. After studying chemistry in Paris, he began investigating nitroglycerine in 1863 and invented a detonator in the same year which revolutionized the explosive and mining industry. He later worked for the Russian Army and established factories in 1872 across Europe which manufactured nitroglycerine. Nobel led a lonely life in Paris in later life, and left his vast fortune of 33,000,000 crowns to establish a trust to award Nobel Prizes in chemistry, physics, medicine, literature and peace. The first series of Nobel Prizes were awarded in 1901.

Nobel Prize *See Nobel, Alfred.*

Nobili, Leopoldo (1784–1835) Italian physicist, born in Trassilico and became professor of physics in Florence. He invented a thermopile to measure radiant heat.

Noble, Daniel (1810–1885) Born in Preston, practiced medicine at Manchester during a typhus epidemic and in charge of the arrangements to control it. He published *Influence of Manufactures upon Health and Life* (1843), and *The Human Mind in its Relationship with Brain and Nervous System* in 1858.

Nocard, Edmond Isidore Etienne (1850–1903) French veterinarian who did pioneering studies on filterable agents in animals. He discovered bovine pleuropneumonia and demonstrated that the tubercle bacillus could be transmitted to man through milk and meat.

Nocardiosis Diseases caused by a genus of actinomycete, *Nocardia*, which affect patients with underlying ill health. Described by John Tindal Cuttino (b 1912) and Anne McCabe of America in 1949. It was named *Nocardia intercellularis*, in honor of French veterinarian, Edmond Isidore Etienne Nocard (1850–1903).

Node of Tawara Atrioventricular node of the heart discovered by Japanese anatomist, Sunao Tawara (1873–1952), a pupil of Ludwig Aschoff (1866–1942) in Germany in 1906.

Nodes of Ranvier Interruptions in the medullary nerve fiber sheath described by Louis-Antoine Ranvier (1835–1922), a neurologist from Paris in 1878.

Noguchi Reaction Diagnostic skin test, a modification of the Wasserman reaction using human instead of sheep corpuscles. Devised by Japanese-born American

bacteriologist, Hideyo Noguchi (1876–1928), of the Rockefeller Institute, New York. He also demonstrated the role of spirochetes of syphilis and cultured *Treponema pallidum*. He died during his studies on yellow fever in West Africa, having shown the viral nature of the disease.

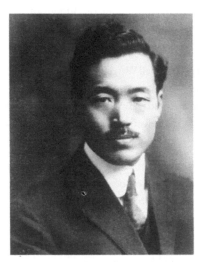

Hideyo Noguchi (1876–1928). Courtesy of the National Library of Medicine

Nollet, Jean Antoine (1700–1770) French abbé and physicist who became the first professor of physics at the Collège de Navarre in Paris. In 1748 he gave an explanation of osmosis and he also invented an early electroscope. *See osmosis.*

Nomenclature [Latin: *nomen*, name + *calare*, call] Scientific system of classification. Founded by Swedish botanist and physician, Carl Linnaeus (1707–1778). One of the earliest English anatomy books on the subject *A New Anatomical Nomenclature* was published by a lecturer in anatomy at Edinburgh, John Barclay (1758–1826) in 1803. The single-word nomenclature in the American Pharmacopoeia was introduced by Boston surgeon, Henry Jacob Bigelow (1816–1890) in 1820.

Non-Disjunction Abnormality of the sex chromosome during meiosis was discovered by Colin Blackman Bridges (1889–1938) in 1913.

Nonsteroidal Anti-inflammatory Drugs (NSAID) *See anti-inflammatory drugs.*

Noonan Syndrome Congenital heart defect, web neck and chest deformity with hypertelorism and mild mental retardation. Similar in appearance to Turner syndrome, but with a normal karyotype. Observed by O. Kobylinski while a medical student at the Estonian University at Dorpat in 1883. It is named after Jacqueline A. Noonan (b 1928) who described it in 1963.

Noorden, Carl Harko von (1858–1944) Viennese co-worker with Bernard Naunyn (1839–1925) in the study of diabetes. Both laid down the principles of the antidiabetic diet before the insulin era.

Nordau, Max Simon (1849–1923) Hungarian physician who moved to Paris in 1886 and wrote several books on moral and social issues including, *Conventional Lies of Society* (1883), and *Degeneration* (1895).

Norepinephrine Studied by George Barger (1878–1939) and Henry Dale (1875–1968) at the National Institute for Medical Research in 1911. It was discovered to be the main transmitter of sympathetic nerve impulses by Swedish pharmacologist and Nobel Prize winner, Ulf Svante von Euler (1905–1983) in 1946. Release of norepinephrine was demonstrated by W S. Peart in 1949. It was studied in detail by Nobel Prize winner Julius Axelrod (b 1912) head of the National Institutes of Mental Health. *See adrenaline, epinephrine.*

Normal Distribution Curve [Latin: *norma*, rule] Devised by French mathematician, Abraham de Moivre (1667–1754) of Vitry, Champagne in 1721. He came to England in 1686 and published *Doctrine of Chances*, based on probability theory in 1718 and a normal distribution curve in 1733. His fundamental law on complex numbers is known as de Moivre theorem.

North American Blastomycosis *See Gilchrist, Thomas.*

Northnagel Sign State of paralysis of facial muscles occurring in thalamic tumors. Described by German physician, Herman Northnagel (1845–1905).

Northrop, John Howard (1891–1987) American biochemist born in Yonkers, New York and educated at Columbia University, before becoming professor of bacteriology at the University of California, Berkeley in 1949. He crystallized pepsin and demonstrated it to be a protein in 1930. He also isolated chymotrypsinogen in 1935, and diphtheria toxin in a crystalline form. He shared the Nobel Prize for Chemistry with James Batcheller Sumner (1887–1955) and Wendell Meredith Stanley (1904–1971) in 1946. Northrop wrote *Crystalline Enzymes*, published in 1939.

Nose Surgery or rhinoplasty Affixing a new nose is an ancient surgical technique first practiced in India in the time of Susruta. Two English surgeons, James Trindlay and Thomas Cruso saw this operation in 1792 done on a bullock-cart driver of the English Army in India and later described it. *See plastic surgery, rhinoplasty.*

Nosology [Greek: *nosos*, disease + *logos*, discourse] System of classification of diseases by symptoms. William Cullen

(1710–1790) of Edinburgh applied it to human diseases in *Synopsis Nosologiae Methodicae* in 1769.

Nostalgia [Greek: *nostos*, return home + *algos*, pain] Inordinate desire to return to one's native land which if ungratified leads to melancholy or madness. William Cullen (1710–1790) classed it as a disorder of the mind along with bulimia and satyriasis in 1772. Thomas Arnold (1742–1816), a physician from Edinburgh at the Leicester Infirmary, listed it as pathetic insanity. It was considered essentially a disease of foreigners in England. Robert Hamilton (1749–1830), an English army·physician from Ipswich, wrote a treatise on it in 1787.

Nostradamus, Michael (1503–1566) Astrologer and physician from France who graduated from Montpellier. He published his predictions of the future, *Prophetical Centuries*, based on astrology, in 1555. He was also physician to Charles IX.

Nothnagel, Carl Herman Wilhelm (1841–1905) German physician and professor at Jena (1874), and Vienna (1882). He described unilateral oculomotor paralysis associated with ipsilateral ataxia, due to lesions of the superior cerebral peduncle of the brain.

Notochord [Greek: *noton*, back + *chorde*, cord] *See chordata.*

Nott, C. Josiah (1804–1873) Born in Columbia, South Carolina and graduated in medicine from the University of Pennsylvania in 1824 before establishing an obstetric practice at Mobile, Alabama. He was one of the first to suggest the involvement of the mosquito in yellow fever in 1840.

Novocaine Local anesthetic discovered by German chemist, Albert Einhorn (1856–1917), in the early 20th century and introduced to medicine by Heinrich Friedrich Wilhelm Braun (1862–1934). In 1916 during World War 1, the Americans took over the patent and marketed it as procaine. Braun later added adrenaline to the preparation to prolong the effect of local anesthesia.

NSAID Abbreviation for nonsteroidal anti-inflammatory drug. Refers to all drugs other than steroids which are capable of reducing inflammation. *See anti-inflammatory drugs*

Nuck Canal Tubule of the peritoneum descending from the uterus into the inguinal canal in young females. Described by Dutch anatomist, Anton Nuck (1650–1692), in 1691. He also published *De Vasis Aqosis Oculi, De Ductu Salivali Novo*, and *Operationes et Experimenta Chirurgica*.

Nuclear Fission Term used by Austrian–British physicist, Otto Robert Frisch (1904–1979) who worked on the

Atomic Bomb project at Los Alamos. He based his experiments on the findings of Lise Meitner (1878–1968) in 1939. *See atomic energy.*

Nuclear Magnetic Resonance Scan *See magnetic resonance imaging (MRI).*

Nuclear Medicine Use of isotopes to investigate function and diseases of organs. Georg Charles von Hevesy (1885–1966), a Hungarian-born professor of chemistry at Stockholm, initiated the use of radio isotopes in the study of living tissues. In 1935 he demonstrated that body tissues such as bone existed in a dynamic state giving up and taking in atoms. He was awarded the Nobel Prize for Chemistry in 1943. Herman Ludwig Blumgart (1895–1977) and Soma Weiss (1898–1942) introduced radioactive substances in evaluation of cardiac function and velocity of blood flow in 1927. Benedict Cassen (b 1902) and co-workers in the 1950s produced clinical images of an organ (thyroid). Study of pulmonary circulation and lung ventilation using xenon was introduced around 1963. The large crystal scintillation camera was developed by H. O. Anger in 1958. Technetium-99, a radioisotope with a short half-life, was introduced by Harper in 1962. Thallium-201 was used for myocardial perfusion imaging by Lebowitz in 1973. *See isotopes.*

Nuclear Reactor The first nuclear reactor for controlled chain reactions was built by an Italian, Enrico Fermi (1901–1954) from Rome, at the University of Chicago in 1942. He moved to America immediately after receiving his Nobel Prize for Physics at Stockholm in 1938 and was appointed as professor at Columbia University in 1939.

Nucleic Acid [Latin: *nucleus*, kernel] Johann Friedrich Miescher (1844–1895) in 1868, extracted a previously unknown substance from the nuclei of pus cells and the heads of salmon spermatozoa (1872) and named it 'nuclein'. The term was replaced by nucleic acid in 1889. An intensive study was done by Swiss-born German chemist, Albrecht Kossel (1853–1927). Russian-born American biochemist, Phoebus Aaron Theodor Levene (1869–1940) demonstrated that they contained ribose sugar in 1909, and further investigation of the substance was undertaken by Walter Jones (1865–1935) who identified ribonuclease in 1920. Nucleic acid was isolated from tobacco mosaic virus by Wendell Meredith Stanley (1904–1971) at the Rockefeller Institute in Princeton in 1935. X-ray diffraction was applied to the study of nucleic acids by English X-ray crystallographer, William Thomas Astbury (1889–1961) in 1937. Research on their synthesis was done by a Spanish-born American biochemist, Severo Ochoa (b 1905) who solved the genetic code and determined the number of

codons. He was awarded the Nobel Prize (with Arthur Kornberg, b 1918) in 1959. Another Nobel Prize was awarded to Sir Alexander Todd (b 1907) of England in 1957 for his work on the structure and synthesis of nucleotides.

Nucleolus Discovered by Gabriel Gustav Valentin (1810–1883), an Italian pathologist and botanist, in 1836.

Nucleus [Latin: *nucleus*, kernel] Described by Robert Brown (1773–1980), a Scottish physician and botanist, in 1831.

Nuel Space Between the outer rod of Corti and the adjacent row of hair cells. Described by Jean Pierre Nuel (1847–1920), professor of otology at Louvain in Belgium, in 1873.

Nuffield Foundation Established for medical, scientific and social research by the motor magnate and philanthropist, William Richard Morris Nuffield (1877–1963), in 1943. He started with a cycle repair shop and went on to making Morris motor cars at Cowley, Oxford. He acquired a vast fortune by mass-producing cars and gave part of it to hospitals, Oxford University and charities. Nuffield College at Oxford was established in 1937.

Nuhn Glands Anterior lingual glands named after German anatomist, Anton Nuhn (1814–1889).

Null Hypothesis [Latin: *nullus*, none] States that there is no difference between control and test systems under study. Devised and explained by English statistician and geneticist, Sir Ronald Aylmer Fisher (1890–1962) of East Finchley, London in *The Design of Experiments* published in 1942. He also studied the Rhesus factor in blood.

Nupercaine Trade name for preparations of dibucaine. Synthesized by Meischer in 1929, and first used as a spinal anesthetic in England by Howard Jones of Charing Cross Hospital in 1930.

Nuremberg Code *See Nuremberg trials.*

Nuremberg Trial Established after World War ll to try Nazi War criminals for unethical treatment and cruel experiments on humans. The first document which outlined ethical regulations on human experimentation based on informed consent was set up in 1947 following the trials. This Nuremberg Code laid down 10 standards to which physicians were expected to conform when carrying out research on humans. The next most important document on human experimentation, the Declaration of Helsinki, was passed by the World Medical Assembly in Helsinki in 1964. It contained further guidelines on biomedical research involving human subjects.

Nurses Agency Act To register and regulate agencies that supplied nurses, passed in 1957.

Nursing in America Elizabeth Bayley Seton (1774–1821) at Emittsburg, Maryland founded the Sisters of Charity in 1809 to provide nursing care for the poor. The Sisters of Charity of Nazareth was established in 1812 in Louisville. The Irish Sisters of Mercy arrived in America in 1846. Until 1860 no training existed for nurses in America. Rebecca Taylor, head nurse at the Massachusetts General Hospital for 34 years, was one of the finest examples of dedication to nursing before formal training was instituted. The first American medical graduate, Elizabeth Blackwell, pioneered training in America by sending volunteers to Bellevue Hospital around 1859. Dorothea Dix was appointed as superintendent during the Civil War. Clara Barton, known as the Angel of the Battlefield, is considered as an American Nightingale of the Civil War. A Polish–German immigrant doctor, Maria Elizabeth Zakrzewska (1829–1902), trained nurses at the New England Hospital for Women and Children in 1860. Her assistant, Susan Dimock, who visited the Kaiserwerth Institute in Germany, began a one-year graded course for the nurses in 1872. The first trained nurse in America was Linda Richards, a graduate of this program and she became the first nurse in charge of the Boston Training School for Nurses at Massachusetts General Hospital, in 1873. The training school at Bellevue preceded the Boston School by a few months and that at New Haven Hospital opened later in the same year (1873). The American Nurses Association was established by incorporating the Associated Alumnae of the nurses of Bellevue, Illinois and Johns Hopkins, in 1911. The *American Journal of Nursing* was published in 1900 and the first textbook *New Haven Manual of Nursing* was published in 1879. The first training school in a hospital for the mentally ill was established at the McLean Hospital in Boston in 1882.

Nursing [Middle English: *norture*, nurse] The Irish Sisters of Charity, founded by Mother Mary Aikenhead from Dublin in 1815, was the first to reorganize hospital nursing in the English-speaking countries. During the early 19th century almost all nurses were recruited from the domestic servant class. Working conditions were appalling and nurses often had to sleep in wards and cook their own meals. Nursing sisters were from a higher social class and matron's duties were mostly of an administrative nature. Reform of the profession began in the latter half of the 19th century with the introduction of training. The Institute of Kaiserswerth near Düsseldorf, where Florence Nightingale spent three months in 1851, played an important role in this. The Institute was established in 1833 by Pastor Theodor Fliedner as a home for female ex-convicts and later came to include a hospital, lunatic asylum, orphanage and school. Organized training in England commenced at St John's House in 1848, under the supervision of clergymen. Pupil nurses attended King's College from 1856. The Nursing School at St Thomas' Hospital was founded by Florence Nightingale in 1860. A rapid expansion of paid professional nursing staff occurred after 1866 and the first professional association, the British Nurses Association, was founded by Ethel Gorden Manson (1857–1947), matron at St Bartholomew's Hospital, in 1886. The College of Nursing was proposed in 1916 by Arthur Stanley chairman of the Joint War Committee of the British Red Cross Society. The pioneer of nursing in Australia was Elizabeth Kenny (1886–1952) who started nursing in the bush and later established clinics providing physical therapy to polio victims in several parts of the world.

Nussbaum Cells Found in the pyloric gastric glands. Described by Moritz Nussbaum (1850–1915), a professor of biology and histologist at Bonn in 1877.

Nutrition [Latin: *nutrx*, nurse] Aulus Cornelius Celsus (25 BC–AD 50) wrote on the role of food in maintaining health. The value of lemon juice in protecting against scurvy was pointed out by the naval surgeon John Woodall (1556–1643) in 1611. A metabolic treatise on food in relation to body weight and excretion was written by Sanctorio Sanctorius (1561–1636) in 1614. Controlled trials with lime against scurvy were performed by James Lind (1716–1794), a British naval surgeon in 1747. Frederick Accum (1769–1838), a German chemist from Buckeburg raised the issue of adulteration of food in 1820 in *Treatise on Adulteration of Food and Culinary Poisons*. He also wrote *Culinary Chemistry*, on the scientific principles of cooking. Accessory food factors, vitamins, were propounded by Sir Frederick Gowland Hopkins (1861–1947) in 1906. The first of these, to prevent beriberi, was discovered by Polish-American biochemist, Casimir Funk (1884–1967), in 1911. Henry Russell Chittenden (1856–1943), an American physiologist from New Haven, Connecticut founded physiological chemistry and nutrition in America. He wrote *Physiological Economy in Nutrition* (1905), and *Nutrition of Man* (1907). The role of amino acids was studied by William Cumming Rose (1887–1984), an American biochemist from Greenville, South Carolina. He discovered threonine (1936), and nine essential amino acids, including methionine (1937), and valine (1939). Severe protein malnutrition in children, 'kwashikor', was described by British pediatrician, Cicely Williams (1893–1992) in 1934. Poor nutrition is still the major cause of death in the world. *See vitamins.*

Nuttall, Thomas (1786–1859) English-born American naturalist from Yorkshire who migrated to Philadelphia in 1808. He wrote *Genera of North American Plants* in 1818. Nuttall served as the curator of the Botanical Garden at Harvard from 1822 to 1833.

Nux Vomica Seed from *Strychnos Nux-vomica*, a plant indigenous to India and the Malay archipelago, was introduced into medicine by the Arabs. The first description was given by Valerius Cordus (1515–1554) of Hesse in 1540, and *De Nuce Vomica* giving an account of its toxic effects on animals, was published by J. Lossius in 1682. It was used in England in the 17th century as a pest poison. The poisonous action is due to the alkaloids, brucine and strychnine. Brucine was isolated from bark by French pharmacist, Pierre Joseph Pelletier (1788–1842), in 1819.

Nyctalopia [Greek: *nyx*, night + *alaos*, blind + *opia*, eye] Night blindness. William Briggs (1642–1704) gave an account of the condition in England in 1684. A classical description was given by William Heberden (1710–1801) in 1768. *See night blindness.*

Nylander Test Detects dextrose in the urine. Devised by Swedish chemist, Claes Gabriel Wilhelm Nylander (1835–1907).

Nymphomania [Greek: *nympha*, bride + *mania*, madness] A state of insatiable sexual desire or auto-eroticism in the female. *Nympha* was used in ancient Greek writings to refer to the clitoris. An early treatise *Nymphomania, or a dissertation concerning the furor uterus,* translated from the French by English physician Edward Sloane Wilmot was published in 1785. *See furor uterinus.*

Nystagmus [Greek: *nystagmos*, drowsiness] The occurrence in multiple sclerosis (Uhthoff sign) was described by German physician and ophthalmologist, Wilhelm Uhthoff (1853–1927) of Breslau. *See Wernicke encephalopathy, miner's nystagmus, Barany chair.*

Nystatin Antifungal agent produced from the soil bacterium, *Streptomyces noursei*, by Elizabeth Hazen (1885–1975) of New York State Department of Health in 1950. Specifically effective against *Candica albicans*. It was developed and marketed by E. R. Squibb and Sons who patented it in 1951.

Nysten, Pierre Hubert (1771–1818) Physician from Liége in Belgium at the Foundling Hospital in Paris. He wrote *Recherches de Physiologie et Chemie Pathologique* and several other medical works.

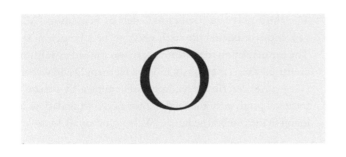

O Antigen Somatic antigens were first identified in cases of *Salmonella typhi* infection by Polish bacteriologist Arthur Felix (1887–1956) in 1924.

O'Beirne Sphincter Band at the junction of the colon and the rectum, first described by Irish surgeon, James O'Beirne (1786–1862).

Oat Cell Carcinoma Cancer of the mediastinum and hilum of the lung. Described by William George Barnard (1892–1956) of London in 1926. He used the term oat cell, as the tumor consisted of small oval cells resembling oats.

Obermayer Test Detects indican in urine, using lead acetate as a reagent. Devised by Austrian physiological chemist, Friedrich Obermayer (1861–1925).

Obermeyer Spirillum (Syn: *Borrelia obermeyeri*, *Borrelia recurrentis*) Causative spirochete of relapsing fever transmitted by the human louse. Discovered by German physician, Otto Hugo Franz Obermeyer (1843–1873) in 1868.

Oberst Operation Done for ascites. A flap of skin is projected into the abdomen to provide drainage of ascitic fluid. Devised by a German surgeon, M. Oberst (1849–1925).

Oberth, Herman Julius (1894–1990) Hungarian-born physician who gave up medicine for astrophysics. He is considered the founder of the science of space rockets. *Rocket to Interplanetary Space* was published by him in 1923.

Obesity [Latin: *obesus*, fat] Overeating was denounced by most of the ancient philosophers and physicians, including Hippocrates (460–377 BC) and Aristotle (384–322 BC). One of the best work on the subject, by Athelme Brillat-Savarin (1755–1826) of France was *Physiologie du Gout* published in 1825. He described obesity as that state of fatty congestion where, 'without the person being ill, the limbs grow little by little in volume and lose their natural shape and harmony'. George Cheyne (1671–1743), an eminent Scottish physician, changed his eating habits on moving to London and gained weight, reaching over 32 stones. He embarked on a diet of vegetables and regained his normal weight and published *An Essay on Health and Long Life*, an important practical work on obesity, in 1724.

Obstetric Chair [Latin: *obstetrix*, midwife] Used during childbirth for thousands of years until the French obstetrician, François Mauriceau (1637–1709) dispensed with it and started delivering his patients in bed.

Obstetric Forceps [Latin: *obstetrix*, midwife] *See forceps.*

Obstetric Ultrasonography [Latin: *obstetrix*, midwife] Sonar or ultrasound was first developed by a French scientist Paul Langevin (1872–1946) in 1915 for ships to detect icebergs. Application for fetal examination *in utero* was first done by Ian Donald (1910–1987), professor of obstetrics at Glasgow University in 1958.

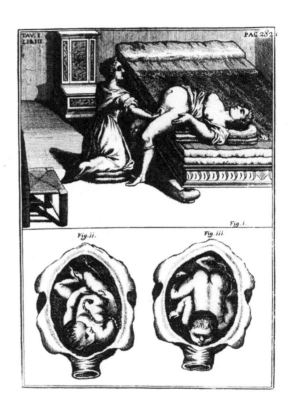

Illustration from S. Melli (1766), *La Comare*, showing the position for obese patient (top) and correction of abnormal fetal positions

Obstetrics [Latin: *obstetrix*, a midwife] Obstetrics was practiced during ancient Greek times by female midwives. Physicians such as Galen (AD 129–200), Rufus of Ephesus (AD 110–180), Soranus of Ephesus (AD 98–138) and Aretaeus the Cappadocian (AD 81–138) were familiar with the problems related to pregnancy, and puerperal fever is mentioned in the aphorisms of Hippocrates (460–377 BC). François Mauriceau (1637–1709), an eminent French obstetrician, dispensed with the obstetrical chair and delivered his patients in bed. His *Des Maladies des Femmes Grosses et Accouchees* was translated into English by Hugh

Chamberlen (1632–1720). Geronimo Scipione Mercurio (1550–1616), professor of medicine at Bologna and Pisa, wrote a book on obstetrics in 1586 in which he advocated cesarean section in cases of contracted pelvis. The contagious nature of puerperal fever was noted in 1795 by Alexander Gordon (1750–1799), an obstetrician from Aberdeen. He advocated disinfection of the clothes of the midwife and doctor before they attended the mother. An illustrative book, *The Anatomy of the Human Gravid Uterus*, was written in 1774 by William Hunter (1718–1783), accoucheur to the Queen. The combined method of internal and external podalic version was described in 1860 by John Braxton Hicks (1823–1897) of Rye in Sussex, an obstetric physician at Guy's Hospital. Chloroform was used successfully in 1847 by Sir James Young Simpson (1811–1870), a Scottish obstetrician. John Snow (1813–1858), the first physician to specialize in anesthesia, popularized the use of chloroform in obstetrics by administering it to Queen Victoria. The first incision of a rigid perineum which was likely to tear during delivery (episiotomy) was performed by Dublin man-midwife, Fielding Ould (1710–1789), and the procedure was introduced into America by Valentine Taliaferro (1831–1888) in 1851. Operative delivery in obstetrics using a spinal block was performed by A. Kreis in 1900, and Achile Mario Dogliotti (1897–1966) introduced epidural anesthesia in 1931. The application of ultrasound was first done by Ian Donald (1910–1987), professor of obstetrics at Glasgow University in 1979. One of the most comprehensive historic accounts on the subject is given in the *Eternal Eve* published by Harvey Graham in 1950. *See antenatal care, labor, cesarean section, forceps, puerperal fever, maternity hospitals.*

Obstructive Airway Disease *See emphysema, asthma.*

Obstructive Cardiomyopathy *See hypertrophic cardiomyopathy.*

Occipital Lobe [Latin: *ob*, against + *caput*, head] Lobe of the brain in the back part of the head. The laminar structure of the cerebral cortex was shown in the occipital lobe by Francesco Genneri (1750–1797) of Parma in 1782. Lesions of the occipital cortex leading to cortical blindness were demonstrated by a veterinary physiologist at Berlin, Hermann Munk (1830–1912), in 1881.

Occipital Puncture Puncture of the cisterna magna to obtain a sample of cerebrospinal fluid for diagnostic purposes was first done by American neurologist, James Bourne Ayer (1882–1963), in 1920.

Occulomotor Nerve [Latin: *oculus*, eye + *motor*, mover]

The third nerve of the brain. Galen of Pergamon (AD 129–200) considered the sixth nerve to be a branch of it. The eye in relation to the third nerve was studied by Johann Gottfried Zinn (1727–1759) in 1755. Herman David Weber (1823–1918) described a syndrome of hemiplegia with contralateral paralysis of the oculomotor nerve secondary to a lesion in the cerebral peduncle (Weber syndrome), in 1863.

Occult Blood Test Advocated as a routine diagnostic test in gastroenterology by German gastroenterologist, Ismar Isidor Boas (1858–1938). He and Anton Ewald (1845–1915) introduced the test meal for measuring gastric secretion.

Occupational Cancer Cancer of the scrotum in chimney sweeps due to chronic exposure to soot was described by Sir Percivall Pott (1714–1788) in 1770. The same disease was described by S. R. Wilson of the Royal Infirmary Manchester in 1906 in cotton spinners, caused by prolonged contact with lubrication oil. Adenocarcinoma from chronic chromate exposure was described by D.A. Newman of Glasgow in 1890. Deaths from aplastic anemia after exposure to radium were reported by J. C. Mottram in 1921. He also observed a low red cell count in 'anemia radiotoxica' on exposure to radiation. Leukemia from radium exposure was observed by P. E. Weil and Antoine Marcelin Lacasagne (b 1884) in 1925. In 1927 20 deaths occurred due to blood dyscrasia caused by radium in luminous dial painters in New Jersey. Cancer of the bladder in fuchsin manufacture was described by Ludwig Rehn (1849–1930) in 1895. Its relation to the dye industry was demonstrated by Leuenberger of Basel in 1912. Several workers, including Hans Curshmann (1875–1950) of Germany (1920), R. Oppenheimer (1926) and M.W. Goldblatt (1949), demonstrated the carcinogenic properties of aniline and related compounds on the bladder. *See occupational diseases.*

Occupational Diseases Georgius Agricola (1494–1555), a physician in the mining town of Joachimsthal in Bohemia, established the scientific study of occupational diseases in the mid-16th century. The first monograph on mine and smelter workers was written by Paracelsus (1493–1541) and published posthumously as *Von der Bergsucht und anderen Bergkrankheiten* in 1567. *De Morbis Artificum Diatriba* was written by Italian, Bernardini Ramazzini (1633–1714) from the University of Padua in 1690. Scrotal cancer in chimney sweeps was described by Sir Percivall Pott (1714–1788) in 1770. The same cancer from chronic contact with tar and mineral oil was observed by S.R. Wilson of Manchester Royal Infirmary in 1892. The first book in England was written in 1832 by Charles Turner Thackrah (1795–1833), a pioneer of industrial medicine in England and founder of the Leeds Medical School. Thomas M. Legge (1863–1932) was the first medical inspector of factories in England in 1898, and was responsible for the decline in lead poisoning in industry. Compulsory notification of industrial poisoning and diseases was introduced by the Home Office in England in 1901. *See chimney sweeps, coal miner's disease, silicosis, pneumoconiosis, radiation injury, glass blower's cataract, vibration injury, farmer's lung.*

Occupational Therapy First used to treat mental disorders by Seneca (4 BC–AD 65). Galen (AD 129–200) commented 'employment is nature's best physician' in AD 172. Simple activities were used successfully in a mental hospital in Philadelphia by Benjamin Rush (1745–1813) in 1798. Occupation as a form of treatment for mental illnesses was also proposed by Samuel Tuke (1784–1857) of York in 1815 and John Conolly (1794–1866) at the Hanwell Asylum in London in 1843. It was introduced into other medical specialties in the 19th century.

Oceanography Pytheas of Marseilles (360–290 BC) was the first Greek to interpret the tide and associate its movements with the moon and its phases. The theory of tides was explained by Johannes Kepler (1571–1630) in 1598 and Sir Isaac Newton (1642–1727) in 1683. *Physical Geography of the Sea* was published by an American naval officer, Matthew Fontaine Maury (1806–1873) in 1855. Deep-sea dredging was introduced by Scottish zoologist, Sir Charles Wyville Thompson (1830–1882) in 1868 and revealed life at the bottom of the ocean. Christian Viktor Hensen (1835–1924) of Kiel laid the foundation for 'oceanic bionomics' or the study of the economics of life of the ocean. He used the word 'plankton' (Greek: *planketon*, drifting) in 1888 to denote the floating life forms in the ocean.

Ochoa, Severo (b 1905) American geneticist, born in Spain and worked in Heidelberg and Oxford before emigrating to the USA to take up a post at Washington University Medical School. He later moved to the New York University School of Medicine. He isolated two enzymes from the Krebs cycle and polynucleotide phosphorylase, determined a number of genetic codons, studied protein synthesis and initiating factors in binding of N-formylmethionine. He was awarded the 1959 Nobel Prize for Physiology or Medicine, together with Arthur Kornberg (b 1918). *See nucleic acids.*

Ochsner, Albert John (1858–1925) American surgeon of Swiss descent, born in Wisconsin, and obtained his medical degree from Rush Medical College, Chicago in 1886. After postgraduate study in Vienna, Berlin and London he returned to Chicago as chief surgeon to the Augustana Hospital in 1889. He was professor of clinical surgery at the University of Illinois College of Medicine in 1900, wrote a book on appendicitis, and served as president of the American College of Surgeons from 1923 to 1924.

Ochsner Sphincter Found in the duodenum, below the opening of bile duct. Described by Albert John Ochsner (1858–1925), professor of surgery at the University of Illinois in 1906.

Octogenarians [Latin: *octageni*, 80 each; Greek: *okta*, eight + *genos*, descent] Luigi Cornaro (1467–1566) from Venice wrote a book on preserving good health in old age in 1550 and proposed rules for maintaining health and prolonging life. He again wrote on the rules for maintaining health and prolonging life when he was 86 years. His third book on the joys of old age was written at the age of 95 years and he died in his ninety-ninth year. The British philosopher and scientist, Herbert Spencer (1820–1903) worked until his death at 83 years. The Prussian scientist, Baron Alexander von Humboldt (1769–1859) completed one of his important works at the age of 89 years. Abraham Jacobi (1830–1919), the founder of pediatrics in America and the first president of the American Medical Association, had an active practice at the age of 90 years.

Oculist [Latin: *oculus*, eye] *See eye, ophthalmology.*

Oddi Sphincter Bile duct at the entrance to the duodenum. Described by Francis Glisson (1597–1667) in 1654. It was redescribed by Italian physician, Ruggero Oddi (1845–1906) of the University of Perugia in 1887.

Odier, Louis (1748–1815) Physician from Geneva who studied at Edinburgh and Leiden Universities, and introduced vaccination. He published *A Manual of Practice of Medicine* in 1790.

Odling, William (1829–1921) *See oxygen.*

Odo of Meune (d 1161) Medical writer of Arab influence. He wrote *De virtutibus herbarium* or *Macer Floridus*, that describes the therapeutics of some 77 simples and is the oldest extant Scandinavian medical text.

Odometer (Syn: pedometer, way-measurer, perambulator) Instrument to record the distance traveled. Originally called 'hodometer' and described by Roman architect, Vitruvius around AD 10. The 'odometer', to count the steps of a person while walking, was invented in the 15th century. John Fernel (1497–1558), physician to Catherine of Medici, used a similar instrument to measure distances in 1550. Another form was devised by Paul Pfinzing of Nuremberg in 1554.

Odontology [Greek: *odontos*, tooth + *logos*, discourse] Science of teeth. Richard Owen (1804–1892) discovered the connection between the vascular and soft parts of the tooth tissue and the hard substance in 1839. He published one of the first illustrated books in 1840, *Odontology*. *See dentistry.*

Oeder, George Christian (1728–1791) Botanist and physician from Anspach, Germany who studied under Albrecht von Haller (1708–1777) at Göttingen, before becoming professor of botany at Copenhagen. He published *Flora Danica* and *Elementa Botanica*.

Oedipus Complex Sexual attraction to one's mother. Described by Austrian psychiatrist, Sigmund Freud (1856–1939), in his *Three Essays on the Theory of Sexuality* published in 1905. The term derives its origin from Greek mythology where Oedipus was raised by foster parents and unwittingly killed his real father and married his mother, not knowing that he was her son.

Oehl Layer Stratum lucidum of the epidermis described by Eusebio Oehl (1827–1903), professor of histology at Pavia in Italy in 1857.

Oersted, Hans Christian (1777–1851) Danish professor of physics at Copenhagen. He discovered the magnetic effect produced by an electric current on a needle in 1819. He also isolated aluminum in 1826.

Oertel Treatment Use of natural methods such as massage, diet, mountain climbing and exercise for treatment of heart diseases. Proposed by a Munich physician, Max J. Oertel (1835–1897).

Ogilvie Syndrome Functional obstruction of the large bowel in elderly patients. Described by London surgeon, Sir William Heneage Ogilvie (b 1887) of Guy's Hospital in 1948.

Ogston, Alexander (1844–1929) Surgeon and regius professor at Aberdeen who discovered *Staphylococcus* bacteria in 1881. The imaginary line (Ogston line) used in surgery that extends from the tubercle of the femur to the intercondylar notch, was described by him in 1876.

Ogston Operation Involves removal of the inner condyle of the femur for knock-knee, was described by Scottish surgeon Alexander Ogston (1844–1929).

Ogston–Luc Operation Incision at the edge of the orbit for frontal sinus disease. Devised around 1885 by Scottish surgeon Alexander Ogston (1844–1929) and French surgeon Henry Luc (1855–1925).

Oguchi Syndrome Characterized by night blindness and grayish appearance of the fundus. Observed in Japan by ophthalmologist, Chuta Oguchi (1875–1945) in 1912.

Ohara Disease Tularemia (named after the county of Tulare in California where it was first described) is an infectious disease found in rodents and other wildlife but which affects humans with plague-like symptoms. It is known as Ohara disease in Japan following description of the condition by Shoichiro Ohara in 1930. *See tularemia.*

Ohm, George Simon (1789–1854) German professor of physics at Nuremberg (1833–1849). He published his law relating to voltage, current, and electrical resistance in 1827. The unit of resistance in electricity is named after him.

Oil of Wintergreen Ancient remedy for rheumatism obtained from *Gaultheria procumbens*. Its active principle, methyl salicylate, is a glucoside and was first isolated in 1819.

Okazaki, Reiji (1930–1975) Japanese biochemist and professor at Nagoya University. He worked with bacteria and bacteriophages and identified DNA–RNA fragments which are named after him. Together with Arthur Kornberg (b 1918), he was the first to show that there was a primer sequence of RNA attached to DNA and detached by the 'Kornberg enzyme'. Okasaki was awarded the 1970 Asahi Prize for his work. *See deoxyribonucleic acid.*

Oken, Lorenz (1779–1851) Naturalist and professor of medicine at Jena (1807–1816). He founded a controversial journal called *Isis* which led to his resignation. He became a professor at Munich in 1828, and at Zurich in 1832. He proposed that the skull is a modified form of the vertebra, which was later disproved.

Olbers, Heinrich Wilhelm Matthäus (1758–1840) German physician and astronomer who discovered seven minor planets and calculated the velocity of falling stars.

Old Age The first book on therapeutics in old age, *The Cure of Old Age*, was written by Roger Bacon (1214–1292). Another, on preserving good health in old age was written by a Venetian, Luigi Cornaro(1464/6–1566) in 1550. Hieronimus Cardanus, an Italian physician in the 16th century, described indicators of long life: a family history of long life, a cheerful easy disposition, and the ability to sleep long and sound. Anselmus Aurelius, chief physician to the Duke of Mantua in the 16th century, published *Gerocomice sive de fenum regimine* (1606) in which he considered old age to be the most important stage in life as it excelled in prudence and understanding. Another treatise, *a gerocomice de senum conservatione, et senilum morborum curatione*, was published by François Ranchin (1560–1641), a professor at Montpellier in 1625. Counseling was started in San Francisco by an American psychiatrist, Lilien J. Martin (1851–1943) who lived to 92 years and wrote *Salvaging old Age* (1930) and *Handbook for Old Age Counsellors* (1944). *See geriatrics, octogenarians, psychogeriatrics.*

Oldham, Richard Dixon (1858–1936) Geologist and seismologist born in Dublin, and educated at Rugby. He was director of the Indian Museum in Calcutta and made an important report on the Assam earthquake of 1897. He described the Earth's core using seismographic records in 1906.

Olefin [Latin: *oleo*, oil + *facere*, to make] Unsaturated aliphatic hydrocarbon with one or more double bonds, prepared by French chemist, Marcellin Berthelot (1827–1907), in 1862.

Olfactory Nerve [Latin: *olfacere*, to smell] Caspar Bartholin (1585–1629), the Elder, a physician from Copenhagen in Denmark, described the functions of the olfactory nerve in 1611. Extensive experiments to locate the olfactory sense in animals were performed by Conrad Victor Schneider (1614–1680) of Prussia in 1650 and published in 1655. A further description was given by Italian surgeon, Antonio Scarpa (1747–1832), in 1789. Olfactory mucous membranes and cells (Schultz membrane and cells) were described by Maximillian Johann Sigismund Schultz (1825–1874), professor of anatomy at Halle and Bonn.

Olfactory Seizure The brain center for olfactory function was studied by Sir David Ferrier (1843–1928) in 1874. A tumor in the right temporosphenoidal area causing olfactory seizures was described by John Hughlings Jackson (1835–1911) in 1890.

Oligocene [Greek: *oligos*, few + *kainos*, recent] Part of the Tertiary period in Earth history identified by Heinrich Ernst Beyrich in 1854.

Oligodenroglia [Greek: *oligos*, little + *denron*, tree + *glia*, glue] A group of neuroglial cells within the central nervous system. First demonstrated and named by Spanish neurologist, Pio del Rio Hortega (1882–1945) in 1921.

Olitsky, Peter Kosciusko (1886–1964) Worked with Albert Bruce Sabin (1906–1993) to isolate a pure culture of the poliomyelitis virus in 1936.

Olive Oil From fruit of the tree, *Olea europea*, was important to the ancient Hebrews and is mentioned in the Bible. In ancient times the olive was known as 'bak' and was a symbol of goodness and purity. Romans preserved olives in brine, Egyptians used the oil for beautification, and the Greeks

used olives as contraceptives. Palmitic acid was extracted from olive oil by Collett in 1854, and tripalmitin was shown to be the main constituent by Heintz and Kruz in 1857.

Oliver, George (1841–1915) Pioneer in endocrinology. In 1895, while working with Sir Edward Albert Sharpey-Schafer (1802–1880) in England, he demonstrated the effect of injecting extracts of suprarenal gland. The extract produced contraction of arteries and accelerated heart rate, thereby increasing blood pressure. The active substance was named adrenaline in England and epinephrine in America.

Oliver, Sir Thomas (1853–1942) Pioneer in modern trade and occupational diseases who wrote *The Health of the Workers, Occupations as they affect the life of the workers* in 1925. He was the first medical inspector of factories in England.

Oliver Test Detects albumin in the urine using sodium tungstate and citric acid. Devised by English physician, George Oliver (1841–1915).

Oliver, William Silver (1836–1908) British army physician who described the sign of tracheal tug seen in thoracic aortic aneurysm.

Ollier Disease (Syn. multiple enchondromatosis, dyschondroplasia) Consists of nonossified cartilage of the metaphysis and diaphyses of the long bones. Described by French surgeon, Léopold Louis Xavier Edouard Ollier (1830–1901), in 1899. The inner osteogenetic layer of the periostium (Ollier layer) was described by him in 1859.

Olshausen Operation Uterus is sutured to the anterior abdominal wall as treatment for retroverted uterus. Devised by Berlin obstetrician, Robert von Olshausen (1835–1915).

O'Meara, Barry Edward (1786–1836) Irish physician who was doctor to Napoleon and accompanied him to exile on St Helena. He published *Napoleon in Exile* in 1822.

Onanism *See coitus interruptus.*

Oncology [Greek: *onkos*, mass or bulk + *logos*, discourse] Study and treatment of cancer, established as a specialty in America by James Ewing (1866–1943), professor of oncology at the Cornell University Medical College, New York. His work was internationally recognized and he published an important treatise, *Neoplastic Diseases*, in 1919. Denis Parsons Burkitt (b 1907) from Enniskillen, Northern Ireland was a pioneer of chemotherapy in Britain. He introduced cyclophosphamide and methotrexate in 1960 for treatment of Burkitt lymphoma. Work on antimetabolite compounds that inhibit DNA synthesis was pioneered by American biochemist, George Herbert Hitchings (b 1905) of Washington and New York biochemist, Gertrude Belle Elion (b 1918), in the late 1950s. They prepared the anti-leukemic drug, 6-mercaptopurine, in 1954. Further work led to patents on 18 drugs from purines and pyrimidines. They shared the Nobel Prize for Physiology or Medicine with Sir James Whyte Black (b 1924) in 1988. *See Burkitt lymphoma, cancer, cancer therapy, Cancer Act, carcinogenesis, P53 gene.*

Oncogenes [Greek: *onkos*, mass or bulk + *genesis*, production] Play a role in normal growth of mammalian cells, but can cause cancer through mutation. Discovered by American virologist, John Michael Bishop (b 1936) of Pennsylvania. He shared the Nobel Prize for Physiology or Medicine with Harold Elliot Varmus (b 1939) of New York in 1989. Varmus was a medical graduate of Columbia University and professor of microbiology and immunology at the University of California Medical Center, San Francisco, in 1979. The two ways by which retroviral transduction activates oncogenes was discovered by German-born, American microbiologist, Peter Vogt (b 1932), professor of microbiology at the University of Southern California.

Oophorectomy [Greek: *oon*, egg + *pherein*, to bear + *tome*, to cut] *See ovariotomy.*

Operon [Latin: *opera*, work; Greek: *on*] Genetic unit that coordinates expression from DNA to messenger RNA. Discovered and named by François Jacob (b 1920), Sydney Brenner (b 1927), F. Cuzin and Jacques Lucien Monod (1910–1976) of France in 1963.

Ophidism [Greek: *ophidion*, snake] Poisoning by snake venom is common to most tropical countries. In 1898 in India 20,000 persons died from snake bites. The Indian shrub, (*Rauwolfia serpentina*) and the American snakeroot (*Aristolochia serpentaria*) are used as folk remedies and the former was introduced to Europe by French botanist, Plumier, who named it after the 16th century German botanist, Leonhard Rauwolf (1537–1606). Joseph Fayrer (1824–1907), a surgeon to the East India Company, wrote the first book on poisonous snakes in India in 1884, *Thanatophidia in India*. Silas Weir Mitchell (1829–1914) of Jefferson Medical College studied snake venom and published, *On the Treatment of Rattle Snake Bites with Experimental Criticisms upon the Various Remedies now in Use*, in 1861. The pioneers of antiserum therapy were Albert Calmette (1863–1933), a French bacteriologist and Thomas Richard Fraser (1841–1919) from England. Antivenene, an antidote to snake venom, was prepared by Calmette at the Pasteur Institute in Lisle in 1896. One of the first institutes to produce antivenene sera was founded by Vital Brazil (1865–1950) at Sao Paulo in 1911.

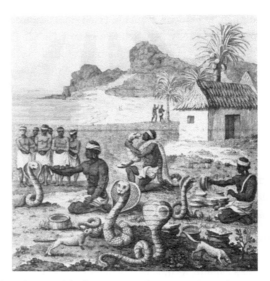

Hindus adoring and feeding serpents. Thomas Maurice, *Indian Antiquites* (1744). W. Richardson, London

Ophthalmia Neonatorum [Greek: *ophthalmos*, eye + *neos*, new; Latin: *natus*, born] Common cause of blindness in the 18th and 19th centuries. A survey by the Ophthalmological Society in England in 1880 showed that 30 to 40% of blindness in all ages was due to ophthalmia neonatorum. Carl Sigmund Franz Crede (1819–1892), professor of obstetrics and gynecology at Leipzig, wrote on prevention in 1884 using silver nitrate. The incidence declined drastically with introduction of sulfonamides and, by 1944, the percentage of blindness had dropped to 9.2%.

Ophthalmology [Greek: *ophthalmos*, eye + *logos*, discourse] Practiced as a separate branch of medicine in ancient Egypt. Philoxenus, who lived around 270 BC, was one of the most celebrated Alexandrian oculists. Aetius of Amida (AD 527–565) wrote an extensive treatise on diseases of the eye in the 6th century. Jesu Haly or Isa ibn Haly (AD 850) was an Arab oculist at Baghdad who wrote *Liber memorialis ophthalmicorum* in three parts. The first contained anatomy and physiology, and parts two and three dealt with external diseases. Demosthenes Philalethes from Marseilles wrote a standard work on the subject that remained extant until AD 1000. The earliest printed book, *De Oculis eorumeque egritudinibus et curis* (1474) was written by Benvenuto Grassi of Salerno. George Bartisch (1535–1606), founder of modern ophthalmic surgery, wrote an illustrated book on eye surgery, *Ophthalmodouleeia*, in 1583. The first English monograph, *A briefe treatise touching the preservation of the eie sight*, was published by Walter Bayley (1529–1592) in 1586. Antonio Scarpa (1747–1832), father of Italian ophthalmology, published an important book in 1801. Another English book, *A Synopsis of the Diseases of the Eye*, was published by Benjamin Travers (1783–1858), a surgeon at St Thomas' Hospital in 1820. The earliest treatise in America was written by George Frick (1793–1873) of Maryland, and the study of the eye was established as a specialty in America by Elkanah Williams (1822–1888) of Cincinnati. Friedrich Albrecht von Graefe (1828–1870) of Berlin, one of the greatest eye surgeons, founded the *Archiv für Ophthalmologie* in 1854, introduced iridectomy as treatment for glaucoma and iritis, and cataract operation in 1855. He operated for strabismus in 1857 and introduced the linear method of cataract extraction in 1868.

Ophthalmology in America The first eye infirmary in the United States was opened in New London by Elisha North (1771–1843) of Goshen, Connecticut in 1800. The earliest treatise, *A Treatise on Diseases of the Eye*, was published in 1823 by George Frick (1793–1873) of Maryland, the first American to specialize in the field. The Baltimore Dispensary for the Cure of Diseases of the Eye was established in the same year. William Gibson (1788–1868) of Philadelphia operated for strabismus in 1818. The Massachusetts Eye and Ear Infirmary was founded by E. Reynolds and J. Jefferies (1796–1876) in 1827. The specialty was established by Henry W. Williams (1821–1895) with his lectures in 1850. He was appointed as professor of ophthalmology at Harvard in 1871. His brother, Elkanah Williams (1822–1888), was also an eminent professor in the same field at the Miami Medical College. The ophthalmic clinic at the New York College of Physicians and Surgeons was established by Rea Agnew (1830–1888) in 1866. He was professor of ophthalmology in the same institute in 1869.

Ophthalmoscope [Greek: *ophthalmos*, eye + *skopein*, to view] *See funduscopy.*

Opical Rotation *See stereochemistry.*

Opie, Eugene Lindsay (1873–1971) American pathologist from Staunton, Virginia who graduated from the Johns Hopkins University in 1897. He suggested the presence of an antidiabetic substance in the islets of Langerhans of the pancreas in 1903, while professor of pathology at the Johns Hopkins. He was professor of pathology at Washington University (1910–1923), The University of Pennsylvania (1923–1932) and Cornell University.

Opisthotonos [Greek: *opistho*, behind + *tonos*, tension] Spasm consisting of extreme hyperextension of the body. *See tetanus.*

Opium Extract of the opium poppy, *Papaver somnifera*. Known to the ancient Sumerians 5000 years ago. An alabaster figure of an Assyrian priest carrying opium poppies, dating to 700 BC, is in the Louvre, Paris. The effect of the juice of poppy was mentioned by Nicander around 100 BC. He also proposed wine and honey as treatment for opium poisoning. John Jones (1645–1709) of Windsor gave an accurate description of symptoms from intoxication and withdrawal of opium in *The Mysteries of Opium Revialed* in 1700. It was introduced as Dover Powder into England by Captain Thomas Dover (1662–1742) in 1710. Opium trade flourished in the early 19th century and nearly 3000 tons of poppy juice were imported into China in 1820. Friederich Wilhelm Sertürner (1783–1841), a German pharmacist, crystallized the extract of opium and obtained morphine in 1801. *See morphine.*

Oppenheim Disease (Syn: amyotonia congenita) Form of myopathy accompanied by hypertonicity, weakness, and hyperflexibility. Described by Hermann Oppenheim (1858–1919), a German neurologist, in 1900.

Oppenheimer, Julius Robert (1904–1967) New York pioneer in the field of nuclear physics who graduated from Harvard University in 1925. He joined the atomic bomb project in 1942 and became director of the Los Alamos nuclear laboratory in 1943. He was appointed professor of physics at the Institute for Advanced Study, Princeton University, in 1947.

Opsonin [Greek: *opsonein*, to buy food] Any substance that binds to particulate antigens and induces phagocytosis. The role of serum in stimulating phagocytosis was demonstrated by Sir William Boog Leishman (1865–1926) in 1902. A thermolabile substance in the serum which acted on bacteria during phagocytosis was demonstrated and named 'opsonin' by Sir Almroth Edward Wright (1861–1947) and Stewart Douglas Rankin (1871–1936) of England in 1903.

Optic Atrophy [Greek: *opsis*, sight + *a*, not + *trophein*, nourish] *See Leber optic atrophy, Fuchs atrophy.*

Optic Chiasma [Greek: *opsis*, sight + *chiasma*, two crossed lines] Crossing of fibers within the optic nerve. First illustration was given by Leonardo Da Vinci (1452–1519). Samuel Thomas Sommering (1755–1830) of Holland described it in 1786.

Optic Nerve [Greek: *opsis*, sight] Alcmaeon, a pupil of Pythagoras, who dissected animals and studied their brains around 500 BC, has been credited with the discovery of optic nerves. They were rediscovered by Constanzo Varole (1543–1575), a surgeon of Bologna in 1538. The origin of the optic nerves in the brain was described by Bartholomew Eustachio (1524–1574) around 1550. Samuel Thomas Sommering (1755–1830) of Holland described the crossing of fibers within it in 1786.

Optical Lenses *See spectacles.*

Optics [Greek: *opsis*, sight] The discovery of a convex lens made from rock crystal in the ruins of Nimrud provided evidence that the ancients had knowledge of optics. The oldest convex lens in existence is from the island of Crete, and dates to the Minoan civilization around 1000 BC. The Greeks used burning lens around 424 BC. Early treatises were written by Euclid (300 BC), Ptolemy (AD 90–168), and Alhazen (AD 965–1040). Alhazen's work, *Kitab Al-Manazir* (Book of Optics), included refraction, reflection, and study of lenses, and formed the basis for the invention of spectacles, telescopes and microscopes. Magnifying power was described by Seneca (4 BC–AD 65) in AD 50. The study of optics was introduced into Europe by Vitello of Silesia (Poland), who wrote *Opticae Libridecem* (Ten books of Optics) around 1265. Spectacles are said to have been invented by Savinus Aramatus of Pisa around 1300. The first application of lenses for magnification was by a Venetian, Daniello Barbaro, in 1568. Johannes Kepler (1571–1630) published his *Dioptrice* in 1611, and the law of refraction was discovered by Snellius or Willebrod Snell (1580–1626), professor of mathematics at Leiden in 1624. Vision was explained by Réne Descartes (1596–1650) in *Dioptrique* published in 1637. Scottish physicist Sir David Brewster (1781–1868) invented the kaleidoscope and lenticular stereoscope.

Oral Contraceptives [Latin: *oralis*, mouth + *contra*, against + *ceptor*, receiver] The contraceptive pill was developed following ovarian studies by an Austrian, Ludwig Haberlandt (1885–1932), in 1921. Investigation of progesterone as a contraceptive was done by Willard Myron Allen (b 1904) and George Washington Corner (1889–1981) of America in 1929. Further development was by American endocrinologist, Gregory Goodwin Pincus (1903–1967), who was the first to determine the correct amounts of progesterone to be used in the pill. The risk of blood clots in susceptible women was noted by several English workers in 1968.

Orchiopexy [Greek: *orchios*, testis + *pexis*, fixation] Operation to mobilize the undescended testis. Performed by Charles Bell Robert Keetly (1848–1909) of West London Hospital in 1894. He implanted the testis in the thigh and this method was adopted and perfected by Franz C. Torek (1861–1938) of America in 1908. Another method was devised by Arthur Dean Bevan (1861–1943) of America in 1899. Implanting through the septum of the scrotum was described by C. Walther, a French surgeon, in 1906. Louis Ombredanne (b 1871), a French pediatric surgeon perfected the Walther procedure and used it on 1000 patients. His method was popularized in England by Philip Turner (b 1873) of Guy's Hospital in the 1920s.

Orchitis [Greek: *orchios*, testis + *itis*, inflammation] The first accurate clinical description of orchitis associated with mumps was given by Robert Hamilton (1721–1793) of Edinburgh in 1790.

Organ of Corti Receptor organ of sound which consists of a complex structure of basilar membrane, cochlea, hair cells and other structures of the ear. Described by Italian anatomist, Alfonso Bonaventura Corti (1822–1888), in 1851.

Organ Transplantation [Greek: *organon*] Permanent grafting of animal tissue was demonstrated in the hydra by Swedish biologist, Abraham Trembley (1710–1784) in 1742. Skin grafting was done by Italian surgeon, Guiseppe Baronio (1759–1811), around 1800 and he demonstrated the fundamental principle that an autograft from the same animal would take, while an allograft from another animal was rejected. Experimental physiologist, Karl Friedrich Wilhelm Ludwig (1816–1895), professor at Zurich, kept organs alive by pumping blood through them in 1856. Alexis Carrel (1873–1944), a French-born American biologist, is considered father of modern organ transplantation. He perfected the method of end-to-end arterial anastomosis using triple thread sutures in 1902, and reported the first heart transplantation in a dog in 1905. Growth of nerve fibers from cells outside the organism was demonstrated by Ross Granville Harrison (1870–1959) in 1907. Pioneering work on rejection reactions during transplantation was done by British immunologist, Sir Peter Brian Medawar (1915–1987). Another study on transplantation immunity was done by Georg Schone of Berlin in 1912. Work on histocompatibility commenced a year later by Clarence Cook Little (1888–1971) and Ernest Tyzzer (1875–1966). Little's work, using inbred mouse strains, while founder-director (1929–1956) of the Roscoe B. Jackson Memorial Laboratory at Mount Desert Island, Maine, led to significant advances in transplantation medicine and the study of cancer. Jean Baptiste Dausset (b 1916), a French immunologist from Toulouse, developed the procedure of tissue typing in organ transplantation. The immuno-suppressive properties of azothiaprine, a derivative of 6-mercaptopurine, was demonstrated by R. Schwartz and William Dameshek (1900–1969) in 1959, and introduced as an immunosuppressive agent in organ transplantation in 1962. Jean Borel, a researcher at the Sandoz Institute, noted the immunosuppressive property of cyclosporine, which was introduced to overcome rejection reactions in 1978. *See tooth transplantation.*

Organic Chemistry [Greek: *organon*] The term originally referred to chemistry of 'organized' or living matter.

Swedish chemist Jöns Jacob Berzelius (1779–1848) in 1806 described it as: 'the part of physiology which describes the composition of living bodies, and the chemical processes which occur in them' in *Lectures in Animal Chemistry*. This definition was abandoned following the synthesis of urea from potassium cyanate and ammonium sulfate by Friedrich Wöhler (1800–1882) in 1828, and of acetic acid by Hermann Kolbe (1818–1884) in 1845. Wohler announced, 'I must tell you that I can make urea without the need of kidneys or of any animal whatever' in a letter to Berzelius. John Baptiste André Dumas (1800–1884), an apothecary from Geneva, determined the nitrogen content in organic compounds and determined vapor density in 1823. Marcellin Berthelot (1827–1907) of Paris was first professor of organic chemistry at the College de France and produced benzene and naphthalene in 1851. He published *Organic Chemistry founded on Synthesis* in 1860. The six-carbon ring structure of benzene was proposed by August Kekulé (1829–1896) in 1865. He stated 'We have come to the conviction that no difference exists between organic and inorganic compounds. Therefore we define organic chemistry as the chemistry of organ compounds' in his book on organic chemistry, published between 1859–1860. Three dimensional structure was illustrated by Jacobus Van't Hoff (1852–1911) of Rotterdam in 1874. A complete catalogue of organic compounds, *Handbook of Organic Chemistry*, was published by German chemist, Friedrich Konrad Beilstein (1838–1906) in 1881. *See biochemistry.*

Organic Free Radicles One of the first treatises was written by French chemist, Auguste Laurent (1807–1853) of St Maurice. Their existence was discovered in 1900 by Russian chemist, Moses Gomberg (1866–1947) from the Ukraine who emigrated to America in 1884, while a professor at Michigan University.

Organotherapy [Greek: *organon*, instrument + *therapio*, take care] Treatment with animal organs or extracts has been practiced since ancient times. The Hindu *Ayurveda* describes use of testicular tissue in treatment of impotence. This practice was revived in the 19th century by Édouard Brown-Sequard (1817–1894) who advocated use of testicular extracts for debilitation around 1889. Sir William Osler (1849–1919) attempted to treat Addison disease with glandular therapy at the Johns Hopkins Medical School, Baltimore, in 1891.

Oribasius (AD 325–403) Roman physician to Emperor Julian at Constantinople during the Byzantine period. He compiled an encyclopedia of medicine in 70 volumes. One of his treatises *Medicoe collectiones ad Julianum* was translated by the Arabian physician, Rhazes (850–932). Oribasius's anatomical writings earned him the name of 'The Ape of Galen', but he did describe the salivary glands which had been overlooked by Galen (AD 129–200).

Oriental Sore [Latin: *orientalis*, eastern] *See Baghdad sore.*

Origin of Species [Latin: *origo*, to rise] *See evolution, Darwin, Charles.*

Ormuzd Ahura Mazda was the Persian god of goodness and light who created the world. He delegated the art of healing to a powerful angel, Thrita, who became the god of medicine and healing.

Ornithodoros [Greek: *ornis*, bird + *dorus*, bag] Genus of tick which causes relapsing fever by transmitting the spirochete, *Borrelia recurrentis*. Identified independently by two groups: Philip Ross and Milne in Uganda, and Joseph Everett Dutton (1877–1905) and John Launcelot Todd (1876–1949) in the Congo, in 1904.

Ornithology [Greek: *ornis*, bird + *logos*, discourse] The first printed monograph, containing a description of birds mentioned by Aristotle and Pliny, was written by English naturalist from Cambridge, William Turner (1510–1568) in 1544. Ulysses Aldrovandus (1522–1605), professor of medicine and philosophy at Bologna, wrote *Ornithology* in 1599. Pierre Belon (1517–1574), a medical graduate from Paris, wrote a *History of Birds*, including comparative anatomy. John Latham (1740–1837), a physician from Dartford, published *General History of Birds* (1821–1828) in eleven volumes. English ornithologist, John Gould (1804–1881) from Lyme Regis, published *Birds of Europe* in five volumes (1832–1837), *Birds of Australia* in seven volumes (1840–1847), *Birds of Great Britain* in five volumes (1863–1873), and *Birds of Asia* (1849–1883). The American Ornithology Union was founded by Barney Charles Cory (1857–1921) from Boston. He published *Birds of Bahamas* in 1878, and *Birds of the Americas* in 1918. The Ridgway color system for bird identification was invented by an American ornithologist, Robert Ridgway (1850–1929) of Mount Carmel, Illinois.

Ornithosis [Greek: *ornis*, bird + *osis*] (Syn: parrot fever, psittacosis) The first description of an outbreak of psittacosis was by Swiss physician Jacob Ritter in 1879. Seven cases were reported in a household in Switzerland which kept parrots and other exotic birds, three of whom died. In 1891 Edmund Isidore Nocard (1850–1903) isolated a *Salmonella* which he mistakenly thought was the causative organism and named it *Bacillus psittacosis* (now *Nocardia*). About 1930, Samuel Philips Bedson (1886–1969) and other workers identified a virus as being responsible for the disease. Thomas Milton Rivers (1888–1962), an American virologist at the Rockefeller Institute, established the basis for diagnosing psittacosis by injecting the sputum of the patient into mice in 1938.

Oroya Fever (Syn: Carrion disease) Named after the place in Peru where the first cases were noted. *Bartonella bacilliformis,* the bacteria responsible, were seen in red blood cells by a Peruvian physician, A. L. Barton (1871–1950), in 1915. The organism was named *Bartonella* in his honor by Richard Pearson Strong (1872–1948) and colleagues. Arsphenamine was used in the treatment by J. Arce in 1918. *See Carrion disease.*

Orphan Houses The first house was initiated by the Roman emperor Trajan (AD 52–117) in 105. Emperor Justinian established several in Byzantium under his laws. The first in England was established in 1758 at Hoxton, and it later moved to Haverstock Hill. An asylum for female orphans was established at Lambeth in 1758, and the London Orphan Asylum was formed in 1813. The Royal Albert Orphan Asylum was founded at Bagshot in 1864. *See child care, Barnardo, Thomas.*

Orth, Johannes (1847–1923) German pathologist who described kernicterus in 1875.

Orth Stain Lithium and carmine, introduced into histology by German pathologist, Johannes Orth (1847–1923).

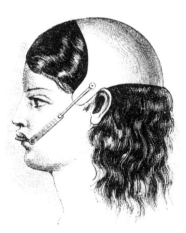

Correction of protruding teeth with a vulcanite plate connected to a skull cap. E.S. Talbot, *Irregularities of the Teeth and their Treatment* (1888). H.K. Lewis, London

Orthodontics [Greek: *orthos,* straight + *odous,* tooth] Practice of correcting irregularities of teeth, started by John Hunter (1728–1793) and Pierre Fauchard (1678–1761). The Orthodontical Society of London was founded in 1856.

Orthodontics was developed in America by Edwin Hartley Angle (1855–1930) of St Louis who published *A System of Appliances for correcting Irregularities of the Teeth* (1890) and *Treatment of Malocclusion of Teeth* (1907). The American Society of Orthodontics was formed in 1901 and the journal *American Orthodontist* first appeared in 1907.

Orthopedics [Greek: *orthos,* straight + *pais,* child] The Edwin Smith papyrus (1500 BC) describes splints used by the Egyptians. Hindu Brahmin surgeons treated fractures with great skill. Paul of Aegina (625–690) defined a fracture as 'a division of the bone, or a rupture, or excision of it, produced by external violence'. Hippocrates (460–377) has dealt with fractures and dislocations in *de Fracturis.* He discussed the anatomy of the bones and joints, physiology of movements, classification of fractures, methods of reducing fractures, immobilizing limbs and various other orthopedic topics. Galen (129–200) used the term 'abruptio' (to take away) to denote fracture of long end of a bone. The first orthopedic hospital was founded in 1790 at Orbe, Switzerland, by Jean-André Venel (1740–1791). Samuel Cooper (1780–1848) in his *Dictionary of Practical Surgery* published in 1809, devoted over 50 pages to fractures. The term was coined by French surgeon, Nicholas Andry (1658–1747) of Lyons in 1741. Pott fracture and spinal caries were described by Sir Percivall Pott (1714–1788) in 1779. The Royal National Orthopaedic Hospital was founded by William John Little (1810–1894) in 1839. The first book in America was published by Samuel David Gross (1805–1884) in 1830, and one of the first surgeons to specialize was John Ball Brown (1784–1862) of Boston. *Lectures on Orthopedic Surgery* was published by Louis Bauer (1814–1898) of America in 1862. Hugh Owen Thomas (1834–1891) of Liverpool was the father of modern orthopedics in England. He came from a family of bone setters and devised various apparatus for treatment of deformities and fractures, including the Thomas splint for compound fractures of the femur. Jacques Mathieu Delpech (1777–1832), professor of surgery at Montpellier, pioneered orthopedic surgery in France and devised a new method of treatment of club foot by subcutaneous section of the achilles tendon, and pointed out the tubercular nature of spinal caries. Gurdon Buck (1807–1877), a leading surgeon from New York, established treatment for fractures of the thigh by applying traction through weights and pulleys in the mid-19th century. In England it was recognized as a specialty in 1898, with the establishment of the British Orthopaedic Society. A pioneer in radiology was Etienne Destot (1864–1918) of Lyon who used it for diagnosis of bone disease two months after Wilhelm Konrad von Röntgen (1845–1923) discovered X-rays in February 1896.

Joseph Lister's (1827–1912) aseptic technique was introduced into orthopedic surgery in America by Lewis Atterbury Stimson (1844–1917) of New Jersey who wrote a treatise on fractures in 1883. The Orthopedic Association in America was formed in 1887, and the American Academy of Orthopedic Surgeons was founded in 1933. The British Orthopaedic Association was established in 1933.

Orthopnea [Greek: *orthos*, straight + *pnoia*, breath]. Difficulty in breathing except when upright, a symptom in cardiorespiratory disease. Defined by Paul of Aegina (625–690) as 'to pant for breath, and from their being obliged to keep the chest erect for fear of being suffocated, they are called orthopnoeic'. Oxford physiologist, John Mayhow (1645–1679) explained the symptom and mechanism in 1668.

Ortner Syndrome Paralysis of the left vocal cord due to enlarged left atrium in mitral stenosis. Described by a professor of medicine at Vienna, Norbert Ortner (1865–1935).

Osborne, Henry Fairfield (1857–1935) American paleontologist from Fairfield, Connecticut who served as professor of zoology at Columbia University. He published *The Age of Mammals* (1910), *Man of the Old Stone Age* (1915), and *The Origin and Evolution of Life* (1917).

Osborne, Thomas Burr (1859–1929) Born in New Haven, Connecticut, he was an eminent biochemist who studied nutrition and demonstrated the importance of glycine and lysine in diet in 1912, together with Lafayette Benedict Mendel (1872–1935) of Yale.

Oscillograph Oscilloscope for recording variation of physical properties over a time period. Invented by a German physicist, Karl Ferdinand Braun (1850–1918) in 1897.

Osgood-Schlatter Disease Painful tibial tuberosity in adolescence. Described independently by an American orthopedic surgeon, Robert Bayley Osgood (1873–1956) of Boston, and a Swiss surgeon, Carl Schlatter (1864–1934), in 1903.

Osiris Egyptian God who left his kingdom to be managed by his wife Isis and her faithful minister Hermes.

Osiris Journal of the history and philosophy of science. Founded by George Sarton in 1936. He was professor of history of science at Harvard in 1940.

Osler, Sir William (1849–1919) Regius professor of medicine at Oxford, born in Devon, Canada. He studied medicine at Montreal and Toronto and was appointed professor of medicine at McGill University, Toronto in 1874, a position he held for 10 years. He described one of the first human cases

of actinomycosis in 1886, effective treatment of Addison disease with fresh hog adrenal extracts in 1896, and hereditary angioneurotic edema in 1888. He was a reformer of American medical education, and in 1889 made a strong appeal for correction. Five medical schools and the staff of the Johns Hopkins Hospital issued a circular in 1890 resolving to improve the system. He described familial hemorrhagic telengiectasis, a condition of multiple telengiectatic lesions of the face and upper gastrointestinal tract associated with bleeding tendency, in 1907. With McCrae, he reported his clinical experience in 150 patients with gastric cancer in 1900. His most important book, *The Principles and Practice of Medicine*, was first published in 1892. A biography, *The Life of William Osler,* was published by the American surgeon, Harvey Cushing (1869–1939), in 1940. *The Great Physician, A short Life of William Osler* was published by Edith Gittings Reid, and *A Year with Osler, 1896–1897* was written by Joseph Pratt in 1949.

Osler Nodes Cutaneous nodules found in subacute bacterial endocarditis. Described by Sir William Osler (1849–1919) in 1908.

Osler–Rendu–Weber Syndrome (Syn: hereditary hemorrhagic telengiectasis) Independently described by Henri Rendu (1844–1902) of Paris in 1896, Frederick Parkes Weber (1863–1962), professor of applied therapeutics at Temple University, Philadelphia in 1904, and Sir William Osler (1849–1919) in 1907.

Osmic Acid First used to stain nerve tissue by Italian histologist, Vittorio Marchi (1851–1908), in 1891.

Osmium Heavy metal discovered by Smithson Tennant (1761–1815), a physician and chemist from Selby, Yorkshire in 1804. The name is derived from the Greek, 'osmum' due to its pungent smell.

Osmolarity [Greek: *osmos*, impulse] Solute concentrations of urine and blood were first compared to assess renal functions by Heinrich Dreser of Germany in 1892. Galeotti in 1902 and Claude Bernard (1813–1878) of Paris used freezing point depression to calculate the concentration of solutes in urine and blood.

Osmosis [Greek: *osmos*, impulse] Discovered by a French Abbe, Jean Antoine Nollet (1700–1770), professor of physics at the College de Navarre in Paris in 1748. René Joachim Henri Dutrochet (1776–1847) re-investigated it and showed in 1835 that water from a weaker solution moved into a stronger solution through a membrane, and named the process osmosis. Diffusion across a membrane was attributed to osmotic pressure by Thomas Graham (1805–1869) in 1854. The semipermeability of the membrane was demonstrated by Moritz Traube (1826–1894), a plant physiologist, in 1867. The process was demonstrated using cane sugar solution in a vessel with semipermeable walls by Wilhelm Friedrich Philipp Pfeffer (1845–1920) of Germany in 1877. Further work was done in the same year by Hugo De Vries (1848–1935) of Holland, and precise measurements was achieved by F. N. Morse and Frazer of America in 1912. An outstanding work on osmotic pressure of proteins was done by Søren Peter Sørenson (1868–1939) in 1917.

Osteitis Fibrosa Cystica [Latin: *osteo*, bone; Greek: *itis*, inflammation; Latin: *fibra*, band + *kytos*, hollow] Rarefaction of bone due to parathyroid tumors. First observed by Gerhard Engel in 1864 and named after Friedrich Daniel von Recklinghausen (1833–1910) of Germany who described it in detail in 1891. This disorder was recognized by Max Askanazy (1865–1940) at Tübingen in 1904. The first successful treatment by surgical removal of parathyroid adenoma was performed by a Viennese surgeon, Felix Mandl (1892–1957), in 1925.

Osteoblast [Greek: *osteo*, bone + *blastos*, bud] Cells responsible for bone growth and formation. Described by Carl Gegenbaur (1826–1903), a comparative anatomist at the University of Würzberg, in 1885.

Osteoclast [Greek: *osteo*, bone + *klan*, to break] Cells responsible for resorption of bone. Described by Charles Phillipe Robin (1821–1885), professor of histology at the Faculty of Medicine in Paris.

Osteoclasis [Greek: *osteon*, bone + *klan*, to break] An instrument used to break the bone in orthopedic surgery was invented by Italian orthopedic surgeon, Francesco Rizzoli (1808–1880) to fracture a normal femur to compensate for shortening.

Osteogenesis Imperfecta [Greek: *osteo*, bone + *gennan*, to produce] Congenital disease characterized by brittle bones due to defective ossification. Described by Swedish physician, Olof Jacob Ekman (1764–1839), in 1788 and Johann Friedrich Georg Christian Lobstein (1777–1835), professor of pathology and clinical medicine at Strasburg, gave another account in 1833, and the syndrome was named after him. It was described independently by Dutch anatomist, Wilhelm Vrolik (1801–1863), in 1854. British dermatologist, Alfred Eddowes (1850–1946), a graduate from the University of Edinburgh in 1873, gave a description and it is known by his name in Britain. He worked at Royal Salop Hospital in Shrewsbury and came to London in 1897 and practiced as a dermatologist at several hospitals.

Osteology [Greek: *osteo*, bone + *logos*, discourse] Galen (AD 129–200) wrote on the bones and recommended dissection of apes for their study. Abu Mohammed Abdul Latif (1162–1231), an Arab scientist in Egypt, was the first to challenge the inaccuracies in Galen's writings on osteology. An early work was by Volcher Coiter (1534–1576), a pupil of Gabriele Falloppio (1523–1562) and a physician at Nuremberg in 1575, and included developmental osteology in an infant with illustrations of the centers of ossification. Clopton Havers (1650–1702), a London physician and anatomist, described the spaces in the compact tissue of the bone (Haversian canals) in *Osteologia Nova, or some observations of the Bones and the Parts belonging to them, with the manner of their accretion and nutrition*, published in 1691, the first complete book on osteology. *Osteographia or Anatomy of Human Bones*, published by William Cheselden (1688–1752) of St Thomas' Hospital in 1733, contained an accurate description of all the human bones with illustrations. A modern 19th century monograph on osteology in England, *Human Osteology, comprising a Description of Bones*, was published in 1855 by Luther Holden (b 1905), a demonstrator in anatomy at St Bartholomew's Hospital.

Osteomalacia [Greek: *osteo*, bone + *malakia*, softness] Jean Louis Petit (1674–1750), director and surgeon at the Academy de Paris, gave an account of osteomalacia. The second description, *An Extraordinary Case in Physic*, was given by Thomas Cadwalader (1708–1779), a pupil of William Cheselden (1688–1752) in 1744. Henry Thomas, a surgeon at the London Hospital, described it in his treatise, *A Remarkable Case of Softness of Bones*, in 1776. It was shown to be due to lack of vitamin D by John Preston Maxwell (1871–1961) in 1929. Pseudofractures in osteomalacia were described by Louis Arthur Milkman (1895–1951) of America in 1930. *See vitamin D.*

Osteometry [Greek: *osteo*, bone + *metron*, measure] Comparative study of the measurements of human and animal bones was founded in 1795 by Charles White (1728–1813) who studied the relationship of the humerus to the forearm. His work was revived by William Lawrence (1783–1867) in 1817. Paul Broca (1824–1880) quoted the work of Lawrence in his own publication on the subject in 1862.

Osteomyelitis [Greek: *osteo*, bone + *myelos*, marrow + *itis*, inflammation] The term spinosa ventosa was first used by Arab physicians to describe the disease of the bone which discharged its contents through the surface of the skin— essentially chronic osteomyelitis. The term was first used by French surgeon, Auguste Nelaton (1807–1873). Samuel Cooper described it and performed a partial but extensive resection of the affected tibia in 1787. Osteomyelitis of the tibia was described by a London surgeon, William Hey (1736–1819), in 1803. John Howship (1781–1841), a surgeon to St George's and Charing Cross Hospitals in London, suffered from osteomyelitis which motivated him to study bone diseases, and publish *On the Natural and Diseased state of the Bones* in 1820. Another account in America was given by Nathan Smith (1762–1829), a surgeon from Connecticut, in 1827. He used trepanning as treatment for bone necrosis. The first successful use of penicillin in osteomyelitis was by Howard Walter Florey (1898–1968) and co-workers in 1941.

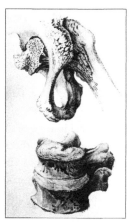

Osteomyelitis of thigh bone and vertebrae. Sir Charles Bell, *A System of Operative Surgery* (1809). Longman, London

Osteopathy [Greek: *osteo*, bone + *pathos*, suffering] Practice evolved through centuries of bone setting. It was named 'osteopathy' by American physician, Andrew Taylor Still (1828–1917) of Kansas. The first American school of osteopathy was established in Kirksville, Missouri in 1892. The American Association for Advancement of Osteopathy (later known as the American Osteopathic Association) was founded in 1897. *See bone setters.*

Osteopetrosis [Greek: *osteo*, bone + *petra*, stone + *osis*] Congenital condition of thick and hard bones due to failure of resorption of intercellular ground substance. Described by a German radiologist, Heinrich Ernst Albers Schonberg, in 1903. It was first known as marble bone disease and later named Albers–Schonberg disease.

Osteotomy [Greek: *osteo*, bone + *tomein*, cut] The first was performed in the United States for ankylosis of the hip joint by John Rhea Barton (1794–1871) of Lancaster in 1826. It was pioneered in England by Henry Albert Reeves (1814–1914), a surgeon to the Orthopaedic Hospital, London, in 1877. He performed 493 osteotomies up to 1885 without a single death.

Ostwald, Friedrich Wilhelm (1853–1932) German professor of chemistry at Leipzig who proposed the law of dilution which bears his name. He invented a process to make nitric acid from ammonia, proposed a new theory of color and defined the catalyst as an agent which accelerates the rate of a chemical reaction. His *Lehrbuch der allgemeinen Chemie*, published in 1885, marked the beginning of physical chemistry. He received the Nobel Prize for Chemistry in 1909.

Otis, Fessenden Nott (1825–1900) American urologist who designed a method for internal urethrotomy and introduced the use of local anesthesia in urology in 1884.

Otolaryngology or otorhinology [Greek: *otos*, ear + *laryngx*, upper part of wind pipe + *logos*, discourse] The first monograph on the diseases of the larynx was written by Giovanni Batista Codronchi (1547–1622) in 1597, and the first clinical manual on the ear was published by Hieronymus Mercurialis (1530–1606) in 1584. The first treatise on the structure, function and diseases of the ear was written by Joseph Guichard Duverny (1648–1730) of Paris in 1683. Armand Trousseau (1801–1867), with Jules Hippolyte Cloquet (1787–1840), published a classic treatise on laryngology in 1837. A British pioneer in otology was Joseph Toynbee (1815–1866) who published *Diseases of the Ear* in 1860 and devised a speculum for examination. Sir Morell MacKenzie (1853–1925), another eminent English otorhinologist, published *Diseases of the Nose and Throat* in 1880. *See larynx, laryngoscope.*

Otorhinology *See otolaryngology.*

Otosclerosis [Greek: *oto*, ear + *sklerosis*, hard] The first account as a clinical entity was given by Adam Politzer (1835–1920) of Vienna in 1895. Fenestration operation was suggested by George John Jenkins of London in 1913, and successful treatment using his method was conducted by Maurice Joseph Louis Sourdille (1885–1961) in 1937. Julius Lempert (b 1890) devised another surgical technique in 1938.

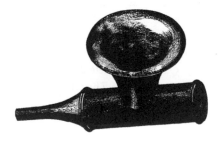

John Brunton's otoscope. George P. Field, *A Manual of Diseases of the Ear* (1894). Balliére, Tindall & Cox, London

Otoscope [Greek: *oto*, ear + *skopein*, to view] Invented by Anton Friedrich von Troeltsch (1829–1890) of Germany in 1860. An improved version was devised by John Brunton (1836–1899) in 1865.

Ott, Isaac (1847–1915) American who did extensive work on nervous regulation of body temperature for over 30 years. His work led to the discovery of the thermoregulatory center in the hypothalamus. He demonstrated the lactogenic property of the anterior lobe with J.C. Scott in 1911.

Otto, John Conrad (1774–1844) Born in Philadelphia, he was a pioneer in the study of hemophilia in America. He graduated from the College of New Jersey in 1792 and obtained his MD from the University of Pennsylvania in 1796. His observations on bleeders in families were published in 1803.

Otto Disease Protrusion of the acetabulum into the pelvic cavity in some cases of osteoarthritis. Described by Breslau surgeon, Adolph Wilhelm Otto (1786–1845).

Otto, Friedrich Wilhelm Robert (1837–1907) Chemist and toxicologist at Brunswick who described a method of identifying organic poisons in biological material.

Ould, Sir Fielding (1710–1789) Born in Galway, Ireland, he was an obstetrician at the Rotunda Hospital in Dublin who wrote *Treatise on Midwifery* in 1742. This includes a description of the mechanism of labor. He also performed an incision on a rigid perineum (episiotomy) which was likely to tear during the delivery of the child.

Ovalocytosis The only mammal which has oval red corpuscles is the camel. Oval red cells in humans were first shown by Melvin Dresbach (1874–1946) in 1904, and are inherited through a dominant Mendelian trait.

Ovarian Tumor [Latin: *ovarium*, ovary] The Krukenberg tumor, a bilateral fibrosarcoma of the ovary, was described by Friedrich Ernst Krukenberg (1871–1946) of Germany in 1896. The Brenner tumor, a peculiar benign neoplasm of the ovary, was described as 'oophoroma folliculare' by another German, Fritz Brenner (b 1877), in 1907. A similar neoplasm of the ovary was described by Ernst Gottlieb Orthmann (1858–1922) in 1899. Arrhenoblastoma, a tumor of the ovary made of convoluted tubules resembling the seminiferous tubules of the testis, was described by E. P. Pick of Berlin in 1905, and G. Schikele described a second case with similar histology in 1906. The term 'arrhenoblastoma' was proposed by Robert Meyer of Berlin to denote the group of similar masculinizing tumors in 1930. The presence of an ovarian tumor associated with ascites and pleural effusion (Meigs syndrome) was described by Joe Vincent Meigs (1892–1963) of America in 1937.

Ovary [Latin: *ovarium*, ovary] Site of egg production in the hen was identified and named 'ovarium' by the Italian anatomist Hieronymus Fabricus ab Aquapendente (1537–1619) in 1600. The Graafian follicle, a structure or sac found on the surface of the ovary, was described by Regnier de Graaf (1641–1673) of Holland in 1672. The first suggestion that the ovary secreted internal substances which had a remote and overall effect on the organism was made by Théophile de Bordeu (1722–1776), a physician from Montpellier, in *Recherches sur Glandes*, published in 1746. It was the first suggestion of hormonal function of the ovary. The mammalian ovum within the follicle was found by Estonian anatomist, Karl Ernst von Baer (1792–1876), in 1827. The effect of the corpus lutea on ovulation was shown by American pathologist, Leo Loeb (1869–1959) in 1911. *See estrogen, corpus luteum, ovariotomy.*

Ovariotomy [Latin: *ovarium*, ovary; Greek: *tome*, cut] The first successful operative treatment of an ovarian tumor was performed by Robert Houston of Glasgow in 1701. He made an incision and evacuated the contents from the cyst. A complete ovariotomy was carried out by Ephraim McDowell (1771–1830) of Kentucky in 1809. Nathan Smith (1762–1829) of Connecticut performed another in 1821, quite unaware of McDowell's earlier achievement. The procedure was greatly advanced in America by Dunlop Atloe and, by 1850, 36 were performed in America with a record of 21 recoveries. Augustus Bozzi Granville attempted the procedure in London in 1826, and Charles Clay (1801–1893) of Manchester commenced in 1842. By 1850 in England, a record of 91 ovariotomies had been done but still with a high mortality of 36%. A successful ovariotomy on a woman of 75 years was reported by E. P. Bennett in 1861. Sir Thomas Spencer Wells (1818–1897) performed a complete ovariotomy in 1858. Wells became an expert and performed over 1000 operations by 1880. Emiline Horton Cleveland (1829–1878), a graduate of the Female Medical College of Pennsylvania (1855) and professor of obstetrics at the Woman's Hospital, Philadelphia, was the first woman in America to perform major abdominal surgery and ovariotomy in 1875.

Overton, Charles Ernest (1865–1933) Botanist who investigated osmosis. *See narcosis.*

Oviduct [Latin: *ovum*, egg + *ductus*, duct] The primordial female genital tract or oviduct (Müller duct) was described by Johannes Peter Müller (1801–1858) of Bonn in 1830. The function of cilia within it in moving the ovum was described by German physiologist, Gabriel Gustav Valentin (1810–1909), in 1834.

Ovulation [Latin: *ovum*, egg] The first account on an anatomical, physiological and pathological basis was given by Regnier de Graaf (1641–1673) of Holland in 1672. Similar work of Jan Swammerdam (1637–1680) was published in the same year. John Beard (1858–1924) suggested in 1897 that the corpus luteum may be an inhibitor of ovulation during pregnancy, and this was confirmed by Auguste Prenant (1861–1927) in 1898. American pathologist, Leo Loeb (1869–1959) found, in 1911, that extirpation of the corpora lutea in guinea pigs accelerated the next ovulation, while extirpation of other parts of the ovary had no such effect. W. L. Williams, in America, found in 1921 that estrus and ovulation could be induced within 48 hours in cows by squeezing out the corpus luteum through rectal manipulation. Edgar V. Allen (1892–1943) and George Adelbert Doisey (1893–1986) of St Louis did valuable work on hormones in ovulation and isolated the active principle of the ovarian hormone, estrogen, in 1923.

Ovum [Latin: *ovum*, egg] Galen (AD 129–200), and Aristotle (384–322 BC) thought that fertilization of the ovum took place through a mystic process called 'aura seminalis'. It was believed that the ovum was complete in itself and was capable of producing an embryo after a suitable stimulus was received. This view, called 'preformation', was held until the 16th century. One of William Harvey's (1578–1657) aphorisms was '*Omni vivum ex ovo*' (every living thing comes from the egg). The germinal vesicles were shown in the ovum of birds by Jan Evangelista Purkinje (1787–1869) in 1825. Karl Ernst von Baer (1792–1876), an Estonian, described the structure of the mammalian ovum in 1827. He announced his findings in *De Ovi Mammalium et Hominis Genesi*. The segmentation of the frog ovum was described by Swiss physician Jean Louis Prévost (1838–1927) in the same year. Martin Barry, an embryologist and surgeon from Edinburgh, observed the union of spermatozoa and ovum in the rabbit in 1843 and published his findings in *Researches in Embryology* in 1849. Carl Gegenbaur (1826–1903), a German comparative anatomist, showed the unicellular nature in all vertebrates in 1861. The zona radiata was described by Theodor Ludwig Wilhelm Bischoff (1807–1882), professor of anatomy and embryologist at Heidelberg, in 1884. Edouard Gérard Balbiani (1823–1899), professor of comparative embryology in France, described the yolk nucleus in 1893. The youngest human embryo, of 13 days, was described by Hungarian gynecologist, Peters Hubert (1859–1939), in 1899.

Owen, Robert (1771–1858) Social reformer from Newtown, Montgomeryshire, who was instrumental in bringing in reforms to improve conditions of factory workers, including children. He founded infant schools in Britain and published *New View of Human Society* in 1814.

Owen, Sir Richard (1804–1892) Born in Lancaster, he was a comparative anatomist and paleontologist, who trained as a physician at Edinburgh University and St Bartholomew's Hospital, where he was a pupil of John Abernethy (1764–1831). He was curator of the Royal College of Surgeons before being appointed as the first superintendent of the natural history department of the British Museum in 1856. He described *Trichina spiralis* and 1835 and the extinct early bird, *Archaeopteryx*. He founded the Royal Microscopical Society of England.

Oxalate Together with citrate solutions were shown to be effective anticoagulants by French physiologist, Nicolas-Maurice Arthus (1862–1945) and C. Pages in 1890, and confirmed by C. A. Peckelharing in 1892. Sodium oxalate was introduced as an anticoagulant for blood and milk by Arthus.

Oxenbridge, Daniel (1576–1642) Physician from Northamptonshire who practiced in London. In 1630 he wrote *General observations and prescriptions in the practice of physick* which contained some case histories in psychiatry. His work was published posthumously in 1715.

Oxford University The first mention of an academy at Oxford was made by Pope Martin in 802. King Alfred founded schools in the city in 879, and a Royal Charter was granted by Henry III in 1249 which marked the foundation of the university. He also founded 'an infirmarie for sicke' in 1233. According to *Anglica Judaica*, a Jewish school of medicine existed at Oxford in the 11th century. The first teacher of medicine at Oxford was Stokes in 1251, who also taught at the Jewish medical school. Oxford became known as the seat of learning after the siege of the castle by King Stephen in 1411. One of the first degrees in medicine was awarded to Thomas Edmonds in 1449, and Thomas Bloxam graduated in medicine from Oxford in 1455. Oxford school was incorporated into a university by Queen Elizabeth l in 1571.

Oxidation Potential Together with reduction potential in a living organism (*Escherichia coli*), was measured by L. J. Gillespie in 1920. American chemist William Mansfield Clark (1884–1964) did further studies determining the acidity of milk and developed titration indicators. Microinjection methods to study oxidation were introduced by English biochemist Joseph Needham (b 1900). Further work was done independently by B. Cohen and R. Chambers in 1933.

Oxygen Therapy First suggested for resuscitation by John Hunter (1728–1793) in 1775. Chaussier used it to resuscitate asphyxiated neonates in 1780. Thomas Beddoes (1760–1808) experimented with the gas (and nitrous oxide) for treating diseases in 1794. Oxygen therapy was popularized by Scottish physiologist, John Scott Haldane (1860–1936), during World War 1. The occurrence of arterial anoxemia in lobar pneumonia was shown by Alvin Leroy Barach (b 1895) and M.N. Woodwell in 1921 and their work formed the basis for oxygen therapy in pneumonia.

Oxygen [Greek: *oxys*, sour + *gennan*, to produce] John Mayow (1640–1679), an English chemist, realized that when substances burnt in air a chemical union with a constituent of the atmosphere took place. He called this gas 'igneo aereum' or 'spiritus nitro-aerius'. His insight into combustion was not accepted, and the erroneous theory of German chemist Georg Ernst Stahl (1660–1734), that when substances burnt they used an essence within them called phlogiston, became accepted. Phlogiston theory was held for over a hundred years until Joseph Priestley (1733–1804), an English chemist, obtained pure oxygen by heating a metal oxide. He called the gas 'dephologisticated air' in 1774. Oxygen was discovered independently by a Swedish apothecary, Carl Wilhelm Scheele (1742–1786), in the same year. In 1775 Antoine Laurent Lavoisier (1743–1794) named the substance responsible for combustion 'acidifying principle' which, in Greek was 'oxygine principle', hence its present name. The atomic weight was calculated at 16 by London chemist, William Odling (1829–1921), who qualified as a physician from London University in 1851. The first commercial preparation of oxygen using fractional distillation of air was achieved by Karl von Linde (1842–1934) in 1895.

Oxytetracycline Teramycin antibiotic isolated from *Streptomyces rimosus* by Alexander Carpenter Finlay (b 1906) and co-workers in 1950.

Oxytocin [Greek: *oxys*, sour + *tokos*, birth] The action of extract of posterior pituitary was demonstrated by British physiologist, Sir Henry Halett Dale (1875–1968), in 1906. William Blair Bell (1871–1936) a Liverpool obstetrician, used crude oxytocin in labor in 1909. The specific hormone from the posterior lobe of the pituitary gland which causes contraction of the uterus was isolated by American biochemist, Oliver Kamm (b 1888) and colleagues in 1928. It was synthesized in pure form by American biochemist, Vincent du Vigneaud (1901–1978), in 1952. He was born in Chicago and became professor at Cornell University Medical College in 1938. He also discovered the metabolic pathway from methionine to homocysteine, and synthesized thiamine (1942) and vasopressin (1953). He was awarded the Nobel Prize for Chemistry in 1955.

Oxyuris [Greek: *oxys*, sour + *oura*, tail] The first differentiation of oxyuris from other intestinal parasites was made by Alexander of Tralles (AD 525–605).

Ozone [Greek: *oze*, stench] In 1785 van Mareum observed a peculiar smell in the air around an electrical machine. This 'electrified air' was used by Cavallo to treat fetid ulcers. It was identified as a form of oxygen by an Irish physical chemist from Belfast, Thomas Andrews (b 1813). In 1840 Christian Friedrich Schönbein (1799–1868), a German chemist who worked in Basel, inferred that the odor was caused by a new gas and he named it 'ozone'. In 1845 Jean Charles de Marignac (d 1894) and De la Rive suggested it was an allotropic form of oxygen. In 1848 Hunt postulated that it was an oxide of oxygen, and the presence of three oxygen atoms was suggested by English chemist William Odling (1829–1921) in 1861. His theory was later proved by Soret in 1866 and Brodie in 1872. The ozone layer in the upper atmosphere was discovered in 1913 by a French physicist, Marie Paul Auguste Charles Fabry (1867–1945).

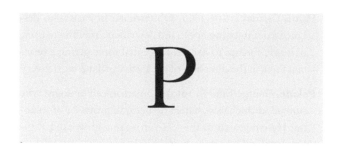

P53 Gene A gene which normally suppresses cancer in man. Identified by the current professor of cancer research at the University of Dundee, David Lane (b 1952) from Purley, Surrey in England. It was observed during research on tumor viruses in cells and was thought to be a contaminant until Lane started investigating it in 1978. His work showed that the abnormality of the gene led to cancer. Lane shared the Paul Ehrlich Award at Frankfurt with his co-workers, Arni Levine of Princeton University, New Jersey and Bert Vogelstein of Johns Hopkins Oncology Center, Baltimore, in 1998.

Pacchioni Bodies Corpuscles forming small prominences of arachnoid tissue under the dura mater. Described in 1692 by Italian professor of anatomy, Antonio Pacchioni (1665–1726) of Rome. Pacchioni also proposed that the dura mater exerted a contractile force on the brain.

Pacemaker *See cardiac pacing.*

Pachon, Michel Victor (1867–1938) French physician from Bordeaux who designed a sensitive oscillometer in 1909 to record arterial pulsation of the extremities.

Pachymeningitis [Greek: *pachys*, thick + *meninx*, membrane + *itis*, inflammation] (Syn. inflammation of the dura mater) The term 'pachy-meningite cervicale hypertrophique' for chronic meningitis of the spinal dura mater was coined by French neurologist, Jean Martin Charcot (1825–1893). *See dura mater.*

Pacini Corpuscle Sensory nerve end organs described by Italian professor of anatomy at Pisa, Filippo Pacini (1812–1883) in 1840. Also described in 1717 by Abraham Vater (1684–1751), professor of pathology and therapeutics at Wittenberg, and known as Pacini–Vater corpuscles. Pacini also described the causative organism of cholera, *Vibrio cholerae*, in 1854.

Padua City in northeast Italy whose famous University was founded in 1222 and rose to prominence during the Renaissance. The anatomical theaters were established during the time of Andreas Vesalius (1514–1564), the greatest anatomist of the period, making anatomy a regular part of the curriculum. Some of the many distinguished students and teachers include: British founder of the Royal College of Physicians, Thomas Linacre (1460–1524); John Caius (1510–1573) who went to study under Montanus (1498–1552); William Harvey (1578–1657) who was taught by Hieronymus Fabricus ab Aquapendente (1533–1619); Giovanni Battista Morgagni (1682–1771) who showed the relationship between anatomy and disease; Galileo Galilei (1564–1642) who taught mathematics and astronomy; and James Gregory (1638–1675) a Scottish mathematician.

Padutin Proteolytic enzyme, now known as serine protease, which activates plasminogen. In 1926 E. K. Frey (b 1888) and H. Kraut isolated a substance from urine which, when injected intravenously into dogs, caused a drop in blood pressure. They named it 'kallikrein' and later changed it to 'padutin'. In 1929 Frey observed that the fluid in a large pancreatic cyst contained the same substance. It has remained non-specific treatment for many conditions including thromboangitis obliterans, indigestion and impotence.

Pagenstecher Ointment Secret remedy consisting of yellow oxide of mercury and prepared by German ophthalmologist, Alexander Pagenstecher (1828–1879). He also defined a method of surface marking the origin of attachment of any movable abdominal tumor.

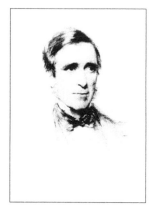

Sir James Paget (1814–1899). Courtesy of the National Library of Medicine

Paget, Sir James (1814–1899) Son of a shipowner and mayor of Great Yarmouth. He studied medicine at St Bartholomew's Hospital where he discovered the parasite, *Trichinella spiralis*, while still a student. He became a surgeon at the same hospital and attended Queen Victoria. He gave an original description of eczema of the nipple and mammary cancer (Paget disease) in 1874. His *Lectures on Surgical Pathology and Clinical Lectures* was published in 1853.

Paget Disease Osteitis deformans is a disease of late life and was described by Sir James Paget (1814–1889) in 1877.

Paget Disease Carcinoma of the nipple accompanied by eczematous changes and carcinoma of the lactiferous ducts. Described by Sir James Paget (1814–1889) in 1874.

Pahvant Valley Fever *See tularaemia.*

Pain [Latin: *poena*] Sensation of discomfort or distress in response to a stimulus, found in all living organisms. Higher animals respond with a natural reaction such as rubbing the affected organ or seeking to avoid the painful stimulus. In man the physical and emotional consequences of pain have affected human history. Prehistoric man learned to avoid harmful stimuli thereby improving chances of survival, and attributed it to gods or devils. Babylonian clay tablets reveal the practice of exorcisms and incantations to relieve pain. The ancient Chinese developed acupuncture and later anesthesia was used for relief. Egyptian papyri describe headaches, toothaches and facial pain and they believed that the seat of pain was the heart and not the brain. Narcotic plants such as madragora, Indian hemp, henbane and poppy were used by Greeks, Romans and Egyptians to overcome pain. Alcmaeon, a pupil of Pythagorus (580–500 BC) was the first to postulate that the brain perceived stimuli. His theory was forgotten for over 200 years until it was revived by Theoprastus (372–287 BC). The earliest form of electrotherapy for neuralgia and headache was practiced with the use of the torpedo fish by Dioscorides (AD 40–90). The modern theory of pain which states that whenever a stimulus is applied in excess it causes pain, was suggested by Erasmus Darwin (1731–1802) and developed by Wilhelm Erb (1840–1921), Friedrich Gustav Jakob Henle (1809–1895) and others. Since then several other theories have been proposed and research and the struggle to conquer pain continues.

Painter's Colic (Syn: lead colic, colica pictonum, French: colique des peintres) Intestinal colic caused by lead poisoning and found in house-painters in the 19th century.

Painting Various maladies such as palsy of the limbs, black teeth, cachexia, and loss of sense of smell occurred in professional painters. In 1700 Bernardino Ramazzini (1633–1714) described causes in *On the Diseases of Tradesmen* and attributed them to materials such as red and white lead, varnish and various oils used in painting. Jean François Fernel (1497–1558), physician to Henry II of France, described palsy of hands and colicky abdominal pains in a painter from Anjou in 1554. These symptoms are now recognized as typical of lead toxicity. *See lacquer poisoning.*

Pajot, Charles (1816–1896) Obstetrician in Paris who designed a decapitating hook, and described a method of using obstetric forceps to exert a tangential force giving a resultant force in the direction of the birth canal during delivery.

Palade, George Emil (b 1912) Romanian cell biologist who studied in Bucharest, where he became professor of anatomy. He emigrated to the USA in 1946 and worked at the Rockefeller Institute in New York before moving to Yale in 1972. In 1990 he became professor of cellular and molecular biology at the University of California at San Diego. He developed cell fractionation methods and described mitochondria, endoplasmic reticulum, ribosomes and the Golgi apparatus. He showed that protein synthesis occurs on RNA strands and that these proteins are carried through the cell wall in vacuoles. He shared the Nobel Prize for Physiology or Medicine in 1974. *See ribosomes.*

Paleobotany [Greek: *palaios*, old] *See paleophytology.*

Paleolithic Age [Greek: *palaios*, old + *lithos*, stone] Term suggested by British politician and biologist, Sir John Lubbock (1834–1913) in 1865 to divide the Stone Age, on the basis of stone artifacts, into the time of rough stone instruments (Paleolithic) and a later stage of polished stone (Neolithic) instruments. The Paleolithic age was later divided into the period of Neanderthal man and the time of appearance of *Homo sapiens* or modern man.

Paleontology [Greek: *palaios*, old + *onto* + beings + *logos*, discourse] Sir Richard Owen (1804–1892) first used the term in 1838 and wrote *Palaeontology* in 1860. It is the study of the origin and development of life on Earth. It started with studies of fossils by Conrad Gesner (1516–1565) in 1565, and was established as a science by Georges Cuvier (1769–1832) of Paris around 1800. The Palaeontographical Society was founded in London in 1843 and published important treatises on Earth's organic remains.

Paleopathology [Greek: *palaios*, old + *pathos*, suffering + *logos*, discourse] Study of ancient diseases through examination of mummies, fossils, osseous remains, Egyptian papyri and Babylonian clay tablets. Coronary atherosclerosis, schistosomiasis, bone tumors, tuberculous abscesses and many other conditions have been found to be thousands of years old through such examination. A pioneer in the field was Sir Mark Armand Ruffer (1859–1917) who studied conditions such as tuberculosis of the spine, arteriosclerosis and gall stones in Egyptian mummies from 3000 BC.

Paleophytology [Greek: *palaios*, old + *phyton*, plant + *logos*, discourse] Branch of paleontology which deals with fossil plants. *Fossil Botany* was written by Solms-Laubach of the

University of Göttingen in 1891, and *Studies in Fossil Botany* was published in 1900 by Henry Scott Dunkinfield (1854–1934), keeper of the Jodrell Laboratory at Kew. Other books including: *English Wealden Flora* (1894), *Jurassic Flora* (1900–1903), and *Plant Life through the Ages* were published by English botanist, Sir Albert Charles Seward (1863–1941) of Lancaster.

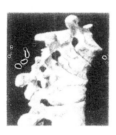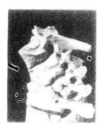

Tuberculosis of the dorsal spine in a New Stone Age skeleton. From Bartels, P. (1970) *Arch. Anthrop.* 34, 243, with permission

Paleozoic Period [Greek: *palaios*, old + *zoe*, life] Era corresponding to the lowest stratified layer of the Earth containing the remains of the earliest forms of life, over 400 million years ago. It was named by the British geologist, Adam Sedgwick (1785–1873).

Palate [Latin: *palatum*, palate] Partition dividing the oral and nasal passages, known to ancient physicians as the 'diaphragma oris'. It was differentiated into the hard and soft palate by Andreas Vesalius (1514–1564) in 1550.

Pale Hypertension Together with red hypertension, were noted by German physician, Franz von Volhard (1872–1950), professor at Halle (1897) and Frankfurt (1927) in 1931. Red hypertension is essential hypertension without renal complications, and pale hypertension is essential hypertension with renal complications and other forms of secondary hypertension.

Palfyn Sinus Space within the crista galli of the ethmoid communicating with the frontal and ethmoidal. Described by Jean Palfyn (1650–1730), professor of anatomy at Paris in 1702.

Pallas, Peter Simon (1741–1811) Son of a German professor of surgery. He studied medicine at Halle, Leiden and Göttingen, but later devoted his career to natural history in England and later in Russia. He reclassified worms, sponges and corals and his methods laid the foundations for modern taxonomy. He published *Miscellania Zoologica* (1766), *Spicelia Zoologica* (1767) and other works. Several species of birds were named after him.

Palmer, David Daniel (1845–1913) Founder of chiropractic medicine in 1895. He was a storekeeper from Toronto and

established his School of Chiropractic Medicine at Davenport, Iowa in 1899. His son B.J. Palmer (1881–1961) helped to promote his system of medicine.

Palmiter, Richard De Forest (b 1942) American molecular geneticist who became professor of biochemistry at the University of Washington in 1981. He produced the first transgenic mice by injecting human growth hormone into a mouse embryo. *See genetic engineering.*

Palmitic Acid Most fats and oils contain it and it was found in margarine by Heintz in 1852 and in olive oil by Collett in 1854. Tripalmitin was discovered to be the chief constituent of olive oil, by Heintz and Krug in 1857.

Palpation [Latin: *palpatio*, to touch] Method of physical examination by touch has no traceable definite time of origin. It was practiced by witch doctors and sorcerers. Hippocrates (460–377 BC) described its application in diagnosis.

Paludism [Latin: *palus*, marsh] Malaria. The term derives its origin from the belief that it arises from the noxious gas in marshes.

Paludrine [Latin: *palus*, marsh] *See antimalarials*

Pampiniform Plexus [Latin: *pampinus*, tendril] The spermatic cord derives its name from its resemblance to vine tendrils.

PAN *See polyarteritis nodosa.*

Panacea [Greek: *panakeia*, to heal] Daughter of the Greek god of medicine Aesculapius, and goddess of health. Her name was given to a mythical herb capable of curing all diseases.

Pancoast, Joseph (1805–1882) New Jersey professor of anatomy and surgery at Jefferson Medical College. He performed a section of the trigeminal nerve at the foramen ovale as treatment for trigeminal neuralgia in 1872. His *A Treatise on Operative Surgery* was published in 1844.

Pancoast Tumor Superior sulcus tumor of the apex of the lung, causing pressure on the chest wall, intercostal nerves and brachial plexus, and differs from other lung tumors. American radiologist, Henry Khunrath Pancoast (1875–1939) of Philadelphia, described it in 1932. He came from a Quaker family and was professor of radiology at the University of Pennsylvania. He described the radiological features of an aneurysm of the thoracic aorta in 1908. *See Horner syndrome.*

Pancreas [Greek: *pan*, all + *kreas*, flesh] Dutch physician, Regnier de Graff (1641–1673) collected pancreatic juice through an artificial pancreatic fistula in a dog in 1664. Polyuria and thirst in dogs after experimental excision of the pancreas was demonstrated by Johann Conrad Brunner (1653–1727) in 1683. The relationship between fibrosis of the pancreas and diabetes mellitus was noted by John Bright in the middle of the 19th century. The first systematic experiments to show that pancreatectomy led to diabetes mellitus were by Josef von Merring (1849–1908) and Oskar Minkowski (1858–1931) in 1889. In 1903 Eugene Lindsay Opie (b 1873) suggested that an antidiabetic substance was present in the islets of Langerhans. The alpha and beta cells in the islets of Langerhans were identified independently by M. A. Lane (1907), and R. R. Bensley (1911), of America. *See insulin, islets of Langerhans.*

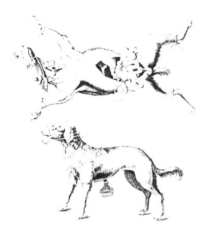

Pancreatic fistula induced by de Graaf

Pancreatic Function In 1902 Sir William Maddock Bayliss (1860–1924) and Henry Ernest Starling (1866–1927) discovered the hormone secretin which travels via the blood stream and causes pancreatic secretion in duodenal mucosa. The suggestion that the secretions depend on a reflex between the duodenal mucosa and vagus was made by Ivan Petrovitch Pavlov (1849–1936) in 1910. Fecal fat estimation as a function of pancreatic insufficiency was devised by Schmidt of Berlin in 1910. In the same year, the estimation of diastase in the urine was used as a diagnostic test by Julius Wohlgemuth (1874–1948).

Pancreatic Juice Shown to breakdown food during digestion in 1844 by Gabriel Gustav Valentin (1810–1883) of Germany.

Pancreatic Resection Carcinoma was treated with resection of the head of the pancreas and the duodenum in 1937 by German-born Chicago surgeon Alexander Brunschwig (1901–1969).

Pancreatic Duct Discovered by Bavarian anatomist Johann Georg Wirsung (1600–1643) in 1631. He was assassinated in a quarrel over the priority of the discovery. His discovery was announced by his pupil J. Vesling (1598–1649) of Padua in 1641.

Pancreatoduodenectomy Involves the excision of the head of pancreas and duodenum in cases of pancreatic cancer and was first performed by Chicago surgeon Alexander Brunschwig (1901–1969) in 1937. He described a one-stage operation in 1943.

Pandemic [Greek: *pan*, all + demos, *people*] Widespread epidemic of contagious disease throughout a continent or country. Black Death in the Middle Ages was one such.

Pander Cell Nerve cells in the subthalamic nucleus described by German embryologist and anatomist, Christian Heinrich Pander (1794–1865) in 1817. He studied medicine in Berlin, Dorpat, Göttingen and Würzburg and obtained his MD in 1817. He discovered the embryonic layers and coined the term 'blastoderm'.

Paneth, Frederick Adolf (1887–1958) Austrian chemist born in Vienna and graduated from Munich. He moved to Britain in 1933 and worked first at Imperial College in London and later at Durham University. After the War he returned to Germany and was director of the Max Planck Institute. He developed radioactive tracers (with George Charles von Hevesy, 1885–1966) and used the method to establish the age of rocks.

Paneth Cells Secretory cells in the mucosa of the small intestine were described in 1887 by Joseph Paneth (1857–1890), professor of physiology at Breslau.

Panizza Foramen Interventricular foramen of the heart normally found in lower vertebrates. Its abnormal presence in mammals was studied in 1844 by Bartolomeo Panizza (1785–1867), Italian comparative anatomist at Pavia.

Pantheon [Greek: *pan*, all + *theos*, god] Temple in Rome to all the gods was built by Agrippa in 25 BC during the reign of Augustus. Also used generally to refer to any public building dedicated to notable people.

Pantothenic Acid A characteristic dermatitis in poultry due to nutritional deficiency was noted by A. T. Ringrose and L. C. Norris in 1930. The deficient factor was identified as the same as 'bios' previously noted (1901) as necessary for reproduction in yeast. It was identified as a B vitamin and constituent of coenzyme A by John Roger Williams (1893–1988) in 1933. The structure of pantothenic acid was elucidated by D. W. Woolley in 1940.

Panum, Peter Ludwig (1820–1885) Danish physiologist from Copenhagen who studied the pathology of embolism in 1868, malformations of the embryo in birds eggs in 1860 and poisonous alkaloids in 1856. During an outbreak of measles in the Faroe Islands in 1846 he made an epidemiological study of it.

Pap Smear *See George Nicholas Papanicolau, cervical smear.*

Papanicolaou, George Nicholas (1883–1962) American anatomist and cytologist who was born in Greece and introduced cytology into diagnosis of cancer. He investigated normal cyclical changes of the vaginal epithelium with Charles Rupert Stockard (1879–1939) in 1917 and described the role of the vaginal smear in cancer in 1928. Papanicolaou and Herbert Frederick Traut (b 1894) published *The Diagnosis of Uterine Cancer by Vaginal Smear* in 1943. He also wrote *New Cancer Diagnosis* (1928), *A New procedure for staining Vaginal Smears* (1942), and *Atlas of Exfoliative Cytology* in 1954. The smear test used in diagnosis of cervical cancer is popularly known as the 'Pap smear'.

Papataci Fever *See phlebotomus fever.*

Papaverine [Latin: *papaver*, poppy] An alkaloid of opium first isolated by Georg Franz Merck (1825–1873) in 1848 and synthesized by Pictet and Gams in 1909.

Papilledema The mechanism of swelling of the optic disc was explained by Viennese neurologist, Ludwig Turck (1810–1868). Its association with headache and brain tumor was noted by Edward Constant Seguin (1843–1898), professor of neurology at the College of Physicians and Surgeons, Columbia University.

Pappenheim, Artur (1870–1916) German professor of hematology at Berlin who founded the journal *Folia Hematologica* in 1904. The Pappenheim stain is a specific test for plasma cells.

Paper Chromatography *See chromatography.*

Paper Said to have been invented in China around 170 BC although the Egyptians used the papyrus reed to make a paper-like material several thousand years previously. In Europe it was made from cotton rags in 1300. The first paper mill was established at Dartford, England in 1494, and coarse white paper was produced by an Englishman of German origin, Sir John Speilman at Dartford in 1590. Continuous paper of indefinite length was produced in 1807, the longest roll being 13,800 feet.

Papilla [Latin: *papillae*, pimple] Term first used by the Romans to refer to the nipple of the breast. Jacopo

Berengario da Carpi (1470–1530), or Berengarius, an Italian surgeon from Pavia, applied the term to renal papillae. Marcello Malpighi (1628–1694) introduced it to describe the papillae of the tongue in 1670.

Papillae *See papilla.*

Papin, Denis (1647–1712) French physician and physicist from Blois who studied medicine at the University of Angers. He came to England in 1675 and worked for a brief period with Robert Boyle (1627–1691). He invented the steam digester with a safety valve in 1681 which he used to dissolve bone and other products under pressure. His principle was later applied to the present-day domestic pressure cooker and autoclave..

Pappenheimer Bodies Iron granules found in erythrocytes in peripheral blood in cases of hemolytic anemia. Described by New York biochemist, Alwin Max Pappenheimer (1878–1955). He introduced treatment of rickets with cod liver oil (vitamin D) in 1920.

Paprika-Splitters' Lung Paprika or red pepper was introduced to Europe for medicinal purposes by Turkish invaders during the 16th century. It later became a prominent industry in Yugoslavia and Hungary and women who split this fruit to remove the mold, *Mucor stolonifera*, developed pulmonary disease which manifested as a cough with thick expectoration from cavities in the lung.

Papyri The Egyptians used the papyrus reed to make a form of paper from which a large part of our knowledge of their civilization and medical practices has been obtained. A mathematical papyrus from 1650 BC, written by Ahmes, was found by Henry A. Rhind (1833–1863) in the 19th century and is now at the British Museum. The Ebers papyrus (1500 BC) was bought by Egyptologist George Moritz Ebers (1837–1898) of Berlin in 1862. It contains details of Egyptian medicine dating back to 3300 BC and was the first papyrus containing descriptions of medical practices, herbal medicines, demonology and mineral medicines. Another medical treatise from 1600 BC was found near Luxor in 1862 by Edwin Smith (1822–1906). It relates to early Egyptian surgery from 2500 BC and contains descriptions of 48 diseases, plasters, splints for broken bones, suturing, cauterization and other ancient but advanced methods of surgical and medical practice. The therapeutic Papyrus of Thebes, which is 65 feet long and dates from 1552 BC, deals with medicine and gives specific remedies for diseases. One chapter is devoted to diseases of children and another to diseases of women. The Hearst papyrus (1500 BC) was discovered at Der-el-Ballas in 1899 and is now at the

University of California. The Brugsch papyrus or the Greater Berlin papyrus, dates from the time of first Egyptian dynasty, and was found near the pyramids of Sakarah at Memphis. It describes the heart, veins and other organs.

Paquelin, Claude Andre (1836–1905) Physician from Paris who, in 1876, introduced a cautery made of platinum heated by passage of a volatile hydrocarbon.

Para-Aminobenzoic Acid The significance of the structural resemblance between the antibacterial substance sulfanilamide, and para-aminobenzoic acid, a bacterial antagonist, was shown independently by British microbiologists, Donald Devereux Woods (1912–1964), and Paul Fildes (1882–1971) in 1940. The Woods–Fildes hypothesis, that para-aminobenzoic acid is an essential metabolite of bacteria and sulfanilamides, by virtue of their structural similarity in blocking bacterial metabolism, formed the basis for research on sulfanilamides as effective antibiotics.

Para-Aminosalicylic Acid (PAS) Benzoates and salicylates increase respiration in bacteria and this observation led to the search for competitive inhibitors for use as antibacterial agents. Jögen Lehman (b 1898) introduced PAS (4-aminosalicylic acid) in 1946, and it became a first-line drug in treatment of tuberculosis.

Paracelsus (1493–1541) Also known as Theoprastus Bombastus von Hohenheim, was a physician, alchemist, philosopher and astrologer from Switzerland. His name means beyond (para) Celsus, after Aulus Cornelius Celsus (25 BC–AD 50) a celebrated physician. Paracelsus was one of the first to discard the ideas of Galen (AD 129–200) and publicly burned the *Canon* of Avicenna (980–1037). He was the founder of chemical therapeutics and introduced mercurials as treatment for syphilis. He also described miner's disease. He advocated teaching in vernacular language (German) instead of Latin, and wrote on a variety of subjects including cosmology, anthropology, sorcery, astrology, philosophy and medicine.

Paracentesis Abdominis [Latin: *para*, side by side + *kentesis*, to puncture] Used as treatment for ascites and dropsy by Hippocrates (460–377 BC) and revived by Paul of Aegina (625–690). Southey tubes with trocar and cannula for paracentesis abdominis were designed in 1879 by Reginald Southey (1835–1899), a physician at St Bartholomew's Hospital. *See ascites.*

Paracentesis Thoracis [Latin: *para*, side by side + *kentesis*, to puncture] Thoracentesis was suggested by Hippocrates (460–377 BC) who recommended making an incision in the chest. This method was later considered dangerous and discouraged by several physicians including Caelius Aurelianus in the 5th century, but Paul of Aegina (625–690) revived it. In 1850 Henry Ingersoll Bowditch (1808–1892) and Morrill Wyman (1812–1903) of the Massachusetts General Hospital were the first in America to remove fluid from the chest through a puncture with a trocar into the chest wall. The suction pump for the procedure was designed by Wyman.

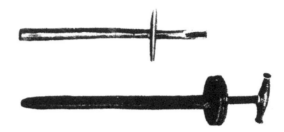

Instruments used for thorcic paracentesis

Paragonimus westermani Lung fluke causing endemic hemoptysis mainly in the Far East and China, described by Kerbert in 1878. The ova were described in a paper *Ueber parasitare Hamaptoe or Gangrenosis pulmonum* by Erwin Otto Edouard von Baelz (1849–1913) in 1880. The life cycle was elucidated by three Japanese parasitologists, K. Nakagawa (b 1919), H. Kobayashi (b 1920) and S. Yokogawa (b 1919).

Paraldehyde Rapid acting sedative introduced into medicine as a narcotic by Vincenzo Cervillo (1854–1919) of Palermo in 1884. It was used in obstetrics by Rosenfield and Leo Max Davidoff (1898–1975) in 1932.

Paralysis Agitans [Greek: *para*, side by side + *lyein*, to loosen; Latin: *agitans*, putting in motion] Shaking palsy was described by London physician, James Parkinson (1755–1824) in 1817 and later named in his honor.

Parangi Peculiar affection of the skin accompanied by ulceration and general debility amongst the people of Ceylon, who believed it to be venereal. Described by Loos in 1868 and later by Dunforth as 'vanni' plague (Vanni: a village in Ceylon) in 1873. A study of the causes was made by W. E. Kynsey, the principal Civil Medical Officer of Ceylon.

Paranoia [Greek: *para*, beside + *nous*, mind] Term used by Hippocrates (460–377 BC) in his classification of mental diseases to refer to a primary form of insanity. Emil Kraepelin (1856–1926) of Germany adopted the term to modern psychiatry in 1886 to denote a state of extreme suspicion.

Paraplegia [Greek: *para*, beside + *plege*, stroke] Paralysis of the body transversely affecting both sides. Sir William Gull

(1816–1890) of Guy's Hospital made postmortem studies of cases in 1856.

Parasitology [Greek: *parasitos*, one who eats at another's expense + *logos*, discourse] Intestinal worms were the first parasites to be identified by ancient physicians as a cause of disease. Examination of tissues from 3000-year-old Egyptian mummies showed the presence of *Trichinella spiralis* and *Schistosoma hematobium*. Hippocrates (460–377 BC) studied parasites and divided intestinal worms into round lumbricae (*Ascaris*), and broad lumbrici (*Taenia*). Intestinal worms resembling earthworms were described by Paul of Aegina (625–690). The first protozoan parasite identified was *Giardia lamblia*, by Antoni van Leeuwenhoek (1632–1723) who noted it in his stools in 1681. The first anatomical description of *Ascaris lumbricoides* was given by Edward Tyson (1650–1708) in 1683. The egg and the reproductive process of the roundworm were described in 1684 by Francesco Redi (1626–1698) of Italy, regarded as the first parasitologist. *Echinococcus* was used for the vesicular hydatid by Karl Asmund Rudolphi (1771–1832) in 1808. Experimental methods started in 1850 when Ernst Friedrich Herbst (1803–1893) succeeded in transmitting *Trichina* by feeding infected meat to animals. Carl Theodor Ernest von Siebold demonstrated that dogs could be experimentally infected with *Echinococcus* in 1854 and its complete life history and morphology was given by Rudolph George Leuckart (1822–1898) in 1860. Theodor Maximillian Bilharz (1825–1862), professor in zoology at Cairo, in 1851 discovered *Schistosoma hematobium* in the blood vessels of patients. Thomas Spencer Cobbold (1828–1886) of London, a leading helminthologist and a friend of Sir Patrick Manson (1844–1922), named *Filaria bancrofti* and *Bilharzia hematobia*. David Gruby (1810–1898) of Hungary proposed the genus Trypanosome after his discovery of the protozoan in blood of frogs in 1844. He also showed transmission of microfilaria infection through blood transfusion. *Dracunculus oculi*, a filarial worm which causes loa loa, was described by E.G. Guyot in 1778, and the larval forms of the parasite in the eye was studied by Patrick Mason in 1891. Sir Joseph Bancroft (1836–1894) discovered *Wuchereria bancrofti*, cause of filariasis in Brisbane, Australia in 1876. The protozoan, *Plasmodium*, that causes malaria was discovered in 1880 by Charles Louis Alphonse Laveran (1845–1922), a French parasitologist, while professor of pathological anatomy at the University of Rome. Laveran received the Nobel Prize for his work on malariology in 1907. M Clifford Dobell (1886–1949), an eminent protozoologist, published the classic works *Amoeba living in Man* (1919), and *Intestinal Protozoa of Man* (1921).

Parasympathetic Nervous System [Greek: *para*, beside + *sympatheticos*, feeling] Term introduced in 1905 by John Newport Langley (1852–1925), a neurophysiologist from Newbury, Berkshire. He also coined the terms 'preganglionic' and 'postganglionic' while he was a professor at Cambridge. *See autonomic nervous system.*

Parathormone *See parathyroid.*

Parathyroid [Greek: *para*, beside + *thyreos*, shield] Glands described in the Indian rhinoceros by Sir Richard Owen (1804–1892) in 1850, and later in man by Rudolph Virchow (1821–1902) in 1863. Following removal of the thyroid, patients were observed to develop agonizing muscular cramps leading to death within a few days. The cause was not identified although the existence of parathyroid glands had been known since 1850. The four small bodies, beside the thyroid glands, were described as accessory thyroid tissues by Swedish anatomist, Ivar Victor Sandström (1852–1889) in 1879. In 1891 French physiologist Marcel Eugène Émile Gley (1857–1930) removed the parathyroid glands while keeping the thyroid intact and demonstrated a fatal tetany. He then removed the thyroid gland while preserving the parathyroids without any serious ill effects thus demonstrating the importance of the parathyroid in preserving life. Parathyroid extract was obtained by Adolf Melancthon Hanson (1888–1959) in 1923, and its active principle was isolated by Canadian biochemist Bertram James Collip (1892–1965) in 1925. A year later Viennese surgeon, Felix Mandl (1892–1957), explored the neck of a patient with osteitis fibrosa cystica and removed a parathyroid tumor which caused an improvement. The association between renal calculi and hyperparathyroidism was noted by Fuller Albright (1900–1969) in 1934, although the association with bone disease had been noted much earlier by Courtial in 1700. S.W. Stanbury performed the first subtotal parathyroidectomy for hyperparathyroidism secondary to uremia and renal failure in 1960. Parathyroid hormone was isolated in pure form by an American, Gerald D. Aurbach (1927–1991) of the National Institute of Health, in 1959. The association between peptic ulceration and hyperparathyroidism was described by L. Pyrah, A. Hodgkinson and C.K. Anderson in 1966.

Paratyphoid Term coined by Émile Charles Achard (1860–1944) of Paris who isolated the *Salmonella* bacillus in 1896.

Paravertebral Somatic Block Injection of local anesthetic close to the vertebral column where the nerve roots emerge from the intervertebral foramina. Introduced by Hugo Sellheim in 1909. Lawen named it 'paravertebral conduction anesthesia' in 1911. Paravertebral block of the eleventh and twelfth thoracic vertebrae in labor was first practiced by J.G.P. Cleland of Oregon in 1933.

Pardee, Arthur Beck (b 1921) American biochemist born in Chicago and trained at the University of California, Berkeley. He was appointed professor of pharmacology at Harvard in 1975. He worked with Linus Pauling (b 1901) on tumor metabolism and antibody reactions, and with Jacques Lucien Monod (1910–1976) on the lac operon of *Escherichia coli*. He discovered feedback control of amino acid synthesis and did important work on DNA repair and synthesis.

Pardee, Harold Ensign Bennett (1886–1972) American cardiologist who described the downward deflection of the T wave in ECG of coronary disease. He was born in New York and graduated from Columbia University. *See myocardial infarction.*

Paré, Ambroise (1510–1590) One of the greatest figures of the Renaissance and undoubtedly it's greatest surgeon. He was born at Bourg-Hersent in France. He was initially opposed by the French Faculties as he was from a simple background and could not read Latin. He overcame this and became the most famous French surgeon of all times. He introduced anatomical discipline into surgery and his contributions include: discovery that gunshot wounds are not poisonous, application of simple dressings to such wounds instead of hot oil, ligature for bleeding after amputation, podalic version of the fetus in utero, artificial limbs, many surgical instruments and implantation of teeth. He held the first judicial postmortem and was surgeon to Francois I, Henry II, Charles IX, Henri III, Henri IV and other members of the French royalty. His work was translated into Latin, German and many other languages.

Parenchyma [Greek: *para*, beside + *chuma*, juice] Used in anatomy in 300 BC by Erasistratus to refer to a gland-like substance of the liver, spleen, kidneys and lungs. It derives from the belief that blood poured like juice into the adjacent (para) organ and became converted into the substance of that organ.

Paresis [Greek: *paresis*, relaxation] Condition of slight or incomplete paralysis. *See general paralysis of the insane.*

Parietal Cell [Latin: *parietalis*, pertaining to walls] Cells of the gastric glands described by Prussian professor of physiology and histology, Rudolf Peter Heinrich Heidenhaim (1834–1897) of the University of Breslau in 1888. Gastric parietal cell antibodies occur in nearly 80% of patients with pernicious anemia, as shown by K. B. Taylor and co-workers in 1962.

Parietal Lobe Syndrome [Latin: *parietalis*, pertaining to walls] Sensory aphasic syndrome accompanied by apraxia and alexia, seen in lesions of the left parietal lobe. Described by Italian psychiatrist, Leonardo Bianchi (1848–1927). Joseph Jules Dejerine (1849–1917) also described it in 1914.

Parieties [Latin: *parietalis*, pertaining to walls] Old term for walls of the abdomen and thorax.

Paris, John Ayrton (1785–1856) Cornish physician from Penzance who proposed that arsenical fumes from industry caused scrotal cancer. His theory was later disproved.

Paris Nomina Anatomica [Latin: *nomen*, name; Greek: *ana*, through + *tome*, cut] Terminology in anatomy (PNA) adopted at the 6th International Congress of Anatomists in Paris in 1955.

Parish Areas in England established by the archbishop of Canterbury, Honorius in AD 636. By the 15th century over 10,000 parishes existed and the Parish Registers which later helped in the study of vital statistics of that period were established in 1538.

Park, Mungo (1771–1806) Edinburgh physician and early explorer of Africa. His first expedition to Niger lasted from 1794 to 1797 and on his return he published *Travels in the Interior Districts of Africa* in 1799. He was killed in Boussa during his second trip to Africa.

Park Aneurysm Arteriovenous aneurysm which communicates with two veins. Described by English surgeon, Henry Park (1744–1831).

Parker Arch Part of the developing skull which completes the occipital portion of the primitive cranium in the lower animals. Described in 1870 by Kitchen William Parker (1823–1890), a general practitioner in London and assistant to Todd at King's College, London.

Parker Incision Incision parallel with the Poupart ligament over the area of maximum dullness due to appendicular abscess. Described by New York surgeon, Willard Parker (1800–1884) who was the first to operate on a case of appendicitis in America.

Parkes, A. Edmund (1819–1876) English sanitary reformer in the 19th century. His name is enshrined in the Parkes Museum of Hygiene instituted in 1876 at University College, London.

Parkes, Sir Alan Sterling (1900–1990) English physiologist, born in Purley, Surrey and educated at the University of Cambridge where he became professor of reproductive physiology in 1961. His main area of research was reproductive endocrinology, and he published *The Internal Secretions of the Ovary* (1929) and other books on the subject.

Parkinson, James (1755–1824) London physician and student of John Hunter (1728–1793). He described perforated appendix, but is famous for his description of paralysis agitans given in 1817. He also recognized ruptured appendix as a cause of death. *See Parkinson disease.*

Parkinson, Sir John (1885–1976) *See Wolf–Parkinson–White syndrome.*

Parkinson, John (1567–1650) Nottingham apothecary who practiced in London. He published a comprehensive English book on plants in 1640, *Theatrum Botanicum,* that contains descriptions of over 3,800 plants.

Parkinson Disease (Syn: paralysis agitans, shaking palsy) Characterized by mask-like facies, tremor and slowness of movements. Described by London physician, James Parkinson (1755–1824) in 1817. Stereotaxic surgery was used as treatment to produce discrete lesions in the basal ganglia by Ernest Adolf Spiegel (1895–1985), H.T. Wycis, M. Marks and A.J. Lee of New York in 1947. Their method was improved by R. Hassler and T. Reichart in 1954, and I. S. Copper and G. J. Bravo in 1958. Implanting of cells from the adrenal gland into the brain as treatment was first proposed by Ignacio Navarro in 1987.

Parham Bands Circular wires used for internal fixation of fractured long bones. Devised by an American surgeon from New Orleans, Frederick William Parham (1856–1927), in 1913.

Parotid Gland [Greek: *para*, besides + *ous*, ear] Term used by Galen (AD 129–200) to denote an inflammatory mass or abscess near the ear. 'Parotis' was first applied by Jean Riolan (1577–1657), a professor of anatomy at Paris in 1640. The excretory duct (Stensen duct) of the gland and its function were discovered by Niels Stensen (1638–1688), professor of anatomy at Copenhagen, in 1682. The first excision was carried out in 1823 by Pierre Augustin Béclard (1785–1825), professor of anatomy at Paris. Auguste Bérard (1802–1846) of Paris published the first monograph on parotid tumors in 1841.

Parotitis [Greek: *para*, besides + *ous*, ear + *itis*, inflammation] *See mumps.*

Paroxysmal Atrial Tachycardia [Greek: *paroxysmos*, excitement; Latin: *atria*, chamber + *tachys*, quick] Described by Léon Bouveret (1850–1929) of Paris in 1889 and named 'atrial tachycardia'. ECG changes were recognized by Sir Thomas Lewis (1881–1945) in 1909, and described in more detail by P.S. Barker and colleagues in 1943. The occurrence in digitalis toxicity was noted by G.R. Herrmann in 1944.

Paroxysmal Hemoglobinuria [Greek: *paroxysmos*, excitement + *haima*, blood + *ouren*, urine; Latin: *globus*, ball] A description was given by Johannis Actuarius, court physician at Constantinople in the 13th century. His *De urinis* was translated by Ambrosio Leoni Nolono in 1529. George Harley (1829–1896) of Haddington in Scotland described two cases in 1865. Suggested to be an autoimmune disease by Julius Donath (1870–1950) and Nobel Prize winner, Karl Landsteiner (1868–1943), in 1903. The similarities between cold urticaria and paroxysmal hemoglobinuria were noted by Thomas Fraser of Edinburgh in 1905. A detailed description of paroxysmal nocturnal hemoglobinuria (Marchiafava–Micheli syndrome) was given by Italian physician Ettore Marchiafava (1847–1935) in 1911. The Ham test showing hemolysis of red cells after incubation with acidified serum was devised by American physician Thomas Hale Ham (b 1905) and H.M. Horack in 1941.

Paroxysmal Nocturnal Hemoglobinuria [Greek: *paroxysmos*, excitement + *haima*, blood + *ouren*, urine; Latin: *nox*, night + *globus*, ball] Marchiafava–Micheli syndrome. *See paroxysmal hemoglobinuria.*

Parrot Fever *See psittacosis.*

Parrot Nodes Nodules on the parietal and frontal bones of the skull in infants with congenital syphilis. Described by French physician Jules Marie Parrot (1829–1883) in 1879.

Parrot Sign Dilatation of the pupils induced by pinching the skin of the neck of patients with meningitis. Described by French physician, Jules Marie Parrot (1829–1883).

Parry Disease Exophthalmic goiter described by English physician, Caleb Hillier Parry (1775–1822) of Bath in 1786. He later published eight more cases and the disease was named after him. Parry also wrote a monograph on arterial pulse.

Parsons, Sir John Herbert (1868–1957) Ophthalmic surgeon at University College Hospital, and curator and pathologist at the Royal London Moorfields Hospital. He published *The Pathology of the Eye* (1904–1908) and other books on ophthalmology.

Parthenogenesis [Greek: *parthenos*, virgin + *genesis*, production] Asexual reproduction or development of an egg without fertilization. Discovered by German zoologist, Karl Theodor Ernest Siebold (1804–1865). The phenomenon was demonstrated experimentally and named by Jacques Loeb (1859–1924), a medical graduate from Strasbourg, in 1884 and further shown in the frog by Eugene Bataillon in 1910.

Partial Gastrectomy *See gastrectomy, Billroth operation.*

Parturition [Latin: *parturio*, bring forth] *See labor, obstetrics.*

PAS *See para-aminosalicylic acid.*

Pascal, Blaise (1623–1662) French mathematician from Clermont-Ferrand and contemporary of Pierre de Fermat (1601–1665). He completed 23 propositions of Euclid at the age 11 and published an essay on cornices at 16. He made a calculating machine in 1617.

Passavant Bar Ridge on the posterior wall of the pharynx, produced by contraction of the palatopharyngeus muscle. Described in 1869 by German surgeon, Philip Gustav Passavant (1815–1893) of Frankfurt.

Passavant Cushion Ridge projecting from the posterior and lateral walls of the nasopharynx at the level of the free margin of the soft palate in cases of atrophic rhinitis. Described by German Surgeon, Philip Gustav Passavant (1815– 1893).

Passive Hypersensitivity Demonstrated to be transferable by Richard Otto (1872–1952) of Berlin in 1906.

Pasteur Institute *See Pasteur, Louis.*

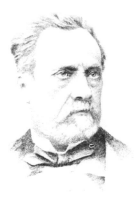

Louis Pasteur (1822–1895). Courtesy of the National Library of Medicine

Pasteur, Louis (1822–1895) French chemist from Dôle and father of modern bacteriology and pasteurization. He showed the presence of living cells in fermentation around 1864. His findings were opposed by several prominent advocates of the spontaneous generation theory. He was appointed professor of chemistry at the Sorbonne in 1867 where his work on tartaric acid led to the discovery of the existence of crystals in two mirror image forms. He postulated the 'germ theory' of disease and showed that the anthrax bacillus could be modified to confer immunity

without producing disease. He used the Latin word, 'vacca' meaning cow, and administered rabies vaccine in 1885. He was the first director of the Pasteur Institute in Paris which was founded with a public donation of 2.5 million francs in 1888.

Pasteurella pestis The first member of the genus was isolated during an epidemic affecting wild hogs and deer by Kitt in 1878. The plague bacillus, *Pasteurella pestis* (or *Yersinia pestis*), was isolated from humans independently by Swiss bacteriologist Alexander Emile Jean Yersin (1863–1943), and Shibasaburo Kitasato (1852–1931) in 1894. The genus was named *Pasteurella* in honor of Louis Pasteur (1822–1895).

Pasteurization a method of partial heat sterilization at 55 to 60°C to prevent fermentation by microorganisms or vinegar formation in wine. Devised by Louis Pasteur (1822– 1895) in 1868.

Patau Syndrome Trisomy 13 syndrome was described by German-born American geneticist, Klaus Patau in 1960.

Patellar Tendon Reflex [Latin: *patella*, shallow dish] *See knee jerk.*

Patent Ductus Arteriosus (PDA) [Latin: *patens*, open + *ducere*, to lead] In 1888 John Cummings Munro (1858– 1910) demonstrated in an infant cadaver that PDA could be ligated, and suggested obliteration in 1907. The characteristic continuous murmur was described by George Alexander Gibson (1854–1913) of Scotland in 1898 and it is known as Gibson murmur. An attempt to close it was made by John W. Strieder in 1937, but closure was incomplete and the patient died. The first successful surgical closure was performed on a 7-year-old girl in 1938 by Robert Edward Gross (1905–1988). *See cardiac surgery.*

Paterson, Donald Ross (1863–1939) *See Plummer–Vinson syndrome.*

Paterson Forceps Bronchoscopic forceps for removal of foreign bodies or biopsy. Designed by British otorhinologist, Donald Ross Paterson (1863–1939) of Cardiff. He also described Kelly–Paterson syndrome in 1919.

Patheticus Oculorum [Greek: *pathetikos*, suffering] The fourth nerve, named by Thomas Willis (1621–1675) in 1650 due to its action of causing downward and outward movements of the eye, giving an appearance of suffering to the face.

Pathognomonic [Greek: *pathos*, suffering + *gnomonikos*, to give judgment] Characteristic sign or symptom of a disease.

Pathological Anatomy *See pathology.*

Pathology [Greek: *pathos*, suffering + *logos*, discourse] The four cardinal signs of inflammation, heat, pain, redness, and swelling were described by Aulus Cornelius Celsus (25 BC–AD 50), a Roman physician. Galen (AD 129–200) devoted six of his books to pathology. Antonio Benivieni (1443–1502), an Italian surgeon from Florence, was one of the first to do autopsies, which earned him the title of the founder of pathological anatomy. The term was introduced in a modern sense by Jean François Fernel (1497–1558), physician to Henry II of France in 1554. The first illustrated book of surgical pathology was published by Marcus Aurelius Severinus (1580–1656) in 1632. One of the greatest pathologists was professor of anatomy at Padua, Giovanni Battista Morgagni (1682–1771). He gave the first descriptions of calcification of coronary arteries, coarctation, endocarditis and carcinoma of the lung. He also correlated clinical findings with autopsy results. An epoch-making study on inflammation, fundamental to pathology, was done by British surgeon John Hunter (1728–1793), and his book *A Treatise on blood, inflammation and gun-shot wounds* was published in 1794. The first American treatise was published by William Edmonds Horner (1793–1853) in 1829. Cellular pathology was inaugurated by Rudolph Virchow (1821–1902), professor of pathology at Berlin. The role of leukocytes in inflammation was studied and explained by William Addison (1802–1881) in 1843. His work on the subject was advanced by German pathologist Julius Friedrich Cohnheim (1839–1884) in 1873, and French zoologist and Nobel Prize winner Elie Metchnikoff (1845–1916) in 1892.

Pathological Society of Great Britain and Ireland Founded in 1906 at a meeting at the University of Manchester. Its founder members were James Lorrain Smith (1861–1931), professor of pathology at Manchester, James Ritchie, professor of bacteriology at Edinburgh and Robert Muir, professor of pathology at Glasgow.

Patin, Guy (1601–1672) French physician and professor of medicine at the College de France who founded the Ecole de Medecin at Paris. He opposed William Harvey's theory of blood circulation.

Paul of Aegina (AD 625–690) Greek surgeon and a physician. His monumental work *Epitomoe medicoe libri septem* in seven volumes was first printed at Venice in 1528. In his sixth book on surgery he gave original descriptions of lithotomy, bronchotomy, tonsillectomy, mastectomy and other procedures. He also freely copied from Galen (AD 129–200), Oribasius (AD 325–403), and Aetius. His complete works were translated into English by Francis Adams (1796–1861) in 1847.

Paul, Theodor (1862–1928) *See antiseptics.*

Paul Sign A feeble apex beat with forcible impulse over the rest of the heart in cases of pericardial adhesions. Described by French physician, Constantin Charles Theodore Paul (1833–1896).

Paul Tube Employed to temporarily drain fecal matter after colostomy in cases of obstruction of the large bowel. Introduced by Frank Thomas Paul (1851–1941), a graduate of Guy's Hospital (1871) and surgeon to the Liverpool Royal Infirmary, in 1892.

Paul–Bunnel Test Detects heterophilic antibodies. Devised by American epidemiologist, John Rodman Paul (1893–1971) and American physician from New Haven, Walls Willard Bunnel (1902–1979) in 1932. It was made specific for glandular fever by the introduction of a differential method by P. H. Walker (1935) and I. Davidsohn in 1938.

Paulesco, Nicholas Constantin (1869–1931) Rumanian physician and pioneer in the study of diabetes. He qualified in medicine from Paris and returned to Bucharest as professor of physiology in 1904. He pointed out the causal relationship between diabetes and lesions of the pancreas.

Pauling, Linus Carl (1900–1994) Eminent American biochemist, born in Portland, Oregon. He was educated at Oregon State College and Caltech and did postdoctoral work in Munich, Zurich and Copenhagen. He wrote *Introduction to Quantum Mechanics* and *The Nature of the Chemical Bond*. He determined the helical structure of large protein molecules in 1951, and was one of the first to study DNA in detail. Pauling was awarded the Nobel Prize Chemistry for his work on chemical bonding and molecular structure in 1954, and the Nobel Peace Prize in 1962 for his opposition to atmospheric nuclear weapons testing.

Paulus Aegineta *See Paul of Aegina.*

Pavlik Harness *See congenital dislocation of the hip.*

Pavlov, Ivan Petrovitch (1849–1936) Experimental physiologist born in Ryazan, a small town in central Russia. He was first attracted to the study of science through reading a Russian translation of George Henry Lewes' *Practical Physiology* at the age of 15. He entered the seminary at Ryazan but he left in 1870 to study at the University of St Petersburg. He passed the state examination in 1879 and became an approved physician although his doctoral thesis in medicine was not completed until 1883. The secretory nerves of the pancreas were discovered by him in 1888, and he was elected professor of physiology at the Military Medical Academy of St Petersburg in 1890. He became director of the Institute of Experimental Medicine in 1913. He worked on the circulatory system, digestive glands and higher nervous activity, and he received the Nobel Prize in 1904. He lectured and worked on conditioned reflexes caused by the involvement of the cerebral cortex in modifying innate reflexes until 1926.

Pavy, Frederick William (1829–1911) English worker on carbohydrate metabolism and diabetes. He correlated hyperglycemia and glycosuria and published *Treatise on Food and Dietetics* in 1874. He described cyclic or recurrent albuminuria (Pavy disease) in 1885, a condition noted in some apparently normal individuals, where albumin is absent in early morning urine samples but appears later in the day. He also described the involvement of joints in typhoid, and introduced ammonia instead of caustic potash in the preparation of Fehling solution.

Pavy Disease *See Pavy, Frederick William.*

Pawlik Triangle Area in the anterior wall of the vagina in contact with the base of the bladder and free of vaginal rugae. Described by Karel Pawlik (1849–1914), a gynecologist at Prague in 1887.

Paxton Disease Involves the hairs of the axilla due to *Tinea*. Described by Francis Valentine Paxton (d 1924) in 1869.

Payr Membrane Fold of the peritoneum over the splenic flexure of the colon. Described in 1910 by Erwin Payr (1871–1947), professor of surgery at Leipzig.

PDA *See patent ductus arteriosus.*

Peacock, Thomas Bevill (1812–1882) Physician at St Thomas' Hospital who wrote a treatise on malformation of the heart in 1858. *See cardiac aneurysm, dissecting aneurysm, Fallot tetralogy.*

Pean, Jules Émile (1830–1898) French surgeon who (unsuccessfully) resected the stomach in carcinoma of the stomach in 1879. He also designed clamp forceps for hemostasis.

Pearson, Karl (1857–1936) British statistician. *See statistics.*

Pechlin, Johannes Nicolaus (1644–1706) Medical graduate from Leiden and professor of surgery at Kiel and Stockholm. He gave original descriptions of several structures of the alimentary canal.

Peckelharing, Cornelius Adrianus (1848–1922) Physiologist from Utrecht who suggested the existence of accessory food substances (1905), later known as vitamins. He also proposed the blood coagulation theory where calcium is released from thrombin to form fibrin from fibrinogen.

Pecquet, Jean (1622–1674) French anatomist and physician, born in Dieppe and graduated in medicine from Montpellier in 1652. He discovered the receptaculum chyli or the thoracic duct while a student at Montpellier in 1647. His *Experimenta Nova Anatomica* was published in 1641.

Pediatric Cardiology [Greek: *pais*, child + *kardia*, heart + *logos*, discourse] The passage of blood through the foramen into the left ventricle in the fetus was first noted by William Harvey (1578–1657), and Jean Baptiste Senac (1693–1770) in 1745 recognized the persistence of the foramen ovale in adult life. The first English monograph on congenital diseases of the heart was written by London physician, John Richard Farre (1775–1862) in 1814. An account of the different types of atrial septal defects was given by Karl Freiherr von Rokitansky (1804–1878) in 1875. Clinical accounts of atrial septal defect were given by: René Lutembacher (1884–1968) in 1916, Maude Elizabeth Abbot (1869–1940) in 1926, and Helen B. Taussig (1898–1986) in 1938. Taussig of Johns Hopkins University was also a pioneer in the surgical intervention of congenital heart diseases. The Blalock–Taussig shunt, the first surgical operation for Fallot tetralogy, was performed by Alfred Blalock (1899–1964) and Helen Taussig in 1945. In England, James William Brown (1897–1958), a member of the editorial board of the *British Heart Journal*, in 1920 joined with D. C. Muir to establish heart clinics for school children. Brown later became a consultant to Grimsby and neighboring hospitals in 1938. His book, *Congenital Heart Diseases*, first published in 1939, was of great importance in establishing cardiac surgery in England. *See atrial septal defect, congenital heart disease, Fallot tetralogy.*

Pediatric Urology [Greek: *pais*, child + *ouron*, urine + *logos*, discourse] Specialty developed in the 1930s. The first monograph was written by Meredith Campbell of America in 1938. The Association of Pediatric Urology of America was formed in 1951, and the first European Congress of Pediatric Urology was held in 1961.

Pediatrics [Greek: *pais*, child] Diseases of children have been a specialty since ancient times. The Therapeutic Papyrus of Thebes (1552 BC), which is 65 feet long, has over 100 pages of hieractic script and a chapter devoted to diseases of children. An early treatise is attributed to the Roman physician, Galen (AD 129–200). However this short manuscript *Liber de Passionibus puero um Galen* was probably written in the 6th century. The first modern treatise was written by Arabian physician Rhazes (850–932). The first printed book, *Libellus de aegritudinibus infantum* (Little Book of the Diseases of Children), based on the works of Avicenna (980–1037) and Rhazes was written by Paulus Begellardus or Bagellaro of Italy in 1472. The first book in England,

Boke of Children, was written by English physician Thomas Phayer (1510–1560) in 1545; another, *Help for the Poor*, was published nearly 100 years later by Robert Pemel (d 1653), a physician from Cranbrook, Kent in 1653; a systematic treatise was written by Nils Rosen von Rosentein (1706–1773) in 1752; and a treatise on care and feeding was published by William Cadogan (1711–1797) in 1748. Modern pediatrics in England was established by Michael Underwood (1737–1820) who in 1793 described a form of childhood paralysis following a brief illness (probably the first scientific account of poliomyelitis), and his book *A Treatise on the Diseases of Children* remained a standard work for 50 years. The French established the Hôpital des Enfants Malades in 1802. French leaders in pediatrics were A.C.E. Barthez (1811–1891) and F. Filliet (1814–1861) and Henri Roger (1809–1891) gave the first lectures. The first American textbook, *A Treatise on Physical and Medical Treatment of Children*, was written by William Potts Dewees (1768–1848) of Philadelphia in 1825. The first American children's hospital was opened in Philadelphia in 1855, and a pediatric clinic was established at New York by Abraham Jacobi (1830–1919) in 1862. J.L. Smith (1827–1897) of Stafford, New York wrote *Treatise on the Diseases of Infancy and Childhood*. An early American journal, *Archives of Pediatrics*, was founded in 1884, and the first meeting of the American Pediatric Society was held in 1889. Thomas Coram, a philanthropist from Lyme Regis in Dorset, established the first Foundling Hospital in England in 1739. George Armstrong (1720–1789) opened a dispensary for the poor in London in 1769 where he treated thousands of poor children at his own expense. This led to similar clinics being set up in other parts of Europe. Armstrong also published *An Essay on the diseases most fatal to Infants* in 1767. The Great Ormond Street Hospital for Sick Children was founded in 1852 at the former premises of Sir Richard Mead (1673–1754), by a London physician, Charles West (1816–1898). The first person to devote time to mentally deficient children was Edouard Séguin (1812–1880) of the Bicêtre Hospital in Paris, who wrote *Traitment Moral, Hygiene et Education des Idiots et des Autre Enfants Arriers* in 1846. Guido Fanconi (1892–1979), Swiss pediatrician at the University of Zurich, described renal tubular dysfunction (Fanconi syndrome) leading to aminoaciduria and cystic fibrosis of the pancreas. Samuel Jones Gee (1839–1911), a physician at the Hospital for Sick Children, Great Ormond Street, described celiac disease in children in 1888. Edouard Heinrich Henoch (1820–1910), a pupil of Johannes Schönlein (1793–1864) and a pioneer in Germany, described Henoch–Schönlein purpura in 1837. George Frederick Still (1868–1898) of Great Ormond Street Hospital was a founder of pediatrics in England and in 1896 wrote *On a form of chronic joint disease in Children* while a registrar. The concept of inborn errors of metabolism was proposed in 1902 by Archibald Edward Garrod (1857–1936), of St Bartholomew's Hospital and the Hospital for Sick Children. *See child psychiatry, pediatric cardiology, Act for Parish Poor Infants, child care, infant mortality rates.*

Pedophilia [Greek: *pais*, child + *philos*, love] Term applied to sexual offenses against children. Swiss psychiatrist Auguste Henri Forel (1848–1931) called it 'pedrosis' and Richard von Kraft-Ebbing (1840–1902), German forensic psychiatrist and expert on sexual pathology, called it 'pedophilia erotica'. A notorious pedophile was French army Marshall, Rais Retz (b 1404) who was tried for his crimes, convicted and was burnt. At the end of the 19th century there was an unfounded belief that gonorrhea could be cured by having sex with a young virgin.

Pel-Ebstein Fever Characteristic pattern of fever in Hodgkin disease. Described independently by two German physicians from Berlin: Pieter Klazes Pel (1852–1919) in 1885 and Wilhelm Ebstein (1836–1912) in 1887.

Pellagra [Italian: *pelle*, skin; Greek, *agra*, rough] First described as *mal de rosa* in the district of Asturia in 1730 by Spanish physiologist, Gaspar Casal (1679–1759) and François Thiérry (b 1719) published an account in 1755. The present name was given by Francisco Frapolli (d 1772) of Italy in 1771. The first description in North America was in 1864, although it was previously known to be widespread. Casimir Funk (1884–1967) proposed that it was a deficiency disease in 1914. Conrad Elvejhem (1901–1962), a biochemist from Wisconsin, demonstrated the effect of nicotinic acid in preventing it in 1938, and it was treated with niacin by English physician, Tom D. Spiers, in the same year.

Pelletier, Pierre Joseph (1788–1842) French chemist and pioneer in extraction of alkaloids from plants. He was born in Paris and qualified as a pharmacist in 1810. He isolated emetine while working with François Magendie (1783–1855) and Joseph Bienaimé Caventou (1793–1877) in 1817. Pelletier and Caventou obtained the alkaloid quinine from the cinchona bark in 1820, strychnine from *Strychnos nux-vomica*, and narceine, an alkaloid of opium with narcotic properties, in 1832. A new alkaloid from pomegranate, discovered later was named 'pelletierine' in his honor in 1877.

Pellucida [Latin: *per*, through + *lucere*, to shine] *See zona pellucida.*

Peltier, Jean Charles Athanase (1785–1845) French physicist from Hain, Somme who developed the thermoelectric method of reduction of temperature, now known as Peltier effect.

Pelvic Peritonitis or pelvic cellulitis [Greek: *pyelos*, oblong basin + *peri*, round + *itis*, inflammation] The first study was made in the mid-19th century by Nonat who described it as 'peri-uterine phlegmon' and the term 'pelvic peritonitis' was introduced Gustav Louis Richard Bernutz (1819–1887), around the same time. Rudolph Virchow (1821–1902) called it 'parametritis', to signify the involvement of other adjacent cellular tissues.

Pelvimetry [Greek: *pyelos*, oblong basin + *metron*, measure] Study of measurement of the pelvis of the mother in relation to childbirth. Henrick van Deventer (1651–1724), a surgeon from Amsterdam, applied orthopedic principles to obstetrics around 1690. He wrote *Operationes Chirugicae Novem Lumen Exibentes Obstricantibus* published in 1701, and an English translation *The Art of Midwifery Improved* appeared later. He described the bony structure of the pelvis and its deformities in relation to labor. Used by British obstetrician William Smellie (1697–1763) in 1752 and Jean Louis Baudelocque (1746–1810) of Paris in 1781. The external conjugate diameter, a measurement often used, is known as Baudelocque diameter. Karl Gustav Carus (1789–1869), professor of anatomy and obstetrician at Montpellier, did further studies in 1820 and defined the 'circle of Carus', with its center at the pubis symphysis and the pelvic outlet as its perimeter or periphery.

Pemphigus [Greek: *pemphix*, blister] (Syn: pompholyx) Skin condition with blebs or bullae which occurs in a variety of dermatological conditions. First large-scale study, involving thousands of patients, was by a dermatologist from Vienna, Ferdinand von Hebra (1818–1880) in 1845.

Pendred Syndrome Inherited disease due to a recessive trait, leading to a defect in binding of iodine by the thyroid gland. Described by Vaughan Pendred (1869–1946) in *The Lancet* in 1896. It is also associated with thyroid goiter and deaf-mutism.

Pendulum [Latin: *pendere*, to hang] Galileo Galilei (1564–1642) of Pisa is credited with the invention in 1639. He first observed the principle from the oscillations of a suspended lamp in the cathedral at Pisa in 1583. His observation that the oscillations were equal in time whatever their range led to its use for measuring time. The principle was employed by Sanctorio Sanctorius (1561–1636) to develop a pulse watch.

Penfield, Wilder Graves (1891–1976) American-born Canadian neurosurgeon, born in Spokane, Washington. He studied at Princeton and Oxford (as a Rhodes scholar) and finished his studies, after war service, at the Johns Hopkins

University. In 1928 he moved to McGill University in Montreal and later became the director of the Montreal Neurological Institute. His research increased understanding of the higher functions of the brain and causes of diseases such as epilepsy.

Pengelly, William (1812–1894) Geologist from Looe in Cornwall. His explorations of the Devonian deposits provided proof for the existence of early forms of man and animals. He has published several papers on the antiquity of man and related subjects.

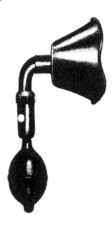

A hand atomiser and mask for penicillin inhalation, used in the treatment of lung conditions. Sir Alexander Fleming, *Penicillin, it's Practical Application* (1946). Butterworth, London

Penicillin [Latin: *penicillium*, brush] Mold as treatment for wounds was used by the ancients. Mycophenolic acid, which inhibited the growth of anthrax bacilli, was obtained in a crystalline state from the *Penicillium* mold by an Italian physician from Rome, Bartolomeo Gosio, in 1896. Another Frenchman, Vaudremer, also experimented with *Aspergillus fumigatus* in 1913 and showed its antagonism to other micro-organisms. A crude preparation was used by Joseph Lister (1827–1912) in Edinburgh to treat an infected wound. When Alexander Fleming (1881–1955) was studying bacterial variation of Staphylococci in 1929, he observed the bacteriolytic effect of *Penicillium notatum* which accidentally contaminated his culture. Its development as an antibiotic is mainly due to the work of Howard Walter Florey (1896–1968) and co-workers at the Sir William Dunn School of Pathology at Oxford in 1939 and Ernest Boris Chain (1906–1979) and colleagues in 1940, and clinical trials by Edward Penley Abraham and co-workers in 1941. It was used in treatment of syphilis in 1943 by John Friend Mahoney (1889–1957) and colleagues of the US Public Health Service. It was produced commercially by Glaxo during World War ll, following the research of

English biochemist, Ernest Lester Smith (1904–1992) of Teddington, Middlesex. Intrathecal administration in treatment of pneumococcal meningitis was introduced by Sir Hugh Cairns (1896–1952) and colleagues in 1944. The molecular structure was elucidated in 1949 by Dorothy Crowfoot Hodgkin (b 1910) an English biochemist who received the Nobel Prize for Chemistry in 1964. *See antibiotics.*

Penicillinase Enzyme produced by *Penicillium* and observed by Edward Penley Abraham (b 1913) and Ernest Boris Chain (1906–1979) in 1940. The crystallized form was obtained from *Bacillus cereus* by M.R. Pollock and co-workers in 1956.

Penis [Latin: *penis*, tail] Peyronie disease or plastic induration of the penis was described by French surgeon, François de la Peyronie (1678–1747) in 1743. The erector mechanism was described by Conrad Eckhard (1822–1915) in 1863. *See phallic phase, phallica.*

Penrose Drain Rubber tube with a gauze wick used in surgery. Devised by American gynecologist, Charles Bingham Penrose (1862–1925) of Pennsylvania in 1890.

Pennsylvania Medical College Started in 1850 as the Female Medical College of Pennsylvania. It changed its name to the Medical College of Pennsylvania in 1969. *See Female Medical College of Pennsylvania.*

Penrose, Lionel Sharples (1898–1972) English geneticist, born in London and educated at St John's College, Cambridge. He qualified in medicine in 1925, and did postgraduate work in Vienna, and his MD thesis was on schizophrenia. In the 1930s he did a major survey of causes of mental illness and in 1945 he was appointed Galton Professor of Eugenics at London University. The increased maternal age as a cause of mongolism or Down syndrome was noted by him in 1938, and he wrote *The Biology of Mental Defect* in 1949 and *An Outline of Human Genetics* in 1960.

Pension Act Established to provide financial help in old age and passed in 1908. The National Assistance Act enacted in 1948 required councils to provide accommodation for the aged in need of attention.

Pentolinium Tartrate Ganglion-blocking drug, similar to hexamethonium but more potent. Synthesized by Libman in 1952 and used in anesthesia by G.H. Enderby in 1954.

Pentose Phosphate Pathway Alternative pathway for carbohydrate metabolism, studied by F. Dickens of England in 1953. Further information on it came from by B.L. Horecker (1954), B. Axelrod and others.

Pentosuria [Greek: *pente*, five + *oureon*, urine] Condition described by Ernst Leopold Salkowski (1844–1923) of Berlin in 1895. Further work was done by H. Aron in 1913. The Bial test for pentose sugars in urine, using hydrochloric acid as one of the reagents, was devised by German physician, Manfred Bial (1870–1908).

Pentothal Sodium Thiopentone was synthesized by Ernest Henry Volwiler and Donalee Tabern in 1932, and used as an intravenous anesthetic by John Silas Lundy (1894–1973) at the Mayo Clinic in 1934. Its rectal use for producing basal narcosis was described by M.L. Weinstein in 1939.

Peppermint The plant *Mentha piperata*, the source of peppermint oil used as a therapeutic agent, an antispasmodic, dyspepsic and carminative was noted by Pliny and the ancient Egyptians and is mentioned in Icelandic pharmacopoeias from the 13th century. John Ray (1627–1705) described it in his *Synopsis Stirpium Britannicarum* in 1696. It is used as treatment for abdominal cramps, nausea, and as a stimulant and was included in the London Pharmacopoeia as *Mentha Piperitis Sapore* in 1721. It is the most extensively used volatile oil.

Pepsin [Greek: *pepsis*, digestion] General name for several enzymes in the gastric juice which catalyze hydrolysis of proteins. Found by German physiologists, Eberle and Theodor Schwann (1810–1882) who named it *pepsin* in 1836. It was crystallized from extract of swine stomach by American biochemist, John Howard Northrop (1891–1987) in 1930. The first X-ray diffraction photograph of pepsin was made by Irish crystallographer, John Desmond Bernal (1901–1971) in 1934.

Peptic Ulcer [Greek: *peptikos*, to digest] William Brinton (1823–1867) of St Thomas' Hospital described it in detail in 1857 with over 7000 postmortem findings. William Prout (1785–1850), a chemical physiologist at Edinburgh, showed the presence of free hydrochloric acid in the stomach. The first operation for a perforated peptic ulcer was performed by Johannes von Mikulicz-Radecki (1850–1905) in 1880. Antacid therapy with frequent milk feeds and compounds such as magnesium hydroxide was popularized by American physician, Bertram Welton Sippy (1866–1924) in 1915. Vagotomy was introduced by Lester Reynold Dragstedt (1893–1975) of New York in 1943. The association of peptic ulcer with hypothalamic lesions was noted by British physician, Harvey Williams Cushing (1869–1939), in 1932. Recurrent peptic ulceration associated with non-insulin secreting islet cell tumors of the pancreas was observed by American surgeons, Robert Milton Zollinger (b 1903) and Edwin Homer Ellison (1918–1970) in 1955. *See duodenal ulcer.*

Peptide Bond The theory of amide linkage or peptide link in a protein, between the α–amino group of one amino acid and α-carboxyl group of another, formed by elimination of one molecule of water was developed German chemists Emil Fischer (1852–1919) and Franz Hofmeister in 1902.

Peptide Small compound yielding two or more amino acids on hydrolysis. Studied by German chemist, Emil Fischer (1852–1919) in 1899. *See amino acids, peptide bond.*

Peptonized Food Term used in the 19th century for artificially digested food.

Percival, Thomas (1740–1804) Medical practitioner from Manchester who devoted his career to the improvement of poor working conditions. He was appointed to an inquiry on this and formed the Manchester Board of Health which supervised medical aspects for workers. He wrote *Medical Ethics* and *Medical Jurisprudence.*

Percussion [Latin: *percussio*, beat] Striking the surface of the body as a method of physical examination was introduced in 1751 by Joseph Leopold Auenbrugger (1722–1809), a Viennese physician. He was the son of an innkeeper and is supposed to have developed percussion while striking barrels to detect the level of the wine. His method was ignored by his contemporaries until it was revived by Jean Nicolas Corvisart (1755–1821) in 1808. *See pleximeter.*

Percutaneous Transhepatic Cholangiography [Latin: *per*, through + *cutis*, skin + *trans*, across; Greek: *hepar*, liver + *chole*, bile, *graphein* + to write] Introduced in 1952 but only used frequently after its value was demonstrated by S. Shaldon, K. M. Barber and W. B. Young in 1962.

Percutaneous Transluminal Angioplasty *See angioplasty.*

Pereira, Jonathan (1804–1853) Born in Shoreditch, he was a physician and professor of chemistry at the London Hospital. He wrote *Selecta e prescriptis* which ran into 18 editions and compiled *Elements of Materia Medica* between 1839–1840.

Pergamon Birthplace of Galen (AD 129–200) and capital of an ancient kingdom of Asia Minor. One of the most celebrated libraries, a rival to the Alexandrian library, was founded at Pergamon by Eumenes in 190 BC

Periarteritis Nodosa or polyarteritis nodosa [Greek: *peri*, around + *arteria*, artery + *itis*, inflammation + *nodus*, knob] The first description was given by Czech physician, Karl Freiherr von Rokitansky (1804–1878), in 1852. An account was given by Adolf Kussmaul (1822–1902) and Rudolf Maier (1824–1888) of Germany in 1886. The

current term was proposed by C. Dickson in 1908. Hypersensitivity as a cause was identified by Arnold Rice Rich (1893–1968) in 1942.

Pericardiocentesis [Greek: *peri*, around + *kardia*, heart + *centesis*, pierce] Performed successfully by Francisco Romero of Barcelona in 1815 and later by Thomas Jowett of Nottingham in 1827. *See tamponade.*

Pericardial Effusion [Greek: *peri*, around + *kardia*, heart] Mentioned by Galen (AD 129–200) after finding it during dissection of a monkey. Dullness to percussion over the right 5th intercostal space was described by Boston physician, Thomas Morgan Rotch (1849–1914). The sign of pulmonary collapse at the left base was described by William Ewart (1848–1929) from the Hospital for Consumption and Diseases of the Chest, England in 1896. *See pericardiocentesis, tamponade.*

Pericardiectomy [Greek: *peri*, around + *kardia*, heart + *ek*, out + *tomnein*, cut] Performed by Paul Hallopeau (1876–1924) of Paris in 1921. Complete excision was performed by Franz Volhard (1872–1950) and Viktor Schmieden (1874–1945) of Germany in 1923.

Pericarditis [Greek: *peri*, around + *kardia*, heart + *itis*, inflammation] Described by Avenzoar (1092–1162), a Jewish physician in Spain. The first autopsy findings were given by Antonio Benivieni (1443–1502) of Italy. Clinical signs were first described by Sir William Broadbent (1835–1907) in 1898, including: diastolic fixation of apex, diastolic shock on palpation, and systolic retraction of the chest wall. Uremic pericarditis in cases of renal failure was observed by Heinrich von Bamberger (1822–1888) of Germany in 1857, and later by Ludwig von Buhl of Stuttgart in 1878. *Clinical and Pathological Notes on Pericarditis* was published by Sir Tennant William Gairdner (1824–1907), professor of medicine at Glasgow in 1860. More recent studies were done by Barach of America in 1922.

Periodic Law *See Medeleeff table.*

Periodic Paralysis (Syn: Westphal syndrome) Rare form of familial intermittent paralysis occurring in early childhood or adolescence, associated with a low serum potassium. Described by Karl Friedrich Otto Westphal (1833–1890) of Berlin in 1885.

Periodic Table [Greek: *periodos*, circuit] The similarity of elements and the constant proportion of each element in different compounds was noted by Joseph Louis Proust (1754–1826) in 1799. His Law of Definite Proportions was explained by John Dalton (1766–1844) in 1800 and calculation of atomic weights of different elements was done by Swedish chemist Jöns Jacob Berzelius (1779–1848) in 1828. Johann Wolfgang Döbereiner (1780–1849), professor of chemistry at Jena, published an account of similarity of elements in groups of three, or triads. This was developed into the Law of Octaves by an Englishman, John Alexander Reina Newlands (1837–1898) in 1863. Dimitri Mendeleef (1834–1907) proposed the periodic table in 1869 which accurately predicted the subsequent discovery of several elements. *See Mendeleef table.*

Periosteum [Greek: *peri*, around + *osteon*, bone] Its role in growth and nutrition of the bone was demonstrated by Joseph Guichard Duverney (1648–1730), professor of anatomy at Paris.

Peristalsis [Greek: *peri*, around + *stalsis*, contraction] Wave-like movement in the walls of the alimentary canal to propel food along. Described by Jean François Fernel (1506–1558) from Mont Didier in France in 1542. Experimental studies were done by F. Martin of Giessen in 1859.

Peritoneal Dialysis [Greek: *peri*, around + *tenein*, to stretch + *dia*, through + *lysis*, loosen] Investigated by Dutch physiologist Hartog Jakob Hamburger (1859–1924) in 1895 and German pathologist Friedrich Rudolf Georg Wegner (1843–1917) in 1877. A specific study was commenced in 1923 by G. Ganter. H. Heusser (1927), E. Haam (1932) and J. Fine (1946) used it as treatment for uremia, and it was later used for reaction to incompatible blood transfusion (1947) and poisoning. In 1950 it was used to treat intractable edema of nephritic syndrome by E. Benhamou and colleagues. It was employed to treat methyl alcohol intoxication by B. J. Stinebaugh in 1960. A plastic conduit for repeated lavage during dialysis was invented by John Putnam Merrill in 1962 and improved by Henderson in 1963. *See pleural dialysis.*

Peritonitis [Greek: *peri*, around + *teinein*, to stretch + *itis*, inflammation] Described by Johann Gottlieb Walter (1734–1818) of Berlin in 1785. The Clark sign, or obliteration of liver dullness due to distension in peritonitis, was described by a New York physician, Alonzo Clark (1807–1887). *See pelvic peritonitis.*

Perityphilitis [Greek: *peri*, around + *typhlon*, cecum + *itis*, inflammation] Old term for inflammation seen around the cecum in cases of appendicitis.

Perkin, Sir William Henry Sr (1838–1907) *See aniline.*

Pernicious Anemia [Latin: *perniciosus*, destructive] Described by James Scarth Combe (1796–1883) in 1824, but its cause and treatment remained unresolved for nearly a

century. The observation that raw or lightly cooked liver could be used for treatment was made by George Hoyt Whipple (1878–1976) and Frieda Saur Robschet-Robbins (b 1893) in 1925, although probably known to the ancients whose writings show raw liver as treatment for various maladies. George Richards Minot (1885–1950) and William Parry Murphy (1892–1987) established the raw liver diet and, together with Whipple, were awarded the Nobel Prize in 1934. The anti-pernicious factor, vitamin B12, was identified and isolated in 1948. American physician, William Bosworth Castle (b 1899) of Cambridge, Massachusetts described the association between achylia gastrica and pernicious anemia in 1929, and introduced use of intravenous liver extract. The structure of vitamin B12 was worked out by Nobel Prize winner, Dorothy Crowfoot Hodgkin (b 1910) of Oxford University, using X-ray crystallography, in 1956. Injections of vitamin B12 were used by Karl August Folkers (b 1906) and Mary Shaw Shorb (b 1907) of America in 1947. The biosynthesis of vitamin B12 was worked out by an English biochemist from Leigh, Sir Alan Rushton Battersby (b 1925), and it was synthesized by American organic chemist, Robert Burns Woodward (1917–1979) who won the Nobel Prize for Chemistry in 1965, and Swiss-born American chemist Albert Eschenmoser (b 1925) in 1976. *See intrinsic factor antibodies, gastric parietal cell antibodies.*

Peroneal Muscular Atrophy [Greek: *perone*, fibula + *myos*, muscle + *a*, without + *trophein*, nourish] *See Charcot–Marie–Tooth–Hoffmann syndrome.*

Peroxidase Crystalline form of the enzyme was obtained from horseradish by H. Theorell in 1942.

Perrin, Jean Baptiste (1870–1942) Lillie physician and professor of physical chemistry at Paris. He discovered equilibrium of sedimentation for which he was awarded the Nobel Prize in Physics in 1926.

Perroncito, Aldo (1882–1929) *See miner's anemia.*

Persian Medicine Developed during the reign of Darius the Great. *Zendevesta*, an ancient book of Persian philosophy devoted several volumes to medicine, one of which is *Venidad*, which states that there are nearly 100,000 diseases affecting mankind. Ahura, or Ormuzd, a mythical god of goodness around 1000 BC, delegated the art of healing to a powerful angel, Thrita, who became the god of medicine and healing. Angra mayanu or Ahriman represented evil and darkness to the Persians around 2000 BC and was opposed by Ormuzd. Persian medicine played an important role during the Mohammedan era and some of its eminent physicians were Rhazes (850–932), Haly Abbas (d 994) and Avicenna (980–1037).

Personality Disorders [Latin: *persona*, person] Aretaeus (81–138) described prepsychotic personality. The writer William Shakespeare explored and described human personalities long before modern psychiatrists and portrayed a compulsive neurotic personality in Hamlet and an insight into jealousy in Othello. French psychiatrist, J. Moreau de Tours (1804–1884) pointed out personality as an underlying cause of mental or psychiatric symptoms. Sigmund Freud's (1856–1939) first work on the general theory of personality, *Ego and the Id*, was published in 1923.

Persoon, Christiaan Hendrik (1761–1836) South African botanist who studied medicine at Leiden and Göttingen, and obtained his PhD from Erlangen in 1799, before he moved to Paris in 1802. He was a pioneer in mycology and wrote *Synopsis Fungorum* in 1801.

Perthe Disease Osteochondritis deformis juvenilis was described by German surgeon at Tübingen, Georg Clemens Perthes (1869–1927). He also used deep X-ray therapy in cancer treatment in 1903.

Pertussis [Latin: *per*, intensive + *tussis*, cough] *See whooping cough.*

Perutz, Max Ferdinand (b 1914) Austrian biochemist, born in Vienna who emigrated to London in 1936, where he became director of the Medical Research Council for Molecular Biology in 1947. He determined the amino acids in hemoglobin, and the alpha helical structure of myoglobin in 1964, for which he shared the Nobel Prize for Chemistry with Sir John Cowdrey Kendrew (b 1917) in 1962.

Peruvian Bark *See cinchona bark.*

Pessary [Latin: *pessarium*, to soften] Ancient physicians used pessaries made of silk, linen, cotton and wool to deliver medicinal substances. These were soaked in medicine and attached to a thread by which they could be withdrawn. They were later made of gums, resins and wax. Towards the latter half of the 18th century they were restricted to treating prolapse of the uterus.

Pestilence [Latin: *pestis*, plague] Term for epidemic diseases which have always plagued mankind. The plague of Athens occurred five centuries before Christ, followed by others in the 2nd and 3rd centuries. Malaria periodically plagued Rome and Emperor Constantine moved his capital to Byzantium in AD 330 partly for this reason. A bubonic plague occurred during the reign of Justinian in AD 542 and struck periodically until the end of the Middle Ages. *See epidemics.*

Peter of Abano (1250–1318) Also known as Pietro d'Abano, was born at Abano, a spa near Padua. He studied medicine and philosophy at Padua and practiced at Constantinople and Paris. He proposed revolutionary ideas such as, that the brain was the source of nerves, and the heart was the source of blood vessels, which raised the suspicions of the Church. He was tried on 55 counts and acquitted. He wrote *Conciliator differentiarum philosophorum et praecipe medicorum* which was printed for the first time at Mantua in 1472.

Peter the Wild Boy In 1725 King George I, while hunting in the forest of Hertswold in Hannover, came across a boy of around 12 years who lived there. His main sources of food were leaves and berries and the only clue to his previous contact with the outside world was the remains of a shirt collar around his neck. He was brought to England in 1726 by the order of Queen Caroline, and was given into the care of Dr Arbuthnot. He failed to talk or write and was given a pension and handed over to the care of one of the Queen's maids. He later moved to a farmhouse in Hertford and died at the age of 72 years.

Peter, Charles Felix Michel (1825–1882) French physician in Paris who described atheroma of blood vessels in his treatise on the heart and blood vessels in 1883.

Peter, Luther Crouse (1869–1942) Philadelphia ophthalmologist who designed an operation for oculomotor paralysis which involved the transplantation of the tendon of the superior oblique muscle.

Peters, Sir Rudolf Albert (1899–1982) English biochemist, born in London and obtained his medical degree from St Bartholomew's Hospital, before being appointed as Whitely professor of biochemistry at Oxford in 1923. He showed the participation of vitamins (thiamin) in the carboxylase cycle, and discovered 2-3-dimercaptopropanol (British Anti-lewisite), an effective antidote for the war gas, lewisite. He demonstrated that fluoride combined organically in bone in 1964.

St Petersburg Academy In Russia, was founded by Peter the Great in 1724.

Peterson, Jacob Julius (1840–1912) Danish medical historian who published a history of therapeutics in 1877.

Pethidine Synthesized by O. Eisleb and O. Schaumann of Germany in 1939. It was first known as Demerol in Canada and America, and Dolantin in South America and Europe.

Petit, Alexis Therese (1791–1820) French physician from Vesoul. The Dulong and Petit Law which states that the product of specific heat and atomic weight is constant for all elements, was proposed by Petit and Pierre Louis Dulong (1785–1838) in 1818.

Petit, François Pourfour du (1664–1741) Pupil of Joseph

Guichard Duverney (1648–1730) at Montpellier who served as an army surgeon and later became a skillful eye surgeon at Paris. He wrote several treatises on comparative anatomy of the eye.

Petit, Jean Louis (1674–1750) Became a surgeon at the age of 16 at the Charité Hospital, Paris and performed the first mastoidectomy. He defined the inferior lumbar triangle (Petit triangle) bounded by external oblique and lattisimus dorsi muscles and the iliac crest.

Petit Canal Encircles the periphery of the lens and was described by French surgeon, François Pourfour du Petit (1664–1741)

Petit Mal Minor form of epilepsy described by Jean Etienne Dominique Esquirol (1772–1840) of Paris in 1815.

Petit Syndrome Mydriasis, exophthalmos and changes in the orbit of the eye, due to irritation of the sympathetic nervous system. Described by French surgeon, François Pourfour du Petit (1664–1741) in 1727.

Petit Triangle Lumbar hernia, bounded by the crest of the ileum, the margins of the external oblique, and latissimus dorsi muscles. Described by Jean Louis Petit (1674–1750), a surgeon in Paris in 1705. He also invented the screw tourniquet and was the first to operate with success on a case of mastoiditis.

Petri Dish Shallow glass dish for use in culturing bacteria, designed by German bacteriologist, Richard Julius Petri (1852–1921).

Pettenkofer, Max Joseph von (1818–1901) German biochemist was born in Neuberg and studied medical chemistry under Justus von Liebig (1803–1873) at Giessen, before he was appointed professor of medical chemistry at Munich in 1745. He was a pioneer in public health and hygiene and was responsible for purifying the water supply to Munich. He was director of the first Institute of Hygiene in the world, in 1879. *See Pettenkofer test.*

Pettenkofer Test For detection of bile, was devised by German chemist Max Joseph von Pettenkofer (1818–1901) in 1844. Paul Ehrlich (1854–1915) devised further such tests in 1883.

Pettigrew, James Bell (1834–1908) Edinburgh curator of the Hunterian Museum in London and the museum of the Royal College of Surgeons in Edinburgh, before being appointed as Chandos professor of medicine at St Andrew's in 1875. He was a pioneer in the study of locomotion in animals including flight in birds.

Petty, William (1623–1687) Hampshire pioneer in statistics who applied statistics to the economy and proposed the first statistical department to record deaths, births, marriages, age, sex, as well as economy, trade and education. He was appointed physician to the army in Ireland in 1652 and took the first census there. He published several books on statistics including *Essays on Political Arithmetic* (1687), and *Political Arithmetik* (1683) which are basic works on modern economics.

Petty, William (1673–1783) Member of the Barber–Surgeons guild in 1739 and elected surgeon-extraordinary to the London Hospital in 1743.

Peutz–Jeghers Syndrome Familial disease due an autosomal dominant trait manifesting as multiple polyps in the gastrointestinal tract associated with pigmentation of the skin and mucosa. Described by John Law Augustine Peutz (1886–1957) of Holland in 1921. Pigmentation was noted by Sir Jonathan Hutchison (1828–1913) in 1896 and F. Weber in 1919. A more complete description was given by Harold Jeghers (b 1904) of America in 1949.

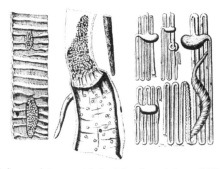

Original figure of Peyer patch by John Conrad Peyer. William Sterling, *Some Apostles of Physiology* (1902). Waterlow & Sons, London

Peyer Patch Nodular lymphatic aggregations in the small intestines. Described by Swiss anatomist, Johan Conrad Peyer (1653–1712) of Schaffhausen. He studied under Joseph Guichard Duverney (1648–1730) in Paris and served as professor of logic and medicine in his hometown.

Peyronie Disease Fibrosis and deformity of the penis. Described by French surgeon, François de la Peyronie (1678–1747) at Montpellier in 1743.

Pfeffer, Wilhelm Friedrich Philip (1845–1920) German pharmacist and botanist, born near Cassel and was professor of botany at Bonn, Basel, Tübingen, and Leipzig. He demonstrated osmosis using cane sugar solution in a vessel with semipermeable walls in 1877. He published his *Handbuch der Pflanzen Physiologie* in 1881.

Pfeiffer, Richard Friedrich Johannes (1858–1945) Polish bacteriologist who discovered *Haemophilus influenzae* in 1892. Between 1893 and 1895 he demonstrated bacteriolysis which provided the first scientific evidence for the presence of antibodies. His work led to the discovery of complement by Jules Jean Baptiste Bordet (1870–1961).

Pfeiffer Disease Emil Pfeiffer (1846–1921) of Germany gave a classic description of infectious mononucleosis under the name 'drusenfieber' in 1889. *See glandular fever.*

Pflüger Cords Linear arrangement of sex cells during the development of the ovary. Described by Eduard Friedrich Wilhelm Pflüger (1829–1910), professor of physiology at Bonn in 1863.

pH Negative logarithm of hydrogen ion concentration, used to measure acidity and alkalinity. Devised by Danish physicist, Søren Peter Lauritz Sørensen (1868–1939) of Copenhagen in 1909. An accurate pH meter was developed by Arnold O. Beckman in 1934. About 80 papers were contributed by Berlin-born American chemist, Leonor Michaelis (1875–1945). *See acidity, buffer.*

Phaenarete Mother of the Greek philosopher Socrates and a midwife.

Pheochromocytoma [Greek: *phaios*, dusky + *chroma*, color + *kytos*, cell] Described by Felix Frankel of Germany in 1886 and named by Ludwig Pick (1868–1935) in 1912. The next description was given by Jacob Pal (1863–1936) in 1905. Ernest Marcel Labbe (1870–1939) described association with paroxysmal hypertension in 1922. A total of 53 patients were identified by A.A. Eisenberg and H. Wallerstein in 1932. The histamine test was devised by Grace Roth and Walter Kvale (b 1907) of America in 1945. A. Engel and Ulf Svante von Euler (1905–1983) of Switzerland found increased catecholamine levels in two patients with the tumor in 1950. The tumor was shown on operation by René Leriche (1875–1955) of Lyon. M. D. Armstrong, McMillan and Shaw observed an increase in levels of vanilmandelic acid (VMA), a metabolite of catecholamine, in urine of these patients in 1956. Both tests are still in use for diagnosis.

Phage *See bacteriophage.*

Phagocytosis [Greek: *phagein*, to eat + *kytos*, cell] Elie Metchnikoff (1845–1916), the founder of cellular immunity, discovered the process, and demonstrated leukocytic function of white cells as scavengers during his research at the Pasteur Institute in Paris in 1901.

Phalanges [Greek: *phalangx*, band of soldiers] Applied to the bones of fingers by Aristotle (384–322 BC) in 350 BC.

Phallic Phase [Greek: *phallos*, penis] Stage in development of the mind during childhood. Proposed and described by Sigmund Freud (1856–1939). It refers to a period of infantile sexual curiosity, usually lasting from three to six years.

Pfannesteil Incision A curved suprapubic incision. Described by gynecologist, Hermann Johannes Pfannesteil (1862–1909) in 1900.

Pharmaceutical Industry *See Allen and Hanbury's, Abbot Laboratories, pharmacy, American Pharmaceutical Association.*

Pharmaceutics *See pharmacy.*

Pharmacognosy [Greek: *pharmacon*, drug + *gnosis*, knowledge] Used by Seydler in 1815 to refer to the science dealing with investigation of crude drugs and other raw materials of vegetable and animal origin.

Pharmacology [Greek: *pharmacon*, drug + *logos*, discourse] The Greek poet Homer and the philosopher Plato (428–348 BC) used the term to denote poisons and remedies. Claudius Galen (AD 129–200) described over 347 herbal remedies which earned him a place as the father of pharmacology. Dioscorides (AD 40–90) used the term materia medica to denote a compilation and description of medical substances. Modern pharmacology studies the nature and physiological action of drugs, and became a specialty only in the mid-19th century. The first laboratory was established at Dorpat by Karl Binz (1832–1912), a pupil of Rudolph Virchow (1821–1902) and Oswald Schmiedeberg (1838–1921). Binz founded the Pharmacological Institute of the University of Bonn in 1869 and published a book on history of anesthesia (1896) and another on materia medica in 1866. The first laboratory in America was founded in Michigan in 1893 and University College in London established one in England in 1905, under Arthur Robertson Cushny (1866–1926), who had been professor of pharmacology at the University of Michigan before returning to London in 1904. He wrote *Pharmacology and Therapeutics* in 1899. *See therapeutics.*

Pharmacopoeia [Greek: *pharmakon*, drug] The first European pharmacopoeia, *Ricettario Florentino,* was published in Florence in 1489. The German pharmacopoeia was written by German physician, Ortolef von Bayrlant in 1477 and was followed by another by Valerius Cordus (1515–1544) at Nuremberg in 1535 and the first German official *Pharmacopoeia Germanica* was published in 1872. The term came into use in 1560, and Ametius Foesius (1528–1595), a physician at Metz, used it in 1561. The first edition of the *Pharmacopoeia Londinensis* was published by the Royal College of Physicians in 1618 and continued into 10 editions until 1851 and the second and third editions were published in 1650 and 1677. These contained strange remedies such as scorpion, spiderwebs, snakeskin, and woodlice. The first official *US Pharmacopoeia* was published in 1821. The *Edinburgh Pharmacopoeia* was published in 1699 followed by *Dublin Pharmacopoeia* in 1793 and these were combined in the *British Pharmacopoeia* published in 1864. The *British Pharmaceutical Codex* (BPC) was published as a complementary volume to the *British Pharmacopoeia* in 1907.

Pharmacy [Greek: *pharmakeus*, druggist] Art of preparing and preserving medicines, practiced since the advent of medicine. It originally involved crude preparations of plants, excreta, urine, and organs of animals and later included metals such as mercury and bromine. The pepperers and spicers in England dominated the practice during the Middle Ages and dealt in crude drugs, spices and commodities such as sugar, dried fruits, salt and oils. The Pepperer's Guild was founded in the 12th century and became the Grocer's Company, to include the apothecaries in 1373. The apothecaries separated themselves in 1617 and dealt specifically with medicines. The Society of Apothecaries, to manufacture drugs on a large scale in England, was established in 1617. The Pharmaceutical Society of Great Britain was founded in 1841.

Pharynx [Greek: *pharyngx*, throat] The Greeks believed that secretions of the brain poured directly into the pharynx. The Rathke pouch, a small diverticulum of the early embryonic pharynx giving rise to the anterior lobe of pituitary gland, was described by a professor at Dorpat, Martin Heinrich Rathke (1793–1860) in 1838. The Seessel's pocket, a diverticulum of the embryonic pharynx found anterior to the cranial attachment of the buccopharyngeal membrane, was described by Albert Seessel (1850–1910), an embryologist and neurologist from Yale. The Waldeyer ring of lymphoid tissue in the pharynx was discovered by German anatomist, Heinrich Waldeyer (1837–1921). The Passavant bridge, a ridge on the posterior wall of the pharynx produced by contraction of palatopharyngeus muscle, was described by a surgeon, Philip Gustav Passavant (1815–1893) of Frankfurt in 1869.

Phenacetin Antipyretic and analgesic synthesized at the Friedrich Bayer Dye Company of Germany under the direction of Carl Duisburg in 1886. It was introduced as a medicine by Oscar Heinrich Daniel Hinsberg (1857–1939) and Alfred Kast (1856–1903) in 1887.

Phenformin Hypoglycemic drug used in treatment of diabetes mellitus. Introduced by Georges Ungar (b 1906) and co-workers in 1957.

Phenol Sulfonaphthalein Test Used extensively to estimate renal functions and devised by Leonard George Rowntree (1883–1959), director of Philadelphia Medical Institute, and another American John Timothy Geraghty (1876–1924) in 1910.

Phenol The antiseptic and disinfectant properties of coal tar were recognized in France in 1817, and phenol was obtained from it by German chemist Friedlieb Ferdinand Runge (1795–1867) in 1834. It was used to preserve cadavers in England in 1851. Carbolic acid derived from it was used at the sewage works in Carlisle and it inspired Joseph Lister (1827–1912) to use it as an antiseptic in 1866. Phenol poisoning in workers who operated the phenol hand spray in operating theaters was described by Sir J. Rickman Godlee (1849–1925) in 1924.

Phenolphthalein Synthetic purgative prepared in America in 1871.

Phenotype [Greek: *phainenin*, to appear] Visible expression of genes first proposed by a Danish professor of genetics at Copenhagen, Wilhelm Ludwig Johanssen (1857–1927), in 1902. He also proposed the term genotype.

Phenylalanine Amino acid isolated from lupin seedlings by Schulz in 1879. It was shown to be essential to growth of rats by American biochemist William Cumming Rose (1887–1984).

Phenylalaninuria Phenylpyruvic oligophrenia. *See phenylketonuria.*

Phenylbutazone Introduced as treatment for rheumatoid arthritis by J. P. Currie, R. A. Brown and G. Will in 1953.

Phenylketonuria Inherited biochemical disorder observed by Norwegian biochemist and physician, Ivar Asbjorn Følling in 1934. He investigated the cause of mental retardation in two children in a family, and found a change in the color of their urine when treated with ferric chloride. He postulated that the disease was due to an inherited error of metabolism and this was proved by G. A. Jervis and R. J. Block who demonstrated in 1940 that it was due to a block in conversion of phenylalanine to tyrosine. Elevation of phenylalanine in the blood with its excretion in the urine amounting to 30 times more than normal was demonstrated by M. Dann in 1943. A simple blood test devised by Robert Guthrie (b 1916) in 1961 that detected the disease in the first few days of life, and screening of newborns was made mandatory in Massachusetts state in 1963.

Phenylpyruvic Oligophrenia *See phenylketonuria.*

Phenytoin Anticonvulsant, also known as hydrantoin was introduced as treatment for epilepsy by Hiram Merrit (1902–1979) and Frederick Ward Putnam (1839–1915) in 1938.

Philadelphia Chromosome Abnormality in patients with chronic myeloid leukemia was observed by P.C. Nowell and D.A. Hungerford in 1960.

Philip, Sir Robert William (1857–1939) From Edinburgh Royal Infirmary, was a pioneer in the study and control of tuberculosis. He established the first tuberculosis dispensary in the world at Edinburgh in 1888, and another in London at Paddington in 1909.

Phillipe, Claudien (1866–1903) Director of the Pathological Anatomy Laboratory at the Sâlpetrière who described the septomarginal tract in the sacral region of the cord in 1901.

Philosopher's Stone The fundamental aim of alchemy was to obtain the 'essence' which would change base metals in to gold and cure all diseases. The guardian or possessor of this mythical essence was said to be the mythical Hermes Trismegistus who probably represented Thot, the Egyptian god of wisdom. According to alchemy traditions, he inscribed the essential secrets of alchemy on an emerald and presented it to Sarah, the wife of Abraham.

Philosophical Transactions of the Royal Society Journal of the Royal Society, first published in 1665. One of its epoch-making treatise, *Principia* by Sir Isaac Newton (1642–1727), was published in 1687. *See Royal Society.*

Philosophy [Greek: *philosophia*, lover of wisdom] Thales who lived around 600 BC is considered the father of philosophy. The term was adopted by Pythagorus who called himself a philosopher around 528 BC. Aristotle (384–322 BC) and Plato (428–348 BC) are two of the best known natural philosophers. The first moral philosopher from the east was Gautama Siddartha Buddha (568–488 BC), a Hindu prince. He proposed the concept of *nirvana* which is a complete withdrawal of interest from the external world to innerself in order to attain a tranquil state devoid of passion. During the 17th century philosophy was classified into: moral or ethical, intellectual and natural or physical. Some eminent British philosophers include Sir Francis Bacon, John Locke, and Herbert Spencer. *See logic, ethics.*

Philtrum [Greek: *philtron*, love portion] Vertical furrow on the upper lip said to have been named due to the association of the mouth with love.

Phimosis [Greek: *phimosis*, muzzling] An operative treatment of the condition by rupturing the mucous membrane of the prepuce was described by American surgeon, Joseph Pancoast (1805–1939) in 1862.

Phlebotomus Fever [Greek: *phlebo*, vein + *tomos*, cut] (Syn: Pappataci fever, sandfly fever) First probable description was given by Alois Pick (1859–1945) in 1886. In 1903, Sir Robert McCarrison (1878–1960) described the three day Chitral fever of the Blue Mountains of Nilgri in India which he thought to be the same. He also suggested that the sand fly (*Phlebotomus papatasi*) was the transmitter of the disease and his theory was confirmed by Robert Doerr (1871–1952) in 1908.

Phlebotomy [Greek: *phlebos*, vein + *tome*, to cut] *See blood letting, cupping.*

Phlegmasia Alba Dolens [Greek: *phlegmone*, inflammation; Latin: *alba*, white] Swelling of the lower extremities in pregnant women was thought to be due to destruction of the maternal lymphatics by Manchester surgeon, Charles White (1728–1813) in 1784, one of the founders of Manchester Royal Infirmary. David Daniel Davis (1778–1841), physician–accoucher to the Queen, was the first to attribute the condition to inflammation of the veins in 1823.

Phlegmone [Greek: *phlegmone*, inflammation] Term used by Galen (AD 129–200) to describe general inflammation or a red resisting painful tumor. It was defined as the 'most violent kind of inflammation' by John Abernethy (1764–1831).

Phlogiston Theory [Greek: *phlogistos*, set on fire] As a cause of burning and rusting was proposed by Georg Ernst Stahl (1660–1734) of Germany in 1697 and upheld for nearly a century until disproved by Joseph Priestley (1733–1804) in 1774. *See oxygen.*

Phocomelia [Greek: *phoke*, seal + *melos*, limb] Congenital abnormality where all four limbs fail to develop in infants born to mothers who took the drug thalidomide before 1960. The drug was introduced as a hypnotic and a sedative in Germany in 1958 and was in extensive use for three years until its withdrawal

Pholcodein Derivative of morphine and sodium ethoxide introduced as an antitussive agent in France in 1950.

Phonocardiography [Greek: *phone*, sound + *kardia*, heart +

graphein, to write] Method of recording heart sounds introduced by Dutch physiologist Willem Einthoven (1860–1927) and M. A. J. Geluk of Germany in 1890. Einthoven published details of his galvanometer in 1907. De Forest invented a triode amplifier in 1906. Huerthle used the microphone to record heart sounds in 1895. Sir Thomas Lewis (1881–1945) did further studies and wrote *The Mechanism and Graphic Registration of the Heart Beat* in 1925.

Phonodeik Apparatus for making photographic recordings of sound waves. Invented by American physicist, Dayton Clarence Miller (1866–1941) of Strongsville, Ohio in 1908.

Phosgene Highly toxic colorless gas prepared by mixing chlorine and carbon monoxide in the presence of sunlight by John Davy in 1812. It was used in chemical warfare by Germans in December 1915. *See gas warfare.*

Phosphatase Hydrolytic enzyme. That found in serum was estimated by H. D. Kay in 1930 and the method was perfected by American biochemist of Russian origin, A. Bodansky (1896–1941) in 1933. *See diagnostic enzymology.*

Phosphate [Latin: *phosphas*, light] A method to estimate inorganic phosphate in blood was devised by R. D. Bell and American biochemist and Nobel Prize winner Edward Adelbert Doisy (1893–1986) in 1920 and it was improved by Alfred Poyner Briggs (b 1888) in 1922. Stanley Rossiter Benedict (1884–1936) modified the method in 1924. A rise in phosphate in the blood in renal failure was observed by Isidor Greenwald (b 1887) of New York in 1915.

Phosphocreatine Substance in muscle contraction discovered independently by two groups of workers: Philip and Grace Eggleton of London and Cyrus Hartwell Fiske (1890–1978) and Yella-Pragada Subbarow (1896–1948) of Boston in 1927. Its role in muscle contraction was studied by A. Szent-Györgi (1893–1986).

Phospholipids The pioneer studies were performed by John Lewis William Thudichum (1829–1901), a German physician who practiced in London. He published his work, *A Treatise on the Chemical Constitution of the Brain*, in 1884.

Phosphorus [Greek: *phos*, light + *pherein*, to carry] Nonmetallic element discovered by Anton Laurent Lavoisier (1743–1794) in 1777, which produces luminescence in the dark. It was isolated from urine by a Swedish chemist, Georg Brandt (1694–1768). Dresden chemist, Kraft suggested that it was present in the human body. Robert Boyle (1627–1691) discovered a way of making it outlined in

Aerial Notiluca published in 1680. The first book on its use in medicine, *De Phosphorhosis: Observationes Quatour, Berolini* was published by J. S. Elsholz in 1680. The phosphoric acid content of bone was shown by two Swedish chemists, Johan Gottlieb Gahn (1745–1818) and Carl Wilhelm Schleele (1742–1786). The effects of phosphorus on animals were studied by Georg Frederick Wegner (b 1843) in 1872 and it was used as a remedy for osteomalacia by W. Busch of Berlin in 1881. Max Kassowitz (1842–1913) prescribed it for rickets in children in 1883. *See red phosphorus, phossy jaw.*

Phosphorylase Enzyme isolated by American couple, Carl Ferdinand Cori (1896–1984) and Theresa Gerti Cori (1896–1957) who were originally from Czechoslovakia. They shared the Nobel Prize for Physiology or Medicine in 1947.

Phosphorylation First step in fermentation, discovered by English physical chemist, Sir Arthur Harden (1865–1940) of Manchester in 1905.

Phossy Jaw Necrosis of the jaw secondary to white phosphorus exposure in industry, first observed in match factories near Vienna in 1844. It was described by Karl Thiersch (1822–1895), professor of surgery at Erlangen in 1867. Finland abolished the use of white phosphorous in the match industry in 1872, and it was prohibited in England in 1910.

Photelometer Photocell linked to a sensitive microammeter for analysis of chemical constituents in small samples of blood and urine. Invented by G. E. Davis and C. Sheard of America in 1927. A photoelectric hemoglobinometer based on the same principle was developed by Sheard and A. H. Sanford in 1928.

Photoelectric Cell Invented by German physicist, Johann Philipp Ludwig Julius Elster (1854–1920) and Hans Friedrich Geitel (1855–1923) in 1896. It consists of an electronic tube with a cathode which is sensitive to light so that it emits electrons. The current generated is proportional to the intensity of light used. The modern cell was developed by Chapin, Fuller and Peterson of the Bell Telephone Company in 1954.

Photography [Greek: *phos*, light + *graphein*, to write] The action of light on chloride of silver was studied by a Swedish apothecary, Carl Wilhelm Scheele (1742–1786) in 1777. In 1839, Louis Jacques Mandé Daguerre (1789–1851) of Cormeilles, France and William Henry Fox Talbot (1800–1877) from Wiltshire introduced a method of using sodium thiosulfate solution to remove unchanged silver iodide in photographic development. In the following year Fox Talbot discovered a negative from which unlimited positives could be made. A carbon process of photographic printing was invented by English chemist, Sir Joseph Wilson Swan (1828–1914) of Sunderland in 1864. He also invented the dry plate in 1871 and bromide paper in 1879. *See photomicrography.*

Photometer Invented by German physicists Julius Elster (1854–1920) and Hans Friedrich Geitel (1855–1923).

Photomicrography [Greek: *phos*, light + *mikros*, small + *graphein*, to write] David Gruby (1810–1898), a mycologist from Hungary, developed photomicrography to illustrate his work. Some of the earliest were published in 1856 by John William Draper (1811–1882), a physiologist from Liverpool who later emigrated to America. Joseph Edwin Barnard (1870–1949) applied it to the study of bacteria and viruses in England in 1925. An American pioneer was George Miller Sternberg (1838–1915) who published a manual. An early modern work, *Handbook of Photomicrography*, was published by Lloyd Hind and Brough Randles in 1913.

Photon Small packets of energy consisting of light particles and proposed by Albert Einstein (1879–1955).

Photosynthesis [Greek: *phos*, light + *synthesis*, putting together] Joseph Priestley (1733–1804) observed that plants use carbon dioxide from the atmosphere and replace it with oxygen. Carbon-14 was used to investigate the metabolic processes by American chemist of Russian origin, Melvin Calvin (b 1911) and he was awarded the Nobel Prize for his work in 1961.

Phototherapy [Greek: *phos*, light + *therapeia*, service to the sick] Mentioned by English physician, Gilbertus Anglicus in the 13th century when he advocated use of red light to treat smallpox. Johann Wolfgang Döbereiner (1780–1849) used light therapy on a scientific basis in 1816. Sir Arthur Henry Downes (1851–1938) and Thomas Porter Blunt in 1877 showed that ultraviolet light killed bacteria. A Danish physician Niels Ryberg Finson (1860–1904) developed a method of treating lupus vulgaris with ultraviolet light in 1890. Infrared light was used as treatment for arthritis, strains and sprains. Phototherapy was introduced as treatment for hyperbilirubinemia by Cremer and his colleagues in 1958.

Phrenic Nerve Palsy [Greek: *phren*, diagram or mind] Sign of thoracic aortic aneurysm described by Scottish surgeon and cardiologist Allan Burns (1781–1813) in *Observations of some of the most Important and frequent Diseases of the Heart* published in 1809.

Phrenitis [Greek: *phren*, mind + *itis*, inflammation] Ancient Greek term for disease of the mind.

Phrenology [Greek: *phren*, mind, *logos*, discourse] External study of the skull as an indicator of mental powers and moral qualities. Hippocrates (460–377 BC) believed that the shape of the body revealed the personality, and Aristotle (384–322 BC) studied the nose, limbs, hair and other parts of the body to characterize people. The concept was proposed by Franz Joseph Gall (1758–1828), a German physician, in 1758. He published a treatise with another German physician, Casper Johan Spurzheim (1776–1832), *Anatomy and Physiology of the Nervous System, and of the Brain in Particular*, in 1800. A popular English treatise, *System of Phrenology*, was published by George Combe in 1819.

Phthisis [Greek: *phthisis*, to decay] *See tuberculosis.*

Phylogeny [Greek: *phylon*, tribe + *genesis*, generation) Study of developmental history of a race or a group of animals.

Physick [Greek: *physikos*, natural] Study and practice of medicine. Many of the physicians from the Middle Ages called themselves doctors of physick.

Physical Chemistry Jacobus Henricus van't Hoff (1852–1911) studied chemical kinetics and Svante August Arrhenius (1859–1927) studied electrolytic dissociation. The application of physics to chemistry was pioneered by Friedrich Wilhelm Ostwald (1853–1932), German professor of chemistry at Leipzig in the 1880s. In his *Lehrbuch der allgemeinen Chemie* published in 1885 he proposed the law of dilution which bears his name. He also discovered and defined the catalyst as an agent which accelerated the rate of a chemical reaction.

Physick Garden [Greek: *physikos*, natural] Botanical garden where medicinal herbs are cultivated. An English garden was established by John Gerard (1545–1612), a London surgeon in 1567, and the Oxford physick garden was founded by the Earl of Danby in 1652. The Chelsea Physick garden was founded by Sir Hans Sloane (1660–1753) and handed to the Apothecaries Company in 1721.

Physick, Philip Syng (1768–1837) Father of American surgery who spent four years with John Hunter (1728–1793) in England, before he returned to America to become professor of surgery at the University of Pennsylvania in 1805. He introduced many operative techniques and introduced absorbable sutures.

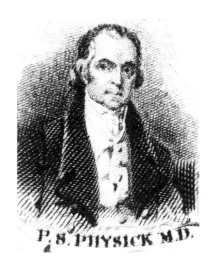

Philip Syng Physick (1768–1837). Courtesy of the National Library of Medicine

Physicotheology [Greek: *physis*, nature + *theos*, god + *logos*, discourse] An attempt to relate nature and god was made by English philosopher and clergyman, William Durham (1657–1735) of Stowton near Worcester in *Physico-Theology* published in 1713. He was chaplain to George I and Canon of Windsor.

Physiognomy [Greek: *physis*, nature + *gnomon*, judge] Art of determining character and disposition by studying facial features. Adamantius of Alexandria (AD 500), a Greek physician wrote one of the earliest works on physiognomy, dedicated to the Emperor Constantine. Giovanni Batista della Porta (1536–1615) of Naples, the father of physiognomy, wrote *De Humana Physiognomia* in 1586. Johann Gasper Lavetor (1741–1801) from Zurich published *Treatise on physiogmony* in 1772.

Physiography *See Salisbury, Rollin*

Physiology [Greek: *physis*, nature + *logos*, discourse] Study of mechanisms of nature, commenced by Aristotle (384–322 BC), and his *De Motu Animalium* contains some basic facts of modern physiology. The term 'physiologia' was first used by a physician, Jean François Fernel (1497–1558) of Paris in 1542. René Descartes (1596–1650) of France published the first physiology book in Europe, *De Homine figuris et latinitate donatus a Florentio Schuyl* in 1622. In England William Harvey (1578–1657) provided experimental proof for circulation of blood in 1628 which was fundamental to physiology. Albrecht von Haller (1708–1777), a Swiss physician and first professor of physiology at Göttingen was one of the greatest physiologists of the 18th century, and introduced the concept of impulse and

irritability of living tissues in *Primae Lineae Physiologiae* published in 1747. Experimental physiology was established by Claude Bernard (1813–1878) of Paris. Some notable contributors include: Edward Sharpey-Schaffer (1850–1935), Henry Ernest Starling (1866–1927), Sir William Maddock Bayliss (1860–1924), Sir Thomas Lewis (1881–1945), Sir Charles Sherrington (1857–1952), Lord Edgar Adrian (1889–1977), Sir Joseph Barcroft (1872–1947) and John Scott Haldane (1860–1936).

Respiratory Physiology *See respiratory physiology, aviation medicine.*

Physiotherapy [Greek: *physis*, nature + *therapio*, take care] A pioneer in the application of physical medicine to diseases of the joints and bones was French surgeon, Amédée Bonnet (1802–1858). He was professor of surgery at l'Hôtel Dieu in Lyon and published *Traite des Maladies des Articulations* (1845) in two volumes, followed by *Traites des Therapeutique des Maladies des Articulations* in 1853. Heinrich S. Frenkel (1860–1931), medical superintendent at the Freihoff Sanatorium at Switzerland, advocated the use of extensive physiotherapy for neurological disease and introduced systematic exercises for tabetic ataxia in 1890. *See occupational therapy.*

Physostigmine Poisonous alkaloid in the Calabar bean (*Physostigma venenosum*) was identified and named by C. Jobst and Hesse in 1863. Hesse also ascertained its structure in 1867. It was introduced as a treatment of myasthenia gravis by Mary Broadfoot Walker (1888–1974) of England in 1934.

Pia Mater [Latin: *pius*, tender + *mater*, mother] Innermost of the three membranes of the brain derives its name from the belief that it protected and nourished the brain like a mother.

Piaget, Jean (1896–1980) Born in Neufchatel, Switzerland, he was a pioneer in child psychology and professor of psychology at Geneva University from 1929 to 1954. His publications include *The Child's Conception of the World* (1936), *The Origin of Intelligence in Children* (1936), and *Early Growth of Logic in the Child* (1958).

Pica [Latin: magpie] The term used to describe an abnormal appetite for a variety of non-nutritive substances, such as earth and coal. Hippocrates (460–377 BC) described it in pregnancy, stating that 'when a pregnant woman longs to eat coal and earth, the likeness of these things appear in the head of the child'. Galen (AD 129–200) gave a detailed description.

Picard, Jean (1620–1682) French astronomer from Anjou who estimated the radius of the Earth by measuring the degree of the meridian in 1660.

Pick, Ludwig (1868–1935) Pediatrician and professor of pathological anatomy at Berlin. He described a disorder of sphingomyelin known as Niemann–Pick disease in 1926.

Pick Cirrhosis Disease of the liver with ascites secondary to constrictive pericarditis. Described by Friedel Pick (1867–1926) of Germany in 1896.

Pick Disease Form of dementia due to cerebral atrophy of the frontal and temporal lobes. Described as 'circumscribed cortical atrophy' by Arnold Pick (1851–1924), a Czech psychiatrist at the University of Prague in 1892. He studied medicine at Vienna and Berlin and was director of the Dobrzau Asylum in 1880 and professor of psychiatry at the German University of Prague in 1886.

Pickering, Sir George White (1904–1980) Born in Northumberland and trained at St Thomas' Hospital. He did clinical research with Sir Thomas Lewis (1881–1945) at University College Hospital for eight years. He was regius professor of medicine at Oxford from 1956, and did pioneering work on essential hypertension. He noted the protein nature of renin and its role in hypertension, and his *Nature of Hypertension* was published in 1960. He also reported a case of internal carotid artery reconstructive surgery in a patient with intermittent hemiplegia or transient ischemic attacks in 1954.

Pickles, William Doctor from Aysgarth in Yorkshire around 1913. He wrote *Epidemiology of a Country Practice* and was a founder member of the Royal College of General Practitioners.

Pickwickian Syndrome Characterized by obesity, breathlessness and cyanosis accompanied by hypoventilation. From a fictional character in *The Pickwick Papers* written by Charles Dickens in 1837. It was introduced into medicine by Sir William Osler (1849–1919).

Picrotoxin [Greek: *pikros*, bitter] Active principle of *Anamirta cocculus*, a plant native to the Malayan Islands, Ceylon and neighboring countries. Known as a poison to Arab physicians including Avicenna (980–1037) and used as a poison in England in 1597 to destroy vermin and fish. It was introduced into medicine by Italian physician Battista Condrochi who wrote *De Baccis Orientalibus* in the 16th century. The substance responsible for its poisonous properties was isolated by Boullay in 1812 and named.

Piedra Black piedra. Fungal disease of the skin noted in Columbia and studied by Nicalou Ozorio in 1876. The causative fungus was named *Trichosporon hortae* by Joseph Emile Brumpt (1877–1951) in 1913. White piedra in Europe, due to *Trichosporon cutaneum*, was described by German physician, Hermann Beigel (1830–1879) in 1865.

Pietro d'Abano *See Peter of Abano.*

Pig One of the earliest treatise on the anatomy of the pig was written by Copho of Salerno in the early 12th century and another, *Anatomia,* was written by Ricardus around the same time.

Pig Aortic Valve G. A. Kaiser and colleagues used it to replace a diseased human aortic valve and published their findings in 1969.

Piles [Latin: *pila*, a ball of any substance] *See hemorrhoids.*

Pilocarpine Alkaloid obtained from the plant *Pilocarpus* which is native to Paraguay and Southern Brazil. It was cultivated in greenhouses in Europe since 1847 and its leaves were introduced as medicine by physician Coutinho from Pernambuco in 1874.

Piltdown Man The greatest scientific fraud so far in history. In 1911, while walking at Piltdown in Sussex, Charles Dawson (1864–1916), a solicitor from Sussex, found a fragment of a skull. He presented it to Arthur Smith Woodward (1864–1944), keeper of the geological department of the Natural History Museum in London, who declared the fragment of the skull to be that of the earliest known ancestor of man and it was hailed as the missing link between man and ape. However, further tests in 1952 by Kenneth P. Oakley proved that the skull was that of a modern man and the jaw belonged to an orangutan. Many eminent paleontologists were suspected to be the perpetrators of the hoax. A trunk belonging to Martin Alister Campbell Hinton, former curator of the zoology section of the museum who died in 1961, was found in the roof of the Natural History Museum and contained bones of animals stained with iron and manganese, in the same proportion as that found at Piltdown, to make them look old.

Pincus, Gregory Goodwin (1903–1967) American physiologist who developed the contraceptive pill. Born in Woodbine, New Jersey and graduated in science from Cornell University in 1924, and undertook postgraduate studies at Harvard, before working in Berlin and Cambridge. He was a pioneer in the study of steroid hormones and began his work on developing a contraceptive pill in 1951. He demonstrated the efficacy and determined the correct amounts of progesterone to be used in 1954.

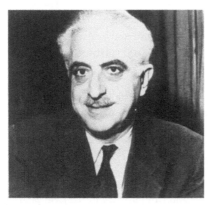

Gregory Pincus (1903–1967). Courtesy of the IPPF

Pineal Body [Latin: *pinea*, pine cone] Part of the brain observed by Galen (AD 129–200) and François Magendie (1783–1855), but its purpose or function was not fully understood. An English account of a pineal tumor was given by Humphrey Ridley (1653–1708) in 1695. Successful removal of a pincal tumor was performed by Hermann Oppenheim (1858–1919) and Fedor Krause (1856–1937) in 1913.

Pinel, Phillipe (1745–1825) Neuropsychiatrist from Languedoc in France who graduated in medicine from Toulouse and worked at Montpellier before becoming head of the Bicêtre in 1793. He identified insanity as an illness and unchained mental patients. He also recognized intellectual deterioration as a separate entity – dementia. His *Traite medico-philosophie sur l'alienation mentale* was published in 1801.

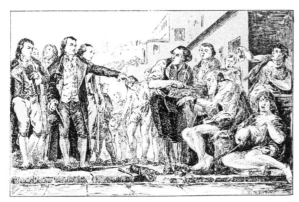

Pinel unchaining the mentally ill. Lucien Nass, *Curiosités Médico-artistiques* (1907). Albin Michel, Paris

Pink Disease Infantile acrodynia, consisting of agitation

and muscular hypotonia of unknown etiology, affecting infants. Described by Emil Feer (1864–1955) of Erlangen in 1921. The name 'pink disease' was given due to the occurrence of erythematous rash on the buttocks and cheeks.

Pinkam, E. Lydia (1819-1883) Massachusetts woman who marketed Pinkam's Vegetable Compound for cure of female weakness in 1872. It was considered the greatest remedy in the world and she became America's first millionairess.

Pinta Tropical dermatitis caused by *Treponema carateum* accompanied by depigmentation. Appeared in Mexico from southern parts of America in 1775. Described by Jean Louis Alibert (1768–1837) in 1829, by Burkehart in Mexico in 1837 and by J. Gastambadie in his history *Mal Pintado* in 1881.

Pirie, George Alexander (1890–1929) Worked at the Royal Infirmary, Dundee and was a pioneer in the use of X-rays in medicine. He suffered from radiation injuries from his work and had to give up his career in 1926.

Pirogoff, Nicolai Ivanovich (1810–1881) Professor of surgery at Moscow who defined the Pirogoff triangle bounded by the intermediate tendon of the digastric muscle, posterior border of the mylohyoid muscle and the hypoglossal. He was also one of the first to use plaster of Paris and rectal anesthesia in clinical surgery. He made a major contribution to military surgery and, following his service in the Crimean War, he published *Principles of General Military Surgery*.

Pirquet, Clemens Freiherr von (1874–1929) Austrian pediatrician and immunologist who coined the term 'allergy' in 1904. The Pirquet test for diagnosis of tuberculosis, where old tuberculin was applied through a needle scratch on the skin, was devised by him in 1907.

Pirquet Test *See Mantoux test, Pirquet, Clemens Freiherr von.*

Pitcairn, Archibald (1652–1713) Scottish physician from Edinburgh and professor at Leiden for a year before returning to Edinburgh in 1693. He was a founder of the Medical Faculty at Edinburgh. His *Dissertationes Medicae* was published in 1701.

Pitcairn, David (1749–1809) Physician at St Bartholomew's Hospital who noted lesions in the heart valves following rheumatic fever. He introduced the term 'rheumatic' in the description of heart disease in 1788. He was a founder of the Medical School at St Bartholomew's Hospital.

Pitcairn, William (1711–1791) Descendant of physician Archibald Pitcairn (1652–1713), founder of the mechanical sect of medicine. He studied at Leiden, graduated from

Rheims and received his doctorate from Oxford in 1749. He was a physician to St Bartholomew's Hospital until 1780 and president of the Royal College of Physicians, London from 1775 to 1785, and holder of its esteemed Gold-headed cane.

Pithecanthropus erectus [Greek: *pithecos*, ape + *oeides*, similar; Latin: *erigere*, to raise up] The teeth, calvarium and femur of a primitive man were discovered in Java by Eugene Marie Dubois, a Dutch physician and paleontologist from Eijsden. He was stationed in Java as surgeon to the Dutch East Indian Army in 1893. His finding gave rise to speculation that Java or Eastern Asia was the place where man evolved and not Africa, as suggested by Darwin. His finding was acclaimed as the missing link, and the primitive man was named *Pithecanthropus erectus*.

Pitres, Jean Albert (1848–1927) Bordeaux physician and contemporary of Jean Martin Charcot (1825–1893) in Paris. He defined several specific areas in the prefrontal cortex known as the Pitres areas.

Pituitary Ablation [Latin: *pituita*, phlegm] Ablation or surgical removal as treatment for carcinoma was pioneered by Rolf Luft and Herbert Olivecrona (1891–1980) in 1952. This procedure, also performed for other conditions, was traumatic before the advent of radioablation. In 1955, A.P.M. Forrest and D.A. Peebles Brown developed a method of destruction by passing a small cannula into the pituitary fossa through the nose and sphenoidal sinus. The second stage of the procedure involved a radon implant through the cannula which imparted a radiation dose and damaged or ablated the pituitary. In 1957 radiation damage to the adjacent structures led to the replacement of radon by yttrium. K. H. Baur and E. Klar improved the access to the pituitary using a transethmoidal route in 1958. A screw to deliver yttrium to the pituitary fossa was devised by Forrest and co-workers in 1958.

Pituitary [Latin: *pituita*, phlegm] Named hypophysis [Greek: *hypo*, below + *physis*, growth] as it was situated directly under the brain and ancient Greek physicians called it 'pituita' in the belief that the mucous secretions of the nose came from it. The pocket of sphenoid bone on which it rests was named 'sella turcica' as it resembled a Turkish saddle. Richard Lower (1631–1691) suggested the endocrine nature of the gland, saying 'fluids from it are poured again into the blood and mixed with it'. Martin Heinrich Rathke (1793–1860) gave an accurate account of the embryological development and an anatomical description of the gland in 1838. Changes in the pituitary following thyroidectomy were demonstrated by N. Rogowitsch in 1889, and the

relationship between acromegaly and pituitary tumor was demonstrated by Oskar Minkowski (1858–1931) in 1887. A rise in blood pressure following injection of pituitary extract was demonstrated by George Oliver (1841–1915) and Sir Edward Sharpey-Schafer (1850–1935) in 1895. Neural connections between the hypothalamus and the pituitary were demonstrated by American neuroanatomist, Stephen Walter Ranson (1880–1942) of Rush Medical College around 1920. *See acromegaly.*

Pituitary Hypothalamic Axis American endocrinologist, Philip Edward Smith (1884–1970), noted that Simmond disease, or panhypopituitarism, could be produced in rats by hypophysectomy. He showed the presence of a gonad-stimulating hormone in the anterior pituitary in 1926, and established that the thyroid depended on the stimulating action of the anterior pituitary, in 1927. *See pituitary.*

Pituitary Tumor *See acromegaly, acromegalic gigantism.*

Pityriasis Rosea [Greek: *pityron*, bran + *iasis*] Skin disease described as a clinical entity by Camille Melchoir Gibert (1797–1866) of Paris in 1860.

Pityriasis Versicolor [Greek: *pityron*, bran + *iasis*] Skin disease described by Carl Ferdinand Eichsted (1816–1892) in 1846 and by T. Sluyter in 1847.

Placenta Previa [Latin: *placentas*, flat cake] The practice of puncturing the amniotic sac to stop hemorrhage in placenta previa was introduced by German midwife, Justine Sigemundin in 1690. An early treatise on uterine hemorrhage was written by Edward Rigby (1747–1821) of London in 1775. The history and treatment were published by Read in 1861, and a paper, *Clinical Lecture on the Treatment of Placenta Praevia* was published in the same year by Robert Barnes (1817–1907) in *The Lancet*.

Placenta [Latin: *placentas*, flat cake] The ancient Chinese used the placenta of humans and animals as a medicine, as did Chinese physician, Chu Chen Heng in the 15th century. The term was introduced by Gabriele Falloppio (1523–1562) in 1561, and Guilio Cesare Aranzi (1530–1589) called it the 'uterine liver' in 1564. The normal mechanisms of placental separation and expulsion were explained by Bernhard Sigismund Schultz (1827–1919) of Freiburg in 1865, and the structure and function were explained by Charles Sedgwick Minot (1852–1914) in 1891. The endocrine nature was recognized in 1904 by Viennese surgeon, Josef Halban (1870–1937).

Plague [Greek: *plaga*, strike] The earliest account is found in the works of Oribasius (AD 325–400), physician to

Emperor Julian. He refers to an earlier description by Rufus of Ephesus (AD 98–117). The first recorded plague in Europe occurred during the period of Justinian in AD 550. *See bubonic plague, pestilence, epidemics.*

Planck, Max Karl Ernst Ludwig (1858–1947) German physicist, born in Kiel and studied at the University of Munich. He introduced the Boltzmann constant into the formula to calculate radiation of heat. In 1900 he proposed the idea that energy is discontinuous and occurs in discrete packets or quanta. He was awarded the Nobel Prize for Physics in 1918.

Plankton [Greek: *planketon*, drifting] Term used in 1888 by Christian Viktor Hensen (1835–1924) of Kiel to denote the microscopic floating life forms in the ocean.

Plantar Reflex *See Babinski reflex.*

Plasma Proteins [Greek: *plasm*, form + *protos*, first] Methods of fractionation of proteins in human blood plasma were developed by Edwin J. Cohn (1892–1953) and colleagues in 1950. *See albumin, globulin.*

Plasmacytoma [Greek: *plasma*, thing molded or formed + *cytos*, cell] *See multiple myeloma.*

Plasmaphaeresis Method by which blood is removed from the body, followed by separation into cells and plasma, before returning the cells to the body. Demonstrated in animals by American biochemist, John Jacob Abel (1857–1938) and co-workers in 1914.

Plasmid Term coined by American geneticist, Joshua Lederberg (b 1925) of New York in 1952. First used to transfer genetic markers from one bacterium to another by William Hayes in 1953. Its role in bacterial resistance to chemicals and toxic metals was demonstrated by Australian-born, British biochemist, Sir Mark Henry Richmond (b 1931), and Eric Johnston in 1964.

Plasminogen Activators Currently used in thrombolytic therapy. Their fibrinolytic effect was demonstrated by S. Sherry, R.I. Lindermeyer and A.P. Fletcher in 1958. A purified form was obtained from pig heart by Fedor Bachmann in 1964.

Plasmodium [Greek: *plasma*, a thing molded or formed + *eidos*, resemblance] A protozoan parasite which caused malaria was discovered by Charles Louis Alphonse Laveran (1845–1922), a French parasitologist, while professor of pathological anatomy at the University of Rome in 1880. Ettore Marchifava (1847–1935) described malaria parasites in red blood cells as 'hemocytozoa' in 1885. Sir Patrick

Manson (1844–1922) proposed the extracorporeal life cycle for the parasite in the mosquito in 1894. His theory was proved by Sir Ronald Ross (1857–1932), who demonstrated its presence in the *Anopheles* mosquito in 1897.

Plaster of Paris Gypsum or sulfate of lime was found at Montmartre, near Paris, and hence its name. Its use for molds was discovered by Andrea del Verrochio in 1466. A starch bandage was used in 1835 by Louis Joseph Seutin (1793–1862), a surgeon at Brussels. Plaster of Paris was introduced as a bandage by Danish military surgeon, Anthonius Mathijsen (1805–1878) in 1852, and in treatment of scoliosis and Pott disease by New York orthopedic surgeon, Lewis Albert Sayre (1820–1900) of America in 1877.

Plastic Surgery [Greek: *plastikos*, to shape] One of the earliest applications was to the nose and face. The work of Aulus Cornelius Celsus (25 BC–AD 50) includes a description of plastic surgery to the face and skin grafting. The art of rhinoplasty was known to the ancient Hindus. Gaspare Tagliacozzi (1546–1599) of Bologna pioneered rhinoplasty in Europe, but his work was opposed by Ambroise Paré (1510–1590) and Gabriele Falloppio (1523–1562) on religious grounds. Carl von Graefe (1828–1870) of Berlin was the founder, with his work on rhinoplasty, blapharoplasty and repair of cleft palate. Frank Hastings Hamilton (1813–1886) treated ulcers by skin grafting in 1854. Transplantation of free skin instead of pedunculated flaps was introduced by Swiss surgeon, Jacques Louis Reverdin (1842–1929) in 1869. Contracture following burns was treated with skin grafts by George David Pollock (1817–1897) in 1871. Sir William Macewen (1848–1924), professor of surgery at the Glasgow Royal Infirmary, whose main interest was study of bones, initiated bone grafts. Skin grafts of intermediate thickness was performed by Louis Xavier Eduard Leopold Ollier (1830–1900) of Paris in 1872, and full thickness skin grafts were advocated by Fedor Victor Krause (1857–1937) in 1893. US army surgeon, Fred Houdlett Albee (1876–1945), employed living bone tissue grafts for internal splints and transplanted the tibia into a diseased spine of patients with Pott Disease in 1915. Vitray Papin Blair (1871–1955) and James Barrett Brown (1899–1971) introduced split skin grafts in 1929. Bone grafts were also used for non-union of a fractured femur neck by Melvin Anderson and co-workers at the Mayo Clinic in 1940s. *See rhinoplasty, nose surgery.*

Platelet Antibodies *See thrombocytopenic purpura.*

Platelets [Greek: *platys*, flat] Discovered in blood by Alfred Donné (1801–1878) of Paris in 1842. An early description was given by Sir William Osler (1849–1919) in 1873.

Georges Hayem (1841–1920), professor of clinical medicine at the University of Paris, gave an accurate account in 1878. The theory that they arise from megakaryocytes in bone marrow was proposed by James Homer Wright (1870–1928) in 1906. Their part in preventing hemorrhage was investigated by American professor of experimental medicine, William W. Duke (1883–1945) at Missouri around 1914.

Platinum In 1557 Scaliger referred to a metal found in Colombia which could not be melted in a furnace. In 1735 Don Antonio de Ulloa, a Spanish naval officer, found the same mineral in Peru and in 1741 Charles Wood, an English metallurgist, sent Brownrigg to Cartagena, Colombia to investigate this metal, known to Spaniards as *Platina de Pinto*. Brownrigg presented his report to the Royal Society in 1750 and described it as a previously undescribed semi–metal. Around 1748 it had no commercial value and the Spanish mined it in Peru to adulterate gold. It was known as 'frog gold' to the British. South American mines were later closed and trade was revived when Russia started exporting it in 1824. The catalytic properties were demonstrated by Bavarian chemist, Johann Wolfgang Döbereiner (1780–1849). It was produced in commercial quantities by Henri Etienne Saint-Claire Deville (1818–1881), a French chemist of West Indian origin, in 1855. Its heat resistance made it useful in chemistry, microbiology and industry in the late 19th century.

Plato (428–348 BC) Athenian philosopher who proposed the Doctrine of Ideas. His original name was Aristocles and he was called Plato because of his large shoulders. He met Socrates at the age of 20 and remained his pupil for eight years. Following Socrates' execution in 399 BC Plato traveled extensively before he retired (387 BC) near Athens and established his school.

Platter, Felix (1536–1614) Born at Basel and graduated in medicine from the University (1556) where he was professor of medicine from 1571 until his death. He was the city physician and director of public health, and displayed great courage in treating plague in 1563. *See cretinism, eye, symptomology.*

Platysma Thin plate-like muscle, named and described by Galen (AD 129–200).

Playfair, John (1748–1819) Scottish mathematician and physicist from Benvie, near Dundee. He was professor of philosophy at the University of Edinburgh in 1805 and a supporter of the Huttonian theory of geology. His *Illustrations of Huttonian Theory*, published in 1802, was a landmark in geology.

Playfair, Lyon, 1st Baron Playfair (1819–1898) Chemist and first scientist in Britain to hold several important public offices. Born in Chunar, India to Scottish parents and studied medicine at Glasgow and Edinburgh Universities. He was a Member of Parliament in 1868, and Deputy Speaker from 1880 to 1883. He helped organize the Great Exhibition in 1851 and was instrumental in establishing the Royal College of Science, South Kensington Science Museum and the Victoria and Albert Museum.

Plegia [Greek: *plege*, stroke] *See apoplexy.*

Pleistocene Period [Greek: *pleo*, more + *cene*, recent] Geological period in Earth's history identified and named by British geologist, Sir Charles Lyell (1797–1875) in 1839.

Pleural Dialysis [Greek: *pleura*, side + *dia*, through + *lysis*, loosening] Treatment for uremia introduced by: V. Gorlitzer, B. DeMorais and J. Hamburger in 1958. Continuous pleural lavage in uremia was reported by Lindholm in 1959.

Pleural Effusion *See thoracentesis.*

Pleural Pressure The importance of the elastic recoil property of the lung in respiration, and the effect of venous return of blood to the heart upon producing a negative pleural pressure, was studied by James Carson (1772–1843) in 1820. *See lung functions.*

Pleurisy [Greek: *pleura*, the side or rib] Paul of Aegina (625–690) described it as 'an inflammation of the membrane which lines the ribs, and is attended with difficulty in breathing, cough, continual fever and pain shooting to the clavicle and hypochondrium'. He recommended venesection, purging, clyster, linctus of pine nuts and bitter almonds as remedies. Venesection was recommended by earlier physicians. Avicenna (980–1037) advocated use of syrup of poppy in protracted cases. London physician Charles Badham (1780–1845) distinguished acute and chronic bronchitis from pleuropneumony and pleurisy. The site and nature of pleurisy was established by Dutch physician, Herman Boerhaave (1668–1738) around 1709.

Pleurodynia [Greek: *pleuros*, side or a rib + *odyne*, pain] Old term for myalgia of the chest wall. Currently used as a synonym for Bornholm disease, an epidemic febrile infectious viral disease that occurred on the Danish island of Bornholm. It was described by Norwegian physician, Ejnar Oluf Sorenson Sylvest (1880–1931) in 1930.

Pleximeter [Greek: *plexis*, stroke + *meter*, measure] Flat instrument applied to the surface of the body to mediate percussion. Invented by a French physician Adolphe Pierre Piorry (1794–1879) who wrote *Traite sur la percussion mediate* describing its use in 1828. His atlas of pleximetry was published in 1851.

Pliny, Gaius Plinius, The Elder (AD 23–79) Roman naturalist and prolific writer who wrote an encyclopedia on natural history, *Historia Naturalis*, comprising 160 books, of which only 37 have survived. His work covered Greek and Roman authors and scientists and provides a valuable insight into culture and science in Roman and earlier Greek times. He was a prefect at the time of the eruption of Vesuvius which destroyed Pompeii and Herculaneum, and he lost his life by trying to get close to the mountain to observe and assist the refugees. The first translation of his work into Latin appeared in Venice in 1469, and an English translation was published in 1601.

Pliny, the Younger Nephew of Pliny the Elder. The first account of the volcanic eruption of Vesuvius was given by him in AD 79.

Plumbism *See lead poisoning.*

Plummer–Vinson Syndrome (Syn: Kelly–Paterson syndrome) Henry Stanley Plummer (1874–1936), professor at the Mayo Clinic in America, described spasm of the upper esophagus and differentiated it from carcinoma in 1912. American physician from Rochester, Minnesota, Porter Paisley Vinson (1890–1959), in 1919 further described a syndrome consisting of glossitis, anemia, and dysphagia, but credited Plummer with the first description. Donald Ross Paterson (1863–1939) of Cardiff and Adam Brown Kelly (1863–1939) of Scotland further described it in the same year.

Plutarch (AD 46–120) Greek historian and philosopher from Chaeronea in Boeotia who was educated at Athens. He mentioned hydrophobia and wrote on the medicinal advantages of wine. He also composed a dialogue on preservation of health.

Plutonium Radioactive element first obtained by Glenn Theodore Seaborg (b 1912) of the University of California at Berkeley in 1940. It was employed in the atomic bomb project which devastated Nagasaki on 9th August 1945.

Pneuma [Greek: *pneumatos*, air] According to Erasistratus (280 BC), it is taken in by the lungs and passes through the heart where it is transformed into vital spirit before it is distributed to other parts of the body, including the brain. This concept was developed by Galen (AD 129–200) and prevailed for over a thousand years.

Pneumatic Drill Uses compressed air to release bursts of impact for drilling earth and concrete. Invented by French engineer, Germain Sommeiller in 1861. D. Hunter, A.I.G. McLaughlin and K.M.A. Perry found that workers who used it suffer from a vascular disease similar to Raynaud syndrome.

Pneumatic Medicine [Greek: *pneuma*, air] Science which treats disease with gases. Established by Thomas Beddoes (1760–1808) in 1798. Sir Humphry Davy (1778–1829) was a pioneer in the field and joined Beddoes's Medical Pneumatic Institution in 1799 and experimented on himself and nearly lost his life. He later demonstrated the effect of inhalation of gases which formed the basis of inhalational anesthesia.

Pneumococcal Vaccine [Greek: *pneuma*, air + *kokkos*, berry; Latin: *vacca*, cow] The antiserum was prepared by Georg Klemperer (1865–1946) in 1891 and active immunization was introduced independently by J.W. Washbourne of England and Pane of Naples in 1896. Polysaccharide antigens were separated by Michael Heidelberger (b 1888) and Oswald Theodore Avery (1877–1955) in 1924, and a vaccine was prepared by Alexandre Besredka (1870–1940) of Paris in 1926. The serum was used extensively until J. M. Anders reviewed the literature in 1904 and concluded that it was ineffective. More purified vaccine was introduced in the mid-20th century for use in immune compromised patients, such as those who have had spleenectomy.

Pneumococcus [Greek: *pneuma*, air + *kokkos*, berry] The infectious nature of lobar pneumonia was described by Theodor von Jürgensen (1840–1907) in 1874, cocci were noted by Karl Joseph Eberth (1835–1926) in 1880, and pairs by C. Talmon in 1882. It was isolated independently by German physician, Albert Fränkel (1848–1916) of Berlin in 1886 and American bacteriologist, George Miller Sternberg (1838–1915). Swelling of the bacterial capsule when treated with antiserum, 'quellung reaction', was observed by Fred Neufield (1861–1945), a colleague of Robert Koch (1843–1910) at Berlin in 1902.

Pneumoconiosis [Greek: *pneuma*, air + *konis*, dust + *osis*, condition] Miner's lung. Georgius Agricola (1494–1555) in his sixth book, *De Re Metallica*, described diseases related to mining. Paracelsus (1493–1541) wrote a monograph on mining and smelting diseases. Bernardino Ramazzini (1633–1714), father of occupational medicine, described miner's lung in his book on occupational diseases in 1700. Thomas Bevill Peacock (1812–1882), a physician at St Thomas' Hospital, established miner's disease as a separate entity and distinguished it from tuberculosis between 1860 to 1866. E. H. Greenhow of Middlesex Hospital carried out a large study of occupational diseases due to mining and manufacture in 1861. The term was coined by F.A. Zenker (1825–1882) in 1866. *See silicosis.*

Pneumonectomy [Greek: *pneumon*, lung + *ektome*, excision] First performed in tuberculosis by David Lowson

(1850–1907) of England in 1893. Total pneumonectomy was done by Evarts Ambrose Graham (1883–1957), professor of surgery at Washington University, St Louis and by Howard Lilienthal (1861–1946) in 1933.

Pneumonia [Greek: *pneumon*, lung] Differentiation between pulmonary collapse and post-operative pneumonia was given by William Gairdner (1824–1907), Regius professor of medicine at Glasgow University in 1854. *See atypical pneumonia, lobar pneumonia.*

Pneumonic Plague Arnoldis Vinarius mentioned cough as a symptom in Black Death in the 17th century. Form of plague accompanied by signs of pneumonia and toxic symptoms and described in detail by L. F. Childe in 1897.

Pneumoren *See retroperitoneal pneumatography.*

Pneumothorax René Laënnec (1781–1826) of Paris clinically recognized and classified it into three categories: simple, due to exhalation from the pleura with no communication with the lung; associated with effusion; and with a fistulous opening to the lung associated with effusion. It was also described by Sigismond Jaccoud (1830–1913) of Paris in 1864. Displacement of the heart was observed as an important physical sign by M. Gaide in 1828. *See artificial pneumothorax.*

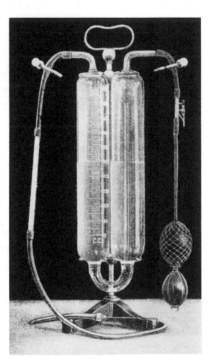

Forlanini's apparatus for artificial pneumothorax. Courtesy of the Wellcome Institute Library, London

Podagra [Greek: *podes*, feet + *agra*, seizing] *See gout.*

Podalic Version [Greek: *pous*, foot] Manual method of turning the unborn child which presents with an abnormal position, practiced by the ancient Hindus. It was revived by French surgeon, Ambroise Paré (1510–1590) during the Renaissance.

Podalirius Son of the Greek god of medicine, Aesculapius.

Podiatry [Greek: *pous*, foot + *iatreia*, healing] *See chiropody.*

Poggendorff, Johann Christian (1796–1877] *See aldehyde.*

Poikilocytosis [Greek: *poikilos*, spotted + *kytos*, hollow + *osis*, condition] Term coined in 1877 by Heinrich Irenaeus Quincke (1842–1922) to denote changes in the shape and size of red blood cells in some cases of anemia.

Poirier, Paul Julius (1853–1907) French surgeon who described the lymphatic gland situated on the uterine artery where it crosses the urethra (Poirier gland).

Poiseuille Law States that the speed of current or flow in a capillary tube is proportional to the square of the diameter of the tube. Proposed by French physiologist Jean Leonard Marie Poisseulle (1797–1869) of Paris.

Poisoning Greek philosopher, Zenophon, in 400 BC states that the practice was so common that it became customary for cup bearers to taste wine before it was offered to the king. Poisons were employed for official executions and Socrates (470–400 BC) was condemned to drink hemlock. King Mithridates of Pontius, who lived around 100 BC, studied the effects on an experimental basis. He tried to immunize himself by taking small quantities of poison and attempted to prepare a universal antidote. Official taste-bearers were appointed during the Middle Ages as poisoning food became very common. During the reign of Henry VIII punishment was death by boiling. Some common poisons used during modern times include arsenic, aconitine and strychnine and murders were even committed by doctors. *See Pritchard, Edward; Palmer, William; Crippen, Harvey and Lamson, George.*

Poisonous Fungi Ancient Greeks and Romans were aware of these and the poet Euripedes lost his wife, daughter and two sons who mistakenly ate some in 480 BC. Nicander mentioned them in his *Alexipharmaca* written around 200 BC. Dioscorides (AD 40–90) divided fungi into edible and poisonous groups. Cultivation of mushrooms began in France in 1707. Paulet studied the incidence of mushroom poisoning in Paris and suburbs and noted that at least 100 deaths occurred from 1749 to 1788. Guillaud recorded at least 100 deaths per annum in the south of France around

1888. The first systematic study was done by French mycologist Bulliard in 1791, and James Sowerby compiled an illustrated work on edible fungi in 1823. Twenty-two varieties of poisonous fungi were described by Cook in *Edible and Poisonous Fungi* published in 1894. The Board of Agriculture in England published an excellent illustrated handbook, *Edible and Poisonous Fungi* in 1910. An historic account was given by William Webber Ford of America in 1909.

Poisson Fossa Infraduodenal peritoneal recess described by French anatomist, Francis Poisson (b 1871) of Calais in 1895.

Poitou Colic *See Devonshire colic.*

Polanyl, Michael (1891–1976) Hungarian-born British physical chemist, born in Budapest and obtained his medical degree from his home university in 1917, and he moved to Manchester as professor of physical chemistry in 1933. He wrote *Science, Faith and Society* (1946), and other books on philosophy and sociology.

Polar Bodies [Greek: *polos*, pivot] Expelled products of the ripe ovum. Shown to be a result of cell division by Otto Bütschli (1848–1920) in 1875.

Polarimeter [Greek: *polos*, pivot + *metron*, measure] *See stereochemistry.*

Polarization of Light [Greek: *polos*, pivot] Related to reflection of light from transparent surfaces and described by French mathematician Étienne Louis Malus (1775–1812) in 1805.

Polio Vaccine The current widely used live attenuated oral vaccine was developed by Albert Bruce Sabin (1906–1993), an American microbiologist of Polish origin, around 1959. It is safe and effective and widely used. The Salk vaccine, made from dead virus, was developed by Jonas Edward Salk (b 1914), a physician and virologist from New York University College of Medicine in 1952.

Polio Virus Scientific evidence for communicability was provided by Otto Ivar Wickman (1872–1914) during an epidemic in Sweden in 1905. It was isolated by Karl Landsteiner (1868–1943) in 1908, and a pure culture was obtained by Olitsky Peter Kosciusko during his work with Albert Bruce Sabin (1906–1993) in 1936. Culture of the virus in human tissues was done by American biologist, John Franklin Enders (1897–1985) of West Hartford, Connecticut, Frederick Chapman Robbins (b 1916), professor of pediatrics at Cleveland, and Thomas Huckle Weller (b 1915). Their work contributed to development of vaccine and they were awarded the Nobel Prize in Physiology or Medicine in 1954.

Poliomyelitis [Greek: *polios*, gray + *myelos*, marrow + *itis*, inflammation] *See acute anterior poliomyelitis, polio virus.*

Politzer, Adam (1835–1920) Hungarian-born professor of otology at Vienna who gave the first account of otosclerosis in 1895. Politzer cone of light, a luminous triangle on the tymphanic membrane, was described by him in 1889. He also designed the Politzer bag to inflate the middle ear for diagnostic and therapeutic purposes. He wrote *Manual of Diseases of the Ear* in 1878.

Pollen [Latin: *pollen*, fine flour] John Elliotson (1791–1868), a professor of medicine at University College London described hay fever and asthma and suggested pollen as a precipitating cause in 1831. Skin reaction to grass pollen in hay fever patients was demonstrated by Manchester physician, Charles Harrison Blackley (1820–1900) in 1873. He also showed that the hay fever can be produced by applying pollen to the eyes. An attempt to produce desensitization by injecting an extract of pollen was made by Leonard Noon (1878–1913) in 1911. A disorder of acute hemolytic anemia mostly in Mediterranean races following ingestion of *Vicia faba* bean or inhalation of its pollen was noted by L. Preti of Germany in 1927. Baghdad spring anemia, an acute form of hemolytic anemia due to inhalation of pollen by atopic individuals, was described by R. Lederer in 1941. Botanical studies were done by Swedish paleontologist, Otta Gunner Elias (1897–1973) who published *An Introduction to Pollen Analysis* in 1943.

Pollination [Latin: *pollen*, fine flour] Experimental work using animal pollinators was done by Joseph Gottlieb Kolreuter (1733–1803) in 1763. A study of fertilization in plants by insects and wind was done by German botanist, Christian Conrad Sprengel (1750–1816) of Brandenberg in 1793.

Pollonium Highly radioactive element discovered by French scientists, Antoine Henri Becquerel (1852–1908) and Marie Curie (1867–1934) in 1893. She named the metal polonium.

Pollution *See air pollution, water pollution.*

Pólya Operation (Syn. Pólya gastrectomy) Operation in which a portion of the stomach is removed and a retrocolic gastrojejunostomy is constructed in an end-to-side fashion to the entire cut end of the stomach. A modification of Billroth II operation devised by Hungarian surgeon, Jenö Alexander Pólya (1876–1944) involved gastrectomy combined with side-to-side anastomosis of the gastric remnant and the duodenum.

Polyarteritis Nodosa [Greek: *poly*, many + *itis*, inflammation; Latin: *arteria*, artery + *nodus*, knob] Described by Karl Freiherr von Rokitansky (1804–1878) in 1852, as periarteritis nodosa by Adolf Kussmaul (1822–1902) and Rudolf Maier (1824–1888) of Germany in 1886. The current term was advocated by C. Dickson in 1908. Its similarity to other immunological conditions, such as SLE and dermatomyositosis, was observed and described by B. M. Banks in 1941.

Polybus Disciple and son-in-law of Hippocrates (460–377 BC) who lived around 410 BC. According to Galen (AD 129–200), one of the Hippocratic treatises *concerning wholesome diet* was written by Polybus.

Polycystic Kidney [Greek: *polys*, many + *kytos*, hollow] Erythrocytosis in polycystic kidneys was described by C.W. Gurney in 1960. A marker was located on chromosome 16 in 1985.

Polycystic Ovary *See Stein-Leventhal syndrome.*

Polycythemia Vera Reported by French physician Henri Louis Vaquez (1860–1936) of Paris in 1892. Sir William Osler (1849–1919) made it more generally known with his papers in 1903. A case in a child of six years was recorded by I. Halbertsma in 1933. Enlargement of the spleen was observed by F. Parkes-Weber (1863–1962) in 1929.

Polygraph [Greek: *poly*, many + *graphein*, to write] A record of arrhythmia on paper was achieved by Sir James MacKenzie (1853–1925) with his polygraph. He developed his own form which simultaneously recorded arterial and venous pulsations in 1897.

Polymerase Chain Reaction Technique which allows tiny quantities of DNA to be copied several million times. Developed by American biochemist, Kary Banks Mullis (b 1944) of Lenoir, North Carolina in the early 1980s. His method has been applied to fields including testing for HIV, forensic medicine and analysis of genetic material in fossils.

Polymorphonuclear Count [Greek: *poly*, many + *morphe*, form] *See Arneth count, agranulocytosis.*

Polymyalgia Rheumatica [Greek: *poly*, many + *myos*, muscle + *algos*, pain] Described as senile rheumatic gout by W. Bruce in the *British Medical Journal* in 1888. Kersley described it in 1951, and it was named by H.S. Barker in 1957. An accurate description was given by J. Forestier and A. Certonciny in 1953.

Polymyxin Generic name for antibiotics obtained from *Bacillus polymyxa* in 1947 by Phillip Gerald Stansly and co-workers, Benedict and Langlykke and Geoffrey Clough Ainsworth and colleagues.

Polyneuritis [Greek: *poly*, many + *neuron*, nerve + *itis*, inflammation] Rudolph Virchow (1821–1902) described it as specific to leprosy. Polyneuritis due to lead poisoning was described by Robert Todd (1809–1860) in 1854. Its occurrence in other cases with no identifiable or specific cause was shown by Dumenil of Rouen in 1864. *See acute infective polyneuritis, alcoholic polyneuritis.*

Polyps A monograph on intestinal polyps was written by Theodor Billroth (1829–1894), professor of surgery at Vienna, who also suggested that they were related to malignancy and should be surgically removed. *See Cronkhite–Canada syndrome, Gardener syndrome, Peutz–Jeghers syndrome.*

Pomegranate Tree indigenous to the Mediterranean, and used as medicine for a variety of conditions. The rind was used as remedy for intestinal worms. Vaginal pessaries were made from it as contraceptives by Aetius of Amida (AD 527–165) and other physicians. It was introduced to Italy by the Greeks in 300 BC.

Pompe Disease Rare disease due to excessive deposition of glycogen in all tissues. Described by Dutch pathologist, Joannus C. Pompe (1901–1945) in 1932 and further studied by M. R. Nihill and his colleagues in 1970.

Pompeii Ancient city in southern Italy buried by an earthquake in AD 63. It was rebuilt but was destroyed again during the eruption of Vesuvius accompanied by an earthquake in AD 79. Pliny the Elder perished in the eruption. The remains were discovered in the 17th century, and the first part was cleared in 1750.

Pompholyx [Greek: *pomphos*, bubble] *See pemphigus.*

Pomponazzi (1462–1525) Physician from Padua who wrote *De immortalite animi* which brought a controversy between catholic physicians and Averroists.

Pons [Latin: *pons*, bridge] Part of the mid-brain described by Costanzo Varoli (1543–1575), an Italian anatomist from Bologna in 1573 and named pons varoli in his honor.

Pontecorvo, Guido (b 1907) Italian-British geneticist, born in Pisa where he studied agriculture. He moved first to Edinburgh and then to the University of Glasgow and became professor of genetics in 1956. He described the parasexual cycle in fungi and proposed that the gene is the unit of function in genetics.

Pope, Sir William Jackson (1870–1939) London chemist, educated at Central Technical College, South Kensington, and appointed professor of organic chemistry at Cambridge in 1908. He was a pioneer in the study of optical properties of compounds, mustard gas and organometallic compounds.

Population Survey The census became a regular feature during the Roman Empire. In England, William I issued a Royal Commission in 1085 to make a survey of the whole of the country except for four northern counties. His survey recorded land ownership for the purposes of taxation. The resulting *Doomsday Book* in 1086 suggests that there were about two million people in England at that time. The first census in Ireland was taken by Sir William Petty (1623–1687) from Hampshire who published a book on statistics, *Essays on Political Arithmetic,* in 1687. The population of England and Wales in 1700 was under 6 million and the entire population of Great Britain in 1801 was just under 11 million. The entire world population in 1863 was estimated to be a quarter of a billion.

Population One of the earliest treatises was written by English clergyman Thomas Robert Malthus (1766–1834). In his *An Essay on the Principle of Population or A View of its Past and Present Effects* published in 1803 he argued that the limits to expansion of population were space and food. *See population survey.*

Porphyria *See acute intermittent porphyria.*

Porphyrin [Greek: *porphyria,* purple] A systematic study of iron-containing hemoglobins or metalloporphyrins was done by German physiological chemist Felix Immanuel Hoppe-Seyler (1825–1895) in 1862. The structure was largely elucidated by Kuster and Hans Fischer between 1910–1940. Formation of hemoglobin from porphyrin and precursors in red cells of bone marrow was shown by B. R. Burmester of Leipzig in 1936. The role of iron was studied by Martin David Kamen (b 1913), Canadian-born American biochemist, in 1948.

Porphyry *See vegetarian diet.*

Porta, Giovanni Batista della (1535–1615) Italian natural philosopher, born in Naples. He wrote on natural magic, occult sciences, crystallography and physiognomy. He demonstrated the camera obscura and was a member of the Academia dei Lincei in Rome 1610. He is also considered the father of physiognomy, because of his *De Humana Physiognomia* of 1586. He wrote a botanical work, *Phytognomonica* in 1583.

Portacaval Anastomosis Between inferior venacava and the portal vein were done experimentally in dogs by the Russian Nikolai Vladimirovich Eck (1847–1908) in 1877. Rosenstein performed the procedure successfully in human portal hypertension in 1912. *See portal hypertension.*

Portal, Antoine (1742–1832) Professor of anatomy at the Jardin du Roi, Paris who gave original descriptions of several anatomical structures. Bleeding due to esophageal varices was observed by him in 1803. He published an important work on epilepsy and a history of anatomy and surgery.

Portal Hypertension Jean Cruveilhier (1791–1874) published his observations on the flow of blood from the dilated portal space at the origin of the left branch of the portal vein within the liver to the anterior abdominal wall in cases of cirrhosis due to portal hypertension in 1835. Bleeding from esophageal varices was observed by Antoine Portal (1742–1832) in 1803, and an account of hemorrhage from dilated esophageal veins in portal hypertension was given by Karl Freiherr von Rokitansky (1804–1878) of Vienna in 1840. Occlusion of hepatic veins leading to cirrhosis and portal hypertension was observed by Rokitansky in 1842, and the condition was further described by George Budd (1808–1882) of England in 1845. It was also described by Hans Chiari (1851–1916) of Austria in 1898. Portal venography for diagnosis was introduced by S. Abeatici and L. Campi in 1951.

Porter, Rodney Robert (1917–1985) English biochemist who studied with Frederick Sanger (b 1918) in Cambridge and developed a method of determining the N-terminus of a protein. He discovered the protease, papain, which cleaves the Y-shaped immunoglobulin and this opened the way for detailed structural studies. He was joint winner of the Nobel Prize for Physiology or Medicine in 1972. *See immunoglobulins.*

Porter Fascia [Latin: *fascia,* band] Pretracheal fascia was described by William Henry Porter (1790–1861), professor of surgery at Trinity College, Dublin in 1826. He succeeded Abraham Colles (1773–1843) to the chair of anatomy in 1836.

Porter Sign Tracheal tug as a physical sign of thoracic aneurysm (Porter sign) was described by William Henry Porter (1790–1861), professor of surgery at Trinity College, Dublin in 1826.

Posadas–Wernicke Disease Coccidiomycosis, described by Argentine pathologist, Alejandro Posadas (1870–1920) of Buenos Aires in 1892. Robert Johann Wernicke (1854– 1922) also described it in the same year..

Positron Microscope The first image using positrons instead of electrons was published by James Van House and Arthur Rich in 1987. *See positron.*

Positron Positively charged particle with same mass as the electron was discovered by New York physicist, Carl David Anderson (b 1905) while working on cosmic rays in a cloud chamber in 1930. His work was advanced by Paul Adrien Maurice Dirac (1902–1984) in 1931. *See cosmic rays, positron microscope.*

Post-Coital Test For motility of sperm, was devised by a urologist at Mount Sinai Hospital New York, Max Huhner (1873–1947), who was born in Berlin, Germany. He wrote *Sterility in the Male and Female and its Treatment* (1913) and *A Practical Treatise on Disorders of the Sexual Function in the Male* (1916). He studied male sterility due to azoospermia using testicular aspiration.

Post-Vaccinal Encephalomyelitis Leading to hemiplegia and recorded by Jacob von Heine (1800–1879) of Germany in 1860, Richardiere in 1870, and Sir William Osler (1849–1919) in 1880. A pathological study was done by H. M. Turnbull in 1912. In the next 20 years 197 cases of encephalitis following vaccination were recorded in England.

Post-Cardiotomy Syndrome [Latin: *post*, after; Greek: *kardia*, heart + *tome*, cut] Also known as Dressler syndrome. A syndrome of pericarditis, pleurisy and fever following pericardiotomy, myocardial infarction, or trauma to the heart was first described by William Dressler (1890–1969) of America in 1955.

Postmortem [Latin: *post*, after + *mors*, death] A judicial postmortem was held by French surgeon, Ambroise Paré (1510–1590) around 1565. Giovanni Battista Morgagni (1682–1771), the founder of morbid anatomy, performed over 600 postmortems and wrote *De sedibus et causis morborum per anatomen indagatis* published in 1761. The postmortem changes in human organs were studied by Maria Francis Xavier Bichat (1771–1802), a physician at Hôtel Dieu in Paris in 1799. He was a founder of microscopic anatomy or histology. Autopsy examinations have shown: emphysema by Matthew Baillie (1761–1823) in 1793, calcific aortic stenosis by Theophile Bonet (1620–1689) in 1679, gastric carcinoma by Morgagni in 1761, hydronephrosis in pregnancy by Jean Cruveilhier (1791–1874) in 1842, acute liver atrophy by Karl Freiherr von Rokitansky (1804–1878), and nephritis by Richard Bright (1789–1858). An extensive treatise of nearly 3000 postmortems was published by Bonet in 1679. William Brinton (1823–1867) of St Thomas' Hospital described the pathology of peptic ulcer disease with over 7000 postmortem findings in 1857. *See autopsy.*

Posterior Columns [Latin: *posterior* after] Charles Frederick Burdach (1776–1847), professor of medicine at Dorpat described the posterior column of the spinal cord in 1819. A treatise was written by Edward Stanley (1793–1862) in 1839. Friedrich Goll (1829–1903), a neuroanatomist from Zurich and contemporary of Rudolph Virchow (1821–1902), described the fasciculus gracilis in 1868.

Posterior Inferior Cerebellar Artery Syndrome Ipsilateral loss of sensation to pain and temperature of the face with the same signs on the contralateral side of the trunk due to vascular occlusion of inferior cerebellar artery. Described by Adolf Wallenberg (1862–1949) of Berlin in 1895.

Potain, Pierre Carl Eduard (1825–1901) French cardiologist, born and educated in Paris where he was a contemporary of Jean Martin Charcot (1825–1893) during his internship. He explained the mechanism and physiology of heart sounds in 1866, the mechanism of the gallop rhythm in 1875 and the opening snap of mitral stenosis (Potain sign). He was a pioneer in aspirating pleural effusions and introduced the Potain aspirator for this purpose in 1869.

Potassium Channel Nerve impulses of the heart were shown to be dependent on diffusible potassium compounds in heart tissue by William Henry Howell (1860–1945), professor of physiology at Johns Hopkins University in 1905.

Potassium Metallic element discovered by Humphry Davy (1778–1829) in 1807. Potassium chlorate was introduced as a remedy for profuse salivation of the mouth and ulcerative lesions of the mouth by Bockh of Griefenhagen in 1840 until Abraham Jacobi (1830–1919) pointed out its tendency to produce hemorrhagic nephritis in 1860. American physician E. J. Fountain experimented on himself by taking 15 grammes of potassium chlorate and died after seven days. An autopsy showed extensive inflammation of the stomach, intestines, bladder and kidneys. Potassium permanganate was introduced as a disinfectant by A. W. Hoffmann in 1859. Microchemical measurement of small quantities in the blood was devised by a Baltimore physician, Benjamin Kramer (b 1887) and F. F. Tisdall in 1920.

Potential Energy [Latin: *potens*, powerful] Term suggested by Scottish scientist from Edinburgh, William John Macquorn Rankine (1820–1872). He applied it to anything which was not in fact energy (kinetic energy) but could be converted into it.

Potential *See membrane potential, injury potential, oxidation potential.*

Pott, Percivall (1714–1788) Surgeon at St Bartholomew's Hospital in London. He described paralysis caused by caries (tuberculosis) of the spine in 1779. He also described the fracture (Pott fracture) involving the lower end of the tibia and fibula which he himself sustained through a fall in 1769. He was an authority on head injuries and described occupational cancer. He gave classical descriptions of hydrocoel, hernia and several other surgical conditions.

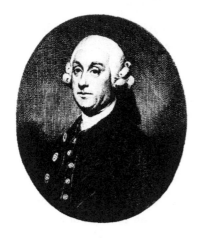

Percivall Pott (1714–1788). Courtesy of the National Library of Medicine

Pott Disease Tuberculosis of the spine has been known for over 3000 years. The mummy of an Egyptian priest of Amon dating from 1000 BC shows evidence of it. Percivall Pott (1714–1788) described the deformity and sequelae due to spinal caries (Pott disease) in 1779, but was probably not aware of its tuberculous nature. Hippocrates (460–377 BC) described it as did Jacques Mathieu Delpech (1777–1832) of France in 1828.

Pott Fracture Fracture of the lower segment of fibula and malleolus of tibia with rupture of the internal lateral ligament of the ankle was described by Percivall Pott (1714–1788) in 1769.

Pottenger Sign Spasm and rigidity of intercostal muscles due to inflammation of the pleura or lung. Described by an American from St Louis, Francis Marion Pottenger (1869–1961) in 1912.

Pouch of Douglas [Old French: *pouche*, bag] Rectouterine peritoneal pouch described by a Scottish physician, James Douglas (1675–1742) who practiced midwifery in London in 1730.

Poultice *See cataplasm.*

Pound Unit of mass in Britain since Saxon times. A standard avoirdupois pound was named after the French

city of Troyes by King Henry II in 1533, where it was used to check the value of coins.

Poupart Ligament [Latin: *ligamentum*, bandage] Ligamentum inguinale was described by Gabriele Falloppio (1523–1562) and redescribed in 1705 by François Poupart (1616–1708), a naturalist and surgeon at Hôtel Dieu.

Power, Sir D'Arcy (1855–1941) Surgeon at St Bartholomew's Hospital and a medical historian. His works on the history of medicine from 1877 to 1930 were compiled by his friends and presented to him in 1930.

Poynting, John Henry (1852–1914) English physicist, born in Monton, Lancashire and professor of physics at Birmingham in 1880. He proposed the 'Poynting factor' in electromagnetic energy following his deduction of James Clerk Maxwell's (1831–1879) hypothesis in 1884. He wrote *of Physics* with Joseph John Thomson (1856–1940) in 1899.

Pratensis, Jason (1486–1558) Born in Zealand, he was a physician who described vertigo as a symptom of brain disease in 1549. He published *De tuenda fanitate* in 1538.

Prausnitz-Küstner Reaction The presence of antibodies in the blood of atopic or allergic individuals was shown by Otto Carl Willy Prausnitz (1876–1973), a British immunologist of German origin, and German gynecologist, Heinz Küstner (1897–1963) in 1921. Prausnitz transferred fish hypersensitivity experienced by his partner Küstner to his own skin by sensitizing himself. This hypersensitive skin reaction was used clinically to diagnose atopic hypersensitivity.

Precipitin Reaction Method of qualitative estimation of antigens and antibodies introduced by Rudolf Kraus (1868–1932) in 1897. It was adapted to quantitatively measure antigen and antibody reactions by Michael Heidelberger (b 1888) and Forrest Kendall (1898–1975) in 1929.

Preformation Theory [Latin: *prae*, before + *forma*, shape] Galen (AD 129–200) and Aristotle (384–322 BC) thought that fertilization of the ovum took place through a mystic power or process called 'aura seminalis'. This view was held up to the 16th century and was revived on a scientific and philosophical basis by Charles Bonnet (1720–1793) of Geneva in 1762. It was first disproved by Caspar Friedrich Wolff (1738–1794) of Berlin in *Theorica Generationis*, a book which opened the field of embryology in 1759.

Prefrontal Leucotomy [Latin: *prae*, before + *frons*, forehead; Greek: *leukos*, white + *tome*, to cut] Trepanning was performed during prehistoric times to extract evil forces. It also probably served as a primitive form of leucotomy.

Experimental work on primates by Sir Victor Alexander Horsley (1857–1916) and John Farquhar Fulton (1899–1960) provided the background for introduction of frontal leucotomy which was first performed by Antonio Egaz Moniz (1874–1955) in 1935. The procedure was introduced into America by Walter Freeman (1895–1972) and James Winston Watts (b 1904) in 1936. A modern technique of using an open skull flap was used on a series of patients at the combined neurosurgical unit of King's College, Guy's Hospital and Maudsley Hospital in 1968. A minimally invasive method known as bilateral stereotactic tractotomy was devised by G. C. Knight and F. Post in 1969. *See lobotomy.*

Pregl, Fritz (1869–1930) Austrian physician and chemist, born in Laibach and studied medicine at Graz University. He pioneered microassay and devised a balance capable of accurately weighing 0.001 milligrams. He was awarded the Nobel Prize for Chemistry in 1923.

Pregnancy Signs The secondary areola of the breast was observed by William Fetherston Montgomery (1797–1859) of London in 1837. The color change in vulvovaginal mucosa is named after Boston gynecologist, James Read Chadwick (1844–1905) who described it in 1887. Contractions of the uterus and their value in diagnosis were noted by John Braxton Hicks (1823–1897) in 1871. Softening of the uterus in the lower region of the lower segment resulting in an increased mobility between the cervix and the corpus was described by Alfred Hegar (1820–1914) and published by his assistant, C. Reinl in 1884. Increased hair growth in pregnancy (Halban sign) was described by a Viennese obstetrician, Josef Halban (1870–1903).

Pregnancy Tests In ancient Egyptian times a woman with a suspected pregnancy was made to urinate over a mixture of wheat, barley, dates and sand. Sprouting confirmed pregnancy, wheat indicated a boy and barley a girl. Estrogens in urine were observed by two German gynecologists, Bernhard Zondek (1891–1966) in 1927 and Selmar Aschheim (1878–1965) who developed the Aschheim–Zondek test in 1930.

Pregnancy [Latin: *praegnans,* with child] *See labor, obstetrics.*

Premenstrual Tension [Latin: *prae,* before + *mensis,* month + *sturere,* to flow] Term coined by R. T. Frank in 1931 to describe a group of psychological and physical symptoms in women from the second week of the menstrual cycle until onset of menstruation.

Prerenal Uremia Azotemia produced by an extrarenal cause such as cholera. Observed by George Froin (1874–1932) and Pierre Marie (1853–1940) of Paris in 1912 and later in the year by Nobecourt. Hemorrhage and sepsis leading to shock were recognized as a cause around the 1930s.

Presenile Dementia [Latin: *prae,* before + *senescere,* to grow old + *de* + *mens,* mind] Deterioration of mental processes from adolescence in certain individuals was observed by French psychiatrist, Augustin Bentoît Morel (1809–1873) who named it 'demence precoce' in 1850. *See dementia.*

Pressure Sores *See bed sores.*

Priapism Paul of Aegina (625–690) defined it as 'a permanent enlargement of the penis, which is swelled both in length and circularly, and there is no venereal appetite attending it'. Caelius Aurelinus (*c* AD 400) distinguished between satyriasis and priapism, the former is acute and the latter chronic. Galen (AD 129–200) and Paul of Aegina recommended antiaphrodisiacal medicines as treatment. *See priapus.*

Priapus Greek god of procreation symbolized by a phallus.

Prickley Heat Skin condition commonly found in the tropics. Explained on the basis of retention cysts caused by blocking of the sweat glands, by Sigmund Pollitzer (1859–1937) in 1893.

Priestley, Joseph (1733–1804) Clergyman and chemist from Fieldhead, Leeds. He established the chemistry of gases as a science in England. He disproved the phlogiston theory by obtaining pure oxygen, 'dephologisticated air', by heating a metal oxide in 1774. He found the composition of ammonia in 1774 and muriatic acid in 1772. He invented the eudiometer to measure the purity or quantity of oxygen in air in 1772. His dissident views led him to emigrate to America in 1794 and he died in Northumberland, Pennsylvania.

Priestly, John Gillies (1879–1941) Born in Yorkshire, he worked with John Scott Haldane (1860–1936) as a respiratory physiologist. He qualified from St Bartholomew's Hospital and did most of his work on respiration and ventilation at Oxford.

Primaquin An 8-aminoquinolone compound introduced as treatment for malaria by Harold John Edgcomb (b 1924) and co-workers in 1950. In 1952 R. S. Hockwald, J. Arnold, J. Clayman and A. S. Alving noted that 5 to 10% of the healthy African-American troops developed hemolytic anemia after treatment. Subsequent studies by P. E. Carson, C. L. Flanagan, C. E. Ickes and Alving in 1956 revealed that the hemolysis was due to a genetically linked deficiency in glucose-6-phosphate dehydrogenase in red blood cells.

Primary Biliary Cirrhosis The presence of mitochondrial

antibodies in 98% of patients with primary biliary cirrhosis was demonstrated by D. Doniach in 1966.

Primates [Latin: *primus*, first] Term coined in 1735 by Carl Linnaeus (1707–1778) to represent the three families of the animal kingdom including: man or *Homo*, ape or *Simia* and sloth or *Bradypus*. A comprehensive history was given by Sir William Edward Clark (1895–1971) in 1949.

Princeton University Fourth oldest university in the United States, founded at Elizabeth, New Jersey in 1746. It later moved to Newark and then Princeton in 1756. It was renamed Princeton University in 1896 and its Graduate School was established in 1901. It became coeducational in 1969.

Pringle Disease *See Pringle, James John.*

Pringle, James John (1855–1922) English dermatologist who described sebaceous adenoma in 1890 (type Pringle) and granularis rubra nasi in 1894. He also edited the color atlas of dermatology, *Dermachromes,* which was produced by Abraham Jacobi (1830–1919).

Pringle, Sir John (1707–1782) Founder of military medicine in Britain, was born in Scotland, and studied medicine in St Andrews and Edinburgh and graduated from Leiden. He proposed that military hospitals on both the English and French side should observe neutrality in care for the wounded and that neutrality should extend to prisoners and those injured in the war. This formed the basis for rules of the Geneva Convention. He used the word 'antiseptic' in his essay *Experiments upon Septic and Antiseptic Substances* published in 1750.

Pringle Band Peritoneal band extending from the mesocolon to the duodenojejunal flexure. Described by Seton Sydney Pringle (1879–1955), a surgeon in Dublin in 1913.

Printer Asthma Caused by sensitivity to gum Arabic used in the printing industry. Described by C. B. Bohner of America in 1941.

Printing A method using a seal and a rotating cylinder was known to the ancient Romans and Greeks. Movable type was known to the Chinese long before its introduction to Europe in the 15th century. The Chinese introduced multicolored printed paper money in 1107. The method of printing prior to this time in Europe was mainly on wooden blocks. The propagator of the movable type printing in Europe, Johann Gutenberg (1397–1468) from Mainz, printed the famous Latin Bible in 1456. The first printer in England was William Caxton (1422–1491) from Kent who published a *History of Troy*. The steam printing press

was invented by Friedrich Konig (1774–1833), a German printer from Eisleben in 1810. Stereotyped plates in printing were put forward by Alexander Tilloch (1759–1829) of Glasgow.

Prinzmetal Angina Unstable angina characterized by transient ischemic changes in the ECG due to spasm of the coronary arteries. Described by American cardiologist, Myron Prinzmetal (b 1908) from Buffalo and who graduated from the University of California, San Francisco in 1933.

Prion An infectious agent consisting of protein and devoid of functional nucleic acid, which resists inactivation by procedures that modify nucleic acids. It causes spongiform degeneration of the brain in various mammalian species. Its transmissibility to mice, rats and hamsters was demonstrated by S.B. Prusiner of San Francisco around 1992. *See prion disease.*

Prion Disease (Syn: spongiform encephalopathy) Disorders of protein conformation that produce neurodegeneration in humans and animals. Scrapie has been known in sheep for over 200 years. Creutzfeld–Jakob disease was described by Hans Gerhard Creutzfeld (1885–1964) in 1920 and Alfons Maria Jakob (1884–1931) in 1921. Kuru was first observed by an American virologist, Daniel Carleton Gajdusek (b 1923) and V. Zigas in 1957. Kuru, scrapie and Creutzfeld–Jakob disease were recognized to be infectious in the 1960s. Spongiform bovine encephalopathy of cattle (BSE) was recognized in England in 1986 and is the result of feeding cattle with meat and bonemeal from sheep infected with scrapie. Such feeding of ruminant-derived proteins to ruminants was banned in England in 1988. After a peak in the BSE epidemic in 1993 the incidence has fallen, consistent with an incubation period of 5 years. Other diseases in the group, such as Gerstmann–Straussler–Scheinker syndrome and fatal familial insomnia were described between 1990–1995.

Pritchard, Edward William (1825–1864) Surgeon from Filey, Yorkshire, who became a member of the Royal College of Surgeons in 1846. He systematically poisoned his wife with antimony in 1864, but was detected and charged with her murder. He was found guilty and hanged.

Pritchard, Urban (1845–1925) London otorhinologist who was the first chair of aural surgery in England at King's College in 1886. The intercellular membrane in the ampulla of the semicircular canals was described by him in 1876.

Private Anatomy and Medical Schools *See anatomy, private schools.*

Procaine Synthesized as novocaine by Alfred Einhorn

(1856–1917) of Germany in 1899. The Americans took over the patent from the Germans during World War l.

Prochaska, Georgius (1749–1820) Moravian professor of anatomy at Prague. He demonstrated the integrated functions of the brain in producing movements of the body in 1779. He also wrote on the heart and blood circulation in 1778.

Proctalgia Fugax [Greek: *proktos*, anus; Latin: *fugax*, swift] Paroxysmal intense pain in the region of the anus and the internal sphincter of unknown etiology. Described in 1917 by Alexander MacLennan, a lecturer in surgery at Glasgow University. It was named after Danish physician, Thornwald Einar Hess Thaysen (1883–1936) who referred to it as 'proctalgia fugax' in 1935.

Proctology [Greek: *proktos*, anus + *logos*, discourse] An Egyptian doctor had his tomb inscribed as 'Keeper of the King's rectum' in 2500 BC. During the Middle Ages, British surgeon John of Ardane (1307–1390) practiced as a specialist in rectal disorders in London and wrote an early illustrated treatise. Sir Charles Bent Ball (1851–1916), a surgeon and proctologist in Dublin, described the rectal valves (Ball valves), which were previously described by Giovanni Battista Morgagni (1682–1771), in *The Rectum and Anus, their diseases and treatment* published in 1887. Elston Charles Blanchard (b 1868) wrote several books including *The Romance of Proctology* (1938), *Epitome of Ambulant Proctology* (1924), *Textbook of Ambulant Proctology* (1928) and *Ambulant Proctology Clinics* (1925).

Profeta, Giuseppe (1840–1911) Sicilian physician in Genoa who proposed the law (Profeta law) that an apparent healthy infant will not be infected by its syphilitic mother.

Progesterone [Greek: *pro*, before; Latin: *gestare*, to bear] Obtained from corpus luteum tissue of sow's ovaries by Adolf Friedrich Butenandt (b 1903) in 1934. *See estrogens.*

Prognosis [Greek: *prognosis*, foreknowledge] Hippocrates (460–377 BC) was a master of prognostics, whose entire system of medicine was based on the observation of favorable and unfavorable symptoms and signs in disease. In his *Prognostics* he stated 'It appears to me a most excellent thing for the physician to cultivate prognosis, for by foreseeing and foretelling, in the presence of the sick, the present, past, and the future, and explaining the omissions which the patients have been guilty of, he will be more readily believed to be acquainted with the circumstances of the sick'. Several signs, such as fixed eyes, profuse sweating, opened mouth, involuntary discharge from the bowels, are described as unfavorable. According to the Arabian physician Rhazes (850–932), it is a bad symptom when a patient loses his modesty and exposes the parts of his body that should be covered. Other ancient physicians including Galen (AD 129–200), Aulus Cornelius Celsus (25 BC–AD 50), Oribasius (AD 325–400), Aetius (AD 502–575), Averrhoes (1126–1198) and Avicenna (980–1037) wrote on favorable and unfavorable signs of disease.

Progressive Bulbar Paralysis (Syn: chronic bulbar paralysis, labio-glosso-pharyngeal paralysis) Described by Louis Dumenil in 1859 and by Guillaume Benjamin Duchenne (1806–1875) in 1860. The current name was given by Wachsmuth in 1864.

Progressive Muscular Atrophy Wasting palsy. *See amyotrophic lateral sclerosis.*

Progressive Multifocal Leukoencephalopathy (PML) Form of demyelinating viral disease in man described by Astrom, Mancall and Richardson in 1958. The causative organism is a human polymavirus found by ZuRhein and Chou in 1965, and named JC virus by Padgett who isolated it in 1971.

Proguanil *See antimalarials.*

Prolactin [Greek: *pro*, before; Latin: *lac*, milk] A hormone from the anterior pituitary which induces enlargement and increased functioning of mammary glands. Isolated by American endocrinologists, Oscar Riddle (1877–1968), R. W. Bates and S. W. Dykshorn, who named it.

Prolan *See APL Hormone.*

Proline Amino acid isolated from cesin by Emil Fischer (1852–1919) in 1901.

Proprioceptor [Greek: *pro*, before + *prios*, early; Latin: *ceptare*, to receive] Highly specialized somatic sensory end organs of muscles, tendons and joints. Described by Sir Charles Sherrington (1857–1952) in 1906.

Prostaglandin The contractile effect of fresh semen on uterine muscle *in vitro* was demonstrated by two New York gynecologists, Raphael Kurzrok (b 1895) and Charles Lieb in 1930. The molecules were detected in human seminal plasma in the same year. Specific activity in contracting the uterus was shown in 1934 by Ulf Svante von Euler (1905–1983) who named them 'prostaglandins' in the belief that they came from the prostate whereas they come from the seminal vesicle. They were isolated in 1960, and inhibition of prostaglandin formation by aspirin-like drugs was demonstrated by Sir John Robert Vane (b 1927) and co-workers in 1970. The purified form was obtained by Swedish biochemists, Sune Karl Bergström (b 1916) and

Bengt Ingemar Samuelsson (b 1934) of Stockholm in the late 1960s, who were awarded the Nobel Prize in 1982, together with Vane. Thromboxane was discovered by M. Hamberg and co-workers in 1975.

Prostate [Greek: *pro*, before + *histanai*, to stand] The term 'prostatei chirsoides' was used by Aristotle (384–322 BC) to denote the seminal vesicles. Herophilus in 300 BC referred to it as 'prostati adenoeides'. Galen (AD 129–200) used the term in AD 180 to describe the prostate, seminal vesicles and associated structures.

Prostatectomy [Greek: *pro*, before + *histanai*, to stand + *ek*, out + *tomnein*, to cut] The Bottini operation where a channel was made through the prostate with galvanocautery for the treatment of enlarged prostate was designed by Italian surgeon, Enrico Bottini (1837–1903), in 1874. Castration for hypertrophy of the prostate was introduced by Philadelphia surgeon, J. William White (1850–1916). Sir William Blizard (1743–1835) of London treated prostatism transurethrally via perineal urethrotomy in 1806. George James Guthrie (1785–1856) described a transurethral instrument for incising inflammatory contracture of the bladder neck in 1834. The technique of removing the prostate thorough the perineum preceded the suprapubic route and was performed by George Goodfellow (1856–1910) and Wishard (1902) in America, and by Nicholl (1894) in England. Suprapubic prostatectomy was performed independently by: William Thomas Belfield (1856–1929) and Eugene Fuller (1894) in America, and MacGill and Sir Peter Johnston Freyer (1851–1921) in England. American urologist, Hugh Hampton Young (1870–1945) modified the method and used an extraurethral approach for ennucleation in 1911. C. H. Chetwood used galvanocautery though the perineum, and Young devised an endoscopic tube for perurethral excision in 1909.

Prostatic Carcinoma New York surgeons, Benjamin Stockwell Barringer (b 1878) and H.O. Woodward, in 1938 showed that the metastatic lesions of prostate cancer caused elevation of serum levels of acid phosphatase. In 1941 Charles Brenton Huggins (b 1901), a Canadian-born American urologist from Nova Scotia, noted that serum levels of acid phosphatase could be further elevated by administering androgens and could be diminished by giving estrogenic substances. Estrogens were shown to be effective in treatment by Huggins and C.V. Hodges in 1941. Acid phosphatase became a diagnostic marker and indicator of therapeutic response. The effect of stilboestrol and orchidectomy was demonstrated on an experimental basis by Huggins in 1941. An initial attempt to localize metastatic lesions using radioisotopes was made by J. P. Hummel and

H.A. Harris in 1956. *See acid phosphatase, prostatectomy.*

Prosthetic Valves [Greek: *prosthetos*, added] *See artificial valves.*

Prostigmine [Greek: *pro*, before + *stigma*, mark] Neostigmine, introduced as treatment for myasthenia gravis by Lazar Remen (b 1907) of Germany in 1934.

Prostitution [Latin: *prostratus*, thrown down] Practiced since the advent of civilization. Germany was one of the first to enforce periodical medical examinations in 1700. A system was introduced to register them in Paris in 1802, in England, the Contagious Diseases Prevention Act of 1864 enforced medical examination and in America a system to examine them every ten days was started in Nashville in 1863.

Protamine Insulin Following the discovery of insulin it was realized that diabetic patients need frequent insulin injections to maintain normal blood glucose, and attempts were made to prepare a long-acting insulin. An insulin combined with protamine protein from salmon roe was prepared by Hans Christian Hagedorn (1888–1971) at the Steno Memorial Hospital in Copenhagen in 1935. A single daily injection was achieved by D.A. Scott of Toronto and Albert Fisher who added zinc to form a relatively insoluble protamine zinc insulin in 1936. A neutral protamine insulin, isophane insulin, containing less protamine, and unmodified zinc insulin was introduced by Hagedorn in 1945.

Protamine [Greek: *protos*, first + *ammniakon*, resinous gum] Class of proteins discovered in sperm cells of fish by Friedrich Miescher (1844–1895) in 1871.

Protein Allergy The fatal effects of injecting albumin into rabbits sensitized to the protein by previous injections was demonstrated by François Magendie (1783–1855) in 1839. This was the first recorded experiment in anaphylaxis. The second was performed by Simon Flexner (1863–1946) in 1894 who showed the fatal effect of a second dose of serum in animals which had previously received a dose of the same serum.

Protein Losing Enteropathy Hypoprotenemia due to loss of proteins through the gastrointestinal mucosa following a variety of diseases was reported by Robert S. Gordon in *The Lancet* in 1959.

Protein Malnutrition *See kwashikor.*

Protein Shock Therapy *See auto-hemotherapy.*

Proteins [Greek: *protos*, first] Term coined by Dutch chemist, Gerrit Jan Mulder (1801–1880) of Utrecht around 1830. He studied nitrogen-containing materials such as silk, blood, egg white and gelatin, and named the complex substance protein. A method of isolating proteins from plant and animal tissues was developed by Heinrich Ritthausen (1826–1912) and Thomas Burr Osborne (1859–1929). Albrecht Kossel (1853–1927), professor of physiology at Hamburg, postulated in 1898 that they were made of polypeptides which consisted of amino acids. Otto Knut Olof Folin (1867–1934), a Swedish born biochemist and professor at Harvard University, demonstrated the importance of amino acids to human digestion and metabolism in 1906. The first amino acid was discovered by Sir Frederick Gowland Hopkins (1861–1947) in 1901. X-ray diffraction photography of a protein, pepsin, was taken by John Desmond Bernal (1901–1971) in 1934. Paper chromatography for separating amino acids was developed in 1942 by London biochemist, Archer John Porter Martin (b 1910) and Richard Laurence Millington Synge (b 1914), a biochemist from Chester, who shared the Nobel Prize for Chemistry in 1952. The number of amino acid residues in a protein molecule was devised in the late 1960s by an American biochemist and Nobel Prize winner, William Howard Stein (1911–1980) at the Rockefeller Institute. *See albumin, amino acids, globulin, plasma proteins.*

Proteus He was king of the island of Pharos in Greek mythology who could change his appearance as will.

Proteus vulgaris Gram-negative bacilli which causes urinary tract infections. Isolated by Gustav Hauser (1856–1935) of Germany in 1885.

Prothrombin Time [Greek: *pro*, before + *thrombus*, clot] The earliest case of bleeding in jaundice was reported by Wedelius in 1683. Armand James Quick (1894–1978) and colleagues in 1933 suggested that the bleeding was due to deficiency of a factor and was identified as prothombin. The two-stage method for determining it was designed by American pathologist, Emory Dean Warner (b 1905), K.M. Brinkhous and H.P. Smith in 1934. A one-stage method for detecting bleeding diathesis was developed by Quick in 1935. *See vitamin K.*

Protonsil Sulfonamide synthesized by Paul Gelmo (1879–1961) in 1908. The bacteristatic properties were recognized by German biochemist Gerhard Domagk (1895–1964), who published his findings in 1935 and received the Nobel Prize for Chemistry in 1939. He is said to have used it on his daughter to prevent her death from a streptococcal infection. It was identified as an effective antibacterial component by Swiss-born Italian biochemist, Daniele Bovet (1907–1992) in 1936, and he was awarded the Nobel Prize for Physiology or Medicine in 1957. Its value in treatment of puerperal sepsis

was established by Leonard Colebrook (1883–1967) and Méave Kenny in 1936. *See sulfonamides.*

Protoplasm [Greek: *proto*, first + *plasma*, plasm] Discovered by French zoologist Felix Dujardin (1801–1860) from Tours in 1835 who named it 'sarcode'. In 1839 a Czech physiologist, Johannes Purkinje (1787–1869), observed the living substance in cells of embryos and renamed it 'protoplasm'. The German botanist, Hugo von Mohl (1805–1872) from Stuttgart, a professor at Bern, showed that the sarcode or protoplasm of living cells was the same in plants and animals in 1846.

Protozoa [Greek: *proto*, first + *zoon*, animal] The first protozoan parasite, *Giardia lamblia*, was identified by Antoni van Leeuwenhoek (1632–1723) in his own stools in 1681. David Gruby (1810–1893) of Hungary proposed the genus *Trypanosoma* after his discovery of it in the blood of frogs in 1844. *Plasmodium* which causes malaria was discovered in 1880 by Charles Louis Alphonse Laveran (1845–1922), a French parasitologist and professor of pathological anatomy at the University of Rome. Clifford Dobell (1886–1949), an eminent protozoologist, published the classic works, *Amoeba living in Man* (1919), and *Intestinal Protozoa of Man* (1921).

Proust Law The Law of Constant Proportions was proposed by French chemist, Joseph Louis Proust (1754–1826) of Angers. He also isolated and identified grape sugar.

Prout, William (1785–1850) Chemical physiologist, born in Horton, Gloucestershire and graduated in medicine from Edinburgh in 1811. He settled in London and established his own laboratory in 1812. He demonstrated the presence of free hydrochloric acid in the stomach in 1823. He analyzed the contents of urine, and isolated urea in 1818. He proposed the law which states that relative atomic weights of all elements are multiples of relative atomic weight of hydrogen.

Prowazek, Stanislaus Joseph Mathias von (1876–1915) German microbiologist who, in 1907, found cell inclusion bodies in conjunctival cells in trachoma and postulated that they were collections of virus enveloped by material deposited from the infected cell. The causative organism of typhus, *Rickettsia prowazeki*, found in lice taken from patients with typhus fever by da Rocha Lima in 1916, was named in honor of the two workers, Howard Taylor Ricketts (1871–1910), and von Prowazek who contracted the disease and died during their research on it.

Pruritis [Latin: *prurire*, to itch] Hippocrates (460–377 BC) stated that it is common in old age. Galen (AD 129–200) ascribed it to external causes such as nettles, lack of cleanliness and sometimes indigestion. Paul of Aegina (625–690) recommended venesection, baths and application of substances such as barley-meal, lupin and a detergent ointment called peponaton, as treatment.

Pseudoxanthoma Elasticum (Syn: Darier disease) Hereditary skin disease with lax or stretched skin associated with cardiovascular and gastrointestinal abnormalities. Described by Jean Ferdinand Darier (1856–1938) in 1896.

Pseudofractures [Greek: *pseudes*, false] Simulated fractures in osteomalacia were described by Louis Arthur Milkman (1895–1951) of America in 1930.

Pseudohypertrophic Muscular Dystrophy [Greek: *pseudes*, false + *hyper*, above + *trophein*, to nourish] *See Duchenne muscular dystrophy*.

Pseudohypoparathyroidism [Greek: *pseudes*, false + *hypo*, below + *para*, beside + *thyreon*, shield] Characterized by chemical changes of hypoparathyroidism but not responding to parathyroid extract. Observed by Fuller Albright (1900–1969) in 1942.

Pseudomonas pyocyanea [Greek: *pseudes*, false + *monos*, alone] (Syn: *P. aeruginosa*) A blue pigment was obtained from organic material, and named 'pyocyanine' by M. Fordos of France in 1860. The bacterial source of the pigment was discovered by French physician, Carle Gessard (b 1850), in 1882. The bacillus was first called 'le microbe pyocynique' by Gessard. The term 'aeroginosa' was first used by J. Schroeter in 1875.

Pseudotuberculoma Silicoticum Foreign body granuloma of the skin simulating tuberculosis, due to accidental implantation of silica material. Described by Samuel George Shattuck (1852–1924) in 1916.

Psittacosis or parrot fever [Greek: *psittakos*, parrot + *osis*] First described by Jacob Ritter in 1879 in Switzerland. A larger outbreak occurred in Paris in 1892 and the source of infection was traced to a consignment of 500 parrots from Buenos Aires. An outbreak in England in 1929 was also due to import of diseased parrots from Brazil. The causative organism was identified by Sir Samuel Philip Bedson of London Hospital in 1930. *See ornithosis*.

Psoas Abscess [Greek: *psoa*, loins] Grafton Elliot Smith (1871–1937) and Sir Mark Armand Ruffer (1859–1917) described it following tuberculosis of the spine in an Egyptian mummy from 1000 BC. Drained through an incision in the loin by Sir Frederick Treves (1853–1923), a London surgeon in 1883. Lord Joseph Lister (1827–1912) treated it with an antiseptic incision followed by insertion of a drainage tube.

Psora [Greek: *psora*, rub to relieve an itch] *See Acarus scabiei*.

Psychiatry [Greek: *psyche*, breath + *iatreia*, healing] The word psyche was adapted to represent the mind or the soul. Cicero (106–43 BC), the Roman philosopher and orator, suggested that body ailments could result from emotional factors and proposed several ideas which are still fundamental to psychiatry and psychotherapy. He disputed the idea of Hippocrates (460–377 BC) that black bile caused melancholia, and attributed the condition to psychological difficulties. Areteaus the Cappadocian (AD 88–138) was a pioneer in establishing psychiatry as a branch of medicine and wrote on melancholia and madness, differentiating senile dementia from mania. St Augustine wrote on introspective psychiatry in *Confessions* in AD 386. In England a book on psychiatry, *A Treatise on Melancholy* was published by Timothy Bright (1551–1615) in 1586. This inspired Robert Burton's (1577–1640) popular book, *Anatomy of Melancholy* published in 1621. A license to practice psychiatry in England was granted to John Freeman in 1600. A book on clinical psychiatry, *Treatise on Madness*, was published by William Battie (1703–1776) in 1758. Benjamin Rush (1745–1813), the first psychiatrist in America, published *Diseases of the Mind* and used occupational therapy in treatment of mental disease. Modern theories and practice of psychiatry were developed in Vienna, Austria and Germany at the end of the 19th century. Eugen Bleuler (1857–1939), professor of psychiatry at the Burgholzli Hospital in Vienna where Carl Gustav Jung (1875–1961) was a student, coined the term 'schizophrenia' in 1911 to include dementia praecox, and the terms autism and ambivalence. Psychoanalysis was introduced by Sigmund Freud (1856–1939) in 1893. Henry Maudsley (1835–1918), an English psychiatrist from Yorkshire advocated the idea that insanity is fundamentally a disease of the body. His *The Pathology and Physiology of the Mind* published in 1867, is a classic in English psychiatry. Two English neurologists, Sir John Charles Bucknill (1817–1897) and Daniel Hack Tuke (1827–1895) advocated removal of physical restraints from institutionalized mental patients. Jean Etienne Dominique Esquirol (1772–1840), a French physician from Toulouse, was one of the first lecturers in psychiatry at Salpêtrière in 1811. Philippe Pinel (1745–1826), a neuropsychiatrist in Paris, identified insanity as an illness and treated patients on a scientific and humane basis around 1800.

Psychoanalysis Josef Breuer (1842–1925), a contemporary of Sigmund Freud (1856–1939), used hypnosis and called this method the 'talking cure'. They published their findings on this new method of treatment in *On the Psychic Mechanisms of Hysterical Phenomena* in 1893. The practice was introduced into England and America by Ernest Jones (1879–1958) of Glamorgan who qualified as a physician from London and was director of the first psychoanalytic clinic in London.

Psychoanalytic Society Organized in Vienna in 1902 by Carl Gustav Jung (1875–1961), Karl Abraham (1877–1925) and led by Sigmund Freud (1856–1939). The New York Society was formed under the chairmanship of Abraham Brill (1874–1928) in 1911 and the American Society was founded in the same year, with James Putnam (1846–1918) as first president. The British Society was founded by Ernest Jones (1879–1958) from Glamorgan.

Psychoasthenia *See Janet Pierre, chronic fatigue syndrome.*

Psychogeriatrics Michel Eugene Chevereul (1786–1889) studied the psychiatric effects of old age. Tom Wilson founded the first psychogeriatric unit at Cornwall in 1948 and showed that the elderly mentally infirm could be maintained in the community. He initiated the collaboration between general practitioners, geriatricians and psychiatrists. Daycare was introduced at the Langthorne Hospital in London by Lionel Cosin in 1948.

Psycholinguistics Developed by Russian psychologist, Lev Semyonovich Vygotsky (1896–1934) who studied social sciences at Moscow University and took up psychology in 1924. His *Thought and Language* published in 1934, became a classic text.

Psychology [Greek: *psyche*, soul + *logos*, discourse] Thomas Hobbes (1588–1679), a philosopher from Westport near Malmesbury, wrote *Human Nature* in 1650 and distinguished between cognition and motive. The term 'psychology' was used in the modern sense by C. Wolff in *Rational Psychology* published in 1734, and David Hartley (1704–1757), a physician from Halifax, in *Observations on Man, His Frame, His Duty and His Expectations* published in 1749. Frederick Eduard Beneke (1824–1825), a founder of systematic psychology in Europe, published *Lehrbuch der Psychologie als Naturwissenschaft* in 1832. Systematic psychology in Britain was founded by Thomas Brown (1778–1820) from Kirkmabreck, who published *Lectures on Philosophy of Human Mind* in 1820. William Benjamin Carpenter (1813–1885) from Exeter, proposed the concept of subconscious mind. Alexander Bain (1808–1903), professor of logic at Aberdeen, published *Senses and the Intellect* (1855) and *Emotions and the Will* in 1859. *Principles of Psychology* (1855) was published by Herbert Spencer (1820–1903) and it classified psychology as a biological science. The first professorship in psychology was created at

the University of Pennsylvania, and James McKeen Cottall (1860–1944) was appointed in 1888. The journal, *Philosophische Studien* was founded by Wilhelm Wundt in 1881, and in America, *The American Journal of Psychology* was started by Granville Stanley Hall (1846–1924) in 1887. William McDougall (1871–1938) from Manchester established a new tradition of psychology at Oxford, and published *Social Psychology* in 1908. Adolf Bastian (1826–1905), an ethnologist from Bremen, founded comparative psychology and studied different races, proposing the theory that folk cultures can be traced to geographical influence. William James (1842–1910) from New York, professor of psychology at Harvard University, proposed the theory of emotion in 1884 and wrote *Principles of Psychology*, published in 1890 and *Textbook of Psychology*, published in 1892. The school of analytical psychology in Vienna was founded by Carl Gustav Jung (1875–1961) at the public mental hospital in Zurich in 1913. *See experimental psychology, sexual psychology.*

Psychology, Feminine *The Psychology of Women, A Psychoanalytic Interpretation* was published by Helene Deutsch (1884–1992) from the Vienna School of Medicine in 1944.

Psychosomatic Disease [Greek: *psyche*, soul + *soma*, body] Plato (428–347 BC) said that body and soul were different entities, but Aristotle (384–322 BC) taught that they were one. Cicero (106–43 BC) suggested that body ailments could result from emotional factors. Aretaeus (81–138) mentioned disorders of the mind and emotion as causes of paralysis. Robert Whytte (1714–1766) of Edinburgh, stated that 'excess fear, grief, joy, and shame have been followed sometimes by death'. J. G. Langerman (1768–1832) suggested that physical diseases were of psychological origin and stressed the need for psychotherapy in 1797. Benjamin Rush (1745–1813) also suggested that some diseases may be psychosomatic in 1786. German psychiatrist, Johan Christian Heinroth (1773–1843) coined the term 'psychosomatic' in 1818. Carl Gustav Carus (1789–1868), professor of anatomy and an obstetrician at Montpellier, proposed the concept of psychosomatic disease. The influence of emotions on the viscera was presented by Sir Clifford Allibut (1836–1925) in his Goulstonian lectures *on the neuroses of the viscera* in 1884. A graduate of Yale Medical School, H. Flanders Dunbar (1902–1959), pioneered psychosomatic medicine in America, and described the accident-prone personality. She founded and edited the journal, *Psychosomatic Medicine* in 1938.

Psychosurgery Treatment for mental diseases proposed by Antonio Egaz Moniz (1874–1955) in early 1930s. He believed that morbid ideas stimulated the neurons and maintained a vicious cycle and any alteration of frontal lobes could interrupt this. His theory was supported by the experiments on frontal lobes of monkeys by John Farquhar Fulton (1899–1960) and C.F. Jacobsen from Yale who noted that monkeys became more manageable after section of their prefrontal lobes. Frontal lobotomy was performed by Moniz and a Portuguese surgeon Almeida Lima in 1935.

Psychotherapy [Greek: *psyche*, soul + *therapio*, take care of] The first modern systematic treatise was published by a German physician, Johann Christian Reil in 1803. Mesmerism was proposed by Franz Anton Mesmer (1734–1815) in 1799 and renamed 'hypnotism' by James Braid (1795–1860), a Manchester surgeon in 1843. The technique was used by Augustine Henry Forel in 1889. Treatment of neurotic diseases with persuasive therapy or psychotherapy was pioneered by Paul Charles Dubois (1848–1918), professor of neuropathology at Bern around 1888. *See group therapy.*

Pterodactyl [Greek: *pteron*, wing] The fossil of a flying lizard was found by the paleontologist, Georges Leopold Cuvier (1769–1832) of Paris.

Pterygopalatine Syndrome Neuralgia of the lower half of the face, nasal congestion and rhinorrhoea secondary to a lesion in the pterygopalatine ganglion. Described by Greenfield Sleuder (1865–1925) of New York in 1908.

Ptolemy, Claudius (AD 90–168) Astronomer and geographer from Alexandria who wrote *Tetrabiblos Syntaxis*, an advanced mathematical work on construction of tables.

Ptomaine Poisonous substance noted in decaying fish by Burrows in 1814. It was shown to consist of putrefactive alkaloids which caused food poisoning by Francesco Selmi who named the group of substances 'ptomaines' in 1872. An Italian chemist Nencki isolated them in 1876.

Public Health Laboratory Service Established in England by the Ministry of Health in 1946. *See public health.*

Public Health The importance of hygiene in relation to health of the society has been known for millennia. Excavations at Mohanjadaro and Harappa in the Indus Valley by English archeologist Sir John Hubert Marshall (1876–1958) of Chester in the 1920s revealed a sophisticated system of sanitation and hygiene existed 5000 years ago. The first subterranean sewers called 'cloacae' were built in Rome around 600 BC. The Aediles, a group of public health officials in Rome around AD 70, looked after cleanliness of public roads, suitability of food items for consumption,

burial methods and other matters. The state of public health deteriorated during the Middle Ages leading to epidemics of plague and other pestilence. The first sanitary legislation in England prescribing a penalty of 20 pounds for casting animal filth into rivers and ditches in urban areas was in effect in 1388. Sewers to drain water from marshes and low lying areas were constructed during the reign of King Henry VIII in 1532 and opened into the river Thames, which became a cesspool and led to appalling sanitary conditions in London by 1840. The earliest design for a mechanical water closet was made by Sir John Harington (1561–1612) in 1596. A system of ventilation to provide fresh air to hospitals, mines, and other crowded places was devised by the British scientist and clergyman Stephen Hales (1677–1761) in 1743. Sir Edwin Chadwick (1801–1890), the great sanitary reformer of England, wrote *Report on the Sanitary Conditions of the Labouring Population* in 1842 that led to the City Sewage Act and the first medical officer in 1848. The Public Health Act was passed in England in 1875 and contained a vast code of sanitary laws in 300 sections. A pioneer in public health in Europe was Peter Johann Frank (1745–1821) of Rotalben who used the term 'medical police' to refer to all preventive aspects. The American Public Health Association was founded in 1872 through the efforts of Lemuel Shattuck (1793–1859) of Boston who presented *Report of the Sanitary conditions of Massachusetts* in 1850. A modern public health campaign in America was launched by Charles Value Chapin (1856–1941), superintendent of health at Providence and president of the American Public Health Association in 1927. William Thompson Sedgwick (1855–1921) of Massachusetts advocated pasteurization of milk and the treatment of drinking water with chlorine.

Puerperal Fever [Latin: *puer*, child + *parere*, bring forth] Childbed fever was mentioned in the aphorisms of Hippocrates (460–377 BC). Epidemics became common during 17th, 18th and 19th centuries, and 200 outbreaks occurred in Europe between 1652 and 1862. Alexander Gordon (1752–1799), an obstetrician at Aberdeen, proposed a contagious nature and advocated disinfection of the clothes of the midwife and doctor in 1795. *An Account of Puerperal fever as it appeared in Derbyshire in 1782* was published by William Butter (1726–1805), a physician from Derbyshire who practiced in London. The initiator of asepsis in prevention was Ignaz Philipp Semmelweiss (1818–1865) of Vienna who demonstrated in 1847 that mortality could be reduced from 18% to less than 2% if hands were washed before examining patients. Oliver Wendell Holmes (1809–1894) preceded Semmelweis in proposing the contagious nature in *On the Contagiousness of Puerperal fever* presented to the Boston Medical Society in 1842. Despite opposition to his work he reiterated his views in *Puerperal Fever as a Private Pestilence* in 1855.

Pulmonary Aneurysm Rupture of an aneurysm into the lung. The first case was published by Fearn in *The Lancet* in 1841. Further cases were described by Carl von Rokitansky (1804–1878) in 1868. The first case of an aneurysm eroding through the wall of the bronchus was presented by Douglas Powell of Brompton Hospital in 1878.

Pulmonary Atresia In association with an intact ventricular septum is an uncommon congenital anomaly. Described by William Hunter (1718–1783) in three patients. Its occurrence together with dextroposition of the aorta was described by Thomas Bevill Peacock (1812–1882) of London in 1858. Surgery was performed by Alfred Blalock (1899–1964) and Helen Taussig (1898–1986) of Johns Hopkins Medical School in 1945.

Pulmonary Circulation Recognized by Al-Nafis, a surgeon from Damascus in the 13th century. Michael Servitus (1511–1553), a native of Aragon in Spain, described it in detail. He also recognized the difference between venous and arterial blood and described his findings in *Restitutio Christianismi* in 1553. Matteo Realdo Colombo (1516–1569), a pupil of Andreas Vesalius (1514–1564), mentioned it in *de Re Anatomica* published in 1559 but he failed to realize the significance of his discovery. William Harvey (1578–1657) called the pulmonary artery 'vena arteriosa' (a vein similar to artery) and the pulmonary vein 'arteria venosa'.

Pulmonary Embolus Migratory clots from peripheral veins. Mentioned by Armand Trousseau (1801–1867) and Dumontpellier of Paris in their paper in 1860. An attempt at pulmonary embolectomy was made by Friedrich Trendelenburg (1844–1924) in 1908. The procedure was successfully carried out 16 years later by Martin Kirschner (1879–1942) in 1924.

Pulmonary Eosinophilia *See Löffler syndrome.*

Pulmonary Functions *See lung functions.*

Pulmonary Osteoarthropathy Clubbing of the fingers and toes associated with arthritis and periostitis of the distal end of the long bones, from secondary anoxemia caused by chronic pulmonary disease or carcinoma of the lungs, was described by Pierre Marie (1853–1940) of Paris in 1890. The condition was re-described by Heinrich von Bamberger (1822–1888) in 1891.

Pulmonary Stenosis An early account was given by James Hope (1809–1841) in his *Treatise on the Disease of the Heart* in 1839. Valvotomy was performed in 1948 by Sir Russell Brock (1903–1980) of Wimbledon, a surgeon at Guy's Hospital.

(a) Pulse tracing of a patient with aortic regurgitation and angina pectoris; (b) Same pulse during temporary relief of pain by amyl nitrite; (c) Tracing of same pulse during severe angina. Thomas Lauder Brunton, *Lectures on the Actions of Medicines* (1897). Macmillan & Co., London

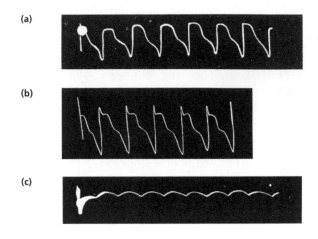

Pulse [Latin: *pulsus*, stroke] Pien Ch'iao of China wrote a treatise on the pulse in 600 BC and the Egyptian physician Imhotep wrote another in 2950 BC. Pulsation of the heart of chick embryo was observed by Aristotle (384–322 BC). Erasistratus (325–250 BC) described it as a wave, but this was disputed by Galen (AD 129–200). Hippocrates (460–377 BC) mentioned it and Herophilus (335–250 BC) studied rhythmic tides produced in arteries by the beating heart around 300 BC. Pliny (AD 23–79) said 'to detect its exact harmony in relation to age and disease, one needs to be a musician and even a mathematician to understand the pulse according to Herophilus'. Paul of Aegina (625–690) described it as 'the movement of the heart and arteries taking place by a diastole and systole'. Aretaeus (81–138) gave a detailed account of the pulse in AD 100. Galen wrote several treatises including: *Liebellus de Pulsibus ad Tirones*, *Pulsuum Compendium* and *Libri Quatuor de Pulsum Differentis*. He recommended the radial pulse for study as it had little flesh over it, is visible, and did not involve taking off the clothes. He divided the pulse into four phases: systole, diastole, presystole and prediastole. The earliest instrument to measure it was designed by Italian physiologist, Sanctorio Sanctorius (1561–1636) and consisted of a lead weight attached to a long thread, the length of which could be adjusted according to the frequency. William Harvey (1578–1657) noted the synchronous nature of it in all arteries in 1628. Counting pulse rate in health and disease was introduced by Sir John Floyer (1649–1734) with his pulse watch in 1707. Slow pulse rate was observed by Marcus Gerbezius (1658–1718) in 1691, Giovanni Battista Morgagni (1682–1771) in 1761 and Thomas Spens of Edinburgh in 1793. Allan Burn of Edinburgh suggested that fits were secondary to a very slow pulse in 1809, and his findings were confirmed by a Scottish physician at St Thomas' Hospital, Robert Reid, in 1824. An important monograph was written by an English physician, Caleb Hillier Parry (1755–1822) of Bath. The sphygmograph, to obtain tracings of the pulse, was used by Karl Vierordt (1818–1884) in 1854. *See dicrotic pulse.*

Pulsus Alterans [Latin: *pulsus*, stroke] Described and differentiated from pulsus bigeminus by Ludwig Traube (1818–1876), professor of pathology at Berlin, in 1872.

Pulsus Bigeminus [Latin: *pulsus*, stroke] A clear description of the condition was given by Ludwig Traube (1818–1876) of Berlin in 1872.

Pulse Deficit [Latin: *pulsus*, stroke] Difference between the apex heart rate and the radial pulse seen in cases of atrial fibrillation. Described by Boston physician, James Jackson, jr (1810–1834).

Pulsus Paradoxus [Latin: *pulsus*, stroke; Greek: *para*, beside + *doxa*, belief or opinion] Decrease in pulse volume during inspiration. Introduced and described as an important physical sign by Adolf Kussmaul (1822–1902) in 1873.

Pupillary Reaction Robert Whytt (1714–1766), a neurologist from Edinburgh, established that it was a reflex reaction in *Essay on Vital and Other Involuntary Motions of Animals* published in 1751, and the reflex (Whytt reflex) is named after him. He described the mechanism and its dilation in death. The effect of spinal injury was described by Douglas Moray Cooper Lamb Argyll Robertson (1837–1909) in 1869. *See Argyll Robertson pupil.*

Purgatives *See laxatives, aperients.*

Purkinje, Johannes Evangelista (1787–1869) Bohemian professor of physiology at Breslau, who observed the living substance in eggs and embryos and named it 'protoplasm' in 1839. He also found that deaf mutes can hear through the bones of the skull in 1821, and this contributed to the study of deafness in mutes. He classified fingerprints in 1832, and the germinal vesicles in the ovum of birds in 1825. Microdissection was suggested by him in 1844, and the reticulated subendocardial fibers of the heart (Purkinje fibers) bear his name.

Purpura [Latin: *purpura*, purple] Avicenna (980–1037) gave a brief description of a chronic form. A modern description of purpura hemorrhagica (Werlhof disease) was given by German physician, Paul Gottlieb Werlhof (1699–1767) of Helmstedt in *Opera Omnia* in 1775. *See thrombocytopenic purpura, Henoch–Schönlein purpura.*

Purves-Stewart, James (1869–1949) Neurologist to Westminster Hospital and the Royal National Orthopaedic Hospital in London. He wrote an important textbook of neurology, *The Diagnosis of Nervous Diseases,* which reached its tenth edition after 41 years and was translated into German, French, Arabic, and Spanish.

Putnam, Frederick Ward (1839–1915) Father of archeology in America. He was professor of archeology at Harvard in 1887 and studied archeological remains of Native Americans. He published over 400 articles.

Putnam, James Jackson (1846–1918) American neurologist, born in Boston and graduated in medicine from Harvard in 1866. He was a founder of American Neurology Association and was professor of diseases of the nervous system at Harvard in 1893. *See subacute combined degeneration of the cord.*

Putnam Disease *See subacute combined degeneration of the cord, Putnam, James Jackson.*

Putrefaction [Latin: *putris*, rotten + *facere*, to make] Investigations were commenced in 1836 by F. Schulz, and Theodor Schwann's (1810–1882) work followed a year later. Schwann said that it was caused by mold and infusoria at the expense of organic substances. This was confirmed by Louis Pasteur's (1822–1895) work on fermentation in 1857.

Putrid Fever Old term for typhoid fever.

Putti, Vitorrio (1881–1940) Professor of orthopedic surgery and medical historian in Bologna. He designed an operation for dislocation of the shoulder.

Pyelitis [Greek: *pyelos*, pelvis + *itis*, inflammation] Pyelonephritis is an inflammation of the kidney and was described in pregnant women by Pierre François Olive Rayer (1793–1867) of Paris in 1841. Sir William Roberts (1830–1899) of Manchester Royal Infirmary observed the presence of rod-shaped bacteria in the urine associated with cystitis following catheterization in 1881. Ernest Leberecht Wagner (1829–1888) of Germany described pyelonephritic kidney and the importance of chronic pyelonephritis in 1882. John Alberton Sampson (1873–1946) of Johns Hopkins Hospital noted that acute pyelonephritis could result from ureteric obstruction or systemic infection in 1903.

Pyelography [Greek: *pyelos*, pelvis + *graphein*, write] Radiological method of visualization of the renal tract introduced by Alexander von Lichtenberg (1880–1949) of Germany in 1906.

Pyelolithotomy [Greek: *pyelos*, pelvis + *lithos*, stone + *temnein*, to cut] First performed by Vincenz Czerny (1842–1916) in 1880.

Pyelonephritis [Greek: *pyelos*, pelvis + *nephros*, kidney] *See pyelitis.*

Pyemia [Greek: *pyon*, pus + *haima*, blood] An account on bacterial endocarditis was given as 'arterial pyaemia' by Sir Samuel Wilkes (1824–1911) in 1870.

Pygmies [Greek: *pugme*, fist] Aristotle (384–322 BC) referred to a race of tiny men the size of a fist. The earliest study was by a French naturalist and ethnologist Jean Louis Armand Quatrefages (1810–1892), professor at the Natural History Museum in 1862, who published studies from the interior of Africa and southmost parts of Asia. J. Kollmann of Basel in his *Pigmaen in Europe* published in 1894, produced evidence for the existence of a European pigmy race in Neolithic times. *See dwarfs.*

Pyknoepilepsy [Greek: *pyknos*, frequent + *lepsy*, I seize] Recurrent attacks resembling petit mal but not epileptiform in nature. Described by Max Friedmann (1858–1925) of Germany in 1906.

Pylorectomy [Greek: *pylorus*, gatekeeper + *ektomnein*, to cut out] Done experimentally on animals by Daniel Carl Theodore Merrem (1790–1859) in 1810. Theodor Billroth (1829–1894) performed a resection of the pylorus for cancer in 1881.

Pyloric Stenosis [Greek: *pylorus*, gatekeeper] Caused by congenital hypertrophy and described by Patrick Blair (1666–1728), a surgeon from Dundee in 1717. It was also described by George Armstrong (1719–1789) of London in 1777 and by Jean Cruveilhier (1791–1874) of Paris in 1829. An account of the disease in infants in America was given by Hezekiah Beardsley (1748–1799) in 1788. German surgeon, Conrad Ramstedt (1867–1963), described an operation for relief of congenital hypertrophic pyloric stenosis. Chronic pyloric ulcer has recently been identified as a further cause.

Pyloroplasty [Greek: *pylorus*, gatekeeper + *plasmein*, to mold] Performed by Italian surgeon Pietro Loreta (1831–1899) in 1882.

Pylorus [Greek: *pylorus*, gatekeeper] Galen (AD 129–200) used the term 'stenotis' to denote the pylorus or narrow part of the stomach. He compared the structure to a gatekeeper or janitor, hence its present name.

Pyocyanine *See Pseudomonas pyocyanea.*

Pyorrhoea Alveolaris Chronic suppurative peridontitis. The study of the jaws of Egyptian mummies dating back to 2800 BC has shown that the disease was present in ancient times.

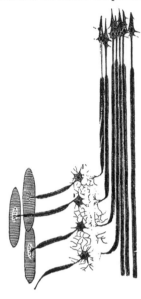

Pyramidal tract system. Jean Martin Charcot, *Lectures on Localisation of Cerebral and Spinal Diseases* (1883). New Sydenham Society, London

Pyramidal Tract Part of the nervous system identified and named by Paul Emil Flechsig (1847–1929) of Leipzig in 1876.

Pyrexia [Greek: *pyressein*, feverish] *See thermometry.*

Pyridoxine (Syn: adermin, antidermatitis factor) Vitamin B6. Deficiency causes dermatitis or acrodynia in rats and was observed by Paul Gyorgy (1893–1976) in 1934. It was named vitamin B6 and synthesized by Staton Avery Harris (b 1902) and Karl Folkers of America in 1939. It was given the name 'adermin' by German chemist and Nobel Prize winner, Richard Kuhn (1900–1967), in 1938, and received its present name 'pyridoxine' from Gyorgy and R. E. Eckhardt in 1940.

Pyrimidine Base in DNA isolated from extract of pancreas by Albrecht Kossel (1888–1956), professor of physiology at Hamburg in 1885. In 1910 he received the Nobel Prize for Physiology or Medicine.

Pyruvate Kinase Deficiency Causes hemolytic anemia and was described by W. N. Valentine, K. Tanaka and S. Miwa in 1961.

Pythagorus (600 BC) Greek philosopher and mathematician, born in Samos around 530 BC and settled in the Greek colony of Crotona in southern Italy. He taught the doctrine of transmigration of souls from one body to another. He founded the study of geology with his observation on the physical changes in the land and its volcanic eruptions. He established the modern system of astronomy, improved geometry and invented the multiplication tables.

Pyuria, Abacterial [Greek: *pyon*, pus + *ouron*, urine] Presence of pus in the urine without growth of bacteria on laboratory culture. It was attributed to renal tuberculosis in 1900. T. Moore in 1943 proposed that it was due to a virus. N. Cooke attributed the condition (as Amicrobic pyuria) to excretion of a toxin in 1944. O. Peters in 1946 proposed that pus in sterile urine was caused by a spirochetal organism. Following his work, intravenous neoarsphenamine was used as a standard empirical treatment during the mid-1940s. Further work reconfirmed that the most common cause of the condition was renal tuberculosis. *See bacteriuria.*

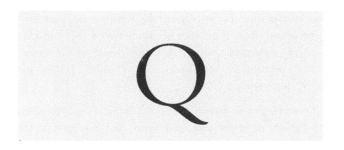

Q Fever Originally named 'Q' to denote query as the causative agent was unknown. Observed by Edward Holbrook Derrick (1898–1976) in 1937 in Queensland, Australia, in an outbreak of febrile illness amongst meat and cattle workers in Brisbane. The causative rickettsial organism, *Coxiella burnetti*, was identified by Sir Frank Macfarlane Burnet (1899–1985). He was one of Australia's greatest scientists who also developed the clonal theory of antibody production which earned him the Nobel Prize in 1960. The same strain of *Coxiella* was recovered from ticks during an outbreak in Montana by Herald Rea Cox (b 1907) and G. E. Davis in 1938. The organism was named for its discoverers, Cox and Burnet.

Quack Medicines *See quackery.*

Quackery Derived from 'quacksalver', a corruption of 'quick-silver' or mercury which was used extensively by quacks. They were present in Roman times, and Charmis, one such physician during the time of Nero, is said to have charged extravagant fees. Many were found in the 15th century, when the practice of medicine began to be regulated by the state and the medical profession. Paracelsus (1493–1541) in his fifth book wrote on banishing them from medicine. Some notable past quacks in England include: Simon Forman (1552–1611) of Wiltshire who practiced in London in 1583 selling love portions and other remedies, William Brodum, one of the most successful quacks of the 18th century in London, James Graham (1745–1794) from Edinburgh who used alternative therapies such as mud baths, and William Reed, a tailor, set himself up as a mender of eyes and was knighted by Queen Anne. Joshua Ward (1685–1761), known as 'spot' due to the birthmark on his face, was exempted from the Apothecaries Act of 1748 by the King and developed a pill, known as 'drop and pill' that contained antimony. Many remedies for amenorrhea were on offer and some abortifacients were camouflaged as treatment for amenorrhea. These included: Dumas Paris pills, Nurse Powell corrective pills, Nurse Mann's remedy, Dr John Hooper female pills, Dr Davis female mixture, Jefferson Dodd corrective, Martin apiol, and Monaid tablets. Consumption cures were also commonly sold in the form of secret remedies for tuberculosis. These include: Tuberculozyme from Derk P. Yonkerman Company Ltd of America, the Brompton Consumption mixture (no relation to the Brompton Consumption Hospital), and Stevens Consumption Cure was claimed by 'Dr' Stevens to contain a herbal medicine from Africa called 'umckaloaba'.

Quadriceps [Latin: *quadri*, four + *ceps*, head] Muscle and name given to the God Janus who had four heads.

Quain, Jones (1785–1851) Lecturer at the Medical School in Aldersgate, and later professor at the new University of London. He wrote an important textbook on anatomy, *Elements of Anatomy*, in 1828 which continued into 11 editions up to 1929.

Quain, Sir Richard (1816–1898) Born in County Cork, Ireland, he was a physician at the Brompton Chest Hospital in London. A form of fatty degeneration of the heart (Quain fatty degeneration) was described by him. He compiled *A Dictionary of Medicine* (1882) in 2 volumes which became one of the most quoted dictionaries of his time.

Quaker The Religious Society of Friends was started in England in 1646 by George Fox (1624–1691) of Leicestershire. They were named 'Quakers' by Justice Bennet of Derby in 1650 because they were said to quake at the Word of God. Some eminent Quaker physicians were: Thomas Young (1773–1829) of Milverton, England, one of the greatest scientists of all times with work on hemodynamics, Egyptology and his undulatory theory of light; Robert Willan (1757–1812) who wrote a monograph *On Cutaneous Diseases* in 1796; and John Fothergill (1712–1780) who gave an original description of diphtheric sore throat in 1748. Quakers also excelled in pharmacy and Allen and Hanburys, one of the earliest Quaker pharmaceutical establishments, was founded by a Quaker, Sylvanus Bevan, grandson of William Bevan, a merchant from Swansea.

Quantitative Analysis [Latin: *quantus*, as much as] Arabian alchemist, Geber, in the 8th century, recognized that a certain quantity of acid was required to neutralize a given amount of base, and in 1699, Wilhelm Homberg of Germany and later Torbern Olof Bergman (1735–1784) of Sweden and Richard Kirwan (1733–1812) of Dublin in 1775 attempted to quantify this, but the crude experimental methods available hindered their success. Methods for study of inorganic compounds were established around 1810 by Jöns Jacob Berzelius (1779–1848), a Swedish physician and a chemist at Uppsala.

Quantum Theory The first suggestion of 'wave' theory of light or energy fundamental to quantum theory was made in 1817 by English physician Thomas Young (1773–1829).

As a result of experiments on thermodynamics by Gustav Robert Kirchhoff (1824–1887) in 1859, Josef Stefan (1835–1893) and Ludwig Boltzmann (1844–1906), the concept that radiation emissions came in packets of quanta was first proposed by the German physicist Max Karl Ernst Ludwig Planck (1858–1947) of Kiel in 1900. Planck quantum theory formed the basis for Albert Einstein's (1879–1955) work on theory of light in 1905 which led to his theory of relativity. It was applied to subatomic physics by Danish physicist, Niels Hendrik David Bohr (1885–1962) in 1913. Wave mechanics were proposed by an Austrian physicist, Erwin Schrödinger (1887–1961) in 1930. The Nobel Prize for Physics was won by Planck in 1918, Einstein in 1921, Bohr in 1922, Schrödinger in 1933, and Werner Karl Heisenberg (1901–1976) of Germany in 1932. American theoretical physicist, David Joseph Bohm (1917–1992) wrote an excellent book on the subject, *Quantum Theory*, in 1951.

Quarantine [Latin: *quadraginta*, forty] Started in Venice in 1127, where all merchants from the Levant were obliged to remain at the House of St Lazarus for 40 days before being admitted to the city. During plague epidemics in England all persons coming from affected areas were confined. Quarantine Acts in England were passed in 1753 and in 1825.

Quarin, Joseph (1773–1814) Viennese physician to Emperor Joseph II who served as the rector of the university on six occasions. He was made a count in 1747.

Quartan Fever [Latin: *quartanus*, fourth] Periodic fevers were classified into quotidian, tertian, subtertian and quartan according to their periodicity by Hippocrates (460–377 BC). The term was used because it occurred every fourth day.

Quastel, Juda Hirsch (1899–1987) British biochemist from Sheffield, who was a pioneer in biochemical aspects of brain disease. He obtained his PhD on bacterial metabolism while working with Frederick Gowland Hopkins at Cambridge. He was staff biochemist at the Cardiff City Mental Hospital where he began his work on mental disease and developed liver function tests for schizophrenia, investigated the effects of amphetamines and synthesis of acetylcholine. During the War he worked at Rothamsted Experimental Station on soil fertility and produced a selective herbicide. He was appointed to the chair of biochemistry at McGill University in Canada in 1947, and after his retirement in 1964, he joined the Kinsman Laboratories at Vancouver where he worked on the role of glutamic acid in metabolism of the brain.

Quételet, Lambert Adolphe (1796–1874) Belgian astronomer and statistician who proposed the concept of an 'average man'. He investigated the development of intellectual and physical qualities of man between 1835 and 1846 and established that the data conformed to the theory of probability. He wrote *Sur l'homme* (1835) and *L'Anthropométrie* (1871).

Quatrefages de Breau, Jean Louis Armand de (1810–1892) French naturalist and ethnologist, and professor at the Natural History Museum in Paris in 1855. Some works include *Unite L'espice Humane* (1861), *Crania Ethnica* (1875–1882), and *Darwin et ses precursieurs Francis* (1892). The English translation, *Metamorphoses of Man and Lower Animals*, was published by Henry Lawson, professor of physiology at Birmingham in 1864. The angle of Quatrefages or the parietal angle used in craniometry was defined by him, and he invented a 'goniometer' for measuring it in 1858.

Quebec Medical Society Canadian society inaugurated in 1826 with Joseph Morrin (b 1794), a graduate of Edinburgh who was born in Dumfries, as its first president.

Queckenstedt Test A block in the flow of cerebrospinal fluid found during lumbar puncture by applying pressure on the jugular vein. Shown by German physician, Hans Heinrich Georg Queckenstedt (1876–1918) of Hamburg in 1916.

Queen Charlotte's Hospital The first lying-in hospital in London was founded by Sir Richard Manningham (d 1759) adjoining his house at Jermyn Street, in 1739. His unit started with 24 beds and became the General Lying-in Hospital in 1752. Queen Charlotte was patron in 1791 and it was renamed Queen Charlotte's Hospital in 1813.

Queen [Anglo-Saxon: *cwen*] Semiramis, queen of Assyria in 2017 BC, was the first woman to hold sovereign authority. She is said to have encouraged men and women to study medicine.

Quellung Reaction Swelling of the pneumococcal bacterial capsule when treated with its antiserum. Observed by Fred Neufield (1861–1945), a colleague of Robert Koch (1843–1910) at Berlin in 1902.

Quenu Hemorrhoidal Plexus A series of lymphatic plexuses in the mucous membrane and skin of the anus. Described in 1893 by professor of surgical pathology at Paris, Edouard André Victor Alfred Quenu (1852–1933).

Quenuthoracoplasty Operation to divide the ribs in order to promote the retraction of chest wall in empyema. Devised by a professor of surgical pathology at Paris, Edouard André Victor Alfred Quenu (1852–1933).

Quevain Disease *See de Quervain disease.*

Quervain Thyroiditis *See de Quervain thyroiditis.*

Quesnay, Francis (1694–1774) Physician and political writer from Montfort l'Amaury, France. He moved to Paris and became physician to Louis XV. He was first permanent secretary to the Academy of Surgery in Paris. He wrote *A Philosophical Essay on the Animal Economy* in 3 volumes. He suggested an arterial cause for gangrene in his *Traite de la Gangrene*, published in 1739.

Quevenne Iron Finely powdered form of reduced metallic iron introduced as a general remedy by French physician, Theodore Auguste Quevenne (1805–1855).

Quick, Armand James (1894–1977) American physician and physiologist who graduated from the University of Illinois and later was professor of biochemistry at the University of Milwaukee. He devised the hippuric acid synthesis test for liver function in 1933. *See prothrombin time, Quick test.*

Quicksilver Liquid state of the poisonous element, mercury. When mixed with fats and various other substances was used as a remedy for skin diseases and a remedy for syphilis. Gabriele Falloppio (1523–1562) opposed its use and wrote *Tractatus de Morbo Gallico* discussing its action.

Quick Test Devised by Armand James Quick (1894–1977), Mary Stanley-Brown and F. W. Bancroft in 1935. Used to measure blood clotting time and monitor anticoagulants, detect severe liver disease and vitamin K deficiency. Studied by American physiologist William Henry Howell (1860–1945) in 1910 and modified into two stages by Emory Dean Warner (b 1905) and co-workers in 1936. *See prothrombin time.*

Quimby, Phineas Parkhurst (1802–1866) Watchmaker from Maine in America who attained national fame for his powers of mesmerism using his medium and student, Lucius Burkmar. Quimby later practiced faith healing or 'mind cure'.

Quincke, Heinrich Iranaeus (1842–1922) German professor of medicine at Bern in Switzerland, who gave (1882) an account of angioneurotic edema. He also distinguished between *Entamoeba histolytica* and *Entamoeba coli*. Therapeutic lumbar puncture performed by Walter Essex Wynter (1860–1945) in 1889, and introduced independently by Quincke in 1891.

Quincy, John (d 1723) London physician in the 18th century whose *Lexicon Physico-medicorum* served as the basis for Dr Hooper's *Medical Dictionary*. He also wrote several other medical treatises and translations.

Quinidine Isomer of quinine used by Karel Frederick Wenckebach (1864–1940) for treatment of atrial fibrillation in 1918. Its effectiveness in auricular fibrillation was conclusively shown by Walter Frey (b 1884) of Germany 1918.

Quinine Alkaloid of cinchona, which suppresses the malarial parasite. The tree bark was brought to Europe by Jesuit missionaries in the 17th century. Used for 'rebellious palpitation' of the heart by French physician, Jean Baptiste Senac (1693–1770) in 1749. It was prepared by Antoine François de Fourcroy (1755–1809) in a crude state from 'quinaquina' or cinchona from Peru in 1792. The pure alkaloid was extracted by Joseph Bienaimé Caventou (1793–1877) and Pierre Joseph Pelletier (1788–1842) in 1820 who named it 'quinine'. *See cinchona.*

Quinism Toxic state due to the use of quinine or cinchona, recognized in the 18th century. Sir Thomas Lauder Brunton (1844–1916) of St Bartholomew's Hospital described the symptoms of deafness, tinnitus, headache, delirium and pyrexia.

Quinquina *See quinine, cinchona.*

Quinsy [Greek: *kynache*, sore throat] According to Paul of Aegina (625–690), 'when the parts within the throat are inflamed the condition is called, 'synanche', and when the parts within the windpipe were inflamed the disease was termed, 'cynanche'. He described acute symptoms accompanied by suffocation in quincy and recommended opening of the vein below the tongue as an emergency measure or application of dog's dung or the dung of wild swallows dried and powdered in honey or throat gargle, application of leeches to the chin and neck, and cupping. If the condition led to suspended animation with foam in the mouth, he stated, no further action was to be taken, which in modern term means 'not for resuscitation'. Similar methods were also described by Hippocrates (460–377 BC).

Quintessence Aristotle (384–322 BC), in addition to the four elements of life, earth, water, fire and air, proposed by Empedocles (c 450 BC), introduced a fifth substance called 'essence'. He thought that individuals of the same species consisted of the same essence but differed in matter. His theory predated the present concept of phenotypic and genotypic characteristics.

Quotidian Fever [Latin: *quotidianus*, daily] Term for ague or malaria in which fever or paroxysms occur at the same hour every day.

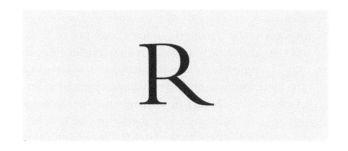

Raabe Test Test to detect albumin in urine using trichloroacetic acid. Devised by German physician, Gustav Raabe around 1905.

Rabbit Woman *See Blondel, James Augustus.*

Rabelais, François (1494–1553) French humanist, Franciscan and later Benedictine monk who studied medicine at Montpellier in 1530 and was a physician and lecturer at the Lyons Municipal Hospital in 1532. His most famous work, published in 1532, was *Pantagruel*, a mixture of theology, law and medicine as satirical and popular tales. It was declared obscene and he was threatened with prosecution.

Rabies Vaccine *See antirabies vaccine.*

Rabies [Latin: *rabere*, to rage] George Gottfried Zinke of Jena proposed that the saliva of the rabid dog was infectious in 1804. This remained unproved until 1879, when Victor Galtier (1846–1908) of Paris managed to produce a paralytic form of rabies in rabbits by inoculating them with infective material. Curare was used to relax the muscles in patients with rabies in 1838. Changes in the central nervous system were reported by Louis Pasteur (1822–1895) and colleagues in 1881, and the first inoculation with antirabies vaccine was performed by him on July 6 1885. Negri bodies, characteristic cell inclusions, were observed by Italian microbiologist, Adelchi Negri (1867–1912) in 1903, but he mistook them for parasitic protozoal organisms. *See hydrophobia.*

Race [French: *race*, family] *See eugenics, ethnology.*

Rachitis [Greek: *rachis*, spine + *itis*, inflammation] Old term for rickets that takes its origin from the belief that it arose from spinal marrow.

Rad Unit of X-ray radiation defined by the British Committee on Radiological Units under the chairmanship on Louis Harold Gray (1905–1965) in 1928.

Radcliffe Infirmary Opened in Oxford in 1770 with funds from a part of John Radcliffe's (1650–1714) estate. The orthopedic department was established in 1918, and anesthesia was fully recognized as a specialty in England by

the creation of the first chair of anesthesia by Lord William Richard Morris Nuffield (1877–1963) in 1922.

Radcliffe, John (1650–1714) Physician from Wakefield who graduated from Oxford and moved to London in 1684, where he established a prosperous practice. He was the first holder of the prestigious gold-headed cane as president of the Royal College of Physicians. He was physician to King William III and Queen Mary and elected a member of parliament in 1713. During the last illness of Queen Ann he sent a message 'her distemper was nothing but the vapors' without visiting her, and for this he was dismissed as physician to the queen. He bequeathed most of the wealth acquired through his practice in London to Radcliffe Observatory and library. Trustees of his will voted to establish the Radcliffe Infirmary with part of the proceeds of his estate. *See Radcliffe Library, Radcliffe Observatory.*

Radcliffe Library Founded at Oxford under the will of John Radcliffe (1650–1714) who left 40,000 pounds to the University of Oxford. The first stone was laid in 1737 and it opened in 1749.

Radcliffe Observatory Named after the physician John Radcliffe (1650–1714) and founded by the Savillian professor of astronomy, Hornsby in 1771. Its publications were started by one of its directors, Manuel J. Johnson in 1842.

Radial Pulse The radial artery was recommended for study of the pulse by Galen (AD 129– 200) as it had little flesh over it, was visible, and did not involve taking off the clothes.

Radiant Heat [Greek: *radians*, to emit] An early work was that of Count Benjamin Thompson Rumford (1753–1814) who proved that its transfer was independent of air or any other medium. His findings were confirmed by Humphry Davy (1778–1829).

Radiation Injury Three months after Wilhelm Konrad von Röntgen (1845–1923) discovered X-rays in 1895, T. J. Edison and William James Morton (1848–1920), a New York physician who introduced dental radiography, suffered radiation conjunctivitis while working with them. Gastrointestinal symptoms due to X-ray exposure were described by D. Walsh in 1897. Ernest Amory Codman (1869–1940) collected 171 cases of X-ray burns in 1902, and the occurrence of cancer following radiation was described by August Franz Albert Frieben in the same year. The first report of cataract due to exposure to X-rays was made by James McDowall Paton in 1909 and the first death occurred in 1914 in a radiologist from Bergamo, Emilio Tiraboschi. (1859–1906), and Marie Curie (1867–1934) suffered injuries during work with radioactive substances three years after the discovery of radium, in 1900. Nobel Prize winner, Irène Joliot-Curie (1897–1956), died from leukemia due to prolonged exposure to radiation during her work. Mutation of genes from radiation was established in *Drosophila* by Nobel Prize winner, Hermann Joseph Müller (1890–1967) of America in 1927. George Alexander Pirie of the Royal Infirmary in Dundee was a pioneer in use of X-rays in medicine until injured by radiation in 1926. An attempt to safeguard those exposed to X-rays was made with the appointment of the Adrian Committee by the Secretary of the State for Scotland and Minister of Health in 1956. Its report, *The Radiological Hazards to the Patients,* was published in 1960. Deaths from aplastic anemia following exposure to radium were reported by J. C. Mottram in 1921. He observed a low red cell count in 'anemia radiotoxica'. Leukemia due to radium exposure was also observed by Prosper Émile Weil (b 1873) and Antoine Marcellin Lacasagne (b 1884) in 1925. In 1927 twenty deaths occurred in luminous dial painters in a company based at New Jersey due to blood dyscrasia caused by radium. The director of the company and a research chemist, S. A. von Sochoky, also succumbed a year later. *See radium.*

Radiation of Heat Measurement of heat loss using a platinum wire was made by Irish physicist, John Tyndall (1820–1893). His work was advanced by a Viennese physicist, Josef Stefan (1835–1893) who proposed that the amount of energy radiated per second from a black body is proportional to the fourth power of the absolute temperature.

Radical [Latin: *radicalis*] Group of atoms which enter into and undergo chemical combination without change in the original constituents of the molecule. Noted by Jöns Jacob Berzelius (1779–1848) in 1828. The definition was given by French chemist Charles Frédéric Gerhardt (1816–1856) around 1850.

Radioactive Tracer The first tracer experiment was done at the Vienna Radium Institute in 1913. Its use in biological research was pioneered by Nobel Prize winner, George Charles von Hevesy (1885–1966) in 1922. Radioactive phosphorus was used to measure blood volume independently by F. A. Brown and R. S. Anderson in 1942. Further work on their use in cellular biology was done by Danish biophysicist, Hans Henrikson Ussing (b 1911), head of the isotope department of physiology at Copenhagen.

Radioactivity [Latin: *radius*, ray] Antoine Henri Becquerel (1852–1908), a French physicist from Paris, discovered that certain substances like uranium salts emitted radiation similar to X-rays in 1895. The phenomenon was named radioactivity by Pierre (1859–1906) and Marie Curie (1867–1934) and these three shared the Nobel Prize in 1903. The hypothesis of atomic disintegration which stated that radioactive elements made of complex particles undergo spontaneous changes or disintegration and discharge high velocity negatively charged electrons or beta rays and positively charged particles or alpha rays was proposed by Lord Ernest Rutherford (1871–1937) and Frederick Soddy (1877–1965) in 1902. The presence of radioactivity in rocks, springs and air was noted by Johann Phillipp Ludwig Elster (1854–1920) of Germany and his colleague, Hans Friedrich Geital (1855–1923), in 1901.

Radioimmunoassay [Latin: *radius*, ray + *immunize*, free] The technique was introduced by S. A. Berson and colleagues in 1956 and refined by American biophysicist, Rosalyn Yalow (b 1921) of New York, for which she was awarded the Nobel Prize for Physiology or Medicine in 1977.

Radioiodine Used in the study of thyroid disease by M. P. Kelsey and co-workers in 1949 and as treatment for thyrotoxicosis by G. W. Blomfield and co-workers in 1951. It was introduced as treatment for leukemia by American hematologist, John Lawrence, of the University of California at Berkeley, in 1936.

Radiology [Latin: *radius*, ray; Greek: *logos*, discourse] Heinrich Daniel Ruhmkorff (1803–1877), a German mechanic from Hannover who lived in Paris, built an induction coil in 1855 that formed the basis for the development of the Geissler tube by German physicist, Heinrich Geissler (1814–1879) of Saxony. This enabled rarefied gases to be visualized when electricity was passed through them. German physicist and chemist Johann Wilhelm Hittorf (1824–1914) noticed a peculiar glow when electricity was passed through a vacuum in a Geissler tube. In 1869 Sir William Crookes (1832–1919) of Cambridge improved the vacuum and observed the effects of passing a current through the tube. The Crookes tube was developed into the cathode ray tube which was used by Wilhelm Konrad von Röntgen (1845–1923) during his work on X-rays. In 1895 while investigating cathode rays, Röntgen noticed that a new ray of greater penetrating power was emitted which he called X-rays. Röntgen announced his findings in 1896 but did not patent his discovery which helped his invention to be freely used in the fields of medicine, science and technology. A pioneer in application of X-rays to orthopedics was Etienne Destot (1864–1918) of Lyon, who used radiology for diagnosis of bone disease two months after Röntgen's discovery. Wolf Becher (1826–1906) of Germany demonstrated that gastrointestinal tract can be outlined by X-rays using lead subacetate in animals in 1896. Further advances were made in the same year including the visualization of blood vessels by injection of a radio-opaque substance by two Viennese, E. Haschek and O. T. Lindenthal. John Macintyre (1857–1928), a laryngologist at the Glasgow Royal Infirmary was another pioneer who established the department of radiology at the Glasgow Infirmary. He initially trained as an electrician before studying medicine, which helped him to construct the first portable X-ray unit before 1900. Walter Edward Dandy (1886–1946), an American neurosurgeon at Johns Hopkins, devised a method of introducing air into the ventricles of the brain to visualize it on X-rays in 1918. The use of X-rays to study the movement of barium in the gastrointestinal tract was pioneered by Walter Bradford Cannon (1871–1945) of Harvard University in 1898. Iodized oil as a contrast medium for use in radiology was introduced by Jean Athanase Sicard (1872–1929) in 1921. Visualization of the gall bladder was made possible in 1924 by Evarts Ambrose Graham (1883–1957) and Warren Henry Cole (b 1898) who used chlorinated and brominated phenolphthalein capable of being excreted by the liver. Iodophthalein, a less toxic compound, was introduced as an oral and an intravenous contrast medium by Whitaker and Miliken in 1929. Pheniodol replaced iodophthalein in 1940. Fluorescein, an early radioisotope used in diagnostic neuroradiology, was introduced by George Eugene Moore (b 1922) in 1947. *See CAT scanner, magnetic resonance scan, ultrasound.*

Radiotherapy [Latin: *radius*, ray; Greek: *therapio*, to care for] Following the discovery of X-rays by Wilhelm Konrad von Röntgen (1845–1923) in 1895, they were used in medicine for deep irradiation of a hairy mole by Leopold Freund (1868–1944) of Vienna in 1896. The first cure by X-rays of a basal cell carcinoma or rodent ulcer of the nose was demonstrated by Thor Stenbeck of Sweden in 1899. The effect of radiation in treatment of cancer was also shown by Tage Anton Ultemus Sjögren (1859–1939) in the same year. An early study on inhibitory effects of X-rays on cancer was done by German surgeon, Georg Clemens Perthes (1869–1927) in 1903. Radium, an element first shown to be radioactive by Antoine Henri Becquerel (1852–1908) in 1896, was used successfully in treatment of cancer by S. W. Goldberg of St Petersburg in 1903. The results of radium treatment for cancer were published by Henri Danlos (1844–1912) in 1904. John Joly (1857–1933), a physicist from Dublin, pioneered use of radium for cancer treatment and devised the Dublin method of radiotherapy. Radium

treatment for cancer of the uterus was developed by Swedish radiologist, Carl Gustav Abrahamson Forssell (1876–1950) in 1917 and by Claude Regaud (1870–1940) in 1933. Another pioneer was Sir Stanford Cade (1895–1973) who wrote *Malignant Diseases and Treatment by Radium* in 1940.

Radium   Pitchblend residue from the Dollar Mine at Jochimstal was allocated to Marie Curie (1867–1934) for investigation following her initial observations. She obtained two radioactive substances, polonium and radium, from it in 1898. Radium was shown to have radioactive properties by Antoine Henri Becquerel (1852–1908) in 1896 and used successfully in treatment of cancer by S. W. Goldberg in 1903. *See radiotherapy.*

Radius Fracture   Fracture of the distal radius of the forearm is known as Colles fracture and was described by Abraham Colles (1773–1843), professor of surgery at Berlin in 1814. John Rhea Barton (1794–1871) described a fracture of the posterior articular margin of the lower end of the radius (Barton fracture) in 1838. Moore fracture involving the lower end of the radius with dislocation of the head of ulna and entrapment of the styloid process within the annular ligaments was described by American surgeon, Edward Mott Moore (1814–1902).

Rae, James (1716–1791) Scottish surgeon from Stirling who advocated lectures on clinical surgery, apart from anatomy. He also pioneered dentistry in Scotland. His son, John Rae, was president of the Royal College of Surgeons in 1804.

Raimondi, Marcantonio (1826–1890) Physician and naturalist from Milan who explored Peru. He proved that isolation was an important factor in speciation. He was professor of medicine in Lima, and later chair of natural history, a post he held for nearly 20 years.

Rainbow   Worshipped by some tribes in Melanesia. The Greek scientist Anaxagoras (488–428 BC) of Ionia explained rainbows and some other natural phenomena. Roger Bacon (1214–1292) also gave a theory of rainbow. In 1611, Antonio de Dominis, the Archbishop of Spalatro suggested that light reflected by raindrops was colored by traversing different thicknesses of water. René Descartes (1596–1650) also gave an explanation in his *Les Meteoros* published in 1637. Sir Isaac Newton (1642–1727) made a small hole in the wall of a darkened room to let in light and placed a prism in its path which resulted in a the fracturing of light into its colors, as seen in the rainbow.

Rainey, George (1801–1844) Demonstrator at St Thomas' Hospital who described ectopic calcifications in tissues, known as Rainey tubes.

Ralfe Test Used for detection of acetone in urine by adding hydroxide and iodide of potassium. Devised by Charles Henry Ralfe (1842–1896), a physician at the London Hospital. He wrote *Urine* (1880) and *Diseases of the Kidney*.

Raman, Sir Chandrasekhara Venkata (1888–1970) Indian physicist from Trichinopoly. He was educated at Madras University and was appointed professor of physics at Calcutta in 1917 where he served for 15 years before becoming the director of the Institute of Science at Bangalore. He was awarded the Nobel Prize for Physics in 1930 for his work on diffusion of light and the discovery of the Raman effect.

Ramazzini, Bernadini (1633–1714) Italian physician and father of occupational medicine, born at Capri near Modena and graduated in medicine from the University of Parma in 1659. He was appointed to the chair of medicine at Padua in 1700 and published *De Morbis Artificum Diatriba* in 1713. This was the first complete treatise on occupational diseases, including miner's lung, farmer's lung, lead poisoning and other occupational diseases.

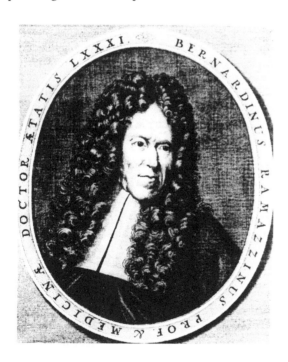

Bernadini Ramazzini (1633–1714). Courtesy of the National Library of Medicine

Ramdohr Suture The upper part of the divided intestine is invaginated into the lower part during intestinal anastomosis. Devised by American surgeon, Caesar A. von Ramdohr (1855–1912).

Ramstedt Operation Used for relief of congenital pyloric stenosis. Devised by German surgeon, Conrad Ramstedt (1867–1963), in 1912.

Ramon y Cajal, Santiago (1852–1934) Spanish physician and histologist who graduated from Zaragoza University in 1873. In 1883 he became professor of anatomy at Valencia, then Barcelona (1886–1892) and finally professor of histology and pathological anatomy at Madrid in 1892. He studied the microstructure of the nervous system and developed many histological stains for this purpose. He shared the Nobel Prize in 1906 with Camillo Golgi (1843–1926) .

Ramsay, Alexander Scottish physician from Forfar in the 17th century. He became a fellow of the Royal College of Physicians of London in 1618 and was appointed physician to Charles I in 1635.

Ramsay, David (1749–1815) Physician and historian from Philadelphia. He practiced at Charleston in South Carolina and became a member of the first Legislative Council in 1776. He wrote *History of American Revolution*, *The History of South Carolina*, and several other works on history.

Ramsay Hunt Syndrome Facial paralysis, painful ears, vesicular eruption of the oropharynx due to herpes zoster infection of the geniculate ganglion. Described by American neurologist, James Ramsay Hunt (1872–1937) in 1917. He graduated from the University of Pennsylvania in 1893 and was made professor at the faculty of the College of Physicians and Surgeons at Columbia University, New York in 1924.

Ramsay, Sir William (1852–1916) Scottish chemist, born and educated in Glasgow. He was professor of chemistry at University College, Bristol in 1880, and moved to London in 1887. He and Lord Rayleigh (1842–1919) discovered argon in 1894. He studied Brownian movement and explained it on the basis of molecular collision in 1879. He was professor of chemistry at University College of London from 1887 to 1912, during which time he was awarded the Nobel Prize (1904) for Chemistry. He wrote *Essays Biographical and Chemical* (1908), *The Gases of the Atmosphere and the History of Their Discovery* (1905) and several other works.

Ramsbotham, Francis Henry (1801–1868) Son of John Ramsbotham, a lecturer in obstetrics at the London Hospital. After graduating from Edinburgh University in 1822, he joined his father and became the first obstetric physician to the London Hospital 1853. He was an opponent of the use of chloroform and published *Principles and Practice of Obstetric Medicine and Surgery* in 1841 which went through 5 editions.

Randacio Nerves Five branches of nerves arising from the spheno-palatine ganglion. Described by a professor of anatomy at the University of Palmero, Francesco Randacio (1821–1903), in 1863.

Ranke Angle In craniometry, was described by Dutch anthropologist and physician, Hans Rudolphe Ranke (1849–1887) in 1883.

Rankine, William John Macquorn (1820–1872) Scottish natural philosopher and engineer, born in Edinburgh and graduated from Edinburgh University in 1838. He defined the terms 'actual' and 'potential' energy. He was chair of engineering at Glasgow in 1855.

Ranula [Latin: *rana*, frog] Old term for a tumor under the tongue, takes its origin due to its resemblance to a frog.

Ranvier, Louis Anthoine (1835–1922) French physician and histologist at the College of France, Paris. He made a special study of peripheral nerves and described the regular interruptions of the myelin sheath (nodes of Ranvier) in 1878.

Raoult Law Defines the relationship between the vapor pressure of a solvent above a solution and the mole fraction of solvent in solution. Proposed by French physical chemist, François Marie Raoult (1830–1901) of Paris. His work provided a reliable method of determining molecular weight.

Rasmussen Aneurysm Branch of the pulmonary artery affected by tuberculous involvement. Described by Danish physician, Fritz Waldemar Rasmussen (1834–1877).

Rat Bite Fever The first report of rat bite fever was given by Whitman Wilcox in 1840, and *Streptobacillus monoliformis* was shown as its cause by Henry Vandyke Carter (1831–1897) in 1887. *See Haverhill fever.*

Rathke Pouch Small diverticulum of the early embryonic pharynx giving rise to the anterior lobe of pituitary gland. Described by a German professor at Dorpat, Martin Heinrich Rathke (1793–1860) in 1838. He graduated in medicine from Berlin in 1818, and also discovered the gillslits and gillarches of birds and mammals in embryonic stage, in 1829.

Rau, J. Johann (1658–1719) Dutch anatomist who discovered the long process of the auditory ossicle, anterior to the malleus, which is named (Rau apophysis) after him.

Rauber Layer Outer cell mass of trophoblastic [Greek: *trophe*, nourishment + *blastos*, rudiment or bud] cells of the blastodermic vesicle. Described by German-born professor of anatomy from Estonia, August Antinous Rauber (1841–1917) in 1880.

Raulin, Joseph (1708–1874) Physician to the king in Paris. He wrote several medical treatises in French including: *Diseases occasioned by Variations in Atmosphere, Vapours in Females, Preservations of Infants* and *Diseases of Lying-in-women.*

Rauwolf, Leonhard (1537–1606) German botanist and physician who traveled extensively in Syria, Arabia and Armenia, before he returned to his native Augsburg in 1576. His catalogue of plants was published at Leiden in 1755. The Indian snakeroot plant used as a remedy for snakebite and for insanity was named after him by the French botanist, Plumier.

Rauwolfia serpentina The Indian snakeroot plant was used as a remedy for snakebite and insanity. French botanist, Plumier described it and named it after the German botanist Leonhard Rauwolf (1537–1606). Five different alkaloids were isolated from it by Indian doctors, S. Siddique and Rafat Siddique in 1931. It was used in the treatment of high blood pressure and psychoses by Indian scientists Ganeth Sen and Katrick Bose, and by 1951, it became established as treatment for hypertension under many names such as reserpine, serpasil, and sandril. Reserpine was the first tranquilizer to be introduced by Robert Wallace in 1951.

Rawson, Sir William (d 1829) Oculist from Cornwall whose original name was Adams. He was apprenticed to a surgeon at Barnstaple where he developed an interest in diseases of the eye. He was appointed oculist to ophthalmology institutions at Bath and Exeter and was later made oculist extraordinary to the Prince Regent.

Ray, John (1628–1705) Born to a blacksmith's family at Black Notley, near Braintree in Essex and educated at Cambridge, where he taught until 1661, before traveling as a naturalist in Britain and abroad. His systems of botanical and zoological classification formed the basis for George Cuvier's (1769–1832) work. His *Historia Plantarum* containing a description of 18,600 plant species, commenced in 1686 and was completed in three volumes in 1704. He also published numerous treatises on a variety of subjects.

Rayer, Pierre François Olive (1793–1867) Physician from Paris and authority on kidney diseases. He described pyelonephritis in pregnant women, in 1841.

Rayleigh, Lord John William Strutt (1842–1919) British physicist, born in Essex and graduated from Trinity College, Cambridge in 1861. He completed his theory of sound in 1878. Sir William Ramsay (1852–1916) and Rayleigh discovered the inert gas helium in 1894. Rayleigh received the Nobel Prize for Physics for his work on gas density in 1904.

Raynaud Disease Described by French physician, Maurice Raynaud (1834–1881) of the Hospital Lariboisière at Paris in 1862. He presented several cases of intermittent cyanosis which occurred on exposure to cold under the term 'local asphyxia of extremities'.

Read, Alexander (d 1680) Scottish physician and anatomist who graduated in medicine from Oxford in 1620 and wrote several medical treatises. One of his most important, *A Description of the Body of Man with practise of Chirurgery, and the use of three and fifty Instruments*, was published in 1615.

Reaumur, René Antoine Ferchault de (1683–1757) French natural philosopher, born in La Rochelle. He invented a thermometer using alcohol and water with a range of zero to 80 degrees. He wrote on insects, *Memoires pour sevir l'historie des Insectes* (1734–1742) in six volumes. He developed a type of porcelain and a method of hatching eggs using artificial heat.

Récamier Operation Uterine curettage devised by French gynecologist, Joseph Claude Anselme Récamier (1774–1852).

Recapitulation Theory States that the series of embryonic stages through which an animal passes during its development represent its evolutionary ancestry. Advocated by Ernst Heinrich Phillipp August Haeckel (1834–1919) in 1866. His theory was supported by Jean Louis Rodolphe Agassiz (1807–1873) a Swiss-American naturalist and glaciologist.

Receptaculum Chyli [Latin: *receptaculum*, store house] Dilatation of the thoracic duct, described in 1647 by Jean Pecquet (1622–1674), a French anatomist, while he was a student.

Recessive [Latin: *recessus*, withdrawn] *See dominance.*

Recklinghausen Disease *See von Recklinghausen disease, osteitis fibrosa cystica.*

Reclus Disease Painless swelling of the mammary glands due to multiple dilation of the acini and ducts. Described by French gynecologist, Paul Reclus (1847–1914).

Recorde, Robert (1510–1558) English physician and mathematician, born in Tenby and graduated from Cambridge in 1545. He wrote a treatise on elementary arithmetic and algebra and introduced the equals sign.

Recorder Leon Scott de Martinville, an American of French origin, made graphic recordings of speech using a vibrating

membrane and stylus around 1865. A patent was obtained by Alva Edison in 1877 and wax discs were used for recording sound by Alexander Graham Bell in 1886. A flat disc phonograph was invented by a German inventor, Emile Berliner (b 1851) in America in 1904.

Rectal Anesthesia Ether was used as rectal anesthesia by Nikolai Pirogoff (1810–1881) and Roux in 1847. Although ether produced excellent narcosis, its use was limited due to damage caused to local tissues. Pirogoff later produced an apparatus, to warm ether and introduced it in the form of vapor. In 1855, Dudley Buxton devised an improved apparatus with a similar function, but again the local side effects predominated. The technique was introduced into France by Daniel Molliere in 1884, but failed to gain acceptance due to severe postoperative colitis. Mixing ether with olive oil was introduced by James Taylor Gwathmey (1865–1944) in 1913. Paraldehyde was used by Vincenzo Cervello (1854–1919) in 1882 and it became widely used as a basal narcotic from 1920 to 1930. Fritz Eicholtz of Germany used avertin or tribromomethyl alcohol in 1926. *See anesthesia, ether, avertin.*

Rectal Biopsy Routine use of rectal biopsy in proctology was established by English surgeon, William Bahall Gabriel (b 1893) in 1948.

Rectal Carcinoma In 1776 H. Pillore a French surgeon from Rouen opened the cecum into the right iliac region through a peritoneal incision for a patient with carcinoma of the rectum. Extirpation was advised by Jacques Lisfranc (1790–1847) in 1830. Early surgical removal was advocated by William Harrison Cripps (1850–1923) in his Jacksonian Prize essay in 1876, and the surgical treatment was revived by Sir James Paget (1814–1889) in England. Perineal excision was performed by Swiss surgeon, Emil Theodor Kocher (1841–1917) in 1875. Excision of the coccyx and the left margin of the sacrum to reach a higher level carcinoma was performed by Paul Kraske (1851–1930) in 1885. Abdomino-perineal resection was established by William Ernest Miles (1869–1947) in 1904. Another radical operation was introduced by William James Mayo (1861–1939) in 1910. A perineal method of excision was developed by Lockhart-Mummery in 1914, and the two stage perineo-abdominal method was described by Paul Turner in 1920. Cuthbert Dukes's (b 1890) analysis of 1000 cases of cancer of the rectum was published in *The Journal of Pathology and Bacteriology* in 1940.

Rectal Diseases [Latin: *rectum*, straight] *See rectal carcinoma, anal fistula, proctology.*

Rectal Feeding Practiced by Spanish physician Avenzoar

(1092–1162). He washed out the lower bowel and then injected milk, eggs and soft food into it, using a goat bladder connected to a rectal tube.

Rectal Prolapse [Latin: *pro*, forth + *laps*, to slip] An operative treatment was described by Polish surgeon, Johann von Mikulicz-Radecki (1850–1905) in 1888.

Rectum [Latin: *rectus*, straight] One of the inscriptions on the Egyptian tomb of a physician from 2500 BC bears the phrase 'Keeper of the King's Rectum'. Hippocrates (460–377 BC) was familiar with the subject and described a rectal speculum. John of Ardane (1307–1390), an English surgeon, specialized in rectal diseases and designed several operations. The O'Beirne sphincter, a band at the junction of the colon and the rectum, was described by Irish surgeon, James O'Beirne (1786–1862). John Houston (1802–1845), a physician from Dublin, described sphincter ani tertius (Houston valve) of the rectum in 1830. Sir Charles Bent Ball (1851–1916), another proctologist from Dublin, described the rectal valves (Ball valves) previously described by Giovanni Battista Morgagni (1682–1771) in his *The Rectum and Anus, their diseases and treatment* published in 1887. *See rectal carcinoma.*

Recurrent Laryngeal Nerves [Latin: *recurrens*, returning; Greek: *laryngx*, upper part of wind pipe] Found on either side of the trachea and were used for experimentation in animals by Andreas Vesalius (1514–1564). He demonstrated that the voice was totally lost by cutting both pairs of nerves.

Red Blood Cell *See red cell.*

Red Blood Corpuscle *See red cell.*

Red Cell Fragility As early as in 1771, William Hewson (1739–1774), a pupil of John Hunter (1728–1793), observed that red cells were destroyed in water but remained normal in salt solution. A salt solution capable of preserving red and other cells was prepared by Sidney Ringer (1835–1910) in 1880. Studies on fragility were done by William Bosworth Castle (b 1897) and G. A. Dalland in 1937, and their work on the subject was followed by that of William Dameshak (1900–1969) and Steven Otto Schwartz (b 1911) in 1938. *See Ham test.*

Red Cell Index Includes mean corpuscular hemoglobin concentration (MCHC), and mean corpuscular volume (MCV). Proposed by American hematologist, Maxwell Myer Wintrobe (1901–1986) during his work on classification of anemias on the basis of red cell morphology in 1930.

Red Cell Probably first seen in 1658 by Athanasius Kircher (1601–1680), a Jesuit priest, while attempting to view the microscopic organism of plague. He used a primitive microscope with a magnification of only x32 and described what he saw as 'worms' of plague in *Scrutium Pestis*. The first definite observation was made by a Dutch naturalist and physician, Jan Swammerdam (1637–1680) in 1658. Antoni van Leeuwenhoek (1632–1723) made microscopical observations of blood in 1674. Georges Hayem (1841–1933), professor of clinical medicine at the University of Paris identified the early stage of generation of red cells and called them hematoblasts in 1877. A classification of anemias based on their morphology was proposed by Maxwell Myer Wintrobe (1901–1986) in 1930 who proposed four types: macrocytic, normocytic, simple microcytic and chronic microcytic. Formation of hemoglobin from its precursor substances within the bone marrow was shown by B. R. Burmester of Leipzig in 1936. The life span of red cells was established by London–born American pathologist, Winifred Ashby (1879–1935).

Red Cross Society The initiator of the movement was a Swiss philanthropist, Jean Henry Dunant (1828–1910) of Geneva. His efforts were motivated by the plight of 40,000 dead or wounded at the battle of Solferino in 1859. He wrote *A Memory of Solferino* in which he pleaded for neutral status for the wounded and for those who cared for them. In 1863 he organized an international Congress in Geneva where his proposals were adapted. The first Relief Society was formed in the same year and it became the Red Cross Society in 1864.

Red Hypertension *See pale hypertension.*

Red Water Fever *See babesiasis.*

Redi, Francesco (1626–1697) Italian physician from Arezzo credited with being the first parasitologist. He refuted the theory of spontaneous generation and demonstrated that maggots developed from eggs laid by the flies. The egg and the reproductive process of the roundworm were described him in 1684.

Reduction Potential *See oxidation potential.*

Reed, Walter (1851–1902) American army surgeon from Virginia who trained in medicine at the University of Virginia and the Bellvue Hospital Medical School. He was head of the Medical Commission in Cuba in 1899 and, together with James Carroll (1854–1907), Aristedes Simone Agramonte (1868–1931) and James William Lazier (1866–1900), studied yellow fever. They worked on the theory proposed by Carlos Finlay in 1881, that the mosquito was the carrier of the disease. Finlay allowed himself to be bitten by mosquitoes during the experiments and survived an attack of yellow fever but his colleague Lazier died of the disease. Further experiments proved that yellow fever was transmitted by a mosquito, *Aëdes aegypti*, in 1900. Reed's work demonstrated that the organism responsible was the same as that described by Martinus Willem Beijerinck (1851–1931) in 1898 and this was the first time that a virus had been implicated in a human disease.

Reed–Sternberg Cell Characteristic cell found in Hodgkin disease and described by Dorothy Reed (1874–1964) of Johns Hopkins Medical School in 1902. These cells were previously recognized by Austrian pathologist, Karl von Sternberg (1872–1935) in 1898.

Rees Test Used for detection of albumin in urine with tannic acid in an alcoholic solution. Devised by English physician, George Owen Rees (1813–1889).

Reflecting Microscope Consists of a reflecting mirror instead of an objective glass. Invented by Giovanni Battista Amici (1786–1863) of Florence in 1812. *See microscope.*

Reflecting Telescope An early instrument was invented by James Gregory (1638–1675), a mathematician from Aberdeen. He described it in *Optica Promota, feu abdita Radiorum Reflexorum and Refractorum Mysteria, Geometrice Enucleata*, published in 1668. Another was built by Sir Isaac Newton (1642–1727) in the same year. John Hadley (1682–1744), an English mathematician and astronomer, perfected it in 1731 and John Mudge (d 1793), a physician and mechanic in Plymouth improved it in 1793. *See telescope.*

Reflection of Heat Known to Pliny (AD 23–79) who described the sacred fire of Vesta which was rekindled using a metallic mirror to reflect the rays of the sun. Giovanni Battiste della Porta (1535–1615), in his seventh book of *Natural Magic,* pointed out that heat and sound could be reflected in the same way as light. Italian professor of mathematics, Bonaventure Calvalieri (d 1647), used a spherical mirror and reflected the heat from burning coal to burn dry substances in 1632.

Reflex Action [Latin: *reflexus*, bent] The involuntary response of the nervous system was observed as early as 1662 by René Descartes (1596–1650) and experiments on the physiology were done by Stephen Hales (1677–1761), a chemist, botanist and clergyman from Teddington in 1730. He noted the reflex withdrawal of the leg in a decapitated frog, and was able to abolish this by inducing a lesion in the spinal cord. The term 'reflex' was introduced by Johan August Unzer (1727–1799) to describe the sensory-motor reaction in 1771. The functions of the dorsal and spinal roots in the reflex arc were described Sir Charles Bell (1774–

1842) in 1811 and François Magendie (1783–1855) in 1822. The segmental nature of the spinal cord and its interface with the higher centers was demonstrated by Marshall Hall (1790–1857) in 1833. Further advances were made by Sir Charles Scott Sherrington (1857–1952) in 1899. Work on the tendon reflex or stretch reflex was continued at Oxford by Edward George Tandy Liddell, a neurophysiologist, and Sir Charles Scott Sherrington in 1924. A comprehensive work, *Reflex Activity of the Spinal Cord,* was published by Sherrington, Sir John Carew Eccles (b 1903), Creed, Derek Denny-Brown (1901–1981) and Liddell in 1932. *See autonomic nervous system, Barbinski reflex, knee jerk.*

Reflux Esophagitis [Latin: *re*, back + *fluxus*, flow + *oisophagos*, gullet + *itis*, inflammation] The presence of hydrochloric acid in the stomach was shown by English chemist and physiologist, William Prout (1785–1850) of Horton. Harvey Williams Cushing (1869–1939) of America used the term 'esophagitis' in relation to pathology found in the esophagus of patients with brain lesions in 1932. The term 'peptic esophagitis' was coined by Asher Winkelstein (b 1894) of America in 1935. Another early account was given by E.B. Benedict and E.M. Dalard in the *New England Journal of Medicine* in 1938. Use of the term to denote inflammation of the esophagus secondary to regurgitation of gastric juices was started by Norman R. Barrett (1903–1979) in 1949.

Refraction [Latin: *refringere*, to break apart] *See optics.*

Refractory Period [Latin: *refractorius*, obstinate] Its existence was observed by a German physiologist of Jewish origin, Moritz Schiff (1823–1896). Refractoriness of a frog's heart during systole was demonstrated by Karl Hugo Kronecker (1839–1914). Francis Gotch (1853–1913) and G.J. Burch in 1899 showed that if a primary stimulus is followed by a second stimulus within 0.008 second, the second stimulus failed to evoke a response. Further investigation were done by Edgar Douglas Adrian (1889–1977) and Keith Lucas (1879–1916) in 1912.

Refrigeration Anesthesia *See regional anesthesia, hypothermia.*

Refrigeration [Latin: *refrigio*, make cool] A mixture of snow and saltpetre was used by an Italian, Zimara, in 1660. Artificial ice was made by freezing water under pressure by Sir John Leslie (1766–1832), professor of physics at Edinburgh in 1810. The invention of steam machines in 1830 and electricity enabled ice to be mass produced and led to establishment of large cold storage rooms. The era of modern refrigeration began with the invention of a compression method, using ammonia, by French engineer, Ferdinand Carre in 1857. His method was improved by a German, Karl Paul Gottfried von Linde (1842–1934) in 1873. Another was invented by Eugène Anatole Demarcay (1852–1903), French chemistry professor in Paris. Freon, a non-toxic and non-inflammable agent for domestic refrigerators, was introduced by American scientist Thomas Midgley (1889–1944) around 1923. *See food industry.*

Refsum Syndrome Congenital condition consisting of retinitis pigmentosa, ataxia, and peripheral neuropathy. Described by F. Thieubaut of Paris in 1939. Another account of the condition was given by Sigvald Refsum (b 1907) in 1945.

Rega, Henry Joseph (1690–1754) Professor of medicine at the University of Louvain in France. He helped the poor and the sick at his own expense and wrote several medical treatises including *De Lymphopathia.*

Regeneration [Latin: *re*, again + *generare*, to produce] *See tissue culture, nerve regeneration.*

Regional Anesthesia Refrigeration anesthesia, by applying cold water or snow, was introduced by Marco Aurelio Severino (1580–1656) of Naples and French military surgeon, Dominique Jean Larrey (1766–1842), used ice to perform amputations in the battlefield in 1807. A freezing mixture of ice and salt was used by James Arnott of Aberdeen in 1847. Benjamin Ward Richardson (1828–1896) used ether spray to produce local refrigeration in 1867. Compression was practiced by James Carrick Moore (1763–1834) of England in 1784. The local anesthetic effect of cocaine on the eye was discovered by Carl Koller (1857–1944) of Vienna in 1884. Neural regional anesthesia was performed by injecting cocaine into the inferior dental nerve for dental extraction by William Halstead (1852–1922) of America in 1884. He also injected cocaine into the meninges and this later paved the way for spinal anesthesia. *See block, local anesthesia, spinal anesthesia.*

Rehabilitation Medicine [Latin: *rehabilitare*, to rehabilitate] Minimizing the effects of incapacitation caused by disease. Occupational therapy was used to treat mental disorders and the physician Seneca (4 BC–AD 65) recommended employment for mental unrest. Galen (AD 129–200) commented that 'employment is nature's best physician'. French surgeon, Ambroise Paré (1510–1590) attempted rehabilitation of amputees with artificial limbs. Simple measures such as gardening, sewing, spinning were used successfully in a mental hospital in Philadelphia by Benjamin Rush (1745–1813) in 1798. Occupation as a form of treatment for mental illnesses was also proposed by

Samuel Tuke (1784–1857), a physician from York in 1815, and by John Conolly (1794–1866) at the Hanwell Asylum in London in 1843. A pioneer in the application of physical medicine to diseases of the joints and bones was French surgeon, Amédée Bonnet (1802–1858). He was professor of surgery at l'Hôtel Dieu in Lyon and published *Traite des Maladies des Articulations* (1845) in two volumes, followed by *Traites des Therapeutique des Maladies des Articulations* in 1853. His works showed the application of physiotherapy in joint disease. One of the first units to treat and rehabilitate spinal injuries in England was Stoke Mandeville Hospital which was started by Sir Ludwig Guttmann (1899–1980) at Buckinghamshire in 1944. In England the Chronically Sick and Disabled Persons Act of 1970 made local authorities responsible for facilities for the disabled.

Reich, Wilhelm (1897–1957) Controversial psychiatrist from Vienna who proposed sexual satisfaction and orgasm as the main theme in psychiatry. He wrote *Function of the Orgasm* in 1929 and was expelled from Germany for his views on sex and politics. He emigrated to America in 1939 and was later prosecuted there for improper practice.

Reichel–Jones–Henderson Syndrome *See Henderson, Melvin Starkey.*

Reichert Cartilage Second bronchial arch described by German professor of comparative anatomy at Dorpat, Karl Bogislaus Reichert (1811–1883) in 1836.

Reichstein, Tadeus (b 1897) Swiss chemist, born in Poland who worked on carbohydrate chemistry. He synthesized vitamin C in 1933. From 1934 he began to work on steroids, isolating and identifying 29, including cortisone and hydrocortisone. He shared the 1950 Nobel Prize for Physiology or Medicine. *See adrenal insufficiency.*

Reid, Alexander (1580–1641) Scottish physician from Aberdeen who lectured at the Barber-Surgeons Hall. He bequeathed his library to Marischal College.

Reid, John (1809–1849) Surgeon at Edinburgh who promoted the study of pathology. He differentiated between typhoid and typhus fever and published several treatises on pathology, anatomy and epidemic fevers of Scotland.

Reid, Thomas (1710–1796) Born in Kincardine and regarded as the founder of the Scottish School of philosophy. He was educated at Aberdeen and was professor of philosophy at King's College and professor of moral philosophy at Glasgow from 1764 to 1781. He wrote *Essay on the Intellectual Power of Man* (1785), *Essays on the Active Power of the Human Mind* (1788) and a number of other treatises.

Reid Base Line Anthropometric measurements defined by Scottish anatomist, Robert William Reid (1851–1939), a demonstrator in anatomy at St Thomas' Hospital, in 1939.

Reil, Johann Christian (1759–1813) Neuroanatomist and physician at Berlin. He described the insula of the cerebral cortex or the lobule of corpus striatum in 1796, known as the island of Reil. He wrote a modern systematic treatise on psychotherapy in 1803.

Reisseisen, Franz Daniel (1773–1828) Anatomist and physician from Strasburg in Germany. He demonstrated contraction of the smooth muscles in the wall of the smallest bronchial tubes during an asthmatic attack in 1808.

Reissner Membrane Membrana vestibularis of the cochlea separating scala vestibuli and scala media. Described by Ernst Reissner (1824–1878), professor of anatomy at Breslau in 1851.

Reiter Disease Characterized by urethritis, conjunctivitis, and arthritis and described by Benjamin Collins Brodie (1783–1862) of St George's Hospital in 1818. A modern description was given by a German bacteriologist, Hans Reiter (1881–1969) of the German Medical Corps in 1916, who mistakenly attributed the disease to a spirochete.

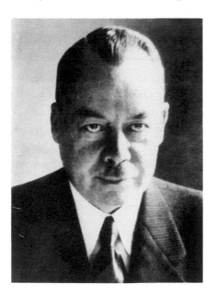

Hans Reiter (1881–1969). Courtesy of the National Library of Medicine

Rejection Reaction Response following autotransplantation of skin was described by Thomas Gibson (b 1915) and Sir Peter Brian Medawar (1915–1987) in 1943. They demonstrated the immunological nature of the phenomenon by showing that the second transplant under similar conditions was rejected more quickly than the first. Nicholas Avrion Mitchison (b 1928) in 1954 showed that transplant immunity could be passively produced by transfusing lymphocytes, thus establishing the fundamental immunological nature of the reaction. The role of 6-mercaptopurine in prolonging survival of kidney grafts in animals was demonstrated by R.Y. Calne in 1960. *See organ transplant, histocompatibility.*

Rejuvenation [Latin: *re*, again + *juvenescere*, to become young] There was an ancient belief that intercourse with a young virgin rejuvenated the body. The alchemist's search for the mythical Philosopher's stone was aimed at attaining eternal youth. Operative procedures were explored in the early 20th century and ligation of the vas deferens was performed as a procedure for rejuvenation by Eugen Steinach (1861–1944). Serge Voronoff (1866–1951), a French physiologist of Russian origin, reported experimental rejuvenation by means of a testicular transplant in 1919. His *Graffes testicularis* (1920) was translated into English as *Rejuvenation by Grafting* in 1925. *See organotherapy.*

Relapsing Fever [Latin: *re*, again + *lapsare*, to slip] Observed and described during the epidemic at the Island of Thasos by Hippocrates (460–377 BC). John Rutty (1697–1775) mentioned it in his treatise on the diseases of Dublin published in 1770. A causative organism, a spirochete (*Borrelia recurrentis*) was discovered by Otto Hugo Franz Obermeier (1843–1873) in 1873. A tick, *Ornithodorus moubata*, was identified in 1904 as a carrier by Hedgeland Philip Ross (1876–1929) and A.D. Milne in Uganda and Joseph Everett Dutton (1877–1905) and John Lancelot Todd (1876–1949) in the Congo. The causative organism of American relapsing fever, the body louse (*Pediculus humanis corporis*), was identified by Frederick George Novy (1864–1957), professor of bacteriology at Michigan. Inoculation with blood from an infected patient or mouse was employed as shock treatment for neurosyphilis around 1920.

Relativity Thomas Young (1773–1829) considered the ether as an invisible medium through which light traveled in waves. Americans, Albert Abraham Michelson (1852–1931) of German origin and Edward Williams Morley (1838–1923) of Newark, New Jersey showed that the velocity of light was the same in all directions and independent of the motion of the Earth. In 1905 Albert Einstein (1879–1955) developed the theory of special relativity which referred to systems in uniform motion relative to each other. His theory of gravitation, the general theory of relativity, was completed on November 25 1915 and submitted to *Annalen der Physik* on March 20 1916. *See Einstein, Albert.*

Remak, Robert (1815–1865) German professor of neurology at Posnán who noted in 1825 that the gray matter of the brain contained cellular tissue. He described the unmyelinated nerve fibers (Remak fibers) in 1838. He observed favus scutula while at the Charité Hospital in Berlin around 1837. He discovered the cardiac ganglia which exert nervous control on the muscular activity of the heart (Remak ganglia) in 1844, and classified the embryonic germ layers into ectoderm, endoderm and mesoderm in 1845. Acetic acid was used to fix nuclei in histology by Remak in 1854.

Renal Acidosis [Latin: *renalis*, kidney] The occurrence of acid intoxication in renal failure was observed by Rudolf von Jaksch (1855–1947) in 1888. Walter Straub (b 1874) and Schlayer in 1912 observed that the carbon dioxide content of alveolar air in uremia was low. Edward Palmer Poulten (1883–1939) and J.H.Ryffel showed that the hydrogen content of the blood was increased in uremia in 1913.

Renal Angiogram [Latin: *renalis*, kidney; Greek: *anggeion*, vessel + *graphein*, to write] Spanish physician, Reynaldo Dos Santos (b 1880), injected a contrast medium directly into the renal arteries in 1937. Injection of a dye into the renal artery via the femoral artery was done by P. L. Farinas in 1949 and Radner used the radial artery for access in 1949. Selective catheterization of renal arteries was developed by H. Tillander in 1951. A modification of the percutaneous technique for catheterization, which allowed the introduction of a catheter of a diameter larger than that of the needle used for initial puncture, was devised by Swedish radiologist, Sven Ivar Seldinger (b 1921) in 1953. A special method for use on the surgically exposed kidney during operation (intra-operative angiogram) was devised by C. E. Alken in 1950.

Renal Artery Stenosis [Latin: *renalis*, kidney] Harry J. Goldblatt (1891–1977) and colleagues demonstrated in 1934 that if both renal arteries were constricted in dogs, hypertension followed. Percutaneous transluminal dilatation of stenosed renal arteries was performed as treatment for renal hypertension by Andreas R. Gruentzig (d 1985) and co-workers in 1979.

Renal Decapsulation [Latin: *renalis*, kidney] Performed by R. Harrison in 1896 and revived by New York surgeon George Michael Edebohls (1853–1908) in 1902.

Renal Dialysis [Latin: *renalis*, kidney; Greek: *dia*, through+ *lysis*, loosening] *See artificial kidney.*

Renal Function A method of estimating creatinine in blood was devised by Max Jaffe (1841–1911) in 1886, and its presence in urine was detected by Max von Pettenkofer (1818–

1901). Jaffe mixed the sample of blood with picric acid and sodium hydroxide, which gave a red color reaction in combination with creatinine (Gaffe method). Danish physiologist, P. B. Rehberg (b 1895) assumed that creatinine was excreted solely through the glomeruli and used its clearance rate as a measure of glomerular filtration in 1926.

Renal Hemangioma [Latin: *renalis*, kidney; Greek: *haima*, blood + *anggeion*, vessel] Rare tumors found by Elexius Thompson Bell (b 1880), professor of pathology at the University of Minnesota, Minneapolis in 1938. He demonstrated only one hemangioma out of 30,000 autopsies performed in his Institute.

Renal Hypertension [Latin: *renalis*, kidney; Greek: *hyper*, above + *tonos*, tone] Profound involvement of the cardio-vascular system with cardiac hypertrophy in cases of renal disease was observed by Richard Bright (1789–1858) in 1827. He also noticed increased resistance of the arteries to injection. Thickening of renal arteries in hypertension was demonstrated by Joseph Tonybee (1815–1866) in 1846. Ludwig Traube (1818–1876) of Berlin found that arterial hypertension was the linking factor between renal disease and hypertension in 1856. The humoral mechanism was demonstrated by Robert Adolf Armand Tigerstedt (1853–1923) and Per Gustaf Bergman (1874–1955). They injected an extract of the cortex of rabbit kidney and produced elevated blood pressure in 1898. They also found that the blood from the renal vein had a similar action and they named the active substance 'renin'. The role of renal ischemia in production of hypertension was demonstrated by Harry Goldblatt (1891–1977) in 1934. The protein nature of renin was suggested by Sir George White Pickering (1904–1982) and Myron Prinzmetal (b 1908) in 1938. Renal changes in malignant hypertension were demonstrated in animals by Clifford Wilson (b 1906) and Frank Burnet Byrom in 1939. *See pale hypertension.*

Renal Osteodystrophy [Latin: *renalis*, kidney; Greek: *osteon*, bone + *dys*, mis + *trophein*, to nourish] *See renal rickets.*

Renal Papillary Necrosis [Latin: *renalis*, kidney + *papilla*, nipple; Greek: *nekros*, dead] The urographic appearance of the kidneys in this disease was described by G. W. Gunther of Stuttgart in 1937. Diagnosis using Gunther's radiological criteria was used by Olle Oleson in 1939.

Renal Rickets [Latin: *renalis*, kidney; Greek: *rachis*, spine] Renal osteodystrophy in patients with chronic renal disease was described by Richard Clement Lucas (1848–1915) of Guy's Hospital in 1883. Conversion of 25-hydroxy-cholecalciferol from the liver to 1-25-hydroxy-cholecalciferol in the kidneys, which explained renal rickets, was discovered by D. R. Fraser and E. Kodicek in 1970.

Renal Stones [Latin: *renalis*, kidney] Substances such as uric acid, calcium and ammonium in urinary stones were shown by English chemist and physician, William Hyde Wollaston (1766–1828) in 1797. A procedure for nephrolithotomy, where the stone was removed through a lumbar incision, was performed by Sir Henry Morris (1844–1926) of London in 1880. An X-ray of renal calculus was taken by John Macyntyre (1857–1928) in 1896.

Renal Transplantation [Latin: *renalis*, kidney] Experimental studies on renal grafts were done by Alexis Carrel (1873–1944) in 1914. A clinical transplant was performed at the Peter Bent Brigham Hospital at Boston in 1955. A series of 9 patients who underwent transplantation from unrelated cadavers was reported by David Milford Hume (1917–1973), John Putnam Merrill (1917–1986) and G. W. Thorn in 1955. Five failed to show any measurable renal function and varying levels of renal functions were obtained from the other four patients for 180 days. The main cause for failure was thought to be an adverse antibody response. A successful renal transplant between identical twins was made by Joseph Edward Murray (b 1919) and co-workers at Peter Bent Brigham Hospital in 1958. The role of 6-mercaptopurine in prolonging survival of kidney grafts in animals was shown by R.Y. Calne in 1960.

Renaudot, Theophrastus (1583–1653) French physician from Lundun who produced the newspaper, *Mercure Francoise* between 1635 and 1643. He was physician to the King at Paris and opened several free clinics for the poor in 1635.

Rendu–Osler–Weber Syndrome (Syn: hereditary hemorrhagic telengiectasis) Multiple telengiectatic lesions of the face and upper gastrointestinal tract with a bleeding tendency. Described by Henri Jules Louis Marie Rendu (1844–1902) of Paris in 1896, Frederick Parkes Weber (1863–1962) professor of applied therapeutics at Temple University, Philadelphia in 1904 and Sir William Osler (1849–1919) in 1907.

Renin [Latin: *renalis*, kidney] A pressor substance in saline extracts of the cortex of rabbit kidney was noted by Robert Adolf Armand Tigerstedt (1853–1923) and Per Gustaf Bergman (1874–1955) in 1898. They injected the extract into animals and found that it increased blood pressure. They also found that blood from the renal vein had a similar action and named the substance 'renin'. Harry Goldblatt (1891–1977), J. Lynch and R.F. Hanzal in 1934 showed that

hypertension could be produced by clamping the renal artery. The protein nature of renin was suggested by Sir George White Pickering (1904–1982), regius professor of medicine at Christ Church College, Oxford and American cardiologist, Myron Prinzmetal (b 1908) of Buffalo in 1938. The enzymatic nature of renin and its action on angiotonin was demonstrated by Eduardo Braun-Menendez (b 1903) from Buenos Aires and Argentinian Nobel Prize winner, Luis Frederico Leloir (b 1906) and colleagues in 1939. Their findings were confirmed by Irwin Heinley Page (b 1901) of Cleveland and O. M. Helmer in 1940. Pure renin was obtained by Goldblatt, Hass and Lamfrom in 1953.

Renogram [Latin: *renalis*, kidney; Greek: *graphein*, to write] A method of assessing kidney function using radioisotopes was introduced by C. C. Winter and G. V. Taplin in 1955. Estimation of renal blood flow using albumin iodine-131 was performed by Perskey in 1957.

Reproduction [Latin: *re*, again + *productio*, production] *See gametes.*

Reserpine *See Rauwolfia serpentina.*

Resonance Theory Theory of hearing that proposed that the transverse fibers of the basilar membrane in the cochlea of the inner ear acted as a tuned resonator. Developed by Hermann Ludwig Ferdinand von Helmholtz (1821–1894) of Potsdam while professor of anatomy and physiology at Bonn in 1855.

Resorcin Bactericidal, fungicidal and antipruritic, 1,3-benzenediol, was obtained in crystalline form by Hlasiwetz and Barth in 1868. A study of the antipyretic properties was done by J. Andreer in 1881, and it remained as a common antipruritic until 1900.

Respiration [Latin: *respiratio*, breathe] Orthopnoea as a symptom of cardiorespiratory disease was described by Paul of Aegina (625–690) as 'to pant for breath and from their being obliged to keep the chest erect for fear of being suffocated, they are called orthopnoeic'. Scientific work on respiratory physiology was done by London physician, John Mayow (1640–1679) who wrote *On Respiration* and *On the Respiration of the Foetus* in 1674. In 1774 Joseph Priestley (1733–1804), a chemist in England, demonstrated that blood became bright red when exposed to oxygen and it turned darker with carbon dioxide. French chemist Antoine Laurent Lavoisier (1743–1794) discovered that it required oxygen in 1775, stating that 'Respiration is therefore a combustion, slow it is true, but otherwise perfectly similar to that of charcoal'. Julien Jean Cesar Legallois (1775–1814), a physician and physiologist from Cherneix, Brittany, discovered the respiratory center in the medulla oblongata in 1812, and Pierre Jean Marie Flourens (1794–1867) identified the bilateral 'vital nodes' of this in 1837. The Hering-Breuer reflex, a neurogenic reflex arising in the lung and controlling the rate and depth of respiration via the vagus nerve, was described by Josef Breuer (1842–1925) and Karl E.K. Hering (1834–1918) in 1868. The part played by the diaphragm was studied by Ludwig Traube (1818–1876) and Le Gros Clark in 1871, and George Minott Garland (1849–1926) of New York in 1878. Other respiratory physiologists include: John Scott Haldane (1860–1936) who investigated the toxic effects of carbon monoxide; John Gillies Priestley (1879–1941) a respiratory physiologist who worked with Haldane; John Hutchinson (1811–1861) who invented the spirometer; Leonard Erskin Hill (1866–1952) who worked on respiratory physiology of caisson disease in 1915; and Sir Joseph Barcroft (1872–1947), professor of physiology at Cambridge who devised an apparatus for blood gas analysis. In cellular respiration, the hydrogen acceptor cytochrome was discovered by MacMunn in 1886. Glutathione, a hydrogen carrier in cellular respiration, was isolated by Nobel Prize winner, Sir Frederick Gowland Hopkins (1861–1947) of Cambridge University in 1921. *See artificial respiration, cellular respiration.*

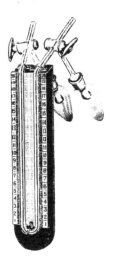

Sir Joseph Barcroft's differential blood gas manometer used for study of tissue respiration. G.V.Anrep and D.T.Harris, *Practical Physiology* (1923). Churchill, London

Respirators *See artificial respiration, iron lung.*

Respiratory Center Julien Jean Cesar Legallois (1775–1814), a physician and physiologist from Brittany in France showed it in the medulla oblongata in 1812. Marie Jean Pierre Flourens (1794–1867) of Paris identified the bilateral 'vital nodes' of the medulla in 1837.

Respiratory Function Tests *See pulmonary function tests.*

Respiratory Physiology Change in blood color in the lungs was noted by a physician and pioneer in blood transfusion, Richard Lower (1631–1691), from Cornwall in 1669. Some physiology experiments on respiration were done by English chemist and physician, John Mayow (1643–1679) who demonstrated the difference between arterial and venous blood in 1674 when a mouse in a closed container died. He named the hypothetical substance in the air 'igneo-aereum' which later was shown to be oxygen. The role of oxygen in respiration was demonstrated by Joseph Priestley (1733–1804), in 1774 and by Antoine Laurent Lavoisier (1743–1794) in 1780. *See respiration, lung functions, aviation medicine.*

Resurrectionist Body snatchers who took bodies from graves to supply for a fee to anatomists for dissection. A famous criminal case was that of Burke and Hare. *See Burke and Hare murders, Anatomy Act.*

Resuscitation *See cardiac resuscitation.*

Reticuloendothelial System [Latin: *reticulum*, net; Greek: *endon*, within + *thele*, nipple] Term coined in 1913 by Ludwig Karl Albert Aschoff (1866–1942) to describe the characteristic cells distributed in the reticulum framework of the spleen, liver and bone marrow which were phagocytotic to dyestuff. Classification of reticuloendothelial diseases was proposed by Maurice Favre (1876–1954), professor of pathological anatomy at Lyons.

Reticulocyte [Latin: *reticulum*, net; Greek: *kytos*, cell] Precursor of the red blood cell identified by Nobel Prize winner, Paul Erhlich (1854–1915), using his own staining method in 1881. A description was given in 1903 by Victor Clarence Vaughan (1851–1929), an American microbiologist and biochemist.

Retina [Latin: *reticulum*, a net] Described as one of the seven layers of the eye by Galen (AD 129–200). The blind spot was discovered by Edeme Mariotte (1620–1684), prior at the Cloister of Saint Martin in France in 1668. Francesco Buzzi, an optic surgeon from Milan, observed and identified the 'yellow spot' or macula lutea and the central fovea in 1782. The layer containing rods and cones was described by Irish ophthalmic surgeon, Arthur Jacob (1790–1874) in 1819. Robert Blassig (1830–1878), the director of the Ophthalmic Hospital at St Petersburg, described the spaces in the anterior part of the retina near the ora serrata in 1863. The theory of vision which ascribed separate functions to rods and cones was proposed by German zoologist, Max Johann Sigismund Schultze (1825–1874) in 1859. Sir David Brewster (1781–1868) published *Optical Study of the Retina* in 1861. *See retinopathy.*

Retinal Detachment [Latin: *reticulum*, net] Mentioned by Charles de Saint-Yves (1667–1733) of Paris in 1722. Histological observations were made by J. Ware in 1805. James Wardrop (1782–1869) in 1818 and Bartolomeo Panniza (1785–1867) in 1826 also commented on the histological findings. Jules Sichel (1802–1868) visualized it through ophthalmoscopy in 1841. A complete description was given by J. Coccius and Adrian Christopher van Tright (1825–1864) in 1853. Albrecht von Graefe (1828–1870) gave an accurate clinical description in 1854. Familial occurrence was pointed out by Treacher Collins in 1892. A new surgical operation was devised by Jules Gonin (1870–1935), a Swiss ophthalmic surgeon, in 1927.

Retinopathy [Latin: *reticulum*, net; Greek: *pathos*, suffering] Retinal changes in hypertension were observed by Ludwig Türck (1810–1868) in 1850, and it was referred to as albuminuric retinitis in *Archives of Ophthalmology* by Richard Liebreich (1830–1917) in 1859. An ophthalmoscopic description was first given by Heymann in 1858. The 'silver wire' appearance of the thickened arteries during ophthalmoscopy was described by Sir William Richard Gowers (1845–1915) in 1876. The study of retinitis in glycosuria was done by Henry Dewey Noyes (1832–1900) in 1869.

Retinoscopy [Latin: *reticulum*, net; Greek: *skopein*, to view] *See skiascopy.*

Retrolental Fibroplasia [Latin: *retro*, backwards + *lens*, lentil + *fibra*, band; Greek: *plasein*, to mold) Found in premature babies and described by Theodore Lasater Terry (1899–1946) of America in 1942. The first cases reported in Europe in 1945 and the signs were explained by W.C. Owens in 1949. A. B. Reece and colleagues demonstrated that the lesion was due to proliferation of endothelial and glial cells in the nerve fiber of the retina in 1952.

Retroperitoneal Pneumatography [Latin: *retro*, backwards; Greek: *peri*, around + *teinenin*, to stretch + *pneuma*, air + *graphein*, to write] Radiological visualization of kidneys by injecting air into the retroperitoneal space was devised by Rossentein and Carelli in 1921. This method carried a high risk of perirenal hematoma and air embolism and it was improved by Riuz Rivas in 1947.

Retroperitoneal Syndrome [Latin: *retro*, backwards; Greek:

peri, around + *teinenin*, to stretch] Term coined by M. Bastos, a Spanish surgeon, and colleagues in the early 1900s to denote the clinical condition of acute hemorrhage into retroperitoneal tissues following abdominal injuries. It was later proved to be caused by involvement of the retroperitoneal ganglia and plexus by hemorrhagic infiltration.

Retroversion of Uterus [Latin: *retroversus*, turned backwards] A description was given by William Hunter (1718–1783) in 1771. A suspension operation was performed by James Alexander Adams (1857–1930) of Glasgow, and William Alexander (1844–1919) of Liverpool in 1881. *An Analysis of the subject of Extra-uterine Foetation, and of the retroversion of the Gravid Uterus* was written by John King of Edisto Island, South Carolina in 1818. The mechanism was explained in detail by German gynecologist, Alwin Karl Mackenrodt (1859–1925) in 1895.

Retzius, Anders Adolf (1796–1860) Swedish anatomist and anthropologist from Stockholm. The ligament of Retzius attached to the extensor retinaculum which acts as a sling to the extensor tendons was described by him in 1841. He described several other anatomical structures.

Retzius, Magnus Gustav (1842–1919) Neuroanatomist at the Karolina Institute in Stockholm. He described the brown lines in the enamel of teeth, known as striae of Retzius, in 1890 and several structures of the brain which are named after him.

Reuter, Baron de (1821–1899) Founder of telegraphic news agency. Born in Kassel in Germany, he emigrated to England in 1851 and established a telegraphic business to convey private messages between England and the continent. In 1858 he persuaded several newspapers to use his agency which he developed into the current international firm (Reuters Agency) for collection and transmission of news.

Reverdin, Albert (1848–1908) Surgeon and cousin of Jacques Louis Reverdin (1842–1929). He demonstrated the fatal effect of excising the thyroid gland in animals.

Reverdin, Jacques Louis (1842–1929) Swiss surgeon in Paris. Transplantation of free skin instead of pedunculated flaps was introduced by him in 1869.

Reverse Transcriptase Viral DNA polymerase enzyme which translates into RNA. Discovered by American molecular biologist, David Baltimore (b 1938) of New York, and virologist, Howard Martin Temin (b 1934) of Philadelphia in 1970. They were awarded the Nobel Prize in 1975.

Review Journals A journal for critical analysis of events and people, *Journal des Scavans*, was published by Denis de Salo of Paris in 1665. Others appeared in Europe including: *Monthly Review* (1749), *Edinburgh Review* (1802), *Quarterly Review* (1809), and *British Quarterly* (1844).

Reye Syndrome Hepatitis, encephalopathy and multi-organ failure in children following an acute mild illness. Described by an Australian physician of German origin, Ralph Douglas Reye (1912–1977) in 1963. Aspirin therapy was identified as the main precipitating cause of the illness in the mid-1980s.

Rh Factor *See rhesus factor.*

Rhazes (AD 850–932) Also known as Mohammed ibn Zakariya al-Razi, was a great Arabian physician who is ranked with Hippocrates (460–377 BC) in his portrayal of disease. He was born at Raj in Khorassan in northeastern Persia, and became a pupil of Hunayn ibn Ishaq (809–873) who made important translations of Galen (AD 129–200) and the *Almagest* of Ptolemy. His *Liber de variolis et morbilis* is the oldest remaining treatise on smallpox and measles. He also wrote on diseases of children, and pioneered genitourinary medicine. He devised catheters with lateral holes in order to drain pus and used lead catheters, instead of inflexible bronze ones. He is credited with 237 works, most of which are now lost. He followed the Hippocratic school of medicine in describing disease and giving a prognosis.

Rheometer [Greek: *rheos*, current + *metron*, to measure] Early form of galvanometer to measure electric current. Invented by André Marie Ampère (1775–1836) in 1820. *See galvanometer.*

Rheostat [Greek: *rheos*, current + *histanai*, to place] Instrument to vary current by regulating resistance. Invented by Sir Charles Wheatstone (1802–1875).

Rhesus Factor (Rh factor) The presence of Rh factor in human erythrocytes was demonstrated by testing human blood against anti-rhesus serum obtained from rabbits after the injection of erythrocytes of rhesus monkeys by Nobel Prize winner, Karl Landsteiner (1868–1943), and Alexander S. Wiener (1907–1976) of Brooklyn in 1940. *See ABO blood groups.*

Rheumatic Fever [Greek: *rheuma*, flux] Mentioned in *Sometyme Rewmatik Humors* by John of Trevesia in 1398. Aortic valve and mitral valve damage were described by Raymond de Vieussens (1641–1715) in 1695. The relationship of acute rheumatism and chorea was noted by Thomas Sydenham (1624–1689). The term 'rheumatism' was used by Guillaume de Baillou (1538–1616). Rheumatic arthritis and

rash were collectively described as 'rheumatic fever' by John Haygarth (1740–1827) of Bath in 1805. In 1797 Matthew Baillie (1761–1823) described the association between rheumatism and heart disease, previously noted by David Pitcairn (1749–1809) in 1788. Rheumatic nodules were described by William Charles Wells (1757–1817), a physician at St Thomas' Hospital in 1810. In 1836 Jean Baptiste Bouillaud (1796–1881) gave the name 'endocardium' to the interlining of the heart and related the occurrence of endocarditis to acute rheumatism. He also described acute rheumatic polyarthritis in 1832 and mentioned the involvement of the mitral valve in articular rheumatism in 1835. The latent period between sore throat and rheumatic symptoms was noted by Haig-Brown in 1886, and bacterial invasion of the throat as an etiological factor was recognized by Mantle in 1887. The characteristic nodular lesions of the heart were described by Ludwig Karl Albert Aschoff (1866–1942) in 1904. The causative bacteria, previously named, *Diplococcus rheumaticus* by Frederick John Poynton (1869–1943) and Alexander Paine, was identified as Streptococcus group A by Rebecca Craighill Lancefield (1895–1981) in 1940.

Rheumatic Gout [Greek: *rheuma*, flux] Old term used for gout and chronic rheumatic diseases.

Rheumatic Heart Disease [Greek: *rheuma*, flux] *See rheumatic fever.*

Rheumatoid Arthritis [Greek: *rheuma*, flux] Described by French physician, Augustin Jacob Landre-Beauvis (1772–1840). The term 'rheumatoid arthritis' was coined by Sir Alfred Baring Garrod (1819–1909) in 1858 to denote a form of arthritis which differed from gout. It was noticed that jaundice had a beneficial effect on rheumatoid arthritis and in 1938 Philip Showalter Hench (1896–1965) attempted to treat it with injection of bile salts and was partly successful. In 1948 he noticed that surgery, pregnancy and starvation, which stimulated the adrenal cortex, also improved rheumatoid arthritis. He suggested that cortical hormones should be tested for anti-rheumatoid activity. Edward Calvin Kendall (1886–1972) supplied a few grams of cortisone to Hench in 1948 to conduct a trial, and a dramatic effect of cortisone on certain cases was published by Hench and co-workers in 1949. Phenylbutazone, one of the first anti-inflammatory drugs, was introduced by J. P. Currie, R. A. Brown and G. Will in 1953. Hench, Kendall and Tadeus Reichstein (b 1897) shared the Nobel Prize for Medicine or Physiology in 1950.

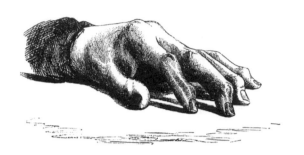

Rheumatoid arthritis involving the hand. Sir Alfred Baring Garrod, *A Treatise on Gout and Rheumatic Gout* (1876). Longmans, Green & Co., London

Rhind Papyrus Oldest surviving mathematical manuscript, thought to be copied from an earlier manuscript by Ahmes who lived around 1650 BC. Also called the Ahmes Papyrus, it was purchased by Scottish Egyptologist, Alexander Henry Rhind (1833–1863) in 1858.

Rhinosporidiosis [Greek: *rhin*, nose + *sporos*, seed] Involving the mucocutaneous tissue of the nose, was noted in Argentina by Alejandro Posadas (1870–1920) of Buenos Aires in 1903. This diseases is also common in India and was described by O'Kinealy in the same year. James Hartley Ashworth (1874–1936) of Edinburgh proposed the genus *Rhinosporidium* as the causative fungus of the disease in 1923.

Rhinolith [Greek: *rhin*, nose + *lithos*, stone] Removal of a rhinolith or nasal calculus was recorded by Gardi in 1502.

Rhinology [Greek: *rhin*, nose + *logos*, discourse] *See otolaryngology*.

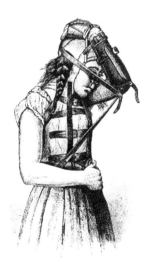

Italian method of rhinoplasty. Sir Frederick Treves, *A Manual of Operative Surgery* (1892). Lee Bros. & Co., Philadelphia

Rhinoplasty [Greek: *rhin*, nose + *plasmein*, to mold] Nose surgery was practiced by ancient Hindu surgeons. A procedure was described by Aulus Cornelius Celsus (25 BC–AD 50) and revived in the 16th century by Gasparo Tagliacozzi (1546–1599), an Italian professor who specialized in plastic surgery at Bologna. A book was published by Carl Ferdinand von Graefe (1787–1840), professor of surgery at Berlin in 1818. An Italian method was introduced to Britain by Sir William MacCormac (1836–1901) of Belfast in 1877. *See nose surgery*.

Rhinoscleroma [Greek: *rhin*, nose + *skeleros*, hard] Nodular hypertrophy of the skin and mucous membrane of the nose. Described and named by Ferdinand von Hebra (1816–1880) and Moritz Kaposi (1837–1902) in 1870.

Rhodes Scholarship Founded by Cecil John Rhodes (1853–1902) from Bishop Stortford who acquired wealth from diamond mines in Africa. His will provided scholarships at Oxford for Americans, Germans and citizens of British colonies.

Rhodium Rare metal in platinum ore discovered by William Hyde Wollaston (1766–1828) in 1804.

Rhodius, John (1587–1659) Danish physician from Copenhagen who wrote several treatises, including one on artificial baths.

Rhodopsin [Greek: *rhodon*, rose + *opsis*, sight] Photosensitive pigment in the retina discovered by Franz Christian Boll (1849–1879) in 1877. Named rhodopsin or 'sehpurpur' (visual purple) by Willy Kuhne (1821–1901) in 1878. Vitamin A in the retina was shown by New York biochemist, George Wald (b 1906) in 1933, and his work led to the discovery of the link between rhodopsin and vitamin A and with night blindness. He shared the Nobel Prize for Physiology or Medicine with Ragner Arthur Granit (b 1900) and Haldan Keffer Hartline (1903–1983) in 1967.

Rhubarb Known for its medicinal properties to the ancient Chinese, and found in the herbal *Pen-King* as Huang-Liang. The name of the genus (*Rheus*) may come from the ancient name of the river Volga, *Rha*, or from the Greek *rheo* meaning 'to flow' referring to its purgative properties. Pliny (AD 23–79), Aulus Cornelius Celsus (25 BC–AD 50), Mesue the Younger (d 1015) and Constantinus Africanus (d 1087) mentioned the plant. Alexander of Tralles (525–605) referred to it. It became an expensive commodity during the Renaissance and was valued 12 times the price of benzoin in Alexandria in 1497. At Ulm in 1596 it was more costly than opium.

Ribbert, Moritz Wilhelm Hugo (1855–1920) A histopathologist in Zurich who initiated the theory of embryonal origin of cancer in 1905.

Ribes, François (1765–1845) Army surgeon from Toulouse who described the uppermost sympathetic ganglion situated on the anterior communicating artery of the circle of Willis, known as the ganglion of Ribes, in 1817.

Ribes Ganglion *See Ribes, François.*

Riboflavin Vitamin B2. In 1932, while investigating oxidation of glucose-6-phosphate by a yeast preparation, Nobel Prize winner, Otto Heinrich Warburg (1883–1970), a German biochemist and director of Kaiser Wilhelm Institute in Berlin, found that the reaction requires the cofactor riboflavin, which he called 'old yellow enzyme'. The important role of this enzyme in oxidation–reduction during respiration was pointed out by Walter Christian (1907–1955) in the same year. It was separated into two components, a protein and a pigment, by the same workers in 1933 and was named vitamin B2. In the same year, another Nobel Prize winner, Richard Kuhn (1900–1967) a professor from Heidelberg University, and Paul Gyorgy (1893–1976) isolated it from several sources and it was renamed riboflavin by the Council of Pharmacy and Chemistry of the American Medical Association in 1937. *See ariboflavinosis.*

Ribonucleic Acid (RNA) Thomas Cech (b 1947) an American biochemist at the University of Colorado, Boulder discovered the ability of RNA to act as a biological catalyst. He also discovered the role of ribosomal RNA in catalyzing its own cleaving and splicing. Canadian biologist Sidney Altman (b 1939), professor of biology at Yale, studied transfer RNA, the amino acid carrier in protein synthesis. Altman and Cech shared the 1989 Nobel Prize for Chemistry for their work. The operon theory of gene regulation and messenger RNA were discovered by French biochemists François Jacob (b 1920) and Jacques Lucien Monod (1910–1976) in 1963 and they shared the Nobel Prize for Physiology or Medicine in 1965. The complete molecular structure of the transfer RNA was worked out by American biochemist, Robert William Holley (b 1922), and American geneticist, Seymour Benzer (b 1921), in 1965. The genetic code found in transfer RNA and involved in assembly of amino acids into proteins under the direction of DNA, was decoded by Indian-born American molecular chemist Har Gobind Khorana (b 1922) and American biochemist Marshall Warren Nirenberg (b 1927). Holley, Khorana and Nirenberg shared the 1968 Nobel Prize for their work.

Ribosomes Subcellular organelles on the endoplasmic reticulum and containing RNA which are the site of protein synthesis. Their function was discovered by American cytologist of Romanian origin, George Emil Palade (b 1912) in 1956. Palade qualified in medicine from Bucharest and migrated to America in 1946. After serving at the Rockefeller Institute, New York (1946–1972), he became head of cell biology at Yale Medical School (1972), and was appointed professor of molecular biology at University of California, San Diego in 1990. In 1974 he shared the Nobel Prize for Physiology or Medicine with Albert Claude and Christian de Duve.

Rice Polishings The pericarp and germ layers, used as a cure for dermatitis induced by vitamin deficiency from eating polished rice. Its action was discovered by H. Schneider in 1930. The active factor in the rice was named 'rice polish factor' by G. C. Supplee and colleagues in 1940. *See thiamin.*

Rich, Arnold Rice (1893–1968) American pathologist from Alabama who worked at the Johns Hopkins Hospital. He described the Hamman–Rich syndrome in 1944. *See Hamman–Rich syndrome.*

Richard, Felix Adolph (1822–1872) Surgeon from Paris who described ovarian fimbria of the ostium of the fallopian tube in 1851.

Richards, Dickinson Woodruff (1895–1973) American cardiologist, born in Orange, New Jersey and educated at Yale. He was a pioneer in application of the cardiac catheter to study blood pressure, oxygen tension and other physiological variables in health and disease. He was a cardiologist at Columbia University (1928–1961) and was professor of medicine there from 1947. He shared the Nobel Prize for Physiology or Medicine in 1956 with Forssman and Cournand, for his work on cardiac catheterization.

Richards, Sir Rex Edward (b 1922) English chemist, graduate of St John's College, Oxford, Vice-Chancellor of the University of Oxford and Director of the Leverhulme Trust. He worked on infrared spectroscopy and nuclear magnetic resonance spectroscopy. He applied NMR to biological problems and contributed to its development as a medical technique.

Richardson, Sir Benjamin Ward (1828–1896) Physician and inventor of ether spray as a local anesthetic. Born at Somerby in Leicestershire and qualified from Glasgow University. He moved to London in 1854 and took up the study of anesthetics in 1865. He also did research on poisons in contagious disease and discovered a bacterial poison called septine in 1865. As an anesthetist, he modified chloroform inhalers and devised a lethal chamber for painless slaughter of experimental animals in 1866. Richardson wrote *A City of Health* and *Biological Experimentation, It's Functions and Limits* (1896).

Richardson, Sir John (1787–1865) Born in Dumfries and graduated from Edinburgh as a physician in 1816. He joined the Naval Medical Service where he served for 48 years and took part in three Arctic expeditions.

Richardson, Sir Owen Williams (1879–1959) English physicist from Dewsbury in Yorkshire. He used the term 'thermionics' to describe emission of electricity from hot bodies. He was professor of physics at King's College, London in 1914 and won the Nobel Prize for Physics in 1928.

Richardson Sign Sign of death was described by Sir Benjamin Ward Richardson (1828–1896). He applied a tight fillet to the arm and if life was present the distal veins swelled.

Richerand, A. (1779–1840) Professor of surgery and physiology in Paris. He was ranked as one of the most skilled surgeons but was unpopular due to his overwhelming ambition, vanity and unpleasant personal traits. He resected the 5th and 6th ribs in 1818.

Richet, Charles Robert (1850–1935) French physiologist, born in Paris and obtained his medical degree there in 1877. He was made professor of physiology at Paris in 1888 and did pioneering work on serum therapy having noted that the blood of animals which are resistant to a harmful bacterium may contain an element that could confer immunity. He coined the term anaphylaxis to denote a form of allergic reaction in 1902, and was awarded the Nobel Prize for his work on allergy in 1913. He also worked on hypnosis, digestion, pain, muscle contraction and animal heat. The International Institute of Metaphysics at Paris was founded by Richet, and Joseph Tessier, professor of medicine at Lyons.

Richet, Louis Alfred (1816–1891) Professor of clinical surgery at Paris. He described the canal for the umbilical vein in the anterior wall of the umbilical canal in 1855.

Richter Scale Measurement of the energy released by an earthquake on a scale of 1 to 9 where an increase of one unit corresponds to 30 times the seismic energy. Invented by American seismologist, Charles Francis Richter (1900–1985) of Hamilton, Ohio and German-born American geophysicist, Beno Gutenberg (1889–1960) in 1932.

Richter Hernia Where only a part of the lumen is protruded. Described by German surgeon, August Gottlieb Richter (1742–1812) of Göttingen in 1785.

Rickets [Greek: *rachitis*, spinal complaint] Observed in Britain around 1620 and described by English physician, Daniel Whistler (1619–1684) of Merton College, Oxford in his *De Morbo puerili Anglorum, quam patrio idiomate indignae vocant* published in 1645. Francis Glisson (1597–1677), regius professor at Cambridge, gave a more complete description in *De Rachitide Sive morbo Purelli qui vulgo, the Rickets Dicteur* in 1650. Decline in fish consumption during the Reformation was probably responsible for the sudden increase in rickets in England, and it came to be known as 'English disease'. Bootius (1600–1654) in 1649 noted its prevalence in Ireland and Robert Darley, an English physician, and Armand Trousseau (1801–1867) in France used cod liver oil as treatment. It became an extremely common disease in smog-choked industrial cities in Europe and the USA at the beginning of the 20th century. Effective treatment was experimentally demonstrated in England by Sir Edward Bland-Sutton (1855–1936) who fed lion cubs in the zoo with crushed bone and cod liver oil in 1889. Between 1908 and 1918 experiments were carried out on dogs in which rickets was induced by diet. Animals which were regularly exercised recovered and a controversy arose as to whether exercise or diet were responsible. In 1890 Palm had suggested the effectiveness of sunlight as a cure and it was later discovered that a chemical reaction producing vitamin D can take place in the skin when it is bared to ultraviolet rays. The increase in the disease was, therefore, attributable to a reduction in light penetration of the smoke-filled atmosphere. Sir Edward Mellanby (1884–1955) produced rickets in dogs by maintaining them on a deficient diet and suggested that the missing nutrient was a fat-soluble substance, vitamin D. He advocated the use of cod liver oil and was responsible for the virtual elimination of the disease. Vitamin D was discovered by American biochemist, Elmer Verner McCollum (1879–1967) and colleagues of Baltimore in 1921 and it was obtained in a crystalline form at the National Institute of Medical Research in London during 1930. *See ergosterol.*

Ricketts, Howard Taylor (1871–1910) Microbiologist from Northwestern University who showed that the causative agent of Rocky Mountain spotted fever was transmitted by ticks. He died in Mexico during his research on the causative organism of Mexican typhus fever, which was named (*Rickettsia muricola*). *See Rickettsia prowazekii.*

Rickettsia burnetii *See Coxiella burnettii, Q fever.*

Rickettsia prowazekii The bacterium found in ticks taken from patients with Mexican typhus fever, by da Rocha Lima (1879–1956) in 1916. Named for Howard Taylor Ricketts (1871–1910), an American pathologist and Stanislas von Prowazek (1876–1915), a German microbiologist, both of whom died during the course of their research on rickettsial diseases.

Ricord, Phillipe (1799–1889) American pioneer in venereology who studied medicine in Paris. He demonstrated the different etiology of syphilis and gonorrhea and described the three stages of syphilis. His work on venereal diseases was published in 1838.

Riddoch Syndrome Inattention to objects in one half of the visual field, with inability to recognize these objects. Described by Scottish neurologist, George Riddoch (1889–1947) in 1917. He graduated from Aberdeen and spent most of his career in London.

Rideal–Walker Test Used to determine the germicidal power of disinfectants. Invented by two English chemists, Samuel Rideal (1863–1929) and J.T. Ainsley Walker (1868–1930) around 1920.

Ridley, Humphrey (1653–1708) English anatomist and physician in London. He described the cerebral vessels of the brain in his *The Anatomy of the Brain* published in 1695. The coronary sinus is named (Ridley sinus) after him.

Riedel Lobe Accessory right lobe of the liver, described by German professor of surgery, Bernhard Moritz Carl Ludwig Riedel (1846–1916) of Jena in 1893.

Riedel Thyroiditis Chronic inflammation of the thyroid leading to a hard mass in the gland. Described by a German professor of surgery, Bernhard Moritz Carl Ludwig Riedel (1846–1916) of Jena in 1896.

Rift Valley Fever Febrile disease caused by a virus carried by mosquitoes and affecting cattle. Described in the Rift Valley of Kenya by Robert Daubney (b 1891) and John Richard Hudson in 1931.

Rig Veda Sacred book attributed to the Hindu god Brahma, containing hymns to the gods.

Rigal Suture Utilizes rubber rings, used instead of thread to close wounds. Devised by French surgeon, Jean Antoine Rigal (1797–1865).

Riggs Disease Pyorrhea alveolaris. Pierre Fauchard (1678–1761) described pyorrhea alveolaris or marginal periodontitis in 1746. It was later named Riggs disease because of a new treatment consisting of scraping the teeth to the roots proposed by American dental surgeon John Mankey Riggs (1810–1885) in 1876. *See dentistry.*

Ringer, Sydney (1835–1910) British physiologist from a Quaker family in Norwich who graduated from University College Hospital, London in 1860. He introduced thermometry in clinical medicine. *See Ringer solution.*

Ringer Solution Sydney Ringer (1835–1910) studied metabolite antagonism in 1883 and found that sodium alone could not maintain the beat of an isolated heart unless balanced by calcium and potassium. He therefore developed a physiological solution consisting of sodium chloride, potassium chloride and calcium chloride, which now bears his name.

Ringworm A parasitic fungus of *Trichophyton* or *Microsporum* that causes tinea. Discovered by Antoine Pierre Ernest Bazin (1807–1878) of France. But initially opposed by some dermatologists including Erasmus Wilson (1809–1884).

Rinnie Test Use of a tuning fork to differentiate between sensorimotor deafness and conduction deafness. Devised by German otologist, Heinrich Adolf Rinnie (1819–1868) in 1855.

Riolan, Jean, Secundus (1580–1657) Leading anatomist of his period and dean of the Faculty of Medicine in Paris. He opposed William Harvey's (1578–1657) discovery of circulation in his *Encheridium Anatomicum* published in 1648. Several anatomical structures described by him in *Anatomia Corporis Humani* (1610) were subsequently named after him.

Riolan, Jean, Primus (1539–1606) French physiologist and the father of the celebrated anatomist, Jean Riolan (1580–1657), Secundus.

Ripault Sign Pressure applied to the eye ball to see if the distortion was permanent – a sign of death. Described by French physician, Louis Henry Antoine Ripault (1807–1856).

Risley Prism Rotating prism in a metal frame with scales. Devised to measure the imbalance of the ocular muscles by Samuel Doty Risley (1845–1920), an ophthalmologist in Philadelphia.

Ritter, Johann Wilhelm (1776–1810) German physicist who studied medicine at Jena. He discovered ultraviolet light through its darkening effect on silver chloride in 1801. He constructed a dry cell battery in 1802 and an accumulator in 1803.

Ritter Disease Dermatitis exfoliativa infantum or staphylococcal scalded skin syndrome. Described by German physician, Gottfried Ritter von Riettshaim (1820–1883) in 1878.

Riva-Rocci, Scipione (1863–1937) Italian physician at the department of pathological medicine in the University of Turin. He improved the sphygmomanometer by using a pneumatic cuff, which was described in *Gazzetta Medicina di Torino* in 1896. He published a further two papers on the technique in the same journal in 1897.

Rivinus, Augustus Quirinus (1652–1723) Professor of physiology and botany at Leipzig. He described the duct of the sublingual glands (duct of Rivinus) in 1678. He also attempted a classification of plants into eighteen groups, based on the morphology of petals or corolla in *Systema Plantarum*. His father, Andreas Rivinus (1601–1656), was also a professor of physiology at Leipzig.

Riverius, Lazarus (1589–1655) Physician in Montpellier and professor of medicine in his native town in 1622, where he remained until his death. He wrote *Institutiones Medicinae, Praxis Medica* and several other treatises.

Rivers, Clive (1872–1929) Physician at the City of London Hospital. Pioneer of artificial pneumothorax in the treatment of tuberculosis. He also advocated the early diagnosis and treatment of pulmonary tuberculosis. *See artificial pneumothorax.*

Rivers, Thomas Milton (1888–1962) American virologist at the Rockefeller Institute who established the basis for diagnosing psittacosis by injecting the sputum of the patient into white mice in 1938.

Rivers, William Halse (1864–1922) British neuropsychiatrist and anthropologist from Kent and member of the Torres Straits expedition who established anthropology on a firm scientific footing by collection of empirical data. His *Instinct and the Unconscious* (1920) challenged Freud's libido theory, and *Medicine, Magic and Religion* in 1924 showed the importance of studying indigenous medical systems in the same context as social institutions.

Riviere Portion A 17th century remedy made of an effervescent solution of citric acid and potassium carbonate. Prepared by French physician, Lazare Riviere (1589–1655).

Riviere Sign Dullness of percussion over the 5th, 6th and 7th dorsal vertebrae indicating pulmonary tuberculosis. Described by an English physician, Clive Riviere or Rivers (1873–1929).

Rivington, Walter (1835–1897) Born in Highgate, he joined the London Hospital as an assistant surgeon in 1863 and became dean of the medical school. His *The Medical Profession* was the first complete account of the history, character and laws governing the medical profession.

Rivini Gland An early description of the sublingual gland was given by August Quirinus Rivenius (1652–1723), a botanist and physician at Leipzig.

Rizzoli Institute Orthopedic institute in Rome founded by F. Rizzoli (1809–1890) of Bologna in 1880.

RNA *See ribonucleic acid.*

Robbins, Frederick Chapman (b 1916) American physiologist and pediatrician from Auburn, Alabama. He worked with John Franklin Enders (1897–1985) and Thomas Huckle Weller (b 1915) at the Infectious Disease Research Laboratory of the Children's Hospital in Boston on improving techniques for culturing viruses. They succeeded in cultivating the poliomyelitis virus, an important step in development of polio vaccine. All three shared the Nobel Prize for Physiology or Medicine in 1954.

Robert of Chester (1110–1160) English scientific writer who wrote an alchemical text in Latin in 1145, translated Al-Kwarizmi's *Algebra* and the *Koran* in 1144.

Robert Ligament Fascicle of fibers arising from the posterior cruciate ligament to the lateral meniscus of the knee. Described by French surgeon, César Alphonse Robert (1801–1862).

Robert Pelvis Rudimentary sacrum with marked narrowing of the transverse and oblique diameters. Described by German gynecologist, Heinrich Ludwig Ferdinand Robert (1814–1874).

Roberts, Richard (b 1943) British molecular biologist who moved to the USA in 1969 to work at the Cold Springs Harbor Laboratory in New York. In 1977 he published his findings on the section of DNA in genes now known as the 'intron' which carry no genetic information. He shared the Nobel Prize for Physiology or Medicine in 1993 with Philip Allen Sharp (b 1944) who had reached similar conclusions.

Roberts Test Used for detection of albumin in the urine with a solution of magnesium sulfate and sulfuric acid. Devised by English physician, Sir William Roberts (1830–1899).

Robertson, Matthew George First professor of mental diseases at the Edinburgh Medical School in 1919.

Robin, Charles Filippe (1821–1885) Professor of histology at the Faculty of Medicine in Paris. He described the lymphatic spaces around the arteries in 1868 (Robin spaces). He also described the osteoclastic cells of bone.

Robinson, Frederick Byron (1857–1910) Surgeon and gynecologist from Wisconsin. He graduated from Rush Medical College in 1882 and practiced in Europe in 1887. He worked with Lawson Tait (1845–1899) at Birmingham before returning to the USA as professor of surgery at Chicago in 1891. Several gynecological structures have been named after him.

Robinson, J. William (1869–1936) Campaigner for birth control in America who protested State interference in distribution of information on contraception. He induced Abraham Jacobi (1830–1919), the first president of American Medical Association, to establish a medical forum for contraception. He wrote *Limitation of Offspring* (1904), and other works on birth control.

Robinson, John (1739–1805) Succeeded Joseph Black (1728–1799) as lecturer in chemistry at Glasgow University in 1766 and was professor of natural philosophy at University of Edinburgh.

Robinson, Victor (1886–1947) Professor of history of medicine at the Temple University School of Medicine in Philadelphia. He wrote *The Story of Medicine* in 1931.

Robinson Circle Formed by the anastomosis of the abdominal aorta, common iliac, hypogastric, uterine and ovarian arteries. Described by American anatomist, Frederick Byron Robinson (1857–1910).

Robison, Robert (1884–1941) British biochemist who studied carbohydrate metabolism. He developed organ culture techniques with Dame Honor Bridget Fell (1900–1986) in 1929. He published on conversion of blood calcium into insoluble calcium in the bone in 1923.

Robot A forerunner, the turtle, was invented by British neurologist, William Grey Walter (1911–1977) who emigrated to America in 1910.

Rockefeller Foundation Established in 1913 by the oil magnate, John Davison Rockefeller (1839–1937), founder of the Standard Oil Company (1870) in Ohio. His foundation donated over 500 million dollars in the first half of the 20th century to various institutions for the development of science and education.

Rockefeller Institute Established in 1902 with funds provided by the oil magnate, John Davison Rockefeller (1839–1937), founder of the Standard Oil Company (1870) in Ohio. Its buildings and laboratory were completed in 1906 on the East River New York, and the microbiologist Simon Flexner (1863–1946) was its first director.

Rocky Mountain Spotted Fever (Syn: blue disease, black fever, spotted fever) Found in the Montana and Idaho districts of America and described by Edward Ernest Maxey (1867–1934) in 1896. The etiology was investigated by Wilson and Chowning in 1902, who mistakenly attributed it to a parasite, *Babesia*, previously known to cause Texas cattle fever. In 1906 A.F.A. King (1841–1914) proposed that it was caused by a tick, *Dermacentor andersoni*, and it was also found to be transmitted by *Rhipicephalus*, *Haemaphysalis*, *Amblyomma* and *Ixodes*. His theory was proved by Howard Taylor Ricketts (1871–1910), who transmitted the disease to a monkey by means of an infected tick in 1909. The causative organism was named *Rickettsia rickettsii*.

Roddick, Sir Thomas George (1846–1923) Canadian surgeon and reformer of medical practice in Canada. He graduated from McGill University and became chief surgeon to Montreal General Hospital. He was instrumental in the establishment of the Medical Council of Canada.

Rodent Ulcer [Latin: *rodere*, to gnaw] Epithelial tumor of the skin described by Charles Hewitt Moore (1821–1870), a pioneer in treatment of cancer in England. A monograph was written by John Collins Warren (1778–1856).

Rodgers, John Kearny (1793–1851) *See humerus.*

Rodgers, David (1799–1877) *See jaw.*

Rodriguez, J.M. (1828–1894) Mexican obstetrician and pioneer in the diagnosis of pregnancy by palpation and auscultation.

Roebuck, John (1718–1794) Physician from Sheffield who studied medicine at Edinburgh University and graduated from Leiden in 1742 but devoted his time to chemistry. He invented the lead chamber process for manufacture of sulfuric acid with Samuel Garbett in 1746 and founded the Carron Ironworks in Stirlingshire in 1759.

Roemer, Olaus (1644–1710) Danish astronomer from Aarhus, Jutland and professor of astronomy at Copenhagen. He calculated the speed of light through space, with impressive accuracy, from astronomical observations in 1695. His most important work *Basis Astronomiae* was published in 1735.

Roesler, Hugo (b 1899) Cardiologist at Temple University Hospital and the Shriner's Hospital for Crippled Children in Philadelphia. He described the rib erosion and aortic knob as radiological signs of aortic coarctation in 1928. His *Clinical Röntgenology of the Cardiovascular System* was published in 1937.

Rogers Sphygmomanometer An early aneroid manometer instead of a mercury one was designed by Oscar Harrison Rogers (1857–1941), a physician from New York.

Roger Syndrome *See maladie de Roger.*

Rogers, Sir Leonard (1868–1962) British physician who worked in Calcutta and wrote *Fevers in the Tropics* and *Bowel Disease in the Tropics.* He gave emetine injections for amebic dysentery and hepatitis in 1912. He advocated intravenous saline solutions in treatment of dehydration due to cholera.

Rogerson, John Physician from Dumfries who emigrated to Russia a year after publishing his doctoral thesis *De Morbis Infantum* in 1765, and became a trusted advisor to Empress Catherine II for 50 years.

Roget, Peter Mark (1779–1869) Huguenot physician at the Manchester Infirmary who compiled *Roget's Thesaurus* from his *Thesaurus of English Words and Phrase* published in 1852. He also contributed to *Encyclopedia Britannica* and wrote a Bridgwater treatise *On Animal and Vegetable Physiology* in 1834.

Rokitansky, Karl Freiherr von (1804–1878) Czech professor of pathology in Vienna, contemporary of Rudolph Virchow (1821–1902), and a founder of modern pathological anatomy. He gave original descriptions of: gastromesentric ilius, spondylolithic pelvis (kyphotic pelvis) (1839), striped muscles in tumor (sarcoma), acute dilation of the stomach (1842), acute yellow atrophy of the liver (1843), a scientific account of hemorrhage from dilated esophageal veins in portal hypertension (1840), and clinical features of congenital transposition of the aorta and pulmonary artery (1875). His work was translated into English and published by the Sydenham Society in 1850.

Rolando Fissure The sulcus centralis of the brain was described by Luigi Rolando (1773–1831), professor of anatomy at Turin. It was named fissure of Rolando by François Leuret of Paris in 1839. Rolando also made a study of the cerebellum and published a series of observations on the effects of experimental removal of the cerebellum in animals. Several other structures of the brain, including Rolandic area and Rolandic convolution, bear his name.

Rolando Fracture Variation of the fracture of the first metatarsal bone. Described by Silvio Rolando, a Milanese surgeon, in 1926.

Roller Nucleus Nucleus lateralis of the accessory nerve. Described by Christian Friedrich Wilhelm Roller (1802–1878), a neuropsychiatrist at Strasburg in 1881.

Rolleston, Sir Humphry (1778–1829) Regius professor of physic at the University of Cambridge and a medical historian. He was physician to King George VI and president of the Royal College of Physicians.

Rollet, Alexander (1834–1903) Austrian professor of histology at the University of Graz, who described the colorless stroma of the erythrocytes (Rollet stroma) in 1880.

Rollier, Auguste (1874–1954) Swiss physician who advocated the use of increasing doses of sunlight in treatment of tuberculosis in 1913.

Roman Medicine The first physicians in Rome were Greeks, as the Romans looked down upon the medical profession and were reluctant to practice. The Aquilian Law made physicians and surgeons accountable for their actions and was enacted in 300 BC. Julius Caesar gave citizenship to Greek physicians and established them as free men in 46 BC. Appointment of physicians was regulated by Emperor Antonius in AD 160. Aulus Cornelius Celsus (25 BC–AD 50) established the four cardinal signs of: inflammation, heat, pain, redness and swelling. Claudius Galen (AD 129–200) from Pergamom in Asia Minor was another Roman philosopher and physician who described over 347 herbal remedies, and earned him the title of father of pharmacology. Dioscorides (AD 40–90) coined the term materia medica to denote his compilation and description of over 600 medicinal substances. Fabiola, a Roman lady who devoted her entire life to working for the poor sick people, is credited with having built the first Christian hospital or nosocomium in Rome around AD 390. Emperor Justinian encouraged the physicians to train pupils in medicine in AD 533 and fixed salaries for physicians. A Roman medicine stamp found at Tranent in East Lothian provided evidence for the existence of Roman medicine in Scotland. The stamp is that of an oculist, Lucius Vallentius, and contains aromatic prescriptions for cicatrices and crocodes used for affection of the eyes. Roman medical instruments have also been located in Scotland and are exhibited at the National Museum of Scotland in Edinburgh.

Romanes, John George (1848–1894) Naturalist and disciple of Charles Darwin. He studied invertebrates and compared the mental development of animals and humans. He wrote *Mental Evolution in Animals*, and the first book on comparative psychology, *Animal Intelligence* in 1883.

Romanovsky Stain Eosin and methylene blue stain for studying blood films. Devised by Dimitri Leonidovitch Romanovsky (1861–1921), a physician from Russia. During his study in St Petersburg, he used the stain to demonstrate that malarial parasites were damaged during treatment with quinine. This was an important landmark in chemotherapy and the first time that a direct effect of chemotherapy on a pathogenic organism was demonstrated on live patients.

Romberg, Moritz Heinrich (1795–1873) German professor of neurology at Berlin who wrote the first formal treatise on nervous diseases, *Lehrbuch der Nervenkrankheiten,* between 1840–1846. He also described the pathognomonic sign in truncal sensory ataxia (Romberg sign).

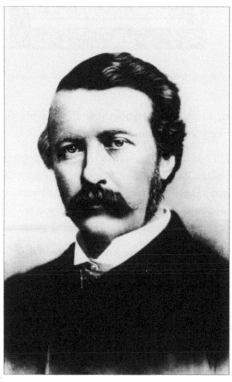

Moritz Heinrich Romberg (1795–1873). Courtesy of the National Library of Medicine

Romberg Sign *See Romberg, Moritz.*

Roemer, Olaus (1644–1710) Astronomer from Copenhagen who invented a transit circle to measure the time of transit across the meridian. He used it to calculate the time it would take for light to traverse the radius of Earth's orbit.

Roemer Serum Early antipneumococcal serum prepared by German professor, Paul Roemer (1876–1916) of Griefswald. He also standardized the old tuberculin method in 1909.

Rondelet (1507–1556) Italian zoologist who studied marine organisms of the Mediterranean. He wrote *Aquatic Animals* in 1554.

Röntgen Rays *See Röntgen, Wilhelm Konrad von, X-ray.*

Röntgen, Wilhelm Konrad von (1845–1923) German physicist who discovered X-rays. Born in Lennep, Prussia, he studied under Kundt (1839–1894) in Zurich and was appointed professor of physics at Giessen in 1879, and at Würzberg in 1888. In 1895, while investigating cathode rays, he noticed a new ray of greater penetrating power emitted from the cathode tube. He accidentally discovered their use when his wife placed her hand on a photographic plate. He announced his findings before the Würzberg Society in 1895 but did not patent his discovery. He was awarded the first Nobel Prize for Physics in 1901.

Rorschach Test Diagnostic procedure in mental disorders and personality tests using standardized ink blots. Devised by Hermann Rorschach (1884–1922), a Swiss neuropsychiatrist at Zurich.

Rose, Edmund (1836–1914) Berlin physician who described cardiac tamponade caused by collection of blood in the pericardium secondary to cardiac rupture.

Rose, William (1847–1910) English surgeon who performed excision of the gasserian ganglion as treatment for trigeminal neuralgia.

Rose, William Cumming (1887–1984) American biochemist from Greenville, South Carolina who studied at Yale and Freiburg Universities. He did research on mammalian nutrition in relation to each of the 20 known amino acids and identified 10 which are indispensable for proper nutrition. He purified threonine (1936), methionine (1937), and valine (1939).

Rosenbach, Julius Friedrich (1842–1923) German surgeon who introduced the name Streptococcus for the cocci found in chains in 1884. He also differentiated between staphylococci and streptococci.

Rosenbach Test Detects bile in the urine using nitric acid as a reagent. Devised by a German physician, Ottomar Rosenbach (1851–1907) in 1876.

Rosenberger Stain Detects spirochetes using aniline oil. Devised by Randal Rosenberger, a bacteriologist in Philadelphia.

Rosenmüller, Johann Christian (1771–1820) Embryologist and professor of anatomy at Leipzig who described the pharyngeal recess (Rosenmüller fossa) in 1805.

Rosenthal, Isodor (1836–1915) Professor of physiology in Germany who described the spiral canal of cochlea (Rosenthal canal).

Roser Line Surface marking from the anterior superior iliac spine to the ischial tubercles. Defined by Wilhelm Roser (1817–1888), professor of surgery at Marburg in 1844.

Rosicrucians Sect of mystical philosophers whose name is derived from *Confessa Rosa Crucis* proposed by Valentine Andreas in 1615. It originated in Germany in the 14th century and was revived in the 17th century. They follow the ancient philosophy of the Chaldeans and Persians.

Ross, Sir Ronald (1857–1932) British physician, born in Nepal and graduated from St Bartholomew's Hospital. He was surgeon major in the Indian Medical Services from 1881 to 1889, and returned to Nilagri mountains in India in 1895 where he identified the mosquito as the carrier of the malarial parasite in 1897. He worked out the life cycle of transmission of malaria through mosquitoes and birds in 1898. He was appointed professor of tropical medicine at the new Liverpool School of Tropical Medicine in 1899, and was awarded the Nobel Prize for Physiology or Medicine in 1904.

Ross, Thomas Arthur (1875–1941) Edinburgh psychiatrist who rejected Freudian psychoanalytic methods. He was president of the psychiatric section of the Royal Society of Medicine in 1936, a member in three BMA Committees on Mental Diseases and served on the committee of Mental Health and Psychoanalysis. He practiced hypnotherapy and psychotherapy and wrote *Common Neuroses* in 1935.

Rossel Test Detects occult blood in feces using Barbados aloin and other reagents. Devised by Swiss physician, Otto Rossel (1875–1911).

Rossetta Stone Ancient Egyptian stone with three scripts inscribed on it. Discovered by Napoleon's soldiers while they were digging near the Rosetta branch of the Nile in 1799. It was brought to England in 1802 and placed in the British Museum. The inscriptions in three kinds of writing (Greek, Demotic or enchorial, and hieroglyphic) were used as a key to Egyptian hieroglyphics by Jean François Champollion (1790–1832) of France who wrote *Precis du Systeme Hieroglyphigue* in 1824.

Rösslin, Eucharius (d 1526) German physician from Worms who later practiced in Frankfurt-am-Main. He wrote a manual on obstetrics, *Rosengarten,* in 1513 which remained as a standard work for nearly two centuries.

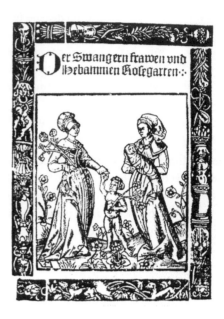

Rösslin's *Rosengarten*. Title page (1513) of one of the earliest obstetrics textbooks

Rostan, Louis Léon (1790–1866) Parisian physician who described cardiac asthma.

Rotch, Thomas Morgan (1848–1914) Philadelphia pioneer of modern pediatrics in America. He graduated from Harvard in 1870 and studied in Berlin and Vienna before he returned to Boston in 1876. He was appointed to the first chair of diseases of children at Harvard in 1888.

Rotch Sign Dullness to percussion over the right 5th intercostal space in pericardial effusion. Described by Boston physician, Thomas Morgan Rotch (1848–1914).

Roth, Moritz (1839–1915) Professor of pathological anatomy at Basel who described the tubercle of epididymis connected with rete testis (Roth vas aberans) in 1877.

Roth Disease Septic retinitis, described by Russian neurologist, Vladimir Karlovitch Roth (1848–1916).

Roth Spots White hemorrhagic spots seen in the retina in cases of bacterial endocarditis. Described by Swiss physician, Moritz Roth (1839–1914) in 1872.

Rothera Test Detects acetone in the urine and was devised by Australian biochemist, Arthur Cecil Hamel Rothera (1880–1915) in 1908.

Rotheram, John (d 1787) Physician from Yorkshire who graduated from Edinburgh. He wrote several treatises, including one on the nature and properties of water.

Rotor Syndrome Congenital form of hyperbilirubinemia

described by Filipino physician, Arturo Rotor in 1948.

Rotunda Hospital *See maternity hospitals.*

Rouget Muscle Circular fibers of the ciliary muscles. Described by French professor of physiology at Montpellier, Charles Marie Benjamin Rouget (1824–1904) in 1856. They were also described by Heinrich Muller (1820–1864) in 1857.

Round Ligaments of the Uterus *See utero-sacral ligaments.*

Roundworm Intestinal colonization was known to the ancients and male fern was used as treatment by Theophrastus (370–285 BC), Pliny (AD 23–79) and Galen (AD 129–200). An anatomical description of *Ascaris lumbricoides* or roundworm was given by Edward Tyson (1649–1708) in 1683. The egg and reproductive process were described by Italian parasitologist, Francesco Redi (1626–1698) in 1684.

Rous, Francis Peyton (1879–1970) American pathologist, born in Baltimore and graduated in medicine from Johns Hopkins University, before he joined the Rockefeller Institute for Medical Research, New York in 1920. His main research was oncogenic viruses for which he was awarded the Nobel Prize for Physiology or Medicine in 1966. *See Rous Sarcoma.*

Rous Sarcoma American pathologist Francis Peyton Rous (1879–1970) of Baltimore discovered a virus which induced a tumor in chickens, capable of being transmitted to other closely related chickens, in 1911. He used his findings to study the behavior of carcinogenic viral agents, and was awarded the UN prize for cancer research in 1962.

Rousette, François (1535–1590) French physician to the Duke of Savoy and a contemporary of Ambroise Paré (1510–1590). He advocated cesarean section and published a series of 15 successful cesarean sections in 1581.

Rousseau, Louis François Emmanuel (1788–1868) French histologist in Paris who described the accessory external lachrymal bone in 1829.

Roussy, Gustave (1874–1948) French pathologist who demonstrated thalamic syndrome due to a lesion of the thalamus in 1906.

Roux, Augustin (1726–1776) French physician from Gascony who graduated from Bordeaux. He wrote several medical and chemical treatises including one on purifying liquors.

Roux, Pierre Paul Émile (1853–1933) French bacteriologist from Charente who served as assistant to Louis Pasteur (1822–1895) before he succeeded him as director of the Pasteur Institute in 1904. He worked on the anthrax and rabies vaccines and did research on syphilis. The pathogenicity of diphtheria toxin produced by the bacteria was demonstrated by Roux and Alexandre Yersin (1863–1943) in 1889.

Roux, Philibert Joseph (1780–1854) Guillaume Dupuytren's (1777–1835) successor at Hôtel Dieu in Paris. He sutured a ruptured female perineum in 1834 and pioneered staphylorrhaphy and repair of cleft palate.

Roux, Wilhelm (1850–1924) German physiologist and anatomist at Halle. He was a pioneer in experimental embryology and recognized germ plasm inheritance from parent to offspring in 1883.

Rowland, Henry Augustus (1848–1901) American physicist and first professor of physics at the Johns Hopkins University in 1875. He advanced thermodynamics and discovered the magnetic effect of electric convection in 1881.

Roxburgh, William (1751–1815) Scottish botanist and physician from Ayrshire who graduated from Edinburgh University. He was director of the botanical gardens at Calcutta and cultivated many economically important Indian plants. He discovered the coloring substance of the lacca insect and wrote *Flora Indica* and *The Plants of the Coasts of Coramandel.*

Royal College of General Practitioners General practice was introduced around 1820 in England to represent the group of medical practitioners who practiced all branches of medicine including surgery, midwifery, pharmacy and medicine. The first attempt to represent them was made with the formation of Associated Medical and Surgical Practitioners in 1826, and a common register was established in 1858. Attempts to establish a college continued and William Pickles from Aysgarth in Yorkshire was an advocate around 1920. He became a founder member of the College. A steering committee was formed in 1952 which led to the establishment of the college in 1961 and it received its charter in 1972.

Royal College of Midwives *See Midwives Institute.*

Royal College of Nursing A rapid expansion of professional nursing occurred after 1860 and the first professional association, the British Nurses Association, was founded by Ethel Gorden Manson, matron at St Bartholomew's Hospital, in 1886. The association received its charter in 1893 and became the College of Nursing in 1916. It was made the Royal College of Nursing through a second charter in 1963.

Royal College of Obstetricians and Gynaecologists
Attempts were made to establish a college for the obstetricians in the early 19th century but the move was resisted by bodies such as Royal College of Physicians on the grounds that the prestige of their college would be diminished. After nearly a hundred years the College of Obstetricians was founded in 1929. It received its charter as the Royal College of Obstetricians and Gynaecologists in 1937.

Royal College of Physicians and Surgeons, Glasgow
Originated in 1599 with a grant from King James VI to two physicians, Peter Lowe (1550–1613) and Robert Hamilton, to regulate medical practice at Glasgow. It was known as the Royal Faculty of Physicians and Surgeons, Glasgow and its present name, Royal College of Physicians, was given to it in 1962.

Royal College of Physicians, Edinburgh An attempt to establish a college was made in 1617 during the reign of King James VI. A second attempt was made in 1630 and the matter was referred to the Privy Council by Charles I but no further action was taken. In 1656, during the time of Oliver Cromwell, a charter was proposed and signed by 16 physicians and presented to Parliament. Again the matter was dropped until efforts by Sir Robert Sibbald (1641–1722), a physician from Linlithgow, in 1681. The College obtained its charter in 1681 with an initial list of 21 prominent members of the medical profession. It acquired its own premises near Cowgate, in 1704. The foundation for new premises was laid at the east end of George Street by William (1710–1790) in 1775 and meetings at the new premises commenced in 1781. A new charter specifying its role was given in 1861.

Royal College of Physicians, Ireland Originally the Fraternity of Physicians, founded in 1654. It was given a Royal charter by Charles II and became the College of Physicians, Ireland in 1667. The present name, Royal College of Physicians, was given in 1890.

Royal College of Physicians, London The first Royal College was established by Oxford physician, Thomas Linacre (1460–1524), under the patronage of Henry VIII in 1518. It was known as College or Commonality of the Faculty of Medicine of London, and was given its present name in 1682. Three volumes of biographical data of all the members were prepared by William Munk (1816–1898) in 1855.

Royal College of Psychiatrists Originally the Association of Medical Officers of Asylums and Hospitals for the Insane, founded in Gloucester in 1841. Its name was changed to Medico-Psychological Association in 1865, and it was given a charter as the Royal Medico-Psychological Association in 1926. The college acquired its present name under another charter in 1971.

Royal College of Surgeons, Edinburgh Barber surgeons of Edinburgh held their meetings at Magdalen Chapel in Cowgate, and their earliest minutes were recorded in 1581. Initially known as the Incorporation of Surgeons, it controlled apprenticeship and practice of surgery in Edinburgh. The Incorporation received a charter in 1778 and became the Royal College of the City of Edinburgh. The college received its present name through another charter in 1851.

Royal College of Surgeons, Ireland The Guild of Barbers existed in Ireland in the 15th century and was granted a charter by Queen Elizabeth in 1577. The surgeons separated themselves from the barbers in 1784 with the formation of the Royal College of Surgeons, Ireland through a Royal charter granted by George III.

Royal Institution of London Founded on 9 March 1799 at a house in Albermarle Street, Piccadilly by Count Rumford and Sir Joseph Banks. It was given a Royal Charter and made The Royal Institution of Great Britain in 1800. Its purpose was defined as 'for diffusing knowledge and facilitating the general introduction of useful mechanical inventions and improvements, and for the teaching by courses of philosophical lectures and experiments, the application of science to common purposes of life'. The first lecture was given in 1801 by Garnett who was the first professor of natural philosophy and chemistry. The second lecture was given by Thomas Young (1773–1829) in 1802. Humphry Davy (1778–1829) was its director in the same year and Michael Faraday succeeded him in 1825.

Royal Jelly First suggested to contain vitamin E, by H. Leonard and E. F. Burnett in their article in *Nature* titled *Fertility of Bees and Vitamin E* published in 1932. This led to its popular use as an aphrodisiac and sexual stimulant.

Royal Medico-Chirugical Society of London *See Royal Society of Medicine.*

Royal National Institute for the Blind The first school for the blind in England was founded in Liverpool in 1791. Edinburgh and London followed in 1799. Louis Braille (1809–1852) devised an alphabet for the blind with varying combinations of six dots in 1834, which is still in use today. An embossed system, based on Roman capitals, was devised in 1845 by William Moon (1818–1894), an inventor from Kent who himself was partially blind. The National Institute for the Blind was established in 1914 and it developed Moon's system for teaching. A Royal charter was given in 1949 and it acquired its present name, Royal National Institute for the Blind, in 1953.

Royal National Orthopaedic Hospital Founded in 1839 by William John Little (1810–1894), a British orthopedic surgeon and known as the Orthopaedic Institution. It was re-named the Royal Orthopaedic Hospital in 1845 and moved to Hanover Square in 1855. After amalgamation of the Royal, the National and the City Orthopaedic Hospitals with the help of King's Metropolitan Hospital Funds in 1905, it became the Royal National Orthopaedic Hospital.

Royal Northern (Central) Hospital, London Founded by S.F. Statham to give medical care to the poor sick of north London in 1856. Originally known as the Great Northern Hospital because of its proximity to the Great Northern Railway Station, Kings Cross. It moved to Holloway in 1888, and after amalgamation with the Royal Chest Hospital in 1924, it was renamed Royal Northern Hospital.

Royal Society of Edinburgh Commenced as the Philosophical Society of Edinburgh in 1739 and became the Royal Society of Edinburgh in 1783. It received a new charter in 1811.

Royal Society of London In 1645 several learned men, including John Wilkins (1614–1672) and John Wallis (1616–1703), started weekly meetings in London. The physicians in their group included Jonathan Goddard, Christopher Merret and Theodore Hawk. The group split in 1649 by the removal of Wilkins, Wallis and Goddard to Oxford. The Oxford group was joined by Seth Ward (1617–1689) and William Petty. Their meetings were held in Wilkins' apartment at Wadham College and later at the house of Robert Boyle (1627–1691). The Philosophical Society of Oxford was formed out of their meetings but only lasted until 1650. The London group continued functioning with its members, Christopher Wren (1632–1723), Laurence Rooke (1622–1662), Lord Brouncker (1620–1684) and several other important men. After the restoration of Charles II it received its Royal Charter in 1662. The Society's publication, *Philosophical Transactions of the Royal Society*, was started in 1665 by Henry Oldenburg at his own expense. Sir Isaac Newton (1642–1727) presented the manuscripts of his *Principia* to it in 1668 and it was published at the expense of Edmund Halley (1656–1742) who was

clerk to the society. Some distinguished presidents include: Sir Christopher Wren (1680), Samuel Pepys (1684), Sir Hans Sloane (1727), Sir John Pringle (1772), Sir Humphry Davy (1778–1829)(1820), and Sir Benjamin Brodie (1858).

Royal Society of Medicine Originated from two institutions in 1907: the Royal Medico-Chirugical Society of London, founded by John Yelloly (1774–1842) and Marcet in 1805, and the Medical Society of London, established in 1773. The society received its Royal charter from King William IV to become the Royal Medical and Chirurgical Society in 1934. It became the Royal Society of Medicine after amalgamation with 17 specialties in 1907 and was given a supplementary charter by Edward VII.

Rubber Gloves Introduced as an aseptic measure in surgery by William Halstead (1852–1922), an American surgeon at Johns Hopkins Hospital. He made bronze casts of his hand upon which the gloves were molded in 1890.

Rubber *See Latex.*

Rubella Vaccine Live attenuated vaccine was developed by Harry M. Meyer in 1966.

Rubella German measles, named by Henry Richard Lobb Veale (1832–1908) in 1866. Experimental proof that it is caused by a virus was provided by Alfred Fabian Hess (1875–1933) of Germany in 1914. Successful transmission in children using filtered nasal washings was demonstrated by Y. Hiro and S. Tasaka in 1938. Experiments on the virus commenced in the 1940s, and Karl Habel of America transmitted it through five consecutive passages in the chorio-allantois of chick embryos in 1942. After the fifth passage the material was capable of producing clinical rubella in rhesus monkeys. The increased risk of congenital heart disease and congenital cataracts during the first trimester of pregnancy was pointed out by Australian ophthalmologist, Sir Norman McAlister Gregg (1892–1966) in 1941. The triad, cataract, congenital heart defects, and deafness (Gregg triad) in children is named after him. Isolation of the virus was achieved in 1962 by Thomas Huckle Weller (b 1915) and Frankelin Allen Neva, and Paul Douglas Parkman, E. L. Buescher and M. S. Artenstein.

Rubidium Alkaline metal discovered by Robert Wilhelm Bunsen (1811–1899) using spectrum analysis in 1861.

Rubini, Peter (1760–1819) Physician from Parma who wrote several treatises on fever. He was archiater and physician to the Archduchess Maria Louisa in 1816.

Rubner, Max (1854–1932) German physiologist and pupil of

Karl Friedrich Wilhelm Ludwig (1816–1895) who held professorships at Munich and Marburg before he succeeded Robert Koch (1843–1910) at Berlin. His main interest was metabolism and he measured the metabolic changes in the body using the animal body as a calorimeter in 1891. He described the specific dynamic action of food.

Rubwunga Disease endemic in northwest Africa and Uganda was shown to be identical to plague by Robert Koch (1843–1910).

Rudbeck, Olof (1630–1702) Swedish anatomist and botanist and a rival to Thomas Bartholin (1616–1680) in his claim to the discovery of the lymphatic system. He was professor of medicine at Uppsala and prepared a large illustrated work on botany with over 3000 woodcuts. His work was destroyed before it could be published, by the great fire of Uppsala in 1702. He was succeeded at Uppsala by his son (1660–1740) of the same name.

Rudin, Ernst (1874–1952) Professor of psychiatry and director of the Kaiser Wilhelm Institute of Psychiatry at Munich. He advocated eugenics during the Nazi period and presided at the third international eugenic congress in New York in 1932. He was the architect of the enforced sterilization program of Nazi Germany.

Rudinger, Nicolaus (1832–1896) Professor of anatomy at Munich who described the muscles internal to the circular fibers of the rectum (Rudinger muscle) in 1879.

Rudolphi, Carl Asmund (1771–1832) Swiss anatomist and helminthologist. He used the term 'echinococcus' to refer to the vesicular hydatid in 1808.

Rudolphine Tables Devised by Johannes Kepler (1571–1630) in 1627, and gave accurate planetary positions and predicted the transits of Mercury and Venus across the Sun. Named in honor of Kepler's patron, Emperor Rudolph II.

Ruffini Corpuscles The muscle spindle or the stretch afferent which is a neuromuscular end organ of the muscle. Studied by Wilhelm Kühne (1837–1900) in 1862. The sensory nature of the spindle was proposed by Sir Charles Scott Sherrington (1857–1952) in 1894 and described in detail by professor of histology at Bologna, Angelo Ruffini (1874–1929) between 1892 and 1898.

Rufus of Ephesus (AD 98–138) Greek physician and surgeon who lived during the reign of the Emperor Trajan. He gave a description of plague and many anatomical structures in *On Naming the Parts of the Body*.

Ruhmkorf, Heinrich Daniel (1823–1877) German mechanic from Hannover who lived in Paris and built the first induction coil in 1855 which formed the basis for the development of the Geissler tube.

Rumford, Benjamin Thompson, Count (1753–1814) English-American founder of the Royal Institution of London. He came to England in 1776 and spent most of his life there. During his travels in the continent he married the wife of Antoine Laurent Lavoisier (1743–1794), the French chemist who was guillotined during the French Revolution. Rumford suggested that heat is a form of energy in 1796.

Runge, Friedlieb Ferdinand (1795–1867) German chemist, born at Hamburg and studied medicine in Berlin and Jena. He obtained caffeine from seeds of *Coffea arabica* in 1820. Carbolic acid or phenol, a by-product of distillation of coal tar, was discovered by him in 1834. He developed a method of chromatography.

Rupture of Bladder Benjamin Bell (1749–1806) suggested suturing the bladder after rupture in 1789, and the procedure was performed by Willet of St Bartholomew's Hospital. William MacCormack (1836–1901) performed his procedure in 1885 and published two cases in 1886.

Rupture An old term for hernia. *See hernia.*

Rusconi, Mauro (1776–1849) Italian embryologist and comparative anatomist from Pavia who wrote several treatises on embryology.

Rush, Benjamin (1745–1813) American physician who graduated from Edinburgh University in 1768 and was appointed professor of physic at the Medical College of Philadelphia in 1789. He was a statesman as well as a physician and a signatory to the Declaration of Indepe dence. He is regarded as the first psychiatrist in America and wrote the first book on mental diseases in America *Diseases of the Mind*, published in 1821. He introduced occupational therapy in the treatment of mental diseases and wrote other treatises on insanity, cholera infantum and yellow fever.

Rush Medical College Chicago college was chartered in 1837 and began courses in 1843. It became the medical department of the University of Chicago in 1898.

Ruska, Ernst August Friedrich (1906–1988) Inventor of the electron microscope, born at Heidelberg and educated at Munich and Berlin Universities. He developed the electron microscope while he was at the Technical University of Berlin in 1931. He shared the Nobel Prize for Physics with two other workers on electron microscopy, Gerd Karl Binnig (b 1947) and Heinrich Rohrer (b 1933) in 1986. *See electron microscope.*

Russell, Alexander (d 1770) Scottish physician from Edinburgh who wrote a history on Aleppo while he was a physician there in 1755. On his return to England in 1759 he became a physician at St Thomas' Hospital.

Russell, James Burn (1837–1904) Pioneer in public health and preventive medicine in Glasgow. He was superintendent of the Parliamentary Road Fever Hospital, established to relieve the pressure caused by epidemics of typhus and other infectious fevers on Glasgow Infirmary.

Russell, Frederick Fuller (1870–1960) Born in Auburn, he was a pathologist who demonstrated the value of antityphoid vaccination in the US Army in 1910.

Russell, Richard (d 1768) English physician who wrote a treatise on sea waters in the 18th century.

Russell Viper Venom Named after a Scottish physician, Patrick Russell (1727–1805) who was medical officer in the British Army in India. He gave a description of viper venom in *Account of Indian Serpents* (1896–1809). *See ophidism.*

Rust Disease Tuberculous spondylitis of the cervical vertebrae. Described by German surgeon, Johann Nepomak Rust (1775–1840) in 1834.

Rutherford, Daniel (1749–1819) Chemist, botanist and physician in Edinburgh. He was a pupil of Joseph Black (1728–1799) and obtained nitrogen from air in 1772.

Rutherford, Ernest (1871–1937) Pioneer of atomic physics, born at Nelson in New Zealand. He studied at Canterbury College and won a scholarship to England in 1894 where he worked in the Cavendish Laboratory at Cambridge under Sir Joseph John Thomson (1856–1940). He invented a system of wireless telegraphy able to transmit over half a mile, which preceded Marconi. He was professor of physics at McGill University, Montreal in 1898 and continued his research into radioactivity. He named alpha rays, radiation rays emitted from radium, in 1899. He and Frederick Soddy (1877–1965) in 1902 put forward the atomic disintegration hypothesis. He proposed an hypothesis which led to the modern theory of atomic structure in 1911. He conceived the idea of an atom as a miniature replica of our solar system with the Sun as the positively charged central nucleus and the planets as the electrons. He published 150 papers and many books including: *Radioactivity* (1904), *Radioactive Transformations* (1906), *Radioactive Substances and their Radiation*, and *Radiation from Radioactive Substances* (1930).

Rutherford, William (1839–1899) Scottish professor of physiology at King's College London in 1869, who occupied the chair at Edinburgh University (1874). He was

a pioneer in the study of hearing and proposed the theory that the tymphanic membrane, on receiving sound, vibrated like a microphone and imparted electrical impulses to the brain. His lectures on physiology at Edinburgh were very popular and the novelist Conan Doyle was one of his students.

Rutter, John (1762–1838) Edinburgh physician who founded the Liverpool Athenaeum and the Liverpool Medical Institution.

Ruysch, Frederic (1638–1731) Professor of anatomy at Amsterdam who coined the term 'bronchial' to describe the arteries and veins around the bronchi in 1665. The capillaries in the deepest part of the choroid (tunic of Ruysch) were described by him in 1721. His museum collection of over 1300 specimens was bought by Peter the Great and was brought to St Petersburg. The sailors who brought the specimens were found drunk after consuming the alcohol used to preserve the specimens. Ruysch's daughter, Rachel, was also an anatomist and was the first woman director of the anatomical museum at Amsterdam.

Ružička, Leopold (1887–1976) Yugoslavian chemist from Vuvkor who became professor of chemistry at Utrecht in 1926, and Zurich in 1929. He pioneered the study of sex hormones and prepared testosterone artificially from cholesterol, with Wettstein in 1935. He was awarded the Nobel Prize for Chemistry with Aleksandr Mikhailovich Butenandt (1828–1886) in 1939.

Rx Symbol representing the eye of Horus, and used as amulet 5000 years ago by the Egyptians. It has remained as the recipe sign for medical prescriptions. *See Horus.*

Ryder, Hugh (1664–1693) London Naval surgeon and surgeon to James II. He wrote *New practical observations in surgery* in 1685.

Ryle, John Alfred (1889–1950) Physician at Guy's Hospital who in 1921 improved the stomach tube designed by Martin Emil Rehfuss (b 1887) in 1914, making it safer and more comfortable for the patient to swallow. He wrote *Gastric Function in Health and Disease* in 1926. The physicist and radioastronomer, Sir Martin Ryle (1918–1984), was his son. *See stomach tube.*

Ryle Tube *See Ryle, John Alfred, stomach tube.*

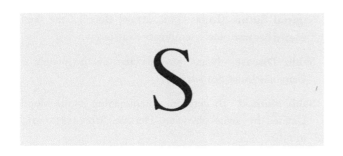

Sabaeism Worship of the sun, moon and stars. In Peru the sacred flame was kept burning throughout the year for the virgins of the Sun. The Coroados tribe of Brazil considered the moon more powerful. Sun and the moon are held as deities by some Indian Hindu tribes.

Sabatier, Paul (1854–1941) French professor of chemistry at Toulouse who worked with Berthelot (1827–1907) at Paris. He researched chemical catalysis with Jean Baptiste Senderens (1856–1936) and discovered catalytic hydrogenation of oils. He shared the Nobel Prize for Chemistry with Victor Grignard (1871–1935) in 1912.

Sabatier Suture Method of approximation of the intestinal wound using cardboard soaked in turpentine. Devised by French surgeon, Raphael Bienvenu Sabatier (1732–1811) of Paris. He performed resection of the head of humerus and amputation at the shoulder joint.

Sabin, Albert Bruce (1906–1993) Polish-American microbiologist who received his medical degree from New York University in 1931. He was professor of pediatrics at the University of Cincinnati in 1946, where he commenced his research on vaccines against Japanese B encephalitis and dengue fever. He developed the live attenuated oral vaccine for polio in 1957. His vaccine was found to be safe and effective and is more widely used than Salk's killed polio vaccine.

Sabin, Florence Rena (1871–1953) Graduate of Johns Hopkins Medical School in 1900 and the first woman to be elected to the National Academy of Sciences in 1925. She studied the maturation of myeloblasts and devised a supravital stain for leukocytes.

Sabouraud, Raymond Jacques Adrien (1864–1938) Born in Nantes, he was an eminent dermatologist at the St Louis Hospital in Paris. He attained a worldwide reputation for his work on ringworm and dermatophytes. His *Les teignes,* published in 1910, is a classic on mycology. He developed X-ray treatment for ringworm in 1904 and devised the Sabouraud culture medium for pathogenic fungi.

Sabouraud Medium Agar for culture of bacteria. Devised by French dermatologist and microbiologist, Raymond Jacques Adrien Sabouraud (1864–1938).

Saccharin [Latin: *sakchar,* sugar] 2,3-dihydro-3-oxobenziso-sulfonazole was the first synthetic sweetener. It was developed in 1879 by two Americans, Constantin Fahlberg and Ira Remsen during their research on coal tar derivatives. It remained a prescription product until the Food and Drugs Administration allowed its use as an industrial food additive in 1938.

Sacher–Masoch, Leopold von (1835–1895) *See masochism.*

Sachs, Bernard Parney (1858–1944) *See Tay–Sachs disease.*

Sachs, Hans (1887–1947) Non-medical follower of Freud and a founder of *Imago* which dealt with application of psychoanalysis to art, mythology, anthropology and literature. He emigrated to America and published a new *Imago* there in 1939.

Sachs, Hans (1877–1945) Serologist in Heidelberg who devised a flocculation test for serodiagnosis (Sachs–Georgi test), with Walter Georgi (1889–1920) in 1919.

Sachs, Julius von (1832–1897) German botanist, born at Breslau in Poland and became a professor at Würzburg in 1868. He proposed that the green pigment was not diffusely present in the plant tissues, but instead was contained in special bodies. His *Lehrbuch der Botanik* (1868) was translated into English in 1875.

Sachs, Willy (1864–1909) Swiss surgeon from Bern who modified Senns plates for suturing intestines.

Sacral Ulcer *See bed sore.*

Sacred Disease [Latin: *sacer,* sacred] The term 'sacred disease' for epilepsy is found in the writings of the Greek philosopher Heraclitus (*c* 500 BC) and the historian Herodotus (484–425 BC). According to Herodotus, the Persian king Cambyses suffered from a strange disease which was called sacred by the others. Plato (428–347 BC) used the name on the grounds that it caused divine revolutions in the head. The term was also applied to leprosy by the ancient Greeks. A monograph on epilepsy, *On the Sacred Disease,* was written by a Hippocratic physician around 400 BC. This gives the first rational approach to epilepsy, placing the brain as the seat of the disease.

Sacroiliac Joint Described by French physician, Joseph Capuron (1767–1850) in 1811. Resection of the joint was performed by German surgeon, Bernhard Bardenheur (1839–1913) in 1899 and French surgeon, Robert Picque

(1877–1927) in 1909. An operation for extra-articular fusion was done by an American orthopedic surgeon, Willis Cohoon Campbell (1880–1941) in 1927. American radiologist, William Edward Chamberlain (b 1892) described X-ray features of the joint in 1932.

Sacrum [Latin: *sacer*, sacred] According to Scottish anatomist Alexander Monro (1697–1767) in 1732, this bone is so named 'from being offered as a dainty in sacrifice or because of its largeness in respect of the other vertebrae'.

Sadism Sexual pleasure obtained through cruelty. Term coined by Richard von Krafft-Ebing (1840–1902) in 1886 and derived from the name of a French novelist, Marquis Donatien Alphonse François de Sade (1740–1814) who was involved in several scandals and acts of cruelty to women.

Sadler Committee Select committee set up by the House of Commons under the chairmanship of a Yorkshire businessman, Michael Sadler (1780–1835), to inquire into working condition of children in the factories in 1831. *See child labor, factory acts.*

Sadlers Wells Medicinal spa built in North London by Sadler in 1683. He entertained patients with a live orchestra in a theater opened in 1765.

Sadomasochism *See sadism, masochism.*

Saemisch, Edwin Theodor (1833–1909) Ophthalmologist from Bonn described serpiginous ulcer of the cornea (Saemisch ulcer) and its treatment in 1870. *See cataract.*

Saenger, Alfred (1861–1921) Neurologist in Hamburg who gave an account of pupils which simulated research on syphilis in 1902.

Safe Period Avoidance of sexual intercourse during receptive times for conception. Described by Avicenna (980–1037). The discovery was by Japanese gynecologist, Kyusaku Ogino in 1929. Herman Knaus of Prague University published similar findings a few months later, on which the modern safe period for contraception is based.

Safety Lamp Devised for miners to detect methane in coal mines. Invented by Sir Humphry Davy (1778–1829) in 1815.

Saffron Medicine, condiment, perfume and dye obtained from *Crocus sativa* stigmas. The name 'krokus' was used for the plant by Homer, Hippocrates (460–377 BC) and Theophrastus (372–287 BC) and the Hebrews called it 'Karcom' and it is mentioned in the Song of Solomon. Saffron tea was used to treat measles and it is still used as a diaphoretic and for chronic hemorrhage of the uterus. The plant was introduced into England during the reign of Edward III around AD 1350.

Sagittal Suture [Latin: *sagitta*, arrow] Bone of the skull, named because of its resemblance to an arrow.

Sahib Disease Name for kala azar by the people of Garo hills, India. *See kala azar.*

Sahli Method To determine hemoglobin in the blood. Devised by Swiss physician, Herman Sahli (1856–1933) in 1902.

Saillant, Charles Jacques (1747–1804) French physician in Paris who wrote a treatise on influenza in 1780.

Saint Triad Consists of gall bladder disease, diverticulosis and hiatus hernia. Described by South African physician at Groote Schuur Hospital, Charles Frederick Morris Saint (1886–1973).

Saissy, Jean Antoine (1756–1822) French physician who wrote a treatise on diseases of the internal ear in 1829.

Sajous, Charles Euchariste de Medici (1852–1929) American physician who wrote an early monograph on internal secretions in 1903.

Sakel, Manfred Joshua (1900–1957) French physician who introduced insulin shock in treatment for schizophrenia in 1937.

Sakharov, Andrei Dimitrievich (1921–1989) Dissident Soviet physicist who graduated from Moscow State University in 1942, and developed the Soviet hydrogen bomb in 1953. He campaigned for civil rights in Russia and proposed a nuclear test ban treaty which led to his house arrest at Gorky. He was awarded the Nobel Peace Prize in 1975, and was released from his arrest in 1986.

Salkowski, Leopold Ernest (1844–1923) Chemist in Berlin who described pentosuria in 1895. He devised tests for purine bases (1894), cholesterol (1872), creatinine (1880), bile pigments (1880), carbon monoxide in blood (1888), glucose in urine (1899) and hematoporphyrin (1891).

Sakushu Fever *See Autumn fever.*

Sal Ammoniac Obtained from camel dung in Ancient Egypt. It was known to Geber, Avicenna (980–1037) called it 'Noshadur' and the Persians called it 'Armeena'. It was employed as a lotion by the surgeons.

Salerno Town near Naples, ancient health resort in the second century BC. Its medical school was renowned in Europe as early as AD 904. The Christian church began monastic medicine in Salerno which developed into a renowned medical center with hospitals and the first medical school in Europe that provided an organized curriculum and awarded doctorates. The Latin poem on the Salernian rules for hygiene and medical treatment, *Regimen sanitatis salernitqanum,* was printed in 1484, and translated into most European languages.

Salicetti, Guilielmo (1210–1277) Italian professor of surgery at Bologna in 1268 who distinguished between arterial and venous bleeding, described crepitus as a sign of fracture, and gave one of the earliest accounts of dropsy caused by diseased kidneys. His *Chyrurgia,* written in 1275, was published in 1476.

Salicin Obtained from the plants wintergreen and white willow and used as a remedy for rheumatism since ancient times. It is a glucoside and was isolated in 1819. The compound was prepared by Raffaele Piria (1815–1865) of Paris in 1839. It was introduced as treatment for acute rheumatism by John Thomas Maclagan (1838–1903) in 1876. *See aspirin, salicylic acid.*

Salicylate *See aspirin, salicylic acid, salicin.*

Salicylic Acid Its clinical use as an antipyretic was demonstrated by Carl Emil Buss of Switzerland in 1875. The anti-inflammatory effects were demonstrated by Said Franz Striker. John Thomas Maclagan (1838–1903) introduced salicylates in the treatment of rheumatic fever in 1876. *See aspirin, salicin.*

Salisbury, Sir Edward James (1886–1978) Botanist from Harpenden in Hertfordshire. He was professor of botany at the University College in 1929 and director of Kew Gardens in 1942. He wrote *The Reproductive Capacity of Plants* (1942) and other works.

Saliva The digestive action of saliva was observed by Italian biologist Lazaro Spallanzani (1729–1799) in 1780. The association between secretions of saliva and gastric juice was proposed by American physiologist, John Richardson Young (1782–1804) of Maryland in 1803.

Salivary Glands *See parotid gland, Walther canal, Mikulicz syndrome.*

Salk Vaccine Killed polio virus vaccine was developed in 1952 by Jonas Edward Salk (b 1914), a physician and virologist at the New York University College of Medicine. His vaccine had to be given by injection and has been largely replaced by Sabin's oral polio vaccine which is more effective and convenient to administer. Salk became the director of the Salk Institute in San Diego, previously known as the Institute of Biological Studies, in 1963.

Salmon, Daniel Elmer (1850–1914) *See salmonellosis.*

Salmon Disease Saprolegnia, a fatal disease of fish, was described by William Arderon, a naturalist from Norwich. He communicated his findings to London microscopist Henry Baker (1704–1774) in 1748, who presented a description to the Royal Society of London later in the same year. The same disease in goldfish was described by Edinburgh physician, J. Hughes Bennett (1812–1875) in 1844. The causative organism, *Salprolegnia monoica,* was identified by English physician, Thomas Henry Huxley (1825–1895) in 1882.

Salmon, William (1644–1713) So-called professor of physick, practiced near St Bartholomew's Hospital where he attended patients who were not admitted to the hospital or discharged uncured. In his *The Practice of Curing Diseases* (1694) he discussed several case histories including one of senile dementia. He was instrumental in introducing digitalis into the London Pharmacopoeia, which he translated into English from Latin. His other works include *The Complete Physician* and *Universal Herbal Folio.*

Salmonella The organism was named after Daniel Elmer Salmon (1850–1914), a veterinary pathologist from Cornell University who isolated American hog cholera bacillus while working with Theobald Smith (1859–1934) at the US Bureau of Animal Industry in 1885. The discovery that the dead virus could be used to induce immunity was made by Salmon and Smith in 1884. *See salmonellosis.*

Salmonella typhimurium Cause of meat poisoning isolated by German bacteriologist Friedrich August Johannes Löffler (1852–1915) in 1892. Another bacillus was identified as the cause of the outbreak by de Nobele during an epidemic of meat poisoning at Aertrycke, Belgium in 1897. It was independently isolated by Herbert Edward Durham (1866–1945) of England and named *Bacillus aertrycke* and later found to be identical with the bacteria isolated by Löffler and renamed, *Salmonella typhimurium.*

Salmonellosis The causative organism of enteric fever, *Salmonella typhi,* was discovered in 1880 by Carl Joseph Eberth (1825–1926), professor of pathology at Halle. The name was given to this group of enteropathogenic organisms in honor of Daniel Elmer Salmon (1850–1914) who isolated the American hog cholera bacillus in 1885. Georg Theodor Gaffky (1850–1918), a German bacteriologist from Hannover, obtained a pure culture of *Salmonella typhi* in 1884 and demonstrated it caused typhoid. Theobald Smith (1859–1934) of America established the bacteria as enteropathogenic in 1893. An important landmark in the study of bacterial food poisoning was the discovery of *Bacillus enteritidis* as a cause of meat poisoning by Austrian physician, Gustav Gaertner (1855–1921), during an outbreak at Frankenhausen in 1888. This organism was later renamed *Salmonella enteritidis*. Sir William George Savage (b 1872) and Bruce White in England contributed to the investigation of salmonella infection in England during the 1920s. The O antigens or somatic antigens of the typhoid bacillus were identified by Polish bacteriologist Arthur Felix (1887–1956) in 1924. In 1934 an International Salmonella Center at the State Serum Institute, Copenhagen was established. J. Wilson in England studied outbreaks in chicks in 1944 and suggested that the presence of bacillus in the egg shell is the cause and considered the possibility of infection of the egg contents by penetration of the shell.

Salpêtrière Hospital Founded in Paris in 1656, mainly for the care of women and children. The hospital was revived in the 19th century and Jean Martin Charcot (1825–1893) was appointed as a physician in 1862.

Salpingitis [Greek: *salpinx*, tube + *itis*, inflammation] Inflammation of the fallopian tubes in live patients and several cases at postmortem were described by Sir James Young Simpson (1811–1870) in 1860. Lawson Tait (1845–1899) opened the abdomen and took out the ovaries and fallopian tubes as treatment.

Salpingography [Greek: *salpinx*, tube + *graphein*, to write] Method of assessing the patency of the fallopian tubes. Devised by William Hollenback Carey (b 1883) of America in 1914. It was discovered independently by New York gynecologist Isador Clinton Rubin (1883–1958) in 1915, who used tubal insufflation for treating sterility resulting from occlusion of the fallopian tubes, in 1920.

Saltatoric Spasm [Latin: *saltatio*, to jump] Condition of inability to stand still due to springing or jumping movements. Described by Heinrich von Bamberger (1822–1888) of Vienna in 1859.

Salter, Henry Hyde (1823–1871) *See asthma.*

Salter Line Incremental lines in the substance of dentine in teeth. Described by Sir Samuel James Salter (1825–1897) of Guy's Hospital in 1865.

Salvarsan The magic bullet, arsphenamine, developed and used in treatment for syphilis by Paul Ehrlich (1854–1915) in 1910. It was later found to be effective in the treatment of relapsing fever and trypanosomiasis. *See side-chain theory, chemotherapy.*

Salvation Army Founded in 1865 by William Booth (1829–1912) of Nottingham, a minister at the Wesleyan Methodist Church. It opened at a Whitechapel public house under the name East London Christian Society and was renamed the Salvation Army by Booth.

Samos Island on the west coast of Asia Minor, colonized by the Ionians in 1043 BC. Epicurus (341–270 BC), the Greek philosopher who founded the Epicurean School, and Pythagorus (580–500 BC), philosopher and mathematician, were born in Samos.

Sampson, John Albertson (1873–1946) Gynecologist from Troy, New York who graduated from Johns Hopkins University in 1899 and later became professor of gynecology at Albany Medical College. He described chocolate cysts of the ovary (Sampson cyst) in 1921. He gave an account of pelvic lymphatics in relation to radical surgical treatment of cervical cancer in 1904.

San Joaquin Valley Fever (Syn: Desert rheumatism) A disease with respiratory symptoms, joint pains and erythema multiforme in California and investigated by Myrnie A. Gifford in 1936. It was recognized as a milder form of coccidiomycosis by E.C. Dickson and Myrnie Gifford in 1938. *See coccidiomycosis.*

Sanatorium [Latin: *sanatorius*, conferring health] Cold, pure air was introduced as treatment for consumption by George Bodington (1799–1882) in 1840. A sanatorium for tuberculosis was established by Gustav Adolf Robert Hermann Brehmer (1826–1899) in Germany in 1859. Another at Nordach, Black Forest was started by Otto Walther in 1888. The King Edward VII Sanatorium at Midhurst in England was founded in 1903.

Sanchez, Francisco (1550–1623) Portuguese professor of medicine at Toulouse in 1612. He was a critic of experimental knowledge and published *Quod Nihil Scitur* which opposed Aristotle's views, in 1581.

Sanctorius Sanctorius or Santorio Santorio (1561–1636) Inventor of the clinical thermometer and Italian physician. He graduated in medicine from Padua in 1582 and practiced in Poland from 1587 for 14 years. He was appointed professor of medicine at Padua in 1611, but resigned in 1629 and settled in Venice where he continued his scientific studies. He designed a balance to calculate the weight in relation to food intake, excretion, perspiration and breathing. His work, *Ars de statica medicina*, was published in 1614. It was probably the first treatise on metabolism and was translated into English by John Quincy in the 18th century. He also designed the earliest instrument to measure pulse rate, which he called pulsilogium. It consisted of a lead weight attached to a long thread, the length of which could be adjusted according to the frequency of the pulse. He probably learnt the principle which is similar to that of a pendulum, from Galileo.

Sandblasting Method of cleaning and correcting irregularities on the surface of metals by projecting sand particles with the use of steam or compressed air, introduced in 1904. Workers in this industry showed a high incidence of fatal silicosis and it was prohibited by the Blasting Special Regulations Act of 1949.

Sanderson, John Scott Burdon (1828–1905) Professor of medicine at Oxford who investigated cattle plague in 1865. He pioneered electrophysiology and devised an improved rheotome with which he made a detail study of electrical changes in the ventricles of the frog and tortoise around 1870.

Sandfly Fever *See phlebotomus fever.*

Sandifort, Edouard (1742–1814) Dutch physician who described congenital cyanotic heart disease in 1771. His work on pathological anatomy (1777–1781) is held equal to that of Giovanni Battista Morgagni (1682–1771).

Sandow Term sometimes used to denote a strong man, takes its origin from Eugene Sandow (1867–1925), a Russian from Königsberg. He was the world's strong man at the Chicago World Fair in 1893 and later opened a Health Institute in London.

Sandstrom, Ivar Victor (1852–1889) *See parathyroid.*

Sanger, Frederick (b 1918) English biochemist who unraveled the complete sequence of amino acids in insulin in 1951 and provided a sequence of amino acids for a protein. He was the son of a physician from Gloucester and was educated at St John's College, Cambridge, before he joined the Medical Research Council Laboratories in 1951. He also did work on the structure of DNA and RNA and became the first person to be awarded two Nobel Prizes for Chemistry in 1958 and 1980.

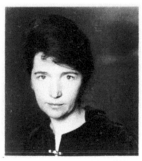

Margaret Sanger (1883–1966). Courtesy of the New Haven Colony Historical Society

Sanger, Margaret Higgins (1883–1966) Pioneer of birth control in America who started her career as a nurse in the poor lower East Side of New York around 1910. She began her crusade on the prejudice against birth control and published *Family Limitation*, but had to leave the country as a result of threatened court action. She returned to America and established the first contraceptive advice station at Brooklyn in 1916. Her other contributions include: the publication of the first radical periodical for women, *The Women Rebel*, the foundation of National Birth Control League in 1917 (later the American Birth Control League) under her presidency, and the organization of the World Population Conference in Geneva in 1927.

Sanger Operation Cesarean operation where the upper part of the uterus is widely opened. Revived and described by Max Sanger (1853–1903) of Bayreuth in 1882.

Sanitation [Latin: *sanitas,* health] *See public health.*

Sanskrit Language of Brahmins of India. Related to Latin, Greek, Celtic and Scandinavian. Horace Hayman Wilson (1786–1860), professor of philology at Oxford, translated the *Rig Veda,* the sacred hymns of the Hindus, and published a dictionary of Sanskrit in 1852. Max Muller (1823–1900) published a history in 1859. *See Aryans.*

Sansom, Arthur Ernest (1838–1907) Wiltshire physician, educated at King's College London, and became physician to the London Hospital in 1890. He wrote *The Antiseptic System* and *Diseases of the Heart.*

Santonin Principle constituent of the plant *Artemisia maritima,* known to the Greeks, Romans and Arabians as a wormicide. Dioscorides (AD 40–90) mentioned seeds which he used as treatment for Ascarides and Lumbrici around AD 60. Alexander of Tralles (525–605) advocated its use against intestinal worms. It is a derivative of naphthalene and was isolated in 1829 by Kahler from Dusseldorf. Augustus Alms, a druggist's assistant at Penzlin, independently isolated it and named it santonin in 1830. It was a popular remedy against *Ascaris lumbricoides* in the 19th century.

Santorini, Giovanni Domenico (1681–1737) Italian anatomist and a pupil of Marcello Malpighi (1628–1694). He described the accessory duct of the pancreas (Santorini duct) and several other structures in his *Observationes Anatomicae* (1724). Some structures have been named after him.

Santorio, Santorio *See Sanctorius.*

Saphenous Vein [Greek: *saphenes,* manifest] Avicenna (980–1037) used the term al-safin (hidden) for the vein in his

Canon written around AD 1010. The Arab physicians used blood letting and found the saphenous vein difficult to find as it was visible only through a small part of its course. According to some, the vein was so named because it stood out as a result of its tortuosity and varicosity. Rene G. Favaloro from La Plata, Argentina performed a successful coronary artery bypass graft using a saphenous vein graft in 1967.

Sappey Vein Found in the venous plexus of the falciform ligament of the liver. Described in 1859 by Marie Philibert Constant Sappey (1810–1896), chair of anatomy at Paris in 1865.

Sapphism Lesbianism, derives its name from the Greek poetess Sappho who lived at Lesbos, around 600 BC.

Sarcoidosis [Greek: *sarkos*, flesh] Benign sarcoid syndrome was described by Norwegian dermatologist Peter Caesar Moeller Boeck (1845–1917) in 1899. French dermatologist Ernest Besnier (1831–1909) gave an account of lupus pernio and other features in 1889. The systemic nature was described by Jorgen Nilson Schumann (1879–1953). An intradermal diagnostic skin test using saline suspension of sarcoid tissue was devised by R. H. Williams and D. A. Nickelson in 1935. Elevation of serum calcium was noted by G. T. Harrell and S. Fisher in 1939. Norwegian pathologist Ansgar Morten Kveim (b 1892) gave a comprehensive evaluation of the skin test in diagnosis in 1941, and the test bears his name. The beneficial effect of adrenocorticotrophic hormone was demonstrated by L. E. Shulman and co-workers in 1952. The condition of bilateral hilar lymphadenopathy was first noted by P. Kerley in 1942.

Sarcoma [Greek: *sarkos*, flesh] Viennese professor, Baron Karl Freiherr von Rokitansky (1804–1878), described a tumor of striped muscles known as sarcoma. Pigmented sarcoma of the skin (Kaposi sarcoma) was described by Moritz Kaposi (1837–1902), a Hungarian dermatologist in 1872. Leo Loeb (1869–1959) was an early experimenter and managed to transmit cystic sarcoma of white mice though 40 generations in 1910. Sarcoma of the bone was described by Samuel Weissel Gross (1837–1899) of America in 1879. James Ewing (1866–1943), professor of oncology at the Cornell University Medical College, New York City, gave a detailed account of the endothelial tumor of the shaft of long bones in 1920 (Ewing sarcoma). *See Rous sarcoma.*

Sarcoptes scabiei [Greek: *sarkos*, flesh + *koptein*, to cut] *See Acarus scabiei.*

Sarsaparillae [Spanish: *zarza*, briar + *parillae*, vine] Plants in the genus Smilax have been used as a remedy for various conditions, including syphilis. It was introduced into Seville from South America by a physician, Nicolas Monardes (1493–1588) of Seville in 1536. A specific account was given by Pedro de Ciezo in *Parte Primera de la Chronica del Peru* in 1553. Its successful use in conditions including rheumatism was given by Portuguese physician of Jewish origin, Joao Rodriguez de Castello Branco in *Curationum medicinalium centuriae quatuor* published in 1556. A preparation known as Zittmann decoction became a popular treatment for chronic syphilis in the first half of the 17th century. William Hunter (1723–1789) promoted it for the treatment of bubo or syphilis, but William Cullen (1710–1790) declared it to be of no value.

Sattler Gland Ciliary glands described by ophthalmologist, Hubert Sattler (1844–1928) of Salzburg in 1877. They were described by Dutch ophthalmologist Jacob Antonius Moll (1832–1914) in 1857.

Saturnine Palsy [Latin: *saturnus*, lead] Lead palsy. *See lead poisoning.*

Satyriasis Abnormal, extreme, insatiable, sexual desire in the male.

Saucerotte, Nicolas (1741–1814) *See acromegaly.*

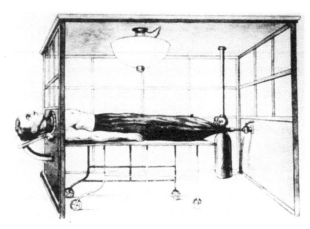

Ferdinand Sauerbruch's negative pressure chamber. Courtesy of the National Library of Medicine

Sauerbruch, Ernst Ferdinand (1875–1951) German cardiothoracic surgeon who held the chairs of surgery at Munich, Zurich and Berlin. He invented the negative pressure chamber which allowed the chest to be opened without loss of respiration or collapsing the lung. He operated for cardiac aneurysm in 1903, and thymectomy as treatment for myasthenia gravis was introduced by him in 1912.

Saunders, John Cunningham (1773–1810) London surgeon who devised a special cutting needle for cataract operation.

He published a treatise on the anatomy of the human ear in 1806.

Saussure, Horace Bénédict de (1740–1799) Swiss geologist and physicist from Geneva who introduced the word 'geology'. He climbed Mont Blanc in 1787 and wrote *Voyages dans les Alps* in 1779 and *Dissertation Physica de Igne*. His son, Nicholas Théodore de Saussure (1767–1845), was a geologist, physician and botanist.

Saussure, Nicholas Théodore de (1767–1845) Physician and botanist from Geneva and son of Horace de Saussure. He studied plant nutrition and showed the role of carbon dioxide in photosynthesis. His wrote *Recherches chimiques sur la vegetation*, published in 1804.

Sauvages, François Boissier de la Croix de (1706–1767) Professor of medicine and botany at Montpellier and member of the Royal Society of London. His publications include *Theoria Febris, Nosologiae Methodicae*, Translations of Hales Essays from English and several other works.

Savage, Henry (1810–1900) A founder and gynecologist at the Samaritan Hospital in London. He described the perineal body between the anus and the vulva (Savage perineal body) in 1863.

Savart, Félix (1791–1841) French physician and physicist who invented the Savart quartz plate for measuring polarization of light and the Savart wheel to measure tonal vibrations. He discovered the law related to the intensity of a magnetic field produced at a given point near a long straight current-carrying conductor with Jean-Baptiste Biot (1774–1862) around 1820.

Savilian Chair Mathematics and astronomy chair at Oxford, founded by Sir Henry Savile (1549–1622), an English scholar from Bradley who was Greek tutor to Queen Elizabeth in 1619.

Saw According to Pliny (AD 29–79), it was designed to resemble the jaw of a serpent by Talos. Abaptiston, an ancient surgical circular saw, was described by Galen (129–200), Fabricius ab Aquapendente (1533–1619) and Johann Schultes (1595–1645) used it for trephining the cranium. A saw for osteotomy was devised by English surgeon, Adams Williams (1820–1900) in 1871. New York surgeon, Fred Houdlett Albee (1876–1945) designed one for cutting bone grafts in 1915. Frank Huntington Bosworth (1843–1925), a New York otorhinologist, devised a saw for removing spurs in the nasal septum. An electric bone saw was constructed by New York surgeon, John

Joseph Moorhead (b 1874) in 1925 and a similar one with a drill was devised by Los Angeles surgeon, James Vernon Luck (b 1906) in 1941. A string saw was used by Robert Abbe (1851–1928) of New York for dilating esophageal stricture.

Saxer Cells Primitive leukocytes in embryonic mesenchymal tissues. Described by Fritz Saxer (1864–1906), a pathologist at Leipzig, in 1896.

Saxon Medicine *See Anglo-Saxon medicine.*

Sayre Apparatus Used for suspending the patient during application of a plaster of Paris jacket. Designed by an American surgeon, Lewis Albert Sayre (1820–1900) from New Jersey.

Sayre, Lewes Albert (1820–1900) American orthopedic surgeon from New Jersey who did the first complete resection of the hip joint and creation of an artificial joint in 1863. *See Sayre apparatus.*

Scabies *See Acarus scabiei.*

Scaliger, Julius Caesar (1484–1558) Italian sign painter who graduated in medicine from Padua. He wrote several works on Theophrastus, Aristotle and Hippocrates.

Scalinus Anticus Syndrome *See thoracic outlet syndrome.*

Scalpel Used in dissection and surgery during the time of Andreas Vesalius (1514–1564). Until this time razors were the sole instruments available in dissections.

Scanners *See CAT scanner, magnetic resonance imaging.*

Scapula [Latin: *scapula*, shoulderblade] Congenital upward displacement of the scapula was described by Dresden surgeon, Otto Gerhard Carl Sprengel (1852–1915) in 1891. The sign of triangular swelling corresponding to the outline of the scapula in cases of fracture was described by Italian surgeon, Antonio Comolli (b 1879) in 1932.

Scarification [Greek: *skariphismos*, scratching up] Method of making little punctures or cuts in order to let out blood and fluid from anasarcous infections or infection with swelling. Practiced from ancient times up to the early 20th century. Instruments called scarifiers were devised for this purpose.

Scarlatina Old name for scarlet fever. There was an epidemic of the disease in Sicily in 1543. An account was given by Daniel Sennert (1572–1637), a German physician and medical writer in 1676. Thomas Sydenham (1624–1689) described it in his book on fevers around 1683. *See scarlet fever.*

Scarlet Fever Long-chain streptococci were noted in the early days of bacteriology and 700 such cases were proved by A. Baginsky and P. Sommerfeld of Berlin in 1900. American parasitologist, Ludwig Hektoen (1863–1951) in 1903 isolated streptococci from blood in 12% of his patients with scarlet fever. Serological identification of hemolytic streptococcal infection was introduced by Paul Moser (1865–1924), a Viennese pediatrician, and Clemens von Pirquet (1874–1929) in 1902. A skin test, the Dick test, was devised by George Frederick Dick (1881–1967) and his wife Gladys Rowena Dick (1881–1963) of Johns Hopkins Medical School in 1924. *See scarlatina, beta hemolytic streptococci.*

Scarpa, Antonio (1747–1832) Italian surgical anatomist and a medical artist. He studied under Giovanni Battista Morgagni (1682–1771) and made several important contributions to surgery. The first comparative study of the organs of hearing in man and other animals was made by Scarpa in 1789, and he also wrote a monographs on hernia, *Traite des Hernies,* in 1814. The membranous labyrinth of the ear was discovered by him in 1772. He is considered the father of Italian ophthalmology and published an important book on the eye in 1801. An accurate account of congenital club foot was given by him in 1803.

Scarpa Triangle Femoral triangle, described by Antonio Scarpa (1747–1832), Italian anatomist, around 1724. *See Scarpa, Antonio.*

Scarpa Fascia Fibrous layer of the superficial fascia of the abdomen, described by Antonio Scarpa (1747–1832). *See Scarpa, Antonio.*

Scatology [Greek: *skatos*, dung + *logos*, discourse] Study or preoccupation with feces..

Scatophagy [Greek: *skatos*, dung + *phagein*, eat] Coprophagia or dung eating has existed since ancient times, especially amongst fanatics.

Sceptic Philosophical sect who carefully analyze everything, doubt all the results and never make conclusions. It was founded by Pyrrho in 336 BC.

Schaafhausen, Hermann (1816–1893) Anthropologist and scientist from Bonn who described a Neanderthal skull in 1858. *See Neanderthal man.*

Schacher Ganglion *See ciliary ganglion.*

Schäffer Reflex Extension of the great toe on pinching the achilles tendon. Described by a German physician, Max Schäffer (1852–1923).

Schally, Andrew Victor (b 1926) Polish-born American biochemist who developed an assay for corticotrophin-releasing hormone, isolated thyrotropin-releasing hormone and luteinizing hormone. He shared the Nobel Prize for Physiology or Medicine with Rosalyn Yalow (b 1921) in 1977. *See thyrotropic hormone.*

Schamberg Disease Progressive pigmentary disorder of the skin, often affecting the lower limbs. Described by American dermatologist, Jay Frank Schamberg (1870–1934) of Philadelphia in 1901.

Schatz Pessary Shell-shaped pessary with perforations. Devised by German gynecologist, Christian Friedrich Schatz (1841–1920).

Schaudinn, Fritz Richard (1871–1906) German zoologist and microbiologist, born in East Prussia, and educated in Berlin. He was director of the Protozoological Research Institute for Tropical Diseases at Hamburg in 1904. He discovered the spirochete, *Treponema pallidum,* the causative organism of syphilis in 1905. He inoculated himself with *Entamoeba histolytica* during his studies on tropical dysentery and demonstrated the amebic cause of the disease in 1903. He also demonstrated that hookworm infection occurs through the feet and described several other groups of protozoans, including *Balantidium* species.

Schaumann, Jorgin Nilson (1879–1953) Dermatologist from Stockholm who described the systemic nature of sarcoidosis (Besnier–Boeck–Schaumann disease) in 1922.

Schauta, Friedrich (1849–1919) Viennese gynecologist who devised a radical vaginal hysterectomy for carcinoma of the cervix (Schauta operation) in 1908.

Schede Method Scraping away all dead tissue in bone necrosis, permitting a blood clot to fill the cavity, and covering it with aseptic gauze and rubber. Practiced by Max Schede (1844–1902), a surgeon in Bonn.

Scheele, Carl Wilhelm (1742–1786) Swedish chemist who was apprenticed to an apothecary at Gothenburg at 14 years old. During his apprenticeship he learned most of his chemistry from books. He moved to Uppsala in 1770 and in 1775 he purchased an apothecary shop in Köping. The phosphorus content of bone was demonstrated Johan Gotlieb Gahn (1745–1818) and Scheele. Scheele also discovered chlorine gas in 1774, and molybdenum in 1778. His other contributions include: a detailed study of hydrogen sulfide, discovery of barium (1774), glycerin (which he called the 'sweet principle of fats', 1779), nitrous acid (1774), Schlee's green, or copper arsenate, uric acid and oxygen (1774). The action of light on silver chloride was studied scientifically by him in 1777. His investigation of Prussian blue in 1782 led to the discovery of hydrocyanic acid, and he was the first to prepare lactic acid from sour milk. His work on combustion predated that of Joseph Priestley (1733–1804) and Antoine Lavoisier (1743–1794) and he wrote *On Air and Fire* in 1777. His work was fundamental to the development of organic chemistry.

Schenck, John Graffenburg de (1531–1598) Swiss physician at Freiburg who wrote *Observationum medicorum* and several other works. His son, John George Schenck, was also a physician and wrote *De Formandis Medicinae Studiis* and *Monstrorum Historia.*

Schenck Disease *See sporotrichosis.*

Schenkius, John Theodore (1619–1671) Professor of medicine at Jena. He wrote *Observationes Medicinae, De Sero Sanquinis* and a catalogue of plants in the medical garden at Jena.

Scheuchzer, John James (1672–1733) Physician and professor of mathematics at Zurich. He wrote a treatise on mineral waters of Switzerland and other works on botany and natural history.

Scheuermann Disease Necrosis of the epiphyses of the vertebrae leading to osteochondrosis in kyphosis. Described by Danish radiologist from Copenhagen, Hoger Werfel Scheuermann (1877–1960) in 1921.

Schick Test Skin test for determining the susceptibility to diphtheria. Devised by Béla Schick (1877–1967), a Hungarian pediatrician in New York in 1911.

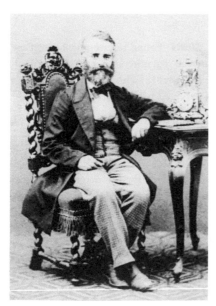

Moritz Schiff (1823–1896). Courtesy of the National Library of Medicine

Schiff Cycle Bile salts secreted into the intestine are reabsorbed and returned to the liver. Described by Moritz Schiff (1823–1896), a German physiologist of Jewish origin, in Geneva. Schiff also investigated the nervous system and defined the pathways for touch and pain sensations in the spinal cord.

Schiff Test Used to detect carbohydrates in urine with sulfuric acid, glacial acetic acid and alcohol. Devised by German chemist, Hugo Schiff (1834–1915) who worked in Florence.

Schiller Test Test for carcinoma, where the cervix is painted with Gram stain to detect unstainable areas of possible carcinoma. Devised by Austrian pathologist, Walter Schiller (1887–1960) of Vienna. After working in various parts of Europe and the Middle East, he joined the Jewish Memorial Hospital in New York in 1937 and later worked at the Cook County Hospital, Chicago from 1938 to 1944.

Schilling Test Test for vitamin B12 absorption by oral administration of radioactive vitamin B12 and urinary excretion of radioactivity. Studied by American hematologist, Robert Frederick Schilling (b 1919) in 1953. This was later developed into the standard Schilling test for the diagnosis of B12-related anemia.

Schilder Disease Induration of cerebral substance due to slow inflammatory reaction was observed by Phillipe Pinel (1822), John Abercrombie (1836), Ernst Gustav Adolf Gottfried von Strümpell (1878) and Dèsirè Magloire Bourneville (1897). Paul Schilder (1886–1940), an American psychiatrist of German origin, identified a subclass where extensive lesions of white matter occurred in both hemispheres. He noticed that the diseased zones had nerve fibers denuded of myelin while their axons were preserved to a variable extent, similar to multiple sclerosis. He described it as 'encephalitis periaxialis diffusa' in 1912.

Schindler, Rudolf (1888–1968) *See gastroscopy.*

Schiøtz Tonometer Instrument for measuring intraocular tension. Devised by Norwegian physician, Hjalmar Schiøtz (1850–1927).

Schirmer Test Test for tear formation using filter paper. Devised in 1896 by German ophthalmologist, Otto Wilhelm August Schirmer (1864–1917).

Schistosoma hematobium [Greek: *schisto*, split + *soma*, body] Discovered by Theodor Maximillian Bilharz (1825–1862), German professor of zoology in Cairo. He located the worms in the portal system of blood vessels of the patients with schistosomiasis in 1851. Wilhelm Griesinger

(1817–1868) later demonstrated the fluke in the veins of the mesentery of the bladder and other parts. The endemic status of the disease in the Cape of Good Hope was noted by John Harley in 1864.

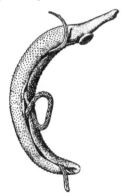

Schistosoma hematobium. Sir Patrick Manson, *Tropical Diseases* (1914). Cassell & Co., London

Schistosoma japonicum [Greek: *schisto*, split + *soma*, body] Endemic disease associated with hepatosplenomegaly and cachexia was noted in Hiroshima, Japan. Autopsy revealed an unidentified helminth in their liver. In 1904, Fujiro Kasurada (1867–1946) found larvae similar to those of *Schistosoma hematobium* in the stools of these patients. A few months later he discovered eggs, similar to those found in man, in the portal system of cats, and he named the new nematode, *Schistosoma japonicum.* The parasite was discovered in the colon of a man from China, by Catto at the St Johns Quarantine Island in Singapore in 1904.

Schistosomiasis [Greek: *schisto*, split + *soma*, body] *See Schistosoma japonicum, Schistosoma hematobium.*

Schizophrenia [Greek: *schizein*, divide + *phren*, mind] The term 'demence precoce' was coined by Austrian psychiatrist, Augustin Bientôt Morel (1809–1873) in 1856, and adapted to psychiatry by Emil Kraepelin (1856–1926) in 1901. Carl Gustav Jung (1875–1961) in 1908 pointed out that 'the name dementia is a not a very happy one, for the dementia is not always precocious nor in all cases is there dementia'. His work, *The Psychology of Dementia Praecox,* was published in 1906. In 1911 Eugen Bleuler (1857–1939), a professor of psychiatry at Burgholzli Hospital, noted that these people were not demented and that they may recover, and renamed the condition 'schizophrenia'. Treatment with electroconvulsive therapy was introduced by Lucio Bini (1908–1964) and Ugo Cerletti (1877–1963) in 1938.

Schlatter Disease Pain in the tibial tuberosity at the point of insertion of the ligamentum patellae, thought to be due to

the avulsion of the tongue-shaped projection of the tubercle. Described by Carl Schlatter (1864–1934), Swiss surgeon in Zurich around 1895.

Schleiden, Matthias Jacob (1804–1881) *See cell.*

Scheiner, Christophorus (1575–1650) Jesuit priest in Vienna who devised a test to demonstrate accommodation and refraction in the eye, in 1619.

Schlemm Canal Found at the junction of the cornea and sclera and described by a professor of anatomy, Friedrich Schlemm (1795–1858) of Berlin in 1830.

Schlling Count *See leukocyte count.*

Schlesinger Test Detects urobilin in the urine using Lugol iodine. Devised by Viennese physician, Wilhelm Schlesinger (b 1869).

Schmerling, Phillipe Charles (1791–1836) Dutch physician from Delft who provided evidence for the antiquity of the human race. He published findings on human bones and extinct animals in 1833.

Schmidt, Alexander (1831–1894) German physiologist who demonstrated that blood coagulation involved a sequence of reactions, in 1892.

Schmidt-Rimpler, Hermann (1838–1915) German physician and pioneer in routine screening of children for eye defects. He devised one of the earliest forms of optometer.

Schmidt, Johann Adam (1759–1809) Oculist in Vienna who described inflammation of the anterior portion of uveal tunica or iris due to syphilis and named it iritis. He founded the first journal of ophthalmology, *Ophthalmologische Bibliothek* in 1801.

Schmidt Clefts Found intersegmentally in the medullary sheath of the peripheral nerves. Described by Henry Schmidt (1823–1888) who was a pathologist at the Charity Hospital in New Orleans in 1874.

Schmidt Syndrome Adrenal insufficiency and hypothyroidism. Described by Martin Benno Schmidt (1863–1949) of Germany in 1926.

Schmidt Test Used for the detection of bilirubin in the feces, with mercuric chloride as reagent. Devised by Adolf Schmidt (1865–1918) who was a physician at Halle.

Schmiedberg, Johan Ernst Oswald (1838–1921) Professor at Dorpat (1870) and Strasburg (1872) who investigated the effects of various poisons and drugs on the frog's heart in 1871. He determined the formula of histamine and nucleic acids.

Schmiedel Ganglion *See inferior carotid ganglion.*

Schmorl Nodes Small cartilaginous intervertebral disc protrusions believed to be degenerative in nature, found during postmortem examination. Described by a German professor of pathology, Christian Georg Schmorl (1861–1932) of Dresden in 1926.

Schneider, Conrad Victor (1614–1618) German anatomist at Wittenberg who wrote a treatise on the membranes of the nose, *De Catarrhis,* in 1660. His work on the organ of sensation of odor published in 1655 led to the naming of the mucous membrane of the nasal cavities as the Schneider membrane. He disputed the prevailing idea that mucus from the nose originated in the pituitary gland.

Schoemaker Line Connects the greater trochanter of the femur to the anterior superior iliac spine. Described by a Dutch surgeon from the Hague, Jan Shoemaker (1871–1940). He described a modification of the Billroth operation for gastroduodenostomy.

Scholer, Heinrich Leopold (1844–1918) German ophthalmologist who described an operative treatment for detachment of the retina in 1889.

Schönbein Test Uses hydrogen peroxide and tincture of guaiac to detect traces of blood. Designed by German chemist and physician, Friedrich Christian Schönbein (1799–1868) in Basel. He was a pioneer in chromatography. Gun cotton which is a highly explosive mixture of nitric acid and sulfuric acid was invented by him in 1846. *See ozone.*

Schonheimer, Rudolf (1898–1941) German-born American pioneer of modern biochemistry who wrote *Dynamic State of Body Constituents.* He used deuterium to trace biochemical pathways and showed the steady degradation and replacement of fat, protein and bone. He distinguished the pathways of saturated and unsaturated fatty acids. He devised a method of estimating cholesterol in the blood.

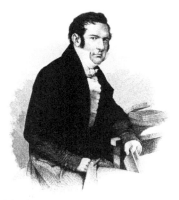

Johannes Lucas Schönlein (1793–1864). From Schönlein's *Pathologie und Therapie,* (1841), St Galen. Courtesy of the National Library of Medicine

Schönlein, Johannes Lucas (1793–1864) German professor of pathological anatomy at Würzburg. He introduced the terms hemophilia and tuberculosis and described peliosis rheumatica (Schönlein disease or purpura rheumatica). He discovered the organism responsible for favus (*Trichophyton schonleinii*).

Schönlein Disease Peliosis rheumatica was described by German physician, Johannes Lucas Schönlein (1793–1864) in 1837. This was the first description of purpura rheumatica.

Schönlein–Henoch Purpura *See Henoch–Schönlein purpura.*

Schott Treatment Treatment for heart disease using warm saline baths with exercise. Advocated by Theodor Schott (1850–1921), a physician at Nauheim, Germany.

Schottmuller, Hugo (1867–1936) German professor of medicine at Hamburg who isolated *Streptococcus viridans* in blood of patients with bacterial endocarditis in 1910. He described paratyphoid in 1900.

Schreger Line Bending of dentine tubules near the surface of the dentine. Described by Danish anatomist, Christian Heinrich Theodor Schreger (1768–1833) of Wittenberg in 1800.

Schroder Operation Method of colporrhaphy designed by German gynecologist, Carl Ludwig Schroder (1838–1887). He wrote a textbook on obstetrics in 1874.

Schroeder Test Used for urea, with a solution of bromine in chloroform. Devised in 1882 by German physician, Woldemar von Schroeder (1850–1898).

Schroeder Van Der Kolk, Jacob Ludwig Conrad (1797–1862) Physician in Utrecht who made microscopic studies of the medulla of the brain in 1859. The fibers of the reticular formation of the medulla are named after him.

Schuchardt, Karl August (1856–1901) German surgeon, born and qualified in medicine at Göttingen. He practiced extended mediolateral paravaginal incision (Schuchardt incision) in vaginal surgery in 1893.

Schüller Disease *See Hand–Schüller–Christian syndrome.*

Schultes, Johann or Scultetus (1595–1645) Surgeon from Ulm who wrote one of the most important illustrated works on surgery in the 17th century, *Armamentarium chirugicum,* in 1653 which went into several editions.

Schultz Angina Necrotic ulceration of the throat following complete disappearance of polymorphonuclear cells in the blood. Described in four patients by German physician, Werner Schultz (1878–1944) of Berlin in 1922.

Schultz Cells *See olfactory nerve.*

Schultz Membrane *See olfactory nerve.*

Schultze, Bernhard Sigismund (1827–1919) German gynecologist in Berlin who demonstrated that the remains of the yolk sac are normally incorporated into the placenta.

Schultze Method Revives asphyxiated neonate by inverting and swinging the infant. Described a German gynecologist, Bernhard Sigismund Schultze (1827–1919).

Schultze, Max Johann Sigismund (1825–1874) German zoologist who in 1861 defined the cell as the building block of a living organism, containing a nucleus and surrounded by protoplasm. He introduced osmic acid as a stain for nervous tissue and demonstrated the different nerve endings of cones and rods in the retina. *See olfactory nerve, retina.*

Schultze, John Henry (1687–1745) Professor of medicine at Halle who wrote *Physiologia Medica, Pathologia generalis et specialis, Historia a Medicinae a rerum initio ad annum et urbis Rome, de Materia Medica* and other works.

Schuster, Sir Arthur (1851–1934) British physicist born in Frankfurt whose major interest was terrestrial magnetism. He designed the Schuster–Smith magnetometer to measure the Earth's magnetic field. He also pioneered spectroscopy.

Schütz, Johann Wilhelm (1839–1920) *See glanders.*

Schwalbe, Gustav Albert (1844–1917) German neuroanatomist who described the vestibular nucleus and several other structures of the brain which are named after him.

Schwann, Theodor (1810–1882) German physiologist who is famous for his classic cell theory (1839). He was born in Neuss and graduated in medicine from Berlin in 1834. He described the neurilemma (sheath of Schwann) in 1839. The striped muscle in the upper part of the esophagus is named after him. He moved to Belgium and was professor of anatomy and physiology at Louvrain in 1838 and Liège in 1848. He showed that air is necessary for development of the embryo, that putrefaction is produced by living bodies and cannot occur in sterile broth, and discovered the organic nature of fermentation in yeast. He isolated pepsin during his work with Johannes Müller (1801–1858) in 1835, and demonstrated that bile is essential to digestion. He proved that the tension of muscle contraction varies with its length.

Schwarz Sign Fat at the apex of the heart causing confusion with enlargement of the heart on a chest X-ray. Described by German radiologist, Gottwald Schwarz (b 1880) in 1910.

Schwartze Operation Mastoid cells in disease of the middle ear, opened with a hammer and chisel. Described in 1873 by German otologist, Hermann Hugo Rudolf Schwartze (1837–1910).

Sciatica [Greek: *ischiadikos*, gout in the hips] A classic descriptions was given by Domenico Cotugno (1736–1822), professor of anatomy at Naples in 1764. Sciatic pain induced by adduction of the thigh was described by French surgeon, Amédée Bonnet (1802–1858) in 1845. The early study and review involving 1000 cases was done by E. Valentine Gibson at the Devonshire Hospital in 1893. A case due to rupture of the intervertebral disc was described by George Stevensen Middleton (1854–1928) of Scotland in 1911. Boston orthopedic surgeon, Joel Goldthwait (1867–1961), described an operation for lumbar disc prolapse in the same year. American neurosurgeon, Walter Edward Dandy (1886–1946) of the Johns Hopkins University operated on what he thought was loose cartilage from the intervertebral disc in 1929. William Jason Mixter (1880–1958) and Joseph Seaton Barr (1901–1963) of Massachusetts General Hospital showed it to be due to disc prolapse in 1934. A scientific study on the cause and mechanics of lumbar disc degeneration was done by Stein Freeberg and Carl Hirsh (1913–1973) of Stockholm in 1950.

Sea Richard Russell (d 1768), an English physician, wrote a treatise on sea waters in the 18th century. Iodine was prepared from seaweed by Bernard Courtois (1777–1838), a manufacturer of nitre in 1811. Sea bathing was advocated as treatment in the 18th century and the Royal Sea-bathing Hospital at Margate in England used this form of treatment.

Sea Sickness Treatment with atropine and strychnine was described by American naval surgeon, Conrad Alfred Girard (1841–1914) in 1906.

Scientific American American scientific magazine for the general reader, founded by Alfred Beach in 1845.

Scientist [Latin: *scientia*, knowledge] Term used by English scholar, William Whewell (1794–1866) of Lancaster, at a meeting of the British Association for the Advancement of Science in 1833. He wrote *History of Inductive Sciences* in 1837 in which he popularized his new term.

Sclavo, Achille (1861–1930) Italian bacteriologist in Rome who developed an antiserum for anthrax in 1895.

Scleroderma [Greek: *scleros*, hard + *derma*, skin] Confused with leprosy and other skin conditions for centuries. An early attempt to differentiate it was made by Italian physician, Carlo Curzio. The term scleroderma was coined by E. Gintrac in 1847.

Sclerosis *See disseminated sclerosis.*

Sclobetoplaga [Latin: *sclopetum*, gun + *plaga*, wound] Synonym for gunshot wound. *See gunshot wounds.*

Scoliosis [Greek: *skolios*, twisted] Known to ancient physicians and during Hippocratic times traction and countertraction were applied on the Hippocratic bench, the scamnum. The earliest study on its pathological anatomy was done by Francis Glisson (1597–1677) in 1650. He thought that all cases were due to rickets and devised an appliance for axillary and head suspension. Ambroise Paré (1510–1590) used a corset of thin iron sheets to treat it. Prevention and treatment of abnormal spinal curvature was described in the first book on orthopedics written by Nicolas André (1658–1742) in 1741. Tuberculous etiology of humpback was noted by German physician, Johann Zaccharias Platner (1694–1747) in 1744. A method of wiring the spinal process in Pott disease or tuberculosis of the spine was introduced by Berthhold Ernst Hadra (1842–1903) of America in 1891. Anterior spinal fusion in treatment of Pott disease and Pott paraplegia was employed by Russell Aubra Hibbs (1869–1933) of Kentucky and Fred Houdlett Albee (1876–1945) of Maine in 1906.

Scopolamine Anticholinergic alkaloid derived from several solanaceous plant species, isolated by German chemist Albert Ladenburg (1842–1911) in 1871 and used in combination with morphine for anesthesia by Schneiderlinn in 1900.

Scopoli, Johann-Antoni (1723–1788) Italian physician from Cavalese in the Tyrol and a naturalist who wrote *Annus I Historico-Naturalis* in 1769. The genus *Scopolia* which have similar properties to hyoscyamus and belladonna, is named after him.

Scorbutus (Syn. scurvy) *See scurvy.*

Scott, John (1799–1846) British inventor of the Scott dressing used by surgeons worldwide in the 19th century. He studied medicine at the London Hospital and became surgeon to the Royal Ophthalmic Hospital, Moorfields in 1828. He was assistant physician to the London Hospital in 1828, where he advocated treatment of diseased joints through passive movement.

Scot, Reginald (1538–1599) English Justice of the Peace and Member of Parliament who associated witchcraft with mental illnesses. In *The discoverie of witchcraft* (1584) he pointed out that melancholy was mistaken for witchcraft.

Scrapie Form of spongiform encephalopathy in sheep and goats was noted in 1755 by Lincolnshire farmers who petitioned Parliament to make it illegal for affected animals to be mixed with healthy animals. The name was given because diseased animals scrape themselves against objects. Understanding came mainly in the present century and its causative agent was fully described by Hunter and Millson in 1977. The most remarkable property of the infectious agent is that it resists boiling and ultraviolet radiation. *See prion disease.*

Scribonius, Largus Roman physician in the first century who accompanied Claudius during his attempt to conquer Britain in AD 47. He wrote *Compositiones Medicamentorum* which was first published by Ruel at Paris in 1529.

Scrofula [Latin: *scrofula*, brood sow] The earliest mention of this disease of inflammatory swelling of lymph glands in the neck, armpit and groins is found in the writings of the School of Salerno. Its effects on children are described in the Hippocratic writings. Galen (AD 129–200) used the name to denote the scirrous hardness which followed the disease. It is also mentioned in several passages of Constantinus Africanus (d 1087). The tuberculous etiology was established with the discovery of tubercle bacillus by Robert Koch (1843–1910) in 1882. *See struma.*

Scrotal Cancer [Latin: *scrotum*, bag] Cancer of chimney sweeps due chronic exposure to soot was described by Percivall Pott (1714–1788) in 1770. It was also described in cotton-mule spinners due to prolonged contact with lubrication oil on spindles by S. R. Wilson of the Royal Infirmary Manchester in 1906.

Scrotal Elephantiasis [Latin: *scrotum*, bag] Described by a Canton physician called Wong in 1858 and by Vandyke Carter (1831–1907) in 1861. A larval nematode was isolated in the chylous fluid of the tunica vaginalis in a case of hydrocele by Jean Nicolas Demarquay (1814–1875) in 1863. The same organism was later found in a number of cases of chyluria by a German physician working in Brazil, Otto Heinrich Wucherer (1820–1873) in 1866. In its male and female form it was found in blood of a Bengali patient by Edward Gayer in Calcutta in 1877. His specimens were later examined and identified by Timothy Richard Lewis who was already familiar with the organism, and he named it *Filaria sanguinis hominis* in 1872.

Scrub Typhus (Syn: Japanese flood fever) Observed in Japan in 1878 and originally known as Shima-mushi or island insect disease. It was first believed that it was caused solely by a trombiculoid red mite, akamushi or tsutsugamushi. Chinese literature of the 16th century describes a similar disease caused by the sandmite. Shibasaburo Kitasato

(1852–1931) in 1893 successfully transmitted it to monkeys. The rickettsial cause was demonstrated by M. Nagayo and colleagues in 1930, and they named it *Rickettsia orientalis*. It was renamed *Rickettsia tsutsugamushi* by N. Ogata in 1931.

Scudamore, Sir Charles (1779–1849) Third son of William Scudamore, a medical practitioner from Kent. He graduated in medicine from Glasgow in 1814 and became a member of the Royal College of Physicians and honorary member of Trinity College Dublin. He was also physician to Prince Leopold and the Duke of Northumberland. He wrote several treatises on mineral water, gout, blood and coagulation, auscultation, pulmonary disease and other subjects. He was an authority on gout who popularized hydrotherapeutics.

Scurvy [Latin: *scorbutus*] A deficiency disease of sailors, known as 'spoyle'. Jean de Joinville (1224–1319) described it in 1250. French clergyman, Jacques de Vitry, gave an account at around the same time. Naval Commander, Sir Richard Hawkins (1562–1622), gave an account on prevention with lemon juice during his voyage to the South Sea in 1593. An early book on naval medicine, *The Surgeons mate*, of 1617 by John Woodall (1556–1643) of the East India Company, contains the suggestion that lime could be used as a cure. James Lind (1716–1794) proved the effect of lemons and oranges in prevention by conducting the first controlled trial on record on HMS *Salisbury* in 1747. His *A Treatise on Scurvy* was published in 1757. It was also found in prisoners during the 19th century and was described by George Budd (1808–1882) who gave a lecture series on 'Disorders arising from defective nutrition'. *See ascorbic acid.*

Scutari Site of a hospital for the Anglo-French army during the Crimean War. Florence Nightingale (1820–1910) and a team of 38 nurses worked there and succeeded in producing a drastic reduction in morality.

Scythia Ancient region of Asia and southeast Europe north of the Black Sea. The Greek historian Herodotus (484–425 BC) mentioned the Scythians who inhaled the vapor of hemp to become intoxicated.

Seborrheic Eczema Unna dermatosis was described by Paul Gerson Unna (1850–1929), a dermatologist in Hamburg.

Secret Remedies Various common ingredients were camouflaged and used in the preparations, mostly by quack physicians and companies. In 1775 Louis XVI paid 18,000 francs to the widow of the Swiss surgeon Nuffer to obtain a secret remedy against tapeworm, which later turned out to be mainly felix mas fern. Frederick the Great similarly obtained a remedy (also male fern extract), after granting an

annuity and the title of councilor to a Swiss apothecary called Matthieu. Peruvian bark was used as a secret remedy and was bought by Louis XIV. The secret of Goddard Powder was bought by Charles II, for 5000 pounds. Another secret remedy called Scot's pills made of aloe and jalap was introduced in 1635 and remained popular until 1875. Patrick Anderson, a physician from Edinburgh in the 17th century, published the virtues of his secret pills in *Grana Angelica* in 1635. His daughter Catherine communicated the secret to Edinburgh surgeon, Thomas Weir, and they remained in use for over 200 years until analyzed in 1910. The Royal College of Physicians published a list of commonly used secret remedies in 1910 along with a detailed analysis of their contents. A select committee was appointed in 1914 to deal with abuses related to patent medicines.

Secretin Hormone secreted by the duodenal mucosa which stimulates the flow of pancreatic juice. Discovered by Sir William Maddock Bayliss (1860–1924) and Ernest Henry Starling (1866–1927) in 1905. It was isolated in crystalline form by Swedish pharmacologist Einar Hammarsten (b 1889), E. Jorpes and G. Agren in 1933. *See hormone.*

Sedillot, Charles Emmanuel (1804–1883) *See gastrostomy.*

Seessel, Albert (1850–1910) Medical graduate from Yale and assistant to Wilhelm His (1831–1904) in Germany from 1876 to 1877, before he returned to America to practice in New York. He described the Seessel pocket, a diverticulum of the embryonic pharynx found anterior to the cranial attachment of the buccopharyngeal membrane.

Sefström, Nils Gabriel (1765–1829) Swedish physician and lecturer in chemistry at the Royal Military Academy in Carlsberg who also taught in the School of Mines. He discovered vanadium. *See vanadium.*

Sègalas, Gascon Pierre Saloman (1792–1875) French urologist and pioneer in application of endoscopy to urology. He improved the method described by Phillip Bozzoni (1773–1809) in 1826 and wrote a treatise in 1828.

Seguin, Armand (1765–1865) French chemist in Paris who studied human metabolism on himself and published a treatise on respiration with Antoine Laurent Lavoisier (1743–1794) in 1789.

Séguin, Edouard (1812–1880) American psychiatrist who proposed education for the mentally deficient. *See idiocy.*

Seiler Cartilage Small cartilaginous rod attached to the vocal process of the arytenoid cartilage. Described in 1879 by Carl Seiler (1849–1905), an American laryngologist of Swedish origin.

Seismograph [Greek: *seismos*, earthquake + *graphein*, to write] An early version involved dropping a ball from the mouth of a bronze dragon into the mouth of a bronze frog and was invented by Zhang Heng in China in AD 132. A modern instrument was invented by Italian meteorologist and professor at Naples, Luigi Palmieri (1807–1896), director of the Vesuvius observatory in 1854. Another was described by Robert Mallet in 1858. An America model was installed at the Lick Observatory in California in 1888. The inverted pendulum type was invented by Emil Weichart in 1900. The Earth's core was discovered using seismographic records by geologist and seismologist, Richard Dixon Oldham (1858–1936) of Dublin in 1906. The Richter scale was invented by Charles Francis Richter (1900–1985) of Hamilton, Ohio in 1930. A system of unprecedented seismographic accuracy of 0.1 second was devised by American geophysicist, Victor Hugo Benioff (1899–1968) of Los Angeles.

Seismometer [Greek: *seismos*, earthquake + *metros*, measure] *See seismograph.*

Seldinger Technique A modification of the percutaneous technique for arterial catheterization, which allowed the introduction of a catheter of larger diameter than the needle used for initial puncture, was devised by American radiologist, Sven Ivar Seldinger (b 1921) in 1953. He used the technique for percutaneous angiography and it was later adapted to therapeutic procedures such as cardiac pacing and intra-aortic balloon pumping.

Selenium [Greek: *selene*, moon] Element discovered by Swedish chemist, Jöns Jacob Berzelius (1779–1848) in 1818 and Johann Gottlieb Gahn (1745–1818). It is a potential industrial hazard in glass, photoelectric material and rubber manufacture. Poisoning from industrial waste was described by Madison, an army surgeon from South Dakota, in 1856 and called 'alkalie disease' due to the mistaken notion that it was caused by alkali in waste from factories. Selenium as the cause of disease was identified by K.W. Franke in 1934, although studies in man by D.M. Hadjimarkos in 1952 showed that it caused dental caries, its pathogenicity to humans is doubtful. It was used as anticancer therapy by M. Wasserman and F. Keysser of Germany in 1911 and A.T. Todd in 1928.

Sella Turcica [Latin: *sella*, saddle] Pocket of the sphenoid bone on which the pituitary gland rests. Named 'sella turcica' due to its resemblance to a Turkish saddle. Enlargement of this on a skull X-ray in a case of acromegaly was shown by Hermann Oppenheim (1858–1919), a neurologist in Berlin in 1899.

Selye, Hans Hugo Bruno (1907–1982) Canadian physician, originally from Vienna and who studied medicine in Prague, Paris and Rome. He worked with Collip on hormonal interactions involving the adrenal and pituitary glands and the hypothalamus on osteoblast multiplication, bone formation, gonadal stimulation and blood sugar level. He developed the general adaptation syndrome in which a physiological mechanism raises resistance to stress, anxiety and their biochemical consequences in disorders such as hypertension, rheumatism and nephrosclerosis. *See stress.*

Semeiology [Greek: *semeiotikos*, symptom + *logos*, discourse] (Syn. symptomatology)

Semen [Latin: *semen*, seed] Gardinius postulated the existence of particles in the semen capable of effecting fertilization, in 1623. Antoni van Leeuwenhoek (1632–1723) observed particles similar to tadpoles under the microscope in semen and this led to the discovery of spermatozoa in 1677.

Semicircular Canal [Latin: *semi*, half + *circulus*, circle] Part of the ear discovered by Gabriele Falloppio (1523–1562), a pupil of Andreas Vesalius (1514–1564). The apparatus of the middle ear including the cochlea and semicircular canals were described by Cecilio Foli (1615–1660) in 1645. The intercellular membrane in the ampulla was described by Urban Pritchard (1845–1925), an eminent London otorhinologist, in 1876. Their role and that of otoliths in maintaining equilibrium was demonstrated by Rudolf Magnus (1873–1927) in 1926.

Semilunar Cartilage of the Knee Surgery for displacement was performed on a 30-year-old miner by Thomas Annandale (1838–1909), professor of surgery at Edinburgh in 1884. His work was published in the *British Medical Journal* in 1885. An experimental study on injury and repair of the semilunar cartilage in animals was done by Donald E. King (1903–1987), chief of orthopedics at Stanford University.

Seminal Vesicle [Latin: *semen*, seed + *vesica*, bladder] The term 'prostatei chirsoides' was used by Aristotle (384–322 BC) to denote the seminal vesicles. Galen (AD 129–200) described the prostate gland, seminal vesicles and associated structures. Prostaglandins were detected in 1930 in seminal vesicles.

Seminiferous Tubule Described by Parisian anatomist Jean Riolan (1580–1687) in 1626.

Semmelweiss, Ignaz Phillipp (1818–1865) Hungarian obstetrician and advocate of asepsis for prevention of puerperal sepsis, born in Budapest. He demonstrated in 1847 that mortality due to puerperal fever could be reduced from 18% to less than 2% if students and doctors washed their hands before attending patients. His findings were not accepted and he was ridiculed and persecuted. He was committed to a mental asylum in Vienna and died of sepsis resulting from a wound infection of the finger in 1865.

Semon Sign Retraction or fixation of the umbilicus in upper airway disease. Described by Sir Felix Semon (1849–1921), a German-born laryngologist in London at the Throat Hospital (1874) and St Thomas' Hospital (1882).

Senac, Jean Baptiste (1693–1770) French physician in Paris and physician to the king. He wrote *On the Structure Action and Diseases of the Heart, Reflections on Drowned Persons*, and translated *Heister's Anatomy*. He used quinine in treatment of palpitations.

Senator, Hermann (1834–1911) German surgeon who described a syndrome of splenomegaly and anemia leading to cirrhosis and ascites (Banti–Senator syndrome) in 1901. The disease was described by Guido Banti (1852–1925) in Florence in 1894.

Seneca, Lucius Annaeus (3 BC–AD 65) Stoic philosopher of Greece who wrote *Natural Questions* which gave an account of natural phenomena. He also gave a classical description of chronic alcoholism.

Sengstaken–Blakemore Tube *See Blakemoren–Sengstaken tube.*

Senile Dementia Areteaus the Cappadocian (AD 81–138) studied prepsychotic personalities and differentiated senile dementia from mania. London physician, William Salmon (1644–1713) described symptoms in a patient in 1692 as, *Defects of the Imagination, Reason and Memory in a Man Superannuated.* Phillipe Pinel (1745–1826) recognized intellectual deterioration as a separate entity – dementia. Jean Etienne Dominique Esquirol (1772–1840) of Paris studied different states of dementia in senility in 1838. British physician and anthropologist, James Cowles Prichard (1786–1848), gave an early description under the title, incoherence, in 1835. Alois Alzheimer (1864–1915), during his research on neuropathology at Emil Kraepelin's (1856–1926) Psychiatric Clinic in Munich, studied brains of demented and senile patients and correlated their signs and symptoms with histological findings. Creutzfeld–Jakob disease, a syndrome of dementia accompanied by pyramidal and extrapyramidal signs which usually occurs after middle age and may be due to a slow virus, was described independently by Hans Gerhard Creutzfeld (1885–1964) and Alfons Jakob (1884–1931) in 1921. Binswanger disease, a form of

progressive subcortical encephalopathy leading to dementia in the fifth and sixth decade of life, was described by Otto Ludwig Binswanger (1852–1929) in 1894.

Senility *See geriatrics.*

Senn Bone Plate Made of decalcified bone and used to approximate and suture the divided intestine by American surgeon, Nicholas Senn (1844–1908) of Rush Medical College, Chicago. He also pioneered use of X-rays in surgical diagnosis.

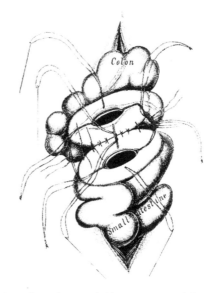

Nicholas Senn's bone plates. Frederick Treves, *A Manual of Operative Surgery* (1892). Lea Bros. & Co., Philadelphia

Senna The extract from leaves or seed pods of plants of *Cassia acutifolia* or senna is an ancient remedy that is currently used as a laxative. Isaac Judaeus, a medical writer from Egypt in the 10th century mentioned that the best senna was brought from Mecca. The Arabian physicians Serapion (339–359) and Mesue (d 1015) introduced it to Europe where it became popular with medieval physicians. It was cultivated as a medicinal plant in Italy in the first half of the 16th century.

Sensory System Thomas Aquinas (1225–1274) of Naples, a pupil of Albertus Magnus (1200–1280), separated the body from the soul and attributed the sensory functions entirely to sensory organs and not the brain. Experiments on the physiology of sensation and reflexes were done by Stephen Hales (1677–1761), a clergyman in Teddington. He noted the reflex withdrawal of the leg in a decapitated frog which he was able to abolish by inducing a lesion in the spinal cord in 1730. The term 'reflex' was introduced by Johan August Unzer (1727–1799) from Halle, to describe the sensory-motor reaction in 1771. Sir Charles Bell (1774–1842) differentiated nerve roots into sensory and motor components in 1811. Pacini corpuscles, end organs of sensory nerves, were described by Italian professor of anatomy at Pisa, Filippo Pacini (1812–1883) in 1840 and by Abraham Vater (1684–1751) in 1717, and were known as Pacini–Vater corpuscles. Krause bulb, sensory nerve end organs, were described by Wilhelm Krause (1833–1910) in 1860. Merkel corpuscles, another form of sensory tactile nerve endings, were described by Friedrich Sigmund Merkel (1845–1919), professor of anatomy at Göttingen in 1880. Ernst Axel Henrik Key (1832–1901), professor of pathological anatomy at Stockholm, described the sensory nerve endings known as the Key bulb. The sensory nature of the muscle spindle was proposed by Sir Charles Scott Sherrington (1857–1952) in 1894, and described in detail by Angelo Ruffini (1864–1929) between 1892 to 1898. Cutaneous areas of the sensory nerve roots related to visceral organs were mapped by Sir Henry Head (1861–1940), a neurologist at the London Hospital in 1893. The proprioceptors, highly specialized somatic sensory end organs of the muscles, tendons and joints, were described by Sherrington in 1906.

Senstaken Tube Inflatable balloon for controlling hemorrhage from esophageal varices. Designed by American surgeon, R. W. Senstaken (b 1923).

Sepsis [Greek: *sepsis*, decay] Commonest cause of fatality following wounds, surgery and childbirth since ancient times. Application of mold to the wound was practiced for centuries and has been rationalized with the discovery of the antibacterial properties of the penicillium mold in 1929. Ignaz Phillipp Semmelweis (1818–1865), a Hungarian obstetrician from Budapest advocated asepsis for prevention of puerperal sepsis. Several other doctors have died of sepsis as a result of accidental surgical wounds. Jacobus Kolletschka, professor of forensic pathology at Vienna, died this way in 1847. Henry Phibrick Nelson, a surgeon at the London Hospital died at the age of 35 years through accidental contamination during surgery. The introduction of the antibacterial sulfonamide compound, Protonsil, by Gerhard Johannes Paul Domagk (1895–1964) in 1935 changed the outlook on sepsis caused by bacteria and revolutionized treatment of bacterial diseases. A 10-month-old infant dying of staphylococcal septicemia was saved by treatment with Protonsil in 1933. Clinical trials in Germany by Domagk and others established treatment of other conditions such as empyema, erysipelas and puerperal fever with sulfonamides.

Septic Abortion An early description of placental bacteremia leading to shock was given by William Emery Studdiford (1897–1964), professor of gynecology at the New York University College of Medicine, and Gordon Watkins Douglas (b 1921) in 1956.

Septicemia A classic account of pyemia or septicemia was given by Sir Samuel Wilks (1824–1911) of Guy's Hospital in 1861. *See sepsis.*

Serapion Junior or ibn Serabi (*c* AD 1070) Arabian physician who wrote many medical treatises including one based on the works of Galen (AD 129–200) and Dioscorides (AD 40–90), *De temparamentis simplicum.*

Serapion of Alexandria (*c* 300 BC) Opponent of Hippocratic medicine. Amongst his unusual remedies he promoted crocodile dung and other excreta, and as a result they became very costly.

Serapion Senior or Yahya ibn Serabi (d AD 930) Syrian physician who wrote two books. A Latin translation by Gerard of Cremona (1147–1187) was published in Venice.

Serenus, Samonicus Roman physician during the reign of Emperor Lucius Septimus Severus around AD 150. He composed a poem on medicine.

Serine Amino acid isolated from the protein, sericin, in silk by Cramer in 1856.

Serology [Latin: *serum*, whey + *logos*, discourse] *See immunology, serum proteins.*

Serpent Used as the physician's emblem since the time of Aesculapius. The grounds of the temple of Aesculapius contained large non-poisonous yellow snakes which were allowed to lick the diseased parts of the body to effect healing. Aesculapius is depicted with a serpent around his staff. *See ophidism.*

Serres Angle Metafacial angle of anthropometry described by Antoine Etienne Renaud Augustin Serres (1786–1868), professor of anatomy and natural history at the Jardin des Plantes, Paris in 1824.

Serres Gland Islands of epithelium present in the gums of infants. Described by Antoine Etienne Renaud Augustin Serres (1786–1868), professor of anatomy and natural history at the Jardin des Plantes, Paris in 1824.

Sertoli Cell Supporting cells of the testicular epithelium described by Enrico Sertoli (1842–1910), professor of experimental physiology at Milan in 1865.

Sertürner, Adam Frederick Wilhelm (1783–1841) German chemist from Hannover who isolated morphine from opium in 1801. *See morphine.*

Serum Proteins Ernest Henry Starling (1886–1927) discovered the functional significance of serum proteins. A calorimetric method of estimating them was devised by California biochemist, David Morris Greenberg (b 1895) in 1929. Another method for total protein content of human plasma and serum was described by American physician, Benjamin Milton Kagan (b 1913) of Baltimore in 1938. Their study was advanced by the development of electrophoresis by Arne Wilhelm Kaurin Tiselius (1902–1971) in 1930. He showed the gammaglobulin components, and globulins and classified them according to mobility.

Serum Sickness [Latin: *serum*, whey] An early description was given by a pediatrician and immunologist, Clemens von Pirquet (1874–1929), of Austria in 1877 and another by German physician Franz Hamburger (1874–1954) and Ernst Monro (1874–1951) in 1903. A monograph was written by von Pirquet and Béla Schick (1877–1967) in 1905.

Serum Therapy Used in therapeutics by Emil Adolf von Behring (1854–1917) against tetanus and diphtheria in 1890. He was the winner of the first Nobel Prize for Physiology or Medicine in 1901.

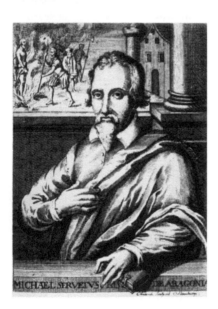

Michael Servetus (1511–1553). William Stirling, *Some Apostles of Physiology* (1902). Waterlow & Sons, London

Servetus, Michael (1511–1553) Spanish physician and probably the first to describe pulmonary circulation saying 'that the mass of blood passes through the lungs by means of

pulmonic veins and arteries'. He also recognized changes from venous blood to arterial blood in the lungs. He was burnt at the stake because he denied the divinity of Christ.

Sesame Oil *See gingili oil.*

Setchenov, Ivan Mickailovich (1850–1898) Considered the father of physiology and neurology in Russia. He described the reflex inhibitory center in the medulla oblongata (Setchenov center) and several other structures of the nervous system.

Seton [Greek: *seta*, bristle] Derived from the use of horsehair to keep a wound open and facilitate discharge of infected material. Silk or linen were used later for this purpose. It was introduced in treatment of ununited fractures by Philip Syng Physick (1768–1837) in 1804.

Seventh Nerve *See facial nerve.*

Severus, Alexander (AD 225–235) Roman physician who established public lecture rooms for teaching medicine in Rome. He granted stipends to teachers who were expected to teach poor state-supported students free of charge.

Sewer [Old French: *sewiere*] Used to drain waste water and other products since ancient times. Sewers to drain water from marshes and low lying areas were constructed in England during the reign of King Henry VIII. They were later opened into the River Thames making it a cesspool. Poor sanitary conditions in London were addressed by Sir Edwin Chadwick (1800–1890) in his report of 1842. The City Sewers Act was passed six years later and the first medical officer of health was appointed. The modern system in London was designed by English pioneer in public health engineering, Sir Joseph William Bazalgette (1819–1891) in 1866. Around the same time, a canal system for Berlin was proposed by Rudolph Virchow (1821–1902). The modern system in Munich was planned by Max von Pettenkofer (1818–1901) in 1869. Impervious drainage pipes replaced the unhygenic brick gullies and brought about a revolution in sanitation, and were invented by Sir Henry Doulton (1820–1897), founder of a pottery factory at Lambeth.

Sex Change The world's first such operation was performed in 1952 on George Jorgenson, who later became known as Christine.

Sex Chromosomes *See accessory chromosome, Barr Murray.*

Sex Determination *See accessory chromosome, Barr Murray.*

Sex-Linked Inheritance Demonstrated in *Drosophila* fly in 1910 by Thomas Hunt Morgan (1866–1945) of Lexington, Kentucky, a pioneer in the field of modern genetics.

Sexology *See sexual psychology.*

Sexual Offenses Act A series of sexual offenses acts were passed in Britain in 1956, 1967 and 1976. The Sexual Offences Act of 1967 removed the prohibition of homosexuality, provided it took place privately between consenting adults.

Sexual Psychology A pioneer was Magnus Hirshfeld (1868–1935), professor of psychiatry at Berlin. He promoted a medical approach to sexual problems and founded the Institute of Sexual Sciences in Berlin. In his *Sexual Anomalies and Perversions* he dealt with homosexuality, sadism and murder in a scientific manner. A British pioneer was Henry Havelock Ellis (1859–1939), a psychologist from Croydon, who published six volumes of *Studies in Psychology of Sex* (1899–1910). Richard von Krafft-Ebing (1840–1902), a German forensic psychiatrist, specialized in sexual pathology. He defined and named many sexual deviations such as masochism and sadism in *Psychopathia Sexualis,* published in 1886.

Sézary Syndrome Exfoliative erythroderma associated with circulation of abnormal lymphocytes. Described French dermatologist, Albert Sézary (1880–1956).

Shaftesbury, Lord, Anthony Ashley Cooper (1801–1885) London reformer responsible for the Coal Mines Act 1842 which prohibited underground employment of women and children under the age of 13. He chaired the Lunacy Commission in 1834 and brought in the Lunacy Act which offered considerable reforms in 1845. A public meeting presided by him in 1861 inspired Thomas Holloway (1800–1883) to build a magnificent sanatorium for the mentally ill at Virginia Waters, Surrey in 1873.

Shaking Palsy *See paralysis agitans.*

Shamanism Religious practices of certain groups in Northern Asia and North America who believe in good and evil spirits. The term is of Siberian origin where shamans worked themselves into a trance inspired by the spirit and were able to foretell the future.

Shampoo Term derived from the Hindu word 'chambon' for washing.

Sharp, Philip Allen (b 1944) American molecular biologist from Kentucky. He was director of the MIT Center for Cancer Research for 1985 to 1991 and co-founder of Biogen. He invented S1 nuclease mapping for detection of unknown RNA molecules and discovered that genes are separated into sections by introns that do not carry genetic information. He was awarded the Nobel Prize for Physiology or Medicine in 1993.

Sharpey, William (1802–1888) Graduate of medicine from Edinburgh University. He studied under Guillaume Dupuytren (1777–1835) and others in Europe before he succeeded Jones Quain (1785–1851) as professor of anatomy and physiology at the University of London in 1836. Sharpey fibers are connective tissue fibers found between the periosteum and the bone. He was the first physiologist in England to devote his entire attention to physiology.

Sharpey-Schäfer, Sir Edward (1850–1935) Pioneer in endocrinology, born in Hornsey, and educated at University College, London where he later became professor of physiology from 1883 to 1899. He was appointed to the chair of physiology at Edinburgh in 1899 and continued in his post until 1933. In 1895, while working with George Oliver (1841–1915) at University College, he demonstrated the effects of extract of suprarenal gland. This was shown to produce contraction of arteries and acceleration of heart rate thereby increasing the blood pressure, and was later named adrenaline. He also investigated the role of the pancreas and what was later to be known as insulin. He wrote *The Essentials of Physiology*, which was considered the most advanced book on physiology in the world for its time, and *Essentials of Histology* in 1885.

Sharpnell Membrane Membrana flaccida of the membrana tymphani. Described by Henry Jones Sharpnell (d 1834) of Gloucestershire, a surgeon to the Royal South Gloucestershire Regiment, in 1832.

Shaver Disease Pneumoconiosis amongst workers in Canada from exposure to corundum or bauxite. Described by Cecil G. Shaver (b 1901) and A. R. Riddell in 1947.

Shaving the Head Formerly used as a method of treating insanity for nearly four centuries. Levinus Lemnius (1505–1568), a clergyman and physician in The Netherlands, in his treatise on complexion published in 1561, considered it to be helpful in allowing vapors that hurt the memory or mind to escape. He also pointed out that shaving the beard lifted the mood.

Shaw, Peter (d 1763) English physician who wrote *Practice of Physic, A course of Chemistry* and an edition of Bacon's work in five volumes.

Shebbeare, John (1709–1788) Physician from Bideford in Yorkshire. He obtained his medical degree from Paris and practiced in London where he was imprisoned twice for violent behavior. He wrote *Letters to the People of England, The Marriage Act,* and several other works.

Sheehan Syndrome Total pituitary failure as a result of post partum hemorrhage. Described by an English physician, Harold Leeming Sheehan (1900–1988) in 1937. He was born in Carlisle and graduated from Manchester University in 1921. He spent his career at Carlisle and Manchester before being made professor of pathology at Leeds in 1946.

Sheffield Royal Infirmary Founded in 1786 mainly through the efforts of William Younge (1762–1838), a medical graduate from Edinburgh University.

Sheldon, John (1752–1808) Son of an apothecary with the same name, from Tottenham Court Road, London. He opened a private anatomy school at Great Queen Street in 1777, and succeeded William Hunter (1718–1783) as professor of anatomy at the Royal Academy in 1782.

Shellfish An outbreak of mussel poisoning occurred in Wilhelmshaven in 1885 resulting in four deaths, and Ludwig Brieger isolated a toxin, Mytilotoxine, from mussels in 1889. Another outbreak occurred in Dublin with five fatalities in 1908. Karl Friedrich Meyer (b 1884) of San Francisco recorded an outbreak of mussel poisoning with six fatalities in California in 1927.

Shen Nung (2820–2697 BC) Chinese emperor, physician and reformer. He organized a system of agriculture, experimented on plants and discovered their medicinal values. The great herbal book *Pen Tsoa*, which describes over 365 drugs is attributed to him.

Sherard, James (d 1737) Apothecary in London who had a garden of unusual plants in Eltham Kent and a catalogue of which was published by John James Dillenius (1687–1747) of Darmstadt in 1732. He qualified as physician during the latter part of his life. His brother, a Fellow of All Souls College Oxford, was a famous botanist who traveled widely and served as tutor to Royalty.

Sherren, James (1872–1945) English surgeon who advocated conservative management for acute appendicitis complicated by peritonitis. He also studied the consequences of injury to the peripheral nerves in man in 1905.

Sherman, Henry Clapp (1875–1955) American biochemist from Ash Grove, Virginia. He was professor of analytical chemistry, professor of organic analysis, professor of food chemistry and Mitchill professor of chemistry at Columbia University. He did research on nutritional requirements for metal ions and vitamins, and in 1920 described the need for calcium in man and the daily requirements, interaction with phosphorus and vitamin D. From 1932 he studied vitamin B requirements in relation to the deficiency disease, polyneuritis. This was followed by vitamin A studies and iron-deficiency anemia.

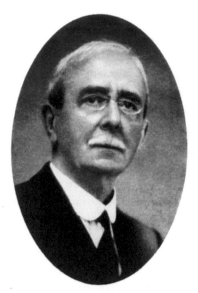

Sir Charles Scott Sherrington (1857–1952). Courtesy of the National Library of Medicine

Sherrington, Sir Charles Scott (1857–1952) Professor of physiology at Liverpool (1895–1913) and Oxford (1913–1935). His contributions to neurology include: the demonstration of decerebrate rigidity by transection of the spinal cord through the upper part of the midbrain in 1897; establishment of knee jerk as a genuine reflex by demonstrating that it was an inherited phenomenon in 1893; demonstration of the sensory nature of the muscle spindle in 1894; description of the proprioceptors which are highly specialized somatic sensory end organs of the muscles, tendons and joints in 1906; and the first use of the term motor unit to denote 'an individual motor nerve fiber together with a bunch of muscle fibers enervated by it' in 1925. He co-wrote a comprehensive work on reflexes, *Reflex Activity of the Spinal Cord*, published in 1932 by Sherrington, Sir Arthur Carew Eccles (b 1903), Creed, Derek Ernest Denny-Brown (1901–1981) and Edward George Tandy Liddell (1895–1981). He shared the Nobel Prize for Physiology or Medicine with Sir Douglas Adrian (1889–1977) in 1932.

Shiga, Kiyoshi (1870–1957) Japanese bacteriologist, born in Sendai on the island of Honshu. He graduated from Tokyo Medical School in 1896 and discovered the bacillus of dysentery (*Shigella shigae*) in 1897. He worked in Germany with Paul Ehrlich (1854–1915) at Frankfurt in 1900 and, on his return to Japan in 1905, became director of the Kitasato Research Institute.

Shigella The first of these bacteria, the *Shigella shigae* group, was described by Kiyoshi Shiga (1870–1957), a Japanese microbiologist, in 1898. Another causative organism of dysentery, *Shigella flexneri*, was discovered by Simon Flexner (1863–1946), an American bacteriologist from Louisville, Kentucky who was the first director of the Rockefeller Institute, in 1900. *Shigella sonnei*, a lactose-fermenting organism and the least pathogenic species, was isolated in Denmark by Carl Olaf Sonne (1882–1948) in 1915.

Shippen, William (1736–1808) Philadelphia physician and son of another physician. He graduated from the College of New Jersey in 1757 and studied medicine under John (1728–1793) and William Hunter (1718–1783) in England. On his return to America he joined John Morgan (1735–1789) in founding the Medical School of the College of Philadelphia in 1765.

Shock A theory based on vasomotor paralysis was proposed by Breslau surgeon, Hermann Fischer (1831–1919) in 1870. Research was done by American surgeon and physiologist George Washington Crile (1864–1943) in 1888. Shock following railway injury was described by London surgeon, Irvine Heinly Page (b 1901). Constriction of peripheral vessels was shown by English surgeon, John David Malcolm in 1893. Avoidance of shock during amputation by nerve block and observation of blood pressure was advocated by Harvey Williams Cushing (1869–1939) in 1902. The theory of exhaustion was suggested by English physician, John Percy Lockhart-Mummery (b 1875) in his Hunterian lectures on shock in 1905. A treatise on the nature and theory was published by New York physician, Samuel Jones Meltzer (1851–1920) in 1908. Intravenous colloids were used as treatment by California physician, James Joseph Hogan (b 1872) in 1915. Fat embolism in traumatic shock was proposed by Boston physician, William Townsend Porter (b 1862) in 1917. The role of capillaries following wounds was described by Sir William Maddock Bayliss (1860–1924) in 1918. Secondary shock due to histamine release was shown by Sir Henry Hallet Dale (1875–1968) in 1919. English physician D. K. Hill studied blood volume during shock in 1941. Shock due to crush injury was demonstrated on an experimental basis by Baltimore surgeon, George Walton Duncan (b 1914) in 1942. Its occurrence in burns and trauma was investigated in the same year by American physician, Sanford M. Rosenthal (b 1897).

Short, Thomas (1789–1843) Medical graduate from Edinburgh in 1815 who was medical officer on St Helena (1815–1821) during the imprisonment of Napoleon, and one of the five medical officers present at his autopsy.

Shorthand Its use in medical work was advocated by William Richard Gowers (1845–1915) of University College Hospital, London, founder of the Society of Medical Phonographers, in 1894. Timothy Bright (1551–1615), a physician, proposed a method of shorthand in *An Arte of Shorte, Swifte and Secrete writing by Character*. A system was invented by Sir Isaac Pitman (1813–1897), an educationist from Trowbridge, Wiltshire and his *Stenographic Sound Hand* was published in 1837. He later established a Phonetic Institute at Bath for teaching shorthand in 1839. His system was introduced into America by his brother Benjamin Pitman (1822–1910) in 1852, who also formed the Phonetic Institute at Cincinnati in 1853. The German system was invented by a civil servant, Franz Xavior (1789–1848) of Munich around 1830. A new system was developed by an Irishman, John Robert Gregg (1867–1948) from Shantonagh, Monaghan who emigrated to America in 1893 and wrote *Gregg Shorthand Manual* in 1888.

Shoulder Amputation Raphael B. Sabatier (1732–1811) of Paris and Jacques Lisfranc (1790–1847) performed amputation of the arm at the shoulder joint in 1815. The excision of the humeral head was performed in a case of tuberculosis of the shoulder joint by James Syme (1799–1870) in 1826.

Shoulder Dislocation *See dislocation of shoulder joint.*

Shoulder Joint The first prosthetic replacement with an artificial joint of rubber and platinum was performed by Jules Emile Pean (1830–1898) of Paris in 1894. *See dislocation of shoulder joint.*

Shwartzman Phenomenon Local skin reaction to the filtrate of bacillus typhus culture. Described by New York physician, Gregory Schwartzman (1896–1965) in 1928.

Shy–Drager Syndrome Progressive neurological disorder accompanied by postural hypotension, rigidity and tremor. Described by two American neurologists, George Milton Shy (1919–1967) of Colorado, and Glen A. Drager (1917–1967) in 1960.

Siemen SI unit of electrical conductance named after German electrical engineer, Ernest Werner von Siemens (1816–1892). He determined the electrical resistance of several substances, invented the self-acting dynamo, devised several galvanometers, introduced a process of electroplating, and developed the first telegraphic system in Prussia. He also established a factory for making electrical and telegraphic equipment in Berlin in 1847.

Siamese Twins Living conjugated twins. Named after Chang and Eng from Thailand who were exhibited in England in the 19th century. A case was brought to the notice of King James IV (1473–1513) in 1490 and he saw to their care and education. They lived to the age of 28 years.

Sibbald, Sir Robert (1641–1722) Scottish physician and naturalist, born in Edinburgh and graduated in medicine from Leiden in 1661. He was the first professor of medicine at Edinburgh University in 1685 and physician to King Charles ll. He established a physick garden at Edinburgh in 1670, and became the founder of the Royal College of Physicians of Edinburgh in 1681. He wrote *History of Sheriffdom of Fife* (1710), *Scotia Illustrata, Liberty and Independence of the Kingdom and Church of Scotland*, and several other works. The genus of plants, *Sibbaldia*, is named after him

Sibenmann Canal Small vascular canals in the aqueduct of the cochlea, described by an ophthalmologist, Friedrich Sibenmann (1852–1928) of Basel in 1894.

Sibson, Francis (1814–1876) Professor of medicine at St Mary's Hospital in London. He described the Sibson fascia, a septum covering the apical pleura attached to the first rib, in 1846.

Sibthorp, John (1758–1796) Born in Lincolnshire and studied medicine at Edinburgh University, before he succeeded his father as Regius professor of botany at Oxford in 1784. He wrote *Flora Oxoniensis* in 1794.

Sicard, Jean Athanase (1872–1979) French physician and radiologist from Marseilles. He specialized in neurology and the mechanisms of pain. He introduced injection of sclerozing solutions for varicose veins. He introduced Lipidol, a radio-opaque iodized oil for injection into cerebrospinal fluid. *See Collet–Sicard syndrome.*

Sick Sinus Syndrome Term coined by Bernard Lown of Brigham Hospital, Boston in 1967. He came across this condition when the sinus node failed to function after cardioversion for atrial fibrillation.

Sickle Cell Anemia Inherited hemoglobinopathy leading to severe anemia with the presence of sickle-shaped red blood cells. Recognized by James Bryan Herrick (1861–1964) of America in 1910. The name was given by Verne Rheem Mason (b 1889) in 1922. Genetic studies were done by Clyde Graeme Guthrie (b 1880) and John Gardiner Huck (b 1891), of the Johns Hopkins University in 1923. The structural variant of hemoglobin responsible was identified in 1949 by Linus Carl Pauling (b 1901), American molecular biologist. Substitution of the amino acid valine for glutamic acid in hemoglobin of patients was demonstrated by Vernon Martin Ingram (b 1924) of England in 1957.

Side-Chain Theory A few chemotherapeutic agents, such as cinchona, mercury and ipecacuanha, were known before Paul Ehrlich (1854–1915) started working on the side-chain theory, while director of the Institute for Experimental Therapy at Frankfurt in 1898. He proposed that an antigen had two distinct groups 'haptophore' and 'toxophile', and the side-chains in mammalian cells contained receptors which anchored the haptophores. This combination brought otherwise harmless toxophiles close enough to the cell to poison it. He used this principle to develop a manmade chemotherapeutic agent, tryphan red, which cured infected mice with trypanosomiasis in 1904. This was followed by his development of arsphenamine, or salvarsan, in 1910.

Sideroblastic Anemia *See sideroblasts.*

Sideroblasts [Greek: *sideros*, iron + *blastos*, bud] Prussian blue was used to stain iron granules in red cells by Guilio Cesare Bizzozero (1846–1901) in 1883. A more detailed study was made by H. Gruneberg in 1940, who showed stainable granules of iron in erythrocytes of mice with a congenital anemia. Alwin M. Pappenheimer (1878–1955) in 1945 noticed that these granules appeared as basophilic bodies (Pappenheimer bodies) when stained with Romanowsky stain. The term sideroblast was introduced in 1954 by E. Kaplan and co-workers to denote a nucleated red cell containing iron granules, visible under the microscope. In 1953 A. S. Douglas noted that these granules were concentrated in a perinuclear ring in the red cells of patients with anemia. The occurrence of anemia with ring sideroblasts in the bone marrow was later named sideroblastic anemia.

Sidgwick, Nevil Vincent (1873–1951) Theoretical chemist and fellow and tutor at Lincoln College, Oxford. He worked on molecular structure and formulated the theory of valence for which he was awarded the Royal Society Medal in 1937. He wrote *The Electronic Theory* of valence in 1927.

Siebold, Karl Theodor Ernest (1804–1865) German zoologist, studied asexual reproduction or development of an egg without fertilization – parthenogenesis. He demonstrated that dogs could be experimentally infected with *Taenia echinococcus* in 1854

Siebold, Phillip Franz von (1796–1866) German physician and botanist introduced western medicine into Japan. He published several works on the flora and fauna of Japan.

Sigerist, Henry Ernest (1891–1957) Professor at the Johns Hopkins University and director of the Institute of the History of Medicine. He published several important books on history of medicine.

Sight [Anglo-Saxon: *sihth*, sight] *See vision.*

Sigmoid Colon [Greek: *sigmoeides*, 'S'-shaped] Derives its name from its resemblance to the Greek letter.

Silicon [Latin: *silex*, flint] Non-metallic element noted to be suitable for glass making by Johann Joachim Becher (1635–1682), a chemist from Bavaria in 1660. Joseph Gay-Lussac (1778–1850) and Louis Jacques Thénard (1777–1857) obtained silicon in 1809, although in an impure form. Pure crystalline silicon was obtained by Deville in 1854. *See silicosis.*

Silicosis Occupational lung disease described in Schneeberg miners as 'mala metellalorum' by Paracelsus (1493–1541) in 1531. It was described in Joachimsthal in Bohemia by George Agricola (1494–1555). A description of the lung pathology was given in 1672 by Isbrand van Diemerbroeck, professor of medicine in Holland. In his *Anatome Corporis Humane*, he described the mass of sand particles found in lungs of stone cutters. The term silicosis was coined by Visconti in 1870. The carcinogenic potential was demonstrated by Haerting and Hesse in 1879. In 1891 Arnold Knight drew attention to cutlery grinder's asthma in Sheffield, and John Scott Haldane (1860–1936) described it in sand-quarry workers in 1911.

Silkworm Disease The fungal cause of muscardine disease of the silkworm was discovered in 1835 by Italian lawyer, Agostino Bassi (1773–1856) who became a farmer. This is considered to be the first proof for pathogenesis of germs. The fungus was named *Beauveria bassiana.*

Silkworms Brought from China to Europe in the 6th century. A microscopic dissection was performed by Marcello Malpighi (1628–1694) in 1669. *See silkworm disease.*

Silurian Period Period in Earth history identified and named by Scottish geologist, Sir Roderick Impey Murchison (1792–1871) of Tarradale in 1835. Murchison falls in Uganda, and the Murchison River in Western Australia are name after him.

Silva, John Baptist (1684–1744) Physician of Jewish origin in Bordeaux who wrote a treatise on the use of bleeding, and a number of other works.

Silver Salt Silver nitrate was prepared by Geber the alchemist in the 14th century and was used as a remedy by Avicenna (980–1037) and by Paracelsus (1493–1541). Girolamo Cardano (1501–1576) and Ambroise Paré (1510–1590) used it as a hair dye in the 16th century. They were used commonly for hysteria and epilepsy in England in the 18th century but use was condemned by Herman Boerhaave

(1668–1738) in 1738.

Silver Stain Used, among other things, to study nerve endings in the muscles and introduced by Julius Friedrich Cohnheim (1839–1884), a German pathologist from Pomerania, Poland in 1863. The method was improved by the Italian histologist, Camillo Golgi (1843–1926) in 1873.

Simmonds Disease (Syn: pituitary cachexia) Hypopituitarism resulting from atrophy of the anterior pituitary lobe. A case history of post-partum necrosis of the anterior pituitary was first published by Leon Konrad Glinski (1870–1918) of Poland in 1913 and a pathologist from Hamburg, Morris Simmonds (1855–1925) in 1914. The name Simmonds disease was introduced by L. Lichtwitz in 1914. A case in America was reported by D. A. L. Graham and R. F. Farquharson in 1931. Philip Edward Smith (1884–1970) in 1930 noted that it could be produced in rats by hypophysectomy. Harold Leeming Sheehan (1900–1988) in 1939 described it following post-partum hemorrhage.

Simmons, James Stevens (1890–1954) American bacteriologist who prepared a citrate agar medium for culture of bacteria. He established *Aedes albopictus* as the vector of dengue fever in 1930.

Simon, Gustav (1824–1876) Professor of surgery in Rostock (1861) and Heidelberg (1867). He wrote monographs on vesicovaginal fistula (1854), splenectomy (1857) and on plastic surgery (1868).

Simon, Sir John (1816–1904) English surgeon, public health reformer and a lecturer in pathology at King's College Hospital, and later a surgeon at St Thomas' Hospital. He was appointed as the first medical officer of health to the city of London in 1848 and brought in several important sanitary reforms. He showed the advantages of smallpox vaccination. He published *General Pathology* in 1850.

Simon, Theodore (1873–1961) French psychologist in Paris who devised the Binet–Simon tests for intelligence with Alfred Binet (1857–1911) in 1911.

Simons, Samuel Foart (1750–1813) Physician from Sandwich in Kent. He graduated from Leiden, and practiced in London. He was elected physician to the Westminster Dispensary in 1780 and was physician to George III in 1803.

Simpson, George Gaylord (1902–1984) American paleontologist from Chicago who introduced the concept of genetics into paleontology. He wrote *Tempo and Mode of Evolution* (1944), *The Meaning of Evolution* (1949) and several other works.

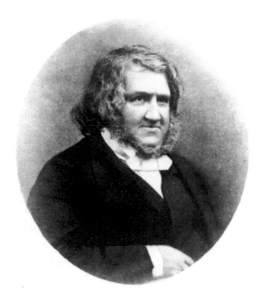

James Young Simpson. H. Laing Gordon, *James Young Simpson and Chloroform* (1897)

Simpson, Sir James Young (1811–1870) Scottish obstetrician from Bathgate, West Lothian who graduated from Edinburgh University in 1830. He was professor of midwifery at Edinburgh in 1840, and used ether as an inhalational anesthetic on a woman in labor in 1840 and later introduced chloroform in 1847. Acupressure, where a pin or needle was passed across the blood vessel to anchor it and apply pressure so as to promote hemostasis to control bleeding during surgery, was introduced by him in 1864. The pin was removed from a few hours to few days after bleeding stopped. He was physician to Queen Victoria and used chloroform in her delivery of Prince Leopold. *See chloroform.*

Sims, James Marion (1813–1883) American gynecologist, born in Lancaster County in South Carolina and graduated in medicine from Jefferson Medical College, Philadelphia in 1835. He practiced as a surgeon in Mount Meigs, Alabama and performed several original operations such as excision of the upper and lower jaw and the repair of hair lip. He developed an interest in vesicovaginal fistula and devised the knee–chest position for gynecology examination. He used a pewter spoon as a vaginal speculum in 1845 which was later developed into Sims duck-billed speculum in 1870. The first successful operation to surgically correct vesicovaginal fistula was performed by him in 1849. His *On the Treatment of Vesico-vaginal Fistula* appeared in the *American Journal of Medical Sciences* in 1852. Around 1850 he moved to New York and worked at the Women's Hospital until 1861. He traveled in Europe and performed his only operation in England which was a repair of vesicovaginal fistula at the Samaritan Hospital, London. He wrote *Clinical Notes on Uterine Surgery* which was published in 1866.

Sims Speculum *See Sims, James Marion.*

Simulated Disease Galen (AD 129–200) was one of the earliest ancient authors to write on simulated disease. He described hemoptysis simulated by cutting the gums and swallowing blood then expectorating it with a self-induced cough. *See Munchausen Syndrome.*

Sinoauricular Node (SA node) The pacemaker of the heart was discovered by Sir Arthur Keith (1866–1955) and Martin William Flack (1882–1931) in 1906. Sir Thomas Lewis (1881–1945) traced excitation from it down the bundle of His to the Purkinje fibers, around 1910.

Sinoatrial Node *See sinoauricular node.*

Sinus Node *See sinoauricular node.*

Sinusitis A method of washing out the antrum of Highmore was described by French surgeon in Paris, Anselme Louis Bernard Berchillet Jourdain (1734–1816) in 1767. George W. Caldwell (b 1866) of New York described the operative treatment for suppuration of the maxillary antrum and other sinuses in 1893. An American laryngologist, Joseph Hammond Bryan (1856–1935) wrote on sinusitis in 1889. English physician, Sir St Clair Thompson (1859–1943) described the symptoms and complications in 1914. Conservative treatment with irrigation was advised by Arthur Walter Proetz (b 1888) of St Louis in 1926 and Melvin Harold Hays (1880–1940) of New York in 1937.

Sipple Syndrome Familial condition of medullary carcinoma of the thyroid, parathyroid adenoma and pheochromocytoma. Described by American respiratory physiologist, John H. Sipple (b 1930) in 1961.

Sippy Diet Antacid therapy with frequent milk feeds and compounds such as magnesium hydroxide for peptic ulcer. Introduced in 1915 by Bertram Welton Sippy (1866–1924), an American gastroenterologist.

Siriasis [Greek: *seiriasis*, disease produced by heat of the sun] Ancient Greek term for inflammation of the brain. Paul of Aegina (625–690) recommended application of egg yoke and oil of roses on the hollow of bregma of the skull as treatment.

Sirkari Disease Another name for kala azar used by people of the Garo hills in India. *See kala azar.*

Sjögren Syndrome Keratoconjunctivitis sicca and xerostomia, enlarged parotid gland with polyarthritis. Described by A. W. M. Houwer in 1927, and J. Iskowitz in 1928. Scandinavian neurologist, Henrik S.C. Sjögren

(1899–1989) noted the additional features of oral, parotid and skin changes in 1933. Further cases were reported by P. Ellman and F. P. Weber in 1949.

Scatological Medicine In his *Scatological Rites of all Nations*, Captain Bourke devoted one section to it. It uses medicines such as ear wax, human flesh, bat blood, mouse dung, rabbit dung, fox dung, sweat of athletes, oil of spider, snake tongue and hundreds of other remedies. The theory may have originated from the belief that nastiness is the sign of efficacy. Hundreds of scatological medicines used since ancient times were mentioned by Pliny (AD 29–79) in his natural history. *See dung.*

Skeleton [Greek: *skeletos*, dried body] *See osteology.*

Skene Gland Paraurethral glands of the female described in 1880 by Alexander Johnston Chalmers Skene (1838–1900), an American gynecologist of Scottish origin. He was professor of gynecology at the Long Island College Hospital in New York.

Skiagram [Greek: *skia*, shadow + *gramma*, writing] Röntgenogram or use of X-rays to obtain photographs.

Skiascopy [Greek: *skia*, shadow + *skopein*, to look] Shadow test to determine refraction of the eye by illuminating the retina with a mirror and observing movements of light and shade of the pupils. Described by Chibret in 1886. It was introduced into clinical medicine by E. Jackson (1856–1942) of Philadelphia.

Skin [Anglo-Saxon: *scinn*, skin] *See dermatology.*

Skin Graft [Anglo-Saxon: *scinn*, skin] Aulus Cornelius Celsus (25 BC–AD 50) included a description of plastic surgery to the face and skin grafting in his writings. Experimental grafting was done by Italian surgeon, Giuseppe Baronio (1759–1811) around 1800. He demonstrated the fundamental principle that an autograft from the same animal worked while an allograft from another animal was rejected. American surgeon Frank Hastings Hamilton (1813–1886) treated ulcers by grafting in 1854. Transplantation of free skin instead of pedunculated flaps was introduced by Swiss surgeon, Jacques Louis Reverdin (1842–1929) in 1869. Contracture following burns was treated with grafts by George David Pollock (1817–1897) in 1871. Grafts of intermediate thickness were performed by Léopold Louis Xavier Edouard Ollier (1830–1900) of Paris in 1872, and full thickness grafts were advocated by German surgeon, Fedor Victor Krause (1857–1937) in 1893. Split skin grafts in plastic surgery were introduced by Vitray Papin Blair (1871–1955) and James Brown in 1929.

Skin Test An early test used in diagnosis of disease was devised by O. H. Salisbury of Ohio. He used suspensions of spores from straw as a test for farmer's lung in 1862. A test for susceptibility to diphtheria was devised by Bela Schick (1877–1967), an Austrian pediatrician in New York, in 1911. The first positive test for house dust extract in allergy was shown by R. A. Kern in 1921. The Dick test to detect susceptibility to scarlet fever was devised by American physicians, George Frederick Dick (1881–1967) and Gladys Rowena Dick (1881–1963) in 1924.

Skin Traction *See femoral fractures.*

Skoda, Josef (1805–1881) Austrian physician from Pilsen, Bohemia. He graduated from Vienna where he spent most of his career. He was a contemporary of Karl Freiherr Rokitansky (1804–1878), and popularized the use of René Laënnec's (1781–1826) stethoscope in clinical medicine and described many auscultatory signs in the chest (Skoda resonance).

Skull [Middle English: *skulle*, cranium] The Cannstadt skull, found in 1700, was one of the earliest of a primitive man. Peter Camper (1722–1789), a surgeon at Leiden, attempted to measure the skull from an anthropological viewpoint. Craniology, study of variation of skull in relation to race, was established by Friedrich Blumenbach (1752–1840) of Göttingen in 1775. Several Neolithic skulls were found in Brittany and other parts of France around 1870. Evidence for primitive man, *Australopithecus*, believed to be three million years old, was found in the Rift Valley in South Africa in 1925. Phrenology, study of the external form of the skull as an indicator of mental powers and moral qualities, was established by Franz Joseph Gall (1758–1828), a German physician, and Casper Johan Spurzheim (1776–1832). Paul Broca (1824–1880) founded anthropometry with his invention of 27 craniometric and cranioscopic instruments. Trepanning is the oldest form of neurosurgery and 19 skulls with trephine holes, from the pre-Incan period were identified by Muniz in 1894. A Neolithic skull with a trephine hole was found in the river Thames in 1864. The calvarium and femur of a primitive man, *Pithecanthropus erectus*, was discovered by Eugene Dubois (1858–1940), a surgeon in the Dutch army while stationed in Java in 1893. Books on comparative anatomy in relation to anthropology include: *Tabulae Craniorum Diversarum Gentium* by Sandifort (1830), *Crania Americana* (1839) and *Crania Egyptiaaca* by Morton (1844), *Atlas de Cranioscopie* (1845) by Gustav Carus, and *Crania Britannica* (1856) by Davis and Thurnum. *See Piltdown man.*

Skull Fracture Percivall Pott (1714–1788) wrote on head injuries and fractures of the skull in 1760. Another English surgeon, William Frederic Teevan (1834–1887), investigated wounds to the skull in 1864 and concluded that fractures occurred in the line of extension and not compression. Symptoms and signs of fracture of the posterior cranial fossa were described by London surgeon, William Henry Battle (1855–1936) in 1890. Cracked-pot note on percussion was described by Sir William Macewen (1848–1924) of Glasgow in 1893. Conservative treatment was advised by New York surgeon, John Fox Connors (1873–1935) in 1934.

SLE *See systemic lupus erythematosus.*

Sleep Described by Hippocrates (460–377 BC) in *De Insominis* and by Aristotle (384–322 BC) in his treatise *Somno et Vigilia*. The aphorisms of Hippocrates state that when sleep is laborious, it is a deadly symptom, when sleep puts an end to delirium it is a good symptom, and both sleep and insomnolency, when immoderate, are bad. Averrhoes of Cordova (1126–1198), Spain, around AD 1150, defined sleep as the recession of the sensorial powers from their organs to the internal part, and stated that those who sleep with their eyes open do not perceive the objects nearest to them. Haly Abbas (930–994) postulated that during sleep animal powers are suspended and the vital and natural powers continue unaffected. Paul Charles Dubois (1848–1918), in 1896, demonstrated that lesions in a specific center near the floor of the third ventricle cause disturbance of sleep. Sleep studies on animals were done by Szymansky in 1918 who observed that animals which depended on tactile and olfactory senses to obtain food had short spells of sleep, and he classified them as polyphasic sleepers, and that animals which used visual sense were monophasic sleepers. The human infant is initially polyphasic in sleep but later becomes monophasic. In 1937 Harvey and Hobart identified five different patterns (delta, delta and alpha, delta, null, and intermittent alpha) using ECG during sleep. Ivan Petrovich Pavlov (1849–1936) experimented on dogs and identified internal inhibition of the internal cortex in 1927. Walter Rudolph Hess (1881–1973), a Swiss physiologist and Nobel Prize winner, worked on the brain as a coordinating organ for the functions of internal organs and sleep.

Sleeping Sickness Terminal presentation of African trypanosomiasis. The presence of trypanosomes in cerebrospinal fluid of patients affected with it was demonstrated in Uganda by Aldo Castellani (1879–1971) in 1902. *See African trypanosomiasis.*

Slit Lamp Used for microscopic study of the living eye. Invented by Swedish ophthalmologist Alvar Gullstrand (1862–1930) in 1903.

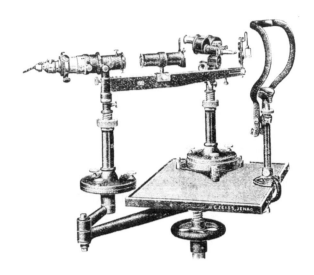

Alvar Gullstrand's slit lamp with corneal microscope. W.V. Freeman, *The British Journal of Physiological Optics*, II, 1927. British Optical Association, London

Sloane, Sir Hans (1660–1753) Physician from Killeleagh in Ireland who studied and practiced in London. He was physician to George II and founded the Chelsea Physick Garden, which he handed over to the Apothecaries Company in 1721. He had over 800 species of plants in his herbarium which he took with him to Jamaica when he was physician to its governor. He was president of the Royal Society in 1727 and advocated immunization for smallpox. His library of over 50,000 volumes and several thousands manuscripts were given to the British Museum.

Smallpox Vaccination *See inoculation.*

Smallpox A treatise on smallpox and measles, *Liber de variolis et morbillis*, was written by Rhazes (AD 860–932) in 910. He mentioned the *Pandects* of Alexandrian physician, Aaron who appears to have been well acquainted with it in the 7th century. It was probably present in India during the time of the *Athara Veda* of the Brahmins and they practiced inoculation. The term variola was used by Constantinius Africanus around 1080. The contagious nature was suggested by the English physician Gilbertus Anglicus in the 13th century, who advocated the use of red light as treatment. Red hangings in treatment were used by John of Gaddesden (1230–1361) and other Anglo-Norman physicians. The pathological differences between smallpox and measles were recognized by Giovanni Filippo Ingrassia (1510–1580). The first American treatise was written by Thomas Thacher (1620–1678) in 1677. Thomas Sydenham (1624–1689) clinically differentiated smallpox from measles in 1685. *See inoculation.*

Smee, Alfred (1818–1877) London surgeon who devised an electric cell made of two plates (one zinc and one platinized silver) in sulfuric acid.

Smegma [Latin: *smegma*, soap]Secretion of the sebaceous glands of the penis that derives its name from its soapy appearance behind the prepuce.

Smell Caspar Bartholin the Elder (1585–1629), a physician from Copenhagen, Denmark, described the functions of the olfactory nerve in 1611. The olfactory apparatus of fish, birds, reptiles and man was studied by Antonio Scarpa (1747–1832) in 1789. The islets of olfactory cells in the hippocampal cortex were described by Julián Calleja y Sánchez (1836–1913), professor of anatomy at Madrid in 1893.

Smellie, William (1697–1763) Scottish surgeon and obstetrician from Lanark. He designed practical straight forceps for use in obstetrics in 1750 and improved longer forceps in 1754. Brachial palsy, later known as Erb palsy, was described by Smellie in 1763. Pelvimetry, study of the measurements of pelvis of the mother in relation to childbirth, was introduced by him in 1752.

Smilax Source of sarsaparilla and the steroid precursor, smilagenin.

Smiles, Samuel (1812–1904) Scottish writer and a medical graduate from Edinburgh University. He was a surgeon in Leeds and later became editor of the *Leeds Times*. His works include: *Physical Education* (1838), *Self Help* (1859), *Thrift* (1875), and *Duty* (1880).

Smith, Sir Alfred Sydney (1883–1969) Forensic medical expert from New Zealand. He was a professor of forensic medicine at Cairo in 1917 and was regius professor of forensic medicine at Edinburgh in 1928. He wrote *Textbook of Forensic Medicine* (1925), and *Mostly Murder* in 1959.

Smith, Eustace (1835–1914) Graduate of University College London who became personal physician to Leopold II, King of Belgium. He returned to London and was appointed physician to the East London Children's Hospital and the London Chest Hospital. He wrote *Wasting Diseases of Infants and Children* in 1868 and *A Practical Treatise on Diseases in Children* in 1884.

Smith Fracture Hand fracture, a reversed Colles fracture, named after Robert William Smith (1807–1873), professor of surgery at Trinity College, Dublin who described it in 1847. His *Treatise on Pathology, Diagnosis, and Treatment of Neuroma* on multiple neurofibromatosis in 1849 preceded Friedrich von Recklinghausen's (1833–1910) description by 33 years.

Smith, Sir Grafton Elliot (1871–1937) Australian neurologist and anthropologist graduated in medicine from Sydney University in 1892. He was professor of anatomy at Cairo in 1900, and occupied the chair of anatomy at Manchester (1909) and University College (1919). He was an authority on brain anatomy and human evolution. He published *Human History* in 1930, and several other works on sociology and evolution.

Smith, Hamilton Othaniel (b 1931) American molecular biologist, born in New York. He graduated from and worked at the Johns Hopkins Medical School. He discovered endonucleases in bacteria that can split DNA of invading phage particles and inactivate them. These endonucleases are known as restriction enzymes and are site-specific and now used in establishing DNA nucleotide sequences. He shared the Nobel Prize for Physiology or Medicine in 1978.

Smith, Henry (1862–1948) British surgeon in the Indian Medical Service who devised the clamp and cautery treatment of hemorrhoids. He described a method of extracting cataracts in the capsule in 1905.

Smith, James Lorrain (1862–1931) Scottish pathologist from Dumfries and pioneer in establishment of the pathological services. After qualifying from Edinburgh University, he was professor of pathology at Belfast, Manchester and Edinburgh. He founded the Pathological Society at Manchester in 1894.

Smith, Sir James Edward (1759–1828) English physician and naturalist from Norwich. He studied medicine at Edinburgh University and graduated from Leiden in 1786. He established the Linnean Society and was its first president. He wrote *English Botany*, *Flora Botanica*, *English Flora*, and *Introduction to Botany*.

Smith, Lester (1904–1992) English biochemist, educated at Chelsea Polytechnic. He worked on dietary requirement for vitamin A, developed the first commercial production of penicillin, isolated vitamin B12 and showed that it contains cobalt and used radiolabeling to distinguish forms of vitamin B12.

Smith, Michael (b 1932) British–Canadian biochemist, educated at the University of Manchester and moved to the University of British Columbia in 1956 and later became professor and director of the Biotechnology Laboratory. He discovered site-specific mutagenesis which is now used in altering the genetic code of organisms to produce useful proteins. He shared the Nobel Prize for Chemistry in 1993.

Smith, Nathan (1762–1829) Surgeon from Connecticut who gave an early account of osteomyelitis in 1827. He also described the contagious nature of typhoid in his treatise, *A Practical Essay on Typhus Fever* published in 1842. He was a founder of the Dartmouth Medical School.

Smith, Nathan Ryno (1797–1879) American surgeon who described an anterior suspensory apparatus for fractures of the lower extremity in 1867.

Smith–Petersen Nail Nail used for fixing fractures of the neck of the femur. Designed by a Boston orthopedic surgeon, Marius Nygaard Smith-Petersen (1886–1953) and colleagues (E.F. Cave and G.W. van Gorder) in 1931. He also described a method of osteotomy for ankylosing spondylitis (which he called rheumatoid arthritis) in 1945.

Smith, Theobald (1859–1934) American microbiologist and immunologist at Harvard University, who was born in Albany, New York. He demonstrated that the tick was the insect vector of Texas cattle fever and distinguished between human and bovine tuberculosis. He also laid the foundation for development of cholera vaccine and improved several other vaccines.

Smith, Sir Thomas (1833–1909) London surgeon who described loss of the femoral head due to acute inflammation in infancy in 1876. He also gave a description of craniohypophysial xanthomatosis (Hand–Schülter–Christian disease) in 1865.

Smith, Thomas Southwood (1788–1861) English physician from Somerset who graduated from Edinburgh University and became a physician to the Fever Hospital in London in 1824. He wrote *Treatise on Fever* in 1830.

Smith Papyrus *See Edwin Smith papyrus.*

Smithsonian Institution Founded by English chemist, James Lewis Macie Smithson (1765–1829), who was the illegitimate son of Sir Hugh Smithson Percy, first Duke of Northumberland. After the rejection of one of his treatises by the Royal Society of London in 1826, Smithson bequeathed a sum of 105,000 pounds to his nephew but stipulated that if he died without heirs the money was to be used to found 'at Washington, under the name of the Smithsonian Institution, an Establishment for the increase and diffusion of knowledge among men'. It was established by Act of Congress in 1846 and the American physicist and inventor of the first electromagnetic motor (1829), Joseph Henry (1797–1878) of New York, was its first secretary.

Smithy, Horace Gilbert (1914–1848) American cardiac surgeon who worked on a surgical treatment for aortic

stenosis. He suffered and died from it before he could find a cure. Charles P. Bailey took up the work and succeed in commissurotomy in aortic valve stenosis in 1950.

Smog A mixture of fog and smoke containing toxic substances from air pollution. It has caused considerable morbidity and mortality. A three-day smog in a small town in Pennsylvania made 6000 persons, or half the population, ill and killed 20 persons in 1948. One of the worst smogs occurred in London in 1952, and deaths exceeded 4000. *See air pollution.*

Smoking Introduced from South America into England by Sir Walter Raleigh in 1565, but the habit of smoking tobacco really started around 1586. King James I tried to stop the habit of tobacco smoking and, in 1602 he issued *Counterblaste to Tobacco* in which he described the habit as 'A custome loathesome to the eye, hateful to the nose, harmeful to brain, dangerous to the lung, and in the black stinking fume therof neerest resembling the horrible Stigian smoke of the pit that is bottomless'. The association of tobacco smoking with angina was noted by J. H. S. Beau (1806–1865) in 1861, and H. Favarger proposed that nicotine constricted coronary arteries in 1882. W. Huchard introduced the term 'tobacco angina' in 1899, and divided it into three groups: functional angina due to coronary artery spasm, organic angina due to nicotine sclerosis, and pseudoangina due to dyspepsia induced by smoking. G. D. Friedman and colleagues showed that angina in smoking was not unique. In 1968 a twelve year follow-up Framingham study demonstrated a positive correlation between heavy smoking and angina. Around the same time, O. Auerbach showed that advanced atherosclerosis of coronary arteries was three times more prevalent in heavy smokers. Dimness of vision due to tobacco was described by William Mackenzie (1791–1868) in England in 1835. A more accurate description was given by Jonathan Hutchinson (1828–1913) in 1864 and the subject was discussed exhaustively by Forster of Germany in 1868. Evarts Ambrose Graham (1883–1957), professor of surgery at Washington University, St Louis, associated smoking with lung cancer. Smoking as a cause of carcinoma of the lung was demonstrated by Sir William Richard Doll (b 1912) and Sir Austin Bradford Hill (b 1897) in 1950. It was listed as a risk factor for stroke by the American Medical Association in 1984. *See tobacco.*

Smollett, Tobias George (1721–1771) Physician from Dumbarton who studied medicine at Glasgow University in 1736 and obtained his MD from Marischal College Aberdeen in 1750. He moved to London in 1738 and wrote his first novel, *Roderick Random,* in 1749. He was a navy surgeon and lived in Jamaica for a short time before he wrote his second novel, *Peregrine Pickle,* in 1751 which criticized Akenside, Fielding and others. He was imprisoned for a short time for writing on the courage of Sir Charles Knowles in the *Critical Review.* His last novel *The Expeditions of Humphry Clinker,* was published in 1771.

Smooth Muscle Antibodies The presence of these in two thirds of patients with active chronic hepatitis, half with biliary cirrhosis, and a quarter with cryptogenic cirrhosis, was shown by G. D. Johnson, E. J. Holborrow and L. E. Glynn in 1965.

Smooth Muscle Contraction of smooth muscles in the wall of the smallest bronchial tubes during an asthma attack was shown by anatomist and physician, Franz Daniel Reinssensen (1773–1828) of Strasburg in 1808. The structure of various specialized cells, such as nerve cells and smooth muscle cells, was described by Theodor Schwann (1810–1882) in 1839. The presence of smooth muscle in the middle coat of smaller arteries was discovered by German histologist, Friedrich Gustav Jacob Henle (1809–1885) in 1844. They were isolated from the tissues by Swiss anatomist, Rudolf Albert von Kölliker (1817–1905) in 1852.

Smyth, James Carmichael (1741–1821) Physician who studied medicine at Edinburgh University and Leiden. He discovered a method of destroying contagion using nitrous oxide, for which he was remunerated by Parliament in 1802. He wrote several pamphlets and an edition of Dr Sark's works.

Snake Bite *See orphidism.*

Snakeroot The plant *Aristolochia serpantaria* was included as a medicine in Gerard's Herbal published by Thomas Johnson, an apothecary in London in 1636. Its use for bites of rattlesnakes was described by Dale (1693) and Geoffrey (1741). It is also used as a stimulant, tonic and diaphoretic.

Sneezing Being aware that it may precede illness, the ancient Greeks said a short prayer to Jupiter, 'help me', every time they sneezed. To stop hiccup Hippocrates (460–377 BC) advised gargling with water and tickling the nose to induce sneezing. Galen (AD 129–200) thought that hiccup was caused by irritation of the stomach leading to violent reaction, and suggested sneezing as a cure. A dissertation, written by Martin Skooskis, was published in the French *Journal des Scavens* in 1665.

Snell, Albert Markley (1896–1960) *See Addison disease.*

Snell, George Davis (b 1903) American geneticist who demonstrated that X-rays can induce mutations in mammals. He worked on the genes responsible for rejection of tissue transplants in mice, the histocompatibility genes or major histocompatibility complex (MHC). He shared the Nobel Prize for Physiology or Medicine with French immunologist, Jean Baptiste Gabriel Dausset (b 1916) and Venezuelan–American immunologist, Baruj Benacerraf (b 1920), for their work in this area. *See histocompatibilty.*

Snell, Simeon (1851–1909) English ophthalmologist.

Snellen Chart Test for visual acuity of the eye devised by Hermann Snellen (1834–1908), a Dutch ophthalmologist at Utrecht in 1862.

Snellius or Willebrord Snell (1591–1626) Professor of mathematics at Leiden who discovered the law of refraction in 1624. The same law was proposed by René Descartes (1596–1650).

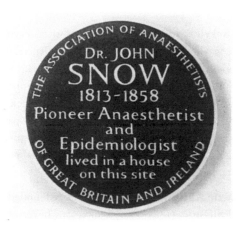

John Snow. Commemorative plaque erected at 54 Frith Street, London

Snow, John (1813–1858) Anesthetist and epidemiologist from York. He started his medical studies in Newcastle Infirmary where he developed an interest in the epidemiology of cholera. He moved to London in 1836 and graduated in medicine in 1844. He was a lecturer in forensic medicine at the Aldersgate School of Medicine until 1849. During the cholera outbreaks of 1848 and 1854 in London, he traced the source of an outbreak to sewage contaminating a well in Soho and he later implicated the river Thames as a source of infection. His work helped to abort the epidemics. As an anesthetist, he invented the ether inhaler and was anesthetist to St George's Hospital in 1847. He virtually put an end to objections to the use of chloroform in obstetrics by administering the agent to Queen Victoria during the delivery of Prince Leopold in 1853. The endotracheal method of inducing anesthesia was tried on animals by him in 1858 and he published *On Chloroform and other Anaesthetics* in the same year.

Snyder, Solomon Halbert (b 1938) American psychiatrist and pharmacologist from Washington who investigated the biochemistry of nervous tissue. He researched catecholamines from different areas of the brain, examined turnover of ornithine decarboxylase and its relation to opiates and psychotropic drugs and found opiate receptors in nervous tissue. He has also investigated cyclic AMP transport and nitric oxide.

Soberheim, Joseph Friedrich (1803–1846) German physician who introduced the word myocarditis in 1837.

Soberheim Method Combined active and passive immunization for anthrax, widely adopted in Germany and South America. Introduced by G. Soberheim of Berlin in 1902. He used a combination of immune serum from cattle and a preparation of attenuated growth of the anthrax bacillus to make his vaccine.

Social Services in Medicine The first social service in the world was started at the Massachusetts General Hospital outpatient department by its physician, Richard C. Cabot (1868–1939) in 1907. He realized the social responsibility of the hospital for those who were affected by sickness and expanded his services to include beds for such patients in 1914. Ida M. Canon was first chief of the Hospital Social Services at the MGH and it became an integral part of the hospital in 1919.

Societé de Anthropologie Paris society founded in 1869 with Paul Broca (1824–1880) as director. The Anthropological Society of London was formed in 1863 and that of New York in 1865.

Society for Psychical Research Founded in London in 1882 under the presidency of Henry Sidgewick, professor of moral philosophy at the University of Cambridge.

Society of Experimental Psychologists American society founded in 1904 by Edward Bradford Titchener (1867–1927), a naturalized American psychologist from Chichester, England.

Socrates (470–399 BC) Athenian philosopher, son of Sophroniscus, a sculptor, and Phaenerete, a midwife. He is regarded as the instigator of inductive reasoning and abstract definitions. He left no writings and most of his works were made known through Plato (428–347 BC) and Xenophon. Plato met Socrates at the age of 20 years and remained his pupil for eight years. Socrates was a censor of public wrongs and private follies and opposed state tyrants, which eventually earned him a death sentence. Hemlock was used in his official execution and described by Plato in

Phaedo. Plato states 'Socrates after swallowing the poison cup walked about for a short time as he was directed by the executioner, when he felt a sense of heaviness in his limbs he laid down on his back, his feet and legs fast lost their sensibility and became stiff and cold, and the state gradually extended towards the heart, when he died convulsed'.

Soddy, Frederick (1877–1956) English radiochemist, born in Eastbourne. He was professor of chemistry at Glasgow, Oxford and Aberdeen. The atomic disintegration hypothesis which stated that radioactive elements made of complex particles undergo spontaneous changes, or disintegrate and discharge high velocity negatively charged electrons or beta rays and positively charged particles or alpha rays, was put forward by Ernest Rutherford (1871–1937) and Soddy in 1902. He used the word 'isotope' to denote elements with identical chemical qualities but different atomic weights. He received the Nobel Prize for Chemistry in 1921. He wrote *Science and Life* (1920).

Sodium Sulfate Glauber salt. *See Glauber, John Rudolph*

Sodium Discovered by Sir Humphry Davy (1778–1829) in 1807. The characteristic spectrum was observed by Irish physicist, Sir George Gabriel Stokes (1819–1903) during his experiments with a prism on the flames produced by a spirit lamp in 1845. Sydney Ringer (1835–1910) studied metabolite antagonism in 1883 and found that cations of sodium could not maintain the beat of an isolated heart unless balanced by calcium and potassium. A reagent for estimating sodium was discovered by H. H. Barber in 1928. A method of estimating it in biological fluids was devised by Albert Macy Butler (b 1894) who worked with Fuller Albright (1900–1969) in describing Albright syndrome. Its importance in diet of patients with Addison disease was demonstrated by Robert Frederick Loeb and G. A. Harrop of America in 1933. A low sodium diet in treatment of heart failure was shown by Henry Alfred Schroeder (1906–1975) in 1941. Dependency of action potential of the cell on sodium concentration was shown by Sir Alan Lloyd Hodgkin (b 1914) and Sir Bernard Katz (b 1911) in 1949.

Soft Chancre *See chancroid.*

Soldier Heart *See Da Costa syndrome.*

Sollmann, Torald Hermann (1874–1965) *See carotid sinus depressor reflex.*

Solution A systematic work on diffusion of dissolved substances and their properties was written by Thomas Graham (1805–1869). He distinguished crystalloid from colloid on the basis of diffusion in 1857. Substances which passed through parchment paper were named crystalloids by him and those which did not were colloids.

Solvent Abuse The habit of sniffing of glue, gasoline, nail polish, plastic cement or similar substances was reported in the United States around 1952.

Somagyi Unit Biochemical assay named after American biochemist, Michael Somagyi (b 1883) of St Louis. He described a method of determining serum amylase, used in the diagnosis of acute pancreatitis, in 1940. A method of measuring reducing sugars in the blood was devised by him in 1926.

Somastatin [Greek: *soma*, body + *statikos*, causing to stand] Inhibitor of hypothalamic hormone isolated and named by Roger Guillemein and colleagues in 1973. It was synthesized later in the same year by D. H. Coy and co-workers at the Tulane University School of Medicine.

Somatotropin [Greek: *soma*, body + *trophein*, to nourish] *See growth hormone.*

Sömmering, Samuel Thomas (1755–1830) German professor of anatomy in Kassel, Mainz, Munich and Frankfurt-am-Main. He described the long pudendal nerve, the suspensory ligament of lachrymal gland and several other structures which are named after him. He also described the crossing fibers of the optic nerves in 1786.

Soranus of Ephesus (AD 98–117) Physician who first practiced in Alexandria and later in Rome, during the reigns of Hadrian and Trajan. He is considered the founder of obstetrics and gynecology. He wrote *On the Diseases of Women*, a standard on the subject for over 15 centuries. He advised contraception with cotton, ointments and fatty substances and denounced mechanical measures for abortion. He also wrote on childhood diseases, hygiene, pharmacology and fractures. Some of his extant works were published in Greek in Paris in 1554.

Sorby, Henry Clifton (1826–1908) Geologist from Woodhouse near Sheffield who introduced the study of rocks with a microscope. His *On the Microscopic Structure of the Calcareous Grit of the Yorkshire Coast* was published in 1851.

Sorcerer Cave paintings have revealed their influence during prehistoric times. They were often called upon to cure diseases which paved the way for them to become medicine men. They practiced trepanning, perforation of the skull and blood letting. Ancient sorcerers also attained considerable knowledge of herbal medicines, poisons and animal products as cures. *See demonology.*

Sørensen, Soren Peter Lauritz (1868–1939) Danish chemist and director of the Carlsberg Research Laboratory in Copenhagen. He described the effect of hydrogen ion concentration on enzyme activity and introduced the pH scale, the word 'buffer' and the general equation for the relationship between acids and bases (the Henderson-Hasselbalch equation). *See buffer, pH scale.*

Sottas, Jules (b 1886) *See Dejerine disease.*

Soubeiran, Eugene (1793–1858) French chemist who discovered chloroform in 1831, independently of Justus von Liebig (1803–1873) and Samuel Guthrie (1782–1848).

South, John Flint (1797–1882) Surgeon who trained in Germany before he was appointed to St Thomas' Hospital. The body of John Hunter (1728–1793) was reburied at Westminster Abbey through his efforts. He published *Household Surgery and Hints on Emergencies*.

Souttar, Sir Henry Sessions (b 1875) *See cardiac surgery.*

Space Medicine Related to physiological and health problems arising out of exploration of space beyond Earth's atmosphere. Interest started with H.G. Armstrong's paper which appeared in the *United States Armed Forces Medical Journal* in 1959. In the same year C.A. Roos produced a bibliography of 446 references. A summary of physiological requirements of man in a sealed cabin was given by R.M. Fenno in 1954. *The pathology of boredom* was published by W. Heron in 1957. A paper on *Potable water recycled from human urine* by J. Sendroy and H.A. Collison appeared in 1958. The implications of radiation in space flight was studied independently by W.H. Langham and H.J. Schaefer in 1959.

Spalding, Alfred Baker (1874–1942) American gynecologist in San Francisco who described an operation for uterine prolapse in 1919.

Spallanzani, Lazaro (1729–1799) Italian physiologist, born in Modena and educated at Bologna before he became a priest. His studies on experimental physiology showed that digestion differed from putrefaction and fermentation in wine and that a sealed vessel of broth did not decay. He showed that blood passes from arteries to veins in a warm blooded animal. He demonstrated that hydrochloric acid was produced by the stomach and established the fact that spermatozoa were essential for fertilization in 1786. He successfully used artificial insemination in amphibians, silkworms and a dog. He wrote *Experiments on the reproduction of Animals*, *Essay on Animalcula in Fluids* and *Microscopical Experiments*.

Spastic Diplegia Cerebral palsy with mental deficiency and muscle weakness in the newborn (Little disease) due to variety of causes such as asphyxia, birth injury and prematurity was described by William John Little (1810–1894), a London orthopedic surgeon in *Deformities of the Human Frame* published in 1843. In his second monograph, *On the Influence of Abnormal Parturition, Difficult Labours etc., upon the Mental and Physical Condition of the Child*, was published in 1862, Little attributed intracranial hemorrhage as the cause in 75% of cases of spastic paralysis.

Specialization Ancient Egyptian physicians specialized in various diseases and records exist of a court physician who called himself the 'Keeper of the King's Rectum' around 2500 BC. At this time Egypt was full of oculists who sometimes specialized in the left or right eye. Herodotus (484–425 BC) commented 'Medicine with them (Egyptians) is distributed so that every physician is for one disease, not for several. The whole country is full of physicians for the eyes, others of the head, others of the teeth, others of belly, and others of obscure diseases'.

Species [Latin: *species*, particular kind] The concept of a group of organisms or species was proposed by French naturalist, Count George Louis Leclerc de Buffon (1707–1788) of Burgundy in 1749. The terms genus and species were used in the system of classification to include every known living thing developed by Carl Linnaeus (1707–1778).

Specific Gravity [Latin: *specificus*, particular kind + *gravid*, heavy] The principle was discovered by Archimedes around 250 BC and he described it in *On Floating Bodies*. Richard Schmaltz, a physician in Dresden, described a method of estimating specific gravity of blood in 1890. A hydrometer for determining it in small volumes of urine was devised by New York physician, George Alexander De Santos (1876–1911) in 1903. The value as an indicator of renal function was advocated by Franz Volhard (b 1872) of Berlin in 1918.

Specific Heat [Latin: *specificus*, particular kind] The concept of quantity of heat required to raise equal weights of different substances through the same temperature was proposed by Irvine, a pupil of Joseph Black (1728–1799). He called it the capacity of heat and it was re-named specific heat by Johan Gadolin (1760–1852) in 1784. The distinction between latent heat and specific heat was made by German-born Swedish physicist, Johan Carl Wilcke (1732–1796) in 1781.

Spectacles [Latin: *spectacula*, to see] Use of magnifying glasses was known to Nero and Seneca (d AD 65), who used ground and polished gems to correct defective sight. Alhazen wrote a book on optics, *Kitab Al-Manazir*, which included refraction, reflection and study of lenses. This was the first step towards the invention of spectacles. Roger Bacon (1214–1294) suggested use of lenses to aid the sight around 1270. The word was used by a Scottish professor at Montpellier, Bernard de Gordon, around 1307 and invented by Savinus Aramatus or Salvino degli Aramati of Pisa around 1300. Some illustrations are found in paintings dating from 1352. They were prescribed for shortsight by Hollorius and others in 1550 and for the near-sighted by Nicholas Krebs of Germany, also known as Nicholas of Cusa, in 1450. They were cumbersome and mounted on wood, metal or leather, but improved during the 15th and 16th centuries. The modern form, with hinged side pieces, came into use in the latter half of the 18th century. A combination of short and long lenses to bring distant objects near was invented by Dutch lensmaker, Hans Lippershey (1571–1619). Use of prismatic and cylindrical lenses was introduced by Dutch ophthalmologist and physiologist, Franciscus Cornelis Donders (1818–1889) of Utrecht.

Spectroscopy [Latin: *spectrum*, image + *skopein*, to view] Robert Wilhelm Bunsen (1811–1899) and Gustav Robert Kirchhoff (1824–1887) in 1859 constructed a prism spectroscope. Sir William Huggins (1824–1910) attached a spectroscope to a telescope and studied lines seen around 40 stars in 1862. He also noted that when a star receded the lines were displaced towards the red end of the spectrum. English astronomer, Sir Norman Lockyer (1836–1920) of Rugby, predicted a new element 'helium', which was discovered by Ramsay in 1895. It was used to determine the chemical composition of the Sun and stars by an Irish physicist, Sir George Gabriel Stokes (1819–1903), professor of mathematics at Cambridge, around 1845. His experiments with a prism on a flame produced by a spirit lamp allowed him to identify the spectrum of sodium and laid the foundation for spectroscopic analysis of various metals and other substances. A spectroscopic survey of stars was done by the Italian astronomer, Angelo Secchi (1818–1878), who catalogued over 4000 stars. Victor Stokes Schumann, an engineer from Leipzig, extended spectroscopy to the ultraviolet spectrum in 1892. The Nobel Prize for Physics for studies on spectroscopic measurement of light was awarded to Albert Abraham Michelson (1852–1931) of America in 1907. *See absorption spectra, dispersion.*

Spectrum [Latin: image] Dispersion of light into its wavelengths. It was shown by Sir Isaac Newton (1642–1727) using a small hole cut in wall of a darkened room with a prism in its path, resulting in the production of intense colors. This principle was used by Robert Wilhelm Bunsen (1811–1899) and Gustav Robert Kirchhoff (1824–1887) to develop their spectrometer in 1859. *See spectroscopy.*

Speculum [Latin: *specula*, mirror] Used for examining internal organs since the time of Hippocrates (460–377 BC). Blepharoxyston or speculum oculi was an ancient instrument used to examine the eye. Hippocrates mentioned a rectal speculum and Paul of Aegina (625–690) devised one with two blades which could be adjusted according to the size of the patient. Soranus of Ephesus (AD 98–117) used a vaginal speculum. The English proctologist and surgeon, John of Ardane (1307–1390), used one to examine the rectum during the Middle Ages. James Marion Sims (1813–1883) of South Carolina used a bent spoon to visualize a vesical fistula in a female in 1845. This was developed into the Sims duck-billed speculum. Another vaginal instrument was designed by Joseph Claude Anthelme Recamier (1774–1852) of Paris. Sir William Fergusson (1808–1877), a Scottish surgeon and pupil of Robert Knox (1791–1862), devised several surgical instruments including a vaginal speculum. The speculum for examination of the ear was invented by British otologist, Joseph Tonybee (1815–1866).

Speech Leon Scott de Martinville, an American of French origin, made graphic recordings of speech using a vibrating membrane and a stylus in 1856. A patent on an apparatus to transmit recorded speech was obtained by Thomas Alva Edison (1847–1931) in 1877. Alexander Graham Bell (1847–1922), Scottish-born professor of vocal physiology at Boston University, was interested in education of deaf mutes and invented an electrical device to transfer speech into a visible form in 1876. His work led to the invention of the telephone in 1876. A voice-operated computer system to interpret speech and answer in a synthetic voice was invented by two Americans, Thomas Martins and R. B. Cox, in 1973. *See speech disorders.*

Speech Disorder Aphasia was described by Carl Linnaeus (1707–1778) in 1745 and the site of the lesion in the brain causing it was suggested by Jean Baptiste Boullaud (1796–1881) in 1825. It was called 'alalia' by Lordet in 1841, Pierre Paul Broca (1824–1880) of Paris re-named it 'aphemia' and Chrysaphis gave it the current name. Pierre Marie (1853–1940) of Paris, during his experiments on the cerebellum, demonstrated the classical symptoms (staggering, tremor and slurring of speech) by ablation of the cerebellum. Henry Charlton Bastian (1837–1915), a British neurologist, described sensory aphasia in 1869. This was called 'word deafness' by Adolf Kussmaul (1822–1902),

and the site of its lesion in the brain was identified by Karl Wernicke (1848–1904). The motor speech center in the brain, the Broca area, was found in the third frontal convolution of the brain of a 21-year-old patient with aphasia during autopsy by Broca in 1861. A collective study on speech defects was done by English neurologist, John Hughlings Jackson (1853–1911) in 1864. Sir Henry Head (1861–1940), a neurologist at the London Hospital, published *Aphasia and kindred disorders of speech* in 1926.

Speed Fusion Operation for malunited fractures of the ankle joint. Devised by American surgeon, James Spencer Speed (b 1890) of Memphis, in 1936.

Speed Operation For recurrent anterior dislocation of the shoulder using a bone graft. Described by American surgeon, Kellog Speed (b 1879), in 1927.

Spemann, Hans (1869–1941) German zoologist, born in Stuttgart and educated at Stuttgart and Heidelberg, and became professor at Rostock in 1908. He showed that the fate of embryonic cells was influenced by adjacent cells and tissues. He wrote *Embryonic Development and Induction* in 1938. He was awarded the Nobel Prize for Physiology or Medicine in 1935.

Spence Axillary Tail Part of the mammary gland extending towards the axilla. Described by James Spence (1812–1882), professor of surgery at Edinburgh in 1871.

Spencer, Herbert (1820–1903) British philosopher, born in Derby. He worked as a railway engineer, teacher, journalist and subeditor before turning to full-time writing. His main interest was evolutionary theory and he wrote *Principles of Psychology* in 1855. He also wrote on ethics and sociology and was an advocate of 'social Darwinism', the idea that societies evolve in competition for resources and that survival of the fittest was morally justifiable. He also wrote: *System of Synthetic Philosophy, Principles of Biology, Principles of Psychology, Principles of Sociology* and *Principles of Ethics. See evolution theory.*

Spencer Wells Forceps Sir Thomas Spencer Wells (1818–1897) was a gynecologist from St Albans, Hertfordshire. He advocated clamping of blood vessels by forceps to arrest bleeding during surgery. He called this 'forci-pressure' and devised forceps for the purpose.

Spens, Thomas (1769–1842) Son of Nathaniel Spens, a physician in Edinburgh. He was a Fellow of the Royal College of Physicians at the age of 25 and gave an account of heart block in 1793. *See heart block.*

Sperm *See spermatozoa.*

Spermatocyte [Greek: *sperma*, seed + *kytos*, cell] *See spermatozoa.*

Spermatozoa [Greek: *sperma*, seed + *zoon*, animal] Gardinius postulated the existence of particles in semen affecting fertilization in 1623. Antoni van Leeuwenhoek (1632–1723) observed particles under the microscope in the semen, similar to tadpoles, and this led to the discovery of spermatozoa in 1677. However, Leeuwenhoek and other scientists of the period continued to believe that the spermatozoa contained the life-giving properties of the embryo and that the ovum merely acted as a nutrient base. Lazaro Spallanzani (1729–1799), an Italian physician, showed that spermatozoa were essential for fertilization in 1786. Their cellular origin was described by Rudolf Albert von Kölliker (1817–1905) in 1841, and evidence that they contained a nucleus was provided by Franz Schweigger-Seidel (1834–1871) and LaValette St George in 1865. *See fertilization.*

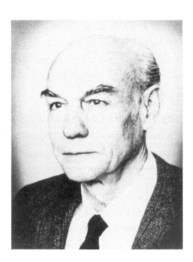

Roger Wolcott Sperry (b 1913)

Sperry, Roger Wolcott (b 1913) American neuroscientist from Hartford, Connecticut. He was Hixson professor of psychobiology at Caltech from 1954 to 1984. He helped establish the way in which nerve cells are wired into the central nervous system and pioneered split-brain experiments. The latter showed that each hemisphere had specific functions. He shared the Nobel Prize for Physiology or Medicine in 1981.

Sphenoid Bone [Greek: *speno*, wedge] Depicted in the first of the seven books of Andreas Vesalius (1514–1564), *De Fabrica Humani Corporis* in 1543

Spherocytosis [Greek: *sphaira*, globe + *kytos*, cell] *See acholuric jaundice, congenital spherocytosis.*

Sphincter of Oddi At the termination of the bile duct.

Described by Francis Glisson (1597–1677) in 1654 and re-described by Ruggero Oddi (1864–1913) from the University of Perugia in 1887.

Sphygmograph [Greek: *sphygmos*, pulse + *graph*, write] *See sphygmomanometer.*

Sphygmomanometer [Greek: *sphygmos*, pulse + *metron*, measure] A mercury manometer to measure blood pressure was devised by Jean Léonard Marie Poiseulle (1799–1869) in 1828 and was known as Poiseulle hemodynometer. A practical method of frequently measuring blood pressure by applying counter pressure to the artery was devised by Karl Vierordt (1818–1884) of Germany in 1854. This was cumbersome due to the attachment of weights, and further improved models using a pneumatic cuff were produced and introduced into clinical medicine by Samuel Sigfried Ritter von Basch (1837–1905) in 1881 and Scipione Riva Rocci (1863–1939), an Italian physician from the department of pathological medicine of the University of Turin, in 1896. A simple portable air machine was devised by Pierre Carl Edouard Potain (1825–1901) in 1889. The Roger sphygmomanometer used an aneroid manometer instead of mercury and was designed by New York physician, Oscar H. Roger, around 1887. A machine for measuring blood pressure in the finger was invented by Angelo Mosso (1846–1910) in 1895. *See blood pressure.*

Spider Naevi *See Bouchard, Charles Jacques.*

Spiegelberg, Otto (1830–1881) German gynecologist from Hannover who studied medicine at Göttingen and graduated in 1851. He accurately described the paraovarian cysts and performed curettage of the uterus for retained tissues. He wrote *Das Compendium der Geburtshilfe*, a popular textbook of obstetrics, at the age of 28 years.

Spighel Lobe *See caudate lobe of the liver.*

Spina Bifida (Syn: hydrorachitis, clove spine) The Arabians attempted to treat this under the impression that it was due to deficient spinous process. Benjamin Bell, a student of John Hunter (1728–1793) and surgeon to the Edinburgh Royal Infirmary, believed that it was a result of spinal marrow disease and that there was no cure. John Abernethy (1764–1831) of St Bartholomew's Hospital, tried applying gentle pressure to cause the fluid to be absorbed. Repeated aspiration as treatment was performed by Sir Astley Paston Cooper (1768–1841) of Guy's Hospital in 1809. English surgeon, Sir Arthur William Mayo Robson (1853–1933), described a method of plastic surgery in 1885. Julius Arnold (1835–1915), a Heidelberg physician, gave an account in 1894. American surgeon, William Wayne Babcock (b 1872) of Philadelphia, devised an operation in 1911 and Wilder Graves Penfield (b 1891), a surgeon in Montreal, described another in 1932.

Spina Ventosa Term used by Arab physicians to refer to a disease of the bone which discharged its contents through the surface of the skin. It is essentially chronic osteomyelitis and was described under that name by Samuel Cooper (1780–1848), professor of surgery at University College London. He performed a successful partial but extensive resection of the affected tibia in a young woman from Richmond for chronic osteomyelitis.

Spinal Accessory Nerve Eleventh cranial nerve (nerve of Willis). Described by Thomas Willis (1621–1675) in *Cerebri anatome*, published in 1664.

Spinal Anesthesia Introduced by a neurologist, James Leonard Corning (1885–1923), of New York in 1885. August Karl Gustav Bier (1861–1949) of Kiel used cocaine in 1899 and Heinrich Irenaeus Quincke (1842–1922) experimented with lumbar punctures on himself and described the procedure in 1891. Successful subarachnoid block using cocaine was performed by Karl Gustav August Bier (b 1861) of Berlin in 1889. It was introduced into Britain by Barker of University College in 1907. In France it was popularized by French surgeon, Marin Théodore Tuffier (1857–1929). Stovain was introduced by Ernest Fourneau (1872–1949) of France in 1904. This was followed by Novocaine or procaine by Russian-born American physician, Max Einhorn (1862–1953), in 1905. Percaine or Nupercaine was synthesized by Meischer in 1929 and used in England by W. H. Jones of Charing Cross Hospital in 1930. *See anesthesia.*

Spinal Caries *See caries of the spine.*

Spinal Cord The ancient Chinese believed that it opened into the testicles and Greek physicians thought that the cerebrospinal fluid poured into the pharynx. Charles Estienne (1503–1564) of Paris described the central canal. Its role in reflex action was demonstrated by Stephen Hales (1677–1761) who noted in 1730 the reflex withdrawal of the leg in a decapitated frog could be abolished by inducing a lesion in the spinal cord. Peter Johann Frank (1745–1821), a Bavarian physician, focused his studies on diseases of the spinal cord in 1792. Charles Frederick Burdach (1776–1847), professor of medicine at Dorpat, described the posterior column in 1819. The role of the ventral and dorsal roots in reflex reaction was discovered by Sir Charles Bell (1774–1842) (1811) and François Magendie (1783–1855) (1822). Its segmental nature and interface with the higher centers was demonstrated by Marshall Hall (1790–1857) in 1833.

Friedrich Goll (1829–1903), a neuroanatomist from Zurich and a contemporary of Rudolph Virchow (1821–1902), described fasciculus gracilis or the posterior column in 1868. Embryonic development was described by Carl Ernst von Baer (1792–1876), a Russian embryologist from Estonia, in 1769. The ciliospinal and genitospinal centers were described by Julius Ludwig Budge (1811–1884), professor of physiology at Bonn, in 1841. A classic work on the conduction pathways was done by French neurologist, Édouard Brown-Séquard (1817–1894), in 1863. Abolition of the tendon reflexes in the lower extremities associated with lesions above the lumbar segment was demonstrated by a British neurologist, Henry Charlton Bastian (1837–1915) from Truro. Muscular rigidity of the body produced by transection of the spinal cord through the upper part of the midbrain was described by Sir Charles Scott Sherrington (1857–1952) of Oxford University in 1897. Sir Victor Alexander Haden Horsley (1857–1916), the founder of neurosurgery in England, removed a tumor in 1888. *Reflex Activity of the Spinal Cord* was published by Sherrington, Sir Arthur Carew Eccles (b 1903), Creed, Derek Ernest Denny-Brown (1901–1981) and Edward George Tandy Liddell (1895–1981) in 1932.

Spinal Curvature The prevention and treatment was described in a book on orthopedics written by Nicolas André (1658–1742) in 1741. The method of anterior spinal fusion was introduced by Russell Aubra Hibbs (1869–1932) of New York and Fred Houdlett Albee (1876–1945) in the treatment of Pott disease in 1906. Their technique was also applied as treatment for scoliosis by Hibbs in 1924.

Spinal Fluid Pressure A water manometer to measure spinal fluid pressure was devised by Boston neurologist, James Bourne Ayer (1882–1963) in 1920.

Spinal Fusion *See scoliosis.*

Spinal Injury An institution for treating them as a specialty in England, the Stoke Mandeville Hospital, was established by Sir Ludwig Guttmann in 1944. The Bradford frame for spinal disorders was devised by American surgeon, Edward Hickling Bradford (1848–1926), in 1890. A classification was proposed by Sir Frank Wild Holdsworth (1904–1969) in 1963. The Halo traction for skeletal fixation of the spine was devised by Vernon L. Nickel, professor of orthopedics at the University of California, San Diego, in 1968. A spring loading device for use in injuries of the spinal cord was introduced by Marian Weiss (1921–1981) from Poland in 1975.

Spinal Nerves Galen (AD 129–200), René Descartes (1596–

1650) and Robert Whytt (1714–1766) suggested the existence of motor and sensory nerves. Sir Charles Bell (1774–1842) established the motor function of the ventral nerve roots in 1811 and the sensory function of the dorsal spinal nerve roots was demonstrated by François Magendie (1783–1855) in 1822. The importance of unmyelinated nerve fibers in the dorsal roots was recognized by Chicago neurologist Stephen Walter Ranson (b 1880) in 1912. *See autonomic nervous system, spinal cord.*

Spinal Puncture *See lumbar puncture.*

Spinal Tuberculosis *See caries of the spine.*

Spinal Tumor The earliest removal was performed by Cline in 1814 and, although his patient died, his treatment aroused considerable interest. Scottish surgeon, Sir William Macewen (1848–1924), reported a successful operation in 1885. British surgeons, Sir Victor Alexander Haden Horsley(1857–1916) and Sir William Richard Gowers (1845–1915), presented a case of successful removal in 1888.

Spinhaler Method of delivery of drugs to the lungs via inhalation, used as treatment for asthma. Developed by a Syrian-born British physician, Edward Collingwood Alyounyan (1922–1987).

Spinning Mule A hybrid between Arkwright's spinning jenny and James Hargreaves water frame was invented by Samuel Crompton (1753–1827) of Bolton, Lancashire in 1779. Scrotal cancer (mule spinners' cancer) due to prolonged contact with lubricating oil in the spindles of the cotton-mule was recognized by S. R. Wilson of the Royal Infirmary Manchester in 1906.

Spinoza, Benedict de (1632–1677) Dutch philosopher and lens maker in Leiden who wrote a treatise on optics in 1671. His doctrine of pantheism, advocating intellectual love of god, was controversial and was published after his death.

Spinster A monograph on gynecological diseases of spinsters was written by Georg Ernst Stahl (1660–1734) in 1724.

Spiranolactone *See aldosterone antagonist.*

Spirillum [Greek: *speira*, spiral] Genus of bacteria, including *Spirillum rubrum*, isolated from a decomposing mouse by E. Esmarch in 1887.

Spirochaete [Greek: *speira*, spiral + *chaite*, hair] Term coined in 1833 by Christian Gottfried Ehrenberg (1795–1876) to denote a large flexible motile microorganism found in water. It was later confined to organisms twisted spirally around their axis. *Borrelia recurrentis*, the causative organism of relapsing fever, was discovered by German physician,

Otto Hugo Franz Obermeier (1843–1873) in 1873. *Treponema vincenti*, found in the throat of patients with Vincent angina, was identified by Jean Hyacinthe Vincent (1862–1950) in 1898. The pathogenic spirochete, *Treponema pallidum*, was discovered in 1905 by Fritz Richard Schaudinn (1871–1906) from Germany who worked as protozoologist at the Institute of Tropical Diseases at Hamburg.

Spirometer [Latin: *spirare*, to breathe + *metron*, measure] Apparatus to measure the vital capacity of the lung. Invented by English physician, John Hutchison (1811–1861) in 1846. *See lung function.*

Spitzka, Edward Charles (1852–1914) New York neurologist who graduated from Vienna. He was editor of the *American Journal of Neurology* and wrote several treatises on neurology. The fibers of the posterior longitudinal bundle connecting the 3rd and 6th nerve cranial nuclei (Bundle of Spitzka) were described by him in 1876.

Spleen [Greek: *splen*, spleen] Described as part of the hepatic system by Averrhoes (1126–1198) who called it the second liver. Aristotle (384–322 BC) in *Historia animalium* compared the anatomical features of hog and human spleen. Paul of Aegina (625–690) described its function as attraction of melancholic humors from the liver without which a black jaundice would intervene. John Zaccharius Acturius of Byzantine in 1300 stated that it attracts melancholic humors. Hippocrates (460–377 BC) described several afflictions in *de Internis affectionibus*. Caelius Aurelianus, a physician in the fifth century, suggested that it should be cut out if it is diseased. Rufus of Ephesus (AD 98–138) considered it to be a useless organ. Italian physician, Guiseppe Zambeccari (1655–1721) at Florence demonstrated that it is not essential for life, in 1680. A splenectomy was performed by Carl Friedrich Quittenbaum (1793–1852) in 1826, but his patient died of shock within six hours. Simon Gustav of Darmstadt, professor at Rostock and Heidelberg, performed the procedure and wrote a monograph in 1857. A spleenectomy in England was performed by Sir Spencer Wells (1818–1897) in 1865, and his patient lived for six days. A successful spleenectomy was done by Jules Émile Péan (1830–1898) in 1867. The immune compromised state following spleenectomy was shown by Deutsch in 1899. Overwhelming sepsis in patients who had a splenectomy was described by H. King and H.B. Shumacker in 1952. Susceptibility of these patients to pneumococcal infection was noted by A. Traub and colleagues in 1987.

Splenic Rupture A case was reported by Leeds surgeon, Edward Atkinson (1830–1905) in 1874. Shifting of dullness in the left flank by clotting of blood in the left paracolic gutter was described by English surgeon, Sir Charles Alfred Ballance (1856–1936), in 1898. Delayed bleeding from the spleen after trauma was noted by London surgeon, Archibald Hector McIndoe (1900–1960), in 1932.

Splint Rigid appliance used for immobilization in cases of fracture or deformity since ancient times. *See Agnew splint, Cabot splint, Gooch splint, Gunning splint, Hodgen splint, Stader splint, Stromeyer splint, Thomas splint, fractures.*

Spock, Benjamin (1903–1998) American pediatrician from New Haven, Connecticut. He graduated from Columbia University in 1929 and became famous through his book, *Baby and Child Care*, written for the general public. He was an opponent of American involvement in Vietnam and was convicted for evading war service in 1968.

Spondylolisthesis [Greek: *spondylos*, vertebra + *olisthanein*, to slip] A description was given by Viennese surgeon, Karl Freiherr Rokitansky (1804–1878), in 1839. Hermann Friedrich Kilian (1800–1863), professor of gynecology at Bonn, pointed out the importance of spondylolisthetic pelvis in pregnancy in 1853. A treatise on the etiology and causes was published by Franz Ludwig Neugebauer (1856–1914) of Germany, in 1885.

Spondylotherapy [Greek: *spondylos*, vertebra + *therapio*, to care for] Method of treating illness by manipulating or applying pressure to specific areas of the spine. Invented in 1910 by Albert Abrams (1863–1924), a physician from Heidelberg, who practiced in San Francisco.

Sponge Kidney *See medullary sponge kidney.*

Spongiform Encephalopathy *See scrapie, Kuru, Creutzfeldt–Jakob disease, mink encephalopathy.*

Spontaneous Generation Attributed to germs from putrefaction. Jan Swammerdam (1637–1682) of Amsterdam opposed the theory. Francesco Redi (1626–1698), a physician from Arezzo in Italy, refuted it with his demonstration that maggots developed from eggs laid by flies. Louis Pasteur (1822–1895) in 1857 proved that microorganisms were the cause of fermentation, thus undermining the theory and introducing the biological theory of germs.

Sporothrix schenckii Also known as *Sporotrichum beurmanni*, fungus isolated from beech bark by Charles Lucien de Beurmann (1881–1955), a French physician, in 1908. The largest epidemic of sporotrichosis occurred in infected timber from mines in South Africa in 1941. *See sporotrichosis.*

Sporotrichosis (Syn: Schenck disease) Avian sporotrichosis, a fatal disease of geese found at stations of the Transcaucasian railway, was described by Sakharoff in 1891. The causative agent was mistakenly identified and named as *Treponema anserinum*. A form was described in 1898 by American pathologist Benjamin Robinson Schenck (1873–1920). A complete description was given by Charles Lucien de Beurmann (1881–1955) in 1912. Asteroid bodies due to the precipitation of antigen–antibody complexes on the cell surface was noted by Alfonso Splendore in 1908. The largest epidemic occurred in South Africa in infected timber from the mines in 1941.

Sports Medicine The Greeks had gymnasiums [Greek: *gymnos*, naked] where they exercised. Galen (AD 129–200) was the first physician to attend to sports injuries through his attendance on the gladiators of Rome. He recommended conservative treatment for wounds, but for cut tendons he recommended uniting them with sutures. An illustrated book on sport and exercise, *Artis Gymnastica apud Antiguos Celliberimae nostris temporibus ignoratae*, was written by Geronimo Mercuriale (1530–1606), professor of medicine at Bologna, Padua and Pisa. Frederick Ludwig Jahn (1778–1852), a physical educationist from Prussia, was the father of gymnastics and founded the first gymnasium at Berlin in 1811. An early treatise on use of gymnastics to treat disease was written by Francis Fuller (1670–1706) in 1705. A modern English treatise was written by Brehmer Charles Heald in 1931.

Sprengel, Hermann Johann Phillip (1834–1906) Physicist from Hannover who emigrated to England in 1859. He invented a high vacuum pump (Sprengel pump) which enabled William Crookes (1832–1919) to construct his cathode ray tube for studying radiation.

Sprengel, P. J. Kurt (1766–1833) German botanist and professor of medicine at Halle. His most important work was on history of medicine.

Sprue Celiac disease due to gluten-induced enteropathy. Described by Samuel Jones Gee (1839–1911) of St Bartholomew's Hospital in 1888 and redescribed by Christian Archibald Herter (1865–1910) in 1908 and Danish physician, Thornwald Einar Hess Thaysen (1883–1936), in 1929.

Spurzheim, Casper Johan (1776–1832) German physician and pioneer in phrenology, which was first proposed by another German physician, Franz Joseph Gall (1758–1828) in 1758. Spurzheim wrote *Anatomy and Physiology of the Nervous System, and of the Brain in Particular* with Gall in 1800. He lectured in England, Ireland and Scotland and settled in America.

Sputum Hippocrates (460–377 BC) commented that, 'if they possess a fetid smell, or sink to the bottom of salt water, they indicate great danger'. Fragments of malignant tissue in sputum was recognized by Walter Hayle Walshe (1812–1892) of London in 1843. Malignant cells were also identified by Lionel Smith Beale (1828–1906) of King's College in 1860 and his finding formed the basis for analysis for malignant cells in diagnosis of lung carcinoma by Leonard Stanley Dudgeon (1876–1938) and C. H. J. Wrigley in 1935. Analysis for malignant cells in diagnosis of lung cancer is currently an established standard.

Spygmograph [Greek: *sphygmos*, pulse + *graphein*, write] Instrument to trace the human pulse, invented by Karl Vierordt (1818–1884) in 1854. An improved form was devised by Etienne Jules Marey (1830–1904) of Paris in 1860. The ink polygraph which measured both arterial pulse and venous pulse was developed by Sir James Mackenzie (1853–1925) around 1900.

Squire, Truman Hoffman (1823–1889) American surgeon who wrote a treatise on the stricture of the urethra (1867) and designed a catheter.

Squint *See strabismus.*

St Anthony Hermit saint from Memphis in the 3rd century, who lived for 104 years on a diet of bread and water. He advocated celibacy and his early followers lived in caves before the monasteries were established. He is the patron saint for ergotism or St Anthony's fire. *See ergotism, erysipelas.*

St Anthony's Fire Ergot poisoning from infected rye or barley occurred in epidemics in the Middle Ages. There was an outbreak in France in AD 857 and several epidemics. Its symptoms of intense irritation and burning leading to dancing were interpreted as demonic possession. In 1085 Pope Urban II designated St Anthony as the saint against of the disease and it was known as 'ignus sacer' (holy fire) or St Anthony's fire. The monastic order of St Anthony nursed those affected and was founded in 1095 by Gaston de Dauphine who believed that his illness (which was probably erysipelas) was cured by Saint Anthony. It has been confused with erysipelas.

St Andrews University First Scottish university, founded in 1411 by Henry Wardlaw, Bishop of St Andrews. Its first degree in medicine was granted in 1696.

St Augustine *See Aurelius Augustinus.*

St Bartholomew's Hospital Oldest hospital to remain at its original site. Founded by Rahere, a public entertainer in 1123. He fell ill on pilgrimage to Rome and vowed that he would build a hospital if cured. St Bartholomew is said to have appeared to him and given him the vision of the hospital. The first Royal Charter was given in 1133 and it was run by the nuns and monks of the priory attached to it. Rahere became prior and master of the hospital until his death in 1144. The priory was closed by the dissolution of monasteries of Henry VIII in 1539, but the hospital remained. Thomas Vicary (1495–1561), surgeon to King Henry VIII, reestablished it, along with Bridewell, St Thomas' and the Bethlehem Hospitals in 1546. It has continued to function at the same site for over 800 years and has had many illustrious medical men such as: William Harvey (1578–1657), David Pitcairn (1749–1809) and Sir James Paget (1814–1899). The medical school was started by John Abernethy (1764–1831) in 1822.

St Benedict *See Benedictine Order.*

St Catherine Hospital Built near the Tower of London and founded in medieval times by Queen Matilda, wife of King Stephen. The Royal Charter was given by Queen Phillipa, the wife of King Edward III.

St Clarw, William (1752–1822) English physician from Preston who specialized in mental diseases. He used a portable electric machine for treating patients.

St Damien *See anarguori.*

St Francis Founded the Franciscan order. He was born to a wealthy cloth-merchant from Assisi in 1182. His dedicated care of lepers earned the title of the nursing saint.

St George's Hospital Lord Lanesborough's house at Hyde Park Corner in London was obtained for the new St George's Hospital and it opened in 1734. It was enlarged to include 200 beds in 1767 and John Hunter (1728–1793) was appointed surgeon in 1768. The hospital was rebuilt in 1824–1834, and by 1890 it had 350 beds. Matthew Baillie (1761–1823) from Larnarkshire also practiced there and attended King George III during his last illness. The first recorded successful blood transfusion was given there by Samuel Armstrong Lane (1802–1892) in 1839. Other important medical men include: Sir Benjamin Collins Brodie (1783–1862), William Cheselden (1688–1752) as a visiting surgeon, Sir Everard Home (1756–1832), Henry Gray (1827–1861) anatomist, and William Stewart Duke-Elder (1898–1978) ophthalmic surgeon to the Queen and founder of the Institute of Ophthalmology at London University in 1948. The move to transfer the hospital to its present site at Tooting started around 1960 and was completed in 1980.

St John Order of Knights Hospitaller Originated during the first Crusade. A monastic hospice mostly run by the

Benedictine order cared for sick pilgrims to the Holy Land and was supported by the Crusaders. The providers and protectors later became the Knights Hospitallers, an order of St John recognized by Pope Paschal II in 1113. They moved to Cyprus, Malta, Rhodes and other parts of Europe and became an influential and wealthy order in the 13th century. In London they established themselves at Clerkenwell but their order was dissolved by Henry VIII during the reformation in 1540. Their power and influence declined in the 17th and 18th centuries and Rome became the headquarters for the Grand Master in the 18th century. The Order was revived in England in 1831 and initiated the modern ambulance service and establishment of the St John's Ambulance Association in 1877.

St John's Ambulance Association *See ambulances.*

St Louis Encephalitis The largest outbreak occurred in St Louis, Missouri in 1933. The causative virus was isolated in the same year by R. N. Muckenfuss and colleagues.

St Mary's Hospital Founded in 1841 in London and it opened to patients in 1851. The medical school was established in 1853. Some of its well known physicians include: Sir Alexander Fleming (1881–1955) who discovered the antibacterial action of *Penicillium* in 1929, Sir William Henry Broadbent (1835–1907) who described the clinical signs in constrictive pericarditis in 1898, and Augustus Desiree Waller (1856–1922) who recorded electrical potential in the human heart in 1887.

St Thomas Aquinas (1227–1274) Dominican monk and architect of Catholic philosophy. He remodeled Aristotelian philosophy to suit ecclesiastical doctrine.

St Thomas' Hospital Originated from the priory of St Mary of the Order of Augustine Canons around 1100, near the Roman bridge of Southwark in London. Most of the priory was destroyed by a fire in 1207 and a soldier named Peter de Rupibus, who became bishop of Winchester, raised a new building through public donations. Beds were established in the hospital around the 13th century and it continued to serve for the next 100 years through generous gifts and donations. By 1507 it was dilapidated and a new building was erected. Following the dissolution of the monasteries in 1540 the hospital closed and remained derelict for 11 years. It was revived by Edward VI with several surgeons on its staff. The first physician was Henry Bull who was appointed in 1556. Modern medicine began with the appointment of Richard Mead (1673–1754) in 1703. Thomas Guy, founder of Guy's Hospital, was a governor of the hospital. Teaching started around 1800 and it had about 450 in-patients. In 1847 the building was compulsorily purchased to make way for a new railway scheme, and its present site was bought for 100,000 pounds. The new hospital facing Parliament was opened by Queen Victoria on 21 June 1871.

St Vitus Dance A form of chorea accompanied by involuntary irregular jerky movements occurring in children and young adults. Described by Thomas Sydenham (1624–1689) in *Schedula Monitoria de Nove Febres Ingressu* (A Sketch by way of warning of the approach of a new fever) and *Processus Integri* in 1686. It is named after St Vitus, patron saint of hysterical and nervous diseases, who lived in Sicily in the fourth century.

Stacke Operation Removal of the mastoid and the contents of the tympanum so that the antrum, tympanum and meatus form a single cavity. Devised by German otologist, Ludwig Stacke (1859–1918).

Stacpoole, Henry de Vere (1863–1951) Irish physician and novelist who wrote *The Blue Lagoon* (1905), *The Pearl Fishers* (1915), and *Green Coral* (1945).

Stader Splint Used in the treatment of fracture of the shaft of long bones and devised by Otto Stader (1894–1962), a veterinarian from Pennsylvania, in 1942.

Staderini Nucleus Nucleus intercalatus, a small nucleus found dorsal to the nucleus of the 12th nerve. Described by Rutilio Staderini professor of anatomy at Siena, in 1894.

Stahl, George Ernst (1660–1734) German scientist who proposed the phlogiston theory. He believed that all substances which burned contained an essence called phlogiston and that they became dephlogisticated after burning. Joseph Priestley demonstrated the role of oxygen in combustion in 1770. He wrote *Experimenta et Observationes Chemicae et Physicae*, *Theoria Medica Vera*, *Fundamenta Chyniae Dogmaticae et Experimentalis* and *Negotium Oliofum*.

Stain Early attempts to stain bacteria with carmine and indigo were made by Wilhelm Friedrich von Gleichen (1717–1783) of Germany in 1778. Some of the best staining methods for bacteria were devised by Carl Weigert (1845–1904) around 1875. Robert Koch (1843–1910) used aniline dyes in 1877. Paul Ehrlich (1854–1915) noted in 1882 that certain bacteria were resistant to decoloration when stained with fuchsin. German bacteriologist, Franz Ziehl (1857–1926), confirmed this and established acid fast staining in 1883. The Rosenberger stain for spirochetes using aniline oil was devised by Randal Rosenberger, a bacteriologist from Philadelphia. Methyl blue was introduced by Ehrlich in 1881. He also used aniline dyes to stain white blood cells in 1877. Orth stain, consisting of lithium and carmine, was introduced into histology by German pathologist, Johannes Orth (1847–1923). Pappenheimer stain, a specific test for plasma cells, was devised by Arthur Pappenheimer (1870–1916), a German professor of hematology in Berlin. The currently used eosin and methylene blue stain for studying blood films was devised by Russian physician, Dimitri Leonidovitch Romanowsky (1851–1921). *See Gram stain.*

Standard Deviation Concept invented by London mathematician Karl Pearson (1857–1936), professor of applied mathematics (1884) and Galton professor of Eugenics (1911) at University College London.

Stanford University Californian university, founded in 1885 by Leland Stanford, a railway magnate, in memory of his deceased son. It was built on Stanford's Palo Alto farm and the founders left an endowment of 21 million dollars for its activities. It opened as a private co-educational institute to 559 students in 1891. The Stanford Food Research Institute was established in 1921 and the Stanford Medical Center was completed in 1959. The Stanford Linear Accelerator Center, funded by Congress, opened in 1961.

Stanier, Roger Yate (b 1916) Canadian microbiologist from Victoria in British Columbia. He researched tryptophan metabolism, discovered the mandelate pathway and the mechanism of streptomycin action.

Stanley, Edward (1791–1861) Surgeon at St Bartholomew's Hospital, London. The retinacular fibers, reflected capsular fibers on the neck of the femur (Stanley cervical ligaments) were described by him in 1818.

Stanley, Wendell Meredith (1904–1971) American biochemist at the Rockefeller Institute for Medical Research in Princeton, University of California and director of the Virus Laboratory at Berkeley. He obtained protein and nucleic acid from tobacco mosaic virus in 1935. He then characterized the shape, amino acid composition, reactive groups and RNA properties of this virus. He shared the Nobel Prize for Chemistry in 1946.

Staphylococcal Food Poisoning J. Denys of Belgium in 1894 isolated *Staphylococcus pyogenes* from meat which had caused an outbreak of diarrhea. An American bacteriologist, Robert W. Goldsborough Owen (b 1882) of Detroit, isolated it from the gastrointestinal tract of patients with food poisoning in 1907. M.A. Barber in 1914 isolated *Staphylococcus albus* from milk, which was responsible for an outbreak of gastroenteritis. Edwin Oakes Jordan (1866–1936) in 1930 showed that man was an important source of enterotoxic staphylococci. G.M. Dack did important studies in the same year. The production of a heat resistant toxin

by staphylococci was shown by C.E. Dolman of Canada and Minet of England in 1938. Dolman and R.J. Wilson of Canada gave the name 'enterotoxin' to the toxin in 1941.

Staphylococcus [Greek: *staphyle*, bunch of grapes + *kokkos*, berry] The bacterium was discovered by Sir Alexander Ogston (1844–1929), regius professor at Aberdeen, who named it in 1881. *Staphylococcus pyogenes* was isolated and described by Anton Julius Friedrich Rosenbach (1842–1923) who divided it into *S. albus* and *S. aureus* in 1884.

Staphylorrhaphy [Greek: *staphyle*, bunch of grapes + *rhaphe*, suture] Surgical treatment for incomplete soft palate. Introduced by American surgeon, John Collins Warren (1778–1856) of Harvard Medical School, in 1828.

Starling, Ernest Henry (1866–1927) One of the greatest British physiologists. He qualified in medicine from Guy's Hospital in 1889 and was professor of physiology at University College London from 1899 to 1923. He devised the heart–lung preparation in 1910, and formulated the law of contraction for heart muscle, known as Starling law of the heart. The concept of hormones and feedback mechanisms was developed by Sir William Maddock Bayliss (1860–1924) and Starling during their work on secretin and other hormones, and the word 'hormone' was coined by Starling. He also discovered the functional significance of serum proteins and demonstrated that kidney tubules could reabsorb water. *See Starling law.*

Starling Law The ability of striated muscle to respond to increased stretch with a proportional increase in contraction was described by Otto Frank (1865–1944) in 1875, and his observation was demonstrated in heart preparations by Ernest Henry Starling (1866–1927) in 1918.

Statistics A book on vital statistics in England was *Natural and Political Observations Upon the Bills of Mortality* by John Graunt (1620–1674). William Petty (1623–1687), a physician from Hampshire and pioneer in statistics, applied statistics to the economy and proposed a department to record deaths, births, marriages, age, sex, economy, trade and education. A census in Ireland was taken by Petty and he published *Essays on Political Arithmetic* in 1687. A lifetable was published by the astronomer, Edmund Halley (1656–1742). Thomas Bayes (1702–1761), a clergyman and mathematician in London, studied statistical inference and wrote *Essay towards solving a problem in the Doctrine of Chances.* Thomas Robert Malthus (1766–1834) wrote *Essay on th Principle of Population* in 1798. A pioneer in medical statistics in France was physician Pierre Charles Alexandre Louis (1787–1872) who also provided statistics on diphtheria, typhoid and yellow fever. Work on vital statistics in England was done in 1839 by William Farr (1807–1883), an official in the General Registrars Office and a general practitioner in London. He related mortality and morbidity in plague and plotted fatality for the smallpox epidemic in 1840. Belgian astronomer, Adolphe Quetelet (1796–1824), applied the theory of probability to humans. Sir Ronald Aylmer Fisher (1890–1962), professor of genetics and a statistician from London, wrote *Statistical Methods for Research Workers* in 1925, which became a standard work on the subject. Physician and mathematician, John Brownlee (1868–1927) from Glasgow University, became director of the Statistical Services of the Medical Research Council and wrote over 80 papers. Statistics was specialty of London mathematician Karl Pearson (1857–1936) who devised the chi-square test of significance and the concept of standard deviation. *See normal distribution curve, medical statistics.*

Status Epilepticus The term 'etat de mal' was used at the Salpêtrière and Bicêtre to denote a series of tonic–clonic attacks of epilepsy. It was translated into 'status epilepticus'.

Stedelman, Ernest (b 1885) A physical chemist from Königsberg who discovered beta-oxybutyric acid in urine in diabetes in 1883.

Stearns, John (1770–1848) First president of the New York Academy of Medicine. He introduced the use of ergot into obstetrics in America in 1807 and published a paper on it in 1822.

Steell, Graham (1851–1942) Son of Scottish sculptor who designed the Scott Monument in Edinburgh. After graduating in medicine from Edinburgh University, he developed an interest in cardiology and became physician to the Manchester Royal Infirmary. He wrote *Physical Signs of Cardiac Diseases* (1181), *Physical Signs of Pulmonary Diseases* (1882), and *Textbook of the Diseases of the Heart* in 1902. *See Graham Steell murmur.*

Stefan, Josef (1831–1893) Viennese physicist who interpreted measurements of the rate of loss of heat from a platinum wire of John Tyndall (1820–1893). He proposed in 1879 that the loss of energy radiated per second from a black body was proportional to the fourth power of the absolute temperature. The Stefan constant or law was incorporated into the formula for calculation of heat.

Steinach, Eugen (1861–1944) Viennese surgeon who proposed the role of hormonal factors in the female reproductive cycle in 1911. He tried experimental ligation of the vas deferens for impotence in 1920.

Stein–Leventhal Syndrome Bilateral polycystic ovaries. Described by two American gynecologists, Irving Freiler Stein (1887–1976) and Michael Leo Leventhal (1901–1971), in 1935.

Steinmann Pin It is inserted through the distal end of the fragment of a fracture and combined with skeletal traction. Introduced by Swiss surgeon, Fritz Steinmann (1872–1932) of Bern, in 1907.

Stellwag Sign Infrequency of blinking and widening of palpebral fissure seen in exophthalmic goiter. Described by Austrian ophthalmologist, Carl von Carion Stellwag (1823–1904).

Steno, Nicolaus or Niels Stensen (1638–1686) Danish anatomist and naturalist from Copenhagen. His *De Musculis et Glandulis Observationum Specimen* on anatomy was published in 1664. He defined the principles behind the formation of the Earth's crust and fossils in 1669. He also discovered the duct of the parotid gland which is named after him. He gave up his medical career for the church, became Bishop of Titiopolis in 1667 and spent the rest of his life trying to convert Northern Europe to Catholicism.

Stenography [Latin: *stenos*, narrow; Greek: *graphein*, to write] The earliest extant system is *Ars Scribendi Charactaris* written around 1412. Timothy Bright (1551–1615) a physician, invented a system of shorthand and published *Characterie An Arte of Shorte, Swifte and Secrete writing by Character. invented by Timothe Bright, Doctor of Phisike* in 1588. Peter Bales published his work in 1590, and John Willis's *Stenographie* was published in 1602. Other systems include those of: Byrom (1750), Taylor (1786) and Pitman (1837). *See shorthand.*

Stensen Duct *See parotid gland, Steno Nicolaus.*

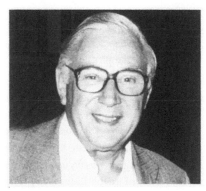

Sir Patrick Christopher Steptoe (1913–1988)

Steptoe, Patrick Christopher (1913–1988) English gynecologist and reproductive biologist from Witney. He graduated from St George's Hospital Medical School and worked at Oldham and District Hospital, Lancashire. He

685

began his work on *in vitro* fertilization with British physiologist, Robert Geoffrey Edwards (b 1925) in 1968 and worked at the Bourn Hall Clinic in Cambridgeshire where he achieved the first birth of a test tube baby in 1978.

Stereochemistry [Greek: *stereos*, solid] The chemical study of spatial arrangement of atoms in molecules and the effect of these arrangements on molecular properties. Scottish physicist, William Nicol (1768–1861), constructed a prism of Iceland spar in 1828 and used it in 1844 to make a polarimeter which facilitated the study of optically active substances. Louis Pasteur (1822–1895) related optical activity and chemical structure in 1848 and stereochemistry originated from his work on tartaric acid in the same year where three tartaric acid isomers were found: one rotated light to the right, one to the left and a third was optically inactive. The explanation was given independently in 1874 by Dutch chemist, Jacobus Henricus Van't Hoff (1852–1911) who suggested that the four bonds of carbon are directed towards a tetrahedron, and French chemist Joseph Achille Le Bel (1847–1930) who wrote on the three dimensional structure of atoms in molecules. The term was coined by German chemist, Viktor Meyer (1848–1897), while studying isomerism of oximes.

Stereoscope [Greek: *stereos*, solid + *skopein*, to see] Instrument that unites two images of an object so as to produce one apparently solid image. Invented by Sir Charles Wheatstone (1802–1875) in 1838.

Stereotaxic Surgery [Greek: *stereos*, solid + *tactus*, touch] Used to produce discrete lesions in basal ganglia as treatment for parkinsonism by E. A. Spiegel, Wycis, Marks and Lee of New York in 1947. Their method was improved by R. Hassler and T. Reichart in 1954, and I. S. Copper and G. J. Bravo in 1958.

Sterilization [Latin: *sterilis*, barren] Method for producing asepsis or removal of microorganisms. An apparatus for automatically regulating steam under pressure (autoclave) for sterilization was used by French confectioner, Nicolas Francois Appert (1749–1841) in 1810. Irish physicist, John Tyndall (1820–1893), wrote *The Floating Matter of Air in relation to Putrefaction and Infection* (1881) proposing a method of applying intermittent heat. Sir John Pringle (1707–1782) published *Experiments upon Septic and Antiseptic Substances* in 1750. Lord Joseph Lister (1827–1912) devised a carbolic spray to sterilize the surroundings during surgery. Sir Arthur Henry Downs (1851–1938) and Thomas Porter Blunt demonstrated the antiseptic effect of sunlight in 1877. *See antiseptics, asepsis, autoclave.*

Sterilization, Female [Latin: *sterilis*, barren] Process of rendering a person incapable of reproduction. Division of the fallopian tubes as a means of female sterilization was suggested by James Blundell (1790–1878) in 1834. S.S. Lungren of Toledo, Ohio recorded his procedure of tying the fallopian tubes during a cesarean section on a patient with a contracted pelvis in 1880. The procedure was popularized by German obstetrician, Max Madlener (1868–1951), around 1919. Ralph Hayward Pomeroy (1867–1925), a New York obstetrician, devised a technique for tying and dividing the fallopian tubes around 1920. A modified method was described in 1924 by another New York obstetrician, Frederick Carpenter Irving (1883–1957). *See vasectomy.*

Sterility *See azospermia, fallopian tubes.*

Sternal Puncture [Greek: *sternon*, breast] *See bone marrow aspiration.*

Sternberg, Karl (1872–1935) Austrian pathologist from Vienna who described Sternberg lymphoma, a mediastinal mass progressing to leukosarcoma. He served as a doctor during World War I and was highly decorated. Later he worked on bowel infection, typhoid and tuberculosis. *See Reed–Sternberg cell.*

Steroids [Greek: *steros*, solid + *oidos*, form] Group of organic compounds related to cholesterol with a cyclopentanoperhydrophenantherine ring were designated steroids according to the suggestion of R. K. Callow and F. G. Young in 1936. An active cortical extract from adrenal glands was prepared by Wilber Willis Swingle (b 1891) and Joseph John Pfiffner (1903–1975) in 1930 who demonstrated the remarkable effect of this extract on adrenalectomized animals. Cortisone was isolated in 1936 by: Tadeus Reichstein (b 1897), Edwin Calvin Kendall (1886–1972) and P. S. Hench (1896–1965), and Oskar Paul Wintersteiner (1898–1971) and Pfiffner. Reichstein elucidated its structure and called it compound F. Research on oxysteroids was commenced in America and dehydrocortisone was synthesized in 1945. Cortisone was first tried as treatment for rheumatoid arthritis by Kendall with remarkable beneficial effect in 1948. O. Hechter and G. Pincus in 1954 made the observation that the amount of cholesterol in adrenal glands markedly decreased when the production and release of hormones is stimulated, and this led to the view that cholesterol is a precursor of adrenal steroid hormones. Fludrocortisone acetate, a 9-halogenated synthetic steroid, was prepared by Fried and Sabo of America in 1953. They became standard treatment for asthma in 1953, and their use in treatment of active chronic hepatitis was suggested by I. R. Mackay and I. J. Wood in 1961. Steroid glycosides are found in *Digitalis* *purpurea, Strophanthus kombe* and other plants. The androgens, estrogens and adrenocortical hormones are also steroids. *See adrenal, estrogen, androgen, Strophanthus.*

Stethoscope. [Greek: *stethos*, chest + *skopein*, to examine] Before its invention in 1819 by French physician, René Theophile Laënnec (1781–1826), physicians applied their ear directly to the chest to listen to chest sounds. He worked at the Necker Hospital and was consulted by an obese woman whose age and sex prevented him from putting his ear against her chest wall as a part of his examination. He rolled a piece of paper and held it against the chest wall of the patient and listened. He published his treatise on auscultation in 1819 and his instrument was later made from wood. Early models were 13 to 18 inches long and were modified into three detachable parts (stem, bell and earpiece) by Judson Dolland. Pierre Piorry (1794–1879) reduced the stem to the thickness of a finger and English physician Charles James Blasius Williams (1805–1889) developed the more popular trumpet-shaped stethoscope. Nicholas Comen devised a flexible monaural stethoscope in 1829. A binaural stethoscope, a wooden chest piece and lead tubes, was made by Williams in 1829. George Camman substituted rubber tubes for lead in 1850 and his model was the prototype of the modern stethoscope. Casper Wistar Pennock (1801–1867) of Philadelphia invented another flexible binaural instrument in 1859 and a diaphragm in the chest piece was introduced in 1894. Howard B. Sprague added the bell-shape to the stethoscope in 1921.

Stevens, William (1786–1868) Surgeon at Santa Cruz who successfully tied the internal iliac artery in a case of aneurysm in 1812.

Stevens–Johnson Syndrome Fever, stomatitis and mucocutaneous eruption. Described by Robert Rendu (b 1886) of Paris in 1916. It was named after two American pediatricians, Albert Mason Stevens (1884–1945) and Frank Chambliss Johnson (1894–1934) who described it in 1922.

Stewart, Alexander Patrick (1813–1883) *See enteric fever.*

Stewart, George Neil (1860–1930) Graduate of the University of Edinburgh who used (with Julius Moses Rogoff) adrenocortical extract for treatment of adrenal insufficiency in 1929.

Stewart, Sir James Purves (1869–1949) English neurologist. *See nerve regeneration.*

Stilbestrol The first estrogen to be chemically synthesized. As naturally occurring estrogens contain a phenanthrene ring, a search for similar compounds were made by Sir Edward Charles Dodds (1899–1973) and co-workers. In 1938

they observed that certain synthetic compounds detected as impurities had an estrogenic effect although they did not have a steroid nucleus. Their observation led to the synthesis of stilbestrol by K. Miescher, C. Scholz and E. Tschopp.

Stiles, Charles Wardell (1867–1941) *See Ancylostoma duodenale.*

Still, Sir George Frederick (1868–1941) Born in London and educated at Cambridge, he started his career as house physician at the Great Ormond Street Hospital for Children. He published *On a form of chronic joint disease in Children* when he was a registrar in 1896. He confined his practice to diseases of children and is considered by some as the founder of pediatrics in England. *His Common Disorders and Diseases of Childhood* was published in 1909.

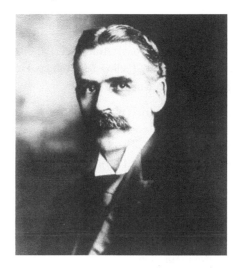

George Frederick Still (1868–1941). Courtesy of the National Library of Medicine

Still Disease Chronic arthritis in childhood. Described by Andre Victor Cornil (1837–1898), a physician at Paris in 1864 and Sir George Frederick Still (1868–1941) in 1896. Still's article, *A form of chronic joint disease in Children* (1896), discussed 22 cases of the disease. Chauffard of Paris described the same condition shortly after Still.

Stiller, Berthhold (1837–1922) Hungarian physician who described general asthenia (Stiller disease) in 1907.

Stilling Root Prolongation of the optic tract extending to the 3rd nerve nuclei, the cerebellum and the pons. Described by Jakob Stilling (1842–1915), professor of ophthalmology at Strasburg in 1882.

Stockard, Charles Rupert (1879–1939) *See carcinoma of cervix.*

Stohr Cells Found in the pyloric gastric glands and named after Philipp Stohr (1849–1911), professor of anatomy at Würzburg who described them in 1887.

Stoichiometry [Greek: *stoicheion*, element] Study and numeric relationships of chemical compounds and elements by mass. Proposed by German chemist, Jeremias Benjamin Richter (1762–1807).

Stoics Disciples of Zeno, a Greek philosopher who lived around 308 BC and taught in a portico, or stoa, in Athens. Their concept was that man should be free from passion and accept calmly all occurrences in submission to divine will or natural order..

Stoke Mandeville Hospital Established by Sir Ludwig Guttmann (1899–1980) in 1944 in Buckinghamshire to treat spinal injuries.

Stoker, William (1773–1848) Irish physician who investigated the velocity of sedimentation of blood corpuscles in 1823.

Stokes, Adrian (1887–1927) American pathologist who found the specific virus of yellow fever in 1923. He died of it during his experimentation.

Stokes, Sir George Gabriel (1819–1903) Irish mathematician and physicist who used spectroscopy to determine the composition of the Sun and stars, identified X-rays as electromagnetic waves and formulated the Stokes law on the force opposing a small sphere in its passage through viscous fluid.

Stokes, Sir William (1839–1900) Irish surgeon who described the method of amputation through the articular end of the femur in 1870.

Stokes, William (1804–1878) Irish physician who gave a description of paroxysmal tachycardia in 1854 and heart block associated with syncopal attacks in 1846. He described Cheyne–Stokes breathing in apoplexy in 1854. His *A Treatise on the Diagnosis and Treatment of the Diseases of the Chest* was published in 1837.

Stokes Lens Combination of a concave cylindrical and convex cylindrical lenses used in the diagnosis of astigmatism. Designed by English physicist, George Gabriel Stokes (1819–1903).

Stokes–Adams Syndrome A classical description of heart block associated with syncopy was given by Robert Adams (1791–1875) of Dublin in 1827. William Stokes (1804–1878), another Irish physician, gave an account of heart block with syncopal attacks in 1846. The condition was later named Stokes–Adams attack or syndrome.

Stoll, Maximillian (1742-1787) Austrian epidemiologist in Vienna.

Stoltz Operation Used for cystocele, by denuding a patch on the anterior abdominal wall and running a purse string suture around the edge. Designed by French gynecologist from Strasbourg, Joseph Stoltz (1803–1896).

Stomach Cancer *See gastric carcinoma.*

Stomach Surgery *See gastrectomy, Billroth operation, abdominal surgery, gastroenterostomy and gastrostomy.*

Stomach Tube Used for studying digestion by withdrawal of a test meal from the stomach. Designed by American physician, Martin Emil Rehfuss (1887–1964), in 1914. It contained a metal capsule which sometimes damaged the gastric mucosa. British physician, John Alfred Ryle (1889–1950), improved it in 1921 by covering the entire tip with rubber and providing perforations above the bulb.

Stomach Ulcer *See gastric ulcer.*

Stone Age The earliest known period of human culture, characterized by the use of stone tools. Identified by French magistrate, Gouget, in 1758. It lasted several hundred thousand years. An early depiction of an ancient medicine man is found in the Ariege cave painting in France. It shows a human wearing a skin around the shoulders with deer's antlers on his head. Evidence of Paleolithic culture was found in Abbeville, France by Jacques Boucher de Perthes (1788–1868) in 1805. His finding provided evidence for the existence of man over 30,000 years ago. Sir John Lubbock (1834–1913) in 1865 used the terms Paleolithic and Neolithic to divide it on the basis of stone artifacts found in Western Europe. Rough stone instruments delimited the Paleolithic, and polished stone instruments were Neolithic. The Paleolithic age was further divided into the period of Neanderthal man and the appearance of *Homo sapiens* or modern man.

Stone Operation For ununited fracture of the tibia was described by Boston surgeon, James Savage Stone (1868–1929) in 1907.

Stonehouse, Sir James (1716–1795) British physician from Berkshire who practiced for nearly 20 years in Northampton and founded the Infirmary. He became a clergyman and died in Bristol. He published a book on friendly advice to patients.

Stoney, George Johnston (1826–1911) Irish physicist and professor of natural philosophy at Galway. He calculated the approximate value of the charge on an electron and introduced that term.

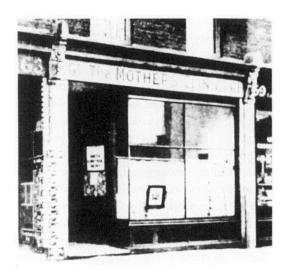

One of the first family planning clinics of Marie Stopes (1880–1938). Reproduced with permission of the IPPF

Stopes, Marie Charlotte Carmichael (1880–1958) Paleobotanist from Dorking, Surrey who graduated from Munich and became the first female science lecturer at Manchester in 1904. In 1916 she became interested in promoting contraception and wrote *Married Love* which was banned in America. She opened the first birth control clinic in England and wrote 70 books on the subject. Her *Contraception: Its Theory, History and Practice*, with an introduction by William Bayliss (1860–1924), was published in 1923.

Stromeyer, George Friedrich Ludwig (1804–1876) German surgeon who performed subcutaneous section of tendo achilles as treatment for club foot in 1830.

Stout, George Frederick (1860–1944) English psychologist from South Shields, Durham. He was professor of logic and metaphysics at St Andrew's from 1903 to 1936. He wrote *Analytic Psychology* (1896), *Manual of Psychology* (1899), and *Mind and Matter* (1931).

Stovaine Amylocaine Discovered by Ernest Fourneau (1872–1949) of France in 1904, and used as a spinal anesthetic by Henri Chaput in 1910. L. H. Maxson in 1938 demonstrated that it was irritable and unsafe as a spinal anesthetic and could produce paralysis.

Strabismus [Greek: *strabismos*, a squinting] Haly Abbas (930–994), a Persian physician, said that it was due to unequal contraction of the eye. Avicenna (980–1037) later remarked that squinting was caused by debility or spasm of some of the muscles of the eye. Paul of Aegina (625–690) recommended wearing blinkers to make the child look forward and also prescribed eye exercises. The amblyoscope, a

stereoscopic instrument to train the eye in order to overcome squint, was designed by Claude Worth (1869–1936) around 1906. The successful operative treatment by severing the tendons of the eye muscles was performed by Johann Friedrich Dieffenbach (1792–1847) of Königsberg in 1829.

Streptococcus [Greek: *strepto*, twisted + *kokkos*, berry] The name streptococcus was introduced by German surgeon, Julius Friedrich Rosenbach (1842–1923) in 1884. He isolated *Streptococcus pyogenes*, differentiated staphylococci and streptococci, and divided staphylococcus into albus and aureus groups. In 1920 James Howard Brown (b 1884) published a monograph in the medical researches of the Rockefeller Institute in 1920 which classified the streptococcal group into A, B, A prime and G, based on the type and degree of hemolysis produced by the bacteria on a blood agar plate. A classification of pathogenic hemolytic streptococci based on serology related to polysaccharides and pathogenicity was proposed by a New York bacteriologist, Rebecca Craighill Lancefield (1895–1981) in 1933. The pathogenic strains of hemolytic streptococci were shown to produce a substance which dissolves human fibrin (fibrinolysin) by American pathologist, William Smith Tillet (b 1892) of Baltimore and R.L. Garner in 1933.

Streptococcus viridans [Greek: *strepto*, twisted + *kokkos*, berry; Latin: *viridis*, green] Isolated from blood of patients with bacterial endocarditis by a German professor of medicine at Hamburg, Hugo Schottmüller (1867–1936) in 1910.

Streptokinase *See thrombolysis.*

Streptomycin Antibiotic obtained from *Streptomyces griseus* by Albert Schatz (b 1920) and co-workers in 1944 and introduced as a first line drug in treatment of tuberculosis by Horton Corwin Hinshaw (b 1902) and Hugh William Feldman (1892–1974) in 1946. Russian-born American microbiologist and Nobel Prize winner, Selman Abraham Waksman (1888–1973), also synthesized it around the same time and used it in treatment of tuberculosis. The structure was worked out by American biochemist, Karl August Folkers (b 1906) and co-workers in 1948. The genetics were elucidated by British geneticist, David Alan Hopwood (b 1933), of Staffordshire, who was John Innes professor of genetics at the University of East Anglia. His work led to development of the technique of genetic manipulation in antibiotic production.

Stress The physiological effects of fear were described by Luis Juan Vives (1492–1540) of Basel as early as 1548. An increase in adrenal output due to emotional stress was observed by American physiologist, Walter Bradford

Cannon (1871–1945) in 1911. A scientific work on stress linking it to biological and physiological consequences in man was done by Hans Hugo Bruno Selye (1907–1982), a Canadian physician of Austrian origin, in the late 1940s. He proposed the stress-adaptation syndrome in 1949.

String Sign Radiology sign where a narrow streak of barium is seen in cases of Crohn disease. Described by New York surgeon, John Leonard Kantor (1890–1947).

String Galvanometer *See electrocardiography.*

Stroke *See apoplexy.*

Stroking Used as a method of healing of diseased parts by many faith healers. A physician who used this method was Valentine Greatrake (1629–1683) from County Cork, Ireland. He became known as 'the stroker' and demonstrated his powers on patients from St Bartholomew's Hospital at the Palace of Whitehall at the request of Charles II.

Stromeyer Splint Two hinged portions which could be fixed at any angle. Devised by German orthopedic military surgeon, George Ludwig Stromeyer (1804–1876).

Strong, Nathan (1781–1837) American physician who described cerebrospinal meningitis in 1810.

Strong, Richard Pearson (1872–1948) American physician from Virginia and a graduate of Yale University in 1893. He was professor at the University of Philippines until 1913 when he became professor of tropical medicine at Harvard University. He organized several expeditions to study tropical diseases and wrote *Diagnosis, Prevention and Treatment of Tropical Diseases.*

Strongyloides stercoralis [Greek: *strongylos*, round] Intestinal parasitic roundworm causing diarrhea. Described by Louis Alexis Normand in Cochin, China in 1876.

Strophanthus [Greek: *strophos*, twisted cord + *anthos*, flower] Seeds of a vine used in Africa to prepare a powerful arrow poison called Kombe. Sir Thomas Fraser demonstrated in 1885 that its action was similar to digitalis in the treatment of dropsy. *See arrow poisons.*

Struma A term used ambiguously to refer to goiter as well as King's evil or scrofula, a condition of induration of glands mainly in the neck and armpits due to tuberculosis. Described by Hippocrates (460–377 BC) who considered the neck as the worst site for it. Galen (AD 129–200) recommended removal with a knife, and application of quicklime and honey was advocated by Paul of Aegina (625–690). Leonides of Alexandria and Antyllus operated on the glands in the 3rd century. Avicenna (980–1037)

practiced bleeding from the site of the lesion for scrofula. *Cinchona,* as a specific treatment, was introduced by John Fordyce in 1755. The tuberculous nature of the disease became known only in the late 18th century. Sea bathing was advocated as treatment, and the Royal Sea-bathing Hospital at Margate used this form of treatment in the 18th century. *On Scrofulous Diseases of the External Lymphatic Glands* was written in 1861 by P.C. Price, a surgeon to Great Northern Hospital and the Metropolitan Infirmary for Scrofulous Children at Margate. Lugol iodine, a mixture of iodine and potassium iodide, was introduced as treatment of scrofula by French physician Jean Guillaume Auguste Lugol (1786–1861) in 1829. The term struma lymphosa refers to Hashimoto disease of the thyroid gland described by Hakaru Hashimoto (1881–1934) in 1912. *See scrofula, thyroid goiter.*

Strümpell–Bechterew–Marie Syndrome *See ankylosing spondylitis.*

Strümpell Disease Polioencephalomyelitis was described by German neurologist, Ernst Gustav Adolf Gottfried von Strümpell (1853–1925) at Leipzig in 1891.

Struthers Ligament Attached to the medial condyle of the humerus. Described by Sir John Struthers (1823–1899), professor of anatomy at Aberdeen, in 1849.

Struthius, Josephus (1510–1578) Hungarian and physician to Sigismund August, King of Poland. His *Ars sphigmica* (1555) was an important work on the action of the heart and diseases of the blood vessels.

Strychnine Seed from *Strychnos Nux-vomica,* which is indigenous to India and the Malay archipelago, is said to have been introduced into medicine by the Arabians. A description was given by Valerius Cordus (1515–1544) of Hesse in 1540, and *De Nuce Vomica,* giving an account of its toxic effects, was published by J. Lossius in 1682. It was used as a pest poison in England in the 17th century and its poisonous action was later proved to be due to its alkaloids, strychnine and brucine. Strychnine was extracted by Pierre Joseph Pelletier (1788–1842) and Joseph Bienaimé Caventou (1795–1877) in 1817.

Stukeley, William (1687–1765) Physician from Lincolnshire, obtained his MB degree in 1709 and then took holy orders in 1729. He wrote a dissertation on the spleen and was a founder of the Egyptian Society in 1741.

Sturge–Weber Syndrome Angioma of the leptomeninges [Greek: *leptos* + slender, *meningx*, membrane] and ipsilateral portwine stain on the face in the region of trigeminal distribution. Described by English Quaker physician, William

Allen Sturge (1850–1919) of Bristol in 1879. An account was also given by Friedrich Weber-Liel (1832–1891) in 1922.

Sturtevant, Alfred Henry (1891–1970) American geneticist from Jacksonville, Illinois. Educated at Columbia University and spent his career at Caltech as professor of genetics and later as professor of biology. He developed chromosome maps of *Drosophila* and provided the background for gene mapping experiments and established the basis for the chromosomal theory of heredity. *See chromosomes.*

Stutter Speech problem described by H. Klencke in *The Cure of Stuttering* published in 1860. He recommended breathing exercises and systematic exercises of organs of speech as cure. A French teacher, Claudius Chervin (1825–1896), did pioneering work on the subject.

Subacute Combined Degeneration of the Spinal Cord (Syn: Dana syndrome, Putnam disease) Degenerative changes in the spinal cord associated with pernicious anemia. Described independently by Charles Loomes Dana (1852–1935) from Vermont, and another American, James Jackson Putnam (1846–1918) of Boston in 1891. A review was given by Ludwig Lichtheim (1845–1928) of Germany in 1897. Another classic description in relation to pernicious anemia was given by English neurologist, Frederick Eustace Batten (1865–1918) of Queen's Square, James Samuel Riesien Russel (1861–1939) and James Stansfield Collier (1870–1935) in 1900.

Subacute Bacterial Endocarditis (SABE) An early description was given by George Hilaro Barlow (1806–1866) and George Owen Rees (1813–1889) in 1843. Norwegian Emanuel Frederick Hagbarth Winge (1838–1921) suggested a microbial cause in 1869. A definitive account was given by Sir Samuel Wilkes (1824–1911) in 1870 under the name, arterial pyemia. The occurrence of peripheral emboli due to valvular vegetations was recognized by William Senhouse Kirkes (1823–1864) of England in 1842. Hematuria with focal glomerular lesions in the kidney due to minute bacterial emboli from endocardial vegetations was observed by Max Hermann Friedrich Loehlein (1877–1921) of Leipzig in 1907. It was already known as hemorrhagic nephritis to Harbitz of Germany in 1899. American physician, Emanuel Libman (1872–1946), referred to these lesions as 'embolic glomerular lesions of subacute bacterial endocarditis' in 1923. The Janeway lesions, which consist of nodular hemorrhagic spots in the palms and soles of patients with subacute bacterial endocarditis, were described by Edward G. Janeway (1841–1911) in 1899, and the cutaneous nodules (Osler

nodes) found were described by Canadian physician, Sir William Osler (1849–1919), in 1908. Roth spots or white hemorrhagic spots seen in the retina were described by Swiss physician, Moritz Roth (1839–1914) in 1872. *Streptococcus viridans* was isolated in cases by Hugo Schottmüller (1867–1936) of Germany in 1910. Effective treatment with penicillin was demonstrated on 269 patients by Ronald Victor Christie (b 1902) in 1948.

Subarachnoid Hemorrhage [Latin: *sub*, under; Greek: *arachnoides*, spider + *haima*, blood + *rheein*, to flow] An early account was presented to the Academie des Sciences, by Joseph Guichard Duverney (1648–1730) who was professor of anatomy at Paris in 1682. In his description he stated that a large clot was found in the theca. The description of the death of King Henry II by Ambroise Paré (1510–1590) is consistent with a subarachnoid hemorrhage and Prince Charles of Sweden died suddenly while riding from a subarachnoid hemorrhage in 1810. An extensive account was given by Giovanni Battista Morgagni (1682–1771) in *De Sedibus et Causis Morborum per antomen indagatis* published in 1761. The suggestion that it was related to aneurysm was made by Sir William Henry Withey Gull (1816–1890) in 1859. From 1800 to 1880 over 86 papers related to it were published. A classical case of rupture of an aneurysm at the bifurcation of the middle cerebral artery was reported by Sir William Osler (1849–1919) in 1877. Byrom Bramwell (1847–1931) associated it with rupture of an intracranial aneurysm in 1886. Sir Charles Putnam Symonds (1890–1978), a neurologist to Guy's Hospital and National Hospital for Nervous Diseases in Queen's Square, reviewed 124 cases in 1923 and concluded that rupture of the intracranial artery was the commonest cause. The presence of blood in the cerebrospinal fluid in cases of meningeal hemorrhage was noted by several workers including George Ferdinand Isidore Widal (1862–1929) (1903), Georges Froin (1874–1932) (1904), and Ingvar (1913).

Subbarow, Yella Pragada (1896–1948) *See phosphocreatinine.*

Subclavian Artery Ligation [Latin: *sub*, under + *clavis*, key] Abraham Colles (1773–1843), a leading Dublin surgeon, tied the subclavian artery in 1811, Wright Post (1766–1822) of Long Island treated a case of brachial aneurysm by tying it in 1816 and Guillaume Dupuytren (1777–1835) performed the same procedure in 1819. An aneurysm of the axilla was successfully treated by tying by Charles Aston Key (1793–1849). An American vascular surgeon, Valentine Mott (1785–1865), treated an aneurysm of the subclavian artery by tying it within the scleni muscles in 1833. Sir William Fergusson (1808–1877), Scottish surgeon and a pupil of

Robert Knox (1791–1862), tied it. *A Successful ligation of Subclavian Artery* was published by Richard James Mackenzie (1821–1854), an anatomist and surgeon at the Edinburgh Royal Infirmary. New York surgeon, William Stewart Halstead (1852–1922), performed a successful ligation of the left subclavian artery in America in 1892.

Subcortical Dementia [Latin: *sub*, under + *cortex*, bark + *de*, down + *mens*, mind] An early form of subcortical encephalopathy leading to a classic picture of dementia in the fifth and sixth decade of life was described by Otto Ludwig Binswanger (1852–1929) in 1894. Another form due to progressive lenticular degeneration was described by Samuel A.K. Wilson (1877–1937) in 1912. The term was used to denote progressive supranuclear palsy by M.L. Albert and colleagues in 1974. The affection of subcortical structures such as basal ganglia, thalamus, hypothalamus, midbrain and cerebellum have since been identified in a variety of conditions including Parkinson disease, Huntingdon chorea and AIDS dementia complex.

Subcutaneous Fluid Injection Devised by Francis Rynd (1801–1861) at the Meath Hospital, Dublin in 1844. He gave an accurate description of the instruments used in 1845 and used the method mainly to treat neuralgias.

Subcutaneous Tenotomy [Latin: *sub*, under + *cutis*, skin + *tendere*, to stretch; Greek: *tomos*, to cut] A method of treatment for clubfoot by subcutaneous section of the achilles tendon was introduced in 1816 by Jacques Mathieu Delpech (1777–1832), professor of surgery at Montpellier. It was applied as treatment for most deformities arising out of muscular defects by German orthopedic surgeon, Georg Friedrich Ludwig Stromeyer (1804–1876) around 1836. It was performed in France by a surgeon, Amédée Bonnet (1802–1858) in 1841.

Subdural Hematoma [Latin: *sub*, below + *dura*, hard; Greek: *haima*, blood] *See chronic subdural hematoma.*

Subhyaloid Hemorrhage [Latin: *sub*, under; Greek: *hyalos*, glass + *haima*, blood + *rheein*, to flow] Described in a 21-year-old man with subarachnoid hemorrhage by Hale White (1857–1949) in 1895 and caused by a ruptured aneurysm of the internal carotid artery.

Submaxillary Gland A description was given by English anatomist, Thomas Wharton (1614–1673), in *Adenographia* published in 1656.

Substantia Nigra [Latin: *substantiae*, substance + *nigresecere*, to turn black] A crescent-shaped grayish black nuclear material lying in the midbrain between the pedunculi and tegmentum. Identified and named by Samuel Thomas

Sömmering (1755–1830) in 1800.

Succinyl Chloride Introduced as a muscle relaxant by Italian pharmacologist, Daniel Bovet (1907–1992).

Succussion Splash [Latin: *succussio*, shaking from beneath] It was used as a physical sign in cases of hydropneuomothorax by Hippocrates (460–377 BC).

Sudden Death A large number occurred in Rome in 1705 which caused public panic. A treatise, *De Subitaneis Mortibus* (1707), which included autopsy findings of five cases, was written by Giovanni Maria Lancisi (1654–1720), professor of anatomy at the Collegio de Sapienza and physician to the Pope. He also wrote *De Motu Cordis et Aneurysmatibus* which contained essays on physiology and the motion of the heart, and on aneurysms of the heart and blood vessels.

Sudeck Atrophy Form of bone atrophy, giving a washed out spotted appearance to the distal bones on X-rays, and accompanied by swelling and tenderness of the tissues overlying it. Described in 1923 by Paul Hermann Martin Sudeck (1866–1938), professor of surgery at Hamburg.

Sudeck Critical Point Highly vasculated area on the colon, between the colic and superior rectal arteries. Described in 1923 by Paul Hermann Martin Sudeck (1866–1938), professor of surgery at Hamburg.

Sudhoff, Karl Friedrich Jakob (1853–1938) German physician and medical historian who occupied the first chair for the history of medicine at Leipzig. He wrote *Bibliographia Paracelsica* (1884–1889) and other works on the history of medicine.

Sue Ryder Foundation Established at Cavendish near Sudbury, Suffolk to promote residential care for the sick, disabled and homeless by English baroness and philanthropist, Sue Ryder from Leeds, in 1953.

Sugar The best sugar is produced from sugar cane and Alexander the Great's admiral, Nearchus, became familiar with it in India. It was used as a beverage in Pompeii. Pliny (AD 29–79), refers to it as saccharum, and Galen (AD 129–200) prescribed it as medicine. Dioscorides (AD 40–90) referred to a concrete honey found in canes in India and Arabia. It was brought to Europe from India around AD 1150 and the Portuguese and Spaniards introduced it into America in 1510. The process of refining sugar was started in Europe by a Venetian trader in 1503 and it was introduced into England in 1659. It was extracted from sugar beet by German agricultural chemists, Andreas Sigismund Marggraf (1709–1782) in 1747 and Franz Karl Achard (1753–1821) in 1799.

Suicide [Latin: *sui*, of himself + *caedere*, to kill] It was considered a crime by most philosophers of Rome and Greece and the hand of the victim was burnt separately from the body. Zeno (362–264 BC) of Citium in Cyprus, founder of the Stoic sect, committed suicide by strangling. Eratosthenes (274–194 BC), librarian at the University of Alexandria, who made significant contributions to the field of mathematics, was blinded by an eye disease and committed suicide. The Roman Catholic Church forbade suicide and denied church services for self-murder. Until 1824 the body of a suicide was buried at a crossroad. An extensive treatise in English on suicide, *Lifes preservative against self-killing*, was written by an Essex clergyman, John Sym (1581–1637) in 1637. He recognized that mental illness may lead to suicide. Antoine Louis (1723–1792) of France wrote on the differential signs of murder and suicide in cases of hanging in 1763.

Sulkowitch Test Used for detecting calcium in urine and devised by Boston physician, Hirsh Wolf Sulkowitch (b 1906).

Sulfa Compounds *See sulfonamides.*

Sulfadiazine Introduced as an antibiotic by Maxwell Finland (b 1902) in 1941. It was used as a local application for burns in 1945 by American surgeon, Kenneth Leroy Pickerell (b 1910) of Baltimore.

Sulfapyrimidine An early antibiotic, developed in 1937 by London chemist, Arthur James Ewins (1882–1957).

Sulfonamides Protonsil was the first such compound to be synthesized by Paul Gelmo (b 1902). Its bacteriostatic property was recognized in the azo-compounds by Gerhard Johannes Paul Domagk (1895–1964) who demonstrated its clinical effectiveness against cocci in 1935. In 1936, English physician Leonard Colebrook and Meave Kenny showed excellent results against puerperal fever and septic abortion, which were both previously fatal. Sulfapyridine was synthesized by Arthur James Ewins (1882–1957) and Phillips in England in 1937 and found to be more effective against pneumococci but also more toxic. Sulfathiozole was introduced in 1940 and was found to be more effective than any previous sulfonamides for staphylococcal infections. The significance of the structural resemblance between the antibacterial substance sulfanilamide and para-aminobenzoic acid was noted independently by Donald Devereux Woods (1912–1964) and Paul Gordon Fildes (b 1882) in 1940. The Woods–Fildes hypothesis contended that para-aminobenzoic acid was an essential metabolite of bacteria and that sulfonamides, by virtue of their structural similarity, blocked their metabolism. Sulfamethazine was introduced by Donald William Macartney in 1942. A number of other compounds of sulfapyrimidine have been synthesized. *See antibiotics.*

Sulfur [Latin: *sulfuris*] Homer and Pliny (AD 29–79) mentioned the use of the pungent fumes produced by burning sulfur for cleansing the air. Valentinius, a Benedictine monk and alchemist in the 15th century, was familiar with its production from green vitriol.

Sumerian Medicine The Sumerian civilization was established in the Mesopotamian riverlands of the Tigris and Euphrates around 3000 BC. It was the world's first empire and cradle of civilization. Their medical knowledge is revealed in the cuneiform writings on clay tablets. They considered blood as vital to all organs and activities and the liver was held sacred as it served to store blood. Marduk was their god of science and medicine and had a temple erected to him which later developed into a school of medicine. Evil spirits were also thought to cause illness. They had considerable knowledge of astronomy and based some of their medicine on interpretation of the stars. *See Mesopotamian medicine.*

Summation [Latin: *summa*, total] Accumulation of effects of a number of stimuli on a muscle or nerve. Evidence that the refractory period is succeeded by increased excitability so that a stimulus of less intensity is required to propagate electrical disturbance in a nerve was provided by Edgar Douglas Adrian (1889–1977) and Keith Lucas (1879–1916) in 1912. It is known as the Law of Summation.

Sumner, James Batcheller (1887–1955) American biochemist, born in Canton, Massachusetts and educated at Harvard. In 1926 he crystallized urease and showed that it was a protein, determined its kinetic and chemical properties and found the reactive sulfhydryl groups on it. He also purified other oxidative enzymes, including monoamine oxidase. He shared the Nobel Prize for Chemistry in 1946. *See urease.*

Sun Pythagorus (580–500 BC) believed that it was one of the twelve spheres. His plan of the solar system placed the Sun in the center and described elliptical movements of the other planets around it. Hicetas of Syracuse in 344 BC suggested that the Sun and moon were motionless and the Earth moved around them. The distance between the moon and the Sun was calculated geometrically by Aristarchus in 280 BC. The English astronomer Edmund Halley established the motion of the Sun around its axis in 1696. *See sunlight, Sabaeism.*

Sunlight Short wavelength rays that show least amount of penetration of tissues were identified as ultraviolet and English physician, Sir Arthur Henry Downes (1851–1938) and Thomas Porter Blunt in 1877 showed that they were capable of killing bacteria. Danish physician, Niels Ryberg Finson (1861–1904) of Copenhagen also demonstrated the bactericidal effect of sunlight. Use of ultraviolet light improved the photomicrographic study of the structure of bacteria and was also used for therapeutic purposes in the 19th and early 20th century. The effectiveness of these rays in curing rickets was demonstrated by Kurt Huldschinsky (1883–1941) of Berlin in 1919. *See Kantor string sign.*

Sunstroke or Heat Stroke A description was given by Georg Horst in 1660. Sir Thomas Longmore (1816–1895), a British army surgeon in India, gave a detailed description in 1859. Another English army surgeon, Alexander Barclay (1822–1874), gave an account in 1860. The mechanism and pathology were explained in 1872 by a neurologist, Horatio Charles Wood (1841–1920) of the University of Pennsylvania.

Superego Sigmund Freud's (1891-1960) first work on the general theory of personality, *Ego and the Id*, was published in 1923. He divided the mind into three parts: ego, id and superego. He described superego as that which developed after ego as a result of education and identification with parents.

Superior Vestibular Nucleus Found in the cranial nerve and described in 1885 by a Russian neurologist, Vladimir Mikhailovich Bekhterev (1857–1927) from a small village, Surali near the Ural mountains and educated at the Military Medical Academy at St Petersburg.

Suppository Frequently mentioned by Hippocrates (460–377 BC) in his works. John Zacharias Acturius, physician to the Court of Constantinople in AD 1300, recommended mild purgatives and suppositories for obstruction in the rectum. Paul of Aegina (625–690) advocated suppositories made of salted honey and nitre. The Arabian physicians, Avicenna (980–1037), Rhazes (AD 850–932) and others mentioned suppositories as treatment.

Suprapubic Cystotomy Procedure performed by French surgeon, Pierre Franco (1500–1561) in 1556.

Suprapubic Prostatectomy *See prostatectomy.*

Suprarenal Glands [Latin: *supra*, above + *ren*, kidney] Jean Riolan (1580–1687) called these capsulae suprarenalis in 1621. They were illustrated and described by Bartolommeo Eustachio (1520–1574), professor at Rome in 1564. Archangelus Piccolomineus (1562–1605) described them in 1586 and Caspar Bauhin (1560–1624) gave a further account

in 1588. They were shown to be essential for maintaining life by Édouard Brown-Séquard (1817–1894) in 1856. The occurrence of an active vital substance in the adrenal medulla was demonstrated in the same year by Edmé Felix Alfred Vulpian (1826–1887) of Paris. *See Addison disease, adrenal insufficiency, adrenaline.*

Supraspinatous Tendon Rupture [Latin: *supra*, above + *spina*, spine] Diagnostic symptoms were described in 1906 by Ernest Amory Codman (1869–1940), a Boston orthopedic surgeon. He also pioneered application of X-rays to orthopedics and wrote *The use of X-rays in the Diagnosis of Bone Disease* in 1905. A method of operative treatment for rupture of supraspinatous tendon of the shoulder was described by him in 1911.

Supraventricular Tachycardia *See tachycardia.*

Suramin *See Bayer 205.*

Surface Tension Property used in the process of emulsification and production of soap. Known since Thomas Graham did research on solutions in 1835. An early work in England was done by Samuel Sugden (1892–1950), a chemist from Leeds. A simple experiment to demonstrate it was devised by van der Mensbrugghe in 1866 and apparatus to measure it was devised by Röntgen and Schneider in 1886. The law describing the relationship between surface tension, molar volume and temperature of liquids was proposed by Hungarian physicist, Baron Roland von Eötvös (1848–1919) of Budapest around 1870. A chapter was devoted to it in William Maddock Bayliss' *Principles of Physiology* published in 1918. *See emulsification.*

Surgery [Greek: *cheir*, hand + *ergon*, work] The oldest extant surgical treatise is the Edwin Smith Papyrus written around 1600 BC, a copy of an earlier treatise from 3000 BC. It contains an account of injuries to the head, nose and other organs along with methods of bandaging. Hippocrates (460–377 BC) wrote on fractures and dislocations around 400 BC. Susruta, the Brahmin surgeon who lived around AD 500, described over 120 surgical instruments and wrote on operations such as amputation, cesarean section, rhinoplasty, lithotomy, excision of tumors and cataract extraction. Paul of Aegina (625–690) devoted his sixth book, *Epitome*, entirely to operative surgery. An important textbook, *Altasrif*, was written by Albucasis around AD 980. Some important surgeons of the Middle Ages include: Roger of Palmero (1200), Guilelmus da Saliceto (1201–1277), Henri de Mondeville (1260–1320), Guy de Chauliac (1300–1367) and John of Ardane (1307–1380).

Ambroise Paré (1510–1590) of France and Andreas Vesalius (1514–1564) were notable surgeons during the Renaissance. Other eminent surgeons of this period include Hildanus Fabricius (1560–1634) and Lorenz Heister (1683–1758) from Germany. A German book, *Bundt-Ertzney*, was written by Heinrich von Pfolspeundt in 1460. During the 18th and 19th centuries, Britain produced surgeons who made significant advances including: Percivall Pott (1714–1788), Benjamin Bell (1749–1806), John Bell (1763–1820), Sir Charles Bell (1774–1842), John Abernethy (1764–1831), Samuel Cooper (1780–1848), Sir Astley Paston Cooper (1768–1841), and James Syme (1799–1870). Not-able surgeons in Europe at this time were: Guillaume Dupuytren (1777–1835), Alfred Armand Velpeau (1795– 1867), Auguste Nelaton (1807–1873) of Paris, and Theodor Billroth (1829–1894) of Germany. In America, notable surgeons include: John Collins Warren (1778–1856), Philip Syng Physick (1768–1837) and Ephriam McDowell (1771– 1830) *See surgical instruments, Barber surgeons, Royal College of Surgeons.*

Surgical Instruments [Greek: *cheir*, hand + *ergon*, work] The state and practice of surgery was more advanced and scientifically based than other areas of medicine during ancient times. According to Pliny, the saw was designed after the jaw of serpent by Talos. The ancient Greeks used forceps to extract teeth and the antiquity of surgical instruments has been revealed by the discovery of flint saws in the Egyptian ruins of Kahun dating back to 5000 BC. Aborigines of Darling River in New South Wales used fine bone needles for boring the septum of the nose. Susruta, the Brahmin surgeon, described over 120 surgical instruments in AD 500 in his description of operations including amputation, cesarean section, rhinoplasty, lithotomy, excision of tumors and cataract extraction. Albucasis in *Altasrif*, written in the tenth century, gave a remarkable illustration of an array of surgical instruments. His book also described surgical operations for fractures, dislocations, bladder stone, gangrene and other conditions and remained a standard for nearly 500 years.

Surgical Hernia Occurs following surgical incision of the abdomen. A method of closure was described by American surgeon, Arthur Marriot Shipley (b 1878) of Baltimore in 1925.

Surgical Shock [Greek: *cheir*, hand + *ergon*, work] Pioneering work was done in 1888 by American surgeon and physiologist, George Washington Crile (1864–1943) of Cleveland, developed his interest following the death of his

friend, and made several important contributions to treatment. He used blood transfusion and adrenaline in treatment and advocated monitoring of blood pressure during surgery. His monograph was published in 1899, and his other works in the field include *Blood Pressure in Surgery* (1903) and *Anemia and Resuscitation* (1914).

Sutherland, Earl Wilbur (1915–1974) American biochemist from Burlingame who studied at Washington University School of Medicine in St Louis. He was director of the pharmacology department of the Western Reserve University from 1953. He researched the conversion of glycogen to glucose and its stimulation by glucagon and epinephrine. He showed that cyclic AMP promotes activation of phosphorylase and suggested that glucagon and epinephrine induce the cell to produce cAMP. He discovered the 'second messenger' principle of hormone action. In 1971 he was awarded the Nobel Prize for Physiology or Medicine. *See AMP.*

Sutton Law Application of the most likely diagnostic test or procedure to give a positive result. Named after an American bank robber, W. Sutton (1901–1980) of Brooklyn.

Sutton Prize Pathology prize at the London Hospital, awarded in memory of Henry Gawen Sutton (1837–1891) who was a physician there.

Suture [Latin: *sutura*, seam] The ancients used bone needles for suturing and some have been found in Paleolithic deposits in France. An ingenious method of bringing the wound edges together using ants was practiced by ancient Africans and Brazilians. The termites or ants bite the edges together with their powerful jaws acting like modern-day clips. The Masai tribe of Africa used thorns to suture wounds. Galen (AD 129–200) recommended uniting tendons with sutures. Absorbable sutures made from animal tissues were introduced during the 18th century by the American surgeon, Philip Syng Physick (1768–1837). New York surgeon, William Stewart Halstead (1852–1922), pioneered circular sutures for intestines in 1887. Benjamin Bell (1749–1806) suggested suturing the bladder for rupture in 1789, and the procedure was performed by Willet of St Bartholomew's Hospital. End-to-end suture of the femoral artery was performed by John Benjamin Murphy (1857–1916) of America in 1896. The modern technique of arterial suture was described by Alexis Carrel (1873–1944) in 1902. Catgut sutures treated with carbolic acid to promote antisepsis were introduced by Lord Joseph Lister (1827–1912) in 1869.

Svedberg, Theodor (1884–1971) Swedish chemist who

studied chemistry at the University of Uppsala and remained at the university for the next 45 years. He was director of the Gustav Werner Institute of Nuclear Chemistry from 1949 to 1967. His early work was on colloid chemistry and he then investigated radioactivity. He developed the ultracentrifuge as a means to follow sedimentation of particles too small to be seen with an ultramicroscope. He received the Nobel Prize for Chemistry in 1926 for this work. He later worked on use of the cyclotron in medicine.

Swaine, A. Clara (1834–1910) American medical missionary who graduated from the Woman's Medical College, Pennsylvania in 1869. She went to India in 1870 and opened the first medical hospital for women in India at Bareilly in 1874, known as Clara Swaine Hospital.

Swallowing The reflex involved in the act of deglutition was described by a German physiologist, Hugo Krönecker (1839–1914) in 1880. The role of the eustachian tube was described in 1861 by Joseph Toynbee (1815–1866), the first aural surgeon to St Mary's Hospital in London. Fluoroscopy was used to study the act of deglutition in animals by Walter Bradford Cannon (1871–1945) of Harvard University in 1898.

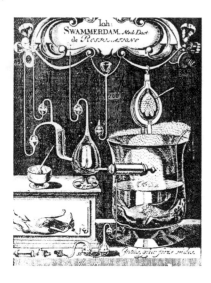

Frontispiece fron Jan Swammerdam's *De Respiratione*. William Stirling, *Some Apostles of Physiology* (1902). Waterlow & Sons, London

Swammerdam, Jan (1637–1680) Dutch naturalist, born in Amsterdam and graduated in medicine from Leiden, although he never practiced as a physician. He observed the red blood cells under the microscope in 1658, and discovered the valves in lymphatic vessels. He devised a system of classification for insects and laid the foundation for the science of entomology with *Historia insectorum generalis*, published in 1669.

Swamp Fever (Syn: mud fever) Once widespread in Eastern Europe in the early 20th century. Identified as due to *Leptospira grippotyphosa* by G. Korthof in 1932.

Swan–Ganz Catheter Use of a flow-directed balloon tip for cardiac catheterization was devised by Harold James Charles Swan (b 1922) and William Ganz (b 1919) in 1970.

Sweating Sickness Unexplained fatal illness accompanied by fever, sweating and prostration that first appeared amongst the troops of King Henry VII in England in 1485, followed by another epidemic in 1507. A third epidemic started in London in 1517 and spread to most parts of England within 6 months. The illness claimed its victims within 24 hours and thousands of people in London died during the five outbreaks. Oxford University and several other institutions had to close during these epidemics. A treatise on the disease was written in 1529 by Euricius Cordus (d 1538), a botanist, poet and physician whose real name was Henry Urban. A description in England was given by John Caius (1510–1573) during the fifth and last epidemic at Shrewsbury in 1552 in his book, *A Boke of Conseill against the Disease commonly called the Sweat or Sweating Sickness*, and he attributed it to lack of personal hygiene.

Swediaur Disease Inflammation of the calcaneal bursa. Described by Austrian physician, François X. Swediaur (1748–1824) in 1790.

Swieten, Gerard van (1700–1772) *See Van Swieten, Gerard.*

Swiss-Type Agammaglobulinemia A few cases of severe lymphopenia and extensive candida infection in infancy were described in Switzerland in 1950. In 1952 a sex-linked familial condition of agammaglobulinemia with recurrent infection was reported in an eight-year-old boy by American pediatrician, Ogden Carr Bruton (b 1908). Both were later classified under the name, 'severe combined immunodeficiency'.

Sydenham Society Founded by an English physician, Sir John Forbes (1787–1861).

Sydenham, Thomas (1624–1689) Called the 'English Hippocrates' due to his observation and classic description of diseases. He was born at Wynford Eagle on the family estate and was sent to Oxford at the age of 18 years. He interrupted his studies in 1642 to serve as an officer in the Parliamentary army during the Civil War. He returned to Oxford in 1646 and was made bachelor of medicine in 1648. He also studied at Montpellier and began practicing in London where he commenced his observations on diseases in 1661. An early work was *Methodus Curandi Febres, propriis observationibus superstructa*. His other works include: *Dissertatio Epistolaris ad Gulielmum Cole* (1682) which dealt with smallpox and hysterical diseases, *Tractus de Podagra et de Hydrope* (1683) essentially a treatise on gout and dropsy, and *Schedula Monitoria de Nove Febres Ingressu*, published in 1686, in which he gave a description of St Vitus dance or chorea (Sydenham chorea). His *Processus Integri in morbis febre omnibus curandis*, which he prepared for his son William Sydenham (1656–1738) to assist in his medical career, was published posthumously in 1693. Sydenham suffered from gout and renal calculi with progressive frequency and severity during his life and died at his house at Pall Mall. A book on Sydenham's work, *Anecdota Sydenhamiana, Medical Notes and observations by Sydenham*, taken mostly from his manuscripts from the Bodelian Library, was written by William Alexander Greenhill (1814–1894) in 1845.

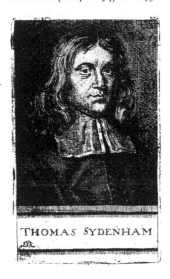

THOMAS SYDENHAM

Thomas Sydenham. Title page of Sydenham's *Opera Omnia* (1696). Courtesy of the National Library of Medicine

Sydenham Chorea St Vitus dance, accompanied by involuntary irregular jerky movements occurring in children and young adults. Described by Thomas Sydenham (1624–1689) in *Schedula Monitoria de Nove Febres Ingressu* published in 1686. It is also named after Saint Vitus, patron saint for hysterical and nervous diseases.

Sylvester, Sir John Baptist, of Aquitaine (d 1789) Graduated from Leiden in 1738 and was appointed physician to the London Hospital in 1749, where he was the first member of the staff to receive a knighthood (1774).

Sylvius, Jacques Dubois (1478–1555) Scholar of classical languages who graduated in medicine from Montpellier at the age of 51 years. He was appointed professor in Paris at the age of 72 years. He taught Andreas Vesalius (1514–1564) and described several anatomical structures which have been named after him.

Sylvius, James (1478–1550) Belgian professor of medicine from Amiens at Paris. His *Opera Omnia* was published in Cologne in 1630.

Sylvius, Franciscus (1614–1672) *See Le Böe, François de.*

Syme, James (1799–1870) Known as the Napoleon of surgery, he was born at 56 Princes Street in Edinburgh. During his boyhood he spent much of his time experimenting in chemistry. A solvent for India rubber and a method to make it waterproof were discovered by him when he was 18 years. This was later patented by Charles Macintosh (1766–1843), a chemist from Glasgow. He graduated from Edinburgh University and succeeded Robert Liston (1794–1847) as lecturer in anatomy at the same institute. An early treatise, *On Caries of the Bone*, was published in 1821 and other publications were *The Excision of Diseased Joints* (1831) and *Principles of Surgery* (1832). After attending the clinics of Guillaume Dupuytren (1777–1835) at Paris in 1822, he returned to Edinburgh and performed several major surgical methods for the first time in Britain. He did the first amputation at the hip joint on a boy of 19 years in 1825, and excised the head of the humerus in a case of tuberculosis in 1826. In 1828 he performed excision of the lower jaw for sarcoma. After being denied a professorship at the Royal Infirmary due to his disagreement with Liston, he established his own hospital at Minto House in Chambers Street. His student, John Brown, immortalized him and his hospital in *Rab and his Friends*.

Symmers, Douglas (1879–1952) American associate professor of pathology at the Bellevue Hospital. He described a new disease with follicular lymphadenopathy and splenomegaly which was later named Brill–Symmers disease.

Symington Anococcygial Body Fibromuscular mass found between the coccyx and the anus in the perineum. Described by Scottish anatomist, Johnson Symington (1851–1924), professor of anatomy at Belfast in 1888.

Sympathectomy Performed for relief of pain due to vascular disease by Mathieu Jaboulay (1860–1913) of Paris in 1900. It was tried as treatment for angina by Thomas Joannesco (1860–1926) of Rumania in 1916. Lumbar sympathectomy was performed through an anterolateral extraperitoneal approach by René Leriche (1879–1955) of Paris in 1933. Boston surgeon, Reginald Hammerick Smithwick (b 1899), performed sympathetectomy for hypertension (1944) and Raynaud disease (1936).

Sympathetic Nervous System [Greek: *syn*, with + *pathos*, feeling] The term sympathetic was introduced by Danish anatomist, Winslow (1669–1760) in 1732. *See autonomic nervous system.*

Symphysiotomy [Greek: *symphysis*, a growing together + *tome*, to cut] Technique described in obstetrics by French obstetrician, Jean René Sigault (b 1740) of Paris in 1777.

Symposium Heraclides of Tarentum, a physician from the school of Herophilus around 75 BC, was one of the first to use the term to refer to his work on dietetics in the form of a dialogue.

Symptomatology [Greek: *symptoma*, any thing that befalls one + *logos*, discourse] A systematic and accurate description of symptoms in various diseases was given by Hippocrates (460–377 BC). Thomas Sydenham (1624–1689) was known for his accurate observations and description of symptoms and signs. An attempt at classification of diseases according to symptoms was made by Felix Platter (1536–1614) of Basel in 1602.

Synapse [Greek: *synapsis*, connection] Word introduced in 1897 by M. Foster and Sir Charles Scott Sherrington (1857–1952) to describe the anatomical relationship between contiguous neurons. The structure was studied in detail by Ramón y Cajal (1852–1954), in 1903. *See synaptic transmission.*

Synaptic Transmission [Greek: *synapsis*, connection] Found in the nervous system and suggested to be more an electrical phenomenon than chemical mechanism by Sir John Carew Eccles (b 1903), an Australian neurophysiologist at Sir Charles Scott Sherrington's (1857–1952) department of physiology at Oxford in the 1920s. Eccles also demonstrated the depolarization of post-synaptic muscle in response to neural stimulus which he named excitatory post-synaptic potential (EPSP). The chemical nature was demonstrated in 1921 by Otto Loewi (1873–1961), a German-born pharmacologist. The chemical substance released was identified as acetylcholine in 1929 by British physiologist, Sir Henry Hallet Dale (1875–1968).

Syncope [Latin: *syncopa*, fainting fit] Cardiac passion is an ancient Greek expression for syncope. Galen (AD 129–200) and other ancient physicians considered it a complication of fever. Caelius Aurelianus described it under morbus cardiacus, and Aretaeus (81–138) used the term syncope for it and recommended venesection as treatment. A report of syncope due to cardiac arrest or heart block was given by Marcus Gerbezius (1658–1718) in 1692. The same condition

was described as 'epilepsy with slow pulse' by Giovanni Battista Morgagni (1682–1771) in 1761 and 'a clear case of syncopal attacks with heart block' was presented by Robert Adams (1791–1875) in 1827.

Syndrome [Greek: *syndrome*, concurrence] The term refers to the clinical picture of a disease made up of several typical symptoms and signs.

Synge, Richard Laurence Millington (b 1914) British biochemist who studied at Cambridge. He developed partition chromatography and counter-current liquid–liquid separation of mixtures. He used powered potato starch packed into columns to separate amino acids. He shared the Nobel Prize for Chemistry with Archer John Porter Martin (b 1910) in 1952.

Synovia [Greek: *syn*, with + *ovum*, egg] Term used by Paracelsus (1493–1541) in 1520, due its resemblance to an egg white. Marie François Xavier Bichat (1771–1802) devoted a chapter in his *Traite des membranes en General et de Diverses Membranes en Particulier* published in 1799. London anatomist, Clopton Havers (1657–1702), considered it as mucus-secreting in nature. Synovectomy as a formal procedure in surgery was introduced by M. Alfred Mignon (b 1854) of Paris in 1899.

Synovial Membrane *See synovia.*

Synovioma Tumor of the synovial membrane described by Robert Fulton Weir (1838–1927), a surgeon from New York, in 1886.

Synthalin The trypanocidal effect of this compound was shown to be due to its action in reducing glucose concentration at cellular levels by Jansco in 1935. This led to a search for similar trypanocidal compounds, and pentamidine was discovered in 1937 as a result.

Synthetic Estrogen After the isolation of natural estrogens it was noted that a 5-steroid group of compounds also had estrogenic activity. A search for similar synthetic compounds was made by Sir Edward Charles Dodds (1899–1973) in 1933. Around the same time, a Harvard-trained biochemist and Nobel Prize winner, Edward Adelbert Doisy (b 1893), started investigating compounds which had estrogenic properties similar to oxidation products of estrodiol. Stilbene, the first synthetic estrogen, was produced in 1936, followed by stilbestrol, synthesized by Dodds in 1938. The most potent oral estrogen, ethinyl estrodiol, was prepared from estradiol by H.H. Inhoffen and W. Hohlweg in the same year. A related chemical to the natural hormone was prepared by K. Miescher in 1944. Total synthesis of estrone was announced by G. Anner and Miescher in 1948. *See estrogens.*

Syphilis Several statements in the *Ayur Veda* suggest that venereal disease was present in India in ancient times. Venereal sores were noted in China before 600 BC and a specific name for it appears in writings from the time of the Tang dynasty around AD 618 to 906. The first Spanish treatise on it was written by Francisco Lopez de Villalobos, physician to King Charles I in 1498. A 15th century Spanish physician, Juan Almonder, published *De Morbo Gallico* in 1502. The term syphilis was coined by Fracastorius (1478–1533) in *Syphilis sive morbus Gallicus* published in 1530. It is said to have been brought to Europe by Columbus' sailors when they returned to Europe in 1493. Treatment with mercury was given by Giorgio Sanmariva of Verona in 1496. Potassium iodide was used as treatment of secondary syphilis by Robert Williams of St Thomas' Hospital in 1831 and its use in tertiary syphilis was popularized by William Wallace (1791–1837) of Dublin in 1835, who also published a treatise on venereal diseases in 1833. The causative organism was discovered in 1905 by Fritz Richard Schaudinn (1871–1906) from Germany, a protozoologist at the Institute of Tropical Diseases in Hamburg. *See Treponema pallidum, venereal disease, genitourinary medicine, neurosyphilis, Lock Hospital.*

Syringe [Greek: *syringx*, pipe] Dominique Anel (1679–1725) in 1712 devised a syringe for the injection of the lachrymal duct. A hypodermic tubular needle and syringe was constructed by French surgeon, Charles Gabriel Pravaz (1791–1853), in 1851. It was developed to give injections by Scottish physician Alexander Wood (1818–1884) in 1855. He used it to give morphine injections to the site of pain or nerves supplying the painful area. It was introduced into America by Foredyce Barker in 1856 and George Thompson Elliot in 1858.

Syringomyelia [Greek: *syringx*, pipe + *myel*, nerve] Morbid cavitation in the spinal cord, first observed by Charles Estienne (1503–1564) in 1546. Theophile Bonet (1620–1689) noted it in 1688. Antoine Portal (1742–1832) related the lesion to paralysis in 1804. The term was coined by Ollivier d'Angiers in 1824. The central canal was shown to be a normal feature by Benedict Stilling (1810-1879) in 1859. Before this time it was thought to be abnormal by d'Angiers and others. A description in England was given by London physician, Sir William Withey Gull (1816–1890) in 1862. Important accounts were also given by Jacob Augustus Lockhart Clarke (1817–1880) and Hughlings Jackson (1834–1911) in 1867. A more detailed and complete account was given by Otto Kahler (1849-1893) in 1888.

Systemic Lupus Erythematosus (SLE) An early descriptions was given by Laurent Theodore Biett (1781–1840), a physician in Paris. Moritz Kaposi (1837–1902), a Hungarian dermatologist, described it in 1872 and it was recognized as a disease entity by G. Pernet of Paris in 1908. The cardiac manifestations were noted by New York physician, Emanuel Libman (1872–1946) in 1911 (Libman–Sacks endocarditis) who published his findings with Benjamin Sacks (1873–1939) in 1924. Nephritis as a common feature was observed by Norman Macdonnell Keith (1885–1976) in 1920 and confirmed by Libman and Sacks in 1924. The wire loop lesions of the kidney were shown by George Baehr (b 1887) and co-workers in 1935. Diffuse collagen disease was described by Paul Klemperer (1887–1964) and colleagues in 1942 and included disseminated lupus erythematosus and diffuse scleroderma. The diagnostic presence of LE cells was discovered by Malcolm MacCallum Hargraves (b 1903) in 1948.

Systolic Blood Pressure [Greek: *systole*, drawing together] A clinical method of measuring it was devised by Samuel Siegfried Ritter von Basch (1837–1905) of Vienna in 1881. He applied external pressure to the artery and felt the pulse beyond the site of pressure, and is still in use today. Pierre Carl Edouard Potain (1825–1901) modified Basch's instrument in 1889 and Scipione Riva Rocci (1863–1939) introduced the air cuff which encircled the limb for measurement of blood pressure in 1890. *See blood pressure.*

Systolic Click When accompanied by a late systolic murmur, it was thought to be extracardiac in origin until 1913 when L. Gallavardin proposed that pericardial adhesions were responsible. The suggestion that it came from the mitral valve due to regurgitation was made in 1963 by J. V. O. Reid and John B. Barlow, professor of cardiology at Witwatersrand, South Africa. It was later attributed to mitral valve prolapse.

Szent-Györgyi, Albert von Nagyrapolt (1893–1986) Hungarian biochemist and Nobel Prize winner (1937) from Budapest who emigrated to America in 1947. He identified the role of vitamin C or ascorbic acid in scurvy in 1928. Adenosine triphosphate was shown to be a key factor in supplying energy for muscle contraction in *in vitro* studies by him in 1938 and he described ATP as a cogwheel in the mechanism of muscle. In 1942 he showed that the proteins, actin and myosin, act together to effect muscle contraction. He said 'to see actomyosin contract for the first time was one of the most exciting experiences of my scientific career'.

Szily, Aurel von (1847–1920) German ophthalmologist who performed chemical cauterization of the choroid in 1934.

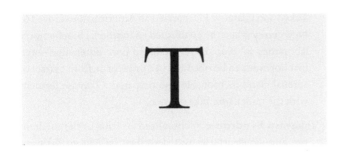

T Cells Suppresser lymphocytes of the immune system. Identified and described by Richard K. Gerson (1932–1983) in 1970.

Tabardillo Spanish term for Mexican or Spanish form of typhus used by Francisco Bravo (1530–1594) of Mexico in his *Opera Medicinalia* published in Mexico City in 1570. This book was the first printed medical book in the New World.

Tabari, Ali Ibn Rabban (*c* AD 600) Christian medical writer from eastern Persia who converted to Islam. He wrote *Firdaus-ul-Hikmat* (Paradise of Wisdom), an early medical encyclopedia. He reported the appearance of smallpox during the siege of Mecca in 569.

Tabby Cat Appearance Characteristic striping of the heart found during postmortem in patients with severe anemia. Described in 1824 by James Scarth Combe (1796–1883), a physician in Edinburgh in his paper *A Case of Anaemia* read before the Medico-Chirurgical Society of Edinburgh in 1822. This description was the first on pernicious anemia, 32 years before Thomas Addison's (1793–1860) account in 1855.

Tabes Dorsalis [Latin: *tabes*, wasting away] (Syn: locomotor ataxia, Duchenne disease) The first account of it involving the spinal cord was given by Sigismund Eduard Loewenhardt (1796–1875) in 1817. The symptoms and signs of locomotor ataxia were described in 1847 by British physician, Robert Bentley Todd (1809–1860). Lesions in the spinal cord were shown by German physician, Moritz Heinrich Romberg (1795–1873) in 1851 and the symptomatology was described by Sir John Russell Reynolds (1828–1896), professor of medicine at University College London, in *Diagnosis of the Diseases of the Spinal Cord and Nerves* in 1855. London physician, Sir William Whithey Gull (1816–1890) presented a series of cases in 1856 and microscopic wasting of the fibers was demonstrated around the same time by Viennese neurologist, Ludwig Türck (1810–1868). It was named locomotor ataxia by Guillaume Benjamin Amand Duchenne (1806–1875) in 1858. Tabetic gastric crises were described by Georges Delamarre of Paris in 1866. The spinal

lesions were also shown by Sir William Richard Gowers (1845–1915) in 1886. Irregular pupils were described by Austrian physician, Emile Berger (1855–1926) in 1889.

Tabetic Crisis Tabetic gastric crisis with paroxysms of severe abdominal pain in patients with tabetic syphilis were described by Georges Delamarre of Paris in 1866. Jean Martin Charcot (1825–1893) and Henri Bouchard (1833–1899) described it later in the same year.

Taboo A term of Polynesian origin which refers to certain practices both sacred and forbidden. Sigmund Freud (1856–1939) in *Totem and Taboo* (1913) proposed a psychological theory for society as a whole.

Taboparesis Neurosyphilis accompanied by symptoms and signs of both tabes dorsalis and general paralysis of the insane. *See tabes dorsalis, general paralysis of the insane.*

Tabor, Robert Sir (1642–1681) English apothecary from Cambridge who became famous through his secret remedy for malaria. He was appointed physician to King Charles II and was later knighted. King Charles had to write to the Royal College of Physicians asking them not to interfere with Tabor's practice. He became famous in France by curing the son of King Louis XIV of malaria. After his death the active ingredient in his secret preparation was found to be the well known cinchona bark which was already in wide use as a cure for malaria. His *Account of the cause and cure of Ague* was published in 1672.

Tachycardia [Greek: *tachys*, speed + *kardia*, heart] Irish physician, William Stokes (1804–1878), gave the first description of paroxysmal tachycardia in 1854 and it was also described by Richard Payne Cotton (1820–1877), from Kensington in London in 1869. Austrian physician Wilhelm Winternitz (1835–1917) showed that supraventricular tachycardia consisted of a series of atrial extrasystoles in 1883. He demonstrated this with the aid of his polygraph. The current name, atrial tachycardia, was given by Léon Bouveret (1850–1929) in 1889. ECG changes were recognized by Sir Thomas Lewis (1881–1943) in 1909, and described in more detail by P. S. Barker and colleagues in 1943. The occurrence in digitalis toxicity was noted by G. R. Herrmann in 1944 and confirmed by Bernard Lown (b 1921), an American electrophysiologist in 1958. *See ventricular tachycardia.*

Tactile Organs [Latin: *tactilis*, pertaining to touch] *See Wagner corpuscle, Meissner corpuscle, Merkel corpuscle.*

Taddeo, Alderotti (1223–1303) Italian physician at Florence who introduced a system of case histories for teaching clinical medicine.

Taenia [Latin: *taenia*, tape] Hippocrates (460–377 BC) divided intestinal worms into round lumbricae (*Ascaris*) and broad lumbrici (*Taenia*) and pomegranate was a popular treatment for both forms. Flatworms were grouped together as *Taenia saginita* and differentiated and described by John Augustus Ephraim Goeze (1731–1786) from Halle in 1782. Karl Asmund Rudolphi (1771–1832) in 1810 divided tapeworms into adult and cystic forms. *Taenia nana*, a common tapeworm, was discovered by Theodor Maximillian Bilharz (1825–1862) in 1852. *Taenia echinococcus* was described by Batsch in 1786 and later by Zeder in 1803. German zoologist, Carl Theodor Ernest von Siebold (1804–1865), demonstrated in 1854 that dogs could be experimentally infected with *Taenia echinococcus* and the complete life history and morphology were given by Karl Georg Friedrich Rudolph Leuckart (1823–1898) in 1860. *Taenia nana* infection in man was shown by Bilharz and named by Thomas Spencer Cobbold (1828–1886) in 1876.

Taenia nana [Latin: *taenia*, tape] Tapeworm infection in man was shown by Theodor Maximillian Bilharz (1825–1862), German professor of zoology at Cairo. The parasite was named by Thomas Spencer Cobbold (1828–1886) in 1876. It is also known as *Hymenolepis nana*.

Taenia saginata [Latin: *taenia*, tape; + *sagitta*, arrow] Beef tapeworm was described in 1782 by John Augustus Ephraim Goeze (1731–1786), a German clergyman and naturalist at Halle.

Taenia solium [Latin: *taenia*, tape; Syrian: *schuscle*, chains] Pork tapeworm was described by Carl Linnaeus (1707–1778) in 1758.

Tagliocozzi, Gaspare (1491–1553) Italian plastic surgeon from Bologna whose work was opposed by Ambroise Paré (1510–1590) and Gabriele Falloppio (1523–1562) on religious grounds. His body was exhumed and reburied in unconsecrated grounds by the church. His *De Curatorum Chirurgia per Infinitonem* was published in 1597.

Tait, Lawson Robert (1845–1899) Surgeon from Edinburgh who settled in Birmingham in 1871. He performed a successful operation for ruptured tubal pregnancy in 1883. He introduced his method of dilating the cervix in 1880 and the flap-splitting operation for plastic repair of the perineum in 1879. He also performed the first hepatotomy in 1880.

Takaki, Kanehiro (1849–1915) *See beriberi.*

Takamine, Jokichi (1834–1922) Japanese-born American chemist from Takaoka who studied chemical engineering in Tokyo and Glasgow. He married an American and moved to New Jersey where he established an industrial biochemistry laboratory in 1890. He crystallized pure adrenaline – the first hormone to be obtained in a pure form, from extract of adrenal gland in 1901. He also prepared a diastase ferment with the tradename Taka diastase.

Takayasu Syndrome Generalized arteritis of the medium size and larger arteries was described by Mikito Takayasu (1860–1938) of Japan in 1908.

Taliafero, Valentine H. (1831–1888) *See episeotomy.*

Talipes [Latin: *talipes*, club foot] *See club foot.*

Tallqvist Scale A color lithographic scale for estimating the percentage of hemoglobin in blood. Devised by a Finnish physician, Theodore Waldemar Tallqvist (1871–1927).

Talma Disease Form of myotonia which develops in adult life following trauma or infection. Described in 1892 by Sape Talma (1847–1918), a physician from Utrecht.

Talmud Ancient Rabbinical writings consisting of the Mishnah and the Gemara and the basis of religious authority for traditional Judaism. Two groups of scholars, one in Babylon, and the other in Palestine started to compile it. It is also an important source of knowledge of Hebrew medicine and contains some of the earliest recordings of animal anatomy, as human dissections were not permitted during that time. The earliest suggestion that a cesarean section could be performed in a live mother is made in the Mishnah. It also mentions contraceptive substances, blood letting and other medical practices.

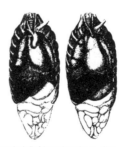

Pericardium not distended (left); pericardium distended with 15 ounces of fluid (right). J. Russell Reynolds, *A System of Medicine* (1877). MacMillan, London

Tamponade [French: *tamponner*, to stop up] An early description of cardiac tamponade caused by collection of blood in the pericardium secondary to cardiac rupture was given by Berlin physician, Edmund Rose (1836–1914). The Beck triad, low arterial pressure, high venous pressure and absent apex beat, was described by American surgeon Claude Schaeffer Beck (1894–1971) of Pennsylvania.

Tapeworm *See Taenia.*

Tanqueral, Planches des (1809-1862) *See lead poisoning.*

Tarantism Dancing mania, started in Apulia in Italy in the latter part of the 14th century. It was believed to have been caused by the bite of Apulian spider or Tarantula. In the 14th and 15th centuries hundreds of people who believed that they had been bitten took to the streets, and their dancing mania spread to many cities and villages in Italy. A description was given by Nicholas Perotti (1430–1480).

Tardi, Claude (1607–1670) French physician who proposed the theoretical basis for blood transfusion from man to man in 1667.

Tardieu Spots Ecchymosis seen on the pleura following suffocation. Described by French physician, Auguste Ambroise Tardieu (1818–1879).

Target Cells Present in iron-deficiency anemia. Observed by Russell Landram Haden (1888–1952) of Kansas, a hematologist and F.D. Evans in 1937. A.M. Barrett named them in 1938.

Tarin, Pierre (1725–1761) French anatomist who studied the brain. He described thickening of the velum medullare at the vermis of the cerebellum (Tarin valve) in 1750. He was also a medical historian.

Tarnier Forceps Axis traction forceps for applying traction along the line of the pelvic axis. Designed in 1860 by French obstetrician, Etienne Stéphane Tarnier (1828–1897).

Tarsus [Greek: *tarsos*, broad flat surface] Term used to denote a variety of flattened objects such as wings of a bird, blade of a saw or rudder of a ship. Galen (AD 129–200) used the term to refer to the flat parts of the skeleton such as the foot, hand or margin of the eyelid.

Tartaric Acid Its salts are used in food preparation and as a cathartic. Produced by Swedish chemist, Carl Wilhelm Scheele (1742–1786) in 1770 and by Justus von Liebig (1803–1873) of Germany in 1846. Stereochemistry originated from Louis Pasteur's (1822–1895) work on three isomers of tartaric acid in 1848. It was developed by Dutch chemist, Jacobus Henricus Van't Hoff (1852–1911) and French chemist Joseph Achille Le Bel (1847–1930) in 1874.

Tattoo [Tahitian: *tatu*, puncture] It was important to the primitive Picts. They, like the Goths, decorated their bodies with various figures using pigments applied with sharp iron instruments. The practice was prohibited for those under 18 in England, following the Tattooing of Minors Act in 1969. It was identified as a mode of transmission of hepatitis B virus in the 1980s.

Tatum, Edward Lawrie (1909–1975) American biochemist from Boulder, Colorado. He worked with George Wells Beadle (1903–1989) on the bread mold, *Neurospora*, and showed the role of genes in biochemical processes. They irradiated the spores with X-rays and examined growth of mutant spores and formulated the 'one gene one enzyme' theory. He collaborated with Joshua Lederberg (b 1925) at Yale in showing that bacteria reproduce by conjunction. All three shared the Nobel Prize for Physiology or Medicine in 1958. He contributed to the subsequent development of genetic engineering by H. Gruneberg, Conrad Hal Waddington (1905–1975) and others. *See genetic engineering.*

Taussig, Helen Brooke (1898–1986) American pediatrician from Cambridge, Massachusetts and a pioneer in surgical intervention for congenital heart disease. She graduated from Johns Hopkins in 1927 and became the first woman professor there. The Blalock–Taussig shunt was the first surgical operation for Fallot tetralogy and was performed by Alfred Blalock (1899–1964) and Taussig in 1945.

Taussig Operation Iliac lymphadenectomy combined with irradiation in cases of cancer of the cervix. Described by American gynecologist, Frederick Joseph Taussig (b 1872) of St Louis in 1934.

Tavel Serum One of the first antistreptococcal sera. Prepared by Ernst Tavel (1858–1912), a surgeon at Bern in Switzerland. He devised a method of gastrostomy in 1906.

Tawara Node Atrioventricular node of the conducting system of the heart. Discovered in 1906 by Japanese anatomist, Sunao Tawara (1873–1952), a pupil of Karl Albert Aschoff (1866–1942) in Germany.

Taxis [Greek: *taxis*, to put in order or arrange] There are several uses for this word: (1) movement of a motile organism in response to an external stimulus; (2) manual replacement of a displaced or injured organ or structure such as a fracture, dislocation or hernia.

Taxonomy [Greek: *taxis*, drawing up in rank or file + *nomos*, law] Used for classification of plants on a morphological basis by Swiss botanist, Augustin Pyrame de Candolle (1778–1841) in 1813 and Carl Linnaeus (1707–1778) in Sweden.

Tay–Sachs Disease Amaurotic familial idiocy with ocular manifestations. Described by Warren Tay (1843–1927), a British ophthalmologist from Yorkshire at the London Hospital in 1880. The cerebral manifestations and its pathology were pointed out by Bavarian physician, Bernard Parney Sachs (1858–1944) in New York in 1887.

Taylor, Alfred Swaine (1806–1880) English forensic scientist and the first chair of medical jurisprudence at Guy's Hospital in 1831. He wrote *Elements of Medical Jurisprudence* in 1836, and *Remarks on Death by Strangulation* in 1852.

Taylor, Alfred Simpson (1868–1942) New York surgeon who described a method of treatment for fracture dislocation of the cervical spine 1924.

Taylor, John Chevalier (1703–1772) Traveling oculist from Norwich and oculist to George II in 1736.

Taylor, Sir William (1843–1917) Medical graduate from Glasgow who became an army physician and served in Canada, Burma and India. He brought several reforms to the British Army after the South African War.

Taylor Apparatus Steel support used in the treatment of Pott disease of the spine. Devised in 1876 by New York orthopedic surgeon, Charles Fayette Taylor (1827–1899).

Taylor Disease Form of idiopathic localized atrophy of the skin described by American dermatologist, Robert William Taylor (1842–1908).

TB *See tuberculosis.*

Tea Taster Lung Caused by the fungus, *Monilia*, and found in Sri Lanka. Described by Marquis Aldo Castellani (1879–1971) of Florence in 1903.

Tea [Latin: *thea*] Infusion from the dried leaves of *Camellia sinensis*, introduced into Europe from the East by the Dutch in 1610. The English diarist Samuel Pepys (1633–1703) mentioned his first cup of tea in 1660. It was imported to England by the East India Company in 1669. The alkaloids caffeine, tannic acid and theophyllin were identified as the active components.

Teacher, John Hammond (1869–1930) Scottish pathologist from Glasgow who reported a case of sciatica due to rupture of the intervertebral disc in 1911. He also wrote an early work on the human embryo.

Teague Agar Used for culture of Ducrey bacillus of chancroid. Devised by New York bacteriologist, Oscar Teague (1878–1923) in 1922.

Teale, Sir Thomas Pridgin (1801–1868) English surgeon from Leeds who wrote a monograph on abdominal hernia in 1846. He also published other treatises on plastic surgery and amputation. *See abdominal hernia*

T Cell Suppresser lymphocytes identified and described by Richard K. Gerson (1932–1983) in 1970.

Technetium Manmade metallic element with no stable isotopes. Produced in 1937 by bombarding molybdenum with neutrons by American physicist of Italian origin,

Emilio Segrè (1905–1989). He shared the Nobel Prize for Physics in 1959. Technetium–99, a metastable isotope with a half-life of 6.03 hours was introduced into nuclear medicine by P.V. Harper in 1962 and is the most commonly used radionuclide in medicine.

Tooth [Anglo-Saxon: *toth*, tooth] *See dentistry, artificial teeth, dental caries, tooth transplantation.*

Teetotaller One who abstains from any form of fermented liquor. Word used by Richard Turner (d 1846) at a temperance meeting in 1833 where he stated 'that nothing but te-total will do'.

Teevan, William Frederic (1834–1887) *See skull fracture.*

Teflon Heat resistant material which prevents clogging and dust settling on it. Discovered by Roy J. Plunkett, an engineer in America in 1938. It is used in many medical appliances including canulae.

Teichmann Plexus Deep and superficial lymphatic plexus found on the wall of the stomach. Described in 1861 by Ludwig Carl Teichmann-Stawiarski (1823–1895), a histologist and professor of anatomy at Cracow.

Telencephalon [Greek: *tele*, far off + *enkephalos*, brain] Term for the anterior part of the developing brain consisting of cerebral vesicles and laminia terminalis.

Telengiectasis [Greek: *tele*, distant or remote + *anggeon*, vessel + *ekteneo*, distend] *See familial hemorrhagic telengiectasis, Campbell de Morgan spots.*

Telephone [Greek: *tele*, distance + *phone*, sound] The inventor of the telephone, Alexander Graham Bell (1847–1922) of Edinburgh, came from a generation of vocal physiologists. His grandfather and father were interested in the education of deaf mutes. It was invented by him while he was professor of vocal physiology at Boston University and patented on February 4th 1876. The first long distance telephone call between Bell and Thomas A. Watson, from New York to San Francisco was made in 1915. The first transatlantic call between Arlington, Virginia and the Eiffel Tower in Paris also took place in the same year.

Telephotography [Greek: *telos*, distant + *photos*, light + *graphein*, to write] The first transmission of a portrait by telephotography was done by Edmund Edward Fournier D'Albe (1868–1933) of London in 1923.

Temin, Howard Martin (b 1934) American virologist from Philadelphia who was educated at Swarthmore College and Caltech. He formulated the provirus hypothesis that genetic material of an invading virus is copied by the host DNA.

In 1970 he isolated reverse transcriptase that transcribes RNA into double-stranded DNA enabling it to be inserted into the host. Such viruses are known as retroviruses. Reverse transcriptase is now used in genetic engineering to copy specific genes. He was awarded the Nobel Prize for Physiology or Medicine in 1975. *See reverse transcriptase.*

Temperament [Latin: *temperamentum*] Inherent predisposition to react to stimuli in a certain manner. Galen (AD 129–200) grouped human differences into nine entities or temperaments. Other writers proposed sanguine, nervous and lymphatic dispositions. Four temperaments, melancholy, sanguine, choleric and phlegmatic, related to the four humors were illustrated in the Guild Book of Barber Surgeons dating from around 1500.

Temperance Abstinence from alcoholic beverages. The first temperance society in America was proposed in 1825 and established in 1826. One of the first temperance movements in England was started by Joseph Livesey of Preston, the editor of *Staunch Teetotaller*, in 1832. The National Temperance Society of England was formed in 1842 and the London Temperance League began in 1851.

Temperature *See thermometer, clinical thermometry.*

Temple Medicine A religious sanctuary from 12,000 BC was found in El Juyo cave in Spain by archaeologists in 1978. Babylonian physicians were priests and known as Assipu priests. They used magic, incantations, religious sacrifices and sometimes drugs. A temple in honor of the Greek god of medicine, Aesculapius, was built at Epidaurus around 600 BC. The grounds contained large non-poisonous yellow snakes which were allowed to lick the diseased parts of the body to effect healing. This led to Aesculapius being depicted with a serpent around his staff. Early practice mainly consisted of mysticism and magic but later gave way to physical medicine with mineral baths, massage, blood letting and therapeutics such as iron, milk and honey. *See Monastic Medicine.*

Templeman, Peter (1711–1769) Physician from Dorchester who practiced in London. He was keeper of the reading room at the British Museum and secretary of the Society of Arts.

Temporal Arteritis (Syn: Horton disease, giant cell arteritis) Inflammation of the temporal and other cranial arteries manifesting as headache and tenderness over the superficial arteries with visual symptoms, mainly during the sixth and seventh decades of life. Described by American physicians, Bayard Taylor Horton (d 1895), T. B. Magath and George Elgie Brown (1885–1935) in 1934. A histological picture of biopsied temporal arteries was described by Horton and Magath in 1937. Severe permanent impairment of vision in temporal arteritis was described by E. W. Shannon and J. Solomon in 1945.

Temporal Bone [Latin: *temporalis*, temple] Cranial bone derives its name due its site where the graying of the hair due to aging is first seen.

Temporal Lobe [Latin: *temporalis*, temple] Auditory radiation to it was traced by Richard L. Heschl (1824–1881) of Vienna in 1878. Its role as the center for olfactory and gustatory sensations was demonstrated by John Hughlings Jackson (1835–1911) in 1889. He also observed the abnormal sensation of smell and taste in a patient with a temporal lobe tumor.

Temporalis [Latin: *temporalis*, temple] Muscle of the cranium which derives its name from its site where the graying of the hair due to aging is first seen.

Tendo Achilles Bursitis Albert disease was described by Eduard Albert (1841–1900) of Austria in 1893.

Tendo Achilles [Latin: *tendere*, to stretch] *See Achilles tendon.*

Tendon Reflex [Latin: *tendere*, to stretch] Term introduced by Johan August Unzer (1727–1799) to describe the sensorymotor reaction in 1771. The role of the spinal roots in the reflex arc was described by Sir Charles Bell (1774–1842) in 1811 and François Magendie (1783–1855) in 1822. The term knee jerk to denote involuntary tendon reflex of the knee was coined by Sir William Richard Gowers (1845–1915), and the physical sign was named patellar tendon reflex by Wilhelm Heinrich Erb (1840–1921), and knee phenomenon by Karl Otto Friedrich Westphal (1833–1941). Erb demonstrated the loss of knee jerk in syphilis of the spinal cord. Reinforcement of the reflex was described independently by Silas Weir Mitchell (1829–1914) and Morris J. Lewis in 1886. Nobel Prize winner, Sir Charles Scott Sherrington (1857–1952), in 1893 demonstrated that it was an inhabitable phenomenon, thus establishing it as a genuine reflex. The segmental nature of the spinal cord and its interface with the higher centers was demonstrated by English physiologist, Marshall Hall (1790–1857) in 1833. Their abolition in the lower extremities associated with lesions above the lumbar segment of the spinal cord was demonstrated by Henry Charlton Bastian (1837–1915) of Truro. Further work was done by Edward George Tandy Liddell (1895–1981), a neurophysiologist at Oxford, and Sherrington.

Tendon [Latin: *tendere*, to stretch] An early reference to surgical repair of severed tendons was made by Galen (AD 129–200), physician to the Roman gladiators. A successful tendon transplantation in a case of paralytic talipes valgus was done by B. F. Parrish of America in 1892. A new method of tendon transplantation, using tendon sheaths to facilitate gliding of tendons, was devised by Leo Mayer in 1916. The proprioceptors, highly specialized somatic sensory end organs of the muscles, tendons and joints, were described by Sir Charles Scott Sherrington (1857–1952) in 1906. *See tendon reflexes.*

Tenesmus [Greek: *teinesmos*, strain] Paul of Aegina (AD 625–690) described it as 'an irresistible desire for evacuation, discharging nothing but some bloody mucus matter'. He recommended injection of honeyed water into the rectum. Galen (AD 129–200) stated that stones were sometimes passed through the anus in such cases. Aulus Cornelius Celsus (25 BC–AD 50) recommended tepid baths.

Tennis Elbow *See elbow.*

Tenon Capsule Fascia bulbi was named after French army surgeon and professor of pathology, Jacques René Tenon (1724–1816) who specialized in ophthalmology, in 1816.

Tenotomy [Greek: *teinein*, to stretch + *tome*, to cut] A new surgical method of treatment for club foot involving subcutaneous section of the tendo achilles was introduced in 1816 by Jacques Mathieu Delpech (1777–1832), professor of surgery at Montpellier. It was applied as treatment for other deformities arising out of muscular defects by German orthopedic surgeon, Georg Friedrich Ludwig Stromeyer (1804–1876) around 1836. It was advocated in France by French surgeon, Amédée Bonnet (1802–1858) in 1841.

Tentorium Cerebellum [Latin: *tentorium*, tent] Name derives from its tent-like appearance over the cerebellum.

Teratology [Latin: *teras*, monster + *logos*, discourse] Term coined in 1822 by Etienne Saint-Hilaire (1772–1844) to denote the study of congenital malformations. He attempted to produce congenital malformations by manipulating chicken eggs. His son, Isidore Geoffrey Saint-Hilaire, named and classified hundreds of specific malformations. Experimental work on malformations especially in birds eggs was done by Peter Ludwig Panum (1820–1885) of Berlin in 1860.

Terminal Care [Latin: *terminus*, end] *See hospice.*

Terramycin *See oxytetracycline.*

Terrier Valve Gall bladder valve found between the gall bladder and the cystic duct. Described in 1891 by Louis Felix Terrier (1837–1908), professor of surgery at Paris.

Terson Gland Conjunctival gland described by French ophthalmologist from Toulouse, Albert Terson (1867–1935), in 1892.

Tertian Fever [Latin: *tertius*, third] Fever occurring every third day in malaria. Described by Hippocrates (460–377 BC).

Tesla Coil Produces a high voltage at high frequency. Invented by Nikola Tesla (1856–1943), an American electrical engineer of Yugoslavian origin, in 1891.

Test Tube Baby Successful *in vitro* fertilization of human gametes was showed by Robert Geoffrey Edwards (b 1925) and Patrick Christopher Steptoe (1913–1988) in 1969. A human test tube baby was born in England in 1978. *See in vitro fertilization.*

Testaceae [Latin: *testa*, shell] Arcellinida, one of the oldest classifications in biology, includes shellfish, oysters and crayfish. Pliny (AD 23–79) distinguished lower animals in water into three classes: crustacea, testacea and mollusca. Their role in dietetics was discussed by Athenaeus of Egypt in *The Deipnosophists*, written during the third century AD.

Testicles [Latin: *testis*] Their tubular nature was discovered by Claude Aubrey who wrote *Testis Examinatus* in 1658. An early account on the structure was given by Regnier de Graaf (1641–1673) in 1668. A modern monograph on structure and diseases was published by Sir Astley Paston Cooper (1768–1841) of Guy's Hospital in 1830. Evidence for the presence of a humoral substance in them which effected an organ remote from its origin was presented by Arnold Adolph Berthhold (1803–1861) in 1849. He transplanted testes to an emasculated rooster and demonstrated normal resumption of male sexual characteristics. Leydig or interstitial cells were described in 1850 by Franz von Leydig (1821–1908), professor of histology and a comparative anatomist at Würzberg. Thomas Blizzard Curling (1811–1888) considered them to be controlled by the brain and sympathetic nervous system in *A Practical Treatise on the Diseases of the Testis*. Testosterone from the testicular tissue was isolated by Dutch pharmacists, K. David, E. Emanse, F. Freud and E. Laqueur in 1933. *See orchidopexy.*

Testicular Reflex Contraction of abdominal muscles on compression of testicles. Described by Swiss surgeon, Theodor Kocher (1841–1917) in 1874.

Testicular Tumor French surgeon, Edme Lèsauvage (1778–1852), gave an account of spermatic cord tumors in 1845. Interstitial cell sarcoma was described by German pathologist, David Paul von Hansemann (1858–1920) in 1895. Seminoma was described by French urologist, Maurice Chevassau (b 1877) in 1906. German physician, Ludwig Pick (b 1868), described arrhenoblastoma in 1905. Radical surgery involving the removal of lumbar lymph nodes and spermatic vein was described by Philadelphia surgeon, John Bingham Roberts (1852–1924) in 1902. Gynecomastia associated with testis tumors was noted by Bennet Judson Gilbert (b 1898) in 1940.

Testis [Latin: *testis*] *See testicles.*

Testosterone [Latin: *testis*, testicle; Greek: *stear*, suet] *See androgens.*

Tetanus Toxoid *See tetanus.*

Tetanus Vaccine *See tetanus.*

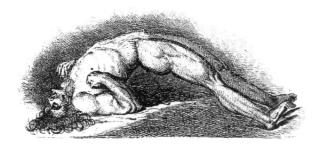

'True opisthotonus'. Sir Charles Bell, *The Anatomy and Philosophy of Expression* (1890). George Bell & Son, London

Tetanus [Greek: *tetanos*, stretched or stiffness] (Syn: lock-jaw) Aretaeus (81–138) observed that the wounds of muscular or nervous part, abortion, and excessive cold caused it, and mentioned the first two causes as fatal. He classified three varieties of spasms: emprosthotonus when the parts of the body are bent forwards, opisthotonus when bent backwards and tetanus when the parts are stretched equally both ways. According to Hippocrates (460–377 BC) it was fatal within four days or recovery occurs. Some remedies recommended by ancient physicians include: oil baths, cupping, purging and antispasmodics such as castor oil and asafetida. The French military surgeon Dominique Jean Larrey (1766–1842) saw numerous cases in the field and wrote on the subject in 1812. He recommended amputation of the limb. Its true cause remained obscure until Antonio Carle (1854–1927) and Giorgio Rattone of Italy demonstrated the transferability of the disease in animals in 1884. In the same year Arthur Nicolaier (b 1862) of Göttingen

showed that it could be produced in guinea pig and rabbit by inoculating them with contaminated earth. A bacillus was observed in a human case by Anton Julius Frederick Rosenbach (1842–1923) in 1886 and it (*Clostridium tetani*) was isolated by Shibasaburo Kitasato (1852–1931) in 1889. Vaccine was developed by Emil Behring (1854–1917) and used during World War l. A formaldehyde-treated toxin was introduced by P. Descombey in 1924. An alum-precipitated toxoid was prepared by Alexander Thomas Glenny (1882–1965), a British bacteriologist in 1930 and used on humans by Leon Gaston Ramon (1886–1963) and Christian Zoeller (1888–1934) in 1933.

Tetany An account of infantile tetany was given by John Clarke (1761–1815) in his treatise on pediatrics, published in 1815. Spasm of the glottis was described by English physician, George Kellie in 1816. It was attributed to the parathyroid gland by Salmon Levi Steinheim (1789–1866) in 1830. Armand Trousseau (1801–1867) named it 'tetanilla' and François Remy Lucien Covisart (1824–1882) described it and introduced the term 'tetanie' in 1852. Trousseau sign of tetanic spasm of the hand on applying pressure to the arm was by described Trousseau in 1861. The Chvostek sign where the facial muscles go into spasms on tapping the facial nerve, a diagnostic sign in tetany, was described in 1876 by Austrian surgeon, Frantisek Chvostek (1835–1884). Parathyroid hormone was used in treatment in 1925 by James Bertram Collip (1892–1965), a biochemist at Alberta.

Tetracycline Antibiotic derived from *Streptomyces aureofaciens* from a Missouri farmyard by a retired botany professor, Benjamin Duggar of Wisconsin in 1948. Aureomycin became the most commonly prescribed antibiotic over the next decades. Oxytetracycline or terramycin was isolated from *Streptomyces rimosus* by Alexander Carpenter Finlay (b 1906) and co-workers in 1950.

Tetralogy of Fallot [Greek: *tetras*, four + *logos*, discourse] Outflow obstruction to the right ventricle, ventricular septal defect, right ventricular hypertrophy and dextroposition of the aorta were described by Etienne-Louis Arthur Fallot (1850–1911) of France in 1888. The Blalock–Taussig shunt, the first surgical operation for Fallot tetralogy, was performed by Alfred Blalock (1899–1964) and Helen Taussig (1898–1986) of Johns Hopkins Hospital in 1945.

Teutonic Order Military knights who attended the sick and wounded of the Christian army during the Crusades. Established at Jerusalem in 1191.

Texas Cattle Fever *See babesiasis.*

Thacher, James (1754–1844) *See Bibliography in Medicine.*

Thacher, Thomas (1620-1678) *See American Medical books.*

Thackeray, William Makepiece (1811–1863) English novelist, born in Calcutta, where his father was in the East India Company. In *Pendennis* he described the life and practice of a typical early 19th century apothecary .

Thackrah, Charles Turner (1795–1833) Pupil of Sir Astley Paston Cooper (1768–1841) at Guy's Hospital. A founder of provincial medical education in England. He formed the Leeds School of Anatomy in 1826 which developed into the Leeds University School of Medicine. He was also a pioneer of industrial medicine and wrote the first book in England on occupational medicine in 1832.

Thaddeus of Florence (1223–1303) Physician who taught anatomy at Bologna where he encouraged dissections. He helped translate some Greek medical classics into Latin.

Thalamic Syndrome Contralateral spontaneous pain, transient hemiplegia, ataxia and choreoathetoid movements due to thrombosis or other lesions of the thalamogeniculate artery. Described by Joseph Jules Dejerine (1849–1917) and Gustave Roussy (1874–1948) of Paris in 1906.

Thalamus [Greek: *thalamos*, inner chamber] Pliny (AD 23–79) referred to the temple of Apis as thalamus. Thalami cordis for the chambers of the heart and thalami penis for the cavernous spaces of the penis were used before the time of Andreas Vesalius (1514–1564). Galen (AD 129–200) used it for those chambers at the base of the brain which he thought supplied animal spirits to the optic nerves. Thalamic nuclei were described by Henri de Mondeville (1260–1320), an Italian anatomist who referred to it as anchee (buttocks). It was revived in a modern sense by Thomas Willis (1621–1675) in 1664 and details of the structure was elucidated in 1869 by Bernhard Alloys von Gudden (1824–1886), a neuroanatomist and professor of psychiatry at Zurich.

Thalassemia Major [Greek: *thalassa*, sea] Hereditary hemolytic anemia first noted to mainly affect those of Mediterranean origin. Association with bone changes in children due to a hemoglobinopathy, was described by American pediatrician, Thomas Benton Cooley (1871–1945) in 1925. A genetic defect involving deletion of a specific globin gene was shown by British molecular biologist, Richard Anthony Flavell (b 1945), head of the Laboratory of Gene Structure and Expression at the National Institute of Medical Research at Mill Hill from 1979 to 1983.

Thalassemia Minor [Greek: *thalassa*, sea] Relatively mild anemia due to a heterozygous thalassemia trait for a specific

hemoglobinopathy. Described independently by F. Rietti (1925) and E. Greppi (1928).

Thales (624–545 BC) Greek philosopher, astronomer and geometer from the city of Miletus in Asia Minor was a founder among Greek philosophers. He devoted his time to mathematics and measured the height of a pyramid by its shadow. He predicted the exact date of the solar eclipse of 585 BC and determined the number of days in a year as 365. He proposed water as the essence and origin of all things and the electrical properties of amber when rubbed were observed by him. Most of his discoveries have been conveyed through Aristotle's (384–322 BC) works.

Thalidomide Introduced as a hypnotic and sedative in Germany in 1958. Its use over the next three years was associated with a form of congenital abnormality called phocomelia, where limbs failed to develop in infants born to mothers who took the drug. It was withdrawn from the market.

Thallium Scan Used for study of myocardial perfusion with thallium-201 tracer. Introduced by E. Lebowitz and colleagues in 1973.

Thallium [Greek: *thallos*, green shoot] Metallic element discovered through spectral analysis by Sir William Crookes (1832–1919) in 1861 and by Belgian chemist, Claude August Lamy (1820–1878) in 1862. Its salts are active poisons and the 201 isotope is used in diagnostics radiology.

Thanatology [Greek: *thanatos*, death + *logos*, discourse] Medicolegal study of death and conditions affecting dead bodies.

Thannhauser, Josef Siegfried (b 1885) German physician who described familial clustering of patients with xanthomas, hypercholesterolemia and premature heart disease (familial hypercholesterolemia) in 1938.

Thayer, William Sydney (1864–1932) American graduate of Harvard and professor of medicine at Johns Hopkins Hospital. He studied and described the third heart sound. He published a volume of poetry, *America 1917 and other verse* .

Thaysen Syndrome Paroxysmal intense pain in the region of the anus and the internal sphincter and of unknown etiology. Described in 1917 by Alexander MacLennan, a lecturer in surgery at Glasgow University. It is named after Danish physician Thornwald Einar Hess Thaysen (1883–1936) who described it as proctalgia fugax in 1935.

Thebesius, Adam Christian (1686–1732) German anatomist at Leiden who gave a description of venarum minimarum cordis (Thebesius veins) and the coronary sinus of the heart (Thebesius valve) in 1708.

Theelin Estrone preparation obtained by a biochemist and Nobel Prize winner, Edward Adelbert Doisy (1893–1986) of Illinois and C. D.Valer in 1929.

Theile Canal Space formed by the reflection of the pericardium on the aorta and the pulmonary artery. Described by German anatomist, Friedrich Wilhelm Theile (1801–1879).

Theiler, Max (1899–1972) South African-born American bacteriologist from Pretoria, who studied medicine at the University of Cape Town, St Thomas' Hospital Medical School and the School of Tropical Medicine and Hygiene at London University. He joined Harvard Medical School to work on amebic dysentery in 1922 and later worked on yellow fever. He moved to Rockefeller Institute and then was appointed to the chair of epidemiology and microbiology at Yale Medical School in 1964. He attenuated live yellow fever virus in 1939, which led to the discovery of 17D vaccine for yellow fever in 1939. He was awarded the Nobel Prize for Physiology or Medicine in 1951 for his work.

Themison of Laodicea (b 50 BC) Founder of the Methodist school of medicine and a physician and disciple of Aesculapiades of Bythnia (110–40 BC). He explained disease on the basis of a state of relaxation or contraction of pores in the body. His followers named acute disease 'status strictus' to denote a state of contraction, and chronic disease 'status laxus' to indicate a state of relaxation.

Thenar [Greek: *thenar*, hand or palm] Aristotle (384–322 BC) defined it as that part of the hand between the carpus and fingers. Galen (AD 129–200) used the term to denote the hollow of the hand. Its current use denotes the fleshy ball of the thumb and was introduced by Rufus of Ephesus (AD 98–138).

Thénard, Louis Jacques (1777–1857) French organic chemist from Louptiere and a contemporary of Joseph Louis Gay-Lussac (1778–1850). He did a scientific study of the composition of bile in 1803 and he used the word 'picromel' to denote the sweetish bitter substance in it. His discoveries include: Thenard blue for coloring porcelain, sodium and potassium peroxide, boron and silicon.

Theology [Greek: *theos*, god + *logos*, a discourse] *Summa Totius Theologicae*, taken from the manuscripts of Thomas Aquinas, was printed in 1596. Some early English books include: *Analogy of Religion* by Butler (1736) and *Natural Theology* by Paley (1802).

Theophilus *See Johann Gottlieb Walter (1734–1818).*

Theophrastus (372–287 BC) Greek physician and philosopher from Eresus on Lesbos. He was a disciple of Aristotle (384–322 BC) and Plato. He wrote several treatises including *History of Plants, Treatise on Stones,* and *Moral Characters of Men.* He described the fundamental differences between plants and animals and the effects of various scents on body and mind and this formed the basis for aromatherapy. He succeeded Aristotle as a teacher in the Lyceum at Athens and laid the foundations for botany through his work on anatomy, physiology, systematics, pharmacognosy and plant pathology.

Theophylline Methylxanthine compound in tea leaves that has antispasmodic effects on bronchial smooth muscles was described by David Israel Macht (1882–1961) in 1921. Other salts are used as cardiac muscle and nervous system stimulants, bronchodilators and anti-asthmatics.

Theorell, Axel Hugo Theodore (1903–1982) Swedish biochemist and director of the Nobel Institute of Biochemistry in Stockholm. He crystallized myoglobin and determined its molecular weight in 1932. He separated flavin mononucleotide from protein and helped to identify vitamin B2. While at Uppsala University he purified diphtheria toxin, characterized cytochrome C, established the linkage between heme and protein and later studied peroxidases and dehydrogenases. He was awarded the Nobel Prize for Physiology or Medicine for his work in 1955.

Therapeutic Index [Greek: *therapeutikos,* inclined to serve] Ratio of dose tolerated by host to dose that cures the infection. Proposed by German bacteriologist, Paul Ehrlich (1854–1915), a pioneer in the field of chemotherapy.

Therapeutic Substances Act 1956 Controls manufacture, import and sale of drugs in England.

Therapeutics [Greek: *therapeutikos,* inclined to serve] Effective herbal remedies were known in China at the time of Emperor Shen Nung, 5000 years ago. Priests in the temple of Aesculapius practiced medicine through mysticism and magic, which later gave way to physical medicine with mineral baths, massage, blood letting and use of substances such as iron, milk and honey. Bizarre and unusual remedies such as crocodile dung, burnt human bones, blood from a stabbed gladiator, urine of an adolescent boy, owl blood, ass liver and similar substances were used by Greeks and Romans up to the 17th century. Galen (AD 129–200) listed over 300 herbal medicines and Pedanius Dioscorides, a

Greek physician from Anarzaba during the reign of Nero, studied medicinal herbs and described over 600 plants in five books on materia medica. Paracelsus (1493–1541), physician, alchemist, philosopher and astrologer from Switzerland, introduced chemical therapeutics, including mercurials. A landmark in therapeutics was the introduction of cinchona as treatment for malaria by a Spanish physician, Juan del Vego in 1639. Modern pharmacology began in the early 19th century with the discovery and isolation of plant alkaloids such as morphine by Frederick Wilhelm Sertuerner (1783–1841), emetine by Pierre Joseph Pelletier (1788–1842) and quinine from cinchona by Joseph Bienaimé Caventou (1795–1877) in 1824. Chemotherapeutics was established by Paul Ehrlich (1854–1915) with his concept of side chain theory. In 1910 he developed salvarsan or arsphenamine for treatment of relapsing fever, syphilis and trypanosomiasis. The battle against bacteria was won with the discovery of protonsil by Nobel Prize winner, Gerhard Johannes Paul Domagk (1895–1964) in 1935 and penicillin by Sir Alexander Fleming (1881–1955) in 1929 and demonstration of its clinical effectiveness by Sir Ernest Boris Chain (1906–1979) in 1940. They shared the Nobel Prize with Howard Walter Florey (1898–1968) in 1945 for their work on penicillin. Hydrotherapy is still used today. Psychotherapy began with Johann Christian Reil (1759–1813) and was established by Sigmund Freud (1856–1939), Carl Gustav Jung (1875–1961) and others. Occupational therapy was also known in ancient times and Seneca, who lived in 30 BC, recommended employment for treatment of mental unrest. Application of physical medicine to diseases of joints and bones was pioneered by French surgeon, Amédée Bonnet (1802–1858) around 1845. Antimetabolites such as mercaptopurine, methotrexate, and cyclophosphamide are used in cancer and immunosuppressive therapy. Alternative therapies such as aromatherapy, homeopathy and acupuncture are also still in use. *See chemotherapy, pharmacology, alternative therapy.*

Theresa of Calcutta (1910–1997) Roman Catholic nun in India, born in Yugoslavia to Albanian parents. She went to India at 18 to join the sisters of Loretto. She was ordained in 1937 and taught in a convent where she later became its principal. In 1948 she left and went to work in the slums of Calcutta and opened a house for the dying in 1952. She underwent some medical training at Paris in 1948. She started her work with lepers in 1957 and continued it for nearly 40 years. She was awarded the Nobel Peace Prize in 1979.

Theriaca [Greek: *therion*, wild animal] Antidote to poisons of wild animals. A cure-all remedy, Thericae Andromachi,

consisting of 60 to 70 different substances, was invented by Andromachus (AD 60) of Crete, physician to Emperor Nero.

Thermodynamics [Greek: *therme*, heat + *dynos*, power] The laws governing heat, named by Lord Kelvin (1824–1907) in 1850. French engineer, Sadi Carnot (1796–1832), proposed that all perfect engines operating between the same temperatures are equally efficient irrespective of the working substance. Rudolph Clausius (1822–1888), professor of physics at Bonn, demonstrated the interconvertibility of heat and work and postulated the second law of thermodynamics that heat cannot pass from one body to another of higher temperature. He also introduced the term 'entropy'. Experiments on the relationship between heat and work were published by Julius Robert Mayer (1814–1878), a medical practitioner from Heilbronn, Bavaria in 1842. British natural philosopher, James Prescott Joule (1818–1889), showed the relationship between work done and generation of heat. American physicist Henry Augustus Rowland (1848–1901) improved on Joule's work in 1881. The third law of thermodynamics was verified experimentally by a German physicist, Sir Francis Eugene Simon (1893–1956) from Berlin, who worked at the Clarendon Laboratory in Oxford. The principles of thermodynamics were applied to chemistry by American theoretical physicist, Josiah Willard Gibbs (1839–1903), and his work contributed greatly to the development of physical and organic chemistry.

Thermometer [Greek: *therme*, heat + *metron*, measure] An air thermometer was invented by Galileo Galilei (1564–1642) in 1592 and others were invented by Pietro Sarpi (1552–1623) in 1609 and Francis Bacon (1561–1626) described his in *Novum Organon* (1620). The suggestion of a liquid thermometer was made by French physician John Rey in 1632, and constructed in 1650 by Ferdinand II, Grand Duke of Tuscany and founder of the Academia del Cimento at Florence. He used alcohol in a sealed glass tube and this was introduced into England by Robert Boyle (1627–1691). Proposals for two fixed points were made by workers such as Martini, Olaus Roemer (1644–1710), Boyle and Sir Isaac Newton (1642–1727). Swedish astronomer, Anders Celsius (1701–1744), established his own scale in 1736 with zero as the melting point of ice and 100 as the boiling point of water, using a mercury thermometer. German instrument-maker Daniel Fahrenheit (1686–1736), who settled in Amsterdam and produced high quality meteorological instruments, devised an accurate alcohol thermometer and a mercury thermometer. He visited Roemer, who used the temperature of melting ice and the human body as his set points, and set his scale at 32 and 96 degrees for these points. The scale of 80 degrees between freezing and boiling points of water was introduced by René Antoine de Réaumur (1683–1757) in 1730 using a thermometer containing a mixture of alcohol and water. *See Celsius, Anders, clinical thermometry.*

Thermometry *See clinical thermometry, thermometer.*

Thessalus of Cos Son of Hippocrates (460–377 BC) and brother of Draco. Both were physicians who established the dogmatic sect which proposed that investigations should cease as Hippocrates has already stated all the essentials.

Thiamine Vitamin B1. The deficiency disease, beriberi, was observed by Jacobus Bontius (1592–1631) and Nicolas Tulp (1593–1674). It was eradicated in Japanese sailors by Kanehiro Takiki (1849–1915), Director-General of the Medical Department of the Navy, who supplemented the diet of rice with fish, vegetables, meat and barley in 1882. The deficiency factor was discovered in alcoholic extracts of rice polishings in 1897 by Christiaan Eijkman (1858–1930), a Dutch physician with the Dutch East India Company and Nobel Prize winner. Association of alcoholic polyneuritis with thiamin deficiency was noted by Patrick Manson (1844–1922) in 1898. A concentrate was obtained from rice by Polish-born American biochemist, Casimir Funk (1884–1967) in 1911 and later named vitamin B1. The name aneurin was given to the anti-beriberi factor by Dutch chemist, Barend Coenraad Petrus Jansen (b 1884) and Willem Frederik Donath (1889–1957) in Jakarta in 1935. The structure was elucidated by Robert Runnels Williams (b 1886) and co-workers who synthesized it in 1936. Its effectiveness in treating Korsakov syndrome was demonstrated by K. M. Bowman and colleagues in 1939. *See beriberi.*

Thiersch, Karl (1822–1895) German professor of surgery at Erlangen who described a method of operative treatment for epispadias in 1869. He devised the Thiersch method of skin grafting where long broad strips of skin of one half its full thickness are used.

Thioactazone [Greek: *theion*, sulfur] Thiosemicarbazide was shown to be active against *Mycobacterium tuberculosis in vitro* by Peak and co-workers in 1944. Work was continued by Gerhard Johannes Paul Domagk (1895–1964) in Germany and led to its introduction as a mainline drug against tuberculosis.

Thiopental, sodium Used as an intravenous anesthetic by John Silas Lundy (b 1894) at the Mayo Clinic in 1934.

Thiouracil *See antithyroid drugs.*

Third Heart Sound *See cardiac sounds.*

Thiry Fistula Experimental intestinal fistula, used to obtain intestinal juice for research. Developed with dogs by Belgian physician, Ludwig Thiry (1817–1897).

Thoma Ampulla Small terminal expansions of the spleenic pulp of the interlobar artery of the spleen. Described by German histologist, Richard Thoma (1847–1923).

Thomas, Edward Donnall (b 1920) American physician and hematologist from Mart in Texas. He studied chemistry and chemical engineering at the University of Texas in Austin and obtained his MD from Harvard in 1946. He joined the Mary Imogene Bassett Hospital in Cooperstown where he worked on bone marrow transplantation. In 1963 he moved to the Washington University School of Medicine in Seattle where he developed tissue-typing and use of immunosuppressive drugs for treatment of leukemia patients. In 1990 he shared the Nobel Prize for Physiology or Medicine. *See bone marrow transplant.*

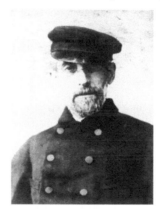

Hugh Owen Thomas (1834–1891). Courtesy of the National Library of Medicine

Thomas, Hugh Owen (1834–1891) Born in Liverpool, was the father of modern orthopedic surgery in England. He came from a family of seven generations of bone setters and devised various devices for treatment of deformities and fractures. The Thomas splint invented in 1876 caused a drastic fall in mortality in compound fractures of the femur.

Thomas, Sir James William Tudor (1893–1976) London surgeon who did pioneer experimental work on corneal transplants on rabbits in 1930.

Thomas, Morgan Educated at Oxford and practiced as a physician in the 16th century. He wrote a book on preserving health, *Haven of health,* based on the works of Galen (AD 129–200) and Hippocrates (460–377 BC).

Thomas Pessary Uterine pessary introduced by New York gynecologist, Theodore Gaillard Thomas (1831–1903).

Thomas, Robert (1753–1835) Physician from Salisbury who wrote *The Modern Practice of Physic* and several other treatises.

Thomas Splint Used for deformities of the hip, knee and ankle joints. Devised in 1876 by Hugh Owen Thomas (1834–1891), English orthopedic surgeon from Liverpool.

Thomas, Theodore Gaillard (1831–1903) American gynecologist from Edisto Island, South Carolina. He practiced in New York and published an important treatise on disease of women in 1868. He performed the first vaginal ovariotomy in 1870.

Thomayer Sign Inflammatory conditions of pelvis where percussion showed tymphany on the right side and dullness on the left side with the patient lying on their back. Described by German surgeon, Joseph Thomayer (1853–1927).

Thompson, Allen (1809–1884) Professor of anatomy at Marischal College. He was professor of physiology at Edinburgh University (1842–1848) and was appointed to the chair of anatomy at Glasgow University in 1877. He was the editor of the seventh edition of *Quain's Anatomy*. *See Thompson fascia*.

Thompson Fascia Yellow fibers covering the inner half of the external abdominal ring. Described by Allen Thompson (1809–1884) of Edinburgh.

Thompson Fascia Iliopectineal fascia described in 1835 by Alexander Thompson (1802–1838), professor of medical jurisprudence at London University.

Thompson, Henry Alexis (1864–1924) Professor of surgery at Edinburgh University. He published two textbooks, *A Manual of Surgery* and *A Manual of Operative Surgery* in collaboration with Alexander Miles in 1904.

Thompson, Sir Henry (1820–1904) English surgeon who described surgical treatment of urinary bladder tumors in 1884.

Thompson, Henry Teacher of Blizard who is said to have been the first to amputate at the hip joint in England, while at the London Hospital around 1752.

Thompson, Sir Henry (1820–1904) Founder and first president of the Cremation Society which was established in 1874. He was a urogenitary surgeon who performed lithotrity on Leopold I and was professor of clinical surgery at University College Hospital.

Thompson Hip Prosthesis Devised in 1952 by American orthopedic surgeon, Frederick Roeck Thompson (1907–1983).

Thompson, John Arthur (b 1899) Scottish zoologist, born in East Lothian. He was chair of natural history at Aberdeen in 1899 and published several works on the evolution of sex.

Thompson, John (1856–1926) Scottish pediatrician at the Royal Edinburgh Hospital for Sick Children. He wrote *Guide to Clinical Study and Treatment of Children* in which he dealt with characteristic differences of diseases in early life. He also recognized congenital hypertrophy of the pylorus.

Thompson, Thomas (1773–1852) Physician and professor of chemistry at Glasgow University. He was the third editor to the *Encyclopedia Britannica* and invented the oxyhydrogen blow pipe.

Thompson, Sir St Clair (1859–1943) Laryngologist from London who designed bayonet-shaped forceps (St Clair Thompson quinsy opener) to drain peritonsillar abscesses. He wrote *Cancer of the Larynx* in 1930.

Thompson, William (1833–1907) American ophthalmologist from Philadelphia who recognized eye strain as a cause of headache. He promoted prolonged rest as treatment for functional neuroses.

Thomsen, Asmus Julius Thomas (1815–1896) *See Thomsen disease*.

Thomsen Disease (Syn: myotonia congenita) Inability to relax the muscles after contraction, occurring during early childhood. Described by Ernest von Leyden (1832–1910) in 1876. Asmus Julius Thomas Thomsen (1815–1896), a Danish physician who himself had the disease, gave a description in 1876 of 23 patients of whom 20 were from his family. A genealogical survey through seven generations of his family was published by Nissen in 1923.

Thomsonian Medicine *See Thomson, Samuel*.

Thomson, James (1822–1892) Irish–Scottish physicist and engineer and elder brother of Lord Kelvin. He became professor of civil engineering at Queen's College Belfast and later at the University of Glasgow. He studied the effect of pressure on the freezing point of water, and wrote several papers on hydraulics.

Thomson, Sir Joseph John (1856–1940) English physicist, Cavendish professor at Cambridge and the discoverer of electrons. He graduated from Trinity College, Cambridge and was the first scientist to hold the post of Master of Trinity College in 1914. He determined the ratio of the charge on a cathode particle to its mass in 1881 and discovered the new atomic particles which he called 'corpuscles' in 1897. These were later universally accepted as electrons. His work on positive rays in 1911 led to the discovery of isotopes.

Thomson, Samuel (b 1769) Born in New England and self-educated on his family's farm where he learned about plants by experimenting on himself and his friends. He proclaimed that disease was due to excess cold in the body and created the Thomsonian cult. He was tried on 20 December 1809 in USA for questionable methods of treatment but found not guilty. He formulated Thomson's remedies and patented them for various maladies.

Thoracentesis [Greek: *thorax*, chest + *kentesis*, puncture] (Syn: Paracentesis thoracis) It was suggested by Hippocrates (460–377 BC). In cases of collection of fluid he recommended making an incision into the chest. His method was later considered dangerous by other physicians including Caelius Aurelianus (fifth century AD) who discouraged the practice. It was revived by Paul of Aegina (625–690). In modern times it was performed by Henry Pickering Bowditch (1840–1911) of Boston who carried out 325 procedures until 1875. The apparatus consists of needle, tube and suction pump to draw fluid from the pleural cavity and was designed by Boston physician, Morill Wyman (1812–1903) around 1860.

Thoracic Aneurysm *See aortic aneurysm.*

Thoracic Duct [Greek: *thorax*, chest] The receptaculum chyli, which is a dilatation of the thoracic duct, was described in man by French anatomist Jean Pecquet (1622–1674) while a student, in 1647. It was observed in the horse by Eustachio (1520–1574) in 1563. A description of it and the lymphatic vessels was given by Thomas Bartholin (1616–1680) a physician at Copenhagen, in 1652. Discovery was also claimed by Swedish anatomist, Olof Rudbeck (1630–1702) in 1652.

Thoracic Outlet Syndrome [Greek: *thorax*, chest] E. Bramwell pointed out the first cervical rib as a cause of pressure symptoms in 1903. A classic work on the subject was written by William Williams Keen (1837–1932) of America in 1907 and division of the first rib as treatment was performed by T. Murphy in 1910. Other symptoms due to compression of the brachial plexus and blood vessels were recognized by American neurosurgeon Alfred Washington Adson (1887–1951) of Iowa and I. Caffey. Adson recommended division of the scalenus anterior muscle for relief of symptoms in 1947. He also described the Adson sign where the radial pulse became obliterated when the head was turned to the affected side. It was described as scalenus syndrome by American surgeon, Howard Christian Naffziger (1884–1961) in 1937. Pressure from the scelenus anticus muscle, causing acroparesthesia and neuritis of the hands was described by British neurologist, Sir Francis Martin Rouse Walshe (1885–1973) in 1945.

Thoracic Surgery [Greek: *thorax*, chest] *See cardiac surgery, cardiac transplant, coronary artery bypass surgery, cardiopulmonary bypass machine, aortic aneurysm, pneumonectomy.*

Thoracic Sympathetic Block [Greek: *thorax*, chest] Block of thoracic ganglia of the sympathetic chain by paravertebral injection of drugs was performed by Max Kappis (1881–1938) in 1900 and by Hugo Sellheim in 1905. Alcohol was used to prolong the block by Swatlow in 1926.

Thoracoplasty [Greek: *thorax*, chest] Removal of several ribs to collapse the lung was performed as treatment for empyema by Ernest George Ferdinand von Küstner in 1889. Extensive rib resection for empyema was also done by Max Schede (1844–1902) in 1890. Decortication as treatment for empyema was introduced by French surgeon Edmond Delorme (1847–1929) in 1894. It was performed in England by Morriston Davies in 1912.

Thorax [Greek: *thorax*, chest] The Greek term denotes armor or cuirass which protected the chest and abdomen. Aristotle (384–322 BC) and Hippocrates (460–377 BC) used the term to denote both the chest and abdomen. Plato (428–348 BC) restricted its use to the chest, and Galen (AD 129–200) introduced it into anatomy.

Thorel, Christen (1868–1935) German physician in Nuremberg who described the myocardial bundle (Thorel bundle) connecting the atrial and atrioventricular nodes beside the inferior vena cava. He reported talcosis of the lung in 1896.

Thorium Rare metal obtained from a black mineral from the island of Lovon in Norway by Jakob Berzelius (1778–1848) who named it after the Scandinavian god, Thor, in 1828. It was used parentrally in cancer treatment in the United States during the 1920s. Thorium nitrate was introduced as a contrast agent for pyelography by a Kansas urologist, Jonathan Edwards Burns (b 1883) in 1915.

Thorius, Raphael (d 1625) Physician during the reign of James I who wrote a poem on tobacco, *Hynnus Tabaci*, published in 1651. He died of plague.

Thornton, John Roberts (1758–1837) Botanist and physician at Guy's Hospital. He wrote *The Philosophy of Medicine or Medical Extracts on Nature and Health* in 1798 on the Brunonian system of medicine. He is known for his

Temple of Flora or Garden of the Botanist, Poet, Painter, and Philosopher.

Thornwaldt Disease Inflammation of the Luschka tonsil with formation of a cyst containing pus, leading to pharyngeal stenosis. Described by German physician, Gustavus Ludwig Thornwaldt (1843–1910).

Thorpe, John (1682–1750) Physician from Penshurst in Kent who wrote on curious ancient illustrations.

Thorpe, Sir Thomas Edward (1845–1925) English physicist and chemist from Manchester. He pioneered analytical chemistry and was appointed by the British Government to do analytical work on chemical hazards. He was professor of chemistry at Anderson's College, Glasgow and wrote *Dictionary of Applied Chemistry* in 1893.

Thoth Mythical figure of the ancient Egyptians, considered the inventor of science and arts.

Threlkeld, Caleb (1646–1728) English physician from Cumbria who qualified in medicine from Edinburgh in 1709 and became a divine and botanist. He wrote a book on plants of Ireland.

Threonine Amino acid isolated from hydrosylates of fibrin in 1935 by William Cumming (1887–1984), an American biochemist.

Thromboangitis Obliterans [Greek: *thrombos*, clot + *angeion*, vessel + *itis*, inflammation; Latin: *oblitaratus*, erase] Obliteration of the lumen of most arteries of the leg by a chronic proliferative process was described by German physician Felix von Winiwarter (1848–1917) in 1879. He observed a new growth of intima in the blood vessel and named it endarteritis obliterans. It was observed to be caused by occlusion of the blood vessels in secondary thrombosis by New York physician, Leo Buerger (1879–1943) who named it in 1908. He confirmed arteriosclerosis as the cause in 1926.

Thrombocytopenia [Greek: *thrombos*, clot + *kytos*, hollow + *penia*, poverty] See *thrombocytopenic purpura*.

Thrombocytopenic Purpura [Greek: *thrombos*, clot + *kytos*, hollow + *penia*, poverty; Latin: *purpura*, purple] Described as purpura hemorrhagica by German physician, Paul Gottlieb Werlhof (1699–1767). The autoimmune nature of it was realized when Ackroyd demonstrated antiplatelet factors in patients who developed it after taking Sedormoid in 1949. The autoimmune theory was advanced in 1951 by G. Evans who observed that some patients with acquired hemolytic anemia with antibodies to red cells also

developed it. Methods to detect platelet antibodies were developed in early 1950, and W. J. Harrington and colleagues demonstrated platelet agglutinins in 100 out of 132 patients with it in 1956. Spleenectomy remained the first line of treatment in severe cases in the 1950s and was superseded by use of high dose steroids in the 1960s.

Thrombokinase [Greek: *thrombos*, clot + *kinesis*, motion] Term used by Paul Oskar Morawitz (1879–1936) of Germany to denote an important enzyme of the blood clotting system which was later found to convert prothrombin to thrombin. Isolated from lung tissue by New York biochemist and Nobel Prize winner in 1986, Stanley Cohen (b 1922).

Thrombolysis [Greek: *thrombos*, clot + *lysis*, dissolution] Fibrinolytic substance isolated from group A beta-hemolytic streptococcus by a Baltimore physician, William Smith Tillet (b 1892) and R.L. Garner in 1933, who called it streptococcal fibrinolysin. The mechanism of fibrinolysis was elucidated by a microbiologist, L. Royal Christensen, who renamed it streptokinase in 1945. Tillet and A.J. Johnson demonstrated its effectiveness in dissolving intravascular clots in animals in 1947. A purified form was developed and experimentally tried by S. Sherry and A.P. Fletcher in 1958. Its use in dissolving clots in human veins was demonstrated by Johnson and W. R. McCarthy in 1959. Their experiments showed clearance of experimental thrombi in the forearm veins of human volunteers. Similar results were obtained by Johnson using urokinase in 1963. The feasibility of thrombolytic therapy in myocardial infarction was demonstrated by Fletcher and co-workers in 1959. The effectiveness of plasminogen activators in clot lysis was shown by Sherry, Fletcher, and R.S. Lindermeyer in the same year. Infusion of streptokinase directly in to the site of coronary thrombus was performed by P. Rentrop and co-workers in 1979.

Thromboplastin Generation Test [Greek: *thrombos*, clot + *plassein*, to form + *genos*, descent] Allows detection and localization of defects in clotting factors in the blood. Developed by R. Biggs and A. S. Douglas in 1953. It was developed into a quantitative method by Biggs, J. Eveling and G. Richards in 1955.

Thromboplastin [Greek: *thrombos*, clot + *plassein*, to form] Potent tissue extract with anticoagulant activity was found by F. Rauschenbach of Dorpat in 1882 and Leonard Charles Woolbridge (1857–1889) of England. It was called thrombokinase by Paul Oskar Morawitz (1879–1936), implying that it was an enzyme. It was renamed by William Henry Howell (1860–1945) of Johns

Hopkins University in 1912.

Thrombosis [Greek: *thrombos*, clot] Term used in 1848 by Rudolph Karl Virchow (1821–1902) to denote the formation of blood clots.

Thrombotic Thrombocytopenic Purpura [Greek: *thrombos*, clot + *kytos*, hollow + *penia*, poverty; Latin: *purpura*, purple] Diffuse thrombotic vascular lesions in arterioles and capillaries was described by American physician, Eli Moschcowitz (1879–1964) in 1925.

Thromboxane [Greek: *thrombos*, clot + *oxane*, ring] Inducer of platelet aggregation, discovered by M. Hamberg and co-workers in 1975. *See prostaglandins.*

Thrush Candidiasis was described by Hippocrates (460–377 BC) and Aulus Cornelius Celsus (25 BC–AD 50) mentioned it in his account on apthae. Samuel Pepys in his entry on 7 June 1665 has recorded it as one of the terminal symptoms of Admiral Sir John Lawson. Scientific evidence for a fungal etiology was presented by David Gruby (1810–1898) of Paris in 1843. *See candidosis.*

Thucydides (469–391 BC) Greek historian from Athens who wrote a history of the Peloponnesian War, giving a detailed account of a mysterious epidemic illness later known as Athenian plague which struck Athens around 430 BC. It was present in the south of Egypt and Ethiopia and later spread to Libya, Persia and Athens.

Thudichum Test Detects creatinine using ferric chloride as reagent. Devised by John Lewis William Thudichum (1829–1901), a German physician who practiced in London. He was the first lecturer in chemistry at St Thomas' Hospital in 1865 and a pioneer in biochemistry.

Thunberg, Carl Peter (1743–1828) Swedish botanist who studied medicine at Uppsala and was ship's surgeon to the Dutch Government in South Africa in 1770. He did botanical studies in Japan and Sri Lanka and on his return was professor at Uppsala. His *Flora Japonica* was published in 1784.

Thurston, Louis Leon (1887–1955) Professor of psychology at Chicago University (1927–1952). His main interest was intelligence testing and he devised several tests. He wrote *Vectors of Mind* (1935) and *Multiple-factor Analysis* in 1947.

Thymectomy [Greek: *thymos*, thymus + *ektome*, excision] *See thymus.*

Thymus Genus of herbs native to central Europe. The name was used by Hippocrates (460–377 BC) to denote a dry cough. The ancients referred to an aromatic plant which was used in sacrificial burning of the gland.

Thymus [Greek: *thymos*, thymus] Galen (AD 129–200) used the word to describe skin. An account of the gland was given by Jacopo da Carpi Berengario (1470–1530), an Italian surgeon from Pavia in 1521. William Hewson (1739–1774), a London hematologist, demonstrated the origin of white blood cells or leukocytes from lymphatic glands and thymus in 1774. Sir Astley Paston Cooper (1768–1841) wrote *The Anatomy of the Thymus Gland* in 1832. The concentric corpuscles of the thymus were described in 1846 by Arthur Hill Hassall (1817–1894), an English physician from Teddington. The presence of multiple abscesses in it in cases of congenital syphilis was described by Paul Dubois (1795–1871) of Paris in 1850. An association between myasthenia and thymus was found by Karl Weigert (1845–1904) in 1901. Thymectomy was performed as treatment for myasthenia by Ernst Ferdinand Sauerbruch (1875–1951) of Germany in 1912 and revived by American surgeon, Alfred Blalock (1899–1964). Its immunological nature was demonstrated by French-born Australian immunologist, Jacques Albert Francis Pierre Miller (b 1931) in 1961. A syndrome (DiGeorge syndrome), characterized by congenital absence of the thymus and parathyroid glands leading to recurrent infection, was described by American pediatrician, Angelo Mario DiGeorge (b 1921) and co-workers in 1967.

Thyroglobulin [Greek: *thyreos*, shield; Latin: *globus*, ball] Chemical investigation was suggested by Hermann Lebert (1813–1878) in 1862. Thyroglobulin, an iodine-containing protein, was isolated by English pediatrician, Sir Robert Hutchison (1871–1960) in 1896.

Thyroid Antibodies [Greek: *thyreon*, shield + *anti*, against] An unusually large amount of circulating gammaglobulin with abnormal flocculation tests in the sera of patients with Hashimoto thyroiditis was observed by G. A. Fromm, E. S. Lascano and G. Burr of Argentina in 1953. Their findings were confirmed by R. W. Luxton and R. T. Cooke of England in 1956. The suggestion that these may represent circulating antibodies to thyroglobulin was made by Deborah Doniach, R. Hudson and I. M. Roitt in the same year. A condition similar to Hashimoto thyroiditis was produced in rabbits by injecting extract of thyroid by N. R. Rose and E. Witebsky in 1956. The presence of agglutinating antibodies in 30% of patients with hyperthyroidism was demonstrated by S. G. Owen and G. A. Smart in 1960.

Thyroid [Greek: *thyreon*, shield + *eidos*, form] Used by Galen (AD 129–200) to refer to the four-sided cartilage which made up the larynx. It was named in the present context by English physician, Thomas Wharton (1614–1673) in 1646.

The function was doubted by many physicians until the 19th century. They believed that it secreted lubricants for the trachea and served no useful function. In 1883 Emil Theodor Kocher (1841–1917), a Swiss surgeon and Nobel Prize winner, developed surgical treatments for thyroid disorders which helped elucidate its function. He also developed treatment with thyroid extract. Adolf Magnus-Levy (1869–1955), a German physiologist in America, gave thyroid extracts from animals to men in 1895 and found that their basal metabolic rate was elevated. Iodine, long known to have beneficial effects on cretinism, was shown to be present in the thyroid by Eugen Baumann (1846–1896) of Berlin in 1896. American Nobel Prize winner, Edward Calvin Kendall (1886–1972), isolated pure extract from thyroid in 1914 and named it thyroxin. *See thyroxin, thyroid goiter, thyrotoxicosis.*

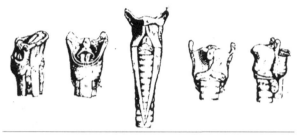

Thyroid gland, drawn by Vesalius in the 16th century

Thyroid Goiter Pliny (AD 23–79), Juvenal, Vitruvius, and Vulpian made statements which indicate that they were aware of the condition in people from the Alps who presented with a stout neck. Marco Polo observed the same condition in central Asia around 1270. Chinese used extracts of thyroid gland to treat goiter in the 7th century. A medical description was given by Arnold of Villanova (1234–1311) who observed it in Lucca and advocated the use of seaweed. Surgical removal of enlarged thyroid was recommended by Guy de Chauliac (1300–1367). The definite relationship of goiter and cretinism was shown by Paracelsus (1493–1541) who observed it in Salzburg. A scientific inquiry was commenced by Michele Vincenzo Malacarne (1744–1816) who also wrote a book on it in 1789. Endemic goiter in Africa was observed by Mungo Park (1771–1806) in the mountains of Congo and Niger. Iodine deficiency in air and water as the cause was proposed by Swiss physician Jean Louis Prévost (1838–1927) and Maffoni, and by Chatin in 1853. *See thyroid, thyrotoxic goiter, Basedow disease, cretinism.*

Thyroid Stimulating Hormone (TSH) *See thyrotrophic hormone.*

Thyroidectomy [Greek: *thyreos*, shield + *ektome*, excision] Partial thyroidectomy was done by Joseph Henry Green (1791–1863), a surgeon at St Thomas' Hospital in 1825. His patient died 15 days later due to sepsis. A total excision was done by Paul Auguste Sick (1836–1900), a German surgeon, in 1867. Another case was reported in 1874 by Sir Patrick Heron Watson (1832–1907), a surgeon at the Edinburgh Royal Infirmary. The pioneer in thyroid surgery was Swedish surgeon, Emil Theodor Kocher (1841–1917), who performed over 2000 operations.

Thyrotoxicosis [Greek: *thyreos*, shield + *toxikon*, poison] (Syn: Graves disease, Parry disease) Exophthalmic goiter resulting from thyrotoxicosis was described by Caleb Hillier Parry (1755–1822), a physician from Bath in 1786, who published eight more cases later. Robert James Graves (1796–1853), a Dublin physician, gave an account of three cases in 1835, and Karl Adolph von Basedow (1799–1854) from Merseberg near Leipzig, described four cases in 1840. Albrecht von Graefe (1828–1870), an eye surgeon in Berlin, described the stationary nature of the eyelid (lid lag sign) in thyrotoxicosis, the Graefe sign. Julia and Cosmo Mackenzie of Johns Hopkins Hospital identified the antithyroid properties of thiourea in 1930 while experimenting with products to induce intestinal suppression of bacterial flora. Phenyl thiourea was discovered about the same time by Curt Richter. Effectiveness of thiourea in humans was established around 1940 by Edwin B. Astwood (b 1909) of Boston, who used thiourea and thiouracil as treatment for hyperthyroidism in 1943. Radioiodine was used in the study of thyroid disease by M. P. Kelsey and co-workers in 1949 and introduced as treatment for thyrotoxicosis by G. W. Blomfield and co-workers in 1951.

Thyrotropic Hormone [Greek: *thyreos*, shield + *trophein*, to nourish] The relationship between the pituitary and thyroid glands was suggested by N. Rogowitsch in 1888. Philip Edward Smith (b 1884), of California, established conclusively that the thyroid depended on the stimulating action of the anterior pituitary in 1927. Harvey Williams Cushing (1869–1939) in the same year noted that hypopituitary patients had a lower metabolic rate. Thyroid stimulating hormone which caused thyroid hyperplasia was discovered in the anterior pituitary of pigs independently by Loeb and Aron in 1929. The structure of thyrotropin releasing hormone (TRH) was elucidated by Lithuanian-born American biochemist and Nobel Prize winner, Andrew Victor Schally (b 1926) at Tulane University in 1969.

Thyroxin The active extract of the thyroid was isolated by Edward Calvin Kendall (1886–1972) of Detroit who named it while he was at the Mayo Institute in 1914. The structure and empirical formula of tetraiodothyronine and its precursor, 1-tyrosine, were determined in 1926 by Sir Charles Robert Harington (1897–1972) of University College Hospital Medical School. A synthetic preparation from coal tar was obtained by Harington during his work with George Barger (1878–1939) in 1927. Harington's *The Thyroid Gland, its Chemistry and Physiology* was published in 1933. *See thyroid, antithyroid drugs.*

Tibia [Latin, *tibia*, a pipe] The word originally referred to ancient musical instruments made of shin bone of animals and birds. The shin bone itself later acquired the name.

Tic Douloureux *See trigeminal neuralgia.*

Tick-Borne Diseases Several forms have been identified. Aka mushi (Japanese: red insect), a seasonal fever occurring along rivers of certain regions in Japan, was one of the first to be described by Palm in 1878. The trombeculoid tick was identified as the transmitter. The tick was shown to be the vector in Texas cattle fever in 1893 by Theobald Smith (1859–1934), professor of microbiology at Harvard University. The causative organism of Q Fever, *Coxiella burnettii*, was recovered from ticks during an outbreak in Montana by Herald Rae Cox (b 1907) and G. E. Davis in 1938. *Borrelia duttoni*, a spirochete causing African relapsing fever was identified by Joseph Everett Dutton (1877–1905) and John Lancelot Todd (1876–1949) in 1905. *Ornithodorus*, a genus of tick which cause relapsing fever by transmitting *Borrelia recurrentis*, was identified by two independent groups, Philip Hedgeland Ross (1876–1929) and A.D. Milne in Uganda, and Dutton and Todd in Congo in 1904. The causative agent of Rocky Mountain spotted fever was shown to be transmitted by ticks by Howard Taylor Ricketts (1871–1910), a microbiologist at Northwestern University in 1906.

Tidy Test Detects albumin in the urine using phenol and glacial acetic acid as reagents. Devised by English physician, Charles Meymott Tidy (1843–1892).

Tiedemann Nerve Plexus of nerve fibrils around the central artery of the retina arising from the central ciliary nerves. Described by Friedrich Tiedemann (1781–1861), professor of anatomy at Heidelberg.

Tietze Syndrome (Syn: costochondral junction syndrome) Painful swellings at the costochondral junction of the sternum, of unknown etiology. Described by German surgeon, Alexander Tietze (1864–1927) of Berlin in 1921.

Tigerstedt, Robert Adolf Armand (1853–1923) *See renin, renal hypertension, cardiac output.*

Tilingius, Matthias (d 1615) Physician from Westphalia who wrote several medical treatises including *De Febribus, De llaudano Opiate* and *Cinnabaris Mineralis*.

Tillet, William Smith (b 1892) *See thrombolysis.*

Tilli, Michael Angelo (1655–1740) Physician and botanist from Florence. He was professor at Pisa and physician to the Duke. He wrote *Catalogue Horti Pisani* in 1723.

Tilney, Frederick (1875–1938) Father of the New York School of Neurology. He was educated at Yale University and studied medicine at Long Island College Hospital before he was elected professor of neurology at Columbia University. His *The Brain from Ape to Man* is considered a classic on modern evolution. He also wrote *The form and functions of the central nervous system* with Henry Alsop Riley (1887–1966) in 1921.

Timaeus of Locria Greek philosopher and disciple of Pythagorus, who thought that there was a universal motion in nature. His treatise on the nature of the soul and of the world is mentioned by Plato (428–348 BC) .

Tinea cruris [Latin: *tinea*, grub] Acute or chronic fungal infection generally seen in males and affecting the groin, perineum and perineal area. A description of this fungal disease was given by Friedrich Wilhelm Felix von Barensprung (1822–1864) in 1854.

Tinea imbricata [Latin: *tinea*, grub] Chronic tropical skin disease found in the Malay Archipelago and Southeast Asia. Described in the Philippines by English navigator, Sir William Dampier (1652–1715), during his voyages in 1686. It was later noted in Polynesia and named Tokelau disease. It was described as *On Tokelau Ringworm and its Fungus* by T. Fox in *The Lancet* in 1874. Patrick Manson (1844–1922) identified the causative fungus and named it in 1879. Another treatise, *Le Tokelau et son parasite* was published by Bonnafy of Paris in 1893. The fungus was renamed *Trichophyton concentricum* by Raphael Blanchard (1857–1919) in 1896.

Tinea rubrum [Latin: *tinea*, grub] The fungus was identified and named by Marquis Aldo Castellani (1879–1971) from Florence while he was in Sri Lanka in 1910.

Tinel Sign In carpel tunnel syndrome, tapping over the carpel tunnel causes paraesthesia over the median nerve distribution of the hand. Described by French neurologist, Jules Tinel (1879–1952) from Rouen who practiced at Paris.

Tinnitus [Latin: ringing] Noise in the ear was discussed by Galen (AD 129–200) who considered indigestion, excess of wine, violent vomiting, increased sensibility and improper application of medicines to the ear as some of the causes and prescribed local injections of the juices of madragora and poppy into the ear. Aulus Cornelius Celsus (25 BC–AD 50) suggested special attention to diet and recommended injections of castor oil with vinegar, oil of iris, oil of bay and myrrh with nitre. Haly Abbas (930–994), an Arabian physician, proposed that if all the above local measures failed, the cause was probably from the brain or auditory nerve.

Tiselius, Arne Wilhelm Kaurin (1902–1971) Swedish chemist from Stockholm who was educated and worked at Uppsala. He developed a method of determining diffusion constants of proteins and introduced moving boundary electrophoresis for examining protein purity. He isolated several viruses and separated and identified amino acids, sugars and other molecules using activated charcoal, silica, cellulose and ion exchange chromatography. He worked with Frederick Sanger (b 1918) on insulin. He was awarded the Nobel Prize for Chemistry in 1948. *See gammaglobulin, antibody, immunoglobulin.*

Tissot, Simon August Andre (1747–1834) Physician from Lausanne who was professor of medicine in his home town. He wrote *Avis au Peuple sur la Sante ou Traites des Maladies* in 1760, which went to 9 editions and was translated into many languages. Other treatises include: *Variolation* (1754), *Treatise on epilepsy* (1770), *Nervous diseases* (1782), *Onanism* (1760) and *Diseases of men of the world* (1770).

Tissue Culture Growth of cells *in vitro* was shown by American biologist, Ross Granville Harrison (1870–1959) in 1907, who showed regeneration of separated embryonic nerves of a frog when they were preserved in lymph. Alexis Carrel (1873–1944) perfected the technique in 1911 by growing embryonic heart muscle in culture for over 25 years. In 1911 fibroblasts from chick embryos were taken at the Rockefeller Institute and were maintained in culture until 1928. German physiologist Wilhelm Roux (1850–1924) and Leo Loeb (1869–1959) did further experiments and in England T. S. P. Strangeways of Cambridge, and Albert Fisher of London were pioneers.

Tissue [French: *tissu*, woven] Twenty-one different tissues in animals, including bone, blood, and muscle were described in 1797 by Maria François Xavier Bichat (1771–1802) of the Hôtel Dieu in Paris. He is considered a founder of microscopic anatomy. *See histology.*

Titanium Element known in the 17th century from black sand or menakite and described by William Gregor, a priest at Menachen in Cornwall. Martin Henry Klaproth (1743–1817) of Germany studied it in detail and named it in 1795.

It is remarkable for its light weight and was initially used to make artificial teeth. It is currently a popular metal for spectacle frames and a fracture fixative.

Titchener, Edward Bradford (1867–1927) American psychologist, born in Chichester, England. He founded the Society of Experimental Psychology in America in 1904 and wrote *Experimental Psychology* (1901–1905) in 4 volumes.

Tobacco Amblyopia Dimness of vision due to tobacco smoking. Described by William Mackenzie (1791–1868) in England in 1835. A more accurate description was given by Jonathan Hutchinson (1828–1913) in 1864, and an exhaustive account by Forster of Germany in 1868.

Tobacco Derives its common name from the Haitian word for the pipe in which it was smoked. The Latin name, *Nicotiana tabacum*, derives from the Portuguese, Joan Nicot, who introduced it to Europe. King James I realized the ill effects of tobacco smoking and in 1602 and he issued *Counterblaste to Tobacco* in which he described the habit as 'A custome loathesome to the eye, hateful to the nose, harmeful to brain, dangerous to the lung, and in the black stinking fume therof neerest resembling the horrible Stigian smoke of the pit that is bottomless'. Cultivation was prohibited by Charles II in 1684. Catherine de Medici introduced the use of tobacco snuff for headaches to her court. Inhalation or smoking of tobacco was learnt from the Indians and few people smoked it in England until the habit was popularized by Ralph Lane in 1586. *See smoking.*

Tobacco Mosaic Virus First virus identified and studied by Martinus Wilhelm Beijerinck (1851–1931) in 1898. It was given the name mosaic as the infected leaves contain dark and light green mottling. It was isolated by American biochemist, Wendell Meredith Stanley (1904–1971) of the Rockefeller Institute for Medical Research at Princeton in 1935. The presence of ribonucleic acid in the virus was shown by an English botanist, Frederick Charles Bawden (b 1908) in 1937, and the infectivity was found to be due to its RNA by Alfred Gierer and Gerhard Schramm in 1956. Heinz Fraenkel-Conrat (b 1910), a German-born American molecular biologist, proved that it could be reconstituted from protein and nucleic acid, thus raising the possibility of a 'living chemical' in molecular biology. *See virus.*

Tobias, Phillip Valentine (b 1925) South African anatomist and physical anthropologist from Durban, who qualified in medicine from Witwatersrand University in 1950. He described several hominid species and named *Homo habilis.* He published over 800 papers on evolution and anthropology.

TOCP *See triorthocresyl phosphate.*

Tod Muscle Located at the posterior aspect of concha and described by London otologist, David Tod (1794–1856), in 1832.

Todd, Alexander Robertus (b 1907) Scottish chemist who synthesized vitamin B1 or thiamin in 1937. He was born at Glasgow in 1907 and was professor at Manchester (1938) and Cambridge (1944) before he became the first chancellor of the new University of Strathclyde in 1978. He was awarded the Nobel Prize for his work on vitamins in 1957.

Todd, Robert Bentley (1809–1860) British physician at King's College. He edited a *Cyclopedia and Anatomy* in 1833 and *Physiological Anatomy and Physiology of Man* from 1845 to 1859, which remained the standard textbook for many decades. He was also a co-worker of Sir William Bowman (1816–1892) who described the capsule of the kidney.

Todd Paralysis Epileptic hemiplegia affecting the epileptic side. Described by Robert Bentley Todd (1809–1860) who was an English physician and professor of physiology at King's College, in 1856.

Toilet The Romans introduced the chamber pot around 300 BC and it remained in household use for two thousand years. The water closet with mechanical means of disposal was proposed by Sir John Harington (1561–1612), an English writer from Kelston near Bath. His water closet was installed at the Richmond palace of Elizabeth I, his godmother. He described it in *The Metamorphosis of Ajax* published in 1596.

Tokelau Disease *See Tokelau itch.*

Tokelau Itch Tokelau disease was described from the island of Tokelau in the South Pacific by Sir William Dampier (1652–1715) during his voyages in 1686 and later noted in Polynesia. Patrick Manson (1844–1922) identified a fungus as its cause and named it *Tinea imbricata* in 1879. It was renamed *Trichophyton concentricum* by Raphael Blanchard (1857–1919) in 1896.

Tokology [Greek: *tokos*, birth + *logos*, discourse] *See obstetrics.*

Tolbutamide Sulfonylurea compound introduced as treatment in diabetes by Helmut Maske of Germany in 1956.

Toledo Known as Toletum to the ancients, and capital of the Visigothic kingdom of Athanagild in AD 554. The University at Toledo was founded in 1499.

Tommaselli Disease Pyrexia and hematuria due to excessive use of quinine. Described by Italian physician, Salvatore Tommaselli (1834–1906).

Tomes Fibers Dentinal fibrils described in 1850 by a London dental surgeon, Sir John Tomes (1815–1895), father of Charles Sissimore Tomes (1846–1928) of the London Hospital.

Tomes Process Ameloblast processes on the enamel cells of teeth. Described in 1897 by Charles Sissimore Tomes (1846–1928), an anatomist and dentist at the London Hospital.

Tomography [Greek: *tomo*, cut + *graphein*, to write] Technique for recording internal body images at a predetermined plane using X-rays. Described by German physician D. L. Bartelink in 1933.

Tonegawa, Susumu (b 1939) Japanese molecular biologist who studied chemistry at the University of Kyoto and received his PhD from San Diego in 1968. He then moved to the Institute for Immunology at Basel, Switzerland and worked on restriction enzyme and recombinant DNA techniques in relation to the origin of antibody diversity. He confirmed that in formation of antibody-manufacturing cells (B lymphocytes) genes undergo changes that allow them to produce a new and wide range of antibodies. In 1981 he was appointed professor of biology at MIT and examined the workings of T lymphocytes. In 1987 he received the Nobel Prize for Physiology or Medicine.

Tongue [Anglo-Saxon: *tunge*, tongue] The word 'papilla' to denote microprojections on the tongue was introduced by Marcello Malpighi (1628–1694) in 1670. The Webers glands, or the lateral glands of the tongue, were described by Ernest Heinrich Weber (1795–1878), professor of physiology at Leipzig. Meyer glands beneath the tongue, in the hypoglossus muscle, were described in 1871 by Georg Hermann von Meyer (1815–1892), professor of histology at Zurich. Serous glands of taste papillae were described in 1873 by Victor Ebner von Rofentein (1842–1925), Austrian professor of histology at Innsbruck. Magenta-colored smooth tongue devoid of papillae is a feature of riboflavin deficiency and was observed by English physician, Hugh S. Stannus (b 1877) in 1911.

Tonic Pupils The term was coined by Gordon Holmes (1876–1965), who described it in 19 female patients as 'partial irridoplegia associated with other diseases of the nervous system' in 1931. An independent account of pseudo-Argyll Robertson pupils with absent tendon reflexes was given in the same year by William John Adie (1886–1935).

Tonometer [Greek: *tonos*, tension + *meter*, measure] Apparatus for tuning musical instruments invented by H. Scheibler of Crefeld in 1834. An instrument to measure intra-ocular pressure using the lever principle was invented by Norwegian physician, Hjalmar Schiotz (1850–1927) in 1881 and introduced into clinical practice in 1905. Another with a spring, based on the aneroid principle, was introduced by J. M. Albarenque in 1917. A mercurial tonometer, where the displacement of the piston was measured in millimeters of mercury, was invented by M. Cohen in 1921. A simple and practical instrument was designed by P. Bailliart in 1923. Several models were invented by Friedrich Wilhelm Ernst Albrecht von Graefe (1828–1870), Franciscus Cornelis Donders (1818–1889), Hermann Snellen (1834–1908) and others.

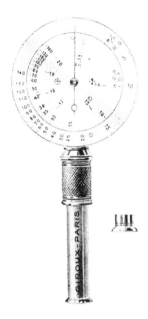

Bailliart tonometer. W. Stewart Duke-Elder, *Recent Advances in Opthalmology* (1927). J & A Churchill, London

Tonsillectomy [Latin: *tonsilla*, tonsil; Greek: *ektome*, excision] *See tonsillitis.*

Tonsillitis [Latin: *tonsilla*, tonsil; Greek: *itis*, inflammation] Aretaeus (81–138) has given an accurate and detailed account of inflammation of the tonsils and the uvula. He also noted the childhood predisposition to it, that was endemic in Syria and Egypt. Some of his treatments include: bleeding from the arm, acrid clysters, purgatives, ligature of the extremities and astringent local applications. Aulus Cornelius Celsus (25 BC–AD 50) advocated the use of cataplasms, fumigation and fermentation. Aetius of Amida, around 600 AD, recommended opening of the abscess when the tonsils suppurate. Tonsillectomy was described by Ambroise Paré (1510–1590) and Fabricius Hildanus

(1560–1634). A modern tonsillotome was designed by American surgeon from Philadelphia, Philip Syng Physick (1768–1837) in 1828. Removal of tonsils by blunt dissection was introduced by George Ernest Waugh (1875–1940) in 1909. Bernard Schlesinger (1896–1984) and Frederick John Poynton (1869–1943) noted that post-streptococcal arthritis following tonsillitis was due to an allergy to bacterial products rather than bacterial toxins, in 1931.

Toothache Galen (AD 129–200) wrote on diseases of teeth in his fifth book and recognized that the tooth was a sensitive organ and described the throbbing nature and intensity of tooth pain. He prescribed strong applications of vinegar as treatment. Archigenes, a Greek surgeon who lived around 100 AD, listed several treatments including spirit of nitre, hot fermentation with vinegar and heated linseed. He recommended filling the hole in the tooth with hot wax. Aulus Cornelius Celsus (25 BC–AD 50) advocated diet and food which did not require mastication and judicious use of wine. Aetius of Amida (502–575) wrote on removing teeth using red arsenic. Eustachio (1520–1574) attributed the exquisite sensitivity of teeth due to the abundant nerve supply.

Tooth, Howard Henry (1856–1925) English physician, born in Brighton and educated at Rugby and St John's College, Cambridge. He graduated in medicine from St Bartholomew's Hospital in 1880 where he became a physician in 1906. He described the peroneal form of progressive muscular dystrophy (Charcot–Marie–Tooth–Hoffmann syndrome) in 1886.

Tooth Transplantation The practice was mentioned by Ambroise Paré (1510–1590) in 1564, and became a vogue in the 18th century. It was the first instance of exploitation of humans in organ transplantation. The poor and young were enticed to part with teeth in return for money. John Hunter (1728–1793) did numerous transplants and popularized the practice. It was introduced into America in 1781 by French surgeon, Pierre le Mayeur. He advertised a fee of two guineas for anybody willing to part with a tooth. In 1784 he claimed to have done 123 successful transplants.

Topinard, Paul (1830–1912) Anthropologist from Paris who described the Topinard line and several other landmarks in anthropometry.

Torek, Franz (1861–1938) *See esophageal carcinoma, orhidopexy.*

Torricelli, Evangeliste (1608–1647) Italian mathematician, born in Faenza and worked with Galileo during the last three months of Galileo's life. He developed the theory of atmospheric pressure, and discovered that the unit in each column of water or mercury in a tube was a measure of pressure exerted by the atmosphere. Based on his finding he worked with Vivianni (1622–1703) and constructed the first barometer in 1643.

Torsade de Pointes 'Fringe pointed tips' was coined in 1966 by F. Dessertenne to denote a form of atypical ventricular tachycardia with altered polarity and varying amplitude of the QRS complexes. However, its electrocardiographic features had been recognized in 1922 by L. Gallavardin.

Torsus Aorticus Prominence of the medial wall of the right atrium of the heart caused by the aorta. Described in 1929 by T. Walmsley in *Quain's Element of Anatomy*.

Torti, Francesco (1658–1741) Italian physician who introduced cinchona into Italy. He used the term 'malaria' (bad air) for ague (malaria) in his *Therapeutica Specialis ad febres quasdam pernisiosa* published in 1712.

Torticollis [Latin: *tortus*, twisted + *collum*, neck] *See wry-neck.*

Total Body Irradiation X-rays were shown to suppress antibody response by American pathologist, Ludvig Hektoen (1863–1951) in 1915. *See immunosuppressive agents.*

Total Gastectomy *See gastrectomy.*

Total Hip Replacement *See artificial hip joint.*

Tourette Disease Violent muscular jerks of the shoulders, extremities and face, beginning in childhood with explosive grunting or coprolalia. Samuel Johnson is thought to have suffered from it. Described in 1885 by French neurologist, Georges Edouard Albert Brutus Gilles de La Tourette (1855–1909).

Tourniquet [French: *tourner*, to turn] Instrument for stopping flow of blood into a limb by applying pressure. Many surgeons, including Fabricius Hildanus (1560–1624) and James Yonge (1646–1721), were familiar with it. Morel devised one at the siege of Besancon in 1674. The screw tourniquet was invented by Jean Louis Petit (1674-1750) of France in 1718. One made of rubber was invented by German surgeon, Johannes Friedrich August von Esmarck (1823–1908) in 1869. A modern tourniquet was devised by English physician, L. Dougal Callander in 1940.

Towne View *See acoustic neuroma.*

Townsend, Joseph (1740–1816) Physician and clergyman, educated at Caius College, Cambridge and studied under William Cullen (1710–1790). He wrote *Physician's Vade Mecum, A Guide to Health* and other works on religion and travel.

Townsend, Sir John Sealy Edward (1868–1957) Irish physicist from Galway who made the first measurement of the electric charge in the electron in 1897. He was professor of physics at Oxford in 1900.

Townsend Mixture Remedy containing potassium iodide and mercuric oxide prepared by an English physician and clergyman, Joseph Townsend (1740–1816).

Toxicology [Greek: *toxin*, poison + *logos*, discourse] A treatise was written by Nicander in *Alexispharmaca* around 150 BC which described various plant, mineral and animal poisons and discussed the antidotes. The Persian king, Mithridates, is said to have self-experimented on poisons and developed a state of immunity by taking small nonlethal doses in 80 BC. Dioscorides (AD 40–90) also gave an account on the subject. A printed book written by Petrus de Amano (1250–1315) was published in 1472. French physician, Matthieu Orfila (1787–1853) a founder of modern toxicology, wrote *Traité des Poisons* in 1814 which systematized the subject. An English book on the effects of poison on the body was published by Thomas Addison (1793–1860) and John Morgan (1797–1847) in 1829. *A Treatise on Poison* was written in 1829 by Sir Robert Christison (1797–1882), professor of jurisprudence at Edinburgh. He also self-experimented to study the poisonous effects of calabar bean seed from tropical Africa in 1876 and, on finding it to be intensely poisonous, he recommended it for official executions. An American book was written by Theodore George Wormley (1826–1897) in 1867.

Toxoid [Greek: *toxico*, poison + *eidos*, form] Resembling a poison. *See tetanus.*

Toxoplasma [Greek: *toxin*, poison + *plasmein*, form] Genus of coccidian protozoa. Charles Louis Alphonse Laveran (1845–1922), a French parasitologist and Nobel Prize winner, described it in 1900. It was suggested to be a human pathogen by Marquis Aldo Castellani (1879–1971) of Florence in 1911. Human toxoplasmosis was established as a disease by Abner Wolf (b 1902) and David Cowen (b 1909) in 1937.

Toynbee, Joseph (1815–1866) Aural surgeon to St Mary's Hospital, London in 1852. He described the corneal corpuscles (Tonybee corpuscles) in 1841, and explained the role of the eustachian tube during swallowing in man, in 1861.

TPHA *Treponema pallidium* hemagglutination assay, for diagnosis of syphilis was devised by Tara Rathlev in 1967.

Trace Elements Elements important for growth and

function of all life. In 1860, Louis Pasteur (1822–1895) demonstrated that yeast will grow only in a culture medium which contained such compounds. Julius von Sachs (1832–1897) and Wilhelm Knop demonstrated this in higher plants in the same year. Their importance in diet of higher animals was established by Thomas Burr Osborne (1859–1929) and Lafayette Benedict Mendel in 1919. A review, *Trace Elements in Plants and Animals,* was published by W. Stiles in 1946.

Trachea Aristotle (384–322 BC) used the term to refer to arteries, in the belief that they contained air. 'Arteria leia' was used for arteries and 'arteria trachea' referred to the wind pipe.

Tracheobronchoscopy Direct bronchoscopy was performed by German laryngologist, Gustav Killian (1860–1921) in 1898, and a book on endoscopy which included tracheobronchoscopy was written by Chevalier Jackson (1865–1958) in 1907. He removed an endobronchial tumor using a bronchoscope in 1917.

Tracheoesophageal Fistula Described by Thomas Gibson in 1697 in association with esophageal atresia in a two-year-old baby. However, William Durston has been credited with the first description of it in 1670. But his case was of conjoined females and the esophageal lesion only vaguely resembled that described by Gibson. Occurrence of it without atresia was recognized by D. S. Lamb of Philadelphia in 1873. Primary end-to-end anastomosis of the esophagus as treatment was performed by Cameron Haight (1901–1970) and Harry Townsley in 1941. P.M. Engel and co-workers in 1970 reported an unusual case in a woman who survived to adulthood and gave birth to a daughter with an identical lesion.

Tracheostomy [Greek: *tracheo* + *stomoun,* to make an opening] Pierre Fidéle Bretonneau (1778–1862) of Tours, France performed it for croup. Armand Trousseau (1801–1867) of the Hôtel Dieu, Paris pioneered intubation and performed a tracheostomy in 1851. It was used as treatment for a foreign body stuck in the glottis by John Hepworth of England in 1861. Friedrich Trendelenburg (1844–1924), a German surgeon, administered endotracheal anesthesia through a cannula after a tracheostomy in 1869.

Tracheotomy Incision of the trachea.

Trachoma [Greek: *trachoma,* roughness] Form of granular conjunctivitis known in ancient Greece and Rome and caused by *Chlamydia trachomatis.* The contagious nature was noted by French military surgeon, Dominique Jean Larrey (1766–1842) in 1800. Transmission of the infective agent from animals to humans was demonstrated by German

neurologist, Karl Wernicke (1848–1905). C. Hess and P. Romer did the first transmission of trachoma to animals in 1906. Cell inclusion bodies in conjunctival cells were shown by German zoologist, Stanislaus Joseph Matthias von Prowazek (1875–1915) in 1907. Sulfanilamide was used in the treatment by Heinmann in 1937.

Trajan (AD 52–117) Roman emperor who established an asylum and school for orphans in AD 105.

Trall, R. T. (1812–1877) American writer on sex and related issues, such as contraception. He wrote *Sexual Physiology* (1866) and *Hydropathic Encyclopedia* (1853).

Alexander of Tralles (AD 525–605) Physician from Lydia, an ancient country in Asia Minor, practiced phlebotomy and treated gout with catharides. Some of his medical treatises were printed in Basel and Paris centuries after his death.

Trallianus *See Alexander of Tralles.*

Tranquilizer [Latin: *tranquillus,* calm] In 1947, French surgeon Laborit at Val de Grace at the Military Hospital in Paris investigated use of antihistamines to inhibit the reaction of the autonomic nervous system to physical stress in surgery. He was impressed by the effect of promethazine in calming and relaxing patients and started investigating the phenothizine group of drugs with the help of Parisian anesthetist, P. Huguenard, in 1949. Charpentier produced a phenothiazine, code named RP 4560, in 1950 and Laborit found that this induced tranquillity without clouding consciousness and persuaded a group of psychiatrists, Hamon, Paraire and Velluz at Val de Grace Hospital, to try it. The drug was evaluated by Jean Delay and Pierre Deniker at the nearby St Anne's Hospital in 1952 and introduced as chlorpromazine into mental hospitals in France in the same year and England in 1953. Another early tranquilizer was mephenesin, which was serendipitously discovered by F. M. Berger and Bradley of England during their search for a preservative for injections in 1946. Meprobamate was synthesized by Berger around 1952. Librium was synthesized by Lowe Randall of America in 1960.

Transaminase Enzymes that catalyze the transfer group of an amino acid from a donor to an acceptor. *See diagnostic enzymology.*

Transduction [Latin: *transducere,* to lead across] Method of genetic recombination in bacteria where DNA is transferred between bacteria by a bacteriophage leading to reconstitution of a second organism. This is basic to the field of genetic engineering and was discovered by American geneticist, Joshua Lederberg (b 1925) of New Jersey who shared the Nobel Prize for Physiology or Medicine in 1958 for his discovery.

Transfer RNA The molecular structure of the transfer ribonucleic acid was worked out by American biochemist and Nobel Prize winner, Robert William Holly (b 1922) of Cornell Medical School, in 1965. The genetic code is involved in the assembly of amino acids into proteins under the direction of RNA, and was decoded by Ya-Ming Hou and Paul Schimmel in 1988.

Transfusion [Latin: *transfusio*, to pour over] *See blood transfusion, blood bank, ABO blood groups.*

Transfusion of Plasma [Latin: *transfusio*, to pour over] Substitute for blood transfusion in cases of emergency. Described by American surgeon, Walter Low Tatum (b 1899) in 1939.

Transient Ischemic Attacks *See apoplectiform cerebral congestion.*

Transistor Tiny electrical device which replaced the thermionic valve. Invented by John Bardeen (b 1908), Walter Houser Brattain (b 1902) and William Bradford Shockley (1910–1989) in 1947. It paved the way for the development of implantable defibrillators for ventricular arrhythmias.

Transpiration [Latin: *trans*, through + *spirartio*, exhalation] Discharge of air, sweat or vapor through the skin. Shown in plants by a professor of physick at Gresham College, John Woodward (1665–1728), a pioneer in plant physiology. It was also described by Muschenbroeck, professor at Leiden, and French physician and botanist, Jean Etienne Guettard (1715–1786).

Transplantation [Latin: *trans*, across + *plantare*, to plant] *See organ transplantation, renal transplantation, rejection reaction, cardiac transplant, cadavers, tooth transplantation.*

Transposition of Viscera [Latin: *trans*, across + *positio*, placement] A complete transposition in the abdomen and chest in a woman of 85 years, who was previously well, was described at postmortem, by Edward Parker Young of England in 1860.

Transsacral Block Use of local anesthetics to block the sacral nerves through the posterior sacral foramina was performed by Pauchet and A. Läwen in 1909.

Transurethral Prostatectomy *See prostatectomy.*

Transversalis Fascia Described by Sir Astley Paston Cooper (1768–1841) in 1807, who discussed the importance of the fascia in relation to hernia.

Trapezius [Greek: *trapezion*, an irregular four-sided figure] Used to refer to the present muscle of the upper trunk by

Jean Riolan (1580–1657), professor of anatomy at Paris in 1630.

Trapp Formula Used to calculate the amount of solids in a liter of urine by multiplying the last two figures of its specific gravity by a constant (Trapp coefficient). Devised by Russian pharmacist, Julius Trapp (1815–1908).

Traube, Ludwig (1818–1876) German pathologist and brother of Moritz Traube (1826–1894). He became professor at the Berlin Friedrich-Wilhelm University and developed experimental pathology using animals. He also worked on the pathology of fever and effects of drugs on muscular and nervous activity. He used digitalis in management of heart disease and described rhythmic variations in tone of the vasoconstrictor center (Traube–Herring waves). He also studied the part played by the diaphragm in respiration and gave a clear description of pulsus bigeminus in 1872.

Traube, Moritz (1826–1894) German wine merchant from Rabitor, brother of Ludwig Traube (1818–1876), was also a plant physiologist and chemist. He worked on fermentation and in 1858 proposed the idea of an enzyme in yeast that was responsible. He studied various enzymes and showed the permeability of a membrane containing cupric ferrocyanide to water but not other solutes in 1867.

Traube Space Area over the chest where the resonance of the stomach could be elicited. Described in 1868 by Ludwig Traube (1818–1876), professor of medicine in Berlin.

Trauma *See trauma surgery.*

Trauma Surgery [Greek: *trauma*, wound] Galen (AD 129–200), physician to the gladiators of Rome, managed trauma by conservative methods. Ambroise Paré (1510–1590) introduced ligature in trauma surgery, where amputation and cautery were the mainstay of treatment for limb injuries. Ambulances were introduced by Dominique Jean Larrey (1766–1842) of Paris, a military surgeon, to provide first aid for the wounded. These were two or four wheeled carts drawn by the horses. Mining and industrial accidents became an important cause of trauma in the 19th century and road traffic accidents in the 20th century. An accident service was started in England with the establishment of the Birmingham Accident Hospital in 1941 which later expanded to include other emergencies. Reattachment of a completely severed human arm was performed by Ronald A. Malt and Charles McKhann of America in 1964. *See abdominal injuries.*

Traumatic Tenosynovitis Observed by Alfred Armand Louis Marie Velpeau (1795–1867) in 1818 and the French named it 'cellulite peritendonitis' around 1840.

Travers, Benjamin (1783–1838) Surgeon at St Thomas' Hospital. He described bruit in auscultation of the cranium in a cases of caroticocavernous fistula in 1809, and performed carotid artery ligation for berry aneurysm in 1811. He wrote a monograph on intestinal anastomosis, *An Inquiry into the Processes of Nature in Repairing of the Intestines* in 1812.

Travers, Morris William (1872–1961) English chemist from London and professor at Bristol University (1903–1937). He discovered the inert gases krypton and neon with Scottish chemist, Sir William Ramsay (1852–1916) in 1898.

Treatment *See therapeutics.*

Treitz Hernia Retroperitoneal hernia through the duodenojejunal recess. Described by Wenzel Treitz (1819–1872), professor of pathological anatomy at Prague.

Treitz Ligament Suspensory ligament of the duodenum described in 1853 by Wenzel Treitz (1819–1872), Czech professor of pathological anatomy at Prague and Cracow.

Trelat Sign Small yellowish spots near tuberculous ulcers of the mouth. Described by French surgeon, Ulysses Trelat (1828–1890).

Trematoda [Greek: *trematodes*, pierced] *See flukes.*

Trench Fever Louse-borne rickettsial disease, common during World War 1. A case was reported by John Henry Graham (1868–1957) in 1915 and it was named by Herbert Hunt (1884–1926) and Allan Coates Rankin (1877–1959) in the same year. Outbreaks also occurred on the Russian and German fronts during World War ll. The causative organism, *Rickettsia quintana*, was isolated from the lice of patients with trench fever by German physician Hans Töpfer (b 1876) in 1916 and from a patient in Yugoslavia in 1948 by H. Mooser and co-workers.

Trench Foot Caused by prolonged exposure of feet to water and described by French Army surgeon, Dominique Jean Larrey (1766–1842) in 1812.

Trendelenburg, Friedrich (1844–1924) German surgeon who was professor of surgery at Rostock, Bonn, and Leipzig. He administered endotracheal anesthesia thorough a tracheostomy with an inflatable cuff in 1869. He described the Trendelenburg position used in surgery and anesthesia, Trendelenburg sign for congenital dislocation of hip and Trendelenburg test for varicose veins.

Trendelenburg Gait Caused by paralysis of the gluteal muscles causing waddling. Described by Friedrich Trendelenburg (1844–1924) of Germany in 1895.

Trendelenburg Operation *See embolectomy.*

Trendelenburg Position Patient supine on a table tilted at 45°, with feet and legs over the edge. Described by German surgeon, Friedrich Trendelenburg (1844–1924) in 1880. It was popularized in America by his pupil Willy Meyer (1859–1932) of New York, in 1884.

Trendelenburg Sign Congenital dislocation of the hip, described by Friedrich Trendelenburg (1844–1924) of Germany in 1895.

Trendelenburg Test Test for varicosity and incompetence of the valves by raising the leg above the level of the heart. Devised by German surgeon, Friedrich Trendelenburg (1844–1924).

Trepanning *See trephining*

Trephine [Latin: *trephina*, a borer] A saw used for trepanning. *See terephining.*

Trephining [Latin: *trephina*, a borer] Skulls of primitive man found in various parts of the world has shown that trepanning is the oldest form of neurosurgery. Studies by Pierre Paul Broca (1824–1880) in 1876 showed evidence of healing in these skulls indicating that it was performed on live subjects. It was also an accepted form of treatment by Hippocrates (460–377 BC), Paul of Aegina (AD 625–690) and other ancient physicians. Studies amongst races from Melanesia and Algeria in the 19th century have shown that it was done to cure conditions such as epilepsy, head injury and demonic possession.

Treponema Immobilization Test Test for diagnosis of syphilis devised by Robert Armstrong Nelson (b 1921) and Manfred Martin Mayer (b 1916) in 1949. The Treponema hemagglutination test was devised by Tara Rathlev in 1967. *See Treponema pallidum.*

Treponema pallidum [Greek: *trepein*, to turn + *nema*, thread; Latin: *pallidus*, pale] Causative organism of syphilis discovered and named by Fritz Richard Schaudinn (1871–1906) from Germany and a protozoologist at the Institute of Tropical Diseases at Hamburg. Erich Hoffman (1868–1959), a German dermatologist who worked with Schaudinn, prepared the serum from a genital lesion which led to the discovery in 1905. The dark field method for detection of the spirochete was devised by Karl Landsteiner (1868–1943) in 1906, and the Wassermann serology test for diagnosis for syphilis was devised in the same year by a German bacteriologist, August Paul von Wassermann (1866–1925). The organism was isolated from the syphilitic aorta by Karl Otto Reuter (b 1873) in 1906, and a pure culture was obtained by Japanese pathologist, Hideyo Noguchi (1876–1928), while working in New York, in 1911. He also devised the Noguchi test, using human corpuscles instead of sheep corpuscles, as a modification of the Wasserman reaction.

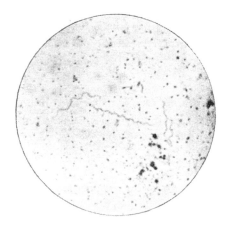

A film of syphilitic material from the inguinal glands, prepared by E. Hoffmann and photographed by Fritz R. Schaudinn. F. Schaudinn and E. Hoffmann, *Selected Essays on Syphilis and Small-Pox* (1906). New Sydenham Society, London

Treponema vincentii Spirochete found in the throat of patients with Vincent angina and identified by Jean Hyacinthe Vincent (1862–1950) in 1898.

Treves, Sir Frederick (1853–1923) Surgeon from Dorchester, England. He wrote several works on surgery and reported a case of true hemophilia in a female in 1886. His *Manual of Surgical Anatomy* (1881) was translated into several languages. He received the Jacksonian Prize for an essay on intestinal obstruction in 1884. He also wrote *The Elephant Man and other Reminiscences*, the true story of Joseph Merrick (1860–1890), a grossly deformed man suffering from neurofibromatosis. In 1902 he saved the life of King George V by diagnosing and operating for appendicitis, for which he was appointed surgeon to the king and baronet. *See elephant man.*

Treviranus, Gottfried Reinhold (1776–1837) German biologist and anatomist from Bremen, and brother of Ludolf Christian Treviranus (1779–1864). He studied medicine and mathematics at the University of Göttingen and became professor of mathematics at Bremen. He wrote *Biologie* (1802–1822), all that was known at the time about living systems, and which introduced the term to the public.

Treviranus, Ludolf Christian (1779–1864) German anatomy

professor at Bremen and Breslau, who discovered intercellular spaces in tissues.

Triad [Latin: *trias*, group of three] Association of three typical signs in syndromes. *See Merseberg triad, Beck triad, Gregg triad, Jacod triad, Francis triad, Charcot triad, Hutchinson triad.*

Triassic Period [Greek: *tria*, three] Early part of Mesozoic era in history. Identified and named by Friedrich August von Alberti in 1834.

Triboulet, Henri (1864–1920) French physician who isolated streptococci from patients with acute rheumatism in 1898. He also devised a fecal test for intestinal tuberculosis, which is now obsolete.

Tricarboxylic Acid Cycle *See Krebs Cycle.*

Trichinella spiralis [Greek: *trichinos*, hair; Latin: *spira*, coil] Parasitic nematode found in meat. Calcified cysts in muscles, later identified to be due to trichinosis, were described by Friedrich Teidmann in 1821. *Trichinella spiralis* was described by John Hilton (1804–1878) in 1833, and the parasitic nature of the worm was pointed out by Sir Richard Owen (1804–1892) in 1834. Sir James Paget (1814–1889) discovered it independently while a student at St Bartholomew's Hospital. Rudolph Leuckart (1823–1898) described it in 1860 and the clinical diagnosis of trichinosis was established by Nicholaus Friedrich (1825–1882) in 1862.

Trichiniasis [Greek: *trichinos*, hair] *See Trichinella spiralis.*

Trichloroethylene Discovered by E. Fisher in 1864 and used as a fat solvent in dry cleaning. It was used to treat trigeminal neuralgia by Herman Oppenheim (1858–1915) of Berlin in 1915 and as an anesthetic agent by American pharmacologist, Dennis Emerson Jackson (b 1878) of Cincinnati, in 1934. Large-scale use as an anesthetic was documented by Cecil Striker in 1935.

Trichomonas vaginalis [Greek: *trichinos*, hair + *monas*, unit] Parasitic flagellated protozoan found in the vagina and male urinary tract. It was recognized by Alfred Donné (1801–1878) of Paris in 1836.

Trichophyton concentricum [Greek: *trichinos*, hair + *phyton*, plant] Fungus that attacks skin, hair and nails. Described by Patrick Manson (1844–1922) in 1879 and named by Raphael Blanchard in 1896. *See Tokelau disease.*

Trichophyton rubrum [Greek: *trichinos*, hair + *phyton*, plant; Latin: *ruber*, red] Fungus that attacks skin, hair and nails. *Epidermophyton rubrum* was described by Marquis Aldo Castellani (1879–1971) during his work in Sri Lanka in 1910.

Trichophyton violaceum [Greek: *trichinos*, hair + *phyton*, plant] Fungus that attacks skin, hair and nails. Described by E. Bodin of Paris in 1902.

Trichuriasis [Greek: *trichinos*, hair + *oura*, tail] Caused by an intestinal nematode parasite, *Trichura*, described by Spanish physician, Alexo de Abreu (1568–1630) in 1623. It was identified and described by Johann Georg Roederer (1727–1763) in Germany in 1760.

Trichuris *See trichuriasis.*

Tricuspid Incompetence [Latin: *tri*, three + *cuspis*, point] Reference was made to it by Robert Adams (1791–1875) in his treatise on diseases of the heart, published in 1827. John Hunter (1728–1793) gave a classic description based on specimens of diseased mitral and aortic valves in his museum. Accentuation of the murmur during inspiration (Carvallo sign) was noted by Mexican cardiologist, J.M. Rivero Carvallo. *See tricuspid valve.*

Tricuspid Valve [Latin: *tri*, three + *cuspis*, point] Terminology for heart valves was established by William Cheselden in *Anatomy of the Human Body* published in 1713. He stated that 'over the entrance of auricles in each ventricle are placed valves to hinder the return of blood, when the heart contracts. Those in the right ventricle are termed tricuspides and those in the left, mitrales'. *See tricuspid incompetence.*

Trigeminal Neuralgia or tic douloureux [Latin: *tri*, three + *geminus*, twin] Described by Quaker physician from Yorkshire, John Fothergill (1712–1780) as 'a painful affection of the face' in 1773 and it was known as Fothergill disease. Injection into the deep foramina of exit of the main fifth nerve from the skull as treatment was performed by Jean Albert Pitres (1848–1927) and Henry Verger of Paris in 1902 and independently by Joseph Louis Irenée Abadie (1873–1946). Gabrielle Ferdinand Lévy (1886–1935) and A. Baudouin devised an approach for the injection from outside the cheek to the foramen ovale and foramen rotundum in 1906 and this became established over the previous route. Alcohol injection of the Gasserian ganglion through the sigmoid notch was performed by Wilfred Harris (1869–1960) of St Mary's Hospital in 1910. Vascular compression as a cause was suggested by American neurosurgeon, Walter Edward Dandy (1886–1946) of Johns Hopkins in 1930. He performed partial resection of the sensory root of the trigeminal ganglion (Gasserian ganglion) as treatment in 1934. The microvascular surgical method of decompressing the vessel and replacement with a piece of teflon was devised by W. J. Gardner and M. V. Miklos in 1959. Thermocoagulation of the affected division of the trigeminal ganglion by a percutaneous method was described by W. H. Sweet and J. G. Wepsic in 1974. *See Gasserian ganglion.*

Triglycerides Hypertriglyceridemia was placed under type IV phenotype of hyperlipoprotenemias by D.S. Frederickson and R.I. Levy in 1972. Diabetic and genetic forms were differentiated by J.D. Brunzell and co-workers in 1975. Familial hypertriglyceridemia of autosomal dominant origin was described by H.N. Neufield and U. Goldbourt in 1983.

Triiodothyronine One of the thyroid hormones, discovered by Jack Gross (b 1921) and Rosalind Venetia Pitt Rivers (b 1907) in 1953.

Trimethylene *See cyclopropane.*

Trinitritin Nitroglycerin was prepared by Italian chemist Ascanio Sobrero of Turin in 1847. Alfred Nobel of Sweden attempted to use it as an explosive in 1864. It was introduced as treatment for angina by William Murrell (1853–1912) of University College, London, in 1879.

Trinity College, Cambridge Founded by Henry VIII in 1546.

Trinity College, Dublin A grant to the Augustine Monastery of All Saints was conferred by Queen Elizabeth in 1591 and the first stone was laid by Thomas Smith, mayor of Dublin, in 1593. It received a new charter in 1637 and the library was erected in 1732.

Trinity College, Oxford Founded in 1554 by Sir Thomas Pope on the foundations of a previous institution, Durham College.

Trinity Hospital, Edinburgh Founded by Queen Mary in memory of her husband, James II, in 1466. It closed and gave way to the railway in 1845.

Triorthocresyl Phosphate (TOCP) A plasticizer agent known as lindol in industry. Also used as an additive to petrol for smooth performance of automobile engines. It was found to be a toxic contaminant in the food industry and in certain medications. Six cases of neuritis were reported in patients who took it as treatment for tuberculosis, by C. Lorot of Paris in 1899. An epidemic occurred in the United States due to contamination of Jamaica Ginger beverage in 1930. Out of 316 cases admitted to Cincinnati General Hospital, 60 men were permanently crippled by its neurotoxic effect. Since then several epidemics have occurred across the world. It was shown to be a cholinesterase inhibitor by H. Block in 1941.

Trismus [Greek: *trismos*, grinding] Tetanic spasm affecting the muscles of the jaw following tetanus. *See tetanus.*

Trisomy 18 Syndrome Associated with soft tissue defects, mental retardation and cardiac abnormalities. Described independently by English medical geneticist at Oxford, J.H. Edwards (b 1928) and K. Patau, in 1960. The occurrence of chromosome 18 in triplicate was demonstrated by Patau in 1961.

Trisomy 21 Chromosome abnormality and cause of Down syndrome, described by Jerome Lejeune in 1959. *See Down syndrome.*

Trobondeau, Adrian Louis Matthew Frederic (1872–1918) French naval physician who in 1906 proposed the theory (with Jean Bergonie, 1857–1925) that the sensitivity of the cells to radiation varied according to reproductive capacity and differentiation.

Trocar [French: *trois quarts*, three quarters] Sharp pointed surgical instrument for piercing, used with a cannula and invented by Sanctorio Sanctorius (1561–1636) of Padua. He also invented a thermometer and did work on human metabolism.

Trochanter [Greek: *trochanter*, a runner] Bony protuberance below the neck of the femur, derives its name due to its motion in running. It was introduced into anatomy by the Roman physician, Galen (AD 129–200).

Troichobezoar Concretion of hairs formed in the intestine. *See bezoar.*

Troisier Sign Enlargement of the lymph gland above the clavicle in cases of intra-abdominal malignancy. Described by French physician, Charles Emile Troisier (1844–1919). He is supposed to have observed it on himself.

Trojan War Homer's *Iliad,* written around 900 BC, is an important source of knowledge on ancient Greek medicine, mainly through its description of the Trojan war around 1200 BC. It contains descriptions of 141 war wounds of the neck, chest, bladder, spinal cord and femur, including their treatment. Homer also used 150 anatomical terms.

Tröltsch Space Found between the two pouches of the mucous membrane in the upper part of the middle ear. Described by German aural surgeon, Anton Friedrich von Tröltsch (1829–1890). He invented a modern otoscope in 1860 and devised a new method of mastoidectomy in 1861.

Trombiculoid Mite *See tsutsugamushi.*

Trommer Test Detects dextrose in urine using sodium hydroxide and copper sulfate as reagents. Devised by German chemist, Karl August Trommer (1806–1879) in 1841.

Tronchin, Theodore (1709–1781) Physician from Geneva who studied at Cambridge and later under Herman Boerhaave (1668–1738) in Leiden. He practiced in Geneva and Paris and published a dissertation on colica pictonum and other medical works.

Trophoblast [Greek: *trophe*, nutrition + *blastos*, germ] The Langhans layer, or cytotrophoblast, which covers the chorionic villi beneath the syncytial layer was described by a German pathologist, Theodor Langhans (1839–1915) of Bern, in 1870. The Rauber layer, an outer cell mass of trophoblastic cells of the blastodermic vesicle, was described by a professor of anatomy at Dorpat, August Antinous Rauber (1841–1917) in 1880.

Tropical Disease *See tropical medicine.*

Tropical Medicine A European book on tropical medicine, mainly on India, was written by Garcia D'Orta (1501–1568) in 1563, an English book by George Whetstone (1545–1588) (published in 1598) and a Dutch book by Jacob de Bontius (1592–1631), who described beriberi followed. *An Essay on Diseases Incidental to Europeans in Hot Climates* was published by James Lind (1716–1794) in 1768, who also introduced lemon juice as the cure for scurvy. Louis Daniel Beauperthuys (1803–1871) from the West Indies and who graduated in medicine from Paris, is one of the forgotten pioneers of tropical medicine. He investigated virulent outbreaks of yellow fever in Venezuela and the West Indies and pointed out the causal relationship of mosquitoes in the marshes to such epidemics. Sir Patrick Manson (1844–1922) from Fingask, Aberdeen made several important contributions which have earned him the title of father of tropical medicine. He worked in Formosa and China and, on his return, founded the London School of Tropical Medicine in 1898. He proposed the extracorporeal life cycle for the malarial parasite in the mosquito in 1894 and described the periodicity of the filarial parasite and the *Anopheles* mosquito as its vector in 1879. Nobel Prize winner, Sir Ronald Ross (1857–1932), surgeon major in the Indian Medical Services, while working at the Nilagri mountains in India, identified the mosquito as the carrier of malarial parasite in 1897 and showed the transmission of malarial disease to birds by bites of infected mosquitoes in 1898. He was professor of tropical medicine at Liverpool in 1899. The London School of Tropical Medicine was incorporated into the University of London in 1905 and amalgamated with the School of Hygiene in 1925 to become the London School of Hygiene and Tropical Medicine. William

Whiteman Carlton Topley (1886–1944) was the first professor of bacteriology and immunology.

Tropical Pulmonary Eosinophilia A syndrome of cough and asthma accompanied by eosinophilia and X-ray changes in the lungs. Described amongst the Indians, by R.J.Weigarten in 1943.

Tropical Sprue (Syn: Indian sprue, chronic tropical diarrhea, cachectic diarrhea) Mentioned by William Hillary (1697–1763) in Barbados and described by Colin Chisholm (1755–1825) of London in 1822.

Trotter, Robert (1648–1727) Scottish physician who graduated from Leiden. On his return to Edinburgh he was president of the Royal College of Physicians on two occasions, in 1694 and 1700.

Trotter, Thomas (1760–1832) Scottish physician from Roxburghshire who graduated in medicine from Edinburgh University. He was physician to the Royal Hospital at Portsmouth in 1793 and to the navy in 1794. He wrote *Medica Nautica, or an Essay on the Diseases of Seamen, Essay on Drunkenness, a Review of the Medical Department of British Navy* and other works. He retired to Newcastle and practiced as a physician.

Trotter, Wilfred Batten Lewis (1872–1939) English neurologist who studied the pathology and symptoms of post-head injury status and defined concussion in 1924. In 1911 he described Trotter syndrome, associated with deafness, palatal paralysis and facial neuralgia due to nasopharyngeal carcinoma.

Trotter Syndrome *See Trotter, Wilfred Batten.*

Trotula (*c* 1125) Midwife from a noble family in Salerno during the medieval period. She is supposed to have written *De passionibus mulierium.*

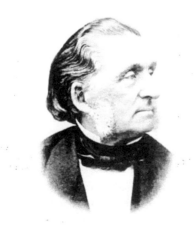

Armand Trousseau (1801–1867). Courtesy of the National Library of Medicine

Trousseau, Armand (1801–1867) Eminent physician and clinical teacher at the Hôtel Dieu, Paris. He performed a tracheostomy in 1865 and was a pioneer of intubation. He received the prize of the Academy of Medicine for his treatise on laryngeal phthisis in 1837. His lectures were translated into English by Victor Bazire, and published in 5 volumes in 1868. *See Trousseau sign.*

Trousseau Sign Indication for hypocalcemia involving tetanic spasm of the hand on applying sufficient pressure to the arm. Described by Armand Trousseau (1801–1867) of Paris in 1861.

Trudeau, Edward Livingston (1848–1915) New York physician who was a pioneer in the study of tuberculosis in America.

Trueta, José (1897–1977) Spanish surgeon who worked in the Military Hospital in Barcelona during the Civil War (1936–1939). He emigrated to England in 1939 and succeeded Herbert Seddon (1903–1977) as professor of orthopedics at the Nuffield Orthopaedic Centre in Oxford in 1949. He developed the closed plaster method for treating wounds and was one of the first to use penicillin for osteomyelitis.

Truncus Arteriosus [Latin: *truncus*, stem] A successful operation for truncus arteriosus was conducted by D.C.McGoon and G.C.Rastelli in 1967.

Truss One of the first – a transverse spring truss for use in hernia or ruptures – was invented and patented by Robert Brand in 1771.

Trypan Blue Introduced as treatment for trypanosomiasis by Maurice Nicolle (1862–1932) and Felix Mesnil (1868–1938) in 1906. Its effectiveness in the treatment of babesiasis was demonstrated by American physician, George Henry Faulkner Nuttall (1862–1937) and S.Hadwen in 1909.

Trypan Red Paul Ehrlich (1854–1915), director of the Institute for Experimental Therapy at Frankfurt and originator of the side-chain theory, produced the first man-made chemotherapeutic agent, tryphan red, in 1904, which cured infected mice with trypanosomiasis.

Trypanosoma cruzi Carlos Chagas (1879–1974), a physician at the Osvaldo Cruz Institute, Rio de Janeiro, discovered the causative agent of American trypanosomiasis (Chagas disease), a pathogenic protozoan and its insect vector in the state of Minas Geras in Brazil, in 1909. The life cycle of the parasitic protozoan was described by Alexandre Joseph Emile Brumpt (1877–1951) in 1912.

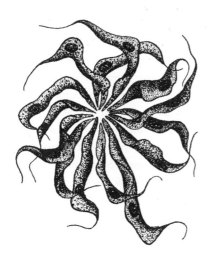

Agglutinated *Trypanosoma lewsi* in blood. Sir Patrick Manson, *Tropical Diseases* (1914). Cassell & Co, London

Trypanosomiasis Sleeping sickness. Deaths in cattle following tsetse fly bites in Africa were noted in 1857 by the missionary surgeon, David Livingstone (1813–1873). English Naval surgeon, John Atkins (1685–1757), mentioned a fly disease of African horses known as 'nagna' in 1734. The first accurate description, called *kondee* in Africa, was given by an English doctor, Thomas Masterman Winterbottom (1765–1859) who practiced in Sierra Leone. The causative agent was identified in the blood of the diseased animals by Sir David Bruce (1855–1931) in 1894. The first trypanosome to be identified was in a salmon by Gabriel Gustav Valentin (1810–1909) in 1841. The name for the genus of the protozoal etiological agent was proposed by Hungarian mycologist, David Gruby (1810–1898), following his discovery of the organism in the blood of frogs in 1844. British parasitologist, Timothy Richard Lewis (1841–1886), found *Trypanosoma lewisi* which infected rats in Calcutta in 1879. A case of human trypanosomiasis was described by Joseph Everett Dutton (1877–1905) in 1902 and named *Trypanosoma gambiense*. *Trypanosoma rhodisiense*, cause of sleeping sickness, was discovered by John William Watson Stevens (1865–1946) and Harold Benjamin Fanthom (1875–1937) in 1910. *See Trypanosoma cruzi, trypanosomicidal drugs.*

Trypanosomicidal Drugs The African explorer, David Livingstone, used arsenic in the treatment of African horse disease and arsenic preparations were found to cure 'Surra' in horses in India by Lingaard in 1899. Atoxl (p-amino-phenyl arsenate) was shown to cure human African trypanosomiasis by Thomas and Breinl of England in 1904. The effectiveness of antimony tartrate in treating it in experimental animals (maladie du sommeil) was demonstrated by London physician, George Henry Plimmer

(1856–1915) and J.D.Thompson in 1908. Bayer 205 (suramin, Germanin), a synthetic remedy, was first introduced in 1920 and tested by Ludwig Hadel and Wilhelm Jotten of Germany in the same year. A trial on human trypanosomiasis was done by German physician, Peter Muhlens (1874–1943) and W. Menk on a German affected by *Trypanosoma gambiense* in 1921. BR Compounds (BR 68,34), the prototype arsenic compounds linked to heterocyclic rings, were introduced by A. Binz and C. Rath in 1927.

Trypsin Alimentary enzyme discovered by Aleksander Danilevsky (1838–1923) in 1862 and isolated by a German biochemist, Wilhelm Friedrich Kühne (1837–1900). Kühne also coined the term enzyme in 1878 to denote organic substances which activated chemical reactions. A crystalline form was obtained by American biochemist, John Howard Northrop (1891–1987) of New York in 1932. Chymotrypsinogen was isolated by Northrop in 1935, who wrote *Crystalline Enzymes* in 1939.

Trypsinogen *See trypsin.*

Tryptophane The first essential amino acid to be identified was isolated by William Sydney Cole (1877–1952) of Trinity College Cambridge and Sir Frederick Gowland Hopkins (1861–1947) in 1901.

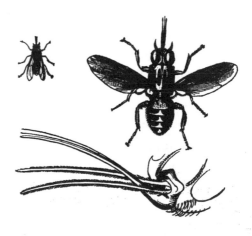

Illustration of tse tse fly, life size and magnified, and proboscis. David Livingstone, *Missionary Travels and Researches in Africa* (1858). Harper, New York

Tse Tse Fly Deaths in cattle following tse tse fly bites in Africa were noted by the explorer, David Livingstone, in 1857. The intermediate host status of the fly was demonstrated by Friedrich Karl Kleine (1861–1950) in 1909. *See trypanosomiasis.*

TSH *See thyroid-stimulating hormone.*

Tsutsugamushi Disease originally known as Shimamushi,

or island insect disease. The trombiculoid mite, Aka mushi, was observed as its cause in Japan in 1878. Chinese literature from the 16th century describes a similar disease caused by the sand mite. Active research on the subject was commenced by Baron Shibasaburo Kitasato (1852–1931) in 1893 and he successfully transmitted the disease to monkeys in 1918. The rickettsial cause was demonstrated by M. Nagayo and colleagues in 1930, who named the organism, *Rickettsia orientalis*. It was renamed *Rickettsia tsutsugamushi* by N. Ogata in 1931.

Tswett, Mikhail Semenovich (1872–1919) *See chromatography.*

Tubal Ligation *See sterilization.*

Tubercle Bacillus [Latin: *tuberculum*, small hump] The bacillus of mammalian tubercle was discovered by Robert Koch (1843–1910) in 1882 and was the first bacteria attributed to a human disease. The avian tubercle bacilli was discovered independently by several workers including Rivolta, Angelo Maffucci (1847–1903), Roger and Sibley in 1890. The peculiar property of acid fastness of the bacillus was demonstrated by Theodor Albrecht Edwin Klebs (1834–1913) in 1896. Transmission to man through milk and meat was shown by French biologist, Edmond Isidore Etienne Nocard (1850–1903). A seroagglutination test was devised by French physician, Saturnin Arloing (1846–1911) in 1898.

Tubercle [Latin: *tuberculum*, small hump] Gaspard Laurent Bayle (1774–1816), a physician from Provence who practiced in Paris, established in 1810 the pathological nature of the lesion, previously known as tubercle. Jean Antoine Villemin (1827–1892) used the term in his *Etudes sur la Tuberculose*, published in Paris in 1868.

Tuberculin Test For diagnosis of tuberculosis. Devised by Austrian physician, Clemens Freiherr von Pirquet (1874–1929) in 1907, who applied old tuberculin to the skin with a needle scratch. Subcutaneous injection of a controlled amount of tuberculin for the test was introduced by French physician, Charles Mantoux (1877–1947) in 1910.

Tuberculosis Disease affecting the lungs, known as phthisis or consumption before the discovery of the tubercle bacillus, *Mycobacterium tuberculosis*, by Robert Koch (1843–1910) in 1882. Percivall Pott (1714–1788), a surgeon at St Bartholomew's Hospital in London, described spinal caries in 1779 but probably did not realize its tuberculous nature. A description of the pathological appearance of the tubercle in the lung was given by Matthew Baillie (1761–1823) in *Morbid Anatomy of Some of the Most Important Parts of the Human Body* published in 1793. Gaspard Laurent

Bayle (1774–1816), a physician from Provence who practiced at Paris, gave pathological findings in *Recherches sur la Phthisie Pulmonaire* published in 1810. Before the identification of a bacterium, various remedies, such as sea air and warm climate, were recommended as treatment. Induction of artificial pneumothorax as treatment was introduced by James Carson (1772–1843) of Liverpool in 1821 and used for the next 100 years. Other forms of collapse therapy, such as phrenic crush, apicolysis and thoracoplasty, were also used. Secret remedies were common before the advent of chemotherapy and included Tuberculozyme, Brompton Consumption mixture and Steven's Consumption Cure. The infectious nature was demonstrated by French physician, Jean Antoine Villemin (1827–1892) who inoculated an animal with material taken from the lung of a patient with tuberculosis in 1865. A tuberculosis dispensary was established at Edinburgh by Sir Robert William Phillip (1857–1939) of Edinburgh Royal Infirmary in 1888. He pioneered study and control and established a tuberculosis dispensary in London at Paddington in 1909. Creosote, obtained from wood, was a popular remedy for the next 50 years and was revived as a specific remedy by Charles Jacques Bouchardt (1837–1915) in 1877. The drug Iproniazid was used in treatment in 1910 and streptomycin was introduced as first-line drug by Hortin Corwin Hinshaw (b 1902) in 1946. Isoniazid was used by Edward Robitzek in 1952 and given in combination with pyrazinamide by Walsh McDermott and colleagues in America in 1954. Cycloserine was introduced by P. B. Storey in 1958, and ethionamide was added by Noel Rist in 1959. Ethambutol was used by J. P. Thomas and co-workers in 1961. *See BCG vaccine, collapse therapy, tubercle bacillus, tuberculous meningitis, intestinal tuberculosis, Ghon focus.*

Tuberculous Lymphadenitis *See scrofula.*

Tuberculous Meningitis Scientific study was done in 1764 by Robert Whytt (1714–1766), a neurologist at Edinburgh. Drainage of cerebrospinal fluid as a therapeutic measure was tried by Walter Essex Wynter (1860–1945) in 1889 who described four patients. Lumbar puncture was advocated by Heinrich Irenaeus Quincke (1842–1922) in 1891.

Tuberculous Spondylitis [Latin: *tuberculum*, small hump + *sphondylos*, vertebra + *itis*, inflammation] Affecting the cervical vertebrae and known as Rust disease was described by Austrian surgeon, Johann Nepomuk Rust (1775–1840) of Berlin in 1834.

Tuberous Sclerosis [Latin: *tuberculum*, small hump; Greek: *skleros*, hard] (Syn: adenoma sebaceum, Bourneville disease,

Pringle disease) Condition associated with skin growths. Described by Désiré Magloire Bourneville (1840–1909) of Paris in 1880 and English dermatologist, John James Pringle (1855–1922). A detailed description of these skin tumors and their association with mental retardation and epilepsy (epiloia) was given by John Thompson in 1913.

Tuffier, Theodore (1857–1929) *See aortic stenosis, spinal anesthesia, lobectomy of lung, artificial respiration.*

Tuke, Daniel Hack (1827–1895) Great grandson of William Tuke (1732–1822). He qualified in medicine from St Bartholomew's Hospital and specialized in psychiatry. He was a lecturer in mental diseases at Charing Cross Hospital from 1892. He wrote *A Manual of Psychological Medicine* (1852) and *Dictionary of Psychological Medicine* (1892).

Tuke, Sir John Battey (1835–1913) A member of the Tuke family of psychiatrists, and lecturer in mental diseases at Edinburgh. He advocated abolishing physical restraint for the mentally ill.

Tuke, Samuel (1784–1857) Grandson of William Tuke (1732–1822). He published *Description of the Retreat* which included a classic account of moral therapy given at his grandfather's Retreat at York.

Tuke, William (1732–1822) Tea and coffee merchant from York who became a great British philanthropist. He was a reformer of the care for the mentally ill and founded the Retreat for the Insane at York.

Tularemia (Syn: Pahvant Valley fever, Ohara disease, deer fly fever) Plague-like illness amongst rodents was first observed at Tulare in California by George Walter McCoy (b 1876) in 1911. In the following year he and C.W. Chapin isolated the causative organism of the disease (named *Francisella tularensis* in 1921) from guinea pigs after inoculating them with infective material. It was observed in Norway by Collet in 1895, who called it the lemming fever. The first human case transmitted by deer ticks was observed in California in 1914. The disease is known as Ohara disease in Japan where it was described by Japanese physician Shoichiro Ohara in 1930.

Tully Powder Remedy containing morphine, prepared by American physician, William Tully (1795–1859).

Tulp Valve *See Tulp, Nicolas.*

Tulp, Nicolas (1593–1674) Dutch anatomist who is the central figure in Rembrandt's painting, the Anatomy Lesson. He was the mayor of Amsterdam and defended the city against the French in 1672. The iliocelic valve of the large intestines bears his name.

Tumor [Latin: *tumere*, to swell] *See cancer.*

Tungsten [Swedish: heavy stone] Brittle metal element isolated by Karl Wilhelm Schleele (1742–1786) in 1781 and obtained in pure form by the du Layart brothers of France in 1786. It was used in construction of the first X-ray fluoroscope by Alva Edison (1847–1931), and exhibited at the New York City electrical exhibition in 1896.

Tungsten Lamp Lamp filled with gas invented by American chemist, Irving Langmuir (1881–1957) of Brooklyn, New York.

Tuning Fork Instrument which gave a pure musical tone of constant pitch, invented by John Shore in 1711.

Tunnicliff, Ruth (1876–1946) Born in Chicago, she specialized in bacteriology and researched on streptococci and anaerobes.

Tupper, Sir Charles (1821–1915) Physician from Edinburgh who settled in Canada and became a powerful figure in Canadian politics. He was elected first president of the Canadian Medical Association in 1867, but later devoted his time to politics. He was High Commissioner for Canada in London in 1884, and on his return to Canada he was appointed as the Minister of Finance.

Türck Cell Abnormal leukocyte, resembling a plasma cell. Described by Austrian physician, W. Turck (1871–1916).

Türck, Ludwig, (1810–1868) Viennese neurologist and laryngologist who devised a laryngoscope in 1857. He described the micropathology of the spinal cord in tabes dorsalis, the direct pyramidal tracts known as the Türck column in 1856, and observed the retinal changes in hypertension in 1850.

Turing, Alan Mathison (1912–1954) London mathematician who made an outstanding contribution to computer science. He proposed the Turing Machine in 1936, a logical machine capable of calculating any calculable number. The first programmable computer was based on his concept.

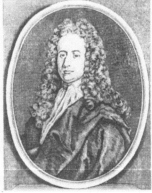

Daniel Turner (1666–1741). Courtesy of the National Library of Medicine

Turner, Daniel (1666–1741) English physician who wrote a book on dermatology, *De Morbis Cutaneis* in 1717.

Turner, Edward (1797–1837) Born in Jamaica and graduated in medicine from Edinburgh University. He was professor of chemistry at University College, London in 1828 and wrote several treatises including *Elements of Chemistry including recent Discoveries* and *Doctrines of the Science*.

Turner, George Grey (1877–1951) Surgeon from Newcastle-upon-Tyne who reported successful resection of the thoracic esophagus in 1933. He wrote *The Hunterian Museum, yesterday and tomorrow* (1946), and *Rutherford Morison and his Achievement* (1948), a biography of James Rutherford Morison (1854–1940) who was a surgeon at the Royal Infirmary at Newcastle. The Turner sign is local discoloration of the skin of the loin 2–3 days after an attack of acute pancreatitis.

Turner, Henry Hubert (1892–1970) American physician from Illinois who studied in Vienna and London and became professor of medicine at the University of Oklahoma. He was a founder of the Endocrine Society and its first president. *See Turner syndrome.*

Turner, Peter (1542–1614) Medical graduate of Heidelberg and physician at St Bartholomew's Hospital. His *Plea for a madwoman* (1606) to prevent her child being taken from her because of her melancholie (depression), was one of the earliest recorded human approaches to psychiatric patients in England.

Turner Sulcus Interparietal sulcus of the brain described by Sir William Turner (1832–1916) of Edinburgh University.

Turner Syndrome XO syndrome, characterized by sexual infantilism, short stature and webbing of the neck in phenotypic females. Described by American endocrinologist, Henry Hubert Turner (1892–1970) of Illinois in 1938. He included seven cases with the above features. The same condition, known as status Bonnieve–Ullrich in Europe, was described by Otto Ullrich (1894–1957) in 1930. A sex chromosomal defect was shown to be the cause by C.E. Ford in 1959.

Turner, Thomas (1793–1873) Surgeon to the Manchester Infirmary who was a founder of the Manchester School of Medicine.

Turner, Sir William (1832–1916) English surgeon from Lancaster who qualified from St Bartholomew's Hospital in London and succeeded John Goodsir (1814–1867) as professor of anatomy at Edinburgh University in 1867. He

described the subzonal membrane of the amnion within the chorionic vesicle in 1872, and wrote *The Convolutions of the Human Cerebrum Topographically Considered* in 1864.

Turner, William (1510–1568) English naturalist from Morpeth, Northumberland who studied at Pembroke Hall, Cambridge. He wrote *Libellus de Herbaria* in 1538 and the first printed monograph on birds in 1544, containing a description of birds previously mentioned by Aristotle (384–322 BC) and Pliny (AD 23–79).

Turyn Sign Patient feels pain in the gluteal region if the great toe is bent, in cases of sciatica. Described by Felix Turyn (b 1899), a physician from Warsaw.

Tuthill, Sir George (d 1835) English physician who confined his practice to diseases of the brain.

Tuttle Proctoscope Rectal speculum with an electric light attached to its extremity and capable of inflating the rectal ampulla. Designed by New York surgeon, James Percival Tuttle (1857–1912).

Twilight Sleep Form of narcosis induced by morphine and scopolamine during labor. Introduced by Richard von Steinbuchel in 1902. German physician, Carl Joseph Gauss (b 1875) advocated it in 1906. It was widely used in obstetric practice until the 1940s.

Twinning Pill Compound of calomel and ipecacuanha for gastrointestinal symptoms, introduced by British surgeon, William Twinning (1813–1848), who worked in India.

Twort, Frederick William (1877–1950) English bacteriologist from Surrey who studied medicine in London and became professor of bacteriology in 1919. He developed methods of culturing acid-fast staining organisms and extracted vitamin K from dead tubercle bacilli. He also discovered a 'transmissible lytic agent' which was later named by F.H. D'Hérelle as the bacteriophage, thus heralding the beginnings of molecular biology.

Twort–D'Hérelle Phenomenon Lysis of bacterial colonies in a culture and the agent responsible was first observed by Frederick William Twort (1877–1950), a British microbiologist, and later observed by Félix Hubert D'Hérelle (1873–1949), a Canadian bacteriologist working in France, in 1917, who named it the bacteriophage.

Twyne, Thomas (1543–1613) Physician from Canterbury who graduated from Cambridge. He practiced astrology, wrote poetry and translated several books of *The Aeneid* into English.

Tylor, Sir Edward Burnet (1832–1917) Born in Camberwell,

London, he was a one of the first British anthropologists who wrote *Researches into History of Mankind* in 1865. He was the first professor of anthropology at Oxford 1896 and regarded as the founder of the systemic study of human culture. His other important works include *Primitive Culture* (1871) and *Anthropology* (1881).

Tympanum [Greek: *tympanon*, drum] First used to describe the ear drum by Gabriele Falloppio (1523–1562) who was a pupil of Vesalius. The theory that the tympanic membrane of the ear, on receiving the sound, vibrated like a microphone and imparted electrical impulses to the brain was put forward in 1869 by William Rutherford (1839–1899), a Scottish professor of physiology at King's College London and pioneer in the study of the mechanism of hearing.

Tymphanic Membrane *See tympanum.*

Tyndall, John (1820–1893) Physicist, born in County Carlow, Ireland and moved to Preston in Lancashire around 1843, where he became a member of the Mechanics Institute. He studied in Marburg under Robert Bunsen (1811–1899) for three years and when he returned to England he succeeded Michael Faraday (1791–1867) as president of the Royal Institution in 1867. He wrote *Radiant Heat in its relation to Gases and Vapours* and *On the sounds produced by Combustion of Gases in Tubes.* He later investigated acoustic properties of the atmosphere and behavior of light. He discovered the Tyndall effect of scattering of light by colloidal particles in solution and suggested that the blue color of the sky was caused by such scattering. His contribution to medicine, *The Floating Matter of Air in relation to Putrefaction and Infection,* was published in 1881.

Typhoid [Greek: *typhodes*, like smoke, delirious] A description of an epidemic typhoid fever was given by Thomas Willis (1621–1675) in his *De febribus* in 1659. Early records in Europe were made by John Rutty (1697–1775) during an epidemic at Dublin in 1739, and John Huxam (1692–1768) in England in the same year. A confirmed description in German literature was given by Riedel in 1748 and an accurate description of the intestinal lesions in typhoid in France were given by Prost (1804) and by Petis and Serres in 1813. The name 'fievre typhoide' was coined in 1829 by Pierre Charles Alexandre Louis (1787–1872), physician and medical statistician in Paris, who also described the rose spots as a sign. The contagious nature was noted by American physician, Nathan Smith (1762–1829) in *A Practical Essay on Typhus Fever,* published in 1842. The term 'enteric fever' was given by Charles Ritchie (1799–1878) of England in 1846. A clear differentiation between typhus and typhoid was made by Alexander Patrick Stewart

(1813–1883) in 1840. Pierre Fidèle Bretonneau (1778–1862) of France gave a classic pathological description in 120 patients at autopsy and showed the characteristic features of Peyer patches. A clear picture in England resulted from work on continued fevers (1849–1851) by Sir William Jenner (1815–1898). William Budd (1811–1880) of Devon, brother of George Budd (1808–1882), suggested excreta as a source of typhoid in *Typhoid Fever: Its nature, mode of spreading and Prevention* published in 1873. Karl Joseph Eberth (1835–1926) of Würzberg, a pupil of Rudolph Virchow (1821–1902) and professor of pathology at Halle, showed that *Salmonella typhi* was the causative organism in 1880.

Typhoid Bacillus *Salmonella typhi*, causative agent of enteric fever. Described by Karl Joseph Eberth (1835–1926) of Würzberg in 1880 and isolated by German bacteriologist, George Gaffky (1850–1918) in 1884. *See typhoid.*

Typhoid Vaccine English bacteriologist, Sir Almroth Edward Wright (1861–1947), observed that inoculation with dead typhoid bacilli caused the patient to acquire immunity. He developed the first vaccine based on this. It was superseded by a mixed prophylactic vaccine, anti-paratyphoid–typhoid vaccine (TAB) in the 1930s. Typhoid vaccine was also used in conditions such as neurosyphilis to induce protein shock therapy around 1900. It was previously used intravenously to induce fever and vasodilatation in treatment of thromboangitis obliterans.

Typhus [Greek: *typhos*, stupor arising from fever] An early reference to the disease was made during an epidemic at the monastery of la Cava near Salerno in 1083. A description was given by Girolamo Fracastoro (1478–1553) in his *De Morbis Contagiosis* who called it 'lenticulae' or 'peticulae' in 1546. It was confused with typhoid until the middle of the 19th century, when it was clearly differentiated by Alexander Patrick Stewart (1813–1883) in 1840. The body louse was identified as a transmitter by Charles Jules Henri Nicolle (1886–1936)), a French physician, Nobel Prize winner and pupil of Louis Pasteur (1822–1895) in 1911. It was the first rickettsial disease to be identified and named *Rickettsia prowazekii* after Howard Taylor Ricketts (1871–1910) and Stanislas Joseph von Prowazek (1875–1938), who died from the disease during their research, by Henrique da Rocha Lima (1879–1956) in 1916. Polish bacteriologist, Arthur Felix (1887–1956), while working with Edmund Weil (1880–1922) in Eastern Galicia, devised an agglutinin reaction for diagnosis in 1916. During their research they noticed the presence of a proteus-like organism in the urine of a patient and demonstrated that this organism, proteus X, agglutinated sera of other patients with typhus. This formed the basis for the use of the proteus test to differentiate various rickettsial diseases. *See factory fever, murine typhus, scrub typhus.*

Tyrell Fascia Prostatoperitoneal aponeurosis. Described by Frederick Tyrell (1793–1843), a surgeon at St Thomas' Hospital and nephew of Sir Astley Paston Cooper (1768–1841), in 1824.

Tryon, Thomas (1634–1703) London merchant who called himself a student of physick and denounced the exposure of patients at the Bethlem Hospital to the public. He wrote a treatise on dreams and visions in 1689 which pointed out the psychological factors leading to mental disease.

Tyrosine Amino acid observed as a product of pancreatic digestion by Justus von Liebig (1803–1873) of Germany in 1846. An inborn error of metabolism of the acid (tyrosinosis) was described by Grace Medes (1886–1967) in 1932.

Tyrothricin First commercially produced antibiotic obtained from the soil bacterium, *Bacillus brevis*. Discovered in 1939 by French-born American bacteriologist René Jules Dubos (1901–1982) of the Rockefeller University, New York.

Tyson, Edward (1651–1708) English physician and anthropologist from Bristol who was educated at Magdalen Hall, Oxford. He practiced in London and was appointed physician to Bridewell and Bethlehem Hospitals. He considered that comparative anatomy would reveal the underlying structural unity of nature. He studied the anatomy of an orang-utang and suggested that it was intermediate between man and ape and wrote *The Anatomy of the Pigmy compared with that of a Monkey, an Ape and a Man* (1698) and several other works.

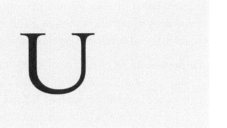

Udránsky Test   Detects bile using furfurol as reagent. Devised in 1890 by László Udránsky (1862–1914), a physiologist at Budapest.

Uffelmann Test   Detects lactic acid in gastric juice using ferric chloride and phenol as reagents. Devised by German physician, Julius August Christian Uffelmann (1837–1894).

Uhthoff Sign   Occurrence of nystagmus in multiple sclerosis. Described by German ophthalmologist, Wilhelm Uhthoff (1853–1927) from Breslau.

Ukambine   Crystalline alkaloid and constituent of African arrow poison, similar to strophanthine but more potent. *See arrow poisons.*

Ulcer   [Latin: *ulcus*, a sore] Defined as 'a solution of continuity' by Hippocrates (460–370 BC). John Hunter (1728–1793) in his treatise on inflammation, noted that pressure, irritation of stimulating substances, weakness inutility of parts or organs and the death of tissue are causes of ulcers. E. Home (1756–1832) wrote a monograph in which he has prescribed application of hemlock, argentum and arsenic. *See duodenal ulcer, Marjolin ulcer, rodent ulcer, gastric ulcer, Helicobacter pylori.*

Ulcerative Colitis   [Latin: *ulcus*, a sore; Greek: *kolon*, colon + *itis*, inflammation] Chronic relapsing condition of the colon described as 'acute extensive ulcerations of the colon' by Sir William Henry Allchin (1846–1912) of London in 1885. The first sulfonamide derivative, sulfanilamide (Protonsil), was used in treatment by Bannick, Brown and Foster in America in 1937. Toxicity of sulfanilamide led to a search for a safer compound and neoprotonsil was introduced in 1938.

Ulcerative Gingivitis   *See Vincent angina.*

Ullrich Syndrome   Congenital variant of Oppenheim disease, consisting of kyphoscoliosis, contractures of the large joints and immobility of proximal joints with hypermobility of distant joints. Described by Otto Ullrich (1894–1957) in 1930.

Ullrich–Turner Syndrome   *See Turner syndrome.*

Ultraviolet   [Latin: *ultra*, beyond] Observed in the spectrum by William Hyde Wollaston (1766–1828) in 1802. Short wavelength ultraviolet rays showed least amount of penetration of tissues and Sir Arthur Henry Downes (1851–1938) and Thomas Porter Blunt in 1877 showed that these were capable of killing bacteria. Use of ultraviolet light greatly improved photomicrographic study of the structure of bacteria and were also used for therapeutic purposes. Their effectiveness in curing rickets was demonstrated by Kurt Huldschinsky (1883–1941) of Berlin in 1919. *See bacterial structure.*

Ultracentrifuge   [Latin: *ultra*, beyond + *centrum*, center + *fugere*, to flee] A centrifuge capable of very high speed was invented by Swedish physical chemist, Theodor Svedberg (1884–1971) in 1923 and used to study colloid particles. He was awarded the Nobel Prize for Chemistry in 1926.

Ultrafiltration   [Latin: *ultra*, beyond; French: *filtrer*, to strain] Performed by Charles J. Martin in 1896 using a filter consisting of porous clay coated with gelatin. He fixed the filter in a gunmetal case and applied a pressure of 30 atmospheres through a nozzle to effect the filtration. It was developed by Bechold who named it ultrafilter in 1907. *See artificial kidney.*

Ultralente Insulin   *See insulin.*

Ultramicroscope   [Latin: *ultra*, beyond; Greek: *mikros*, small + *skopein*, to view] Devised by Siedentopf and Richard Adolf Zsigmondy (1866–1930) around 1848. Their instrument projected light from a source on suspended particles in solution which were then viewed on a dark background through the microscope. It was improved by F.H. Wenham who added a dark-field condenser in 1850.

Ultrasonic Doppler   *See Doppler phenomenon.*

Ultrasonography   [Greek: *ultra*, beyond + *sono*, sound + *graphein*, to write] Ultrasound was first applied to marine work in the Sound Navigation and Ranging System (SONAR) during World War 1. Ian Donald, professor of obstetrics at Glasgow University, applied the principle to medicine by using it to examine a fetus *in utero* in 1961.

Ultzmann Test   Detects bile pigments in urine using potassium hydroxide as reagent. Devised by German urologist, Robert Ultzmann (1842–1889).

Umbilical Cord   [Latin: *umbilicus*, navel] The vessels of the umbilical cord which form valve-like projections were described in 1669 by Nicolas von Hobokoen (1632–1678), professor of anatomy at Harderwick. French surgeon, Raphael Bienvenu Sabatier (1732–1811) of Paris proposed that oxygenated blood from the placenta was brought by the umbilical vein, passed through the heart without mixing and supplied the head. Anatomical evidence to support this was provided by Caspar Friedrich Wolf (1733–1794) in the 18th century. The study of fetal physiology was advanced in 1927 by A. Huggett who showed that it was possible to deliver the fetus while it was attached to the mother through an intact umbilicus. The canal for the umbilical vein in the anterior wall of the umbilical canal was described in 1855 by Didier Dominique Alfred Richet (1816–1891), professor of clinical surgery at Paris.

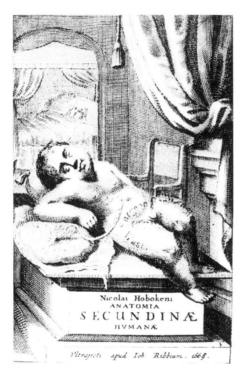

Frontispiece from Hobokoen's *Anatomia Secundinae Humanae* (1669)

Umbilical Hernia A description of a surgical procedure for treatment of umbilical hernia was given by Sir Astley Paston Cooper (1768–1841) in 1807. A radical operation was devised by William James Mayo (1865–1939) in 1901.

Umbilicus [Latin: *umbilicus*, navel] *See umbilical cord.*

Umckaloaba Herbal medicine from Africa used in the early 1900s as treatment for tuberculosis.

Unconscious As a state in psychiatry, was suggested by J. Moreau de Tours (1804–1884). It was used by Karl Gustav Carus (1789–1869) to refer to a conscious mental component from the past which later became unconscious to the person. Unconscious and subconscious states of the mind were investigated by Rudolph Hermann Lotze

(1817–1881) in 1852. Sigmund Freud (1856–1939) studied and demonstrated unconscious phenomena between 1895 and 1920 and developed psychoanalytic methods.

Underwood, Michael (1737–1820) London pediatrician who established modern pediatrics in England. He described a form of paralysis following a brief illness in children in 1793 which was probably the first scientific account of poliomyelitis. His *A Treatise on the Diseases of Children* also contained an account of congenital heart disease and was a standard work on pediatrics for 50 years.

Underwood Disease Scleroderma neonatorum was described by Michael Underwood (1737–1820) of London, a pioneer in pediatrics.

Undescended Testis *See orchidopexy, cryptorchism.*

Ungulant Fever *See brucellosis.*

Undulatory Theory of Light Proposed by Christian Huygens (1625–1695) in *Treatise in Light* published in 1690. His theory was supported by Robert Hooke, and Isaac Newton (1642–1727) proposed his corpuscular theory as an alternative. Huygen's theory was verified by a physician, Thomas Young, in 1802.

Unguentum Neapolitanum Ointment made from mercury and used in treatment of syphilis in Naples in the early 16th century.

Unipolar Leads *See electrocardiography.*

Universalists Sect who believed in the final salvation of all men, arose from the doctrine proposed in the Talmud by Origen in 230 AD. It was formed in Britain in 1760 by James Relly and in America by John Murray in 1770.

University The Alexandrian University, formed by Alexander the Great in 331 BC, attracted scholars from all over the world, such as Euclid the mathematician, Archimedes the physicist, Herophilos the anatomist, and Erasistratos the physiologist. It had four departments: literature, mathematics, astronomy and medicine, and its library was the largest in the world with over 400,000 volumes. Cambridge University is said to have been founded by King Sigebert of East Anglia in AD 630. Oxford University was mentioned by Pope Martin in 802. The three oldest Scottish universities are: St Andrew's University founded in 1411, University of Glasgow founded in 1451, and Aberdeen University founded in 1494. The University of Bologna in Italy began around AD 422 and is considered to be the oldest university in Europe. The dates of establishment of other important universities: Naples, Italy (1224); Toulouse,

France (1229); Cologne, Germany (1385); Louvain, Belgium (1426); Toledo, Spain (1499); Venice, Italy (1592); Montpellier, France (1289); Vienna, Austria (1365); Cracow, Poland (1364), Geneva, Switzerland (1368); Heidelberg, Germany (1386); Leipzig, Germany (1409); Florence, Italy (1439); Basel, Switzerland (1460); Uppsala, Sweden (1496); Strasburg, Germany (1538); Königsberg, Germany (1544); Leiden, Holland (1575); Edinburgh, Scotland (1582); Dublin, Ireland (1591); Dorpat, Germany (1632); Utrecht, Holland (1636); Halle, Germany (1694); Erlangen, Germany (1743); Berlin, Germany (1810); Bonn, Germany (1818); Zurich, Switzerland (1832); Munich, Germany (1826); and Bern, Switzerland (1834).

University College, London Founded by Lord Brougham, Thomas Campbell and others in 1826. The medical school opened in 1828 with Sir Charles Bell (1774–1842) as professor of surgery. The teaching hospital attached to the university was opened in 1834. It changed its name to University College London through a charter in 1836, and at the same time the University of London was established through another charter. Names of some of the famous medical men who taught at the University College include: John Elliotson (1791–1868), professor of medicine who described hay fever and asthma; Samuel Cooper (1780–1848) author of *A Dictionary of Surgery*; Sir Thomas Barlow (1845–1945) who described infantile scurvy; and Sir William Richard Gowers (1845–1915), who gave the name knee jerk to the tendon reflex of the knee and introduced the colorimetric method of estimation of hemoglobin. The college has a strong tradition in physiology including: Archibald Vivian Hill (1886–1977) who measured heat produced in a muscle; Albert Frank Stanley Kent (1863–1958) who described cardiac tissue at the atrioventricular junction; Ernest Henry Starling (1886–1927) who devised the heart–lung preparation and proposed the concept of hormones; Sir William Maddock Bayliss (1860–1924) who did classic experiments on physiology with Starling; Otto Loewi (1873–1961), German-born pharmacologist who found the neurotransmitter, acetylcholine; Sir Thomas Lewis (1881–1945), pioneer in the application of the electrocardiography; Sir Bernard Katz (b 1911) who elucidated the mechanism of release of acetylcholine by nerve impulses; Sir Edward Sharpey-Schafer (1850–1935) who demonstrated the effects of the extract of suprarenal gland; and Sydney Ringer (1835–1910) who introduced thermometry in clinical medicine. Other graduates include: Lord Joseph Lister (1827–1912), the founder of the antiseptic system of surgery; Henry Maudsley (1835–1918), psychiatrist who advocated the idea

that insanity is a disease of the body; and William Murrell (1853–1912) who introduced nitroglycerin as treatment of angina.

Unna Dermatosis Seborrhoeic eczema described by Paul Gerson Unna (1850–1929), a dermatologist from Hamburg, in 1887. He also introduced the use of icthyol, resorcin and zinc oxide paste into dermatology.

Unsaturated Fatty Acids *See essential fatty acids.*

Unverricht Disease A rare form of familial epilepsy known as myoclonus epilepsy, where clonic spasm of a group of muscles occurred in paroxysms. Described by German physician, Heinrich Unverricht (1853–1912) in 1891.

Unzer, Johan August (1727–1799) German physiologist who introduced the term reflex in 1771 to describe the sensory-motor reaction.

Ur Chaldean town in Mesopotamia founded in 4000 BC. Some of the oldest known clay tablets have been found in its remains.

Uranism Term for homosexuals in Europe, coined by Carl Heinrich Ulrich in 1850.

Uranium German chemist, Martin Heinrich Klaproth (1743–1817), purified uranium and named it in 1781. Its radioactivity was discovered by Antoine Henri Becquerel (1852–1908) in 1896. The isotope, uranium 235, was discovered by a Canadian, Arthur Jeffrey Demper (b 1896) in 1935. *See radium.*

Uranoplasty [Greek: *ouranos*, palate + *plassein*, to mold] Plastic surgery of the palate. *See plastic surgery.*

Urates [Greek: *ouron*, urine] *See uric acid.*

Urea Clearance Test Test for renal functions devised by a Paris physician Leo Ambard (b 1876), American physician Franklin Chambers McLean (b 1888) and San Francisco physician Thomas Addis (b 1881), and further refined by Eggert Hugo Möller, J. F. McIntosh and Donald Dexter Van Slyke (1883–1971) in 1928.

Urea Concentration Measure of function of the kidneys devised by Hugh Maclean (1879–1957) and Owen Lambart de Wesselow in 1920.

Urea [Greek: *ouron*, urine] End product of animal metabolism described by English physician William Cruikshank (1745–1800) in 1773, and its properties were investigated by William Prout (1785–1850) in 1815. Synthesis of urea from potassium cyanate and ammonium sulfate by German chemist, Friedrich Wohler (1800–1882) in 1829 signaled the beginnings of organic chemistry. He qualified in medicine from Heidelberg in 1823 and specialized in gynecology but never practiced. He became professor of chemistry at Göttingen in 1837.

Urease A crystalline form of the enzyme was prepared by American biochemist and Nobel Prize winner, James Batcheller Sumner (1887–1955) of Canton, Massachusetts in 1926. He was a graduate of Harvard and he became professor of biochemistry at Cornell University in 1929.

Uremia [Greek: *ouron*, urine + *haima*, blood] Intoxication due to poor kidney functioning was described by French physician, Pierre-Adolphe Piorry (1794–1879) of Poitiers in 1840. *See azotemia, prerenal uremia, urea.*

Uremic Pericarditis [Greek: *ouron*, urine + *peri*, round + *kardia*, heart + *itis*, inflammation] Occurs in cases of renal failure and was studied by Heinrich von Bamberger (1822–1888) of Vienna in 1857 and Ludwig von Buhl (1816–1880) of Stuttgart in 1878. More recent studies on the subject were done by Alvan Leroy Barach of New York in 1922.

Ureter [Greek: *oureter*] *See ureteric calculi, ureteric catheterization.*

Ureteric Calculi Demonstrated with the use of X-rays and an indwelling opaque catheter by Geza von Illyes (b 1870) of Budapest in 1901. Dilatation of ureteral orifice as treatment was performed by a Baltimore urologist, Howard Atwood Kelly (1858–1943) in 1900. Sign of maximal tenderness below the McBurney point on both sides was shown by Boston urologist, James Dellinger Barney (b 1878) in 1938. Lumbar ureterolithotomy as treatment was described by Frederic Eugene Basil Foley (b 1891) in 1935.

Ureteric Cancer A case of primary cancer of the ureter established by microscopic diagnosis was reported by Swedish physician, P. Johann Wising (1842–1912) in 1878.

Ureteric Catheterization Performed in a woman by Sir John Simon (1816–1904) around 1850 and under direct vision by Joseph Casimir Grynfeltt (1840–1909) in 1876. Catheterization of a male ureter was performed by James Brown (1854–1895) of Johns Hopkins Hospital in 1893.

Urethral Catheter Ancient version were made of silver and bronze tubes. Rhazes (850–932) an Arabian physician, devised bronze models with lateral holes to drain pus. He also used lead catheters whenever flexibility was needed. Flexible catheters made of woven silk covered with gum were devised by M. Bernard, a silversmith from Paris in the second half of the 18th century, and manufactured by Walsh of London. A double channeled urethral catheter was

designed by American surgeon, Nathan Bozemann (1825–1905).

Urethral Stricture Rhazes (850–932) from Persia, showed that hematuria was a symptom of bladder disease and he wrote at length on urethral stricture. French surgeon, Ambroise Paré (1510–1590) recognized their existence and called them 'carnosities'. He also devised two instruments introduced through the urethra to scrape off urethral granulations around the stricture. Urethrotomy, or internal longitudinal incision, was performed by American surgeon, Philip Syng Physick (1768–1837) of Philadelphia in 1795. English surgeon, Claudius Galen Wheelhouse (1826–1909) designed a form of external urethrotomy, where the stricture was identified with a probe before cutting the urethra in front of it. Open urethroplasty was introduced by Johanson in 1953. Physick's method was revived with modifications and performed under direct vision through a urethroscope by Sachse in 1971.

Urethrotomy *See urethral stricture.*

Uric Acid One of the first substances to be linked to organic disease was discovered in 1776 by Carl Wilhelm Scheele (1732–1786), a Swedish chemist. Accumulation of uric acid or urates in the blood of patients with renal disease was shown by Alfred Baring Garrod (1819–1909) using his 'thread test' in 1848. A colorimetric method of measuring uric acid in blood was devised by Otto Folin (1867–1934) and Willey G. Denis in 1912. The rise of uric acid in the blood which precedes the rise of urea in renal failure was noted by Victor Carlyl Myers (b 1883) in 1916.

Urinary Calculus Calculus in Greek means little stone or pebble. Hippocrates (460–377 BC) stated that stones in the kidney are formed from phlegm which has been converted to sand due to preternal heat in a bladder with a thick and turbid state of urine. He recognized that surgery was the only treatment for well formed stones. Lithotomy during his time was already established as a separate branch of surgery. Galen (AD 129–200) thought that the only certain remedy for stones was lithotomy but advocated lithotriptics such as pepper, galbanum, ammoniac, apronitrum, asarabaca and herbs in the early stages. Aetius of Amida (AD 527–165) recommended goat's blood as treatment. Hippocrates, Aetius and other ancient physicians observed that intake of milk predisposed to stone. Pierre Franco (1500–1561) of France was one of the best lithotomists of the 16th century who introduced a suprapubic approach, while Frere Jacques (1651–1714) performed over 5000 operations. William Cheselden (1688–1752), a famous lithotomist in England, was known for his precision and speed in such surgery. The variable composition of urinary stones was noted by William Hyde Wollaston (1766–1828), in 1797. A kidney stone was visualized using X-ray by John McIntyre (1857–1928) at Glasgow in 1896.

Urinary Cast Cylindrical structure of microscopic size observed in urine by Simon of Vienna and Hermann Nasse (1807–1892) in 1843. They were shown to arise from the kidneys, from postmortem by Gustav Jakob Henle (1809– 1885) of Germany in 1844.

Urinary Diversion An operation where the ureters were implanted into the rectum in ectropia vesicae. First performed by Sir John Simon (1816–1904) in 1852.

Urine Examination Cryoscopic analysis of urine was introduced by Hungarian physician, Alexander von Sandor Korànyi (b 1866) in 1895. Chicago surgeon, Malcolm LaSalle Harris (1862–1936) described a method for obtaining urine samples separately from each kidney in 1898. A method of estimating specific gravity of small amounts of urine was described by New York physician, George Alexander de Santos (1876–1911) in 1903. A quantitative method of estimating urinary sediments was devised by San Francisco physician, Henry Gibbons (b 1906) in 1934. *See albuminuria, bacteriuria, glycosuria.*

Urine Osmolarity *See osmolarity.*

Urine [Greek: *ouron*, urine] The urine of diabetics was noted to attract insects due to its sugar content by ancient Brahmins who called it honey urine. Hippocrates (460–377 BC) noticed the 'white clouds' in urine which are now known to be albumin. Uroscopy, a chart containing various colors and conditions of urine in disease with written advice for physicians for each finding, was used during the Middle Ages. Urine of humans and animals has been used as medicine since ancient times. It was taken after childbirth for constipation. The Arabian physician Haly Abbas (930–994) advised a draught containing lentils, fennel and the urine of a boy not come to puberty as treatment for jaundice. Greeks differentiated between the urine of prepuberty and adolescence and this has been proved with the isolation of sex hormones which are now in use in treatment of various hormone-sensitive cancers such as those of the prostate and breast.

Urodynamics A study of the mechanics and pattern of urine flow was done by the Italian physiologists, Angelo Mosso (1846–1910) and Pellcani in 1881. They devised a manometer capable of recording the intravesical pressure at rest and during micturition. A clinical cystometer for measuring the intravesical pressure was devised by

Harry Rose (1906–1986) in 1927. A catheter, manometer and a moving strip of bromide paper to measure and record bladder and sphincter behavior was designed by Derek Ernest Denny-Brown (1901–1981) and Robertson in 1933. Stewart developed this into a cystometer in 1942.

Urogenital Surgery *See urology.*

Urokinase [Greek: *ouron*, urine + *kinein*, to move] *See thrombolysis.*

Urology [Greek: *ouron*, urine + *logos*, discourse] Lithotomists were the earliest surgeons and were well established during Hippocratic times. Ammonius (283–247 BC), a surgeon of Alexandria, described the method of extraction of stone. Rhazes (850–932), an Arab physician, devised bronze and lead catheters with lateral holes to drain the pus. Urological surgery was established as a specialty around 1790 by Pierre Joseph Desault (1744–1795) and François Chopart (1743–1795) of Paris. Leopold Ritter von Dittel (1815–1898), professor of surgery at Vienna, specialized in urology, and described enucleation of the enlarged lateral lobes of the prostate through an external incision in 1860. Joaquín Dominguez Albarrán (1860–1912), Cuban-born French professor of medicine, wrote on surgery of urinary passages in 1909. An electrically-lit cystoscope was invented by Max Nitz (1848–1906) of Berlin in 1877, and use of anesthetic in urology (cocaine) was introduced by Fessenden Nott Otis (1825–1900) in 1884. Jean Casimir Felix Guyon (1831–1920), professor at Paris, published his lectures on urology in 1881 and a treatise on the surgical diseases of the bladder and prostate in 1888. James Brown (1854–1895) of Johns Hopkins Hospital catheterized male ureters in 1893. A double channeled urethral catheter, Bozemann catheter, was designed by American surgeon, Nathan Bozemann (1825–1905).

Urquhart, Patrick (1642–1725) Aberdeen clinical teacher and successful medical practitioner who also practiced embalming.

Urso of Calbaria Physician who lived in the 13th century and wrote several treatises including *De Effectibus Qualitatum* and *De Effectibus Medicinae.*

Urticaria [Latin: *urtica*, nettle] *See angioneurotic edema.*

Urticaria Pigmentosa [Latin: *urtica*, nettle] Nettleship disease, chronic urticaria leaving brown stains on the skin. Described by London ophthalmologist, Edward Nettleship (1845–1913) in 1869.

Uterine Cancer *See carcinoma of cervix.*

Uterine Fibroid *See fibroid.*

Uterine Inversion *See inversion of the uterus.*

Uterine Prolapse [Latin: *pro*, in front + *laps*, to slip] An early method of surgical treatment was devised in 1919 by an American obstetrician and gynecologist, Alfred Baker Spalding (1874–1942). He was educated at Columbia University and became professor of obstetrics at Stanford University in 1912. The Manchester operation, where high amputation of the cervix is done with repair of the anterior and posterior vaginal walls, was devised by Archibald Donald (1860–1937) and William Edward Fothergill (1865–1926) of Manchester in 1890 and modified by Fothergill in 1915. The Gilliam operation of ventrosuspension was devised in 1900 by David Todd Gilliam (1844–1923) of America.

Uterine Sound Instrument for exploration, dilatation and measurement of the cavity of the uterus. Invented by James Marion Sims (1813–1883) a gynecologist from South Carolina.

Uterosacral Ligaments [Latin: *uterus*, womb + *sacrum*, sacred + *ligamentum*, band] Posterior round ligaments of the uterus, described by Antoine Petit, professor of anatomy at Paris in 1760. The posterior aponeurosis of the broad ligament was described in 1897 by French gynecologist, Paul Petit.

Uterus Named after the Roman goddess, Uterina, who guarded the womb. The Ebers Papyrus refers to it as an independent animal within the body. Aristotle considered it to be the most important organ in the body. Mondino de Luzzi (1276–1328), professor of anatomy at Bologna, described it in 1315. An accurate anatomical description was given by Bartholomew Eustachio (1520–1574), professor at Rome in 1552. An accurate description of the innervation was given by Scottish gynecologist, Robert Lee (1793–1877) in 1841.

Uvea The choroid, iris and ciliary body were together called 'chiton rhagoides' by Galen (AD 129–200) because of their resemblance to a grape with the stalk torn off. The present term is derived from the Greek word 'uva', a grape.

Uveoparotid Fever Heerfordt syndrome, a form of sarcoidosis involving the parotid glands, was described by Christian Frederik Heerfordt (1872–1953) in 1909.

Uvula [Greek: little grape] Term used by Aulus Cornelius Celsus (25 BC–AD 50) to denote the structure. The present term for the distal fleshy part of the soft palate came into use in 1695.

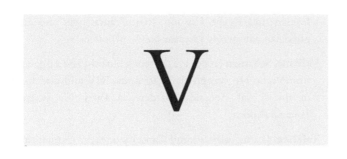

Vaccination in America   Boston physician, Zabdiel Boylston (1680–1766), inoculated his son in 1721 with the material taken from the pustule of a person with smallpox. Benjamin Colman (1673–1747) of Boston wrote a book on smallpox vaccination in the same year. Other American treatises include those of Coleman (1722), Increase Mather (1721), Benjamin Franklin (1706–1790) in 1759 and Benjamin Rush (1745–1813) in 1781. Benjamin Waterhouse (1754–1846), professor of medicine at Harvard, inoculated his four children in 1800 with a smallpox obtained from a physician named Haygarth of Bath, England. The Vaccine Institute was established at Baltimore by James Smith in 1802.

Vaccination   [Latin: *vacca*, cow] Term coined by Louis Pasteur (1822–1895) in 1881. The Royal Jennerian Institution was founded in 1803 and vaccination was made compulsory in England in 1853, in Ireland and Scotland in 1863. *Papers on the History and Practice of Vaccination* was edited by John Simon and was published by the Board of Health in 1853. *See inoculation, immunology.*

Vaccine Therapy   Following the introduction of fever therapy for syphilis and other diseases by Austrian psychiatrist, Julius Wagner-Jauregg (1857–1940) in 1877, several vaccines, such as tuberculin, typhoid and rabies, were introduced as shock therapy for syphilis in the early 1900s.

Vaccine   [Latin: *vacca*, cow] *See typhoid vaccine, antirabies vaccine, BCG, cholera vaccine, measles vaccine, pneumococcal vaccine, polio vaccine, smallpox, inoculation.*

Vacuum   [Latin: *vacuus*, empty] Aristotle studied it and conclude that it did not exist. Torricelli (1608–1644), Galileo's assistant, was the first to create a vacuum around 1644. A practical way of producing a vacuum became possible with the invention of the air pump by Otto van Guericke (1602–1686), the mayor of Magdeburg in Prussia, in 1656. His device was developed by Robert Boyle (1627–1691) for his experiment on gases.

Vagabond Disease   Discoloration and excoriation of the skin caused by scratching secondary to human pediculosis.

Described by Edward Headlam Greenhow (1814–1888) of London in 1876.

Vagabond   *See vagrant.*

Vagadasastir   Ancient Hindu book which deals with demonology and medicine. It describes the human body as having 100,000 parts and 17,000 vessels.

Vagal Syncope   *See carotid sinus syndrome.*

Vaghbata   Hindu Brahmin physician who lived in the seventh century.

Vagina   [Latin: *vagina*, a scabbard or sheath] The term was coined by Gabrielle Falloppio (1523–1562), a pupil of Andreas Vesalius (1514–1564). He also described the tubes of the ovaries which are named after him.

Vaginal Agenesis   Two cases of congenital absence of vagina treated by plastic surgery were reported by American gynecologist, Carl Henry Davis (b 1883) of Milwaukee in 1928.

Vaginal Contraceptive Devices   Vaginal pessaries made of pomegranate seed were mentioned as contraceptives by Aetius of Amida (AD 527–165). Various other forms of vaginal caps and diaphragms were used in the 19th century. The douche and vaginal sponge were advocated as contraceptives by a physician, George Drysdale, in his treatise on sex education, *Elements of Social Science*, published in 1854. *See birth control, contraceptive devices.*

Vaginal Hysterectomy   [Latin: *vagina*, sheath; Greek: *hystera*, womb + *ektome*, to cut out] Performed in 1507 by Italian surgeon, Jacopo Berengario da Carpi (1470–1530) of Pavia. A successful operation was performed by Sauter in 1822, and the modern surgical method of removing the uterus for cancer through the vagina, was introduced in 1878 by Vincenz Czerny (1842–1916), Czech professor of surgery at Heidelberg. His procedure was further developed by Christian Albert Theodor Billroth (1829–1894), German professor of surgery in Austria, and Polish surgeon, Johann von Mikulicz-Radecki (1850–1905). Radical vaginal hysterectomy for uterine carcinoma was introduced by Friedrich Schauta (1849–1919) in 1902.

Vaginal Speculum   Use of the speculum to visualize internal organs such as the rectum, vagina and ear, was known in the time of Hippocrates (460–377 BC) and Soranus of Ephesus (AD 98–138), an early gynecologist, used it. James Marion Sims (1813–1883) of South Carolina used a bent spoon to visualize a vesical fistula in 1845. His device was later developed into Sims duck-billed speculum. Another was designed around the same time by Joseph Claude Anthelme Recamier (1774–1852) of Paris. Sir William Fergusson (1808–1877), a Scottish surgeon and a pupil of Robert Knox (1791–1862), devised several surgical instruments, including a vaginal speculum around 1860.

Vaginismus Condition of painful spasm of the vaginal muscles during sexual intercourse described by James Marion Sims (1813–1883) in 1861. He recommended removal of the hymen, incision and subsequent dilation of vaginal orifice as treatment.

Vagrant [Latin: *vagari*, to wander] In the Middle Ages they were marked with the letter V. In 1530 they were whipped and returned to the place where they were born or last lived for over three years.

Vagus [Latin: *vagor*, wandering] The nerve derives its name from the observation that it supplied an array of organs. Thomas Willis (1621–1675) described a branch of the vagus supplying the aorta as a wandering nerve, in 1664. Inhibition of the heart by stimulating the vagus nerve was demonstrated by Alfred Wilhelm Volkmann (1800–1877) of Dorpat in 1838, and redescribed by Eduard Friedrich Weber and Ernest Heinrich Weber (1795–1878) in 1845. Volkmann experimentally induced bronchospasm by stimulation in 1844. Other inhibitory nerves in the autonomic nervous system were discovered by German physiologist, Edward Friedrich Wilhelm Pflüger (1829–1910) in 1864. In 1869 Friedrich Leopold Goltz (1834–1902) experimented on decerebrated frogs and showed that their heart could be stopped by tapping the stomach. Experimental research on the action of vagus and cervical sympathetic nerves on the heart, respiration, stomach, ear, and pupils was done by Auguste Desire Waller (1856–1922) in 1861. The neurogenic reflex arising in the lung which controls the rate and depth of respiration via the vagus nerve was described by Josef Breuer (1842–1925) and Karl Hering (1834–1918) in 1868. German-born Nobel Prize winner, pharmacologist and physiologist, Otto Loewi (1873–1961) of Strasburg, demonstrated in 1921 that a substance liberated from the stimulated vagus nerve ending, when perfused on to a second heart, was capable of slowing the rate of heart beat. This substance was the first neurotransmitter to be isolated and it was later identified as acetylcholine. The suggestion that secretions of the pancreas depended on a reflex between duodenal mucosa and vagus was made by Russian Nobel Prize winner, Ivan Petrovich Pavlov (1849–1936) in 1910.

Vaillant, John Foy (1632–1706) French physician and historian from Beauvais who published history on Rome,

Caesars and Egypt. His son, John Francis, was also an physician who wrote a treatise on use of coffee.

Vaillant, Sebastian (1669–1722) French botanist and surgeon from Vigny. He was physician to Louis XIV and director of the Royal Botanical Gardens at Paris. He wrote *Botanica Pariense*.

Valence [Latin: *valere*, strong] Capacity of every element to combine with other elements was proposed by an organic chemist, Sir Edward Frankland (1825–1899) of Churchtown, Lancashire in 1852. He was a pupil of Baron Playfair (1819–1898) in London, Robert Wilhelm Bunsen (1811–1899) in Marburg and Justus von Liebig (1803–1873) in Giessen. He was professor of chemistry at Owen's College, Manchester and later became lecturer at St Bartholomew's Hospital, London in 1857. Further research was done by American physical chemist, Gilbert Newton Lewis (1875–1946) of Weymouth, Massachusetts. He was educated at Harvard and worked with Wilhelm Ostwald (1853–1932) at Leipzig and Walther Hermann Nernst (1864–1941) at Göttingen, before his appointment at the University of California, Berkeley. He wrote *Valence and the Structure of Atoms and Molecules* in 1923.

Valentin Cords Linear arrangement of female sex cells in the developing ovary described by a pupil of Johannes Evangelista Purkinje (1787–1869) and comparative anatomist, Gabriel Gustav Valentin (1810–1883) in 1838. Valentin was professor of physiology at Bern for 45 years.

Valentin Ganglion On the superior dental nerve. Described by a professor of physiology at Bern, Gabriel Gustav Valentin (1810–1883) in 1839.

Valentine, Basil Pseudonym for a German Benedictine monk who wrote on alchemy in the 17th century, including *Currus Triumphalis Antimonii* (1671), and other treatises. He obtained alcohol completely free of water.

Valentine, Michael Bernard (1657–1929) Professor of medicine at Giessen who published several works including *Cynosura materiae Medicae* and *Medicina Nova-Antiqua*.

Valentine Position Patient supine at the edge of the table with legs hanging down, used for irrigating the urethra. Described by New York surgeon, Ferdinand C. Valentine (1851–1909).

Valerius Cordus *See Cordus Valerius.*

Valine Amino acid isolated by Gorup-Besanez from extract of pancreas in 1856. It was isolated from the hydrolysate of casein by Fischer in 1901.

Valium *See benzodiazepine.*

Valla, George (d 1460) Italian physician and professor at Venice who wrote *De Expetendis et Fugiendis rebus* in two volumes.

Valleix Points Tender points in a nerve causing neuralgia. Described by French physician, François Louis Valleix (1807–1855).

Valli, Eusebius (1762–1816) Italian physician from Pistroia who was well known for his self experimentation on disease. He tried the efficacy of plague vaccine on himself and survived, but succumbed to yellow fever in Havana.

Vallisnieri, Antonio (1661–1730) Tuscan naturalist and professor of medicine at Padua. He studied the reproductive system of insects and wrote treatises on the ostrich (1712) and chameleon in 1715.

Valsalva, Antonio Maria (1666–1723) He succeeded Marcello Malpighi (1628–1694) as professor of anatomy at Bologna. Several anatomical structures including, the aortic sinuses, anterior ligament of the auricle and the muscle of tragus, are named after him.

Valsalva Maneuvre Inflation of the eustachian tube by closing the nose and the mouth during forcible expiration. Described by a professor of anatomy at Bologna, Antonio Maria Valsalva (1666–1723).

Valverda, John de Spanish physician in the 16th century who accompanied the cardinal of Toledo to Rome. He wrote a treatise on anatomy which was published in Venice in 1589.

Valves [Latin: *valvae*, fold] Described as outgrowths of the veins by Jacques du Bois (1473–1555) in 1555. Their function in maintaining a unidirectional flow of blood in veins was observed by Fabricius (1533–1619), a teacher of William Harvey (1578–1657). *See artificial valves, mitral valves, tricuspid valves.*

Valvotomy [Latin: *valva*, fold; Greek: *tome*, cutting] Sir Lauder Brunton (1844–1916) proposed the idea of splitting open the commisures of the mitral valve to relieve symptoms of severe mitral stenosis in 1902. A valvotomy for stenosis was done on the pulmonary valve by E. Doyen (1859–1916) in 1913 but was unsuccessful. Elliot Carr Cutler (1888–1947) of Western Reserve University of Cleveland, Ohio performed one for a severe mitral stenosis through the transventricular approach in 1923. Cutler and Samuel Levine's (1891–1966) work 'Cardiotomy and Valvulotomy for Mitral Stenosis' was published in the *Boston Medical and Surgical Journal* in 1923. Sir Henry Sessions Souttar (1875–1964) pioneered a procedure by introducing his fingers through the left atrium and splitting the mitral commisures in a case of mitral stenosis in 1925. Valvotomy through the right ventricle in a case of pulmonary stenosis was performed by Russell Claude Brock (b 1903) of Guy's Hospital in 1948.

Valvular Heart Disease *See rheumatic fever, aortic stenosis, mitral stenosis, valvotomy, subacute bacterial endocarditis.*

Vanadium Element discovered in 1801 by Spanish mineralogist, Andrés Manuel Del Rio (1764–1849) of Madrid. Swedish physician and chemist, Nils Gabriel Sefström (1765–1829) in 1830 named it after the Scandinavian goddess, Freya Vanadin. It was isolated in Cheshire mines by English chemist, Sir Henry Enfield Roscoe (1833–1915) in 1865. It is used to make a steel alloy. Its anhydride was shown to be a strong respiratory irritant by F. Molfino in 1938. Vanadium poisoning due to its toxic dust was described by H. Synmanski in 1939.

Van Buren Disease Hardening of corpora cavernosa, described by American surgeon, William Holme Van Buren (1819–1883).

Vandale, Anthony (1638–1708) Dutch trader who studied medicine and became professor at Harlem. He published on a variety of subjects outside medicine.

Van Deen Test Test for blood in gastric juice, using guaiac acid and glacial acetic acid as reagents. Devised by a Dutch physician, Izaak Van Deen (1804–1869).

Van Den Bergh Test Detects unconjugated bilirubin using diazo reagent. Described in 1900 by Dutch physician, A.A. Hymans Van Den Bergh (1869–1943).

Vander-Monde, Charles Augustine (1727–1762) Physician born in Macao to European parents. He practiced in Paris and wrote a dictionary on health, a treatise on surgery and on methods of perfecting the human species.

Van Der Waals Equation Defines the physical state of gas and liquid. Proposed by Dutch professor of physics at Amsterdam, Johannes Diderik Van Der Waals (1837–1923) in 1873. He also proposed the concept of weak attraction between molecules (Van Der Waals force) and was awarded the Nobel Prize for Physics in 1910.

Van Der Waals, Johannes (1837–1923) Dutch physicist who graduated from Leiden in 1865 and did extensive studies on the nature of gases. He proposed his equation on temperature, volume, and pressure relationship of gases in 1873. His

The Continuity of the Liquid and Gaseous States was published in the same year and he was made professor of physics at Amsterdam University in 1877.

Vane, Sir John Robert (b 1927) English biochemist and co-winner of the Nobel Prize for Physiology or Medicine in 1982. He studied pharmacology at Birmingham and St Catherine's College Oxford, and taught at Yale (1953–1955) and London. He studied adrenergic receptors of the nervous system and the role of the lung in drug uptake and metabolism. He described the inhibition of prostaglandin synthesis by aspirin and similar drugs with his co-workers in 1970. He also discovered prostacyclin, the short-lived antagonist of platelet aggregation which is crucial for the control of thrombus formation.

Van Gehuchten Method Fixing method for histologic tissue in a mixture of glacial acetic acid and chloroform. Devised by Belgian anatomist, Arthur Van Gehuchten (1861–1914).

Van Gieson Stain Histological staining method for tissues, using alum-hemotoxylin. Devised by neuropathologist, Ira Van Gieson (1865–1913) of New York.

Vanquelin, Louis Nicholas (1763–1829) French analytical chemist and professor of chemistry at Paris. He isolated the amino acid asparagine from asparagus in 1806. The elements chromium and beryllium are two of his other discoveries.

Van Slyke, Donald Dexter (1883–1971) American biochemist at the Rockefeller Institute and pioneer in the study of the acid–base balance. He devised an early apparatus for analysis of blood gases in 1924. He also proposed a minimal pH level of 6.95 below which coma occurs. He demonstrated in 1934 that urea clearance paralleled blood flow though the kidneys, which later formed the basis for the urea clearance test for kidney function.

Van Swieten, Gerard (1700–1772) Pupil of Herman Boerhaave (1668–1738) at Leiden who founded the Vienna School of Medicine and prevailed on the government to rebuild Vienna University. He wrote *Commentary on the Aphorisms of Boerhaave.*

Van't Hoff, Jacobus Henricus (1852–1911) Eminent chemist, born in Rotterdam and graduated from Utrecht in 1874. He was professor of chemistry at Amsterdam in 1878 and moved to Berlin in 1896. He is considered the founder of stereochemistry and physical chemistry and proposed the tetrahedral structure of carbon in 1874. He also pointed out that solutions and gases behaved similarly and proposed the dissociation theory related to electrolytes in solution in 1877.

Vaquez–Osler Disease *See polycythemia vera.*

Varenius, or Bernhard Varen (1622–1650) Dutch physician and geographer who wrote *Geographia Generalis,* a standard work in geography for more than a century. It was improved and enlarged by Isaac Newton in 1672.

Varicella [Latin: variegated or spotted] Chicken pox was differentiated from scarlet fever by Giovanni Filippo Ingrassia (1510–1580) of Italy in 1553. A gangrenous form was described by Sir Jonathan Hutchinson (1828–1913) in 1882. Occurrence through contact with *Herpes zoster* was observed by J. von Bokay of Germany in 1892. The presence of inclusion bodies in skin lesions of varicella were observed by Ernest Edward Tyzzer (1875–1965) in 1905.

Varices [Latin: enlarged] Hippocrates (460–377 BC) recommended puncture of a vein in the leg as treatment. Paul of Aegina (625–690) ligated the affected veins and Aetius of Amida (AD 527–165) and Albucasis (936–1013) described operations. *See esophageal varices, varicose veins.*

Varicocele [Latin: *varix,* dilation; Greek: *kele,* tumor] A method of subcutaneous ligation of veins for varicocele was devised by French surgeon, Auguste Theodore Vidal de Cassis (1803–1856). Another operative method for radical cure was described by H. Lee in *The Lancet* in 1861. George Heaton (1808–1879), a Boston surgeon, described a surgical cure in 1877. English surgeon, Sir William Henry Bennett (1852–1931) published a monograph in 1891.

Varicose Vein [Latin: *varix,* dilation] Surgical treatment was described by Aulus Cornelius Celsus (25 BC–AD 50). Ligation of veins as treatment was described by Aetius of Amida (AD 527–165), physician to Emperor Justinian. Ambroise Paré (1510–1590), the legendary French surgeon, considered that varicosity was associated with conditions such as melancholia and disturbance of menstruation and he revived ligation of the veins below the knee as treatment. John Hunter (1728–1793) in 1786 and Sir Everard Home (1756–1832) in 1803 practiced ligation of veins above the knee. Injection of sclerosing agents was introduced by Charles Gabriel Pravaz (1791–1853) in 1851 and Paul Linser (b 1871) of Tübingen used mercurial chloride in 1911.

Varmus, Harold Elliot (b 1939 American molecular biologist, born in New York and educated at Amherst College, Virginia, Harvard University and Columbia University. He was appointed professor of microbiology and immunology at the University of California Medical Center in 1979. He received the Nobel Prize for Physiology or Medicine in 1989 (together with Michael Bishop, b 1936) for his discovery of oncogenes, which have been of vital importance in understanding the mechanisms of cancer. *See oncogenes.*

Varolio, Constanzo, or Varolius (1543–1575) Italian professor of anatomy at Bologna and Rome. He described the fluid in the brain and the pons (pons varoli) in 1573.

Vas Deferens Chicago surgeon, William Thomas Belfield (1856–1929) performed vasotomy as a therapeutic procedure in 1884. Ligation of it was experimentally performed for impotence by Eugen Steinach (1861–1944) in 1920. Excision of whole or part of the vas deferens (vasectomy) was commenced to induce male sterility in the 1930s.

Vascular Surgery [Latin: *vas*, vessel] *See aortic aneurysm, cardiac surgery, cardiac transplant, embolectomy, coronary artery bypass graft, valvotomy.*

Vascular System [Latin: *vas*, vessel] *See blood circulation, capillary circulation, heart, cardiology, veins, arteries.*

Vasectomy *See vas deferens.*

Vasovesiculography Used to visualize the male reproductive organs on X-ray. Devised by Chicago surgeon, William Thomas Belfield (1856–1929) in 1905. He also described vasotomy in 1884.

Vasoconstriction [Latin: *vas*, vessel + *constringere*, to draw tight] A study of nervous control of the circulatory system was performed by Claude Bernard (1813–1878) around 1843. He was convinced that contraction of the arteries was under nervous influence. In 1851 he cut the sympathetic nerve on one side in a rabbit and observed dilation of blood vessels on the same side. This led to discovery of the vasomotor nerves in 1858. Charles Brown-Séquard (1817–1894) performed a similar experiment and demonstrated vasoconstriction of blood vessels by stimulating the cut peripheral sympathetic trunk in 1852.

Vasodilation [Latin: *vas*, vessel + *dilatus*, separate] Claude Bernard (1813–1878) extended his studies on nervous control of blood vessels in 1858 and discovered the vasodilator fibers in the chorda tympani. By stimulating this nerve he demonstrated an increase in blood flow to the area. *See vasoconstriction.*

Vasomotor Nerves [Latin: *vas*, vessel + *movere*, to move] *See vasoconstriction.*

Vasomotor Reflex [Latin: *vas*, vessel + *movere*, to move] Discovered by Russian physiologist, Elie de Cyon (1842–1912) and German physiologist, Carl Friedrich Wilhelm Ludwig (1816–1895) in 1866.

Vasomotor Rhinitis or hay fever (Syn: Bostock catarrh, catarrhus aestivus, allergic rhinitis, vasomotor rhinitis) Described by John Bostock (1773–1846) of Guy's Hospital in 1817. *See pollen, hay fever.*

Vasopressin *See antidiuretic hormone.*

Vater, Abraham (1684–1751) Professor of botany, anatomy, pathology and therapeutics at Wittenberg. In 1720 he described the duodenal papillae and the ampulla of the bile duct which are named after him. He also described the pacinian corpuscles.

Vatican Founded on the Mons Vaticanus hill of Rome. Its palace containing 7000 rooms was built by Liberius, and its library containing valuable books and manuscripts was founded by Pope Nicholas V in 1448.

Vattier, Pierre (1623–1667) French physician from Orleans who wrote historical works on Muslims and a medical work, *Avicennae de morbis mentis*, in 1659.

Vaughan, William English medical writer who lived during the latter half of the 16th century. He wrote *Directions for Health*, with an apology for not being a physician in 1608.

Vectius, Vallens Roman physician and follower of Themison (*c* 100 BC). He improved the Methodist system of medicine proposed by Themison.

Vector [Latin: *vehere*, to carry] The culex mosquito was identified as the vector in filaria by Sir Patrick Manson (1844–1922) and Sir Joseph Bancroft (1836–1894) in 1878. A tick was shown to be a vector in Texas cattle fever in 1893 by Theobald Smith (1859–1934), a professor of microbiology at Harvard University. *Xenopsylla cheopsis*, a genus of flea, was shown to be a vector of plague by Masanori Ogata (1852–1919) in 1897. Italian physician, Amico Bignami (1862–1929), while working with Ettore Marchiafava (1847–1935), identified the role of the *Anopheles* mosquito as a vector in transmission of malaria. The mosquito, *Aedes aegypti*, was shown to be a vector in transmission of dengue fever by Thomas Lane Bancroft (1860–1933) in 1906.

Vectorcardiography [Latin: *vehere*, to carry; Greek: *kardia*, heart + *graphein*, to write] The concept of representing the electrical forces of the heart by recording the vector forces from the surface of the body was proposed by Willem Einthoven (1860–1927) and G. Fahr in 1913. The vector loop cardiogram was developed by Hubert Mann (1895–1975) while a medical student in 1920. The vectorcardiogram was introduced into clinical medicine by Fritz Schellong of Germany in 1939. The term vectorcardiogram was suggested by Frank Norman Wilson (1890–1952) and F.D. Johnston in 1938.

Veda Ancient Brahmin (Sanskrit) term for learning or

knowledge. The Vedas, or the sacred book of the Hindus, was written in Sanskrit around 1000 BC. *See rigveda, ayurveda.*

Veddahs Sri Lankan, pre-Dravidian tribe who have features common to Australian aborigines, suggesting a common ancestral origin since the Stone Age. An early account is given in Knox's *An Historical Relation of Ceylon* published in 1681. Further ethnic studies were done by J. Bailey in 1863 and later by Davy and Sir James Emerson Tennant. They were considered to be barbarians on the basis of their personal hygiene, had no names and did not bury the dead. Studies done by Fritz and Paul Sarasin revealed quartz implements comparable to those of the Paleolithic age, and their findings were described in *polia Zeyandica* (1919). *The veddas (Ceylon)* was published by English anthropologist and physician from London, Charles Gabriel Seligman (1873–1940) in 1911.

Vegetarian Diet Porphyry of Tyre (AD 233–304), a disciple of Plotinius (203–270), protested violently against use of meat as food in *Concerning Abstinence from Animal Food.* The book is addressed to Firmus Castricius who was a vegetarian, and it suggested that murderers and tyrants were flesh eaters. The Vegetarian Society in England was founded in London in 1847.

Vein [Latin: *vena*, vein] The Greek physician Erasistratus dissected human bodies around 300 BC and postulated that arteries contained air or 'breath of life' and veins carried nutrients. He believed that the valves of the heart directed blood towards veins. Fabricius (1533–1619) in 1608 noted that valves in veins opened towards the heart, but he offered no explanation. In 1628 William Harvey (1578–1657) observed that these valves prevented venous reflux and John Hunter (1728–1793) in 1785 noted that veins accommodate the excess blood when arteries contracted.

Vella Fistula Artificial fistula created by dividing the intestine in two places and fixing both pieces to the abdominal wall. Described by Italian physiologist, Luigi Vella (1825–1886).

Velpeau, Alfred Armand Louis Marie (1795–1867) Professor of clinical surgery at the Paris Faculty. Several anatomical structures have been named after him including: the inguinal canal, ischiorectal fossa, and tela subserosa around the kidney. He wrote a comprehensive surgical treatise and attempted operative treatment of aneurysm.

Vena Cava [Latin: *vena*, vein + *cavus*, hollow] Described in 1850 by John Marshall (1818–1891), professor of surgery at University College London. A precise description of the

thoracic portion of the inferior vena cava was given in 1862 by Hubert von Luschka (1820–1875), professor of anatomy at Tübingen.

Venel, Jean Andre (1740–1791) *See orthopedics.*

Venereal Disease Act 1917 Prohibits unqualified persons from treating sexually contacted diseases in England.

Venereal Disease Morbus venereus was used to denote syphilis and gonorrhea by French physician, Jacques de Berthencourt of Rouen in 1527. The Ebers Papyrus contains a description which suggests that gonorrhea existed around 2500 BC. Aulus Cornelius Celsus (25 BC–AD 50) and Galen (AD 129–200) also described gonorrhea. Syphilis was only described in the 15th century and two theories exist, one proposing that it was endemic in Europe, and the other that it was brought from America after the discovery of the New World. French physician, Jean François Fernel (1497–1558) suggested that gonorrhea and syphilis were two distinct diseases, whereas John Hunter (1728–1793) believed them to be the same and tried to prove it by inoculating himself. Unknown to him, the inoculum contained both gonorrhea and syphilis and he contacted syphilis and falsely confirmed his original belief. Hunter published *A Treatise on Venereal Diseases* in 1786. The difference between syphilis and gonorrhea based on the response to mercurial treatment was shown by Benjamin Bell (1749–1806) of Dumfries, a pupil of Hunter, in 1793. The two diseases were shown to be definitely different by Phillipe Ricord (1799–1889) of Paris in 1838. Condylomata acuminata, or genital warts, have been known for 2000 years. Condylomata lata, or syphilitic warts, were differentiated from genital warts by Gabrielle Falloppio (1523–1562). *See Contagious Diseases Act, genitourinary medicine, syphilis, herpes genitalis.*

Venesection [Latin: *vena*, vein + *sectio*, cutting] Established as a remedy during the time of Hippocrates (460–377 BC). It continued to be practiced for over 2000 years until questioned in the 19th century. In England much of the battle against venesection was fought at Edinburgh, and Hughes John Bennett (1812–1875) produced scientific evidence against it in 1856. *See bloodletting.*

Venidad [Persian: law against devils] Volume in the Persian philosophy *Zendevesta.* It describes three groups: doctors, surgeons, herbalists and magicians, and deals with demonic aspects of disease. *See Persian medicine.*

Venner, Tobias (1577–1660) English physician from Petherton in Somerset, and educated at Oxford. He practiced at

Bridgewater and later at Bath. He wrote *Vis recta ad Vitum longam* and a treatise on Bath waters.

Venom [Latin: *venenum*, poison] *See ophidism.*

Venous Pulsation Tracings of the jugular vein were recorded by French cardiologist, Pierre Carl Eduard Potain (1825–1901) in 1867 and in 1892 by Sir James Mackenzie (1853–1925) with his ink polygraph.

Venous Thrombosis *See deep vein thrombosis.*

Ventilator Stephen Hales (1677–1761) described his invention to the Royal Society in 1741. Neil Arnott (1788–1874) an English inventor and physician wrote a treatise on them in 1838, and a commission on ventilation and warming was appointed to prepare a report in England in 1859. *See artificial respiration.*

Ventricle [Latin: *ventriculus*, small cavity] The Roman physician Galen (AD 129–200) proposed that blood from the left ventricle reached the right side of the heart via pores in the interventricular septum. His teaching was accepted for over a thousand years until William Harvey (1578–1657) announced his discovery of the circulatory system in 1628. He calculated the volume of blood ejected from the left ventricle into the aorta by estimating the change in size.

Ventricular Aneurysm Result of myocardial infarction. Treated surgically by Denton Cooley and co-workers in 1959.

Ventricular Fibrillation An account of death due to ventricular fibrillation was given by Alexander John MacWilliam (1857–1937), a professor at the University of Aberdeen in 1889. Swiss physicians Jean Louis Prévost (1838–1927) and L. Batelli induced ventricular fibrillation in a dog's heart in 1899 by applying a small current and terminated the arrhythmia by giving a larger dose of the current. These studies were followed by W. B. Kouwenhouven, D.R. Hooker and O. R. Langworthy in 1932. Induction of sinus rhythm by countershock was demonstrated by the same workers in 1933. Countershock to a fibrillating human heart leading to recovery was performed in 1945 by Claude Schaeffer Beck (1894–1971) and colleagues of America. Paul Maurice Zoll (b 1911) and co-workers terminated it in four patients in 1956 by applying alternating countershock current. The advantage of direct current (DC) was noted and a DC capacitor discharge capable of depolarizing the myocardium transthoracically was developed by B. Lowen and R. Amarasingham in 1962.

Ventricular Septal Defect Treatment by surgical closure was demonstrated by Herbert Edgar Warden and colleagues

in 1954. *See congenital heart diseases.*

Ventricular Tachycardia Experimentally demonstrated in 1862 by Danish physiologist Peter Ludwig Panum (1820–1885) by injecting tallow into coronary arteries. An ECG recording was made by George Robinson (b 1922) and G. Herrmann in 1921.

Ventriculography Introduction of air into the cerebral ventricles to visualize them radiologically was practiced by Walter Edward Dandy (1886–1946) in 1918. A special technique to minimize the air introduced, using 12 projections, was designed by Erik Lysholm (1891–1947) in 1935. *See air ventriculography.*

Ventriloquism [Latin: *ventriculus*, a small belly + *quism*, speak] Some famous ventriloquists of the 18th and 19th centuries include: Baron Mengen and M. St Gille of France (1772), and Thomas King (1716) and Charles Matthews (1824) of England.

Verapamil Calcium channel blocker that dilates coronary arteries and decreases myocardial oxygen demand. *See calcium channel.*

Verdier, Caesar (d 1759) French surgeon from Avignon who practiced in Paris. He wrote treatises on anatomy, surgery and midwifery.

Verga, Andrea (1811–1895) Italian neurologist from Milan who in 1856 described a small tunnel in the petrous temporal bone which now bears his name. It is a space between the corpus callosum and the body of Fornix.

Verheyen, Phillippe (1648–1710) Belgian theologian who became interested in anatomy after amputation of his foot following an accident. He became professor of surgery at Louvain in 1693 and wrote *De Corporis Humani Anatomia* and *De Febribus.* The venae stellata of the kidney are named Verheyen stars.

Vermiform Appendix [Latin: *vermis*, worm + *forma*, shape] Called the worm of the bowel by physicians in ancient Egypt and cecum intestinum around 1600. A description was given in 1521 by Italian surgeon, Jacopo Berengario da Carpi (1470–1530) of Pavia. *See appendicitis.*

Vermifuge [Latin: *vermis*, worm + *fuge*, expel] *See antihelmintics.*

Verneuil Disease Syphilitic involvement of the bursae. Described by French surgeon, Aristide August Stanislaus Verneuil (1823–1895). He founded the *Revue de Chirurgerie* in 1881 and introduced iodoform as treatment for cold.

Verney, Ernest Basil (1894–1967) *See antidiuretic hormone.*

Vernier Scale Subdivision of ordinary scale designed to give a more accurate reading. Invented by French instrument maker, Pierre Vernier (1584–1638) in 1631.

Veronal Barbiturate synthesized by Emil Fischer (1852–1919) and Josef von Mering (1849–1908) in 1902 and named after the Italian city of Verona.

Veronensis, Antonius Fumanellus Italian physician in the 16th century. He wrote a book on preservation of health, *De fenum regimine,* in 1540.

Verruga Peruana (Syn: bartonellosis, Oroya fever, Carrion disease, Peruvian wart) Infection with *Bartonella bacilliformis,* transmitted by sandflies and found in small areas of Peru, Ecuador and Colombia. A description was given by Augustin Zarate, Chancellor of Lima, in his history of the conquest of Peru published in 1543. A medical description was given by Archibald Smith of Edinburgh in 1842, Tschudi (1846), Oriosola (1858), Salazar (1860), Dounon (1871), Fournier (1874) and Bourse (1871). *See Oroya fever, Carrion disease.*

Vertebra *See astragalus, atlas, axis.*

Vertebrata [Latin: *verto,* I turn] Subphylum of the Chordata containing all animals with a true backbone. Classified by a lecturer on animal morphology, Francis Maitland Balfour (1851–1882) of Edinburgh in *Treatise on Comparative Embryology* published in 1880.

Vertebral Disease *See ankylosing spondylitis, Calvé disease, Pott disease, sciatica, Kümmell disease, Rust disease, intervertebral disc prolapse, caries of the spine, Scheurmann disease, spinal injuries, spondylolisthesis.*

Vertebral Deformity *See kyphosis, scoliosis.*

Vertebrobasilar Insufficiency A description was given by Galen (AD 129–200) in his treatise on old age. He stated that those suffering from giddiness must not take any exercise in which they must bend often or turn around.

Vertigo [Latin: *vertigo*] Galen (AD 129–200) in his treatise on old age stated that those suffering from giddiness must not take exercise in which they must bend often or turn around. Vertigo as a symptom of brain disease was described by Jason Pratensis (1486–1558) of Zealand in 1549. Irritation of the semicircular canals as a cause was shown by German physiologist Friedrich Leopold Goltz (1834–1902) in 1870. It was studied in detail on a physiological basis in 1906 by Austrian physician and Nobel Prize winner, Robert Bárány (1876–1936).

Vesalius, Andreas (1515–1564) Father of anatomy who developed his interest as a child by dissecting a variety of animals. He studied medicine at the University of Paris but was dissatisfied with the lack of dissection of human bodies. He then started dissecting bodies which he recovered from executions and burial grounds and observed that many of Galen's (AD 129–200) statements were incorrect. Vesalius returned to his home town Louvain in 1536 and taught anatomy in the University where he obtained permission to dissect human bodies. He moved to the University of Padua in Italy as professor of anatomy at the age of 23 years and, after ten years of hard work, he published his seven books of *De Fabrica Humani Corporis* in 1543. Disillusioned by opposition to his work, he abandoned his academic pursuits and became personal physician to King Charles V in Brussels. When the King retired Vesalius left the Court and traveled extensively. He was shipwrecked on a Greek Island and died of exhaustion.

Vesicovaginal Fistula [Latin: *vesica,* bladder + *vagina,* sheath + *fistula,* pipe] Surgical treatment was pioneered by Johann Friedrich Dieffenbach (1792–1847), professor of surgery at Berlin. Montague Gosset (1792–1854) used a silver gilt wire to repair it in 1834. An early successful operation was performed by John Peter Mettauer (1787–1875) in 1840. The operative treatment was popularized by James Marion Sims (1813–1883) in 1852 and Washington Lemuel Atlee (1808–1878) in 1860.

Vesling, Johann (1598–1649) Professor of anatomy at the University of Padua. The linea media scroti, described by him in 1641 is named for him.

Vestibular Nerve [Latin: *vestibulum,* passage] The superior nucleus of the vestibular nerve was described by Vladimir Beckhterev (1857–1927) in 1898.

Vestigeal Organ [Latin: *vestigium,* footprint] A phylogenetically redundant organ.

Vesuvius The cities of Pompeii and Herculaneum were destroyed by the eruption of mount Vesuvius in AD 79. 200,000 people, including Pliny the Elder, died.

Veterans Administration Formed as the result of a program to look after former members of the military who took part in the American War of Independence. Initially it provided homes to care for the elderly and disabled. The Veterans Hospitals were established in the early 20th century. The multiple agencies responsible for care of veterans were amalgamated in 1930 to form the Veterans Administration.

Veterinary Medicine [Latin: *veterinarius,* diseases of beasts]

In Arab medicine animals are treated with the same methods as humans. Rock inscriptions in Girnar, near Junagarh in India, attributed to the Aryan king Asoka (273–232 BC) contain an edict on medicine for animals. Paintings from the Middle Ages show maladies of dogs being treated by humans. A book devoted to animal anatomy and veterinary medicine was written by Carlo Ruini (1531–1598) of Italy in 1598. An early veterinary school in Europe was established by a French veterinary surgeon Claude Bourgelat (1712–1799) at Lyons in 1761. The first veterinary school in London was established in 1791, and Charles Vial de St Bel, a graduate of the Lyons school was appointed first principal. The second veterinary school, was established at Edinburgh in 1818 by William Dick, son of a farrier. *The Veterinarian* was founded in 1828 and continued until 1902. The first veterinary school in America was founded by a Frenchman, Alexandre Liautard at New York in 1875. The leading institute for veterinary research in America, the US Bureau of Animal Industry, was established in 1883 and was responsible for the discovery of the causative organism of Texas cattle fever in 1888.

Vi Antigen Antigen of the typhoid bacillus discovered by Arthur Felix (1887–1956) and Margaret Pitt in 1934.

Vibration Injury A case of vascular lesion due to use of vibration tools was recorded by Loriga in 1911. Alice Hamilton (1869–1970) described it in 1918 amongst Indian workers who used pneumatic tools to cut stones.

Vibrio [Latin: *vibrare*, to vibrate] Genus of bacteria responsible for cholera and paracholera, classified by Christian Gottfried Ehrenberg (1795–1876) in 1838. The causative organism of cholera, *Vibrio cholerae*, was discovered by an Italian professor of anatomy at Pisa, Filippo Pacini (1812–1883) in 1840.

Vicary, Thomas (1495–1561) Surgeon from Maidstone who revived St Bartholomew's Hospital under the patronage of King Henry VIII in 1548. He is featured in a painting by Holbein illustrating the Act of Incorporation of the Company of Barber–Surgeons by Henry in 1541. He wrote an early anatomy book, *A Treasure for Englishmen, containing the Anatomie of Man's Body* in 1548.

Vicq D'Azyr, Félix (1748–1794) French physician and comparative anatomist in Paris and physician to Marie Antoinette. He described the mammilothalamic tract in 1786 which bears his name. He succeeded Louis Leclerc de Buffon (1707–1788) as secretary to the French Academy.

Victorius, Benedict (1481–1520) Italian physician and professor of medicine at Bologna. He wrote *De Morbo*

Gallico, a treatise on diseases of children and several other works.

Vidal Disease Neurodermatitis was described by French dermatologist, Jean Baptiste Emil Vidal (1825–1893) of Paris.

Vidal Operation Subcutaneous ligation of the veins in varicocele. Devised by French surgeon, Auguste Theodore Vidal de Cassis (1803–1856).

Vidian Artery *See Vidianus.*

Vidian Nerve *See Vidianus.*

Vidianus (1500–1569) Also known as Guido Guidi. Born in Florence and was professor of medicine at the University of Pisa. He described the nerve of the pterygoid (Vidian nerve) and its artery (Vidian artery) in 1611. He published a large volume on health.

Vienna The University of Vienna was founded in 1365. The Vienna School of Medicine was founded by Gerard van Swieten (1700–1772) whose efforts prevailed on the government to revive the university.

Vierordt, Karl (1818–1884) German clinician who made several important contributions to medicine including: discovery of a method of calculating circulation time of blood in 1842; invention of the hemacytometer for determining the number of corpuscles in a given volume of blood in 1852; discovery of a practical method of frequently measuring blood pressure in humans by applying counter pressure to the artery in 1854; and invention of sphygmograph in 1854.

Viesseux, Gaspard (1746–1814) Physician in Geneva who described cerebrospinal meningitis in 1805.

Vieussens, Raymond de (1641–1715) French anatomist from Montpellier, described the pathological state of the diseased mitral valve in 1705. He made an antemortem diagnosis of an aortic aneurysm around 1700, and described several structures including: the anterior medullary velum, ansa subclavia of the sympathetic nerves, and the central canal of cochlea columella, all of which are named after him.

Vignal, Guillaume (1852–1893) French histologist who studied under William Rutherford (1839–1899) at Edinburgh and later worked at the histological laboratory of the College of France in Paris for most of his life. Vignal cells are embryonic connective tissue on the axis cylinders of the fetal nerve fibers described by him in 1889.

Vigneaud, Vincent du (1901–1978) American biochemist, born in Chicago and studied in the USA, Berlin and Edinburgh. He was head of the George Washington School of Medicine and departmental head at Cornell Medical College. He studied amino acid interconversion, dietary requirements of sulfur amino acids and discovered the metabolic pathway from methionine to homocysteine. He found the relationship between choline, lecithin and methionine and showed the dietary importance of thiamin. He was awarded the Nobel Prize for Chemistry in 1955. *See oxytocin.*

Vigo, de Johannis (1460-1520) Italian surgeon from Genoa who came to Rome during the time of Michelangelo and was surgeon to Pope Julius II in 1503. He gave an account of the first epidemic of syphilis in Europe in *Practica in arte chirurgica copiosa* printed in 1515 and running to 52 editions.

Villaret Syndrome Unilateral paralysis of the 9th, 10th, 11th and 12th cranial nerves following lesions in the retro-parotid space. Described by Maurice Villaret (1877–1946) of Paris in 1916.

Villemin, Jean-Antoine (1827–1892) French surgeon and medical graduate from Paris (1853) demonstrated the infectious nature of tuberculosis by transferring it from man to rabbit in 1868.

Villemin Sphincter Sphincteric fibers at the termination of the duodenum were described by French professor of anatomy at Bordeaux, Fernand Villemin in 1922.

Villerme, Louis Rene (1782–1863) Parisian physician and public health reformer. He investigated the causes of premature death in humans and wrote *Tableau de l'etat physique et moral* in 2 volumes, on vital statistics, in 1840.

Vollmer, Herman (1896-1959) New York pediatrician who devised a tuberculin patch test in 1937.

Vinblastine Alkaloid of periwinkle, *Catharanthus roseus*, was introduced as treatment for Hodgkin disease by Irving Stanley Johnson (b 1925) and colleagues in 1963.

Vinca Alkaloids *See vincristine, vinblastine.*

Vincent Angina *Treponema vincentii*, a spirochete found in the throat of patients with Vincent angina was identified by French bacteriologist, Henri Vincent (1862–1950) in 1898.

Vincent, Henri (1862-1950) French bacteriologist in the Military Service, born in Bordeaux and graduated in medicine from Paris in 1887. He was posted to Algiers in 1891 and isolated the causative organism of madura foot, *Nocardia madurae*, while he was there in 1894. *See Vincent angina.*

Vincristine Alkaloid of periwinkle, *Catharanthus roseus*, was introduced as treatment for acute leukemia in children by Irving Stanley Johnson and colleagues in 1963.

Vinson, Porter Paisley (1890-1959) *See Plummer–Vinson syndrome.*

Viomycin Antibiotic isolated from *Actinomyces vinaceus*, *Streptomyces puniceus* and *S. floridae*. It was introduced as first line treatment for tuberculosis by Alexander Carpenter Finlay (b 1906) and colleagues in 1951.

Viral Hepatitis An epidemic following parentral transmission of the virus occurred during inoculation of workers for smallpox at Bremen, Germany in 1883, where 191 shipyard workers developed jaundice due to hepatitis. The nonparentral form of infective hepatitis A was shown by W. P. Havens, R. Ward and V. A. Drill in 1944.

Virchow, Rudolph Ludwig Karl (1821–1902) Eminent German pathological anatomist, born in Schievelbein, Pomerania and graduated in medicine from Berlin. He established cellular pathology and coined pathological terms such as: leukocytosis (1858), leukemia (1845), neuroglia (1854), thrombosis (1848) and amyloid (1854). The analysis of diseased tissues on the basis of cell formation and cell structure was given by him in *Die Cellularpathologie*, published in 1856. He was also a politician and administrator and proposed a sewer system for Berlin in 1866.

Virus [Latin: *virus*, poison] Viral diseases such as smallpox were known in 1700 BC in China. Scientific evidence for the existence of living particles smaller than bacteria was presented by Dmitri Iosofich Ivanovski (1864–1920) in 1892. He investigated the tobacco mosaic virus and discovered that the sap of the diseased plant was capable of transmitting the disease despite filtration through a bacterial filter. His finding was not taken seriously until Martinus Willem Beijerinck (1851–1931) revived interest in 1898 in his *Ueber ein Contagium Vivum Fluidum* which provided further evidence of the filterability of the virus. Friedrich Löffler (1852–1915) and Paul Frosch (1860–1928) demonstrated the filterability of the organism producing foot-and-mouth disease and this was the first instance where a virus was demonstrated to be the cause of animal disease. Yellow fever was the first human disease to be identified as caused by a virus.

Viscera [Latin: *viscera*, organs in the abdomen] Illustrations were given by Magnus Hundt (1449–1519) in his *Anthropologium de Homis Dignitate, natura, et propriatatibus*, published in 1501.

Viscosity *See blood viscosity.*

Vision [Latin: *videre*, to see] Ancient Greeks considered the lens of the eye was the center of the 'pneuma' or visual spirit. They also postulated that the eye emitted rays by which the objects were perceived. The Arab scholars Hunain ibn Ishak (809–877) and Alhazen, around AD 900, advanced other theories. The mechanism of accommodation of the lens was explained by English physician, Thomas Young (1773–1829), in 1792. The link between rhodopsin in the retina and vitamin A was established by American biochemist and Nobel Prize winner, George Wald (b 1906) in 1933. Understanding of color vision was developed by American, Edwin Herbert Land (1910–1991) of Bridgeport, Connecticut in 1947. Work on the neurophysiology of vision was done by Torsten Nils Wiesel (b 1924), Roger Wolcott Sperry (b 1913) and David Hunter Hubel (b 1926), for which they were awarded the Nobel Prize for Physiology or Medicine in 1981. *See visual cortex.*

Visual Cortex Pierre Jean Marie Flourens (1794–1867) established that vision depended on the integrity of the cerebral cortex, in 1823. Bartolomeo Panniza (1785–1867) localized the visual function to the posterior part of the cerebrum in 1855. German neurologist, Eduard Hitzig (1838–1907) did further work on the localization in 1874. The occurrence of unilateral homonymous hemianopia in monkeys following experimental unilateral ablation of the occipital cortex was demonstrated by E.A. Schafer (1850–1935) in 1888. The visual pathway was further clarified by Lithuanian physician, Oskar Minkowski (1858–1931) working in Breslau in 1917.

Vital Statistics The first book, *Natural and Political Observations Upon the Bills of Mortality,* was published by John Graunt (1620–1674) of Hampshire in 1662, and a life table for life insurance was published by Edmund Halley (1656–1742) in 1693. Sir William Petty (1623–1687) studied mortality rates and his work was advanced by Gregory King (1648–1712). French mathematician, Pierre Simon Marquis de Laplace (1749–1827) of Normandy wrote *Theorie analitique des probabilitis* in 1812, which was another important landmark. The study of vital statistics was established on a scientific basis by physician and statistician, William Farr (1807–1883) of Kenley, Shropshire, in 1839. *See mortality.*

Vitali Test Used for detection of alkaloids with the reagents, potassium hydroxide and sulfuric acid. Devised by Italian physician, Dioscoride Vitali (1832–1917).

Vitalism Concept of the existence of a vital energy of psychological or spiritual nature in all living organisms. Proposed by German zoologist and philosopher, Hans Adolf Eduard Driesch (1867–1941).

Vitamin In 1873 Forster demonstrated that animals died

when fed only with protein, fat, carbohydrates, water, and salt. In 1881 Nikolai Ivanovic Lunnin (1853–1937) proved that adding milk to their diet increased survival. Sir Frederick Gowland Hopkins (1861–1947) extended the studies in 1912 and proved the existence of accessory food factors, later named vitamins. The first was identified by a Polish chemist, Casimir Funk (1884–1967), in 1911 and prevented beriberi. He named it 'vitamine'. The second, a fat soluble product which prevented eye changes, was discovered by Elmer Verner McCollum (1879–1967) from the University of Wisconsin in 1913 and named 'fat soluble A'.

Vitamin A The ancient Chinese and Egyptians recommended liver for eye problems around 1600 BC. Jacques Guillemeau (1550–1613) of France described night blindness and recommend liver in the 16th century. Cod-liver oil was used to treat juvenile conjunctivitis by M. Mori in Japan in 1904. A deficiency of a fat-soluble factor was recognized as a cause of conjunctivitis by American biochemist Thomas Burr Osborne (1859–1929) and Lafayette Benedict Mendel (1872–1935) in 1913. Elmer Verner McCollum (1879–1967) and N. Simmonds recognized the similarity of xerophthalmia in rats and conjunctivitis in children with a deficient diet. Carotene was shown to be the main source of vitamin A by T. Moore in 1930. Further research led to the conclusion that vitamin A gave protection against infection and reduced morbidity and mortality. The chemical structure and function was established by Russian-born Swiss chemist and Nobel Prize winner, Paul Karrer (1889–1971) in 1931. Synthesis was achieved by German chemist and Nobel Prize winner, Richard Kuhn (1900–1967) and C.J. O.R. Morris in 1937 and a more pure form from fish liver oil was obtained by Harry Nicholls Holmes (1879–1958) and Ruth E. Corbet later in the same year. Its presence in the retina was shown by New York biochemist, George Wald (b 1906) in 1933 and led to the discovery of a link between rhodopsin in the retina and vitamin A. He shared the Nobel Prize for Physiology or Medicine with Ragnar Granit (b 1900) and Haldan Hartline (1903–1983) in 1967. The daily requirement was established by American biochemist, Henry Clapp Sherman (1875–1955) of Columbia University in 1934.

Vitamin B Complex Vitamin B was believed to be a single entity until M.I. Smith and E.G. Hendrik showed in 1926 that it consisted of two factors, a thermolabile antineuritic factor and a thermostable growth promoting factor. These were called vitamins B and F in America and B1 and B2 in England. The thermolabile factor was discovered to contain riboflavin (later known as vitamin B2), vitamin B6 or Ademin (1935), nicotinic acid (1937), pantothenic acid

(1939), folic acid (1942), biotin (1940) and inositol (1940).

Vitamin B1 *See thiamin, beriberi.*

Vitamin B2 *See riboflavin.*

Vitamin B6 *See pyridoxine.*

Vitamin B12 *See pernicious anemia.*

Vitamin C *See scurvy, ascorbic acid.*

Vitamin D Rickets was demonstrated to be a deficiency disease by Sir Edward Mellanby (1884–1955) in 1913 and shown to be curable with sunlight by Kurt Huldschinsky (b 1883) of Germany in 1919. H. Chick of London demonstrated that sunlight and cod-liver oil cured rickets during his work on post-war famine in Vienna in 1928. The active substance was detected by Elmer Verner McCollum (1879–1967) at the Johns Hopkins School of Hygiene in 1922. Activation of ergosterol by sunlight forming vitamin D2 was discovered by German chemist and Nobel Prize winner, Adolf Windaus (1876–1959). *See rickets, cod-liver oil.*

Vitamin E Discovered by Herbert McLean Evans (1882–1971) of California and K. J. Scott in 1922. Its antisterility property was demonstrated by Evans and Katherine Scott Bishop (1889–1976) in the same year.

Vitamin K A hemorrhagic disease in chicks fed on a diet poor in fats was observed in 1929 and a vitamin deficiency as a cause was proposed by Danish professor of biochemistry at Copenhagen and Nobel Prize winner, Carl Peter Henrik Dam (1895–1976) in the same year. The fat-soluble nature of this factor was shown by W.D. McFarlane in 1931, and Dam named it vitamin K in 1934. A progressive fall in prothrombin in blood of chicks fed with a vitamin K deficient diet was observed by Armand Jacques Quick (b 1894) in 1937. Deficiency in man was shown in 1939 and it was obtained in pure form by Russian-born Swiss chemist and Nobel Prize winner, Paul Karrer (1889–1971) and Dam in the same year.

Vitello (1220–1270) *See optics.*

Vitruvius, Markus Pollio Roman architect who designed Rome at the time of Augustus just before the Christian era. He wrote a book on architecture titled *De Archtectura, Libri Decem,* in ten volumes. The gold amalgam, a preparation of gold in mercury, was first described by Vitruvius in AD 27.

Vitus, St *See St Vitus Dance.*

Vivisection [Latin: *vivus,* living] *See antivivisectionists.*

VMA Vanilmandelic acid. *See pheochromocytoma.*

Vocal Cord Paralysis due to recurrent laryngeal nerve lesion was studied by Berlin physician, Carl Adolf Christian Jacob Gerhardt (1883–1902) in 1863. American surgeon, Jacob DaSilva Solis-Cohen (1833–1927) used a laryngoscope to remove a polyp on the vocal cord in 1867. German physician, Ottomar Rosenbach (1851–1907) explained the mechanism of paralysis in 1880. An operation to restore its function was described by American surgeon in Seattle, Brian Thaxton King (b 1886) in 1939 and a New York otorhinologist, Joseph Dominic Kelly (b 1888) in 1941. Pittsburgh surgeon, John Wesley Shirer (b 1899) modified King's operation in 1944.

Voelcker, Friedrich (1872–1955) *See esophagectomy.*

Vogt, Peter (b 1932) German-born American microbiologist, educated at the University of Tübingen and moved to the University of Colorado as an assistant professor, later becoming professor. He also worked at the Universities of Washington and Southern California. He studied oncogene transduction by retroviruses and showed two ways in which the oncogene could be activated by alteration in the genetic sequence. *See oncogenes.*

Vogt Angle Found between the nasobasilar and alveolonasal lines. Defined by German neurophysiologist, Karl Vogt (1817–1895).

Vogt Point In the skull where trephination can be performed for traumatic meningeal hemorrhage. Defined by German surgeon, Paul Frederick Emmanuel Vogt (1847–1885) of Griefswald.

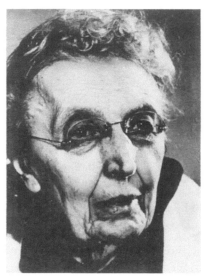

Cécile Vogt (1875–1962). Courtesy of the National Library of Medicine

Vogt Syndrome Athetosis, emotional lability and rhythmic oscillation of the limbs due a lesion in the corpus striatum.

Described by French physician, Cécile Vogt (1875–1962) and German neurologist, Oskar Vogt (1870–1959) in 1920.

Voigt, Christian August (1809–1890) Austrian professor of anatomy at Vienna who described the hair tracts known as Voigt lines in 1857.

Voit, Max (b 1876) German embryologist and professor of anatomy at Göttingen. A branch of the ramus anterior of the acoustic nerve, Voit nerve, was described by him in 1907.

Voit Nucleus   Cerebellar nucleus accessory to the corpus dentatum. Described by German physiologist, Karl von Voit (1831–1908) of Munich. He was also a pioneer in animal metabolism.

Volhard, Franz von (1872–1950) *See pale hypertension.*

Volkmann Canal   Found in bones which carry blood vessels from the periosteum. Described in 1873 by German professor of physiology and anatomy, Alfred Wilhelm Volkmann (1800–1877) of Dorpat.

Volkmann Contracture   In fingers and wrists following ischemia secondary to injury at the elbow or improper application of tourniquet. Described in 1881 by a German surgeon, Richard von Volkmann (1830–1889), professor of surgery at Halle. He also identified industrial tar and paraffin as carcinogens in 1875 and performed an excision of the rectum for cancer in 1878.

Volt   Unit of electricity named after the Italian inventor of electric battery, Alesandro Volta (1745–1827).

Voltolini Disease   Acute purulent inflammation of the internal ear leading to violent pain, delirium and unconsciousness. Described by Friedrich Edward Rudolf Voltolini (1819–1899), an otorhinolaryngologist at Breslau.

Volvulus   [Latin: *volvere*, to twist around] An operation for it was performed by Adolf Frederick Linstedt (1847–1915) and Johann Anton Waldenström (1839–1879) in 1878. A successful operation in England was performed by Henry Edward Clark (1845–1909) in 1883.

Vomiting   [Latin: *vomitare*] Originates from the word for a Roman plow which threw up the earth to either side. Twenty causes were described by S.O. Habershon of Guy's Hospital in 1861. He published a book in gastroenterology, *Diseases of the Stomach, the Varieties of Dyspepsia, their Diagnosis and Treatment* in 1865. *See emesis.*

Von Gierke Disease   (Syn: hepatomegalia glycogenica) Caused by an inborn error of glycogen storage and accompanied by hepatomegaly. Described in two children by Edgar Otto Konrad von Gierke (1877–1945) in 1929. A detailed description was given by S. van Creveld in 1932.

Von Graefe   *See Graefe, Friedrich Wilhelm Ernst Albrecht von.*

Von Jaksch Disease   Form of pseudoleukemia in children described by Rudolf von Jaksch (1855–1947) in 1889.

Von Recklinghausen Disease   Multiple tumors of the nerve with cafe-au-lait-spots in the skin, known as neurofibromatosis. Described by Robert William Smith (1807–1873), a surgeon at Dublin in 1849. A classic description was given in 1882 by Friedrich Daniel von Recklinghausen (1833–1910), professor of pathology at Königsberg. *See elephant man.*

Von Willebrand Disease   Congenital hemorrhagic disease characterized by epistaxis and bleeding from gastrointestinal tract with normal platelets. Described by Finnish physician, Erik A. von Willebrand (1870–1949) in 1933.

Voronoff, Serge (1866–1951) Russian physiologist, educated in Paris and became director of experimental surgery at the College of France. He developed a theory connecting glandular secretions to longevity and pioneered endocrinological surgery. *See rejuvenation.*

Vries, Hugo Marie de (1848–1935) Dutch physiologist and geneticist, born at Haarlem. He studied osmosis in 1877. The theory that a new species can arise by a single mutation was put forward by him while he was professor of botany at Amsterdam in 1890. He attained worldwide recognition as a pioneer in the study of mutation with his work *Die Mutationstheorie*, published in 1901. *See mutation.*

Vrolik Syndrome   Form of rapid fatal congenital osteogenesis imperfecta. Described by Dutch anatomist, Willem Vrolik (1801–1863) in 1854.

Vulcanization   Process of molding rubber by treating it with sulfur, discovered independently by Charles Goodyear (1800–1860) in America, and Thomas Hancock (1786–1865) in England, in 1844. Their invention helped to bring in large-scale use of condoms, rubber catheters, tourniquets, air mattresses and other surgical appliances.

Vulpian, Edmé Felix Alfred (1826–1887) Physician in Paris who demonstrated the presence of an active vital substance in the adrenal glands in 1856, later named adrenaline. Also remembered in Vulpian atrophy, a progressive muscular dystrophy. *See nerve regeneration.*

Vulva   According to Isidorus, in AD 600, the external female genitalia were named due their likeness to the wings of a folding door.

Vulvectomy   Total surgical removal of vulva was done by French surgeon, Antoine Basset (1882–1941) in 1912.

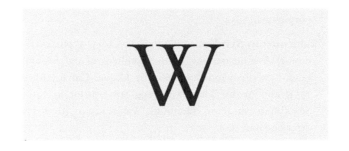

Waage, Peter (1833–1900) Norwegian chemist who studied medicine at Christiana University, Oslo in 1854, but changed to science. He established the Law of Mass Action governing the effects of reactant concentration on rate of reaction, with his brother-in-law, Cato Maximillian Guldberg (1836–1902) in 1864.

Waalich, Nathaniel (1786–1854) Danish botanist graduated in medicine from Copenhagen and became surgeon to the Danish colony at Serampore in India. He was superintendent of botanical gardens in Calcutta in 1815. He brought back over 8000 botanical specimens from India.

Waardenburg Syndrome (Syn: Vogt syndrome) Parrot-beaked nose, hypertelorism, cleft palate, and congenital heart defects. Described by Swiss ophthalmologist Alfred Vogt (1879–1943) in 1933 and by Dutch physician, Petrus Johannes Waardenburg (1886–1979) in 1934.

Wachendorf Membrane Membrana pupillaris. Described by Bernard Albinus in 1737 and in 1758 by Eberhard Jacob Wachendorf (1703–1758), professor of surgery at Utrecht.

Waddell, Laurence Austin (b 1854) Glasgow physician in India who edited the *Indian Medical Gazette* for several years. He published *The Buddhism of Tibet* (1895), *The Tribes of Bramaputra Valley* (1900), *Excavations at Paliputra* (1903) and several other works.

Waddington, Conrad Hal (1905–1975) English embryologist and a pioneer in genetic engineering. He was professor of animal genetics at Edinburgh University (1947–1970). He studied the effects of chemical messengers on embryonic cells during development and examined the effects of genes and environment. He published *Organizers and Genes* (1940), *Principals of Embryology* (1956), *Ethical Animal* (1960), and *Biology for the Modern World* (1962).

Wadham College Oxford college founded by Nicholas (1536–1610) and Dorothy Wadham in 1613. It was the regular meeting place for the founders of the Royal Society prior to 1658.

Wafer, Lionel English naval surgeon and an explorer in the 17th century. During his travels with Dampier they quarreled and he was left at Darien where he managed to survive amongst the Indians due to his medical skills. He was rescued by an English vessel and published his experiences in 1690.

Wagener, Henry Patrick (b 1890) American ophthalmologist from Rochester, Minnesota who described various grades of hypertension based on the funduscopic appearance of the retina.

Wagner, Ernest Leberecht (1829–1888) German physician who wrote a treatise on uterine cancer in 1858. He described dermatomyositis in 1863.

Wagner, John James (1641–1695) Swedish physician and city librarian at Zurich. He wrote *Historia Naturalis Helvetiae Curiosa*.

Wagner Corpuscle Tactile nerve endings described in 1852 by Georg Meissner (1829–1905) and Rudolf Wagner (1805–1864), professors of physiology and comparative anatomy, respectively, at Göttingen.

Wagner Operation Osteoplastic resection of the skull. Described by German surgeon, Wilhelm Wagner (1848–1900) in 1889.

Wagner Spot Nucleolus of the ovum. Described in 1836 by Rudolf Wagner (1805–1864), professor of comparative anatomy and physiology at Göttingen.

Wagner-Jauregg, Julius (1857–1941) Austrian neurologist and psychiatrist, educated in Vienna. He investigated the relationship between cretinism and goiter and treated late stage paralysis in syphilis by inducing malarial fever. He received the Nobel Prize for Physiology or Medicine in 1927. *See artificial fever.*

Wagstaffe Fracture Causing separation of the internal malleolus. Described by English surgeon, William Warwick Wagstaffe (1843–1910).

Wahl Sign Distention of the proximal portion of obstructed bowel. Described by German surgeon, Eduard von Wahl (1833–1890). He described the systolic murmur over an injured artery in 1885.

Waitz, Theodor (1821–1864) German anthropologist and psychologist. He was professor of philosophy at Marburg and published on psychology and education, including *Anthropologie der Naturvolker* (1859–1871).

Wakley, Thomas (1795–1862) British physician and founder of the longest surviving weekly medical journal, *The Lancet*. He was the member of Parliament for Finsbury (1835–1852) and a coroner. His work on analysis of food led to the Adulteration of Food and Drink Act in 1860.

Waksman, Selman Abraham (1888–1973) American biochemist, born in the Ukraine. He moved to America in 1910 and became a citizen in 1917 and graduated from Rutgers University in the same year. He spent most of his working life at Rutgers and was professor of microbiology. He worked on breakdown of organic substances in the soil by microorganisms, and their classification. From 1939 he searched for antibacterial substances of medical importance and discovered streptomycin in 1944, neomycin in 1949 and stretocin. He received the Nobel Prize for Physiology or Medicine in 1952. His published works include *Enzymes* (1926), *Principles of Soil Microbiology* (1938), and an autobiography titled *My Life With Microbes* (1954). *See antibiotics.*

Walbum, John Julius (1724–1799) German physician and naturalist who practiced at Lubeck and wrote on natural history.

Walcher Position A position in obstetrics with legs hanging down during delivery. Described by Arab surgeon, Albucasis (936–1013) and revived by German gynecologist in Stuttgart, Gustav Adolf Walcher (1856–1935) in 1889.

Wald, George (b 1906) American biochemist from New York who studied in New York and Berlin. He was professor of biology in Harvard and worked on visual purple in the retina and its conversion on illumination to vitamin A. He established the relationship between night blindness and vitamin A deficiency and shared the 1967 Nobel Prize. *See vitamin A.*

Walden Inversion Optical activity of a compound in which substitution occurs on an enantiomer causing inversion of the configuration. Discovered in 1895 by Latvian chemist, Paul Walden (1863–1957).

Waldenström Disease Acute thyrotoxic encephalopathy. Described by Swedish professor of medicine at Uppsala, Jan Gosta Waldenström (b 1906) in 1945.

Waldenstrom, Johann Anton (1839–1879) *See volvulus.*

Waldenström Macroglobulinemia Dysproteinemia with raised IgM paraprotein in the serum, and systemic effects of hyperviscosity of blood. Described by Swedish professor of medicine at Uppsala, Jan Gosta Waldenström (b 1906) in *Acta Medica Scandinavia* in 1944. He described acute

porphyria in 1934.

Waldenstrom Syndrome (Syn: Calvé–Legg–Perthes syndrome) Aseptic necrosis of the epiphysis of the femoral head. Described independently by Jacques Calvé (1875–1954) and Arthur Thornton Legg (1874–1939) in 1910. Stockholm surgeon, Henning Waldenstrom (b 1877) described it in 1909.

Waldeyer Ring Ring of lymphoid tissue in the pharynx. Named after its discoverer, Heinrich Wilhelm Gottfried von Waldeyer (1836–1921), a German anatomist.

Waldeyer-Hartz, Heinrich Wilhelm Gottfried (1836–1921) German histologist and anatomist who made several contributions to medicine. He was the professor of pathological anatomy at Breslau (1868), Strasburg (1872), and Berlin (1883). He did histological classification of cancers showing that carcinomas come from epithelial cells and sarcomas from mesodermal tissue. He suggested the terms 'chromosome' and 'neuron' and discovered the germinal epithelium in 1870. *See motor neuron, Waldeyer ring.*

Walker, Sir James (1863–1935) Scottish professor of chemistry, born in Dundee and pioneer in the study of amphoteric electrolytes and ionization.

Walker, John (1759–1830) English physician and geographer, born in Cockermouth, Cumbria. He was head of the London vaccine institution and wrote several works on geography.

Walker, J.T. Ainsley (1868–1930) *See Rideal–Walker test.*

Walker, Mary Edwards (1832–1919) American surgeon, educated at the Syracuse Medical College, New York in 1855 and was a surgeon for the Union Army during the Civil War. She was the first woman to be appointed Assistant Surgeon to the United States Army in 1864, and she is commemorated in a postage stamp issued by the United States Postal Service in 1982.

Walker, Mary Broadfoot (1888–1974) *See myasthenia gravis.*

Walker, Sir Norman (1862–1942) Scottish dermatologist who succeeded William Allan Jamieson (1839–1916) at his school of dermatology in 1916. He translated Paul Unna's (1850–1929) work on dermatology in 1896.

Wall, John (1708–1776) English physician, born at Powick in Worcestershire and educated at Merton College, Oxford. He wrote a treatise on Malvern waters.

Wallace, Alfred Russel (1823–1913) Welsh naturalist and pioneer of the theory of evolution, born at Usk in Monmouthshire. He commenced his study of species with his first exploration to the Amazon in 1848. He corresponded with Darwin on his discoveries and was inspired by his *Origin of Species* and called his own book on the subject *Darwinism* which was followed in 1870 by *Contributions to the Theory of Natural Selection*. He has also made a remarkable comparative study of the flora of the Malay peninsula where he spent eight years and published *The Malay Archipelago* in 1869.

Wallace, William (1791–1837) *See lymphogranuloma venereum.*

Wallenberg Syndrome Ipsilateral loss of pain and temperature sensations in the face, with contralateral hypoesthesia for pain and temperature of the trunk due to occlusion of the posterior inferior cerebellar artery. Described in 1895 by German neurologist, Adolf Wallenberg (1862–1949) at Berlin.

Waller, Augustus Desire (1856–1922) Son of Augustus Volney Waller (1816–1870) and an eminent English physiologist, born in Paris and graduated from Aberdeen University in 1878. While working at St Mary's Hospital London he conceived the idea of measuring the variation in action currents in the living heart using electrodes attached to moist skin and connected to a galvanometer that measured the movements in a fine column of mercury and were photographed on a moving plate in 1887. This principle was later developed into the electrocardiograph.

Waller, Augustus Volney (1816–1870) English physiologist who graduated from Paris. He did research at Bonn (1851–1856) and Paris (1856–1858) before he was appointed professor of physiology at Birmingham in 1858. He demonstrated in 1850 that the axis cylinder, if cut off from the nerve cell, will undergo degeneration while the central stump will remain viable for a longer time. This was based on experiments on the glossopharyngeal and hypoglossal nerves and is known as the Law of Wallerian degeneration.

Wallerian Degeneration A sequence of events in the distal portion of a severed nerve described by Augustus Volney Waller (1816–1870) in 1850.

Wallgren, Arvid Johan (1889–1973) *See aseptic meningitis.*

Wallis, John (1616–1703) English mathematician and Savillian professor at Oxford, born in Ashford, Kent and graduated from Cambridge. He was a founder of the Royal Society, and made several important contributions to mathematics. He made a general statement on logarithms. His *Arithmetica Infinitorum*, which contained the essence of differential calculus, was published in 1655.

Walsh, Edward (d 1832) Irish physician, educated at Edinburgh and spent most of his career as an army physician in the West Indies, Europe and Canada. He published *A Narrative of the Expedition to Holland*.

Walshe, Walter Hayle (1812–1892) London physician who recognized fragments of malignant tissue in sputum in 1843. He also described the presystolic component of the murmur of mitral stenosis.

Walshe, Sir Francis Martin Rouse (1885–1973) British neurologist at the National Hospital for Nervous Diseases, Queen's Square, London (1921) and later at University College Hospital. In 1945 he described the symptoms of acroparesthesia and neuritis of the hands caused by pressure from the scalenus anticus muscle in thoracic outlet syndrome.

Walter, Friedrich Augustus (1764–1826) Son of German anatomist, Johann Gottlieb Walter (1734–1818). He was director of the anatomical museum at Berlin and in 1805 the first medical counselor.

Walter, Johann Gottlieb or Theophilus (1734–1818) Professor of anatomy at Frankfurt and later at Berlin. He dissected over 800 cadavers and collected over 3000 anatomical specimens which he sold to the King of Prussia. The smallest branch of the splanchnic nerve passing through the renal plexus bears his name.

Walter Nerve *See Walter, Johann Gottlieb.*

Walther Canal Duct of the sublingual salivary gland. Named after August Friedrich Walther (1688–1746), professor of pathology at Leipzig, who described it in 1724.

Walther, Phillip Franz von (1782–1849) German physician who described corneal opacity in 1845. He advocated the application of physics, chemistry and natural sciences to medicine.

Walton, George Lincoln (1854–1941) American surgeon who described a method of reducing dislocation of cervical vertebra in 1895.

Wanley, Nathaniel (d 1690) Clergyman from Coventry who was was educated at Trinity College Cambridge, and wrote *General History of Man*, collected from the writings of historians, philosophers, and physicians of all ages and countries.

Wangensteen, Owen Harding (1898–1981) American surgeon at Minneapolis who in 1932 devised a suction technique via a nasal catheter for management of intestinal obstruction. He described a technique for intestinal anastomosis in 1940.

War Injuries *See abdominal injuries, army medicine and surgery, Geneva Convention, gunshot wounds.*

Warburg, Otto Heinrich (1883–1970) German biochemist from Freiberg and professor of biochemistry in his home town and in 1931 director of Kaiser Wilhelm Institute for cellular pathology in Berlin. He discovered the role of iron in oxidase enzymes leading to the discovery of the heme protein, and developed the gas manometer. He was awarded the Nobel Prize for Physiology or Medicine in 1931. He was prevented from accepting it by Hitler as he was a Jew. *See riboflavin, cytochrome oxidase.*

Ward, Frederick Oldfield (1818–1877) Sanitary reformer who graduated from King's College Hospital. He published *Outlines of Human Osteology* while a medical student. The triangular area which intervenes amongst the trabeculae of the cancellous tissue of the neck of the femur is named after him. He was appointed commissioner of sewers in London in 1854.

Ward, James (1843–1925) English psychologist from Hull who popularized psychology by publishing several articles in the *Encyclopedia Britannica* from 1886. He was professor of Philosophy at Cambridge in 1897, a post he held until his death. He wrote *Naturalism and Agnosticism* (1899), *Psychological Principles* (1918), *A Study of Kant* (1922) and several other works.

Ward, Joshua (1685–1761) *See quackery.*

Ward, Nathaniel Bagshaw (1791–1868) London physician known for his contributions to botany. He invented the Wardian case for transporting live plants on long voyages. He wrote *On the Growth of Plants in closely glazed cases* in 1842.

Ward, Seth (1617–1689) Born in Hertfordshire, he was Savillian professor of astronomy and a founder of the Royal Society. He was the bishop of Exeter from 1662 to 1667, and later of Salisbury.

Ward Triangle *See Ward, Frederick Oldfield.*

Wardrop, James (1782–1869) Scottish surgeon from Torbane who graduated in medicine from Edinburgh University and settled in London in 1809. He resected the lower jaw and advocated distal ligation of an artery (Wardrop operation) for aneurysm. *See keratitis.*

Ware, James (1756–1815) British surgeon and oculist from Portsmouth. He was a demonstrator at Cambridge before establishing his own practice there in 1791. He wrote *Observations on Ophthalmy, Remarks on Fistula lachrymalis* and *Chirurgical Observations.*

Warfarin *See dicumarol.*

Waring, Edward John (1819–1891) British physician who compiled the Indian pharmacopoeia in 1868. He also published a bibliography of therapeutics in 1879.

Warren, Jonathan Mason (1811–1867) American surgeon and son of John Collins Warren (1778–1856). He revived the Hindu method of rhinoplasty in the United States in 1837.

Warren, John Collins (1778–1856) American surgeon, born in Boston and graduated from Harvard where his father was professor of anatomy and surgery. He succeeded his father to the chair and was dean to the medical school in 1816. He performed an operation for strangulated hernia in 1846 and removed a tumor in the neck of a patient after administering ether, at the suggestion of Morton, on 17th October 1846 which was one of the first demonstrations of ether as an anesthetic. He was a founder of the *New England Journal of Medicine and Surgery* in 1812.

Warren, John (1753–1815) *See Harvard Medical School.*

Warren, Samuel (1807–1877) Medical student from Edinburgh who gave up his studies to become a lawyer. He became Queen's Counsel in 1851 and was the member of Parliament for Midhurst from 1865 to 1869. He was also a novelist, and wrote *Passage from the Diary of a late Physician* which fictionalized the experiences of a pompous and ineffective doctor.

Warren Theory Lymphatic spread of carcinoma of the prostate to the bones. Proposed by American physician, Shields Warren (b 1898) in 1936.

Wartenberg Sign The little finger is held in adduction in ulnar paralysis. Described by German-born American neurologist, Robert Wartenberg (1887–1956).

Warthin Sign Exaggerated pulmonary sounds in cases of acute pericarditis. Described by American pathologist, Aldred Scott Warthin (1867–1931) from Indiana and professor of pathology at Michigan.

Wart [Dutch: *werte,* wart] Produced in humans through experimental inoculation by Josef Jadassohn (1879–1921) in 1896. Filterable agents were shown to be the cause by Guiseppe Ciuffo of Italy in 1907. Kingery in 1921 used extract of wart passed through a Berkefeld filter to produce warts in humans, thus confirming the role of filterable agents.

Wasserman, August Paul von (1866–1925) German bacteriologist born in Bamberg and graduated in medicine from Strasburg in 1888. He was director of the Institute of

Experimental Therapy in Berlin and discovered the complementation test for diagnosis of syphilis (Wasserman test) in 1906.

Wasserman Reaction   *See Treponema pallidum, Wasserman, August.*

Waste Water   *See sewers.*

Wasting Palsy   *See amyotrophic lateral sclerosis.*

Water Cure   Established by a Silesian patient called Vincent Priessnitz (1799–1851). He recovered completely from injuries sustained in an accident by applying wet compresses and drinking large quantities of water. It became a popular form of remedy in the 19th century.

Water Excretion Test   Devised as a test for adrenal function by L.J. Soffer and J.L. Gabrilov in 1952. Water excreting power is estimated before and after a loading dose of oral cortisone. In cases of adrenal insufficiency impaired water excretion was improved after taking cortisone.

Water Load Test   *See Albarran test.*

Water Pollution   Sewers for draining water from marshes and low lying areas were constructed in England during the reign of King Henry VIII and later opened into the River Thames, making it a cesspool. Such poor sanitary conditions in London were addressed by Sir Edwin Chadwick (1800–1890) in a report in 1842. In 1848 the City Sewers Act was passed and the post of medical officer of health was created. The idea that disease could be waterborne was developed by John Snow (1813–1858), an English physician from Yorkshire.

Water Purification   Chlorine was used to purify water by William Cruikshank of England in 1800. William Thompson Sedgwick (1855–1921) of Massachusetts, a pioneer of public health in America, advocated the treatment of drinking water with chlorine and has become a standard worldwide. Use of charcoal filters to purify water to prevent the spread of cholera was described by English surgeon, John Parkin (1801–1886) in 1832. American army surgeon, Carl Rogers Darnall (1867–1941) devised a filter for drinking water in 1908. A bacterial system of sewage and water purification was described Joseph William Dibdin (1850–1925) of London in 1897. Another method was described by American army surgeon, William John L. Lyster (1869–1947) in 1917.

Water Hammer Pulse   Characterized by a sudden impact and rapid fall in aortic insufficiency (Corrigan pulse). Described by Sir Dominic Corrigan (1802–1880) in 1832 and named after a Victorian toy, which worked on the water hammer principle.

Water   Thales (624–545 BC) of Miletus, a Greek philosopher, proposed water as an essence and origin of all things. Empedocles of Agrigentum (*c* 450 BC) and Alcmaeon (*c* 520 BC), pupil of Pythagorus (580–500 BC) and a physician, enunciated the doctrine of the four elements: earth, water, fire and air. It continued to be considered an element until English chemist, Henry Cavendish (1731–1810), demonstrated that it is a compound.

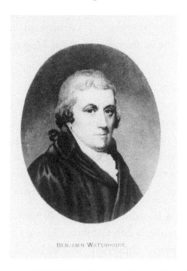

Benjamin Waterhouse (1754–1846). Courtesy of the National Library of Medicine

Waterhouse, Benjamin (1754–1846) American physician who studied medicine at Edinburgh and Harvard Universities. He was the first professor of medicine at Harvard in 1803. He introduced inoculation for smallpox in America and his book, *History of Kinepox* (1800), is a classic on the subject.

Waterhouse–Friderichsen Syndrome   Circulatory collapse in cerebrospinal meningitis. Described by Arthur Francis Voelcker (1861–1946) in 1895. Suprarenal apoplexy as the cause was shown in 1911 by English physician, Rupert Waterhouse (1873–1958) at the Royal National Hospital for Rheumatic Diseases at Bath. It was redescribed by Danish pediatrician, Carl Friderichsen (b 1886) in 1918.

Waters, Ralph Milton (b 1883) American anesthetist from Madison, Wisconsin who described a closed circuit method for cyclopropane anesthesia in 1934.

Waterson, John James (1811–1883) Scottish natural philosopher and engineer. He studied science and medicine at Edinburgh and served in India as an engineer. He proposed the basis for kinetic theory of gases to the Royal Society in 1845, but his findings were ignored until revived by Lord

Rayleigh in 1892. Waterson also did research on the physiology of mental processes.

Watkin Operation Used for prolapse of the uterus where the bladder is separated from the anterior wall of the uterus so that the uterus is left in position to support the entire bladder. Designed in 1899 by Chicago gynecologist, Thomas James Watkins (1863–1925).

Watson, Francis Sedgwick (1853–1942) Boston surgeon who described median perineal prostatectomy in 1889.

Watson, Henry (1702–1793) Lecturer in anatomy and a surgeon to the Westminster Hospital. He wrote a treatise on the bladder.

Watson, James Dewey (b 1928) American biologist from Chicago who worked with Francis Harry Crick (b 1918) and discovered the structure of DNA at the Cavendish Laboratory in Cambridge, England in 1953. He and Crick received the Nobel Prize for Medicine or Physiology in 1962. He wrote a personal account of the discovery, *The Double Helix* in 1968. *See deoxyribonucleic acid (DNA).*

Watson, John Broadus (1878–1958) American psychologist from Greenville, South Carolina. He was a professor at the Johns Hopkins University where he did research on behaviorism. His *An Introduction to Comparative Psychology* was published in 1913.

Watson, John (1807–1863) New York surgeon who performed esophagotomy for esophageal stricture in 1844.

Watson, Sir Patrick Heron (1832–1908) British surgeon who graduated from Edinburgh (1853) and served in the Crimea. He returned to Edinburgh and was a lecturer in military surgery and venereal diseases. He served on the General Medical Council for 25 years and was also a member of the University Commission. He was a pioneer of thyroid surgery.

Watson, Sir William (1715–1787) English scientist, born in London and educated at the Merchant Taylors School. After his apprenticeship under an apothecary, he set up his own practice in London. He studied electricity and discovered insulating conductors for use in increasing charge and investigated the passage of electricity through a rarefied gas, for which he was awarded the Copley Medal by the Royal Society in 1745. He was given an MD by the University of Halle in 1757 and was physician to the Foundling Hospital in London in 1762. He was admitted to the Royal College of Physicians in 1784 and knighted in 1786.

Watson–Crick Model *See deoxyribonucleic acid (DNA).*

Watt, Robert (1774–1819) Physician from Ayrshire who was president of the faculty of physicians and surgeons at Glasgow. He compiled *Bibliotheca Britannica* (1819) and a *Catalogue of Medical Books* (1812) and wrote several medical treatises.

Watts, James (1736–1819) English scientist and pioneer of pneumotherapy with Thomas Beddoes (1760–1808).

Watts, James Winston (b 1904) *See prefrontal leucotomy.*

Weale, Job Apothecary from Kingston-upon-Thames in the 17th century who became a licentiate of medicine and member of the London Society in 1637.

Weatherall, Sir David John (b 1933) English molecular geneticist who worked at the Johns Hopkins Medical School, the University of Liverpool and became Nuffield professor of clinical medicine at Oxford in 1974. He studied thalassemias and his work greatly improved the clinical outcome and prediction.

Webbed Fingers *See Zeller operation.*

Weber, Adolf (1829–1915) Ophthalmologist from Darmstadt in Germany who described the blockage of the Schlemm canal as a cause of glaucoma in 1877.

Weber, Ernst Heinrich (1795–1878) German physiologist and one of the three brothers who were professors at Leipzig. He showed that digestive juices are products of glands and opened this as an area of research. The inhibitory action of the vagus nerve on the heart was demonstrated by him and his brother Friedrich Weber (1806–1871) in 1845. His other brother, Wilhelm Eduard Weber (1804–1891), was a pioneer in electromagnetism.

Weber, Frederick Parkes (1863–1962) American professor of applied therapeutics at Temple University, Philadelphia. He described Osler–Rendu–Weber syndrome of multiple telengiectasis of the skin and mucous membranes in 1907; Weber–Christian disease of non-suppurative nodular panniculitis associated with phagocytic ingestion of fat cells by macrophages in 1925; and the Sturge–Weber syndrome with right sided congenital hemiplegia accompanied by left side brain lesions in 1922.

Weber, Sir Herman (1823–1918) London physician of German origin who graduated from Bonn in 1846. He described the syndrome of hemiplegia with contralateral paralysis of the oculomotor nerve secondary to lesion in the cerebral peduncle (Weber syndrome) in 1863.

Weber, Wilhelm Eduard (1804–1891) Physicist at Göttingen and brother of Ernst Weber. He built his own laboratory at the University of Leipzig, invented an electrodynometer and made several contributions to electromagnetism.

Weber Artery External auditory artery arising from the tymphanic branch of the external carotid. Described in 1845 by a professor of anatomy at Bonn, Moritz Ignaz Weber (1795–1875) from Bavaria.

Weber–Christian Disease *See Weber, Frederick Parkes.*

Weber Glands Lateral glands of the tongue named after Ernst Heinrich Weber (1795–1878), professor of physiology at Leipzig.

Weber Syndrome *See Weber, Sir Herman.*

Weber Test Test for deafness using a tuning fork. Devised by German otologist, Friedrich Eugen Weber (1832–1891).

Webster, John Clarence (1863–1950) American gynecologist born in Shediac, New Brunswick in Canada and qualified in medicine from Edinburgh University in 1896. He was professor of obstetrics at the Rush Medical College, Chicago in 1899, before returning to Canada in 1919. He described an operation for retroversion of the uterus in 1901.

Wechsler–Bellevue Test *See intelligence tests.*

Weed, Lewis Hill (1886–1952) American neurologist who advanced the theory of cerebrospinal fluid circulation proposed by Gustav Retzius (1842–1919) and showed that the fluid was absorbed by arachnoid villi, in 1914.

Weeks, John Elmer (1853–1949) New York ophthalmologist who discovered the bacillus (Koch–Weeks bacillus, *Haemophilus aegyptius*) of epidemic mucopurulent bilateral conjunctivitis (pink disease) in 1886, independent of Robert Koch's (1843–1910) description (1883).

Wegener Granulomatosis Described by H. Klinger of Germany in 1931. German pathologist, Friedrich Wegener (b 1907) described the pathological and clinical aspects as a variant of polyarteritis nodosa in 1936. It was further described by J. Churg and G.C. Godman in 1954.

Wegner Disease Osteochondritic separation of the epiphyses due to secondary syphilis. Described by German pathologist, Friedrich Rudolf Georg Wegner (1843–1917).

Weichselbaum, Anton (1845–1920) Austrian pathologist who isolated meningococcus or *Diplococcus intercellularis meningitides* from the cerebrospinal fluid of patients with meningitis, in 1887.

Weigert, Karl (1845–1904) German pathologist and a cousin of Paul Ehrlich (1854–1915). He devised some of the earliest

and best staining methods for studying bacteria and histological tissues, such as the myelin sheath (1884) and elastic fibers (1898). He showed the association between myasthenia and the thymus in 1901 and gave an account of myocardial infarction in 1880. A classical description of pathological anatomy in Bright disease was given by him in 1879.

Weil Disease Leptospirosis was described by Jeffrey Alen Marston (1831–1911) in 1863. German physician, Adolf Weil (1848–1916), published four cases of infectious jaundice with hemorrhage in 1886. The causative agent, *Leptospira icterohemorrhagia*, was identified independently in 1915 by Ryukichi Inado (1874–1950) and Yutaka Ido (1881–1919) of Japan.

Weil Test Obsolete test for hemolysis. Based on the observation that erythrocytes of syphilitic patients are resistant to the hemolysing effect of cobra venom. Devised in 1915 by New York physician, Richard Weil (1876–1917).

Weil–Felix Reaction Agglutinin reaction for diagnosis of typhus devised by Prague bacteriologist, Arthur Felix (1887–1956) and German physician, Edmund Weil (1880–1922) in 1916. They noticed the presence of a proteus-like organism in urine of a patient with typhus and demonstrated that this (which they named 'proteus X') agglutinated sera of other patients with typhus. Their test was later applied to differentiate between various rickettsial diseases.

Weill Sign Absence of expansion in the subclavicular region of the affected side in infantile pneumonia. Described by French pediatrician, Edmond Weill (1858–1924).

Weinberg, Robert Allan (b 1942) American biochemist from Pittsburgh who was educated at MIT and became associate professor of the Department of Biology and Center for Cancer Research and then professor of biochemistry there. He works on causes of cancer due to acquisition of cancer-susceptible genes and loss of tumor suppresser genes and discovered the Rb1 suppresser gene responsible for a rare childhood cancer which affects the retina.

Weinberg Test A diagnostic serology test for echinococcus. Described by Paris physician, Michel Weinberg (1868–1940) in 1909.

Weingarten Syndrome *See tropical pulmonary eosonophilia.*

Weir Mitchell Disease Erythromelalgia. Silas Weir Mitchell (1829–1914), a leading American neurologist at Philadelphia, described erythromelalgia associated with painful feet in 1872. He also established a rest cure for psychoneurosis which became popular in the 19th century.

Weir Mitchell, Silas (1829–1914) Born in Philadlphia, he was a graduate of Jefferson Medical College (1851). On graduating, he went to Europe and studied in Paris with Claude Bernard (1813–1878). He did extensive work on arrow poisons and snake venom with William Hammond (1828–1900), William Williams Keen (1837–1932) and Simon Flexner (1863–1946). He was also a leading neurologist who proposed 'rest cure' for psychoneurosis, and identified eye strain as a cause of headache. During the American Civil War he worked at the Turner's Lane Hospital in Philadelphia and wrote *Gunshot Woulds and Other Injuries of the Nerves* which included data on phantom limbs. He also described erythromelagia, post-paralysis chorea and the role of the cerebellum.

Weiss, Soma (1898–1942) *See carotid sinus syndrome.*

Weismann, August Friedrich Leopold (1834–1914) German zoologist from Jena who proposed the chromosome theory of heredity. He observed, in 1892, aggregation of self-propagating hereditary materials which are transmitted to offspring through germ cells.

Weiss Reflex Curved reflex seen with the ophthalmoscope on the nasal side of the disk in the fundus. Described by Viennese physician, Nathan Weiss (1851–1883).

Weiss, Robin (b 1940) English molecular biologist and head of the Imperial Cancer Research Chester Beatty Laboratory. He works on the role of retroviruses in causing cancer and on the HIV virus and its mechanism of entry into the cell.

Weitbrecht, Josias (1702–1747) German professor of anatomy at St Petersburg in Russia. He described several anatomical structures which now bear his name: Weitbrecht fibers, retinacular fibers of the neck of femur; Weitbrecht foramen of ovale which is a gap between the capsule of the shoulder joint and the glenohumeral ligament; and the Weitbrecht ligament or the oblique radioulnar ligament.

Welander Ulcer Chancroid or chancre found in the vulva but of nonvenereal etiology. Described by Edward Wilhelm Welander (1840–1917), a physician at Stockholm.

Welch, Francis Henry (1840–1910) English physician who described syphilitic aortitis in 1876.

Welch, William Henry (1850–1934) American pathologist who graduated from Columbia University in 1875 and worked in Europe before his appointment as a pathologist at Bellevue Hospital, New York. He was the first professor of pathology at the medical school at Johns Hopkins Hospital

in 1889. He identified the causative organism (*Clostridium welchii*) of gas gangrene in 1892.

Welcker, Hermann (1822–1897) Austrian physician and anthropologist who was professor of anatomy at Giessen. He was director of the Anatomical Institute at Heidelberg for a short period before he succeeded Volkman at Giessen. The angle of the basicranial axis, described by him in 1882, bears his name.

Welfare State The concept of providing a complete preventive and curative facility to the people on a national scale was proposed by Johan Peter Frank (1745–1821), a German physician and medical reformer. He outlined his ideas in *System of Complete Medical Police* published between 1779 and 1825.

Wellcome Institute for the History of Medicine Established by Sir Henry Wellcome. Systematic purchasing for the library started in 1897 and its museum was established in 1903. It purchased the William Morris collection of incunabula in 1898, and the library of J. F. Payne, a medical historian, in 1911. It opened its doors to the public in 1949. The library and museum were transferred to the Wellcome Trust in 1960 and reunited under one administration in 1964. The trust was converted to the Wellcome Institute for the History of Medicine in 1968. The library at Euston Road is one of the largest on History of Medicine in Europe.

Wellcome, Sir Henry Solomon (1853–1936) American pharmacist and founder of Wellcome Foundation. In 1880 he and M. Burroughs started Burroughs Wellcome in London. Burroughs died in 1895 and Wellcome became naturalized as a British citizen in 1910. He formed the Wellcome Foundation in 1924 and was knighted in 1932. He endowed the profits of his company in his will to the Wellcome Trust for promoting research in medicine.

Weller, Thomas Huckle (b 1915) American virologist from Ann Arbor in Michigan. He studied zoology at Michigan and did research at Harvard on cell cultivation. He worked at the Children's Hospital in Boston on *Schistosoma* and poliomyelitis cell cultivation. He shared the Nobel Prize for Physiology or Medicine in 1954 for his work on the chickenpox and shingles virus. *See filterable viruses.*

Wells, Horace (1815–1848) American dentist at Hartford, Connecticut who introduced nitrous oxide as an anesthetic. He arranged a demonstration of the gas at the Massachusetts General Hospital on December 12, 1844 which failed and he was subject to ridicule. He continued to use it with success for a few years but became addicted to chloroform and joined a touring troop with performing canaries.

Wells, Sir Thomas Spencer (1818–1897) British surgeon and gynecologist who worked in Malta and the Crimea as a naval surgeon (1841–1848). He joined the Samaritan Hospital in 1854 and performed his first hysterectomy for myoma in 1861. A spleenectomy was performed by him in 1865 and his patient lived for six days. He performed a complete ovariotomy in 1858 and by 1880 he had done over 1000. Forcipressure, a method of crushing blood vessels by forceps to arrest bleeding during surgery, was devised by him using forceps invented for the purpose and later named Spencer Wells forceps. He was surgeon to the royal household in 1863 and knighted in 1883.

Wells, William Charles (1757–1817) American scientist and physician from Charleston, South Carolina. He graduated from Edinburgh University and practiced in London where he was physician to St Thomas' Hospital from 1800 to 1817. His important contributions include: an essays on dew in 1814; a treatise on vision; and suggestions on the theory of natural selection. He also showed that the coloring matter in blood was a complex organic substance of iron in 1797, demonstrated the presence of albumin and blood in the urine of patients with renal dropsy in 1812 and described rheumatic nodules in 1810.

Wellwood, Thomas (1652–1716) Scottish physician from Edinburgh, educated at Glasgow. He became King William's physician in Scotland and practiced in Edinburgh.

Welsh Medicine Initially the practice, like most other nations, was in the hands of the priests or Gwyddoniaid (old Welsh for men of knowledge). During the reign of Prydain, the Gwyddoniaid were divided into three orders, Bards, Druids, and Ovates. Ovates were mainly concerned with the study of natural sciences. Medicine, commerce and navigation were the three civil arts in the laws of Dyvnwal Moelmud.

Welsh Cells Cells of the parathyroid glands were described by Scottish professor of pathology at Edinburgh, David Arthur Welsh (1875–1948) in 1898.

Wenckebach Phenomenon A form of progressive atrioventricular heart block until a drop in ventricular beat occurred. Described by Dutch physician working in Vienna, Karel Frederick Wenckebach (1864–1940) in 1899. He also wrote on the beneficial effects of quinine in arrhythmias.

Wenzel, Carl (1769–1827) German surgeon who used artificial induction of premature labor in 1804.

Wenzel, Joseph (1768–1808) German professor of anatomy and physiology at Mainz. He described ventriculus cerebri primus, Wenzel ventricle.

Wepfer, Johann Jacobus (1620–1695) German physician from Schaffhausen and father-in-law of Johan Brunner (1653–1727) whose name (Brunner glands) is associated with the duodenal glands. Wepfer practiced at Basel and was physician to several German princes. He showed in 1658 that cerebral hemorrhage was a cause of apoplexy (stroke) in four cases at postmortem.

Werder, Xavier Oswald (1858–1919) American surgeon who described a radical method of hysterectomy for cancer of the cervix in 1898. His method involved the total removal of vagina and uterus by suprapubic approach.

Werdnig–Hoffman Syndrome Infantile familial form of progressive spinal muscular atrophy. Described independently by Austrian neurologist, Guido Werdnig (1844–1919) at Berlin and German neurologist Johann Hoffmann (1857–1919) in 1891.

Werewolf *See lycanthropia.*

Werlhof Disease Thrombocytopenic purpura. Described as purpura hemorrhagica by German physician, Paul Gottlieb Werlhof (1699–1767) in 1735. *See purpura.*

Werlhof, Paul Gottlieb (1699–1767) A medical graduate of the University of Helmstedt in 1723 who became physician to the court of Hannover in 1760. He also composed poetry and hymns. *See Werlhof disease.*

Wermer Syndrome Multiple adenomatous hyperplasia of the anterior pituitary gland, parathyroid glands, thyroid gland and multiple tumors of the islands of Langerhans. Described by New York physician, Paul Wermer (1898–1975) in 1954.

Werner, Alfred (1866–1919) Swiss inorganic chemist who demonstrated isomerism in inorganic and organic chemistry. He received the Nobel Prize for Chemistry in 1913. *See isomerism.*

Werner Syndrome Hereditary disorder consisting of cataract, osteoporosis, premature graying of hair, short stature and sexual underdevelopment. Described by German physician C. W. Otto Werner (1879–1936) in 1904.

Werner Syndrome Disorder characterized by polydactyly, absence of thumbs and tibia and reduced knee movements. Described by P. Werner in 1919.

Wernicke Area Sensory speech center in the posterior third of the gyrus temporalis superior. Described by German neuropsychiatrist and professor of psychiatry at Breslau, Karl Wernicke (1848–1905) in 1881.

Wernicke Encephalopathy Ophthalmoplegia, nystagmus and confabulation due to thiamin deficiency. Described by German neuropsychiatrist and professor of psychiatry at Breslau, Karl Wernicke (1848–1905).

Wertheim, Ernst (1864–1920) German gynecologist and director of the gynecology department of the Elizabeth Hospital in Vienna. He devised the method of radical panhysterectomy for cervical cancer in 1898.

Werthheim Ointment Used for chloasma and contains ammoniated mercury and bismuth. Formulated by Viennese physician, Gustav Werthheim (1822–1888).

Wesbrook Classification Applied for diphtheria bacilli. Proposed by American physician, Frank Fairchild Wesbrook (1868–1919) of Minneapolis in 1900.

West, Charles (1816–1898) *See Great Ormond Street Hospital.*

Westergren Method Used for determining erythrocyte sedimentation rate (ESR) and devised by Swedish physician, Alf Wilhelm Westergren (b 1891) in 1921.

Westminster Hospital Founded in 1716 by public subscription and initially situated opposite Westminster Abbey and moved in 1939.

Westphal, Carl Friedrich Otto (1833–1890) German neuropsychiatrist born in Berlin where he studied medicine before he became professor of psychiatry there in 1874. He described agoraphobia in 1871, and demonstrated the absence of knee jerk reflex in tabes dorsalis with Wilhelm Erb (1840–1921) in 1875. The nucleus of the third cranial nerve (Edinger–Westphal nucleus) was described by him in 1887. His son, Alexander Westphal, was a professor of neurology at Heidelberg and Berlin.

Westphal Syndrome *See periodic paralysis.*

Westphal–Strümpell Disease Pseudosclerosis of the brain (probably Kinnier-Wilson disease) was described by Carl Friedrich Otto Westphal (1833–1890) in 1883 and Ernst Adolf Gustav Gottfried Strümpell (1853–1925) in 1898.

Weyer, Johan (1516–1588) *See witchcraft.*

Weyle Test Detects creatinine using sodium nitroprusside as reagent. Devised by French chemist, Theodor Weyle (1851–1913).

Wharton, Thomas (1616–1673) English physician who

remained on duty at St Thomas' Hospital in London during the great plague of 1666. He studied at Oxford and Cambridge and obtained his MD from Oxford in 1647. He discovered the duct of submaxillary glands (Wharton duct) and gave a description of the thyroid gland in 1656. He also described the mucoid connective tissue which forms the basic substance of the umbilical cord (Wharton jelly). His *Adenographia, sive glandularum totius corporis descriptio* was published in 1656.

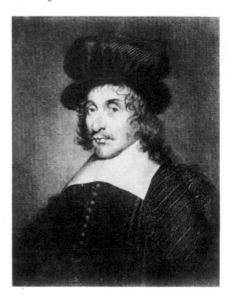

Thomas Wharton (1616–1673). Courtesy of the National Library of Medicine

Wharton Duct *See Wharton, Thomas.*

Wharton Jelly *See Wharton, Thomas.*

Wheatstone, Sir Charles (1801–1875) Physicist from Gloucester. He was professor of philosophy at King's College in 1834, and he invented a sound magnifier, for which he coined the term microphone. He invented the Wheatstone bridge, a device that enabled the galvanometer to measure large electrical current.

Wheeler, Claude Lamont (1864–1916) Editor of *New York Medical Journal* which was published from 1865 to 1925.

Wheeler, John Martin (18791–938) New York ophthalmologist who described several procedures for various eye conditions including glaucoma and ectropion.

Wheelhouse, Claudius Galen (1826–1909) *See urethral stricture.*

Wherry, William Buchanan (1874–1936) American bacteriologist who isolated the causative organism of tularemia in a human in 1914.

Whiplash Injury Noticed in the 19th century with the introduction of high speed railway travel and described in 1866 by Sir John Eric Erichson (1818–1896) of University College, London.

Whipple, Allen Oldfather (1881–1963) New York surgeon who did a pancreatoduodenectomy for cancer of the pancreas in 1935.

Whipple, George Hoyt (1878–1976) American pathologist from New Hampshire who graduated from the Johns Hopkins University where he later served for 9 years. He was appointed professor of pathology at the University of California in 1914. He showed that iron was an important component of red blood cells in 1925 and that eating liver could cure pernicious anemia (with Frieda Saur Robscheit-Robbins, b 1893) and increase hemoglobin in 1925. He shared the Nobel Prize for Physiology or Medicine with George Richards Minot (1885–1950) and William Parry Murphy (1892–1987) in 1934.

Whipple Disease Characterized by deposit of fats and fatty acids in the intestinal lymphatic tissues. Described as 'Intestinal lipodystrophy' in 1907 by American physician, George Hoyt Whipple (1878–1976) of Rochester, New York.

Whipple Triad Hyperinsulinemia with fasting hypoglycemia and recovery after administration of glucose and recurrence of the attack on fasting. Described by New York physician, George Hoyt Whipple (1878–1976).

Whipworm *See trichuris.*

Whistler, Daniel (1619–1684) *See rickets.*

Whitby, Sir Lionel Ernest Howard (1895–1938) Regius professor of medicine at the University of Cambridge. He proved the efficacy of sulfapyridine in treatment of pneumococcal pneumonia in 1938.

White, Anthony (1782–1849) London surgeon who described the excision of the femur for disease of the hip joint in 1838.

White Blood Cell Count *See leukocyte count.*

White Blood Cell *See leukocytes.*

White, Charles (1728–1813) *See dislocation of shoulder joint.*

White, Paul Dudley (1886–1973) American cardiologist who graduated from Harvard. He studied for a year with Sir Thomas Lewis (1881–1945) in London. Almost his entire career was spent at the Massachusetts General Hospital and he wrote his first book on heart diseases in 1931. He treated

President Eisenhower for a myocardial infarction. Wolf–Parkinson–White syndrome (WPW syndrome) due to an accessory conduction pathway which predisposes to cardiac arrhythmia was described by him in 1930. *See Wolf–Parkinson–White syndrome.*

White, William Hale (1857–1949) Physician at Guy's Hospital in 1890 who wrote treatises on materia medica, pharmacy, pharmacology and therapeutics (*Hale-White*) that ran to 26 editions. He also wrote *Great Doctors of the nineteenth century* in 1935 and *Keats as a Doctor and patient* in 1938.

White Disease Keratosis follicularis was described in 1889 by Boston dermatologist, James Clark White (1833–1916).

White Operation Castration for hypertrophy of the prostate. Devised in 1894 by Philadelphia surgeon, J. William White (1850–1916).

Whitechapel Hospital *See London Hospital.*

Whitehead, John (1740–1804) Lancashire physician who graduated from Leiden in 1780 and practiced in London. He attended John Wesley during his last illness and wrote his biography. He also wrote *A Report of a new, easy and successful method of treating Child-bed or Puerperal Fever, made use of by M. Doulcet* in 1783.

Whitehead Operation A one stage procedure for extensive cleft of the hard and soft palate. Devised by New York surgeon, William Riddick Whitehead (1831–1902) in 1871.

Whitehead, Walter (1840–1913) English surgeon who described a method of total removal of the tongue with scissors in 1877.

Whitfield Ointment Benzoic and salicylic acid, used for treatment of fungal infections. Formulated by London dermatologist, Arthur Whitfield (1867–1947). He graduated from King's College in 1892 where he was professor of dermatology in 1906.

Whitley Council Takes its origin from the Committee on the Relations between Employers and Employed set up in England in 1916 under the chairmanship of J.H. Whitley who was later speaker at the House of Commons.

Whitlow 'An abscess forming about the root of the nail' according to Paul of Aegina (625–690). Aetius, Oribasius (325–403) and other ancient physicians also described it and recommended application of astringents such as arsenic, quick lime and flakes of copper. Avicenna (980–1037) described it in detail and recommended immersing the finger into hot vinegar during its early stages. When it is fully formed he advised incision of the abscess.

Whitman, Royal (1857–1946) An orthopedic surgeon at the Hospital for Ruptured and Crippled in New York City who described an operation for ununited fracture of the neck of the femur in 1921. He was also well known for his work on flat-foot.

Whitmore Bacillus Causative organism of melidiosis. Described by Alfred Whitmore (b 1876) and Indian physician, C.S. Krishnaswami in 1912.

Whitnall Tubercle Found on the zygomatic bone and described by Samuel Ernest Whitnall (1876–1950) from Manchester while he was professor of anatomy at McGill University in Canada in 1911.

Whooping Cough Described as 'tussis quintana' by Guillaume de Baillou (1538–1616) in 1578. A clear account where convulsive cough occurred was given by Thomas Willis (1621–1675) in 1675. The causative organism, *Bordetella pertussis*, was discovered by Belgian Nobel Prize winner, Jules Jean Baptiste Vincent Bordet (1870–1961), and French bacteriologist, Octave Gengou (1875–1957) in 1906. Work on a vaccine was done by Patrick Holt Leslie and Arthur Duncan Gardner (b 1884), and an effective vaccine was introduced by Pearl Kendrick (b 1890) and Grace Eldering in 1939.

Whytt, Robert (1714–1766) Scottish professor of medicine at Edinburgh and a pupil of Monroe. He described tuberculous meningitis in children in *Observations on Dropsy of the Brain* published in 1768. He was appointed physician to the king of Scotland and was president of the Royal College of Physicians, Edinburgh.

Whytt Disease Hydrocephalus due to tuberculous meningitis. Described by Robert Whytt (1714–1766), professor of medicine at Edinburgh.

Whytt Reflex *See pupillary reaction.*

Wiart Notch Impression on the pancreas made by the duodenum. Described by French anatomist at Paris, Pierre Wiart (b 1870) in 1899.

Wichmann Asthma Laryngismus stridulus. Described by German physician, Johann Ernst Wichmann (1740–1802).

Wickersheimer Fluid Arsenic trioxide, alcohol and glycerin mixture used for preserving anatomical specimens. Devised by German anatomist, J. Wickersheimer (1832–1896) of Berlin.

Wickman, Otto Ivar (1872–1914) *See acute anterior poliomy-elitis.*

Widal, Georges Ferdinand Isidore (1862–1929) French microbiologist and professor of pathology at Paris who was born in Algeria. He devised the Widal test for typhoid fever based on the agglutination reaction observed previously by Austrian bacteriologist, Max Franz Maria von Gruber (1853–1927) and Herbert Edward Durham (1866–1945) in 1894. Acquired hemolytic anemia, previously described by Georges Hayem (1841–1933) in 1898, was redescribed by Widal in 1907.

Widal Test *See Widal, Georges Ferdinand Isidore.*

Wieland, Heinrich Otto (1877–1957) German chemist who studied at the universities of Munich, Berlin and Stuttgart and received his PhD from Munich, where he spent much of his career. He studied bile acids which aid digestion of lipids and received the Nobel Prize for Chemistry in 1927 for this work. *See bile.*

Wiener, Alexander Solomon (b 1907) *See erythroblastosis fetalis.*

Wiener, Norbert (1894–1964) *See cybernetics, feedback mechanism.*

Wiesel, Torsten Nils (b 1924) Swedish neurophysiologist who graduated in medicine from the Karolinska Institute, Stockholm. He joined the Johns Hopkins Medical School in 1955 and became professor of neurobiology at Harvard Medical School in 1968. He shared the Nobel Prize for Physiology or Medicine for his work on neurophysiology of vision, with Roger Wolcott Sperry (b 1913) and David Hunter Hubel (b 1926) in 1981.

Wiesel Paraganglion Situated in the cardiac plexus of the nerves and described in 1902 by Josef Wiesel (1876–1928), professor of medicine at Vienna.

Wigand Maneuvre Used in breech delivery, described by German gynecologist, Justus Heinrich Wigand (1766–1817).

Wilde, Sir William Robert Wills (1815–1876) Irish surgeon and father of Oscar Wilde. He was an ophthalmologist at Dublin and was appointed surgeon–oculist to Queen Victoria in Ireland in 1853. He described the optical appearance on the external aspect of the membrana tymphani (Wilde cone) in 1853. He wrote *Epidemics of Ireland* in 1851.

Wilder, Russel Morse (1885–1959) *See insulin secreting tumors of pancreas, adrenal insufficiency.*

Wiley, Harvey Washington (1844–1930) American physician from Indiana and food chemist who worked towards the Pure Food and Drug Act of 1906. He published *Not by Bread Alone* in 1915.

Wilkie Artery Supraduodenal artery, described by Scottish professor of surgery at Edinburgh, David Percival Dalbreck Wilkie (1882–1938). He also described stenosis of the same artery complicated by duodenal ulcer (Wilkie syndrome) in 1911.

Wilkins, John (1614–1672) English clergyman from Daventry and a founder of the Royal Society. He married a widowed sister of Oliver Cromwell and was master of Trinity College in 1659. In *Discovery of a World in the Moon,* published in 1628, he discussed the possibilities of traveling to the moon on a flying-machine and inhabitants in the moon.

Wilkins, Maurice Hugh Frederick (b 1916) New Zealand-born British physicist who is known for his work on DNA X-ray crystallography. He was educated at Birmingham and St John's College Cambridge and was director of the Medical Research Council's Biophysics unit at King's College from 1970 to 1972. He shared the Nobel Prize for his elucidation of the structure of DNA with Francis Henry Crick (b 1918) and James Dewey Watson (b 1928) in 1962.

Wilks, Sir Samuel (1824–1911) English physician at Guy's Hospital, London. He was president of the Royal College of Physicians from 1866 to 1899, appointed physician-extraordinary to Queen Victoria in 1897 and was knighted in the same year. Some of his contributions to medicine include: a definite account of (Wilks syndrome) myasthenia gravis (1877); the relationship between renal conditions and nephrotic syndrome (1853); the causes and effects of pyemia or septicemia (1861); and a an account on alcoholic paraplegia (1868). Generalized hypertrophy of superficial and deep lymphatic glands, previously described by Hodgkin, was named Hodgkin disease by Wilks in 1856.

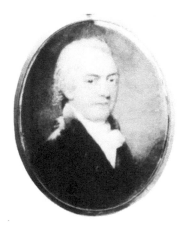

Robert Willan (1757–1812). Courtesy of the National Library of Medicine

Willan, Robert (1757–1812) Quaker physician from Yorkshire who wrote an early monograph, *On Cutaneous*

Diseases, in 1796 which was completed after his death by Thomas Bateman (1778–1821). He classified different kinds of eczema and other skin diseases.

Willebrand, Erik Adolf von (1870–1949) *See von Willebrand disease.*

William of Saliceto (1201–1277) Salicet was an Italian surgeon who wrote an important work on surgery and practiced dissections. He was born in Saliceto and studied medicine at the University of Bologna. He was chief of the local hospital in Verona in 1275 and completed his *Chyrurgia* in the same year, dedicated to his teacher the physician, Dino del Carbo.

Williams, Elkanah (1822–1888) American professor of ophthalmology at Miami Medical College, and younger brother of Henry Willard Williams (1821–1895). He made several significant contributions to his field.

Williams, Francis Henry (1852–1936) American physician who estimated the heart size using a fluoroscope in 1896. This was the first application of X-rays to cardiology.

Williams, Henry Willard (1821–1895) American ophthalmologist at Boston and professor at Harvard in 1871. He designed a special lantern to test color vision. He introduced the method of suturing the flap after cataract excision in 1865.

Williams, John Whitridge (1866–1931) Boston obstetrician who reported a case of choriocarcinoma in 1895. He published a textbook of obstetrics for students and practitioners in 1903.

Williams Sign Dull tymphanitic resonance over the second intercostal space in cases of large pleural effusion. Described by English physician, Charles Williams (1805–1889).

Williamson, Alexander William (1824–1904) London chemist who studied at Heidelberg and Giessen before being appointed professor of chemistry at University College, London in 1849. His main research was on the relationship between alcohol and esters, and catalysts. *See catalysis.*

Williamson, Hugh (1735–1819) Pennsylvania physician who studied medicine at Edinburgh and Leiden. He returned to Philadelphia and served in the revolutionary army after which he was elected to Congress. He wrote *Observations on the Climate of America* and several other works.

Williamson, William Crawford (1816–1895) English paleobotanist and surgeon, born in Scarborough and became professor of geology and natural history at Owen's College, Manchester in 1851. He investigated plant fossils in coal and is regarded as father of paleobotany in England.

Willis, Francis Lincolnshire physician who treated mental disorders in the 18th century. He obtained his MA from Oxford in 1740 and entered holy orders before he took medicine. He established a private asylum for the mentally ill at Greatford in Lincolnshire. He treated King George III during his illness and predicted a good prognosis for the king. His son, Robert Darling Willis (1760–1821) and grandson, Francis Willis (1792–1859) were also physicians who practiced psychiatry.

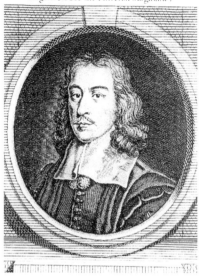

Thomas Willis (1621–1675). Courtesy of the National Library of Medicine

Willis, Thomas (1621–1675) English physician, Sedleian professor of natural philosophy at Oxford (1660), and a founder of the Royal Society, born at Great Bedwyn in Wiltshire. He was educated at Christ Church, Oxford and took his medical degree in 1660. He made several important contributions to medicine including his description of the arterial supply to the base of the brain (circle of Willis) in *Cerebri anatome nervorum que descriptio et usus,* published in 1664; a description of epidemic typhoid fever in *De febribus* in 1659; and of the symptoms in achalasia cardia and its treatment in *Pharmaceutica Rationalis* in 1674. He introduced the concept of 'involuntary' and 'voluntary' or 'volitional' movements in 1664.

Willow Members of the plant genus *Salix,* used since the time of Dioscorides (AD 40–90) who described it in his *Materia medica.* He prescribed leaves mixed with pepper and wine in cases of diseased intestines; fruit for blood spitting; burnt bark with vinegar for warts; and a decoction or fermentation for gout. The bark is a rich source of salicylic

acid (aspirin) and has been used as an analgesic for thousands of years.

Wilms Tumor Embryonic tumor of the kidney described by German professor of surgery at Leipzig, Max Wilms (1867–1918) in 1899.

Wilson, Samuel Alexander Kinnier (1877–1937) Born to Irish parents in America and graduated from Edinburgh. He was neurologist to King's College Hospital and founded the *Journal of Neurology and Psychopathology* in 1920. See *Kinnier Wilson disease.*

Wilson, Charles McMoran (1882–1977) Physician and dean of St Mary's Medical School from 1920 to 1945. He was physician to Winston Churchill and wrote *Winston Churchill, The Struggle for Survival* in 1966.

Wilson, Charles Thompson Rees (1869–1959) Scottish pioneer of atomic and nuclear physics from Glencorse near Edinburgh. He developed the cloud chamber for studying atomic particles in 1897. He was professor of natural philosophy at Cambridge from 1925 to 1934. He shared the Nobel Prize for Physics in 1927 for his work on ionization of water.

Wilson, Edmund Beecher (1856–1939) American zoologist and embryologist from Geneva, Illinois. He studied at Yale and Johns Hopkins Universities and was professor of zoology at Columbia University, New York. He pioneered microdissection and described androgenesis or male parthenogenesis in 1928.

Wilson, Edward Adrian (1872–1912) English physician and explorer from Cheltenham. He took part in the Antarctic expedition with Scott in the *Discovery* from 1900 to 1904. He died with the other crew members on their return journey from the South Pole.

Wilson, James (1765–1821) English surgeon and teacher at Hunter's school of anatomy at Great Windmill Street, London. In 1812 he described the muscle fibers derived from the levator ani surrounding the urethra found above the triangular ligament (Wilson muscles).

Wilson, Sir James Erasmus (1809–1884) London dermatologist who described dermatitis exfoliativa in 1890. He established dermatology as a specialty in England and classified cutaneous disorders. He wrote *Treatise on Diseases of the Skin* (1842), a dermatological atlas (1847) and a dissector's manual in 1838. He donated £5000 to the Royal College of Surgeons to create a chair of dermatology. He paid for the transport of the obelisk known as Cleopatra's needle from Egypt to London.

Wilson Disease Hepatolenticular degeneration due to abnormality of copper metabolism. Described by British neurologist, Samuel Alexander Kinnier Wilson (1874–1937) in 1912. *See Kayser–Fleischer ring.*

Wilson, Louis Blanchard (1866–1943) American physician from Rochester, Minnesota who devised a method of staining sections of live tissue.

Wilson Muscles *See Wilson, James.*

Winckel Disease Characterized by icterus, bloody urine and hemorrhage with a fatal outcome in neonates. Described in 1879 by Munich gynecologist, Franz Karl Ludwig von Winckel (1837–1911).

Windaus, Adolf (1876–1959) Berlin-born German chemist known for his work on the structure of cholesterol, for which he was awarded the Nobel Prize in 1928. He also discovered that light activates ergosterol, converting it to vitamin D2. He also did research on cardiac poisons.

Wine Fermented liquid, generally produced from grapes. Pliny the Elder described 116 different types of wine around AD 50. Plutrach (AD 46–120) said it was the most palatable table medicine. Nicander in 100 BC advocated undiluted wine as a remedy for poisoning by hemlock. It was also used as a stimulant, aphrodisiac, analgesic and anesthetic for centuries. Mandrake wine was used as an anesthetic to perform surgery by Dioscorides (AD 40–90) and was the most popular anesthetic during Middle Ages. Paul of Aegina (625–690) recommended wine for several medical conditions. Arnold of Villanova in the 13th century discussed the role of wine in diet and its use as medication. Brandy obtained by distillation of wine was called the elixir of life by him and he introduced it into pharmacopoeia. *See alcohol.*

Winiwarter, Alexander (1848–1916) *See cholecystenterostomy.*

Winiwarter, Felix von (1852–1931) *See Buerger disease.*

Winslow, Jacob Benignus (1669–1760) Danish anatomist who became professor of physick, surgery and anatomy at the University of Paris and wrote a book in 1733 on descriptive anatomy which disregarded previous hypothetical explanations. The foramen between the greater and lesser sac is named after him. He gave the name 'grand sympathetic' to the ganglion chain and called the smaller branches 'lesser sympathetic'.

Winston, Thomas (1575–1655) English physician who was educated at Cambridge and received his MD from Padua. He established himself in practice in London and was professor of physick at Gresham College. His anatomical lectures were printed in 1650.

Winterbottom, Thomas Masterman (1765–1859) English physician from South Shields who graduated from Glasgow University in 1792 and practiced for 4 years in Sierra Leone, Africa. He described African trypanosomiasis or sleeping sickness in 1803 which he observed during his travels.

Winthrop, John (1588–1649) Governor of Massachusetts, medical reformer and father of paper currency in America.

Winthrop, John (1714–1779) Descendant of John Winthrop (1588–1649) and professor of mathematics at Harvard who founded the first laboratory for experimental physics in America at Harvard in 1746.

Wintrich Sign A change in pitch of the percussion note when the mouth is opened or closed in cases of pulmonary cavity. Described by German physician, Anton Wintrich (1812–1882).

Wintringham, Sir Clifton (1710–1794) Son of a physician from York with the same name who resided in Hammersmith. He wrote *An Experimental Inquiry concerning some parts of the Animal Structure* (1740), *An Inquiry into the Exility of the Human Body* (1743) and other works.

Wintrobe Tube Measures erythrocyte sedimentation rate. Devised by Canadian-born American hematologist, Maxwell Myer Wintrobe (1901–1986) who graduated from the University of Manitoba in 1926.

Wirsung Duct Ductus pancreaticus described by Johann Georg Wirsung (1600–1643) of Bavaria who was professor at Padua in 1642. He was assassinated in 1632 at Padua over the priority of the discovery of the pancreatic duct.

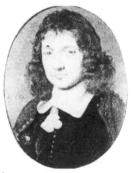

Richard Wiseman (1622–1676). Courtesy of the National Library of Medicine

Wise, Thomas Alexander (1802–1889) Graduated in medicine from Edinburgh in 1824 and wrote *The Pathology of Blood*, *The Hindu System of Medicine*, *Diseases of the Eye*, *Cholera* and *History of Medicine*.

Wiseman, Richard (1622–1676) British surgeon to the

Dutch Navy (1643) who became surgeon to James I and Charles II. He was known as the Pride of England and published *Several Chirugical Treatises* in 1676 and published the first recorded postmortem in the same year, on a patient from the Bethlem Hospital.

Wiseman Syndrome Primary splenic anemia related to congenital hemolytic anemia. Described by American physician, Bruce Kenneth Wiseman (b 1898) of Ohio in 1942.

Wiskott–Aldrich Syndrome Disorder characterized by thrombocytopenic purpura and susceptibility to staphylo-coccal infection due to antibody deficiency. Described by German pediatrician, Alfred Wiskott (1898–1978) in 1937. The familial nature of the disorder due to X-linked recessive trait was shown by American pediatrician, Robert Anderson Aldrich (b 1917) in 1954. He was son of another pediatrician (C.A. Aldrich) at the Mayo Clinic and was professor of pediatrics at the University of Colorado, Denver in 1970.

Wistar Institute Named after American anatomist, Caspar Wistar (1760–1818), who wrote an early book on anatomy.

Witchcraft Superstition and magic prevailed in medical practice for thousands of years until Hippocrates (460–377 BC) established medicine on a rational basis. Insanity was confused with witchcraft during medieval and earlier times, and the insane were subjected to whipping, starving and execution. Reginald Scott (1538–1599), a politician from Kent, identified insanity and depression (melancholy) in 1584 amongst those accused of witchcraft in England. A notorious book on witch hunting, *Malleus Maleficarum*, was written by Johann Sprenger and Heinrich Kraemer in 1497. Although it contained absurd theories it was accepted by the church and was used at the faculty of theology at the University of Cologne. In 1515 about 500 people accused of witchcraft were burnt in Geneva and thousands were sent to death in France. One of the first medical persons to publicly oppose witchhunting was Belgian physician, Johan Weir or Weyer (1516–1588) who published *De Praestigiis Daemonum et incantationibus ac Veneficiis* in 1563. An early treatise on witchcraft was by English physician, William Drage (1637–1669) of Hitchin, Hertfordshire in 1665. Witchhunting continued into the 16th and 17th century and thousands were killed. In America, Cotton Mather (1663–1728) also believed in the evils of witchcraft and 19 were hanged in Salem, Massachusetts.

Withering, William (1741–1799) English physician from Wellington, Shropshire who graduated from Edinburgh with a thesis 'Malignant Putrid Sore Throat' in 1765. He was a great botanist and he wrote *A Botanical Arrangement of all the vegetables Naturally Growing in Great Britain* in 1776. He learnt the value of digitalis in dropsy from a female patient and herbalist, Mrs Hutton from Shropshire, and tried it on patients around 1770. He was a junior physician to Birmingham Hospital in 1775 and continued to use digitalis. By 1779 his cure for dropsy with digitalis became well known and he wrote *An Account of the Foxglove, and Some of its Medical Uses, with Practical Remarks on Dropsy, and other Diseases* in 1785.

Wits Defined by Spanish philosopher, Juan Huarte in 1594 as man's ability for one science but incapability for another. *Concerning the different wits of men* was written by Walter Charleton (1619–1707) of London who was physician to Charles I and II.

Wittgenstein, Ludwig (1889–1951) Professor of philosophy at Cambridge who left Nazi Germany in protest at the Nazi genocide. He gave up his position as a professor at Cambridge and worked as a dispensary porter at Guy's Hospital during the aerial bombings in 1941. He wrote several works on the Nuremberg trials.

Witzel Operation Method of gastrotomy through a thoracic incision. Described by German surgeon, Friedrich Oskar Witzel (1856–1925).

Wölfler Gland Accessory thyroid gland described by German professor of surgery at Graz, Anton Wölfler 1850–1917) in 1880.

Wohler, Friedrich (1800–1882) *See urea.*

Wohlgemuth, Julius (1874–1948) *See amylase.*

Woillez Disease Form of acute idiopathic congestion of the lung described by French physician, Eugene Joseph Woillez (1811–1882).

Wolcot, Erastus Bradley (1804–1880) American surgeon of Benton, New York who was the first to perform nephrectomy in 1861.

Wolff, Julius (1836–1902) German orthopedic surgeon in Berlin who proposed the Wolff law in 1892 which states that all changes in the functions of the bones are accompanied by definite alteration in their internal structure.

Wolff–Parkinson–White Syndrome (WPW syndrome) Electrocardiographic changes of WPW syndrome were described by Paul Dudley White (1886–1973) of Massachu-setts General Hospital in 1930. Other symptoms were described by American cardiologist Louis Wolff (b 1898) and English physician Sir John Parkinson (1885–1976). M. Holzmann explained that the short PR interval and delta wave found in the ECG was due to preexcitation of the ventricle through an accessory or aberrant pathway in 1932. His explanation was based on previous anatomical findings of an atrioventricular pathway by Alfred Frank Stanley Kent (1863–1958). In 1967 D. Durrer devised a method of intraoperative epicardial mapping which provided the electrophysiological evidence for preexcitation through an accessory pathway. H.B. Burchell, in the same year, injected procaine into the atrioventricular groove and temporarily abolished ventricular preexcitation. A leap in treatment was made in 1968 by W. C. Sealy when he surgically divided the accessory pathway and abolished the ECG abnormalities, preventing further attacks of arrhythmia. Electrical ablation of the accessory bundle by transvenous catheter was described by R. Gonzalez in 1981 and by Scheinman in 1982. *See ablation catheter.*

Wolff, Harold George (1898–1962) Professor of physiology at Cornell University who published a study of gastric function in 1943 from a man who had had a gastric fistula since the age of 9 years. A treatise on pain was jointly published by him and Stewart George Wolff (b 1914), an assistant professor at the same university, in 1946.

Wolffian Body Ren primordialis, described by Kaspar Friedrich Wolff (1733–1794) of Berlin, who was professor of anatomy at St Petersburg in 1759.

Wolffian Duct Ureter primordialis described by Kaspar Friedrich Wolff (1733–1794) of Berlin, professor of anatomy at St Petersburg. In 1759 he also proposed the theory of epigenesis which states that new structures arise in the course of development, as opposed to preformation theory.

Wölfler Operation An opening between the stomach and the distal part of the duodenum is created in cases of pyloric obstruction. Devised by Anton Wölfler (1850–1917), a surgeon at Prague.

Wolfring Glands Glands of the lower eyelid conjunctiva. Described in 1872 by Polish ophthalmologist Emilij Franzevic von Wolfring (1832–1906), professor at Warsaw.

Wollaston, William Hyde (1766–1822) British chemist qualified in medicine from Cambridge in 1793 and practiced in London (1797) before turning in 1800 to chemistry. He demonstrated the presence of various substances, including uric acid, calcium and ammonium, in urinary stones in 1797. Ultraviolet rays were observed by him in 1802 and he discovered, palladium in 1803 and

rhodium in 1804. The occurrence of bladder stones in patients with cystinuria was noted by Wollaston in 1810.

Womb [Anglo-Saxon: *wamb*, belly] *See uterus.*

Women Pioneers In Medicine Cleopatra is supposed to be the first woman to have practiced midwifery and medicine. Queen Shubad of Ur ,who lived around 3000 BC, was found buried with surgical instruments and prescriptions. Agnodice, a physician and pupil of Herophilus in 300 BC, practiced disguised as a man. A famous women surgeon during the Middle Ages was Trotula who lived around AD 1050. Several works on midwifery, known as *Trotula* written in the 11th century, have been attributed to her. Abella was a surgeon from the School of Salerno around the same time. In England about 66 women were known to have obtained licenses to practice medicine around 1511. In the following two centuries there was nonuniformity on the role of women as doctors. They were forbidden to be apothecaries in 1615, and in France a decree in 1755 excluded them from practicing surgery. The most famous French woman in midwifery was Louyse Bourgeois (1553–1638) who was a pupil of Ambroise Paré (1510–1590). She published several books based on midwifery. Maria della Donne (1776–1842) was the first woman to obtain a medical degree in France in 1799 and was appointed professor of obstetrics by Napoleon in 1802. The first woman medical graduate from Glasgow University was Marion Gilchrist who obtained her MBCM in 1894. *See Anderson, Elizabeth.*

Wood, Alexander (1817–1884) *See hypodermic injection.*

Wood, Horatio Charles (1841–1920) *See sunstroke.*

Wood, John (1827–1891) Surgeon from Bradford, Yorkshire who contributed several papers on myology while a surgeon at King's College Hospital, London.

Wood, Paul Hamilton (1907–1962) One of the greatest modern cardiologists of England, born in Coonoor India where his father was in the Indian civil service. After schooling in Tasmania and completing his resident post in New Zealand, he returned to England and became house physician at Brompton Hospital in 1933. He was resident medical officer at the National Heart Hospital and Dean of the Institute of Cardiology in 1947. In 1949 he became cardiologist to the Brompton Hospital and contributed to the study of congenital cardiology with his work on atrial septal defect in 1950. He wrote *Diseases of the Heart and Circulation* in 1950.

Wood Vinegar (Syn: acetum pyrolignosum crudum) Made by heating wood in large iron cylinders connected to condensers producing a distillate of wood spirit, acetic acid, water and tarry substances which is further distilled to leave the tarry, creosote-containing substances. It was used in the 19th century as a disinfectant and for cesspools and drains. Justinius Kerner experimented with it on animals in 1820 and creosote was isolated and named by K. Reichenbach in 1832. This became a popular remedy for consumption and digestive disorders for over 50 years.

Woodall, John (1556–1643) British naval surgeon who wrote a book on naval medicine in 1617, *The Surgeons mate,* during his service with the East India Company. He made the first suggestion that lime juice could be used to prevent and cure scurvy. The circular method of amputating the limbs was described by him in 1617.

Woodbridge Treatment An intestinal antiseptic containing calomel used to treat typhoid by American physician, John Elliot Woodbridge (1845–1901).

Woodhead, Sir Sims German (1855–1921) British pioneer in establishing pathology laboratory services in England. After graduating from Edinburgh University he became superintendent of the laboratory services of the Royal College of Physicians there in 1897. He was appointed to the chair of pathology at Cambridge in 1899. He wrote a book on microbiology in 1885, *Pathological Mycology,* with Arthur W Hare, assistant professor of surgery at the University of Edinburgh. His *Practice of Pathology* was published in 1883 and he was the first editor of the *Journal of Pathology and Bacteriology* for 30 years.

Woodville, William (1752–1805) British physician from Cockermouth who graduated from Edinburgh University. He practiced in London and was a physician to the Middlesex Dispensary and Smallpox Hospital. He wrote *Medical Botany* and *History of Smallpox Inoculation.*

Woodward, John (1665–1728) British physician from Derbyshire who was professor of physick at Gresham College in 1692 and wrote *Essay towards the Natural History of Earth* in 1696.

Woodward, Robert Burns (1917–1979) American organic chemist from Boston, Massachusetts. He was professor of chemistry at Harvard University in 1950 and worked on the antimalarial drug, quinine, and penicillin. He synthesized cortisone in 1951, cholesterol, lysergic acid, reserpine, chlorophyll and colchicine and was awarded the Nobel Prize for Chemistry in 1965. He went on to synthesize vitamin B12 and is considered one of the greatest synthetic organic chemists.

Woodward, Sir Arthur Smith (1864–1944) *See Piltdown man.*

Woolner, Thomas (1825–1892) English sculptor and poet who drew the attention of Charles Darwin to the tubercle on the helix of the auricle, commonly known as Darwin tubercle.

Woolsorter Disease *See anthrax.*

Woorali *See curare.*

Word Association Pioneering work was done by Francis Galton (1822–1911) in 1879 and by Carl Gustav Jung (1875–1961) in psychology. Jung developed the word association test where the subject responds with another word to a given word and wrote *Studies on Word Association* in 1906.

Workmen Compensation Act Safeguarded workers in 1897 in England and replaced by the National Insurance (Industrial Injuries) Act in 1946.

World Health Organization Established by the United Nations in 1948.

World Medical Association Coordinates work of various National Medical Associations and was founded at Ferney-Voltaire, France in 1947. Its publications include: *Declaration of Geneva* (1948), *International Code of Medical Ethics* (1949), *Computers and Confidentiality* (1973) and *Declaration of Helsinki* (1964).

Worm, Ole (1588–1654) Danish anatomist and brother-in-law of Casper Bartholin Primus (1585–1629) whom he succeeded as professor of anatomy at Copenhagen in 1624. He described the Wormian bones or ossa suturalia of the skull.

Wormian Bones Sutural bones. *See Worm, Ole.*

Wormwood *See absinthe.*

Worth, Claud (1869–1936) *See amblyoscope.*

Wotton, Edward (1492–1555) Physician and zoologist from Oxford who wrote a Latin treatise, *On the difference of Animals* in 1552, giving an account of the animal kingdom and the animal organism and its parts. He was physician to Henry VIII.

Wound Dressing Wine as a lotion for ulcers was mentioned in a Hippocratic treatise. Arsenic, copper and hellebore were also recommended as cleansing agents for ulcers by Hippocrates (460–377 BC). Aetius of Amida (AD 502–575) used dried plantain, ashes of wood of fig and juice of calamint to treat ulcers containing worms. Applications of bandages for simple ulcers were described by Paul of Aegina

(625–690) as well as wound dressings or 'agglutinants' of juice of plantain, papyrus soaked in wine and pounded new cheese. For larger ulcers he used horsetail and for hollow ulcers he applied extract of snail, aloe and other herbs. *See wound.*

Wound Galen (AD 129–200) gained considerable experience in treating wounds through his attendance on the gladiators of Rome. He recommended conservative treatment, but for cut tendons he recommended, uniting them with sutures. *See wound dressing, trauma surgery.*

WPW Syndrome *See Wolf–Parkinson–White Syndrome; White, Paul Dudley.*

Wreden Sign Gelatinous material found in the external auditory meatus in infants who are born dead. Described as a test for live birth in 1868 by Robert Robertovich Wreden (1837–1893), an otologist at Petrograd in Russia.

Wren, Sir Christopher (1632–1723) English architect, astronomer and scientist, born at East Knoyle, Wiltshire. He was a member of the Invisible College at Oxford which later became the Royal Society. He inaugurated intravenous administration of drugs by injecting opium and *Crocus metallorum* into the veins of dogs using a quill and a bladder in 1656. He was president of the Royal Society from 1680 to 1683.

Wriesberg, Heinrich August (1739–1808) German gynecologist and professor of anatomy at Göttingen. He described several anatomical structures including: internal cutaneous nerve to minor brachi (Wriesberg nerve); cuneiform cartilage of the larynx (Wriesberg cartilage); and a band attached to posterior cruciate ligament of the knee (Wriesberg ligament).

Wright, Sir Almroth Edward (1861–1941) English bacteriologist from Yorkshire and a graduate of Trinity College, Dublin who also studied in Leipzig, Strasburg and Sydney. He was appointed to an army medical school where he developed a typhoid vaccine. He became professor of pathology at St Mary's Hospital, London in 1902 where he worked on parasitic diseases and the protective power of blood against bacteria. His work with Stewart Rankin Douglas (1871–1936) led to the discovery of a thermolabile substance in serum which acted on bacteria during the process of phagocytosis and which was named 'opsonin' in 1903.

Wright Stain Used for megakaryocytes and platelets. Devised by Boston pathologist, James Homer Wright (1871–1928) in 1910. He also prepared special stains for the malarial parasite (1902) and *Treponema pallidum* (1918).

Wright, Thomas (1561–1623) Jesuit priest in England who wrote *The passions of the minde* (1601) in which he raised fundamental issues in psychology and neurophysiology which were later recognized as phantom limb syndrome, localization of cerebral function, coordination of movement and memory in relation to learning. A fifth edition of this appeared in 1630.

Wrist *See carpus, Colles fracture, median nerve compression.*

Wrist Dislocation German professor at Strasburg, Otto Wilhelm Madelung (1846–1926), described congenital dislocation of the wrist in 1878.

Wrist Excision Lord Joseph Lister (1827–1912) performed the operation for caries of the wrist joint in 1865. Scottish surgeon from Edinburgh, James Donaldson Gillespie (1823–1891), described an operation for excision of the wrist in 1870.

Writers' Cramp A classic description was given by Bernadini Ramazzini (1633–1714) in 1713, and another by Sir Charles Bell (1744–1842) in 1830. Sir William Gowers (1845–1915) gave an account of the condition in 1893 and Haupt wrote *On Writer's Cramp with respect to pathology and treatment* (1860) and associated it with squinting, stuttering and other neuroses.

Wroblewski, Felix (b 1921) *See diagnostic enzymology.*

Wryneck Nicolas Tulp (1593–1674), a physician from Amsterdam, gave a detailed description of a 12-year-old boy whose head was drawn towards his left shoulder due to contraction of the scalenus anterior muscle. After failing to treat the condition medically, he approached a surgeon named Minnius who successfully divided the muscle in several stages. Meckren, another surgeon in Amsterdam, recommended a similar operation. Samuel Sharp (1700–1778), a British surgeon, recommended the division of the sternocleidomastoid muscle. A monograph describing over 300 cases was published by Jean René Cruchet (1875–1959) of Paris in 1907.

Wuchereria bancrofti The embryonic form of the filarial worm was observed by a German physician working in Brazil, Otto Eduard Heinrich Wucherer (1820–1873) in 1868, and was shown to be the cause of elephantiasis by British physician Sir Joseph Bancroft (1836–1894) in Brisbane in 1878. The organism was named after Wucherer and Bancroft. The culex mosquito was identified as the vector by Scottish physician, Sir Patrick Manson

(1844–1922) in 1878. *See filariasis.*

Wunderlich, Carl Reinhold August (1815–1877) Professor of medicine at Leipzig who pioneered the application of thermometry to clinical medicine in *Das Verhalten der Eigenwarme in Krankeiten* published in 1868. An English translation by Bathhurst W. Woodman (1836–1877) of Stroud, physician at the London Hospital, was published in 1871.

Wundt, Wilhelm Max (1832–1920) *See experimental psychology.*

Wurtz, Charles Adolph (1817–1884) *See bonds.*

Wyeth Operation Method of amputation at the hip joint using elastic cords and needles to control bleeding. Devised in 1894 by New York surgeon, John Allan Wyeth (1845– 1922).

Wylie Operation Shortening the round ligaments by folding them on themselves and suturing. Used as treatment for uterine retroflexion by a New York gynecologist, W. Gill Wylie (1848–1923).

Wyllie, John (1844–1916) Graduate from Edinburgh (1865), pathologist to the Royal Infirmary in 1875, and a physician there in 1882. He succeeded Sir Thomas Grainger Stewart (1837–1900) as professor of medicine at Edinburgh and wrote *Disorders of Speech*.

Wyman, Morrill (1812–1903) *See paracentesis thoracis.*

Wyndham, Sir Charles (1841–1919) British physician and actor, born in Liverpool and educated at Edinburgh. He obtained his MD from Giessen and was a surgeon in the American Civil War. During his stay in America he acted on the New York stage as Charles Wyndham. He returned to England in 1865 and gained fame on the comedy stage. He opened the Wyndham Theater in 1899 and received his knighthood in 1902.

Wynter, Walter Essex (1860–1945) *See lumbar puncture.*

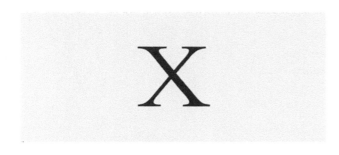

X Chromosome *See accessory chromosomes.*

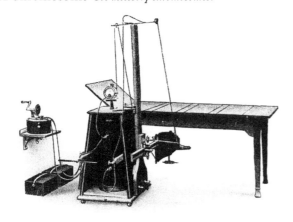

An early portable X-ray installation. Robert Knox, *Radiography, X-Ray Therapeutics and Radium Therapy* (1915). A & C Black, London

X-Ray In 1858 German physicist, Julius Pflucker (1801–1868) used Heinrich Daniel Ruhmkorf's (1803–1877) induction coil to show that when a voltage was passed through two metal electrodes sealed in a glass tube under reduced pressure, sparks were produced. On further reducing the pressure a number of dark spaces appeared. In 1869 German physicist, Johan Wilhelm Hittorf (1824–1914) demonstrated that the dark spaces near the cathode were a form of ray. These cathode rays were investigated by Sir William Crookes (1832–1919) using a high vacuum tube in 1872 and explained by Joseph John Thomson (1856–1940) in 1897. German physicist Wilhelm Konrad von Röntgen (1845–1923) of Würzberg investigated the properties of cathode rays using a Crookes tube and discovered X-rays for which he was awarded the Nobel Prize for Physics in 1901. He discovered their ability to penetrate human tissue and leave an image on a photographic plate quite accidentally. His wife placed her hand between the tube and a photographic plate leaving the first such image. It was found that the rays could penetrate many substances. Progress on the nature of X-rays was made by Charles Glover Barckla (1877–1944), professor of physics at King's College in London, who established their wavelength. A diagnostic X-ray

photograph in America was taken by Michael Idvorsky Pupin (b 1858) of Columbia University in 1896. A prototype of the modern X-ray vacuum tube (Coolridge tube) was invented by American physicist, William David Coolridge (1873–1975) in 1916. He replaced the cold aluminum cathode by a hot tungsten cathode.

X-Ray Crystallography German physicist, Max Theodor Felix von Laue (1879–1960), discovered that X-rays were diffracted by the three-dimensional array of atoms in crystals, for which he received the Nobel Prize for Physics in 1914. Australian-born British physicist, Sir William Bragg (1862–1942) and his son Sir William Lawrence Bragg (1890–1971), used X-rays to discover the positions of atoms in crystals. They established X-ray crystallography which proved to be of immense value in research in many branches of science and they shared the Nobel Prize for Physics in 1915. Powdered crystals in X-ray crystallography were used by Dutch–American physicist Peter Joseph Wilhelm Debye (1884–1966) in 1916, who was awarded the Nobel Prize for Chemistry in 1936.

X-Ray Diffraction The method for analyzing the structure of organic crystals was discovered by William Bragg (1862–1942) and his son Sir William Lawrence Bragg (1890–1971). They constructed the first X-ray spectrometer. Dame Kathleen Lonsdale (1903–1971), an Irish crystallographer at University College London and co-worker with Bragg, used the method to elucidate the structure of hexamethylbenzene and hexachlorobenzene in 1929. D. Crowfoot determined the structure of penicillin in 1949. X-ray diffraction photography of DNA molecules was done by Rosalind Elsie Franklin (1920–1958) of King's College, London in 1953. She shared the Nobel Prize for Physiology or Medicine posthumously in 1962.

X-Ray Injury *See radiation injury.*

X-Ray Protection Transparent lead glass windows for protection from X-rays was introduced in 1900 and aprons, gloves and jackets were invented in 1903. The British X-ray Units Committee was set up under the chairmanship of Sir William Bragg (1862–1942) during the first International Congress of Radiology held at London in 1925. The International Committee on Radiological Protection was formed in Stockholm in 1928. *See radiation injury.*

X-Ray Spectroscopy Developed by Swedish physicist, Karl Manne Georg Siegbahn (1886–1978), who was director of the Nobel Institute for Physics at Stockholm. He produced X-rays of various wavelength and penetrating power and was awarded the Nobel Prize for Physics in 1924. In the same year he showed that they could be refracted by a prism in the same way as light.

Xanthine [Greek: *xanthos*, yellow] Naturally occurring nucleotide discovered in 1817 by Alexander John Gaspard Marcet (1770–1822), a physician and chemist from Geneva.

Xanthomatosis [Greek: *xanthos*, yellow] *See Niemann–Pick disease.*

Xenocrates of Chalcedon (395–314 BC) Philosopher and a pupil of Plato and contemporary of Aristotle, who wrote on natural phenomena, philosophy and astronomy. He taught at Athens and proposed the concept of mind, body and soul.

Xenon [Greek: *xenos*, stranger] Inert gas discovered by Sir William Ramsay (1852–1916) and Morris William Travers (1872–1961) in 1898. Surgical anesthesia using 80% xenon and 20% oxygen was produced by S.C. Cullen and E.G. Gross in 1951. Xenon in metallic form was obtained by Arthur L. Ruoff of Cornell University in 1979.

Xenophanes of Colophon (530 BC) Greek philosopher who was exiled from Ionia after the Persian conquest. He considered the Earth to be fundamental material and made observations on fossils, speculating that the Earth must have been inundated.

Xenopsylla cheopis Genus of fleas some of which were shown to be plague vectors by Masanori Ogata (1852–1919) in 1897.

Xeroderma Pigmentosum [Greek: *xeros*, dry + *derma*, skin] Rare inherited disease characterized by hypersensitivity to ultraviolet light and skin cancer. Described by Hungarian dermatologist Moritz Kaposi (1837–1902) in 1874. The metabolic defect leading to a deficiency in repair mechanisms to DNA in sunlight was demonstrated by J.E. Cleaver in 1968.

Xerophthalmia *See vitamin A.*

Xerostomia [Greek: *xeros*, dry + *stoma*, mouth] *See Sjogrens syndrome.*

XO Syndrome *See Turner syndrome.*

XXY Syndrome *See Klinefelter syndrome.*

Xylocaine *See lignocaine.*

Xylose Excretion Test Measure of renal function devised by Ella S. Fishberg and Friedfeld in 1932.

Xylotherapy [Greek: *xylon*, wood + *therapia*, to treat] Obsolete form of medical treatment where certain woods are applied to the body.

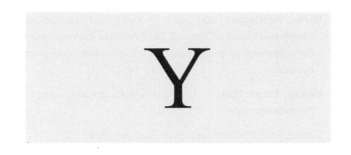

Yale University Third oldest university in America, originated from the Collegiate School of America established at Saybrook, Connecticut with a donation from English administrator, Elihu Yale (1649–1721) in 1701. Yale was born in Boston, Massachusetts and educated in London from 1652. He worked for the East India Company and was governor of Madras in 1687. His donation for the college was realized through sale of his effects in America. The Collegiate School was named Yale College in his honor in 1718 and expanded into Yale University in 1887.

Yalow, Rosalyn née Sussman (b 1921) American biophysicist and the first woman to graduate in physics from Hunter College, New York in 1941. She collaborated with Solomon Berson (1918–1972) in research on diabetes which led to her development of radioimmunoassay (RIA) for measuring minute amounts of biologically active substances, such as hormones and enzymes in blood, in the 1950s. She shared the Nobel Prize for her work on RIA in 1977. She has used her method to investigate insulin, leukemia, neurotransmitters and peptic ulcers. *See insulin antibodies.*

Yamagiva, Katsulsaburo (1863–1930) *See carcinogenesis.*

Yang and Yin In Chinese cosmology, the two forces of nature controlling everything. The feminine, passive and warm, yin determines the outcome by its combination with the cold, moist yang. The principle or Tao (the way) controls the proportion of yin and yang in everything including health. *See acupuncture.*

Yard The word in ancient times denoted the distance from the tip of the nose to the end of the fingers when the right arm was outstretched. The modern yard is defined on the basis of the length of a pendulum with a period of one second at Greenwich, in England, placed by Royal decree in 1824.

Yaws [Caribbean Indian name for the disease] The first reference to it in Europe under the name 'bubas' was made by Gonchlo Fernandez de Ovideo y Valdes (1478–1557) who observed it on St Domingo in 1525. It was described in Brazil by Willem Piso (1611–1678) in 1648 and by Jacobius Bontius (1592–1631) in the East Indies. Peter Labat described

it in the East Indies in 1722, and it was named 'framboesia' (raspberry) by François Boissier de Sauvages (1706–1767) in 1759. The causative organism, *Treponema pertenue*, was discovered by Marquis Aldo Castellani (1879–1971) in 1905.

Yearsley, James (1805–1869) First physician to practice oto-rhinology as a specialty in London. He pointed out that deafness may arise from diseases of the nose and throat and developed the artificial tympanum. The Metropolitan Ear and Throat Hospital at Fitzroy Square was founded by him in 1838. He was an originator of the *Medical Directory* in 1845.

Yeast The role of yeast as a live microorganism in fermentation was shown by Charles Cagniard de Latour (1777–1859) of Paris in 1838. Louis Pasteur's (1822–1895) work on fermentation commenced around 1855 put an end to the theory of spontaneous generation. German wine merchant and chemist, Moritz Traube (1826–1894) of Rabitor, proposed the concept of an enzyme within yeast in 1858. Eduard Buchner (1860–1917), professor of chemistry at Berlin and Nobel Prize winner, extracted zymase from yeast and demonstrated that fermentation of sugar could be effected with it in the absence of living yeast cells in 1897.

Yeki Japanese name for bubonic plague.

Yelloly, John (1774–1842) Born in Alnwick, graduated from Edinburgh University (1796) and was physician to the London Hospital in 1807. He moved to Norwich in 1818 and became physician to the Norwich Hospital in 1820. He founded the Royal Medico-Chirugical Society of London with John Gaspard Marcet (1770–1822) in 1805. *See Royal Society of Medicine.*

Yellow Atrophy *See acute yellow atrophy.*

Yellow Enzyme *See flavoprotein.*

Yellow Fever Vaccine The live virus was attenuated in 1939 by Max Theiler (1899–1972), a South African-born American virologist. Theiler's work led to the discovery of 17D vaccine for yellow fever for which he was awarded the Nobel Prize in 1951.

Yellow Fever Reported in the Antilles by Father J.B. Dutertre in 1635. An epidemic occurred in Spain in 1700 at Cadiz and in Lisbon in 1723. The most virulent epidemic was in the 18th century in America, involving 132 towns where 16,000 people died. One of the first investigators in America was by Baltimore physician, Nathan Potter (1770–1843). He repeatedly inoculated himself with body secretions taken from patients with yellow fever in 1797, but failed to contract it. Italian physician, Eusebius Valli (1762–1816) from Pistroia, died during self experimentation in Havana. Louis Daniel Beauperthuy (1803–1871) from the West Indies who graduated in medicine from Paris, investigated virulent outbreaks in Venezuela and the West Indies, and pointed out the relationship with mosquitoes. *Aedes aegypti* mosquito was suggested to be the carrier by Carlos Finlay (1833–1915) of Cuba in 1881. Walter Reed (1851–1902), an American army surgeon from Virginia, headed a Medical Commission in Cuba in 1898 to study it with his associates James Caroll (1854–1907), Aristede Agramonte (1868–1931), and Jesse William Lazear (1866–1900). Lazier deliberately allowed himself to be bitten and died. Reed's work was subsequently responsible for the eradication of yellow fever in Cuba. William Cedric Gorgas (1854–1920), an American army surgeon from Mobile, Alabama investigated the spread of yellow fever in Havana in 1898. He improved sanitation which resulted in virtual eradication of malaria and yellow fever from Havana. In 1919 Hideyo Noguchi (1876–1928) isolated a virus which he thought was responsible and in 1926 Max Theiler (1899–1972) developed a vaccine. It was the first human disease to be identified as caused by a virus.

Yeo Treatment Used for obesity by giving large amounts of hot drinks and withholding carbohydrates. Formulated by London physician, Isaac Burney Yeo (1835–1914).

Yerkes Scale Used for testing intelligence. Devised by American psychologist, Robert Mearns Yerkes (b 1876) in 1918.

Yersin, Alexandre Émile John (1863–1943) Swiss-born French bacteriologist who worked at the Pasteur Institute at Paris and isolated the bubonic plague bacillus, *Yersinia pestis*, from humans in Hong Kong at the same time as Baron Shibasaburo Kitasato (1852–1931) in 1894. He developed an antiserum for plague and established two Pasteur Institutes in China. He also introduced the rubber tree into China.

Yin and Yang *See yang and yin.*

Yoga [Sanskrit: yoking] Hindu discipline to train the unconscious to achieve spiritual insight. Founded by Patanjali, an Indian philosopher in the third century AD. His four books on Yoga sutra deal with mental discipline to bring about freedom with oneself. A system of exercises, hatha yoga, were developed to promote this state of being.

Yonge, James (1647–1721) Naval surgeon from Plymouth who described the use of turpentine to arrest hemorrhage. He improved the method of flap operation in amputation.

York Retreat Founded by British philanthropist and reformer of the care of the insane, William Tuke (1732–1822). A classic account of moral therapy given at the Retreat at York, *Description of the Retreat* was published by his grandson, Samuel Tuke (1784–1857).

Yorke, Warrington (1883–1943) British parasitologist at the Liverpool School of Tropical Medicine. He experimented with Bayer 205 on a patient with *Trypanosoma rhodesiense* in 1921.

Young, Hugh Hampton (1870–1945) American urologist. *See prostatectomy.*

Young, John Richardson (1782–1804) *See saliva.*

Young, John Zachary (b.1907) English zoologist appointed as the first non-medical anatomy professor in Britain, at University College, London in 1945. He was born in Bristol and studied zoology at Oxford and Naples. He studied the large nerve fiber of the squid which proved useful in neurophysiology research.

Young Operation Used for correction of hammer-toe and claw-toe. Devised by American surgeon, Charles Stephen Young (b 1892) of Los Angeles in 1938.

Young, Robert Bruce (1883–1927) Anatomist who qualified from Glasgow in 1883. He studied the knee joint and described the trapezometacarpel ligament (Young ligament) between the 3rd and 4th metacarpals and the trapezium.

Young, Thomas (1773–1829) Quaker physicist and physician, born in Milverton, Somerset and studied medicine in London, Edinburgh and Göttingen before qualifying in 1800. He was physician to St George's Hospital in 1811 and held the post until his death. He demonstrated the mechanism of accommodation of the lens in vision in 1792. He is considered to be one of the great men of science and his contributions include: classification of diseases in his *Introduction to Medical Literature* in 1813; an essay on consumption in 1815; discovery of the wave theory of light in 1802; physical concepts of energy and work; theory of capillary attraction in 1804; and Young modulus of elasticity. He was also an Egyptologist and deciphered some hieroglyphics.

Younge, William (1762–1838) *See Sheffield Royal Infirmary.*

Yttrium Rare metal found in a quarry at a town called Ytterby by Swedish physical chemist Svante August Arrhenius (1859–1927) who named it. *See pituitary ablation.*

Yudin, Sergey Sergeevich (b 1891) *See blood bank.*

Yule, George Udny (1871–1951) British pioneer in modern statistics. He was a lecturer at University College and Cambridge University and wrote *Introduction to Theory of Statistics* in 1911.

Yvon Test Detects acetanilide in urine with chloroform and mercurous nitrate as reagents. Devised by French physician, Paul Yvon (1848–1913).

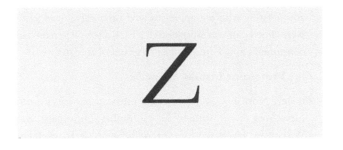

Zacchias, Paolo (1584–1659) Physician to Pope Innocent X at Rome. He wrote on medical jurisprudence, injuries to the eye, insanity and other medical subjects.

Zacharias, Jansen Dutch spectacle maker from Middelburg in Holland in the 16th century, who developed the first compound microscope in 1590 consisting of a double convex lens object piece and a concave eye piece.

Zacutus, Lucitanus (1575–1642) Portuguese physician of Jewish origin who practiced at Lisbon for 20 years and had to leave the city due to a decree against Jews issued by Phillip II. He lived in Amsterdam before his death and wrote several medical treatises.

Zaglas Ligament [Latin:*ligamentum*, bandage] Extends from the posterior superior iliac spine to the second piece of the sacrum. Named after John Zaglas, an assistant to John Goodsir at Edinburgh from 1851 to 1853.

Zahn Lines Corrugations on the free surface of a thrombus formed by the projecting edges of the lamellae of blood platelets. Described by German pathologist, Friedrich Wilhelm Zahn (1845–1904).

Zambeccari, Guiseppe (1655–1721) *See spleen.*

Zander Apparatus Machine to give physiotherapy and apply manipulation to the body. Designed in 1886 by Swedish physician, Jonas Gustav Wilhelm Zander (1835–1920).

Zang Space Area between the two tendons of the origin of the sternomastoid in the supraclavicular fossa. Described by German professor of clinical surgery at Würzburg, Christoph Bonifacius Zang (1772–1835) in 1813.

Zangemeister Maneuvre Used during face presentation in delivery and described by German gynecologist, William Zangemeister (b 1871).

Zanichelli, John Jerome (1662–1729) Italian physician and natural philosopher, born in Modena. He studied fossils and shells and published several treatises on a variety of subjects.

Zannoni, James (d 1682) Italian physician and botanist from Bologna who discovered several plants and wrote *Historia Botanica* (1675).

Zeeman Effect Dutch physicist Pieter Zeeman (1865–1943) demonstrated the splitting of spectral lines into two or three components by observing a sodium or lithium flame in a strong magnetic field in 1896. The theory behind the phenomenon was later elucidated by his teacher, Hendrik Antoon Lorentz (1853–1928).

Zeis Glands Sebaceous glands in the eyelids, described by a professor of surgery at Marburg, Eduard Zeis (1807–1868) in 1835.

Zeiss, Carl (1816–1888) Pioneer in the development of microscopes and lenses. He was born in Weimar, Germany and opened his firm for making optical instruments at Jena in 1846. Ernest Abbe, a physicist and a partner of Zeiss, helped to modernize and produce the microscope on a commercial scale. Their company made the first ground spherical contact lenses for Sulzer in 1892 and in 1936 they started making contact lenses from individual casts of the eyes.

Zeller Operation Used in the treatment of webbed fingers. Devised by Viennese surgeon, Simon Zeller (1746–1816) in 1810.

Zend-Avesta Ancient sacred books of the Parsees, only 3 out of 21 are extant.

Zenker Degeneration Necrosis and hyaline degeneration of striated muscle. Described by Friedrich Albert Zenker (1825–1898), German professor of pathological anatomy at Leipzig (1855) and Erlangen (1862).

Zenker Diverticulum Diverticulum of the upper esophagus, common in elderly males. Described by German professor of pathological anatomy, Friedrich Albert Zenker (1825–1898) at Leipzig.

Zeno of Citium (362–264 BC) Cypriot founder of the Stoic sect. He committed suicide by strangling. *See Stoics.*

Zerfas, Leon Grotius (b 1897) *See amytal sodium.*

Zernike, Frits (1888–1966) Dutch physicist who invented the phase contrast technique in 1935, for which he was awarded the Nobel Prize for Physics in 1953.

Zero [Arabic: *cipher*, zero] Symbol used in India in 876 BC and the goose egg sign for zero appeared in Cambodia and Sumatra in AD 680.

Zeugmatography Method of coupling two fields to an object to produce a magnetic resonance image in radiology. Described and named in 1973 by Paul Lauterbur, professor at the University of Illinois, Chicago.

Ziegler, Alexander Obstetrician at Edinburgh who practiced with his son, William Ziegler. He invented (1830) obstetric forceps in which the Smellie lock was replaced by splitting the shank of one of the shoulder blades to allow passage for the other blade.

Ziegler, Ernst (1849–1905) Professor of pathological anatomy at Zurich (1881) and Tübingen (1882). He founded *Beitrage zur pathologischen Anatomie* while he was professor of pathology at Freiberg in 1886. He published an important work on pathological anatomy in 1881.

Ziegler Forceps *See Ziegler, Alexander.*

Ziegler Operation V-shaped iridectomy for creating artificial pupils. Designed by an ophthalmologist from Philadelphia, Samuel Louis Ziegler (1861–1926).

Ziehl, Franz (1857–1926) *See acid-fast bacteria.*

Ziehl–Neelsen Stain *See acid-fast bacteria.*

Ziemssen Treatment Treatment for anemia using subcutaneous injections of defibrinated human blood. Advocated by Munich physician, Hugo Wilhelm von Ziemssen (1829–1902).

Zieve Syndrome Jaundice, hyperlipidemia, fatty liver and hemolytic anemia related to alcohol intake. Described by American physician, Leslie Zieve (b 1915) in 1958.

Zimmerman, Eberhard Augustus William von (1743–1815) German naturalist who studied at Göttingen and Leiden. He published *Geographical History of Man and Quadrupeds* and other works related to politics.

Zimmerman, Gustav Heinrich Eduard (1817–1866) Graduate of the Medico-surgical Academy at Berlin who described blood platelets (1855) previously observed by Bizzozero in 1852.

Zimmermann, John George (1728–1795) Swiss physician, born at Brug in Bern. He studied under Albrecht von Haller (1708–1777) at Göttingen. He wrote a physiological dissertation on irritability, an essay on solitude, a treatise on dysentery (1767) and other works.

Zinc Element discovered and extracted by Indians in the 14th century. The name 'zinkum' was used by Paracelsus (1493–1541). Zinc salts have mild antiseptic and astringent properties and are used in various medical lotions and applications. *See spelter, zincalism.*

Zinc Carbon Cell Forerunner of the dry cell and battery, invented by French chemist, Georges Leclanche (1839–1882) in 1868.

Zincalism Rare condition with fever, chills, headache and vomiting. An outbreak occurred in Surrey in 1922 where 200 persons who ate apples stewed on a galvanized plate were affected. It was estimated that each affected person had consumed a zinc equivalent to 20 grains of zinc sulfate.

Zinc Protamine Insulin *See insulin.*

Zinder, Norton David (b 1928) American geneticist from New York who studied at Columbia University and Wisconsin. He was professor of genetics at Rockefeller University. He studied mutants of *Salmonella* and described bacterial transduction via a phage. *See genetic engineering.*

Zinjanthropus Hominid fossil skull nearly 1.75 million years old was found in Tanzania by the English archeologist, Mary Douglas Leakey (b 1913) in 1959. It was initially named *Zinjanthropus*, but was later reclassified as *Australopithecus.*

Zinke, George Gottfried *See rabies.*

Zinn, Johann Gottfried (1727–1759) Professor of medicine and director of the botanical gardens at Göttingen. He described the annulus tendineus for the origin of ocular muscles (Zinn ligament) in 1755.

Zinn Artery Central artery of the retina described by German anatomist, Johann Gottfried Zinn (1727–1759). He completed an anatomical study of the eye in 1755.

Zinsser, Hans (1878–1940) American bacteriologist and immunologist and graduate of Columbia University (1901) who was head of the department of immunology at Harvard in 1923. He worked on allergy, virus size, typhus and causes of rheumatic fever. He differentiated epidemic from endemic rickettsial typhus. He wrote *Rats, Lice and History* on typhus fever in 1935.

Zittmann Decoction A preparation of sarsaparilla root introduced into Europe in the first half of the 17th century and a popular treatment for chronic syphilis for nearly two centuries.

Zoll, Paul Maurice (b 1911) *See ventricular fibrillation.*

Zollinger–Ellison Syndrome Recurrent peptic ulceration associated with non-insulin secreting islet cell tumors of the pancreas. Described by two American surgeons at the Ohio State University, Robert Milton Zollinger (1903–1992) and Edwin Homer Ellison (1918–1970) in 1955. They later presented a collection of 75 such cases at the proceedings of the World Congress of Gastroenterology at Washington in 1958.

Zöllner Lines A set of peculiarly arranged lines for testing the eye designed by Dutch physicist, Johann Karl Friedrich Zöllner (1834–1882).

Zona Pellucida [Greek: *zona*, girdle; Latin: *pelluceo*, shine through] Clear zone surrounding the ovum described and named for its transparent nature by Carl Ernst von Baer (1792–1876) in 1827.

Zona Radiata [Greek: *zona*, girdle; Latin: *radius*, ray] Part of the mammalian ovum described in 1884 by Theodor Ludwig Wilhelm Bischoff (1807–1882), professor of anatomy and embryologist at Heidelberg.

Zondek, Bernhard (1891–1966) Israeli gynecologist and endocrinologist, born in Germany who graduated from Berlin Charite and Berlin-Spandau Hospitals. He designed the first reliable pregnancy test with Selmar Aschheim (1878–1965) in 1928. They also discovered the gonadotrophins. He left Germany due to Nazi persecution and was professor of obstetrics and gynecology at the Hebrew University Hadassah Medical School at Jerusalem from 1934 to 1961.

Zoogeography Study of distribution of animals across the world. The first map was published by a German naturalist, Eberhard Augustus William von Zimmerman (1743–1815) in 1777.

Zoology [Greek: *zoon*, animal + *logos*, discourse] Aristotle (384–322 BC) can be considered the first zoologist due to his study of various animals. Galen (AD 129–200) dissected apes and pigs and based his knowledge of anatomy and physiology on these dissections. John Ray (1628–1705) an English biologist from Essex, attempted to classify the plant and animal kingdoms. Zoology became an established science during the 18th century and several chairs were created.

Zoonosis [Greek: *zoon*, animal + *nosos*, disease] A disease of an animal which can be transmitted to man. *See parasitology.*

Zoroaster (628–551 BC) Physician, philosopher and pro-phet of Persia, who proposed the doctrine of good or Ormazd, and evil or Ahriman. The *Zendevesta* on good and evil is based on his philosophy.

Zoster *See herpes zoster.*

Zotterman, Yvunge (1898–1982) Swedish neurophysiologist, educated at the Karolinska Institute and the University of Uppsala. He was attached to the Swedish Royal Navy and spent time each year after his national service in researching problems of deep sea diving. He worked at Cambridge with Edward Douglas Adrian (1889–1977) on recording and analyzing nerve impulses and continued this research on his return to Sweden in 1927. He examined the thermal and pain sensations of the skin and taste. He wrote *Touch, Tickle and Pain*, a two-volume autobiography.

Zsigmondy, Richard Adolf (1865–1929) Austrian chemist and inventor of ultramicroscope. He was also a pioneer in the study of colloidal solutions. His findings were used by Carl Lange (1883–1953) to develop the Lange colloidal gold test for cerebrospinal fluid in 1912. Zsigmondy received the Nobel Prize for colloidal chemistry in 1925.

Zuckerkandl Fascia Retrorenal fascia described in 1883 by Hungarian-born anatomist Emil Zuckerkandl (1849–1910), professor of anatomy at Graz and later at Vienna.

Zuckerman, Solly, Baron (1904–1993) South African-born British zoologist, joined Oxford University as a tutor in 1932, and was made professor of anatomy at Birmingham in 1946. He was a pioneer in the study of origin of human behavior in animals and wrote *The Social Life of Monkeys and Apes* in 1932.

Zuelzer, Georg Ludwig (1870–1949) German research chemist at Berlin. While he was internist in Berlin in 1906 he gave the first subcutaneous injection of the pancreatic extract to a 50-year-old diabetic patient and produced a temporary recovery. After publishing his results in 1908, he took out a patent on his 'Pancreas preparation suitable for the treatment of diabetes' in 1912. However his product was abandoned due to convulsions after its administration which, at that time, were not recognized to be due to hypoglycemia.

Zwinger, James (d 1610) Swiss physician born in Basel who compiled a new edition of his father's *Theatre of Human Life* around 1600. His son Theodore Zwinger (d 1696) was also an eminent physician who published several treatises on medicine and philosophy.

Zwinger, Theodore (1536–1588) Born in Bishofftzel in Turgau and became professor of medicine and philosophy in his home town in 1563. He wrote *Theatre of Human Life* in 1556 which was enlarged by his son James and published around 1600.

Zygote [Greek: *zygotos*, yolked together] Fertilized ovum. *See fertilization.*

Zymase [Greek: *zyme*, leaven] Enzyme extracted from yeast by Eduard Buchner (1860–1917) in 1897.